Management of Medical Problems in Surgical Patients

Management of Medical Problems in Surgical Patients

MARK E. MOLITCH, M.D.

ASSOCIATE PROFESSOR OF MEDICINE
TUFTS UNIVERSITY SCHOOL OF MEDICINE
ASSOCIATE DIRECTOR, CLINICAL STUDY UNIT
PHYSICIAN
DIVISION OF ENDOCRINOLOGY AND METABOLISM
DEPARTMENT OF MEDICINE
NEW ENGLAND MEDICAL CENTER
BOSTON, MASSACHUSETTS

F. A. DAVIS COMPANY · Philadelphia

Printed in the United States of America.

Library of Congress Cataloging in Publication Data
Main entry under title:

Management of medical problems in surgical patients.

Includes bibliographical references and index.
1. Surgery—Complications and sequelae. I. Molitch, Mark E. [DNLM: 1. Intraoperative complications—Therapy. 2. Preoperative care. 3. Postoperative complications—Therapy. WO 178 M725m]
RD98.M355 617'.01 81-9831
ISBN 0-8036-6286-6 AACR2

TO SUSAN, TAMARA AND ETHAN

FOREWORD

With increasing health care costs and the resultant pressure to do as much as possible in the ambulatory setting, patients currently in our hospitals are generally sicker and their management more complicated than ever before. Improvements in technology and life support systems have led to prolongation of life in surgical as well as other patients. In addition, other factors such as the development of a team approach to the care of some patients, for example, those with oncologic diseases or cardiovascular illnesses, have led to greatly increased interaction between all specialties, in particular surgery and internal medicine. It is my opinion that such interaction is positive and has led to improved patient care.

For those of us who, as internists, work predominantly in hospitals, the numbers of consultations and the increasing contact with surgical patients has forced us to improve our knowledge and understanding of surgical problems and the medical aspects of such patients. It is no longer possible, nor proper, for our house officers and fellows to spend all of their time seeing patients only on our medical services or in our ambulatory facilities. We must provide them with experience dealing with medical problems in surgical patients, since those who will practice internal medicine will surely spend considerable time dealing with such problems.

Needless to say, other physicians besides internists and surgeons will need to learn how to approach medical problems in surgical patients. The present book should appeal to a very wide audience. The breadth and scope of this text accurately reflects the diseases and the wide range of problems encountered in practice.

Sheldon M. Wolff, M.D.

Endicott Professor and Chairman
Department of Medicine
Tufts University School of Medicine
Physician-in-Chief, New England Medical Center
Boston, Massachusetts

PREFACE

In this book we have provided information and guidelines for the management of medical problems in patients requiring surgery since such information is otherwise not readily available. In some circumstances such information is present in widely scattered articles in the medical literature, for example the excellent series of articles by Goldman and colleagues on risk assessment in the cardiac patient. On the other hand, much practical information is not available in the literature but exists in the experience of internists, surgeons, and subspecialty clinicians who have seen many such patients. We have tried to cull this scattered literature information and clinical experience into this book so that the busy clinician can have ready access to a single source of information for a vast array of patient management problems. Although some of these management techniques are based upon the personal experience of the authors, they have been careful to avoid dogmatic approaches, and areas of controversy regarding patient management are pointed out in each chapter.

A major difficulty in preparing a book such as this is to prevent it from becoming just another large textbook of medicine. To this end we have tried to confine ourselves to the specifics of patients with medical problems who need surgery, realizing that the clinician presumably has access to standard textbooks of medicine. Each chapter is fully referenced so that for specific instances in which further information is required these references may be utilized.

The book is organized along traditional subspecialty lines, each chapter being written by subspecialty clinicians with experience in managing patients in a surgical setting. These chapters can be referred to directly for specific patient management questions. In addition there are four chapters which affect all patients: Decision Analysis; Fluid, Electrolyte and Acid-Base Disorders; Nutrition; and Anesthesiology. The Decision Analysis chapter is placed first to set the stage for the rest of the book. In it the exciting new techniques of decision analysis are described and are applied to the area of risk assessment and decision making in the patient with medical problems who require surgery. As discussed in this chapter a framework can be structured for assessing risks and benefits for diagnostic tests as well as for therapeutic interventions when faced with a variety of difficult patient problems. The chapter on Fluid, Electrolyte and Acid-Base Disorders discusses the perioperative diagnosis and management of these common disorders. The Nutrition chapter describes how to assess the patient's nutritional status and needs, the risks imposed upon the patient by a poor nutritional status, the catabolic stress of surgery, and the enteral and parenteral techniques of feeding the patient who needs nutritional supplementation. The Anesthesiology chapter discusses specific points about the interaction of anesthesia and medical conditions from the anesthesiologist's point of view.

All of the authors of these chapters either have been or are presently associated with Tufts University School of Medicine and The New England Medical Center. In this way we hope that we have achieved a uniformity of direction in each chapter. The differences in the way different types of diseases interact with the patient needing surgery dictate that the chapters cannot be of uniform style.

Although this book is designed primarily with the medical consultant in mind, we obviously hope that it will prove useful to all caring for the patient in the perioperative period, including subspecialist, surgeon, anesthesiologist, family practitioner, nurse, nurse-practitioner, physician's assistant, in-patient pharmacist and dietician. The ultimate aim of this book is to help the health-care team provide the best possible care of the patient in the perioperative period. This book is meant to be used as a reference work rather than to be read straight through, and the contents and extensive index are designed with this in mind.

I wish to acknowledge the many helpful suggestions and criticisms of my medical and surgical colleagues at New England Medical Center who have read parts of the manuscript. I also wish to thank all of the medical residents who have rotated on the medical consultation service and who have greatly encouraged the production of this book. In particular I wish to express my deep gratitude to Susan Hou, M.D. and Seymour Reichlin, M.D., Ph.D. who encouraged me along the way. Finally, I wish to thank Christine Young and Ruth Wait of F. A. Davis for their very fine efforts and personal touches in enabling this book to be published.

Mark E. Molitch, M.D.

CONTRIBUTORS

Henry Astarjian, M.D.
Associate Clinical Professor of Neurology, Tufts University School of Medicine, Boston, Massachusetts

John S. Banas, Jr., M.D., F.A.C.C.
Associate Professor of Clinical Medicine, Yale University School of Medicine, New London, and Chief, Division of Cardiology, St. Vincent's Medical Center, Bridgeport, Connecticut

Richard S. Blacher, M.D.
Clinical Professor of Psychiatry and Lecturer in Surgery, Tufts University School of Medicine and Psychiatrist, Department of Psychiatry and Cardiothoracic Surgery, New England Medical Center, Boston, Massachusetts

Rita Blanchard, M.D.
Assistant Professor of Medicine, Tufts University School of Medicine, and Assistant Physician, Division of Hematology/Oncology, Department of Medicine, New England Medical Center Hospital, Boston, Massachusetts

David A. Bushinsky, M.D.
Assistant Professor of Medicine, University of Chicago Pritzker School of Medicine, and Medical Associate, Renal Division, Department of Medicine, Michael Reese Hospital and Medical Center, Chicago, Illinois

Ted Butler, M.D.
Instructor, Tufts University School of Medicine, and Assistant-in-Medicine, Department of Medicine, New England Medical Center, Boston, Massachusetts

David Chad, M.D., F.R.C.P.(C.)
Fellow in Neuromuscular Diseases, Department of Neurology, New England Medical Center, Boston, Massachusetts

Jordan J. Cohen, M.D.
Professor of Medicine, Tufts University School of Medicine, and Chief, Renal Division, Department of Medicine, New England Medical Center, Boston, Massachusetts

Johanna T. Dwyer, D.Sc.
Associate Professor of Medicine, Tufts University School of Medicine, and Director, Frances Stern Nutrition Center, New England Medical Center, Boston, Massachusetts

Barry L. Fanburg, M.D.
Professor of Medicine, Tufts University School of Medicine, and Chief, Pulmonary Division, Department of Medicine, New England Medical Center, Boston, Massachusetts

Bruce Furie, M.D.
Associate Professor of Medicine, Tufts University School of Medicine, and Chief, Coagulation Unit, Department of Medicine, New England Medical Center Hospital, Boston, Massachusetts

Sherwood L. Gorbach, M.D.
Professor of Medicine and Microbiology, Tufts University School of Medicine, and Chief, Infectious Disease Division, Department of Medicine, New England Medical Center, Boston, Massachusetts

David Homans, M.D.
Fellow in Cardiology, Department of Medicine, University of Minnesota Hospitals, Minneapolis, Minnesota

Marshall M. Kaplan, M.D.
Professor of Medicine, Tufts University School of Medicine, and Chief, Gastroenterology Division, Department of Medicine, New England Medical Center, Boston, Massachusetts

Paul R. Levesque, M.D.
Associate Professor of Anesthesiology, Tufts University School of Medicine, and Chairman, Department of Anesthesiology, St. Elizabeth's Hospital, Boston, Massachusetts

Daniel S. Matloff, M.D.
Assistant Professor of Medicine, Tufts University School of Medicine, and Staff Physician, Faulkner Hospital, Boston, Massachusetts

Keith P. W. J. McAdam, M.D., M.R.C.P.
Assistant Professor of Medicine, Tufts University School of Medicine, and Assistant Physician, Divisions of Experimental Medicine, Allergy, and Geographic Medicine, Department of Medicine, New England Medical Center, Boston, Massachusetts

James W. McNally, M.D.
Fellow in Cardiology, Division of Cardiology, Department of Medicine, New England Medical Center, Boston, Massachusetts

Mark E. Molitch, M.D.
Associate Professor of Medicine, Tufts University School of Medicine, and Associate Director, Clinical Study Unit, and Physician, Division of Endocrinology and Metabolism, Department of Medicine, New England Medical Center, Boston, Massachusetts

Theodore L. Munsat, M.D.
Professor and Chairman, Department of Neurology, Tufts University School of Medicine, and Neurologist-in-Chief, New England Medical Center, Boston, Massachusetts

Larry Nathanson, M.D.
Professor of Medicine, State University of New York—Stony Brook, School of Medicine, and Director, Oncology-Hematology Division, Department of Medicine, Nassau Hospital, Mineola, New York

Thomas O'Donnell, M.D.
Associate Professor of Surgery, Tufts University School of Medicine, and Director, Non-invasive Vascular Laboratory, Department of Surgery, New England Medical Center, Boston, Massachusetts

John L. Ohman, Jr., M.D.
Instructor in Medicine, Tufts University School of Medicine, and Chief, Allergy Service, Veterans Administration Outpatient Clinic, Boston, Massachusetts

Raymond E. H. Partridge, M.D.
Associate Professor of Medicine, Tufts University School of Medicine, and Physician, Division of Rheumatology and Immunology, Department of Medicine, New England Medical Center, Boston, Massachusetts

Stephen G. Pauker, M.D.
Associate Professor of Medicine, Tufts University School of Medicine, and Chief, Division of Clinical Decision Making and Physician, Division of Cardiology, Department of Medicine, New England Medical Center, Boston, Massachusetts

Stephanie H. Pincus, M.D.
Assistant Professor, Departments of Medicine and Dermatology, Tufts University School of Medicine, and Dermatologist, Department of Dermatology, and Assistant Physician, Department of Medicine, New England Medical Center, Boston, Massachusetts

Richard A. Rudders, M.D.
Associate Professor of Medicine, Tufts University School of Medicine, and Head, Lymphoma Unit, and Physician, Division of Hematology-Oncology, Department of Medicine, New England Medical Center, Boston, Massachusetts

Deeb N. Salem, M.D., F.A.C.C.
Assistant Professor of Medicine, Tufts University School of Medicine, and Director, Cardiac Catheterization Laboratory, Department of Medicine, New England Medical Center, Boston, Massachusetts

Robert S. Schwartz, M.D.
Professor of Medicine, Tufts University School of Medicine, and Director of Division Hematology-Oncology, Department of Medicine, Director of Blood Research Laboratory, and Director of Cancer Research Center, New England Medical Center, Boston, Massachusetts

Francis P. Tally, M.D.
Associate Professor of Medicine, Tufts University School of Medicine, and Physician, Infectious Disease Division, Department of Medicine, New England Medical Center, Boston, Massachusetts

John S. Urbanetti, M.D., (F.R.C.P.)(C.)
Assistant Clinical Professor of Medicine, Yale University School of Medicine, New London, Connecticut

Jay B. Wish, M.D.
Assistant Professor of Medicine, Case Western Reserve University School of Medicine, and Medical Director, Hemodialysis Unit, Department of Medicine, University Hospitals of Cleveland, Ohio

CONTENTS

Chapter 11 PSYCHIATRY 425

Richard S. Blacher, M.D., and Mark E. Molitch, M.D.

Chapter 12 PULMONARY DISEASES 445

John S. Urbanetti, M.D., and Barry L. Fanburg, M.D.

Chapter 1

DECISION ANALYSIS AND CLINICAL DECISION MAKING

Stephen G. Pauker, M.D.*

The physician who manages or provides medical consultations for surgical patients is, in large part, a decision maker. He must help decide which diagnostic tests the patient should have, whether the patient should have surgery, and, if so, when that surgery can be safely performed. As diagnostic test results are obtained, the clinician must interpret the results with respect to the management of the individual patient. Furthermore, modern medical care usually involves several physicians and diverse sources of information. The clinician who is primarily responsible for the case must be able to integrate data from all sources and formulate a coherent plan for patient management.

The physician often conducts his clinical reasoning and management planning on an intuitive, informal basis. In standard, repetitive situations, this approach often provides efficient and correct clinical decisions. Certainly, some common therapies and diagnostic approaches will eventually be shown to be wrong, but the clinician cannot undertake a separate research protocol or detailed analysis for each patient he sees. This chapter will not address such routine clinical problems. Rather, it will consider more complex situations in which the patient is in some way atypical—either the patient's operative risk is high, the diagnosis is uncertain, or the efficacy of alternative therapies is in doubt—and will address the problem of clinical decision making under the condition of uncertainty.

*Dr. Pauker is recipient of Research Career Development Award 1K04GM00349 from the National Institute of General Medical Sciences and is supported in part by grants 1 P41 RR 01096 from the Division of Research Resources and Research Grant 1 PO4 LM 03374 and Training Grant T15 LM 07027 from the National Library of Medicine.

COMMON ERRORS IN CLINICAL REASONING

Before developing a formal approach to such problems, let us consider some common errors which occasionally creep into our informal process of clinical reasoning. One of the most persistent errors concerns the improper interpretation of laboratory test results. The implications of a test result can only be properly understood after due consideration of the sensitivity and specificity of the test *and* the likelihood of disease prior to knowledge of the test result. Sensitivity is the probability of a positive test result in patients who actually have the disease in question, while specificity is the probability of a negative test result in patients who are actually free of the disease. For example, consider the implications of a positive enzyme test for myocardial necrosis in a patient *not* suspected of having an acute myocardial infarction, such as a postoperative patient without clinical findings suggesting infarction. Assume that the sensitivity of the enzyme test is 95 percent and the specificity is 90 percent. Further assume that the likelihood of silent perioperative infarction in this particular patient (given his age and clinical history) is only 1 percent. What is the likelihood that such a patient with a positive enzyme test actually has suffered a myocardial infarction? Most physicians will intuitively say either 95 or 90 percent, although some physicians will suspect that the result may have been a false positive and therefore lower their estimate to 40 or 50 percent. As will be demonstrated, the correct answer is only 8.8 percent!!

A second common error in clinical judgment involves not adequately considering the consequences of diagnosis or therapy. All too often, a clinical presentation will evoke the knee-jerk response of a particular diagnostic work-up being ordered without sufficient thought about the efficacy or even the possibility of therapy in a particular patient. Consider a patient thought to have a pulmonary embolism in the postoperative period. If the likelihood of embolism is high and if the expected complication rate from anticoagulation therapy is low, then it may not be worthwhile to do a pulmonary angiogram—the risk of the angiogram might be greater than the risk of unnecessary anticoagulation therapy in those few high-suspicion patients who do not, in fact, have emboli. Conversely, if the likelihood of emboli is only moderate and the risk of complications of anticoagulation is increased (for example, in a patient with active ulcer disease), then anticoagulation may not be proper even if the angiogram were positive. The point here is not the specifics of these examples but that the clinician must consider his potential actions, based on the various possible results of a diagnostic test. If he would take the same action with a particular patient, irrespective of the test result, then the test may be superfluous and may subject the patient to unnecessary costs and risks.

A third common error involves not fully considering for whom the decision is being optimized. Clearly, medical decisions are made for the express purpose of maximizing the chance of a "good" outcome—but one must first ask "Good for whom?" Although the obvious answer would seem to be the patient, some decisions are optimized for the physician or for society. For example, consider a patient with severe acute coronary artery disease (for instance, one with an evolving myocardial infarction) who develops acute abdominal symptomatology and has findings suggesting colonic perforation. Suppose the anesthesia risk in such a patient is 40 percent, that his late postoperative mortality risk (assuming that he survived surgery) is 20 percent, and that his survival rate without surgery is only 50 percent. Some surgeons would insist on operating, reasoning that they could not live with themselves if he were to die of a treatable disease. Such a statement clearly reflects the doctor's gain from surgery. As far as the patient is concerned, whether he dies from his perforation or from anesthesia, the result is the same. Looking only at survival, we can see that surgery will provide a survival rate of 48 percent (that is, 60% × 80%), whereas medical therapy will result in a 50 percent survival rate. Thus, from the patient's point of view, it would seem that surgery should be declined.

This chapter will present techniques which allow the physician to approach his clinical decisions in a formal and explicit manner. The technique is called decision analysis and relies on a set of tools developed in the field of business administration. The basic premise is that a complex decision can be broken down into a set of simpler ones and those simpler choices can be made more accurately and reproducibly. The simple parts are then integrated into an overall approach to the problem.

AN OVERVIEW OF DECISION ANALYSIS

Clinical decisions are often made under conditions of uncertainty—medicine is not so precise that a given diagnostic or therapeutic plan can always be associated with a known outcome. The definition of the common medical term "prognosis" clearly recognizes this limitation. Stedman's Medical Dictionary defines prognosis as "foretelling of the *probable* course of a disease; a *forecast* of the outcome of a disease" (emphasis author's). Thus, the clinician must consider the array of possible outcomes and the probability or likelihood that each outcome will, in fact, come to pass.

The Decision Tree

The first step in clinical decision making is to structure the clinical problem. Such structure must include the choices which the physician (and the patient) must make and the potential results of each choice. One must clearly separate decisions which the physician can control from chance events which neither the clinician nor the patient can control. For example, consider the choice between pneumonectomy and radiation therapy in a patient with bronchogenic carcinoma. The physician (and the patient) must decide which therapy will be given, but neither can decide the results of that therapy. Those results, that is, the chance that the patient will survive for a given period of time, can be summarized by a survival curve, but the patient has little control over how long he as an individual will live.

As will be explained later, the method of notation which we suggest for providing explicit structure for clinical decisions is the *decision tree.* Such trees can be used to describe the time course of an evolving clinical problem and to summarize the decisions and outcomes to be considered. The major point in structuring clinical problems is to keep the decision tree as simple as possible. Studies in cognitive psychology have demonstrated that the human mind rarely considers more than seven to ten alternatives at a given time, so it is unlikely that physicians actively consider dozens of diagnoses and treatment plans in a given patient. Although the use of pencil and paper relieves this constraint somewhat, it is important, on the other hand, to keep the clinical decision trees from becoming too complex. The lure of completeness and detail often makes the novice consider too many possibilities. The analyst must train himself to deal with the simplest structure which reflects the dynamics of the problem at hand. Consider, for example, the decision between medical and surgical management in a patient with coronary artery disease. When a cardiologist counsels a patient about this therapeutic choice, he speaks of the risks of surgery, the chance of improvement in life style, and the likelihood of survival. The risks of surgery are expressed in terms of the perioperative mortality rate. Nonfatal complications such as cerebrovascular accidents, renal failure, or infection may be mentioned but are not presented in detail. Similarly, if we are to use the decision analytic model effectively, in structuring the problem we must not include excessive detail about minor nonfatal complications of surgery.

Probabilities and Utilities

The next step in this approach to clinical decision making is to consider each potential outcome and develop a measure of the relative likelihood or probability of its occurrence. In many cases, it is simpler and more accurate to compute such probabilities in a stepwise fashion rather then trying to develop a single overall estimate. For example, consider the implications of hematuria in patients taking oral anticoagulants with prothrombin times well within the therapeutic range. It might be difficult to estimate the likelihood that such hematuria is a marker for renal carcinoma and, as such, whether it should be pursued with intravenous pyelography. However, one might estimate the likelihood of anticoagulant-induced hematuria in the absence of renal tumor and then develop a limited estimate of the likelihood that anticoagulation therapy would induce bleeding from a tumor. Such an estimate might be crude but would probably be more accurate than an overall estimate of the likelihood of cancer in patients with anticoagulant-induced hematuria. The final fact required would be the incidence of renal cell carcinoma in patients of the particular age and sex in question. These separate data could then be combined to form an estimate of the likelihood of renal carcinoma in the patient at hand. Again, a convenient shorthand for developing such stepwise estimates of the likelihood of various outcomes is the decision tree—in this case, by diagramming a series of sequential (or conditional) chance events, as will be explained below.

The third step in the decision analytic approach is to attach a relative value, or utility, to each potential outcome. If a clinical problem is sufficiently simple that only two outcomes need be considered (for example, death and survival during the next few weeks), then the value structure is binary (good and bad) and utilities such as one and zero may be used. Unlike this example, in most situations, the problem is not black and white—several outcomes may exist and must be ranked relative to one another. If such rankings, or pair-wise preferences, can be established, then it is usually possible to create a quantitative scale of preferences or utilities which reflects the relative value of each potential outcome. Of course, one question must be answered first: "relative value to whom?" The analyst must first decide whose values and preferences are being considered in the decision making process. The simplest answer is "the patient's," but if that is the case, then the physician must consider mechanisms whereby the patient can express his attitudes or preferences and whereby those utilities can be incorporated into the decision making process.

Analysis

The next step is to calculate the expected value of each possible course of action. Such calculations produce an estimate of the average gain or loss which would accrue if the decision were made repeatedly and if the laws of chance governed the outcome of each repetition. Actually, for a given patient the decision is usually made only once and one particular outcome occurs. Nevertheless, the average outcome measure—the expected utility—is still the best metric of the relative value of each decision option. The choice with the highest expected utility will be the best choice that one can make under the circumstances. Differences between the expected value of the best choice and the other (suboptimal) choices measure the relative cost of making a nonoptimal management decision.

The final phase of clinical decision analysis is to consider the individual data upon which the decision is based and examine whether reasonable variations in such data might lead to a different decision. This process is called *sensitivity analysis* because it tries to determine whether the selection of the apparently optimal choice is sensitive to small changes in the assumptions of the analysis. This step is one of the most powerful tools of the decision analytic technique because it allows the clinician to evaluate the reliability of his decision. He can not only say which diagnostic or therapeutic choice is optimal but how stable that choice is relative to the available data base.

STRUCTURING THE PROBLEM

One of the most important steps in making logical clinical decisions is to organize and structure the problem domain. This process entails considering all the *relevant* decisions and outcomes. The key concept here is the word relevant. Clearly, if one attempted to list all the possible choices and outcomes of even the simplest clinical decision, then the problem would become unmanageable. We as clinicians are taught to hone our clinical choices to their simplest and most straightforward forms. This hard-earned skill should not be abandoned when we approach clinical decision making in a more formal and logical manner. The problem solving tools presented in this chapter are intrinsically quite simple. They are capable of reflecting any level of complexity which the physician wishes to consider, but the tools themselves do not require such complexity. In fact, the physician should strive to represent the clinical choices in the simplest form possible.

Decision Trees

The decision tree is a diagrammatic means of denoting both decisions and outcomes. A *square* node is used to denote a decision point—where the physician or the patient must make a choice. A *circular* node is used to denote a chance event—where neither the physician nor the patient can control the outcome. In such chance situations, the physician may have some idea of the relative likelihood (or probability) of the various potential outcomes of that chance event. Those prognostic estimates are called the branch probabilities of the chance node (Fig. 1).

The customary means of ordering the nodes on a decision tree is based on the time of the event or decision, with progression of time moving from left to right along the tree. Thus, nodes appearing at the proximal or left portion of the decision tree, in general, occur before nodes appearing at the distal or right portion.

Outcomes and the Horizon

The terminal or end branches of the right-most nodes on the tree denote *outcomes*, that is, potential results of the combination of choices and chance events which the tree represents. In this text, an outcome is enclosed within a rectangle. The determination of just what should be called an outcome is dictated by two major considerations—the level of detail included in the tree and the time horizon. For example, in certain clinical situations it may be sufficient to describe an outcome simply as "survives surgery." In other situations, that outcome might be separated into "survives surgery without complications" and "survives surgery with a major complication." In some problems, detail such as "survives surgery with postoperative pneumonia but without neurologic deficit" might be more appropriate. In general, the shorter the time horizon, the less detail is required to represent the problem. Consider the question of surgery for suspected appendicitis: here, a short time horizon of a week or so with outcomes such as "dead," "alive without complications," and "alive after appendiceal rupture" may be quite sufficient. On the other hand, consider the issue of surgery for cancer of the breast: in that case, recurrent cancer may not be manifest for many years, whereas some complications of surgery (such as lymphedema of the arm) may occur far sooner. Here, the tree must be far more detailed to accommodate the broader time horizon.

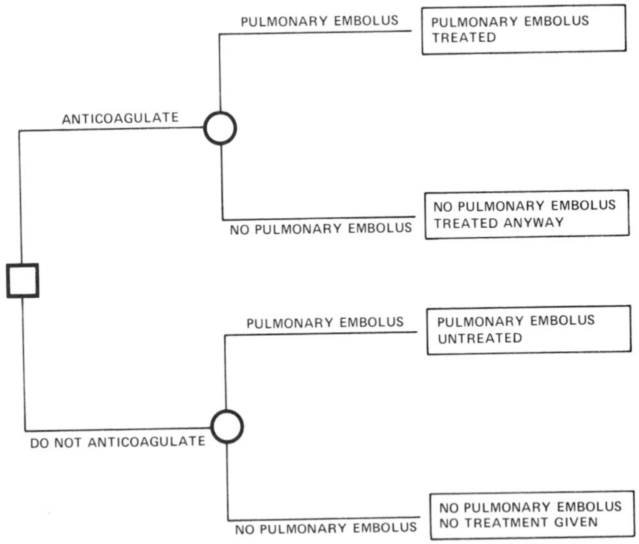

FIGURE 1. A therapeutic decision tree evaluating the use of anticoagulation therapy in patients with possible pulmonary embolism.

The choice of the time horizon, and therefore the choice of the set of outcomes under consideration, is somewhat arbitrary. Most outcomes can be considered to be abbreviations or summaries of further detail in a decision tree. For example, the outcome "alive after appendiceal rupture" as a consequence of postponing surgery in a patient with abdominal pain could be expanded into further "downstream" outcomes such as "adhesions with bowel obstruction" or even "perioperative death after a second operation for the lysis of adhesions." Again the choice between summarization (that is, the designation of a set of consequences as a single outcome) or expansion of an outcome into a detailed tree is dictated largely by the nature of the problem being analyzed.

Let us consider some examples of the use of a decision tree to structure clinical problems. Figure 1 summarizes the simple choice between no anticoagulation and anticoagulation therapy in a patient suspected of having a pulmonary embolus. The square node on the left denotes the choice facing the physician—whether or not to anticoagulate the patient. The two circular nodes denote the chance the pulmonary emboli may (1) be present or (2) absent. The four rectangles at the right denote the potential outcomes of the respective decisions. Sometimes it is helpful to consider these outcomes in more detail, expanding them into branches of the tree as shown in Figure 2. This figure shows that the frequency of anticoagulant complications and the frequency of episodes of re-embolization contribute to each outcome. If further detail is required, the complications can be separated (i.e., fatal, severe, or minor) and the consequences of re-emboliza-

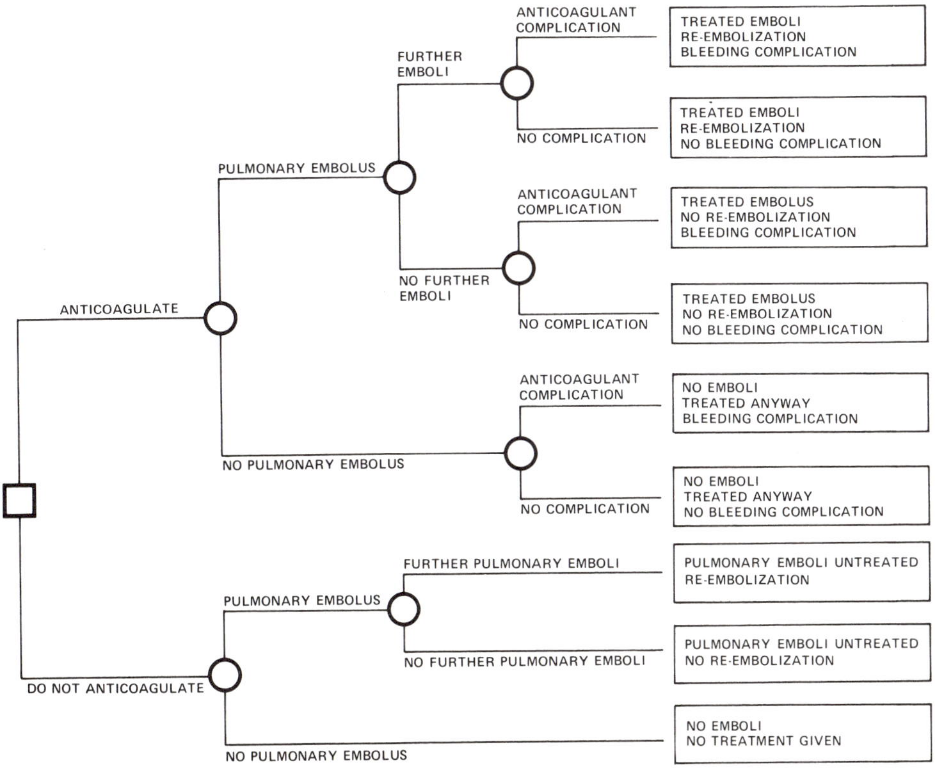

FIGURE 2. An expanded view of the problem displayed in Figure 1.

tion (e.g., death, permanent pulmonary hypertension) can be considered separately. One might also consider *when* each complication occurs (e.g., after 1 week or after 1 month). From this example, it should be clear that the decision tree notational system is quite flexible but that inclusion of excessive detail makes the tree quite dense.

Let us consider several modifications of this problem which might be introduced by the consideration of a diagnostic test. For simplicity we shall consider two extremes of diagnostic testing, extremes which are never really achieved but which are both didactically and clinically useful: a test which is cost or risk-free and a test which provides "perfect" diagnostic information. A lung scan has few complications and risks to the patient but can provide both false positive and (if misinterpreted) false negative results. Figure 3 illustrates the situation of a risk-free but imperfect test and demonstrates several important points. First, the portion of the tree enclosed within the dotted box is identical to Figure 1, that is, the decision whether or not to perform a diagnostic test *depends* on the decision about therapy, but since the diagnostic decision preceeds the therapeutic decision it is placed to the left of the decision tree. Second, the diagnostic test results may be correct (either a true positive or a true negative) or may be in error (either a false positive or a false negative). Since the true state of the patient is not known, therapy is nevertheless based on the test results. If more detail were desired, the chance node depicting the test result could be followed by a decision node (e.g., whether or not to anticoagulate after a positive result). However, if therapy is to be given even after a

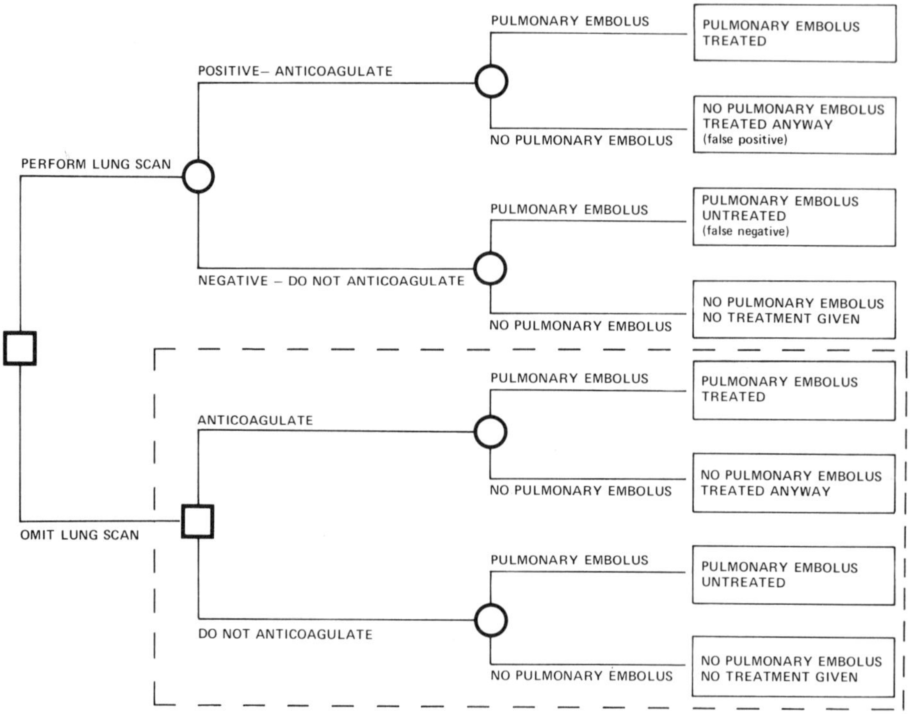

FIGURE 3. A cost-free test—the lung scan.

negative result or omitted even after a positive result, then the test would have been superfluous. Thus, those two implied decision nodes are omitted in Figure 3.

A pulmonary arteriogram is considered the "gold standard" for the diagnosis of pulmonary emboli. If it is done promptly and interpreted correctly, few errors occur. However, pulmonary arteriography is not benign; both fatal and nonfatal complications can occur as depicted in Figure 4. For clarity, the downstream decision about treatment if arteriography is not performed is omitted from this figure. The dotted box should contain Figure 1, as shown in Figure 3 (above). It should be pointed out that the structure of Figure 4 implies that the incidence of complications from arteriography does not depend on whether or not pulmonary emboli are, in fact, present. If this were not the case, then the order of chance nodes in the decision tree should be inverted. For example, consider the problem of whether or not to perform a coronary arteriogram to establish the presence or absence of left main coronary artery stenosis. In that case, the incidence of complications from catheterization (primarily death and myocardial infarction) would be higher if left main obstruction were indeed present. The structure of this latter situation is illustrated by the partial tree in Figure 5.

Some of the most difficult decisions to approach either informally or through formal analysis involve a long time horizon with outcomes expressed as rates. For example, consider surgery for disabling angina in a patient with coronary artery disease. The patient may have marked symptomatic improvement if he survives surgery, but pain can recur or the patient may die at some future time from his coronary disease. Even if the rates of recurrence and survival were well known, providing structure for this problem

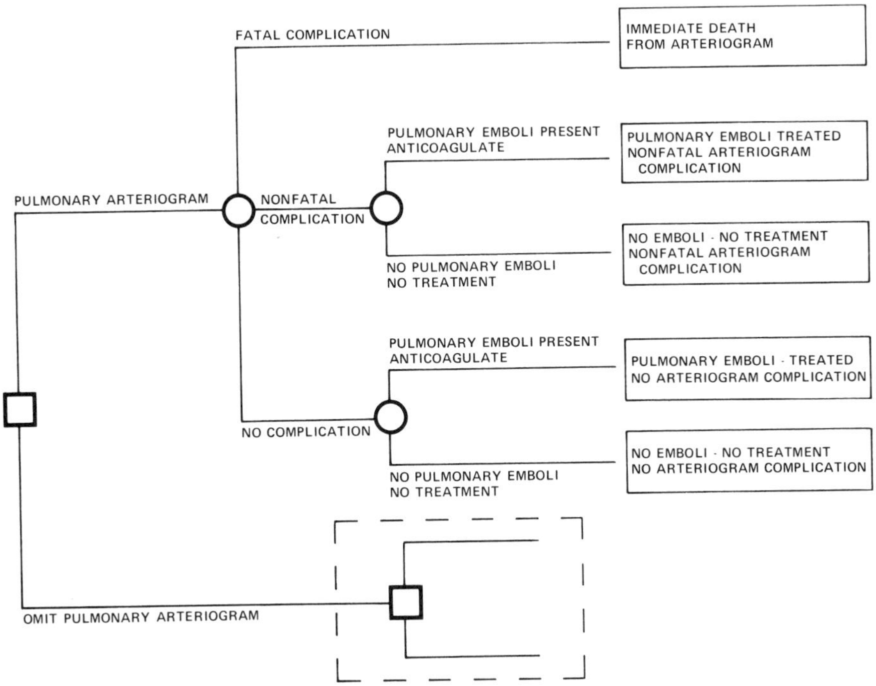

FIGURE 4. A test that provides very accurate information—the pulmonary angiogram.

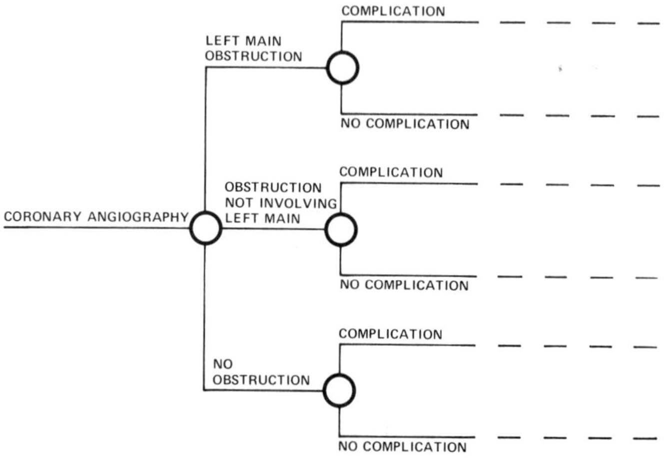

FIGURE 5. A test with complication rates varying with diagnosis.

would be difficult. One might create successive tiers in the tree, with each tier denoting the events of a single year. These tiers might then be arranged sequentially as shown in Figure 6. Unfortunately, the decision tree (or alternatively, our view of the problem) soon becomes unmanageably complex. Two approaches are available for such problems. The simplest solution is to arbitrarily divide the time horizon into several large segments, for example, death in year one, death between one and ten years, and death after ten years. If such crude divisions do not blur the problem unduly, then a rather simple tree might result. Alternatively, one might treat the entire set of recurrent events as a single outcome and summarize a very deep tree with a description of the outcome state. If such outcome states can be compared to one another directly, then again a far simpler tree results. Of course, this approach may simply beg the question, since the comparison of these summary outcome states may require the construction of other decision trees.

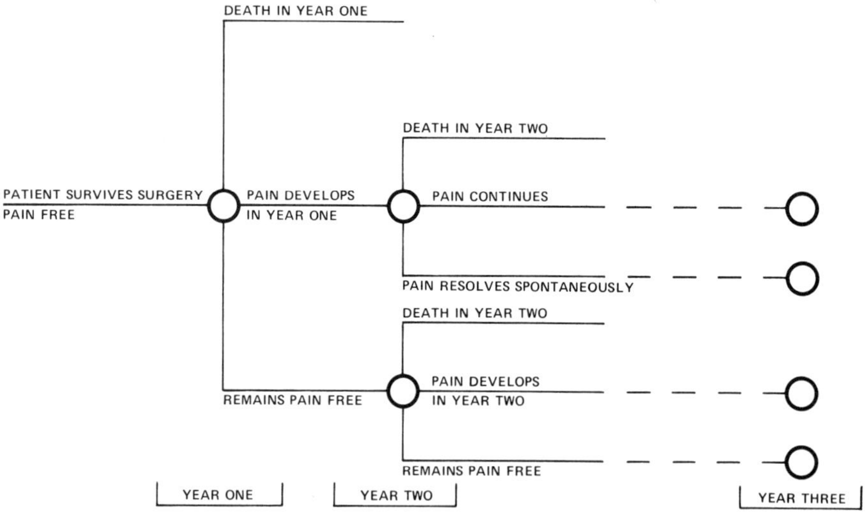

FIGURE 6. Sequential or recurrent set of events.

This brings us to the final issue in designing decision trees—dealing with repetitive sections of a tree. Even if a long time horizon with repetitive events is not present, decision trees (or alternatively, our concepts of a clinical problem) may get quite tangled if descriptions of the consequences of certain treatments and diagnoses are repetitive, differing only in the impact which treatment and diagnosis have on certain prognostic likelihoods. For example, consider the situation in an alcoholic patient with Laennec's cirrhosis, portal hypertension, and esophageal varices who is having recurrent upper gastrointestinal bleeding. If endoscopy is unable to demonstrate unequivocally that the varices are the source of bleeding, then the patient's prognosis depends on the site of bleeding and the therapy given—in this case, either medical therapy or splenorenal shunting. This situation is structured in Figure 7. Actually, this tree is considerably oversimplified; the 17 outcomes at the right are probably inadequate descriptions of the patient's health. For example, late death might be expanded to show when that death occurred; gastrointestinal bleeding and encephalopathy might be expanded to include

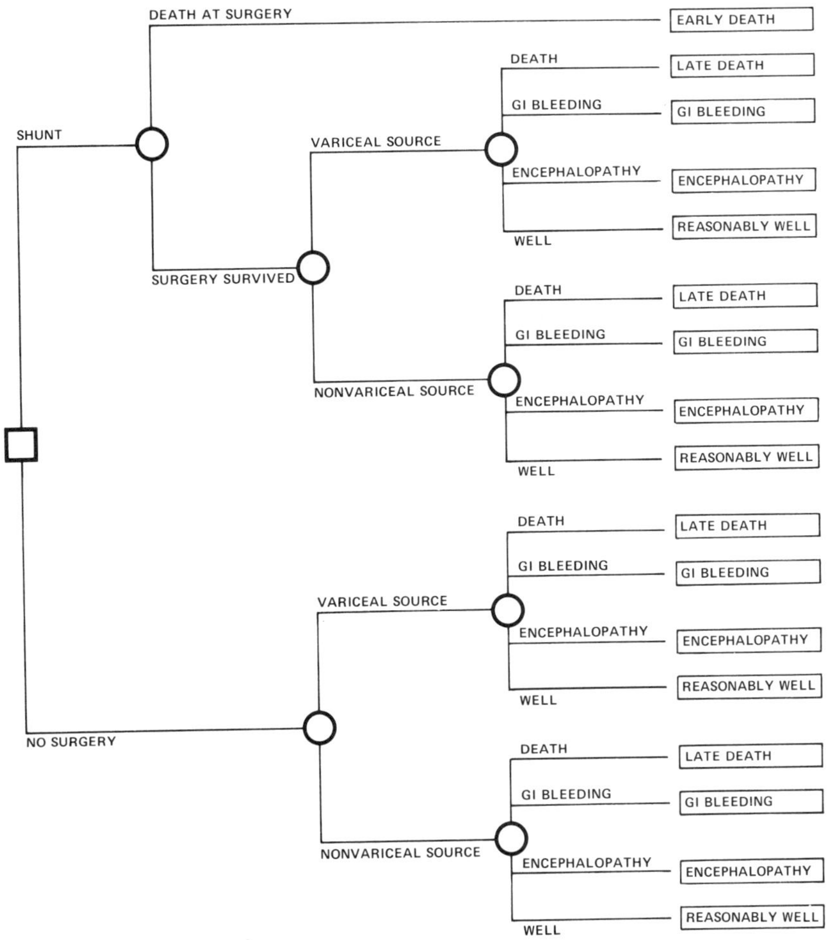

FIGURE 7. A complex tree: Shunt surgery for variceal bleeding.

the frequency, duration, and possible coexistence of those outcomes; and being "reasonably well" must obviously be modified based on other consequences of cirrhosis such as fever, infection, fluid retention, and the like. Nevertheless, the decision tree in Figure 7, although complex, is not an unreasonable representation of the problem. Unfortunately, the effect of shunt surgery, that is, a decrease in bleeding at the expense of an increase in encephalopathy, may lie buried in the complexity of the tree. In contrast, the problem has been restructured in Figure 8, using the notation of a repeated subtree. The tree at the left summarizes the problem only to the extent that the therapy and source of bleeding are specified. The four outcomes in double boxes imply additional tree structures. Those four structures are identical and are shown as the right-hand tree. The only difference among the four subtrees is that the likelihood of bleeding and encephalopathy change. The subtree at the right can be viewed as a function of two variables (i.e., bleeding and encephalopathy) and the values for those variables are specified within each double box. This representation is somewhat simpler than that in Figure 7 and emphasizes the similarities among the prognoses as well as the effect of therapy and bleeding source upon prognosis.

The clinician should now be able to use the decision tree notational system to structure some of the complex problems he faces in patient care. Once he has established the structure, he must turn to the next task—couching the patient's prognosis and the likelihood of various outcomes in terms of probabilities.

OBTAINING AND ESTIMATING PROBABILITIES

First, let us consider the advantages and the limitations of using probabilities to represent the likelihood of various future events. Physicians should be familiar with this concept,

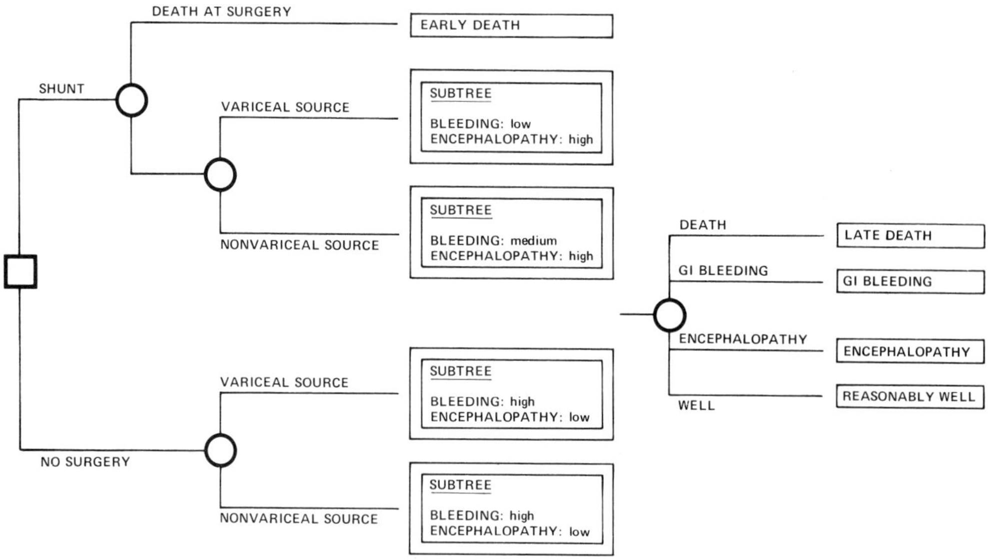

FIGURE 8. The subtree notation: Shunt surgery for variceal bleeding.

although we sometimes become uncomfortable when numerical estimates are used in the care of an individual patient. We often speak of a certain diagnosis or complication as being "common," "unlikely," or "rare." Unfortunately, the meaning of such semiquantitative terms varies from physician to physician. One physician might say that a diagnosis is "probable" and mean that the likelihood of that disease is 95 percent, a physician who reads that statement might interpret "probable" to mean a likelihood of 50 percent. In many cases, a patient with a 95 percent likelihood of a given disease might be treated forthwith, whereas a patient whose chance of disease is only 50 percent might undergo further diagnostic testing. Obviously, such lack of accurate communication might interfere with proper patient management.

The use of numbers to denote relative likelihoods does not imply any greater precision of data—we might consider the numbers accurate only to one significant figure or even less. The motivation for using numbers is to provide information in a consistent form which can be communicated from physician to physician and from the literature to the physician. An additional benefit of using numbers is that they can be combined by well-established rules. For example, if the patient has a 10 percent chance of having pulmonary emboli and if 30 percent of people who have emboli die if they are not anticoagulated, then there is a 10 percent of 30 percent, or 3 percent, chance that this patient will die from untreated emboli. If we had said that emboli were "unlikely" and that death from untreated emboli was "not infrequent," it would be difficult to estimate the likelihood of an embolus-related death.

The particular scale we suggest for representing relative likelihoods is the probability scale, where a value of zero denotes that the event cannot (or will not) occur and where a value of one, or 100 percent, denotes that the event is certain. If we deal with events which are mutually exclusive and exhaustive, then their probabilities must sum to unity. Such is the case for each chance node in a decision tree—the branches denote all possible outcomes, so the probabilities associated with each branch must sum to one. If two events are mutually independent, then the probability of both events occurring equals the product of their probabilities. The probability of an event not occurring is equal to one minus the probability of the event occurring. If two events are mutually exclusive, then the probability of *either* event occurring is equal to the sum of the probability of each event's occurring. For example, if a given surgical procedure has a 5 percent chance of resulting in perioperative death and a 20 percent chance of resulting in a serious nonfatal operative complication, then the chance of either a fatal or nonfatal complication is 25 percent (i.e., the probability of *either* is the sum of 5% and 20%). The chance of no serious complications is 75 percent (i.e., the probability of *neither* is one minus the probability of either). Further assume that the late complication rate is 10 percent in operative survivors. The chance of *only* a late complication will be 10 percent of 75 percent, or 7.5 percent (i.e., the probability of both *no* early and a late complication is the product of the probabilities). The chance of the patient escaping with neither an early nor a late complication is 90 percent of 75 percent, or 67.5 percent. Thus, the chance of either an early or a late complication will be 32.5 percent. It would be improper to just add 25 percent and 10 percent (and get 35%) since 2.5 percent of patients will have *both* early and late complications.

Objections

One argument often raised against the use of probabilities is that the necessary data are just not available as properly controlled studies have not been published. It is important to realize that medical decisions are made every day despite this lack of "adequate" data. In fact, a large part of the art of medicine may be the ability to make critical decisions, upon which lives depend, on the basis of limited, inadequate, and possibly erroneous data. The skilled clinician develops a sense of when data can be accepted and when they should be ignored. Decisions must be made on the basis of information available today. That information may be objective (e.g., published studies) or subjective (opinions of the physician or his consultants based on clinical experience). Clinical decision analysis will neither improve the data upon which decisions are made nor necessarily analyze the problem in greater detail. The main advantages of formal analysis are: providing structure, allowing combination of diverse sources of information, and preventing certain common errors in human reasoning.

Another argument can be made favoring the use of *subjective* probabilities. Patients are all different—one cannot find a patient exactly like patients reported upon in any given series in the literature. For example, many reported series describing the efficacy of lung scanning in diagnosing pulmonary emboli deal with a population in which the average incidence of emboli is 20 to 30 percent. If a particular patient has such a classic history that his likelihood of emboli is far greater, then the import of positive, negative, and suspicious test results would differ markedly from the import in the reported series. Similarly, one might use epidemiologic data to estimate the likelihood of coronary disease in a given patient with chest pain, hypertension, and a history of smoking. Nevertheless, those epidemiologic estimates might need to be modified on the basis of family history, duration of hypertension, and the patient's lifestyle. One can rarely find a report of a series of patients that corresponds *exactly* to a given patient under treatment. Although objective probabilities can serve as an anchor point, ultimately there must always be some degree of subjective adjustment of those estimates to the specifics of each case. Not infrequently a particular case is quite unlike other cases reported in the literature or seen by the physician. In such situations, the *only* available data may be subjective; nevertheless, the clinician should not be inhibited from using quantitative techniques to structure and analyze the problem. It is only through such analyses that the physician can determine the potential impact of the lack of adequate data and thereby address the needs of this patient. This technique is explained in detail in the section on sensitivity analysis later in this chapter.

Another argument often raised against the use of probabilities is that they describe the results expected in a *group* of patients, whereas, in a particular patient, a given result will apply: he will or will not have the disease or suffer the complication. Thus, it is argued, probabilities can be used to describe average results but are quite irrelevant to the management of particular patients. In fact, little could be further from the truth. The assumption that probabilities do not apply and that a given event either will or will not occur is tantamount to saying that all events are equally likely. By this reasoning, a child with pharyngitis either will or will not have an anaphylactic reaction to penicillin. Furthermore, a child who developed urticaria and wheezing when given penicillin in the past also either will or will not develop anaphylaxis. Thus, the risk of penicillin is not increased in patients with prior allergic reactions!? The weakness of this reasoning becomes clear through this hyperbole. Most physicians would not give penicillin to the child who had a prior reaction but would give the drug to otherwise healthy children suspected of having streptococcal pharyngitis. Thus, we implicitly accept that all events are not equally likely but that some are more likely than others. To whatever extent we can distinguish likely from unlikely events, we can use probabilities to express our degree of belief in the likelihood of each event's occurrence.

This view can be expressed slightly differently. Probabilities can be viewed either descriptively or prognostically. As *descriptors,* probabilities denote the observed likelihood of given events in a cohort of patients under examination. To the extent that an individual patient is representative of such a cohort, the probabilities observed in the cohort may be good *predictors* of the state of the patient or of the future events which may befall him. To the extent that an individual patient differs from the observed cohort, the observed probabilities may be poor predictors of the future. The ultimate use of diagnosis and prognosis is to predict and possibly alter future events in a given patient. A fair portion of the physician's implicit training is to allow him to make such predictions with comfort and reasonable accuracy. Probabilities, then, simply become a language in which the clinician can couch his predictions.

Probabilities and Diagnosis

Up to this point, we have used probabilities in two ways: to describe the likelihood of a disease's being present and to describe the likelihood of future events such as complications or morbidity. Let us now consider the use of probabilities in diagnosis. The establishment of a diagnosis involves consideration of many clinical and laboratory data. The usual base or starting point is the frequency of various diseases in a given population. This base rate is then modified by each additional fact learned about the patient. Often such modifications are performed implicitly by the physician, but studies have shown that there are common situations in which such implicit appraisals are fraught with error. Errors commonly arise in the interpretation of laboratory tests, especially when the accuracy of the test has been documented in the literature. In these cases, the physician often ignores or underestimates the importance of other aspects of the case and relies too heavily on the test results and the data in the literature. The physician often does not realize that three separate kinds of probabilities are involved in the interpretation of a diagnostic test result: the prior probability, the conditional probability, and the posterior probability.

Let us consider these three likelihoods in turn. The *prior probability* denotes the likelihood that a given disease is present before a test is performed or the results of the test are known. If the test is to be performed as a screening measure (e.g., an electrocardiogram in an otherwise healthy man about to undergo an elective herniorrhaphy), then the prior probability is the prevalence of the disease (in this case, acute coronary artery disease) in the population of men of the same age. If the patient is in some way different from the general population (e.g., a history of hypertension, smoking, or chest pain), then the population prevalence may no longer be appropriate. Whatever the basis for the estimate, the prior probability should represent the likelihood of the disease, based on all available clinical information, formulated prior to knowledge of the test results.

The conditional probability denotes the likelihood of observing a given test result in patients known to have a particular diagnosis. The two most commonly used descriptors of conditional probability are the sensitivity and the specificity of a test, but those descriptors are only meaningful when a single diagnosis is under consideration and when the test result is binary—either positive or negative. In that case, the conditional probability of a positive test result in patients known to have the disease (the conditioning criterion) is called the sensitivity of the test. The conditional probability of a negative test result in patients known not to have the disease (a different conditioning criterion) is called the specificity of the test. Often several diagnoses are under consideration or several different test results might occur. In such cases, it is best to speak of the conditional probability of a given result in a particular diagnosis. For example, we can speak of the conditional probability of a serum potassium between 3.0 and 3.5 mEq/L in patients with adrenal adenomata as the cause of their hypertension and the conditional probability of a serum potassium between 2.5 and 3.0 mEq/L in untreated patients with essential hypertension.

The posterior probability denotes the likelihood of the patient having a given diagnosis after the results of the test are known. This revised probability is sometimes called the predictive value of the test, but predictive value may be a poor term since the "value" of any clinical information does not rest solely with the likelihood of disease but clearly depends also on the efficacy and risks involved in treating or diagnosing the disease. Therefore, we prefer the term posterior (or revised) probability. In fact, the posterior probability represents the physician's best estimate (after a test has been performed) of the likelihood of disease in a particular patient.

Unfortunately, the practice of medicine is not quite so simple. A particular study can report on a series of patients with a particular diagnostic finding, for example, a strongly positive exercise electrocardiographic test showing over 2 mm of ST depression during mild exercise. Such a study might point out that, *in the cohort of people examined,* 30 percent had significant obstruction of the left main coronary artery. The physician must, however, be cautious in assuming that a particular patient who demonstrates that degree of ischemic exercise response does, in fact, have a 30 percent chance of having left main coronary artery obstruction. That conclusion would only be valid if the clinical characteristics of the patient were *identical* to those of patients included in the study. In other words, the clinician can only accept a posterior probability from a published study if the clinical likelihood of the disease in his patient (before performing the diagnostic test) is the same as the clinical likelihood in patients reported in the study, that is, only if his patient's likelihood of disease equals the disease prevalence in the studied cohort. In general, this condition will *not* be met. Even if the clinician's patient is substantially similar with respect to age, sex, and presentation, the physician usually has far more detailed knowledge of the patient's history, risk factors, and symptoms than would be customarily reported in the literature. Thus, the published series may well serve as an anchor point, but the physician must make certain "adjustments" to insure optimal interpretation of each test result. The only common situation where such adjustments are not needed is when the test is employed as a screening tool (e.g., a preoperative electrocardiogram in a healthy man) because in that situation the patient's likelihood of disease may well correspond to that in a published cohort.

To further illustrate this point, consider the interpretation of a lung scan. Most series of lung scan results are reported on populations that include about 20 to 30 percent of people with angiographically documentable pulmonary emboli (i.e., of all patients submitted to lung scan, 20 to 30 percent can be shown to have positive angiograms). If the physician examines a patient with a long leg cast, hemoptysis, pleuritic chest pain, hypoxemia, and a rub, he will likely conclude that the chance of pulmonary emboli in that patient may be substantially higher than 20 to 30 percent. He would be underestimating the likelihood of embolus in this patient if he were to simply use the posterior probabilities from the reported series.

The goal of the interpretation of a test result is to estimate the posterior or revised probability of disease. The factors which affect that probability are two: the prior probability of each disease and the conditional probabilities of the test result in the various diseases being considered. Those two likelihoods can be combined by Bayes' rule to calculate the posterior probability. The prior probability usually involves some individualized adjustment, with the literature serving as an anchor point. The conditional probabilities can usually be obtained from published reports or expert opinion.

Bayes' Rule

Clearly, there must be a relation among the prior, conditional, and revised probabilities of disease. That relation is described by Bayes' rule which simply states that the revised or posterior probability of disease is the proportion of all patients with the observed finding who also have the disease. In other words, the revised probability equals

$$\frac{\text{probability of finding and disease}}{\text{probability of finding}}$$

For example, if the probability of observing a "high suspicion" result on a lung scan were 30 percent and if the chance of pulmonary emboli being present *and* the lung scan being positive were 20 percent, then the revised probability of pulmonary emboli, *given* a high suspicion scan, would be 20 percent/30 percent, or 0.67. Clearly, both the numerator and denominator of the ratio depend upon the prior likelihood of emboli and on the accuracy of the test. Therefore, the simple ratio must be replaced by a more complex expression to allow for the separate consideration of prior and conditional probabilities.

Most presentations of the use of Bayes' rule as an approach to medical diagnosis involve rather formidable mathematical expressions. Since, in this chapter, we propose the Bayesian approach as a practical tool, we shall offer two alternative techniques for using the approach: one graphical and one tabular. The two methods will provide identical results. The graphic approach provides the physician with a better view of the logic of the interpretive process, whereas the tabular approach is more compact and slightly faster to use.

Let us consider a clinical problem raised earlier in this chapter: the patient shows no cardiac symptoms after routine surgery, but his "screening" enzyme test was positive for myocardial necrosis. In that example, we stated that the likelihood of silent perioperative infarction was 1 percent, that the sensitivity of the enzyme test was 95 percent, and that its specificity was 90 percent. Thus, the prior probability of myocardial infarction is 0.01, the conditional probability of positive enzymes given actual necrosis ($P_{pos/necrosis}$) is 0.95, and the conditional probability of positive enzymes in the absence of necrosis ($P_{pos/no\ necrosis}$) is 0.10.

This situation is shown diagrammatically in Figure 9. The circles denote observations which can be made; the hexagons denote the actual state of the world which, unfortunately, cannot be observed. At the top of the figure, we have shown a cohort of one million patients similar to the patient under examination. We might have used any cohort size or even fractional values. Alterations in the size of the cohort considered would affect the intermediate calculations but not the conclusions. As shown in the hexagons in the second tier, 1 percent of the million patients, or 10,000 patients, will actually have myocardial necrosis and 990,000 will not. Since the conditional probability

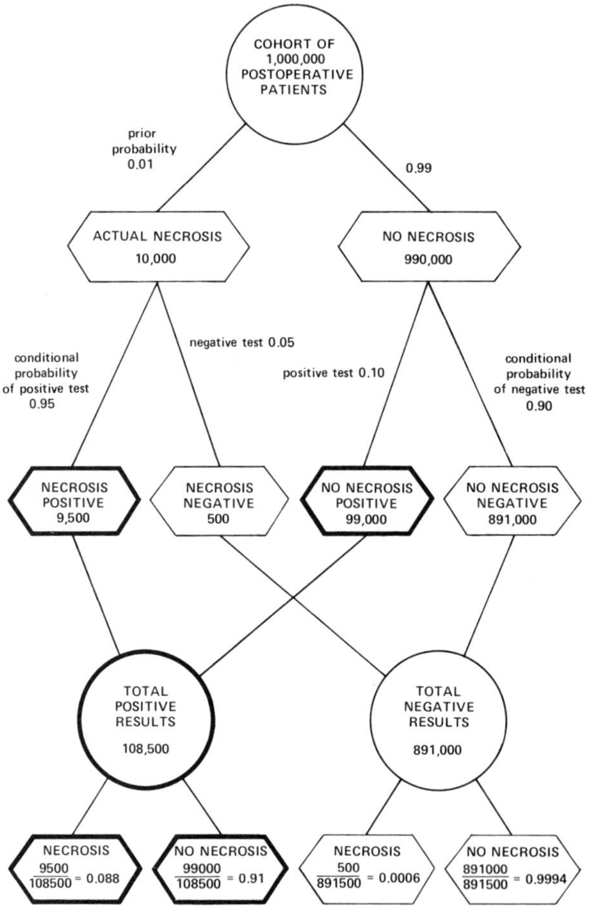

FIGURE 9. Interpreting a diagnostic test: An unexpected abnormal serum enzyme.

of a positive test in patients with necrosis (the sensitivity) is 0.95, 9,500 of the 10,000 patients will have a positive test (denoted by the heavy hexagon in the third tier) and 500 will have (false) negative results (light hexagon in third tier). Similarly, of the 990,000 patients without necrosis, 10 percent or 99,000 will have a (false) positive result (heavy hexagon in third tier) and 891,000 will have a negative result. Thus, the total number of positive results observed after testing the cohort of one million patients will be 108,500 (heavy circle in fourth tier), and the total number of negative results will be 891,500 (light circle in fourth tier). Finally, of the 108,500 positive results, 9,500 or 8.8 percent will be patients who actually have necrosis; of the 891,500 negative results, 500 or 0.06 percent will be patients who actually have necrosis. Thus, a positive result will select a subgroup (heavy circle) in which the probability of necrosis would be 0.088; a negative result will select a subgroup in which the probability of necrosis would be 0.0006.

The alternative method of computation, in this case for a positive result only, is illustrated in Table 1 in which column A lists each diagnostic probability, column B lists the relative likelihood of each diagnosis prior to knowledge of the test result, column C provides the conditional probability of the observed result in each diagnostic category, column D is the product of columns B and C, and column E is the revised or posterior probability of each diagnosis. That revised likelihood is calculated by finding the sum (S) of the entries in column D and then dividing each entry in column D by S. Column B (the prior likelihood) and column C (the conditional likelihood) must each be internally consistent but can be on any scale. For example, as prior likelihoods the physician might use either 1 and 99 or 0.1 and 0.01 or even 10,000 and 990,000. Similarly, the conditional likelihoods could be 95 and 10 or 0.95 and 0.10. Note that the conditional likelihoods will, in general, *not* sum to unity. A product column is then calculated as follows: $1 \times 95 = 95$; $99 \times 10 = 990$. The products are then added, yielding a sum of 1085. Finally, of the 1085 positive results, 95 (or 8.8%) are patients with myocardial necrosis, while 990 of the 1085 (or 91.2%) are patients without necrosis.

To be quite sure that the tabular form of Bayes' rule is clearly understood, let us consider the interpretation of another diagnostic test, in this case, an electrocardiogram.

TABLE 1. Interpretation of a Positive Diagnostic Test for Myocardial Necrosis Using Bayes' Rule

A	B	C	D	E (D/S)
Diagnosis	*Clinical Likelihood or Prior Probability or Likelihood before Test Result Is Known*	*Conditional Probability of Observed Test Result in Patients with Each Diagnosis*	*Product*	*Revised or Posterior Probability or Likelihood after Test Result Is Known*
Myocardial necrosis present	1	95	95	95/1085 = 0.088
No myocardial necrosis present	99	10	990	990/1085 = 0.912
		Sum (S) =	1085	

Imagine that an asymptomatic, normotensive 50-year-old man admitted for elective cholecystectomy was found to have a systolic murmur. Based on the history and the characteristics of the murmur, the admitting physician feels that it is most likely "functional" (probability 0.7) but that aortic stenosis (probability 0.2) and mitral insufficiency (probability 0.1) must be considered. (The choice of probabilities in this example is somewhat arbitrary but nevertheless reasonable.) The routine electrocardiogram demonstrates left ventricular hypertrophy. A consultant suggests that left ventricular hypertrophy occurs in 90 percent of patients with asymptomatic aortic stenosis, 50 percent of patients with asymptomatic mitral stenosis, and 10 percent of normotensive patients with functional flow murmurs. The interpretation of this finding is shown in Table 2: based on clinical presentation and the finding of left ventricular hypertrophy, the likelihood of aortic stenosis becomes 60 percent, of mitral regurgitation becomes 17 percent, and of a functional murmur becomes 23 percent. Of particular note in this example, the addition of a third diagnostic category (compared with the two-category example shown in Table 1) required only the use of one extra line in Table 2.

The two examples given above involve the interpretation of single diagnostic test results. If another test is performed, the revised or posterior probability of one test becomes the prior probability for the next test. For example, if a radionuclide myocardial scintiscan were to be performed on the patient with suspected myocardial necrosis, then the prior probability of necrosis, used for interpreting the scintiscan, would be 0.088, the posterior probability of the enzyme test. The terms prior and posterior refer to the test being interpreted.

Probabilities and Prognosis

As mentioned above, probabilities are also used to describe prognosis, that is, the likelihood that a given set of events or outcomes will occur in the future. These predictions may be based on experience with similar patients, as reported in the literature, or

TABLE 2. Interpretation of an Electrocardiogram Demonstrating Left Ventricular Hypertrophy Using Bayes' Rule

A *Diagnosis*	B *Clinical Likelihood or Prior Probability or Likelihood before Test Result Is Known*	C *Conditional Probability of Observed Test Result in Patients with Each Diagnosis*	D *Product*	E (D/S) *Revised or Posterior Probability or Likelihood after Test Result Is Known*
Functional murmur	70	10	700	700/3000 = 0.23
Aortic stenosis	20	90	1800	1800/3000 = 0.60
Mitral regurgitation	10	50	500	500/3000 = 0.17
		Sum (S) =	3000	

on the subjective impressions of the clinician and his consultants. One of the most common metrics of prognosis is survival. The likelihood of various lengths of survival can be expressed in a variety of ways. The simplest measure is to consider survival after a fixed period of time to be be a discrete event, for example, the one-month survival rate (often used in expressing perioperative risk) or the five-year survival rate (often used in representing the prognosis of patients with cancer). Clearly, these measures are simple to understand, but in their simplicity, they obscure some important details about prognosis. For example, if one considers only the five-year survival rate, then survivals of one year and of four years would be considered equally bad.

To provide additional detail about survival, clinicians have begun to use the crude survival curve or metrics derived from that curve (e.g., the annual mortality rate and the life expectancy) to express prognosis. Appendix A considers the implications of survival curves and the various derived data.

MEASURES OF OUTCOME

Having structured the clinical decision and having estimated the probability of each outcome under alternative therapeutic and diagnostic plans, the clinician must next carefully consider each potential outcome and create a scale of relative values for all such outcomes. The first step in establishing such a rank order is to decide whose interests are to be optimized in the decision making process. The choice of that interested party may well dictate the nature of the outcome scale. Most medical decisions can affect a variety of people in addition to the patient involved: the patient's family, society (in terms of available resources), and the physician. When competing forces come under consideration, some joint measure of the relative value of various outcomes should be employed.

For the remainder of this discussion, we shall assume that the goal of the clinical decision making process is to optimize the chance of a good outcome for the individual patient. Unfortunately, this assumption by itself does not tell us how to rank order the various potential outcomes of a medical management decision. Outcomes might be compared on the basis of many different attributes, for example, length of survival, degree of pain, ability to work. One must first specify which attributes are to be considered and how those attributes should be combined in assigning a relative desirability to each outcome state.

Single Attributes

For simplicity, let us first consider a problem domain in which a single attribute can be used to assign relative values to outcomes. The most straightforward example of such an attribute is survival—outcomes which provide longer survivals are assumed to be preferred over outcomes which provide shorter survivals. If the time horizon of the problem is very short, it may be reasonable to consider just two outcome states: alive and dead, for example, alive after one month and dead after one month. In such simple problems, the clinician's task is elegantly simple—choose the action which provides the greatest chance of the patient's being alive after one month.

In general, the simplest decisions are those involving only two outcomes. The physician acts to maximize the chance of the better outcome occurring. Unfortunately, the analysis rapidly becomes more complex when more than two outcomes are involved, and the underlying philosophy of analysis in such cases is to reduce the problem to an *equivalent* decision in which only two outcomes must be considered. The sections on utility theory presented below are directed toward understanding such simplifications.

Values

Before plunging directly into the complexities of utility theory, let us consider a somewhat simpler subset of choices in which the decision maker considers only the intrinsic value of the outcome and not the uncertainties involved in achieving that outcome. Again, for simplicity, let us consider survival as the attribute upon which the ultimate management decision will be based. It might be reasonable to assign a relative value equal to the average survival or life expectancy achieved by patients reaching that outcome state. On such a *value scale,* immediate death (e.g., a perioperative catastrophe) would have a value of zero, treatment providing a life expectancy of 10 years would have a value of ten, and so forth. If life expectancy is used as the appropriate measure of survival, then the average survival of a given therapy should be an acceptable measure of the value of that therapy. For example, consider the simple decision depicted in the left panel of Figure 10. The upper branch denotes a therapy which will provide a survival of 10 years. The lower branch denotes a therapy which will provide one of two outcomes: survival for 20 years or immediate (e.g., perioperative) death. Assume that the odds of achieving these latter two outcomes are 50:50. If life expectancy were an appropriate measure of survival, then the patient would be expected to be indifferent between the two therapies. This indifference is shown diagrammatically by the balance on the right panel of Figure 10. On one side is a fair gamble between zero and 20 years of survival, whereas on the other side is a certain survival of 10 years (followed by certain death). If the relative values of the two therapies were equal and if the "weight" on the balance were proportional to the value of the therapy, then the scale should be balanced.

Utilities

The attitudes of many patients towards survival demonstrate that the scale would not be balanced. Rather, such patients would be sufficiently worried about the gamble

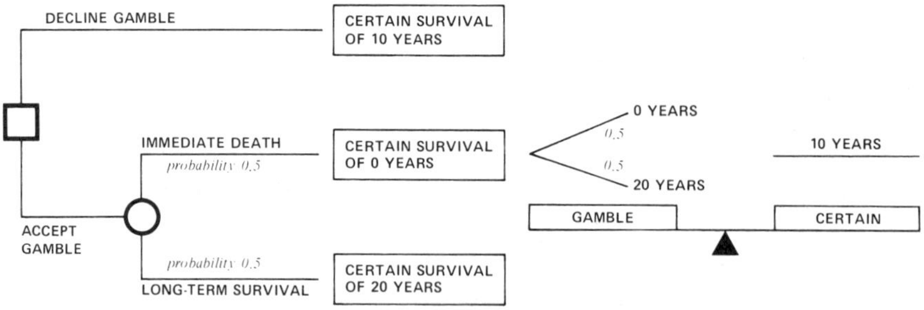

FIGURE 10. The meaning of value.

involved in the second therapy (and the very real possibility that they might die in the immediate future) that they would be willing to "settle" for a certain survival somewhat shorter than 10 years. For these patients, the value or "weight" of the certain outcome would exceed the value or weight of the gamble. That situation is depicted by balance A in Figure 11. One might then ask such a patient if he would "settle" for five years, for example. Suppose that a certain survival of five years was too short, and the weight of the gamble was now greater. That situation is depicted by balance B in Figure 11. By successive approximations, the physician and the patient should be able to identify the period of certain survival which just balances the value of the gamble. This situation is depicted by balance C in Figure 11. For such a patient, it would not be appropriate to use the life expectancy or average survival to compare the relative worth of alternative therapies. In such situations, the physician must develop a different metric (called a "utility" scale) with which he can compare outcome states.

Let us now consider how the clinician can create a *utility* scale. By utility (in the formal sense), we mean a scale which can be applied to decisions made in situations where the outcome is uncertain and which will allow us to apply the "basic decision rule" to be described. If the utility assigned to every outcome is increased (or decreased) by a constant number or multiplied by any positive number, decisions based on those utilities will not be changed as long as the transformation is applied consistently to all utilities. (In general, this same flexibility does not apply to simple value scales.)

Since the utility scale can be linearly transformed without problem, it follows that the top and bottom of the scale can be set arbitrarily. We have customarily used the utility zero to denote the worst possible outcome (i.e., immediate death in the example

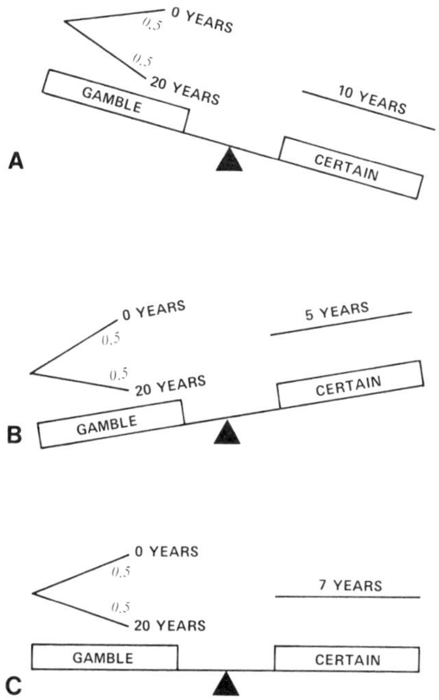

FIGURE 11. Assessing utility for survival.

shown in Figs. 10 and 11) and the utility one to denote the best possible outcome (i.e., survival for 20 years in Figs. 10 and 11).

The basic decision rule is that the utility of a given set of chance events (as represented by a chance node, i.e., circle, in a decision tree) is equal to the *average utility* of the outcomes of the chance event, where average means a weighted average based on the likelihood of each outcome occurrence. Consider, for example, the chance node on the lower branch of the tree in the left panel of Figure 10. The two outcomes both will occur with probability 0.5. Certain survival of 0 years is the worst outcome and is assigned a utility of 0; certain survival of 20 years is the best outcome and is assigned a utility of 1.0. Thus, the chance node has an average, or expected utility of $0.5 \times 0 + 0.5 \times 1.0$, or 0.50. Referring to Figure 11, we see that certain survival for 10 years is preferred to the gamble and thus has a utility greater than 0.50. Similarly, survival for 5 years (balance B) has a utility less than 0.50. The C balance suggests that, for the particular patient whose attitudes are modeled in this figure, a certain survival of 7 years can be assigned a utility of 0.50. Thus, we have developed a utility scale for 3 lengths of survival. The scale may be elaborated in greater detail by asking questions similar to those depicted in Figure 11. For example, consider a hypothetical therapy which results in a 50:50 gamble between survivals of 0 and 7 years. If a certain survival of 2 years were equivalent in value to that gamble, then a survival of 2 years would have a utility equal to the expected utility of that gamble, which would be $0.5 \times 0 + 0.5 \times 0.50$, or 0.25. A sequence of such questions would allow us to develop a general relation between survival and utility, as shown in Figure 12, for an individual patient. Based on that relation, we could determine the utility of any outcome in terms of its survival, for example, a survival of 10 years would have a utility of 0.63. The procedures used for assigning utilities in the above example have involved varying the length of certain

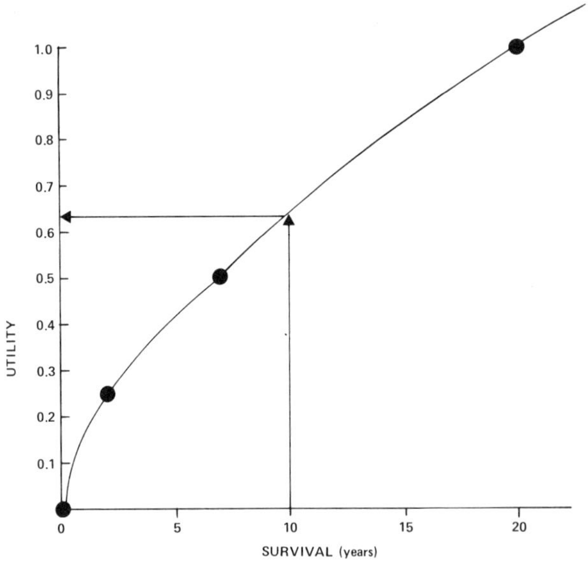

FIGURE 12. A typical survival-utility curve.

survival and holding the odds and outcomes of the gamble fixed. Alternatively, one might have held the certain outcome fixed and varied either the odds of the gamble or the survival produced by either one or both outcomes of the gamble. In theory, all such assessment procedures should be equivalent and should result in identical utility curves for a given patient. In practice, the results show some variations and the physician needs to examine the curve and adjust it to reflect the relative value of the outcomes.

Multiple Attributes

The examples presented thus far in this section have centered around survival as the attribute for comparing outcomes. The same approach might be applied to any other *single* attribute, such as time free of morbidity. In many clinical decisions, however, more than one attribute must be considered. In such cases, we must use what is called a multiattribute or multidimensional utility function. The procedure for formally assessing such functions is too complex to be reviewed here, but some basic principles will be presented. One approach is to create separate utility functions for each separate attribute and then to combine those functions in some manner. The particular technique of combination depends on whether or not the utility functions are independent or interrelated. For example, it would be reasonable to believe that utility functions relating to duration of survival and functions relating to minor morbidity (e.g., the necessity to take medication or see a physician monthly) should be independent, whereas survival is probably not independent of major morbidities (e.g., major neurologic deficits) where life may, indeed, become worse than death. If separate utility functions are assessed and if independence holds, then the two functions may be combined by either addition or multiplication or both, with the use of appropriate scaling factors to relate the survival to the other attributes. For example, consider survival and the necessity to take a medication that causes no side effects. If U_S (years) is the function relating survival to utility and if U_P(pills) is the utility function relating the number of pills required to utility, then the joint function might be of the form

$$(a)\times(U_s[\text{years}]) + (b)\times(U_P[\text{pills}]) + (1-a-b)\times(U_s[\text{years}])\,(U_P[\text{pills}])$$

where a and b are scaling constants. Of course, U_P(pills) decreases as the number of pills increases, since increasing inconvenience is a disutility.

A second approach can be taken in assessing utility functions where more than one attribute is involved by using the *principle of substitution*. By that principle, one replaces complex outcomes with preferentially equivalent (see below) outcomes or simple gambles and then applies the principles of rational decision making to that equivalent problem. For example, consider outcomes described in terms of length of survival and degree of disability where, for simplicity, disability is described as a binary attribute—the patient is either disabled or not. One might consider angina to be such a disability, where various treatment programs may change survival and may leave the patient either with or without disabling angina. (In point of fact, such a problem might be better represented by stratifying the degree of angina into several levels [e.g., absent, mild, severe] and then assessing the impact of each. For clarity, however, in this presentation we assume that angina is either present or absent.) Let us consider the absence of angina to be the reference state for that attribute. For outcomes that do not involve angina (i.e., outcomes where the patient will be pain free), we can simply assess a utility function for length of survival, as explained above. For outcomes which describe a patient disabled by angina, we substitute a preferentially equivalent, but presumably shorter, period of survival without angina and then use the utility of this shorter period of nondisabled years. For example, consider an outcome which results in 20 years of survival and assume that the utility function shown in Figure 12 is appropriate for nondisabled years. In that case, the 20 year outcome would have a utility of 1.0 *if* those 20 years were free of angina. In contrast, if another outcome provides 20 years of disabling angina, we would first ask how many years without angina would be just as good or just as bad as the 20 years with angina. Such a series of questions is shown diagrammatically in Figure 13. Certainly, 20 years without angina is preferable to (has greater utility than) 20 years with angina (balance A). For some patients, however, 20 years with angina might be better than only 10 years free of angina (followed by death), as shown by balance B. Balance C shows that 15 years free of angina might be equivalent to 20 years with angina. If that were the case, then referring to Figure 12 and assuming that those values hold for this patient, we see that 20 years of angina would have a utility of 0.83.

Under certain circumstances, the assignments of multiattribute utilities can be even simpler. Some problems can be structured in terms of a small number of outcomes in which variable duration of survival is not an important factor. For example, the following simplification in the coronary artery surgery decision might be made: since surgery does not affect length of survival, only three outcomes need be considered—immediate death, life with disabling angina, and life free of angina. Clearly, the best outcome would be life free of angina and the worst outcome might be immediate death. Life with angina would have an intermediate utility. To assign that utility, one

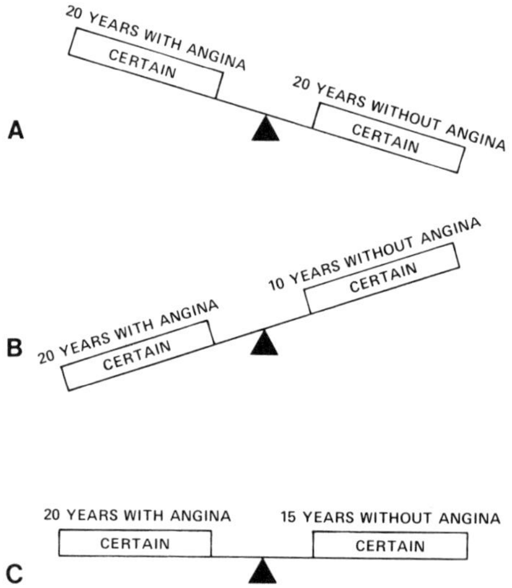

FIGURE 13. Assessing the burden of disability: Angina.

might consider a gamble between immediate death and survival without pain, a gamble for which the probability of the two outcomes was variable. One might then ask at what probability of losing the gamble (i.e., of dying after surgery) would the gamble be preferentially equivalent to life with angina. Suppose that the "break-even" or threshold probability were a 20 percent chance of dying. We might then assign the best outcome (life without angina) a utility of 1.0 and assign the worst outcome (immediate death) a utility of zero. If life with angina were equally preferred to the gamble with a 20 percent chance of perioperative death, then the utility of life with angina would be $0.2 \times 0 + 0.8 \times 1$, or 0.80.

Source and Motivation

The discussion of utilities and values presented thus far has been rather vague about whose attitudes are being modeled by the utility functions. If decision making is designed to optimize the chance of a good outcome, then the utilities should model the attitudes of the person or persons for whom the outcome is being optimized. In most circumstances, that person will be the patient, although benefits and costs to society, the patient's family, and even the physician are sometimes considered. The assignment of utilities is probably most conveniently done by the physician, but assignments made in that manner may not truly reflect the wishes of the patient. Under certain circumstances, it may be appropriate to directly approach the patient and to attempt to assign utilities based on the patient's responses to prestructured questions. Much work remains to be done, however, before such patient utilities can be scientifically and conveniently identified. At present, it is reasonable for the physician to make utility assignments, but in so doing he should try to model, as closely as possible, the attitudes of his patient. In fact, by asking his patient a few questions of the type presented above, he may gain better insight into his patient's attitudes and thereby make more accurate assignments and better management decisions.

Let us review the difference between a value and a utility as a means of describing the relative worth of a potential outcome. Value scales can be established either from objective criteria (e.g., life expectancy, five-year survival, discounted monetary gain or loss) or from a subjective (or personal) view of the potential outcomes. To be a valid value scale, it is only necessary that an outcome with a higher assigned value be preferred to an outcome with a lower assigned value. If the decision can be made without regard to attitudes toward risk, then any such value scale can be employed in the decision making process. Utility scales, on the other hand, incorporate attitudes toward risk (uncertain outcomes) as well as the intrinsic worth of the outcomes. Since utility scales do, in fact, order outcomes by preference, utility scales are also value scales. The converse is, however, not necessarily true—a value scale may not be a valid utility scale if attitudes toward risk are not properly modeled. Utility scales are created in a particular fashion such that the average or expected utility of a set of uncertain outcomes (i.e., a chance node on a decision tree) is preferentially equivalent to the utility of the chance node itself. This is the *principle of substitution* which is the basis for much of decision theory.

Preferential equivalence means the decision maker is indifferent between two potential courses of action. Consider a decision which cannot be made directly, rather, the decision maker must appoint an agent to act in his behalf and must give that agent a set of rules upon which to base the decision. Two actions are preferentially equivalent if the decision maker would tell such an agent that it would make no difference which of those two actions are chosen, that is, they are equally good or equally bad as far as the decision maker is concerned. For example, consider the decision summarized in Figure 14 in which either surgical or medical treatment may be given and in which surgery offers a higher rate of success but might result in a perioperative death. The upper portion of the left panel is a simple decision tree for such a decision. Note that three potential outcomes must be considered: death, disability, and well-being. Assume that a utility scale could be established for these three outcomes and that the utility of being disabled is 0.7, where the utility of death is zero, and the utility of being well is 1.0. The balance at the bottom of the left panel of Figure 14 shows that such a utility assignment is equivalent to saying that the decision maker would be indifferent between a gamble with a 30 percent chance of death and a 70 percent chance of well-being, on one hand, and a certain outcome of disability, on the other. Let us then substitute this exact gamble for each outcome resulting from treatment failure. Since the decision maker is indifferent between certain disability and this 70:30 gamble, such substitutions should not change his attitudes or preferences between the two alternative treatments. The decision tree in the right panel of the figure, therefore, should be strategically equivalent to the tree in the left panel. Note that the effect of substitution has been to reduce the problem to an equivalent decision involving only two outcomes: death and well-being. In general, the effect of using utilities is to make such substitutions throughout a complex problem and to reduce the problem to a choice involving only two outcomes: one good and one bad.

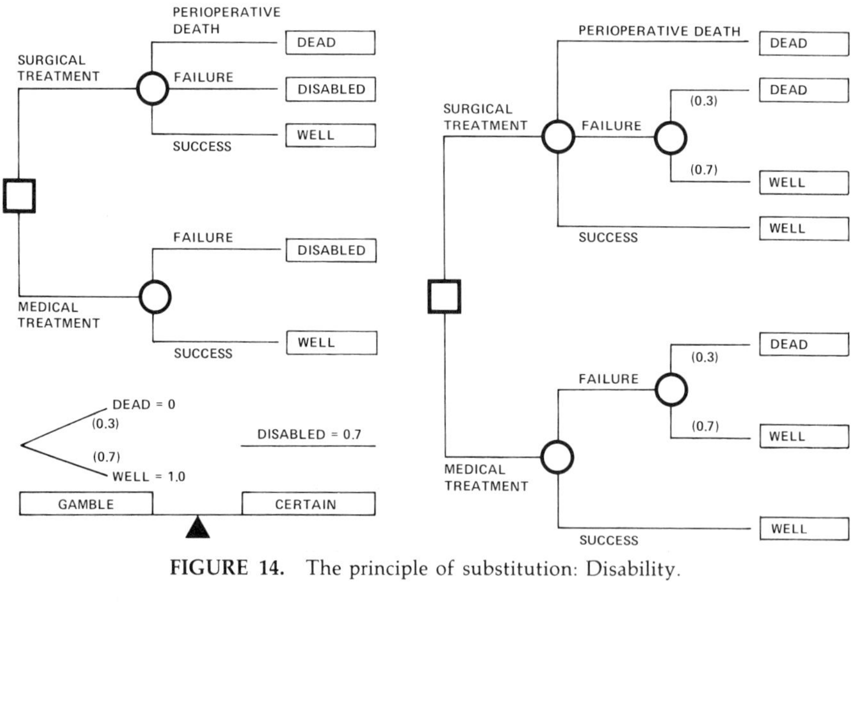

FIGURE 14. The principle of substitution: Disability.

EXPECTATION OF MANAGEMENT PLANS AND THE BASIC DECISION RULE

Having structured the problem domain, estimated the probabilities of potential results of various management strategies, and assigned utilities or values to each possible outcome, the physician should now be in a position to determine which management plan is best. The basic assumption of decision analysis is that the best strategy is the one which, on average, offers the highest chance of a good outcome. This section will first present the mechanics involved in making such choices and then will develop the logic underlying those mechanics.

Folding Back a Decision Tree

Each branch of a decision tree terminates with an outcome, and each outcome has an assigned value or utility. Of course, all such values or utilities will be assigned on a single, consistent scale. Decision trees also contain two kinds of branch points or nodes: decision nodes (denoted as squares) and chance nodes (denoted as circles). The evaluation of a strategy (as opposed to an outcome) is based on the *principle of expectation* which states that logic and probability theory can be used to calculate the *expected value* or *expected utility* of a node. Such calculations proceed from right to left in the decision tree; hence, the process is called "folding back" the decision tree. Once the expected value or utility of a distal node is calculated, that numerical assessment of the worth of the node can be used in evaluating nodes further to the left in the tree. The calculation proceeds node by node.

Decision nodes and chance nodes are handled differently. A decision node represents a choice which the decision maker can make. It is reasonable to assume that a rational decision maker will choose the better action. In a decision analytic context, "better" means having a higher utility or value, and we assume that the decision maker will choose the course of action with the highest expected value or expected utility. Thus, the expected value or utility of a decision node is just the maximum value or utility of its branches. On the other hand, the outcome of a chance node is not under the control of the decision maker, and the average value or utility of such nodes must be calculated. A partial value is found by multiplying the probability of each branch by its associated (expected) value or utility. The sum of all such partial values represents the expected value or expected utility of the chance node.

An example of such calculations is shown in Figure 15 for the choice between medical and surgical therapy in the problem presented in Figure 14. Explicit data about the efficacy of the two therapies has been added: surgery is associated with a 5 percent perioperative mortality rate and a 20 percent failure rate, leaving 75 percent of patients well; medical treatment has a 70 percent failure rate, leaving only 30 percent of patients well. These probabilities are shown in parentheses on the appropriate branches of Figure 15. In addition, the utility of each outcome is shown in the single oval at the end of each branch. First, consider the chance node on the surgical treatment branch. That chance node has three potential outcomes with probabilities of 0.05, 0.20, and 0.75 and with

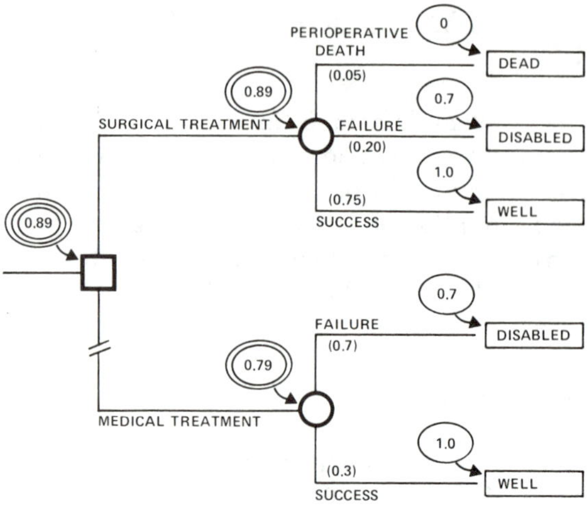

FIGURE 15. The calculation of expected utility: Folding back a tree.

utilities of 0, 0.7, and 1.0, respectively. Thus, the expected utility of the node is $0.05 \times 0 + 0.20 \times 0.7 + 0.75 \times 1.0$, or 0.89. That expected utility is shown in the double oval associated with the node. Similarly, the expected utility of the chance node for medical treatment is $0.7 \times 0.7 + 0.3 \times 1.0$, or 0.79. The rational decision maker, facing such a choice, should opt for surgical therapy since it has a higher expected utility. Thus, the expected utility of the decision node is 0.89 (shown in the triple oval) and the strategy of medical therapy is rejected as indicated by the double slashes through that branch. If further portions of the decision tree existed to the left of the decision node, then the expected utility of 0.89 would be used in those calculations.

Interpreting the Expected Value

Let us now consider the meaning of the calculated expected value or expected utility of a management plan. If the outcomes are compared on a value scale, then that scale will often contain associated units. For example, if the scale is life expectancy, then the associated unit is years of survival. The calculated expected value will be expressed in the same units and in the example, the units for a calculated life expectancy would be years. If the value scale includes consideration of a variety of attributes (e.g., survival and morbidity), then the proper unit for that scale or for the expected value is less clear, although terms like "quality-adjusted years of life" might be used for such a compound unity. On the other hand, if the outcomes are compared on a utility scale or if the scale represents the particular attitudes of an individual patient, then the scale carries no associated units. In such cases, it makes little sense to examine the magnitude of the difference in expected utilities; all that can be said is that the plan with the highest expected utility should be chosen.

When dealing with such utility scales, the physician can get some feeling for the meaning of the expected utilities by using the utility curve to translate each calculated expected utility into a preferentially equivalent, but certain, outcome. For example, suppose that some complex decision was to be made solely on the basis of survival, but that the patient's attitudes toward survival and risk-taking were to be considered. Further assume that the utility curve in Figure 12 represents the patient's attitudes and that the expected utilities of medical and surgical therapy are 0.55 and 0.45 units, respectively. Clearly, medical therapy is to be preferred but by how much? Referring to the figure, we see that 0.55 units is assigned to a certain survival of eight years; therefore, the patient should be indifferent between eight years of certain survival and any therapy with an expected utility of 0.55 units. Similarly, referring to Figure 12, we see that the patient should be indifferent between six years of certain survival and any therapy with a calculated expected utility of 0.45 units. Thus, the strength of preference for medical therapy over surgical therapy should be the same as the strength of preference for a guaranteed certain survival of eight years compared to a guaranteed certain survival of six years. It is important to realize that expected utilities do not describe prognosis alone. Rather, they represent a combination of prognosis and the preferences of an individual patient, making comparison of expected utilities from one patient to another meaningless. Expected utilities are only to be used in comparing alternative management plans for a particular patient.

Theory

If outcomes are compared with a value function with clearly defined units, then the technique of choosing the plan with the highest expected value should be an obvious strategy. Of course, other decision rules might be employed: for example, choose the strategy which minimizes the chance of the worst outcome (e.g., death) without reference to other bad outcomes. By such a strategy, surgery would have been rejected in the problem presented in Figures 14 and 15. In fact, even if the chance of success were zero with medical therapy and the chance of death were one in a million for surgery, the "minimize bad outcome" strategy would still reject surgery. Such examples demonstrate that the expected value criterion is the optimal decision making rule.

On the other hand, if the outcomes are compared on a utility scale without clearly defined units, then the principle of substitution can be used to justify the use of the expected utility criterion. Recall that a branch in a decision tree with a utility used to describe the relative worth of the outcome on that branch is preferentially equivalent to a similar (hypothetical) branch in which the outcome is replaced by a chance node that can result in either the best or the worst possible outcome and in which the hypothetical probabilities of those two outcomes occurring is determined by the assigned utility (see Fig. 14). Thus, the systematic use of a single utility scale is mathematically equivalent to replacing the decision tree with a preferentially equivalent tree which is more complex in structure (i.e., one that has more branches and probabilities) but which contains only two outcomes: the best and the worst. This interpretation of utility scales means that the expected utility of any node in the tree is directly related to the likelihood of winning a hypothetical gamble between the best and the worst outcomes, where those odds are set to make the simple gamble preferentially equivalent to the node in the original tree. Facing a choice between two complex management strategies which can nevertheless result in only two outcomes (with different likelihoods of success for the two strategies), the decision maker should clearly choose the plan with the greatest odds of success. Thus, he should choose the alternative with the highest expected utility.

SENSITIVITY ANALYSIS

At this point, the physician has structured the problem, assessed prognosis under alternative management plans, assigned relative values to the various possible outcomes, and calculated the expected value or expected utility of each plan. From these calculations, he has been able to identify what would appear to be the optimal strategy for treatment. One final step remains. The clinician must now examine the assumptions of the analysis to see whether reasonable modifications in any of those assumptions might result in a different strategy appearing to be optimal. If such analysis shows that the management plan is not altered by any such reasonable variations, then the analysis is said to be *insensitive* to such variations, and the physician can have great confidence in the analysis. If, on the other hand, such analysis shows that the choice of the apparently optimal plan is affected by variations in the assumptions, then the analysis is said to be *sensitive* to such variations, and the physician must be careful in interpreting the results.

It is important to note that the identification of decisions which are sensitive to the assumptions of analysis is the great *power,* and not a weakness, of the decision analytic approach. Clearly, every management decision, whether made implicitly by "clinical judgment" or by formal analysis, *must* depend on such assumptions. In "classic" clinical decision making, such assumptions are implicit and not available for examination, discussion, and modification; in the decision analytic approach, the assumptions are clear and explicit—they can be examined, discussed, and modified. Often this explicitness can be quite disconcerting. When the physician realizes how many assumptions he must make and how "soft" his data are, he becomes worried and annoyed. The immediate reaction is to fault the decision analytic approach for *requiring* such assumptions and data. We must realize, however, that formal analysis does not require any *additional* assumptions; it simply exposes the implicit assumptions that were already being made.

When doing sensitivity analyses, the key concept is that the range of variations in the assumptions must be *reasonable.* Clearly, if prognostic probabilities and utilities are varied over a broad enough range, then every decision will appear sensitive to such variation. For example, consider the decision between surgical and medical treatment outlined in Figures 14 and 15. If the utility of being disabled were not very different from the utility of being well, it is clear that surgery would be less desirable. In fact, if that utility were varied from 0.7 up to 1.0, we would see that whenever the utility exceeds 0.9, surgical treatment would no longer be optimal. On that basis, one could say that the decision is sensitive to the burden of being disabled. However, one must ask whether variation to that level is reasonable. If the disability being considered were, for example, blindness and if the patient's lifestyle were critically dependent on sight (e.g., if he were an artist), then it might be unreasonable to assign a utility greater than 0.9 to being disabled. In that case, the decision would become insensitive to reasonable variations in the utility of blindness. Similarly, consider the operative risk in that example. Medical therapy would become preferable if the operative risk were to exceed 16 percent (compared to the 5% risk assumed in Fig. 15). If the operation being considered were a cataract extraction, it would be most unusual, in normal circumstances, for the operative risk to even approach 16 percent and the decision would appear insensitive to reasonable variations in that parameter. However, if the patient were elderly and had severe cardiac and renal failure, then the decision might become sensitive to operative risk. Whether or not a decision is sensitive to a given parameter is rarely an absolute judgment. It is often a relative statement based on the physician's judgment about what constitutes reasonable variations.

Every problem which the physician faces will depend on several factors and therefore on several assumptions. The clinician must decide which parameters should be subjected to sensitivity analysis. Since such analyses are time consuming, analysis of every parameter is often an unrealistic plan. In general, the physician should choose to examine the parameters of assumptions which are based on the "softest" data and which are, therefore, most subject to variation. Many decisions in medicine involve either performing diagnostic tests to provide data about the presence of a particular disease or administering treatment to patients in whom the diagnosis is not known with certainty. In such settings, one of the softest pieces of clinical information is the clinical likelihood that the patient has the disease in question. As explained above, that clinical likelihood is often called the prior probability of disease. Since that datum is so central to management decisions and since it is often based largely on subjective impressions, it is a prime candidate for sensitivity analysis.

Although the physician may want to subject more than one parameter to sensitivity analyses, the customary approach is to vary one parameter at a time, leaving all other assumptions of the analysis fixed at their most reasonable values. Performing sensitivity analysis in such a "one at a time manner" is equivalent to assuming that variations or errors in the assessments of the various parameters are *independent* of one another. For example, in the analysis performed above we varied the operative mortality and the utility of being disabled quite separately from one another. This is quite proper since there should be no reason to believe that patient attitudes toward disability should be linked to either the surgeon's skill or the patient's anesthesia risk. On the other hand, if we were to consider the two parameters perioperative mortality rate and success rate of surgery, then the independence assumption might be questioned since both parameters would be affected by the skill and experience of the surgical team.

Having motivated the need for sensitivity analyses, we can turn to the practical issues of how such analyses can be performed. Ostensibly, the technique is quite simple: the calculation of expected value or expected utility is performed repeatedly with different values for the parameter(s) in question, and the expected utilities are repeatedly compared to see if the optimal choice is altered. In practical terms, such calculations are burdensome and the long lists of resulting numbers may offer the physician little insight.

We suggest that sensitivity analyses be performed using a combination of algebriac and graphic techniques. The simplest sensitivity analyses consider the effect on the decision of variations in a single parameter, be it a probability or a utility. Such variations in the assumptions of the analysis will result in changes in the calculated expected utilities of various management plans and, under certain circumstances, may affect the choice of the "optimal" plan. The easiest way to visualize such effects is to construct a graph which depicts the relation between a given parameter and the calculated expected utility of each plan. The most straightforward way to prepare such graphs is often to replace the parameter (in the decision tree) with an algebriac variable and then to fold back the tree using that variable. For example, consider the relation between the utility of being disabled (the parameter being subjected to sensitivity analysis) and the expected utility of medical and surgical therapy for the decision problem presented in Figure 15. If we replace the utility of being disabled with the variable "d" (Fig. 16, A), we see that expected utility of surgical therapy becomes 0.75 + 0.20d (rather than 0.89). This function is shown by the solid line in Figure 16, B. Similarly, the expected utility of medical therapy would be 0.3 + 0.7d, as shown by the broken line. The basic decision rule of choosing the strategy with the higher expected utility is equivalent to choosing the strategy corresponding to the higher line. In this analysis, the expected utilities are linear functions of the utility of being disabled. Although this will often be the case, the relation is sometimes curvilinear, as will be seen in the extended example presented later in this chapter. Referring again to Figure 16B, one can see that the solid line (corresponding to surgical therapy) is higher for any patient in whom the utility of being disabled is below 0.9. For all such patients, surgery is the preferable treatment. The two strategy lines intersect at a utility of 0.9, which is therefore a *threshold utility.* All patients for whom the assigned utility is below the threshold should receive surgery, and all patients for whom the utility of being disabled is above the threshold should receive medical therapy.

Figure 17 shows how the relation between the calculated expected utilities of therapy and the probability of perioperative death is derived. In the tree in Figure 17A the operative risk (0.05) is replaced by the variable "m" and the success rate is replaced by the variable "s." If, for the moment, we hold the operative success rate constant at 0.75, we note that the operative risk cannot exceed 0.25 since all the probabilities at the chance node cannot sum to more than 1.0. Thus, the probability of failure is (0.25 − m), and the expected utility of surgery is (m × 0) + ([0.25 − m] × 0.7) + (0.75 × 1.0), or 0.925 − 0.7m. Again, the relation is linear, with the expected utility of surgery decreasing as the operative risk increases. Obviously, the expected utility of medical

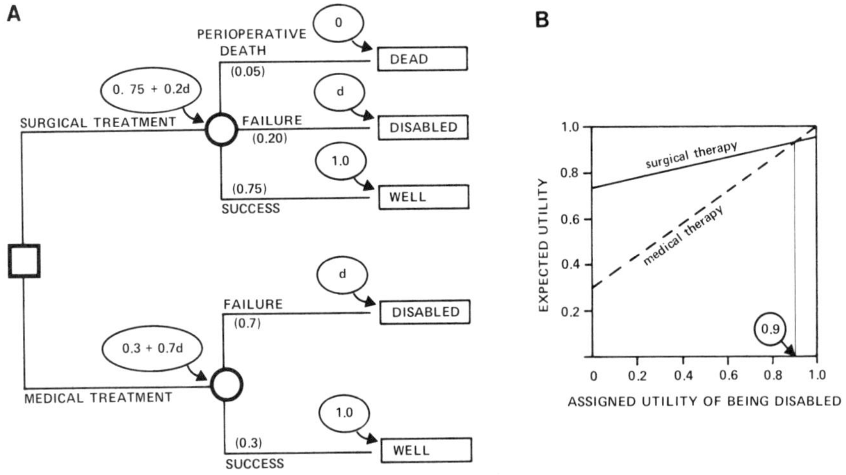

FIGURE 16. Sensitivity analysis under independence: Disability.

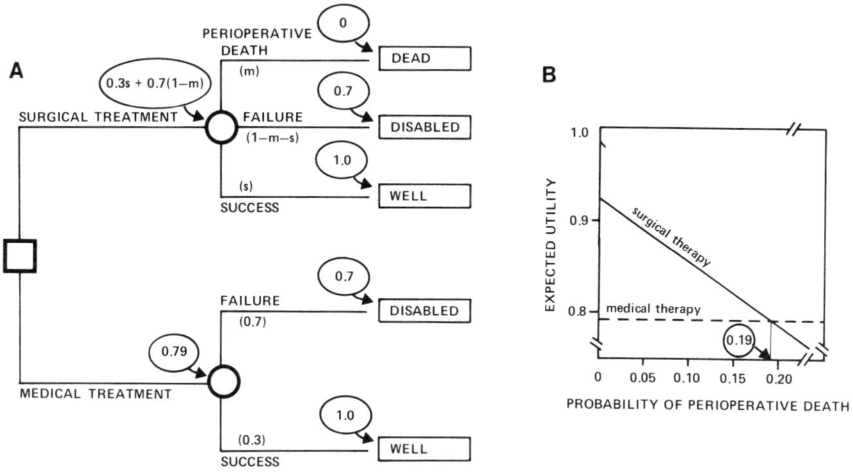

FIGURE 17. Sensitivity analysis under independence: Operative risk.

therapy is not affected by the operative risk. The right panel of Figure 17 shows these relations. Note that the maximum operative risk, under these assumptions, is 0.25. The *threshold probability* for operative risk is 0.19. If the operative risk exceeds that level, surgery should be declined.

The first sensitivity analysis considered the effect of changes in a single utility parameter (d), while the second analysis considered the effect of changes in a *single* probability (m). What if two parameters might be related to one another and therefore cannot be considered separately? Such analyses are called joint sensitivity analyses. For example, consider the operative risk and surgical success rate for the clinical choice shown in Figures 14 and 15. In such situations it is often helpful to consider the relation between one parameter, and the threshold value of the second parameter. In the example under consideration, the operative risk and the surgical success rate clearly both depend on the surgeon's skill and must be considered together. If we continue to use the symbol "m" to denote the operative mortality rate and introduce the symbol "s" to denote the success rate (see Fig. 17, A), then the expected utility for surgical therapy becomes $(m \times 0) + ([1 - m - s] \times 0.7) + (s \times 1.0)$, or $0.3s + 0.7(1 - m)$. The expected utility of medical therapy does not depend on the surgeon's skill and remains 0.79. Note that $m + s$ cannot exceed 1.0, since the sum of the probabilities at a chance node must be one. Setting the expected utilities of medical and surgical therapy equal to one another and solving for s, we find that the threshold value of s equals $0.3 + 2.33m$. This relation is shown by the heavy line in Figure 18, A. Note that since $m + s$ must be less than 1.0, the upper right area of the graph is shaded—all points lying in that area violate that constraint. Clearly, the higher the operative risk, the higher the success rate must be for surgery to remain the optimal choice. For operative risks above 21 percent, surgery would not be optimal therapy even if all surgical survivors were well.

This graph (Fig. 18, A) can be interpreted in a somewhat different way. Consider a pair of numbers which specify the operative risk and the success rate. Such a pair of numbers specify a unique point on the graph. The area above the heavy line corresponds to a set of points for which surgical therapy is preferable and the area below the line

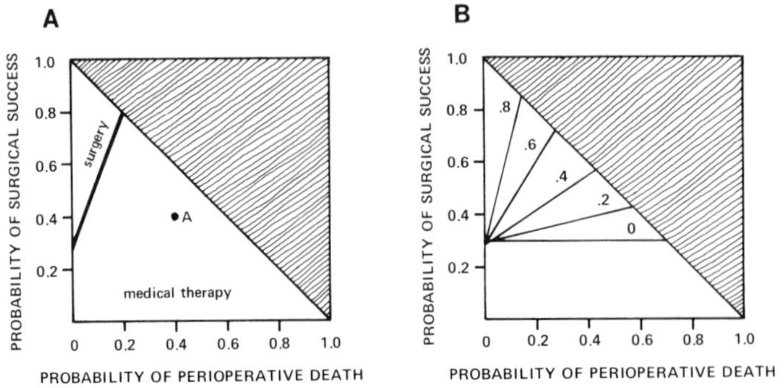

FIGURE 18. Sensitivity analysis without independence: Operative risk and surgical success.

corresponds to a set of points for which medical therapy is better. The area in which a given point lies specifies the optimal therapy. For example, Point A (corresponding to operative risk of 40% and operative success rate of also 40%) lies in the medical area; if the risk and success rate were both 40 percent, then medical therapy is preferred.

The sensitivity analysis summarized in Figure 18, A is based on a utility of 0.7 being assigned to being disabled. Obviously, if the burden of disability were greater (i.e., if the assigned utility were lower), then the patient should be willing to undertake greater risks of surgery. In other words, as the utility of being disabled falls, the area on the sensitivity graph corresponding to surgery should increase. Figure 18, B displays a series of isobars corresponding to different utilities of being disabled. As the utility falls, the area above the corresponding threshold line increases. Note, however, that even if the utility of being disabled were zero (i.e., even if being disabled were tantamount to dying), surgery should be declined if the operative success rate is below 30 percent, since medical therapy provides a 30 percent success rate (see Fig. 14).

A CLINICAL EXAMPLE OF THE DECISION ANALYTIC APPROACH

This section will analyze a common, but difficult, problem that arises in the medical management of surgical patients: the problem of optimal timing for surgery. Clearly, elective surgery should be undertaken only when the patient is stable and when all treatable risk factors have been minimized. In many situations, however, surgery may not be entirely elective, and any delay may expose the patient to risk from his underlying disease. Such a case was described earlier in this chapter when we considered whether to perform a laparotomy in a patient with possible colonic perforation and unstable coronary disease. A similar situation involving vascular surgery will be considered in this section. A generalization of this type of problem will be analyzed in Appendix B.

Case Description

A 70-year-old man presents with increasing abdominal discomfort. Past history reveals long-standing hypertension, stable angina pectoris, and an inferior myocardial infarction three years ago. He has no symptoms of congestive failure. Physical examination demonstrates clear lungs, no murmurs, a soft S_4 but no S_3 gallop and a pulsatile periumbilical mass. Electrocardiogram is unchanged over the past six months, showing only an old inferior infarction and left ventricular hypertrophy. An aortogram reveals a 10 cm fusiform aneurysm, but the patient develops chest discomfort and slight hypotension during the procedure. Electrocardiograms over the next several days reveal an evolving anterior myocardial infarction, a diagnosis confirmed by creatinine phosphokinase enzyme elevations shown to be of the MB fraction. Over the next week his clinical course is uneventful with the exception that his abdominal and back pain continue.

The question is *when* to attempt resection of a huge, enlarging abdominal aortic aneurysm in this 70-year-old man who has sustained an uncomplicated myocardial infarction this week. If the clinical picture were not emergent, one would certainly prefer to wait between three and six months before undertaking a major surgical procedure. In this case, however, the likelihood of an abdominal catastrophe occurring in the next six months is high, and two risks must be balanced: the increasing risk of aortic rupture if surgery is delayed and the decreasing risk from anesthesia at surgery if the patient is allowed to recover from his recent infarction. The following discussion will demonstrate how such a difficult problem can be approached analytically. We hope to demonstrate the *process* of analysis without being sidetracked into lengthy discussions about what those risks are and how they change over time. We shall, therefore, make some arbitrary assumptions about prognosis, but we encourage the reader to question those assumptions and to redo the analysis with his own best estimates of the patient's prognosis if those estimates are at variance with our assumptions.

The Assumptions of Analysis

The assumptions of analysis are:

1. The time frame will be the next six months.
2. The outcome measure will be whether or not the patient is alive at the end of six months.
3. Two causes of death will be considered: anesthesia death and aortic rupture.
4. The anesthesia risk will be assumed to be 40 percent immediately after infarction, 20 percent two months after infarction, 10 percent four months after infarction, and 5 percent six months after infarction, that is, the risk is halved every two months that surgery is delayed.
5. The risk of aortic rupture is assumed to be 50 percent in the next year or 29 percent in the next six months, that is, the risk of rupture is roughly 5.6 percent for each month that surgery is delayed (thus the chance of surviving without rupture for six months is $(94.4\%)^6 = 71\%$; for 12 months we have $(94.4\%)^{12} = 50\%$).
6. All aortic ruptures are presumed to result in death.
7. If the patient survives surgery, then the risk of aortic rupture falls to zero.
8. The possibility of a recurrent myocardial infarction in the next six months which would further delay or increase the risk of surgery is ignored.

Note the explicit nature of each of these assumptions. One could discuss and modify each and then modify the ensuing analysis. However, if the assumptions were not so explicitly stated, arguments about when surgery should be performed would be far less focused than discussions based on formal analysis. For example, one could argue that occasionally people survive aortic rupture, that the anesthesia risk in this patient for such major surgery would be greater than 5 percent even after waiting for six months, or even that the monthly risk of aortic rupture might increase during the next six months, as the aneurysm continued to enlarge. Each of the assumptions could be subjected to sensitivity analysis to see how such changes might affect the decision.

Figure 19 provides a decision tree structure for this problem. The tree in Figure 19, A illustrates several possible waiting periods and uses the subtree notation presented earlier in the chapter. The subtree in Figure 19, B depends on a single variable, the delay before surgery is undertaken. The longer that delay is, the greater is the chance of preoperative aortic rupture, denoted here as the variable r. The longer the delay before surgery, however, the smaller is the perioperative mortality rate, denoted here as m. Figure 20 summarizes the assumed relations between waiting time and the two risks. In graph A, we see that the cumulative risk of preoperative rupture (r) increases with waiting time. In graph B, we see that the operative mortality rate (m) decreases with

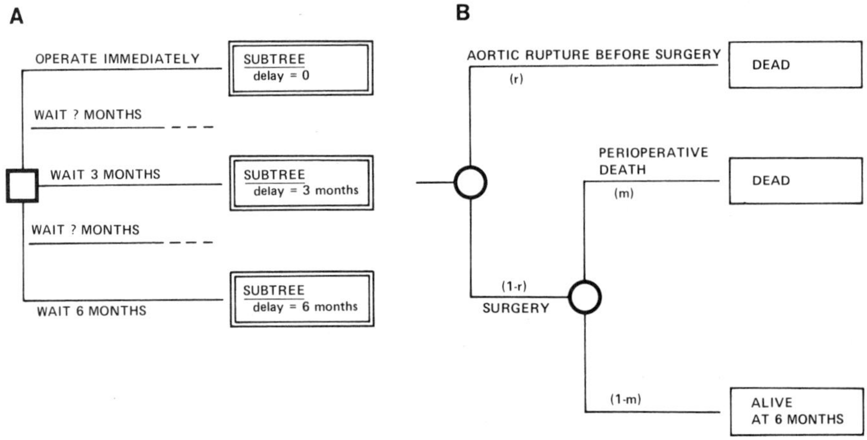

FIGURE 19. A decision tree for choosing optimal timing in patients with acute myocardial infarction and aortic aneurysm.

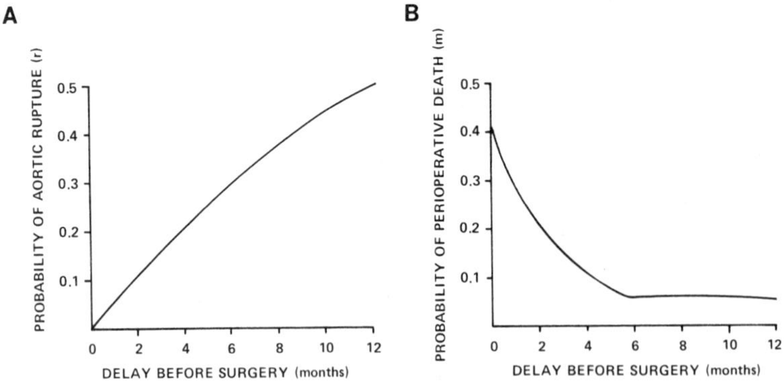

FIGURE 20. Relation between delay and probabilities of aortic rupture and operative risk.

waiting time. For convenience, we have measured waiting time (t) from the myocardial infarction, which according to the case presentation occurred approximately ten days ago. The units of time used in this analysis will be months.

Analysis

In keeping with the choice to measure the relative value of alternative strategies on the basis of whether or not the patient is alive after six months, we shall assign the outcome "dead" a value of zero and the outcome "alive at six months" a value of one. On this value scale, the calculated expected value of a particular management plan will be expressed in units of "probability of six month survival." We have chosen not to consider attitudes toward risk and differences in attitudes toward survival for one month, two months, and so forth, because the time frame is quite short and we assume that surgery will be done within the next six months—the only question is when.

Consider the chance node to the right in Figure 19, B (the outcomes of surgery). Given the utility assignments made above, the expected value of that chance node is $(m) \times 0 + (1 - m) \times 1$, or $(1-m)$. Now consider the other chance node (the possibility of preoperative aortic rupture). The expected value of this node is $(r) \times 0 + (1-r) \times (1-m)$, since $(1-m)$ is the value of the surgical branch. Thus, the expected value of the entire subtree is $(1-r) \times (1-m)$.

Now consider the uppermost branch of the tree in Figure 19, A. That branch describes the strategy of immediate surgery, that is, surgery at time zero. From Figure 20, we can see that, at time zero, r equals zero and m equals 0.4. Thus, the expected value of immediate surgery (that is, the chance that the patient will be alive at six months) is $(1-0) \times (1-0.4)$, or 0.6. Next consider the strategy of waiting three months. From Figure 20 we see that, at time three months, r equals 0.16 and m equals 0.14. Thus, the expected value of delaying for three months is $(1-0.16) \times (1-0.14)$, or 0.72. Certainly, the strategy of waiting three months is better than the strategy of operating in the peri-infarction period. But what about a six month delay? At that time, r would equal 0.29 and m would equal 0.05. The expected value of delaying for six months is $(1-0.29) \times (1-0.05)$, or 0.67. Thus, a six month delay would be preferable to immediate surgery but would not be preferable to a three month delay. Figure 21, A depicts a sensitivity analysis of the delay before surgery performed by plotting expected value (or probability of being alive) as a function of the preoperative delay. Optimal survivals for this particular situation occur if surgery is performed 2.6 months after the myocardial infarction. Note, however, that the curve becomes quite flat in the region of its peak. Thus, if surgery is performed anytime between two and three months after infarction, survivals would be quite similar.

Sensitivity Analysis

To examine the effect of the time horizon, we have extended the curve in Figure 21, A to include delays of up to 12 months. (For delays over six months, the utility scale must be changed. In those cases, survival for the full length of the time horizon is assigned a utility of one.) The extended curve (broken line) shows that the expected value falls

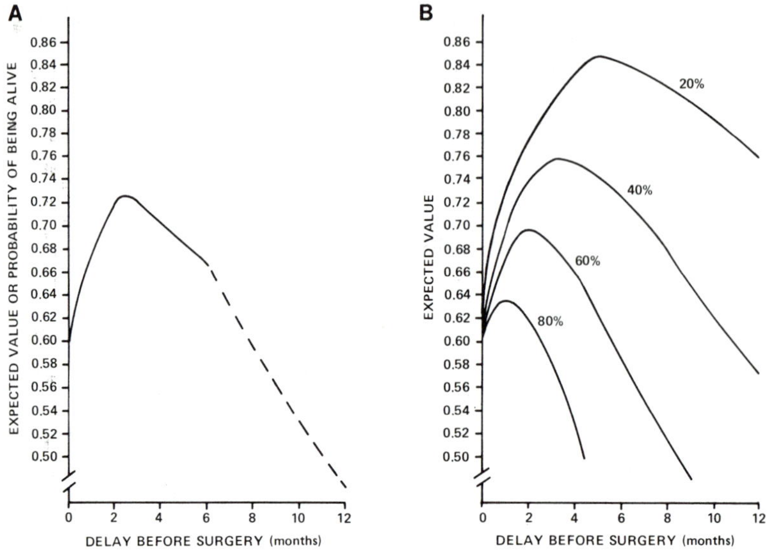

FIGURE 21. Likelihood of survival as a function of delay before surgery.

off quite sharply after six months, and that further delays would not result in improved management. Figure 21, B demonstrates the effect of the likelihood of aortic rupture on the decision. (Recall that we have thus far assumed that the likelihood of rupture is 5.6% per month of delay or 50% per year.) This panel shows the effect of annual rupture rates of 20 percent, 40 percent, 60 percent, and 80 percent. As the likelihood of aortic rupture increases, the probability of being alive decreases, and the optimal delay time for surgery becomes shorter. Thus, if the likelihood of aortic rupture is 80 percent in a year, surgery should only be delayed one month after infarction, whereas if the chance of rupture were only 20 percent in a year, surgery should be delayed five months after myocardial infarction.

It should be noted that few surgically correctable diseases are as life threatening as an expanding aortic aneurysm. It can be shown (see below) that, under the assumptions of this analysis, if the chance of dying in a year from the surgically correctable disease is below 12 percent, then surgery should be delayed a full six months; conversely, if the chance of dying in a year from the correctable disease is above 95 percent, then surgery should be undertaken immediately without regard for the increased anesthesia risk in patients with recent myocardial infarction. An example of such an enormously high risk situation might be an aortic aneurysm which has already ruptured, rendering the patient hypotensive.

The General Case

Having developed an analysis of the optimal timing of surgery for an expanding aortic aneurysm, let us consider the general situation of surgical timing in a patient who has a "correctable" risk factor which increases his risk of surgical catastrophe in the short run but which could be treated to decrease that risk. In other words, we shall address the general issue of delaying surgery to have time to improve the patient's general medical status. The risk factor in the above example was acute coronary disease, but risk factors such as diabetic ketoacidosis, congestive heart failure, or acute infections could be analyzed in a similar fashion. A detailed analysis of this more general situation can be found in Appendix B.

A Note About Data

The purpose of this chapter was to present the techniques of logical decision making in a fashion that the reader could understand and incorporate into his practice. We have attempted to focus on the process of decision making, rather than on particular decisions. For that reason, we have chosen not to emphasize the data upon which the particular examples were based. Most of the illustrations in this chapter were based on subjective estimates of various probabilities and, as such, should not be used as primary sources for such probabilities. The remaining chapters in this book will focus on particular clinical situations and will provide as much data as are currently available on those topics.

SUMMARY

In this chapter we have attempted to present the techniques of decision analysis so that the clinician might use them in appropriately difficult cases. The physician should understand at the outset, however, that using formal decision analysis efficiently requires skill and experience. The casual user will find the techniques both cumbersome and time consuming. With practice, however, the physician will come to rely on this approach in difficult and confusing cases.

It is not unusual for a particularly complex analysis to require several hours to complete. Clearly, the busy physician cannot practice medicine at such a pace. Formal analysis should be reserved for the small subset of clinical situations which are either unusual, confusing, or where counterbalancing risks are clearly at play. As the physician uses this formal approach, he will gain insights into the dynamics of certain generic and common situations. Those insights may well begin to affect his "informal" practice of medicine. For example, he will gain further insight into the fact that information and risk are counterbalancing forces in the consideration of diagnostic procedures. Some errors (false positive and false negative results) might be tolerable if the cost and risk of the test are low (e.g., a stool guaiac test for colon cancer). Similarly, a substantial risk might be tolerated if the test provides highly accurate information (e.g., a pulmonary arteriogram).

Decision analysis can be used to gain insights into the clinical decision making process and can be another tool in the physician's armamentarium for dealing with complex and difficult management problems. The technique is explicit and avoids many of the foibles and errors that plague all implicit human reasoning. The approach is not complex but it is time consuming. It requires that the problem's structure, the clinician's assumptions, and all data be explicitly and quantitatively stated. It allows diverse opinions to be smoothly incorporated into an overall management plan. Among the diverse inputs which it both encourages and utilizes is a direct assessment by the patient of the relative value or relative burden which various health consequences would have. In so doing, the technique allows for greater and more meaningful participation by the patient in the decision making process.

In an era where medical decisions are coming under increasing scrutiny on both economic and legal grounds, the physician must become increasingly concerned with the logic of his decision making process and his ability to both justify and document his reasoning. The use of decision analytic techniques might serve as one means of providing such justification and documentation. By helping the physician avoid unnecessary diagnostic tests and suboptimal therapeutic strategies, this approach might also help limit the cost and improve the quality of medical care.

BIBLIOGRAPHY

1. Bell, DE, Keeney, RL, and Raiffa, H (eds.): *Conflicting Objectives in Decisions.* New York: John Wiley and Sons, 1977.
2. Bunker, JP, Barnes, BA, and Mosteller, F (eds.): *Costs, Risks, and Benefits of Surgery.* New York: Oxford University Press, 1977.
3. Emerson, PA, Teather, D, and Handley, AJ: *The application of decision theory to the prevention of deep vein thrombosis following myocardial infarction.* J Med (New Series) 43:389, 1974.
4. Feinstein, AR: *Clinical biostatistics—XXXIX. The haze of Bayes, the aerial palaces of decision analysis, and the computerized Ouija board.* Clin Pharmacol Ther 21:482, 1977.
5. Feinstein, AR: *Clinical Judgment.* Baltimore: Williams & Wilkins Co., 1967.
6. Galen, RS, and Gambino, SR: *Beyond Normality: The Predictive Value and Efficiency of Medical Diagnosis.* New York: John Wiley and Sons, 1975.
7. Gorry, GA, Pauker, SG, and Schwartz, WB: *The diagnostic importance of the normal finding.* N Engl J Med 298:486, 1978.
8. Hill, PH, Bedau, HA, Chechile, RA, et al.: *Making Decisions: A Multidisciplinary Introduction.* Reading, Mass.: Addison-Wesley, 1979.
9. Jordan, CW: *Life Contingencies.* Chicago: Society of Actuaries, 1975.
10. Kassirer, JP: *The principles of clinical decision making: an introduction to decision analysis.* Yale J Biol Med 49:149, 1976.
11. Kassirer, JP, and Pauker, SG: *Should diagnostic testing be regulated?* (editorial) N Engl J Med 299:947, 1978.
12. Katz, MA: *A probability graph describing the predictive value of a highly sensitive diagnostic test.* N Engl J Med 291:1115, 1974.
13. Keeney, RL, and Raiffa, H: *Decisions with Multiple Objectives: Preferences and Value Tradeoffs.* New York: John Wiley and Sons, 1976.
14. Lusted, LB: *Introduction to Medical Decision Making.* Springfield, Ill.: Charles C Thomas, 1968.
15. McNeil, BJ, Keeler, E, and Adelstein, SJ: *Primer on certain elements of medical decision making.* N Engl J Med 293:211, 1975.
16. McNeil, BJ, Weichselbaum, R, and Pauker, SG: *The fallacy of the five-year survival in lung cancer.* N Engl J Med 299:1397, 1978.
17. Pauker, SG: *Coronary artery surgery: the use of decision analysis.* Ann Intern Med 85:8, 1976.
18. Pauker, SG, and Kassirer, JP: *Clinical application of decision analysis: a detailed illustration.* Semin Nucl Med 8:324, 1978.
19. Pauker, SG, and Kassirer, JP: *Therapeutic decision making: a cost-benefit analysis.* N Engl J Med 293:229, 1975.
20. Pauker, SG, and Kassirer, JP: *The threshold approach to clinical decision making.* New Engl J Med 302:1109, 1980.

21. PAUKER, SP, AND PAUKER, SG: *Prenatal diagnosis: a directive approach to genetic counseling using decision analysis.* Yale J Biol Med 50:275, 1977.

22. RAIFFA, H: *Decision Analysis.* Reading, Mass.: Addison-Wesley, 1968.

23. SAFRAN, C, DESFORGES, JF, TSICHLIS, PN, ET AL.: *Decision analysis to evaluate lymphangiography in the management of patients with Hodgkin's disease.* N Engl J Med 296:1088, 1977.

24. SCHOENBAUM, SC, MCNEIL, BJ, AND KAVET, J: *The swine influenza decision.* N Engl J Med 295:759, 1976.

25. SCHWARTZ, WB: *Decision analysis: a look at the chief complaints.* N Engl J Med 300:556, 1979.

26. SCHWARTZ, WB, GORRY, GA, KASSIRER, JP, ET AL.: *Decision analysis and clinical judgment.* Am J Med 55:459, 1973.

27. SINGER, RB, AND LEVINSON, L (eds.): *Medical Risks: Patterns of Mortality and Survival.* Lexington, Mass.: D.C. Heath and Co., 1976.

28. SISSON, JC, SCHOOMAKER, EB, AND ROSS, JC: *Clinical decision analysis: the hazard of using additional data.* JAMA 236:1259, 1976.

29. U.S. BUREAU OF THE CENSUS: *Statistical Abstract of the U.S.,* ed. 98. Washington, D.C., 1977.

30. VECCHIO, TJ: *Predictive value of a single diagnostic test in unselected populations.* N Engl J Med 274:1171, 1966.

31. WEINSTEIN, MD, AND STASON, WB: *Hypertension: A Policy Perspective.* Cambridge, Mass.: Harvard Univ Press, 1976.

32. WEINSTEIN, MC, AND FINEBERG, HV: *Clinical Decision Analysis.* Philadelphia: W.B. Saunders, 1980.

APPENDIX A: THE CLINICAL IMPLICATIONS OF SURVIVAL CURVES

The simplest representation of prognosis is the effect which time has on survival, often represented as a graph showing the probability of surviving as a function of time. Such curves can have many different shapes: we shall consider several of the most common forms and discuss the implications of each. In trying to understand the information presented in survival curves (sometimes called life-table analyses), we must consider three types of information: cumulative survival rates, mortality rates, and life expectancy.

These survival curves are all based on the observed number of people alive at various time periods after some event, such as surgery or the diagnosis of a particular disease. The fraction of the cohort alive, at any given time, is the survival rate for that time. Unfortunately, in most studies the cohort under observation is larger in the early follow-up years than later in the study because some patients will be "lost to follow-up." For this reason, life-table analyses deal with ever depleting cohorts, but by expressing survival as a probability, such analyses can take advantage of any data which are available. A typical survival curve for the cohort of 40-year-old white males in the United States in 1975 is shown in Figure A-1, A. The survival curve is reasonably flat until the sixth decade and then begins to fall at ever increasing rates. It is important to note that the percentage surviving is the fraction of the *original* cohort and not the fraction of the remaining cohort. For example, consider the thirty-fifth year of follow-up, when the patients would be age 75. In that year, 48.4 percent of the original cohort would be alive whereas 45.1 percent of the cohort would be alive the next year. Thus, 3.3 percent of the original cohort would die in the thirty-fifth year of follow-up. However, at the *start* of the thirty-fifth year of follow-up, 51.6 percent of the original cohort would have already died and therefore would not be at risk for dying in the thirty-fifth

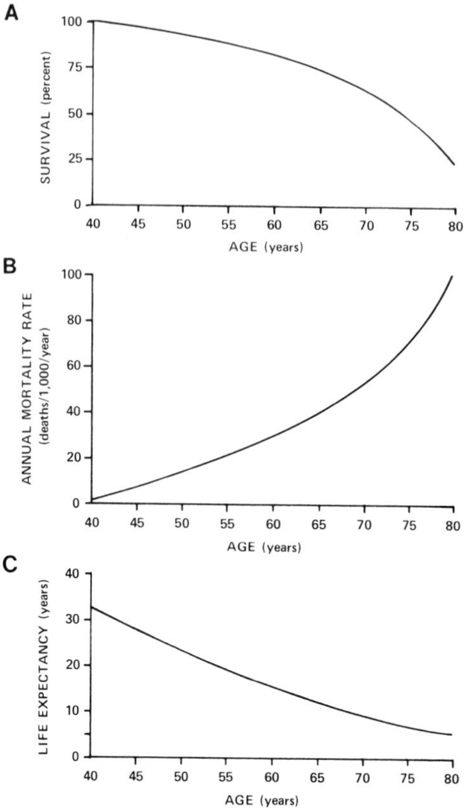

FIGURE A-1. Survival, mortality rate, and life expectancy for white, American males.

follow-up year. Only 48.4 percent of the original cohort were at risk for dying in the thirty-fifth year of follow-up. Hence, the mortality *rate* for that year would be 3.3 percent/48.4 percent, or 6.8 percent. It is customary to express the rate as 68 deaths/1000 patients/year. Figure A-1, B summarizes the effect of age on the mortality rate for the general population of white males in the United States. The annual mortality rate increases exponentially with age and, in fact, roughly doubles with every nine years of added age.

The third common means of expressing survival is the life expectancy or expected survival of a cohort. Life expectancy is a measure of the average length of survival and is calculated by finding the total number of person-years that members of the cohort survive and then dividing that total by the number of people in the cohort. For example, assume we begin with a cohort of 100 men with cancer and that 10 men die each year. The 10 men who die within the first year will have survived for six months, on average. Therefore, in the first year the 10 men will experience a total of 60 months or five years of survival. Another group of 10 men will die in the second year and will have experienced an average of 1½ years of survival each or 15 years total for the group of 10. Thus the total number of person-years of survival for the orginal cohort of 100 men will be 5 + 15 + 25 + 35 + 45 + 55 + 65 + 75 + 85 + 95, or 500 person-years. Since the original cohort contained 100 men, the life expectancy, or average survival, for each man would be 500/100, or five years.

Obviously, this example is trivial, but if the survival curve is not linear, the result may not be obvious. For many survival curves, a convenient *approximation* to the life expectancy is the time period at which exactly one-half of the original cohort remains alive. As we shall see below, however, that value is an approximation only, and if the mortality rate is either constant or decreasing, that approximation will underestimate the true life expectancy.

Figure A-1, C shows the effect of age on life expectancy in white male inhabitants of the United States. In the 40 to 80 year age range, life expectancy appears to decline almost linearly. The regression line for white males between the ages of 30 and 80 has slope −0.7 years of life expectancy/year of age. The important fact is that the slope is *not* unity. If it were unity, we would expect that average survival would decline by ten years for each decade of added chronologic age. In fact, it falls only seven years. In other words, the older the population is, the healthier the people selected from the original cohort. For reference, Table A-1 provides the life expectancy and annual mortality rates for various subgroups of the United States population as of 1975.

As can be seen in the middle panel of Figure A-1, the annual mortality rate of the general population rises sharply with advancing age. A variety of degenerative diseases contributes to this general increase. Certain diseases and "risk factors" elevate the annual mortality rate but do not modify the effect of advancing age. For example, smoking increases the average annual mortality rate by roughly 50 percent, whereas untreated moderate hypertension roughly doubles the rate. Figure A-2 shows the effect of these changes on crude survival, annual mortality rate, and life expectancy for men between the ages of 50 and 65. It is interesting to note that the effect of smoking is to make a cohort of men survive as if the cohort were five years older than its actual age, whereas the effect of moderate hypertension is to make the cohort behave as if it were nine years

TABLE A-1. Summary of Life Expectancy and Mortality Rate per 1,000 Population*

	Life Expectancy (years)				*Mortality Rate/1,000/Year*			
	White		*Nonwhite*		*White*		*Nonwhite*	
Age (years)	*Men*	*Women*	*Men*	*Women*	*Men*	*Women*	*Men*	*Women*
30	42.2	49.0	38.0	45.3	1.62	0.74	4.52	1.60
35	37.6	44.2	33.8	40.7	1.95	1.02	5.56	2.39
40	33.0	39.4	29.8	36.2	2.94	1.67	7.44	3.65
45	28.5	34.8	26.0	32.0	4.90	2.71	10.08	5.62
50	24.3	30.3	22.4	27.9	8.00	4.18	14.45	7.89
55	20.4	26.0	19.2	24.1	12.61	6.38	20.66	11.57
60	16.8	21.9	16.3	20.7	20.30	9.77	29.04	17.29
65	13.7	18.1	13.7	17.5	30.32	13.90	35.50	19.82
70	10.9	14.4	11.3	14.4	45.19	22.17	53.31	36.42
75	8.5	11.2	9.7	12.5	68.08	38.25	74.53	54.06
80	6.7	8.6	8.5	11.0	100.14	62.78	90.65	64.21

*From U.S. Bureau of the Census: *Statistical Abstract of the United States 1977,* ed. 98. Washington, D.C., 1977.

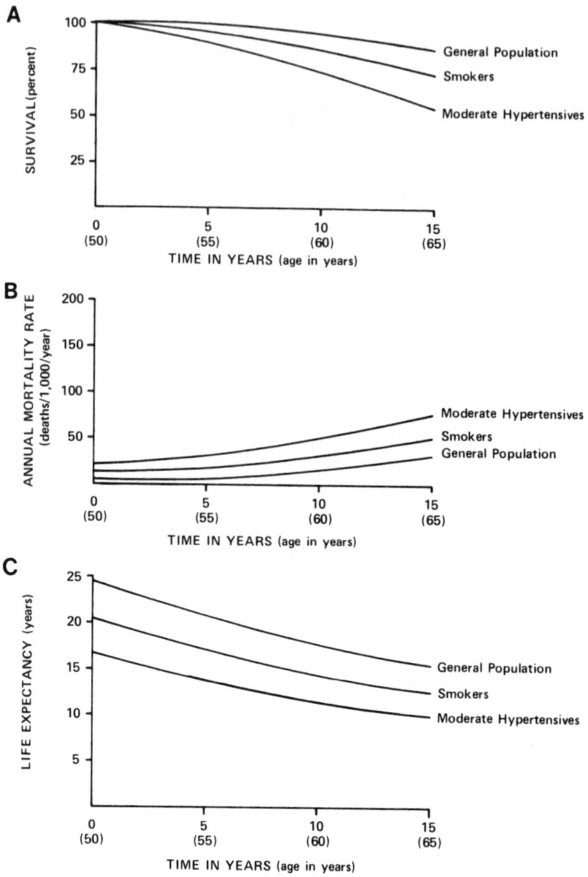

FIGURE A-2. Effect of smoking and high blood pressure on survival.

older. This effect has been well described in the actuarial literature, and various insurance companies assess a penalty for hypertension by adding a fixed number of years to the insuree's chronologic age. This risk factor-adjusted age might be viewed as the physiologic age of the cohort.

Many diseases, such as cancer, have such a profound effect on mortality that they swamp the effect of age (i.e., the development of degenerative processes in other organ systems). Even so, the effect of such severe diseases on mortality may be greater in older populations. To provide some insight into these situations, two further examples of survival curves will be considered—one in which the annual mortality rate is high and constant and one in which the crude survival falls linearly with respect to time. In Figure A-3, B, we have taken the annual mortality rate to be fixed at 150 deaths/1,000 patients/year. As can be seen in Figure A-3, A, the survival curve then becomes a declining exponential. Since the mortality rate does not change with time (i.e., with increasing age, as shown in parentheses for a cohort of 50-year-old men), the life expectancy is also constant (6 2/3 years). In other words, the subgroup of the original cohort which lives

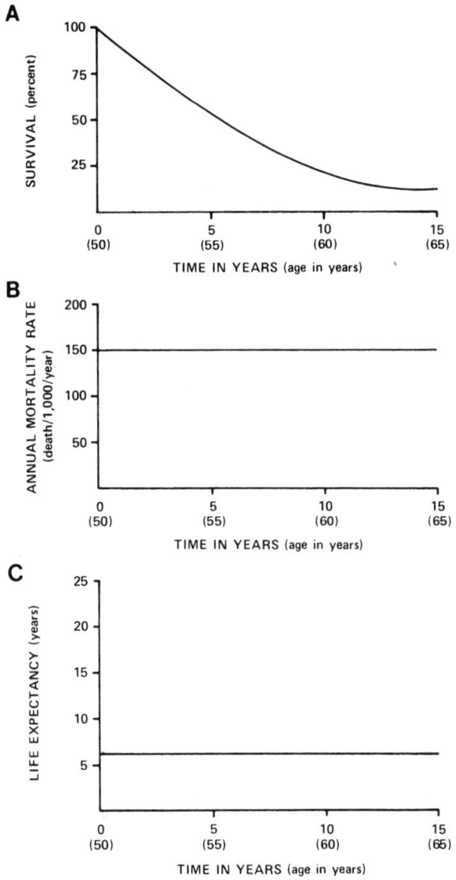

FIGURE A-3. Survival if mortality rate is constant.

to age 60 (i.e., survives 10 years from diagnosis; roughly 20% of the original cohort) will also be exposed to an annual mortality rate of 150/1,000/year and hence will also have a life expectancy of just 6 2/3 years. In the case of a constant annual mortality rate, the life expectancy equals 1/mortality rate. For example, this cohort has a mortality rate of 150/1,000/year, or 0.150. Life expectancy of members of the cohort is 1/0.150 or 6.7 years.

In contrast, the survival curve shown in Figure A-4, A shows a linear drop in the number of survivors, that is, 6.67 percent of the *original* cohort die each year. Since the survivors constitute an ever declining group, the constant 6667 deaths/100,000 patients of the original cohort will result in a sharply *increasing* mortality rate among survivors. For example, after ten years, only one-third of the original cohort will be alive. Thus, if the original cohort were 100,000, there would be 6667 deaths among the 33,333 survivors or an annual mortality rate of 200/1,000/year. Since the survivors are exposed to sharply increasing mortality rates, the life expectancy will decrease with increasing

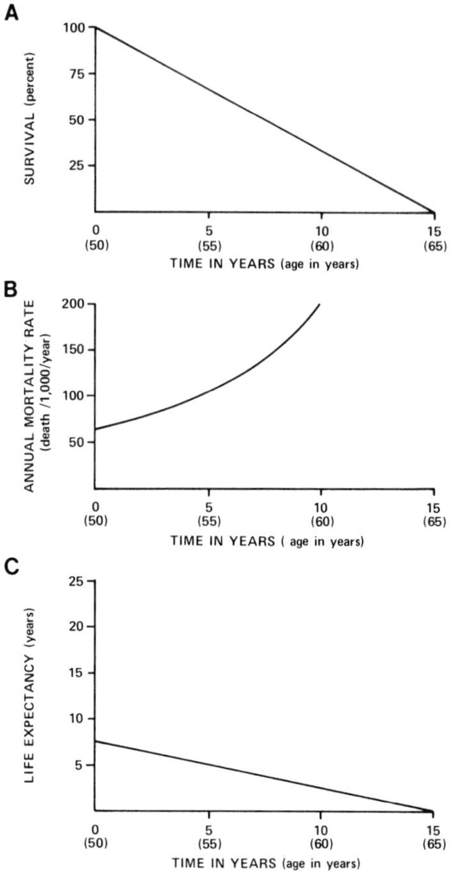

FIGURE A-4. Mortality rate and life expectancy if survival is linear.

age. In this example, as shown in the lower panel, the life expectancy is 7.5 years for the 100,000 people in the original cohort, but is only 2.5 years for the 33,333 people alive at age 60.

APPENDIX B: THE GENERAL CASE OF "CORRECTABLE" OPERATIVE RISK FACTORS

The detailed example presented in the body of this chapter dealt with a patient with an expanding aortic aneurysm who also sustained a recent myocardial infarction. It was assumed that preoperative rupture of the aneurysm would result in death and that the patient would be alive six months after surgery if he survived the perioperative period.

The subtree in Figure A-5 shows the more general situation. In this case, the preoperative catastrophe is not assumed to result in death but results in some level of permanent disability. We assign that level of disability a utility denoted by the symbol k, where utilities range between zero (death) and one (being alive and well). If k is assigned a value of zero, we have the utility assumptions made in the prior example. We

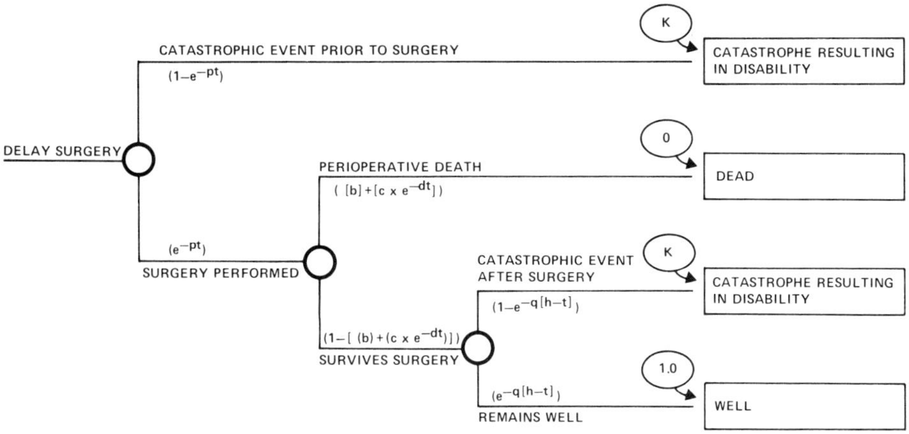

FIGURE A-5. A general tree for choosing optimal time for surgery.

also no longer assume that all patients surviving surgery are guaranteed to be well. Rather, the patient may become disabled after surgery but presumably at a far lower rate. For simplicity we have assumed that such postoperative disabilities have the same utility (k) as preoperative ones. An example of such a disability might be a cerebrovascular accident in a patient being considered for carotid endarterectomy. We assume that the rate of disablement is constant, with rate constant p in the preoperative period and rate constant q after surgery. The efficacy of surgery is measured by the amount by which p exceeds q. Thus, the chance of *not* being disabled before surgery is e^{-pt}, where t is surgical delay time, and chance of a preoperative catastrophe is therefore $(1 - e^{-pt})$. Similarly, the chance of *not* being disabled after surgery is $e^{-q(h-t)}$, and the chance of postoperative disability is $(1-e^{-q[h-t]})$, where h is the time horizon of the analysis and t is the surgical delay time. Note that the quantity $(h-t)$ is the length of time *after* surgery during which the patient is exposed to the postoperative disability rate q. If q equals zero (i.e., if surgery is curative and no postoperative disability can occur), then this model is equivalent to the aortic aneurysm example presented above.

The operative mortality is assumed to decline exponentially from a peak probability if surgery is performed immediately ($t = 0$) to a stable baseline if surgery is delayed to the end of the time horizon ($t = h$). The expression for operative mortality rate is assumed to be of the form: $b + ce^{-dt}$. If $b = 0.05$, $c = 0.35$, and $d = 0.46$/month, then this expression is approximately equal to the mortality rate (m) assumed in the aortic aneurysm case. Figure A-6 illustrates these relations. Figure A-6, A shows the increase in preoperative complications as a function of delay, graph B shows the decline in the operative mortality rate with surgical delay, and graph C shows the decrease in postoperative complications with surgical delay. This last, rather surprising, relation rests on the fact that surgical delay means there is less time available for a postoperative complication to occur. For example, if the time horizon (h) is six months and if surgery is performed after four months delay ($t = 4$), then only two postoperative months are available for complications. If surgery is performed at time h, then, by definition, there can be no postoperative complications *in the time horizon under analysis.* Recall that the utility function

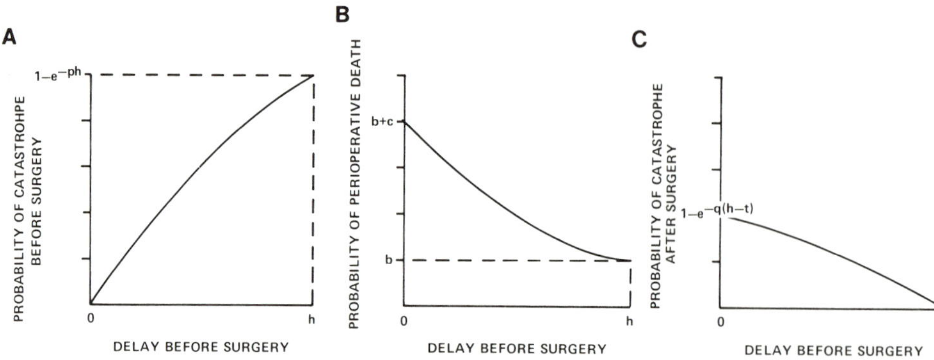

FIGURE A-6. Relation between delay and preoperative, postoperative, and anesthesia risk.

being employed is based on the patient's status at the end of the time horizon, that is, at time h. Complications occurring after time h are not considered since they will occur despite the timing of surgery, assuming that surgery *will* be performed at some time during the horizon of analysis.

One can now fold back the decision tree in Figure A-5 to find the expected utility of delaying surgery for time t. First consider the chance node depicting postoperative catastrophes. The expected utility of that node is $([1-e^{-q(h-t)}]k + e^{-q(h-t)})$ or $(k + [1-k]e^{-q[h-t]})$. Next consider the chance node describing the consequences of surgery. The expected utility of that node is $(0 + [1-(b + ce^{-dt})][k + (1-k)e^{-q(h-t)}])$. Finally, consider the leftmost node in the tree, describing the expected utility of delaying surgery for time t. The calculated expected utility of the leftmost node is expressed as $(1-e^{-pt})k + ([e^{-pt}][1 - (b + ce^{-dt})][k + (1-k)e^{-q(h-t)}])$. This complex expression can be evaluated for various values of surgical delay (t), and the delay which yields the maximum expected utility is the optimal time for surgery.

Sensitivity Analysis

Let us now examine the effect of various parameters on the optimal timing for surgery. First, the effect of the preoperative catastrophe rate (p) will be examined assuming that such catastrophes result in death (i.e., $k = 0$) and that surgery is curative if the patient survives (i.e., $q = 0$). These assumptions are analagous to those made in the aortic aneurysm example described above. If it is further assumed that surgery is being delayed for an acute myocardial infarction with the time course of anesthesia risk described above (i.e., $b = 0.05$, $c = 0.35$, $d = 0.46$/month, and $h = 6$, or a time horizon of six months), then Figure A-7, A shows the relation between the preoperative catastrophe rate and the optimal delay. As was suggested by Figure A-3, higher preoperative catastrophe rates imply that shorter delays would be preferable.

Next, let us examine the effect of the postoperative catastrophe rate (q) on surgical timing, now assuming that the preoperative catastrophe rate (p) is fixed at 0.0578, corresponding to a 50 percent chance of catastrophe if surgery were to be delayed for one year. Figure A-7, B shows that increases in the postoperative catastrophe rate argue for delaying surgery. This is understood if one realizes that the benefit of surgery

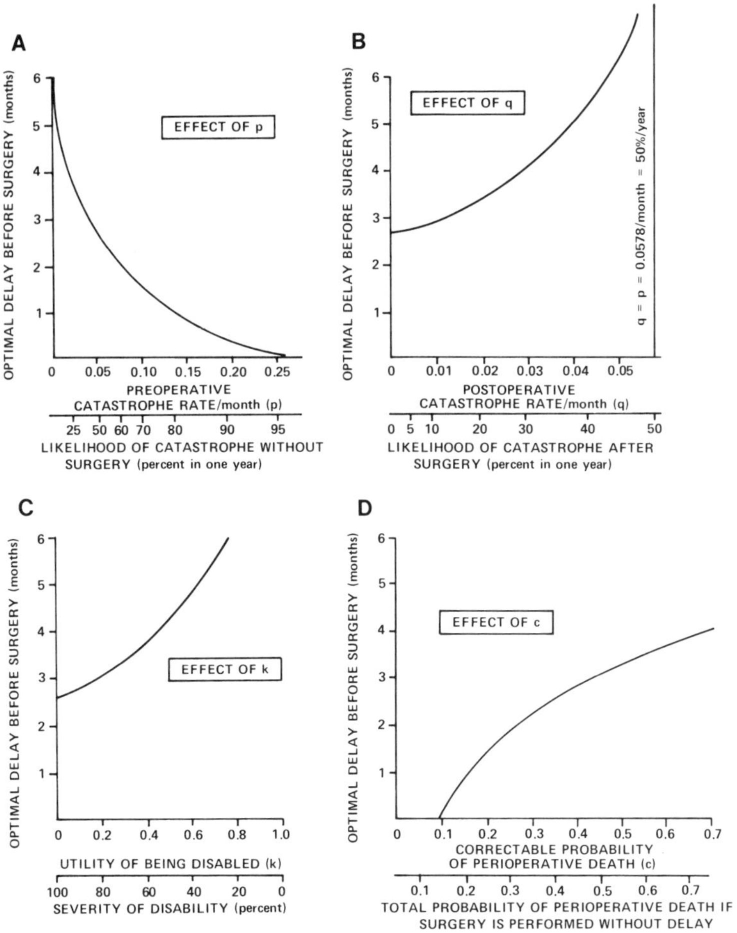

FIGURE A-7. Sensitivity analysis for preoperative and postoperative risk, degree of disability, and anesthesia risk.

depends on the difference between the preoperative (p) and postoperative (q) catastrophe rates. As the postoperative rate increases, that difference, and hence the benefit of surgery, decreases. With less surgical benefit, there would be less reason to push for early surgery in the period after a myocardial infarction. As q approaches 0.0578 (50%/year), optimal delay becomes infinitely large, that is, if there is no benefit, then surgery should not be done at all.

Figure A-7, C summarizes the effect of the degree of disability which a preoperative catastrophe would imply, again assuming that surgery is curative (i.e., q = 0). If the utility of being disabled (k) equals zero, then a catastrophe is assumed to result in death (e.g., aortic rupture); if k is greater than zero, a catastrophe is not as bad as dying (e.g., a cerebrovascular accident); as k approaches unity, the "catastrophic" event becomes increasingly more benign. As can be seen in the graph, increasing values of k (i.e., decreasing levels of disability) argue for longer delays before surgery. Again, this relation is observed because a decreasing degree of disability would imply that the benefit of surgery is less. If a "catastrophic" event resulted in no disability (i.e., if the patient remained well), then there would be little reason to perform surgery at all, and there would certainly be no reason to operate in the peri-infarction period.

Finally, let us examine the effect of changes in the correctable portion of the perioperative risk. Recall that the probability of surgical death was separated, for the purposes of this model, into two parts: a stable baseline risk (b) and a correctable component (ce^{-dt}) which declined with increasing surgical delay. This relation between correctable risk and optimal delay before surgery is summarized in Figure A-7, D. As the correctable portion of the risk increases, the optimal delay increases because more is to be gained (corrected) by delaying surgery. Note that the optimal delay is zero (i.e., surgery should be done immediately) when c is below 10 percent, since surgery should be done urgently if the *marginal* gain in delaying surgery is less than the risk of waiting. For a presumed preoperative risk of 5.8 percent/month, the benefit of delaying surgery disappears when the correctable portion of the surgical risk falls below 10 percent.

A Note on the Mathematics

The formulation of this general model was based on the assumption of exponential decay of operative risk and a constant *rate* of catastrophic complications. The mathematics involved were really quite straightforward: we chose to use exponential functions to express time course. (Of course, an analogous argument could be developed for other functional forms or, indeed, for arbitrary risk relations that can only be described as a graph. The illustrative case developed above shows how such arbitrary relations can be used). Instead of expressing the time courses in terms of e (the base for natural logarithms, equal to 2.718), we could have equivalently used base 2, in which case the preoperative risk ($1-e^{-pt}$) would have been of the form ($1-2^{-st}$) or ($1 - [\frac{1}{2}]^{st}$). From this latter form, it should be clear that s is a rate constant equal to $1/T_{\frac{1}{2}}$, where $T_{\frac{1}{2}}$ is the half-life of decay. Thus, if t equals 0, the risk is 0; if t equals $T_{\frac{1}{2}}$ (i.e., 1/s), then $(\frac{1}{2})^{st}$ equals 0.5 and the risk is 1 − 0.5, or 50 percent. If t equals 2s, then $(\frac{1}{2})^{st}$ equals ¼ and the risk equals 75 percent. To convert from s to p, we only need realize that p = s(1n 2) = 0.69s. Thus, for example, the rate constant for the decline in operative risk (d = 0.46) implies that $T_{\frac{1}{2}}$ = 0.69/0.46, or 1.5 months. (Recall that the risk was assumed to be 40 percent at time zero, 20 percent at time two months, and 10 percent at time four months, and that the baseline risk was assumed to be 5 percent. Thus, the correctable portion was 35 percent, 15 percent, and 5 percent at zero, two, and four months respectively—a half-time of approximately 1.5 months.)

The above sections have dealt largely with acute myocardial infarction as the correctable cause of increased operative risk. This situation was chosen because the timing of surgery after myocardial infarction is a common problem facing the consultant. The same model could be applied to other risk factors. For example, an analogous argument could be developed for patients presenting with an acute infection (e.g., pneumonia). In that case, the correctable portion of the operative risk should decline faster, and hence the time constant (d) would be larger. At the risk of making the analysis seem unduly complex, we have tried to present this section in a general form, thereby providing the reader with insight into the various factors which should influence decisions about surgical timing and how those factors interact. In using this approach the consultant can either refer to the summary graphs in Figure A-7 or can substitute other values in the general formulae given above. The availability of inexpensive, pocket-sized scientific calculators makes the latter approach practical.

Chapter 2

ALLERGIC REACTIONS

Keith P.W.J. McAdam, M.R.C.P., and John L. Ohman, Jr., M.D.

The adjective "allergic" is applied to a wide variety of adverse reactions to drugs and other agents that are "foreign" to the body such as inhaled pollens and dust. While strict medical use of the term allergic implies immunologic mechanisms, it is often loosely applied to many nonimmunologic reactions. This chapter will emphasize reactions having an immunologic basis. Hypersensitivity has been classically divided into four categories:[1] Type I, IgE mediated, immediate hypersensitivity; Type II, cytotoxic reactions; Type III, Arthus or immune-complex type reactions; and Type IV, delayed or tuberculin-type cell mediated reactions. Particular attention will be given here to the immediate hypersensitivity category, which includes a significant proportion of the fatal reactions to drugs and presents the physician with many diagnostic difficulties.

MECHANISMS AND DISEASE CATEGORIES

Immediate Hypersensitivity (IgE Mediated, Anaphylactic)

Immediate hypersensitivity is associated with the production of IgE antibody, which is directed against extrinsic antigens (commonly called allergens). The propensity of bone marrow-derived lymphocytes and plasma cells to form IgE antibody against specific antigens is, at least in part, genetically predetermined. It is regulated by macrophages, which process and present antigen to lymphocytes, and by "helper" and "suppressor" lymphocytes derived from the thymus.

Allergens have a *hapten* portion, against which IgE antibody is directed, and a *carrier* portion that is recognized by immunoregulatory lymphocytes.[2,3] Low molecular weight antigens, such as penicillin, exist as haptens and are poor immunogens in themselves; such haptens must attach to a carrier protein before they can become effective antigens. IgE antibody is always present in relatively low concentration in body fluids. The very high biologic potency of IgE antibody is due to its capacity to bind to tissue mast cells and circulating basophils.

The binding of antigen with cell-bound antibody causes an alteration of the cell membrane, followed by a complex series of intracellular steps that result in the release of various substances that mediate many of the manifestations of immediate hypersensitivity.[4] The mediators of immediate hypersensitivity are directly released or generated as a result of mast cell degranulation. They include: histamine, leukotrienes (slow reacting substances of anaphylaxis), platelet activating factor, and various chemotactic factors. These mediators not only act directly on bronchial smooth muscle and postcapillary venules but also recruit secondary effector cells (eosinophils, neutrophils, macrophages, and platelets) to the site of injury. These recruited cells can greatly amplify tissue inflammatory responses, in part due to release of lysosomal enzymes, and can readily explain the chronicity of allergic reactions.[5]

Eosinophils occur in increased numbers in the blood of patients undergoing allergic reactions. The release of mast cell mediators is associated with the influx of eosinophils into the tissue as the result of several eosinophil chemotactic sustances liberated by the mast cell. Eosinophils tend to modulate the allergic reactions by producing enzymes that degrade inflammatory mediators such as histamine and the leukotrienes which are highly biologically active metabolites of arachidonic acid. Since eosinophilia can occur during allergic reactions to drugs, it can serve as a useful indicator that an allergic reaction has taken place. Its absence, however, does not exclude an allergic reaction. Eosinophilia can also be associated with unrelated conditions such as parasitic infestations.[6]

Elevated eosinophil counts (above 250 cells/mm^3) are found in some situations in which mast cell mediator release does not seem to play an important role. For example, there are forms of nonallergic asthma that are associated with very intense eosinophilia and tissue inflammation. In general, patients with asthma tend to have eosinophil counts in the range of 400 to 1200 cells/mm^3, and occasionally counts of 2500 cells/mm^3 may be reached.

The clinical manifestations of immediate hypersensitivity usually occur within an hour, and often within minutes, following antigenic exposure. The nature of the symptoms depends on the type of exposure (see Table 1). Exposure to airborne pollens, mold spores, and dust results in respiratory allergy consisting of rhinoconjunctivitis and asthma. Ingestion of allergens results in a variety of symptoms related to the gastrointestinal tract as well as more generalized manifestations of anaphylaxis due to systemic absorption of antigens. The latter can be severe and result in laryngeal edema, shock, and death. Such systemic allergic reactions can also occur following the parenteral administration of drugs and insect stings.

Immediate hypersensitivity reactions differ from many other reactions discussed in this chapter in that they are usually initiated by very small amounts of antigen. As little as 10^{-13} gm of ragweed antigen E will produce a wheal and flare response in skin. These

TABLE 1. Immediate Hypersensitivity Reactions

Type of Contact with Allergen	*Examples of Allergens Involved*	*Disease Process*	*Signs and Symptoms*
Topical (on skin)	Animal saliva Dust Grass pollen	Urticaria	Pruritic wheal and flare response at site of contact
		Angioedema	Diffuse swelling when contact is around eyes or mouth
Exposure to airborn particles	Pollens Mold Dust Animal dander	Rhinitis	Nasal pruritis, sneezing, rhinorrhea, nasal stuffiness
		Conjunctivitis	Watering of eyes, injection of conjunctiva
		Asthma	Wheezing, shortness of breath, chest tightness
Ingestion	Foods: nuts fresh fruit shellfish fish, etc. Drugs: penicillin, etc.	Gastrointestinal allergy	Pruritis and angioedema of lips, tongue and pharynx; nausea; vomiting; abdominal cramps
Injection	Insect stings injected drugs (penicillin, etc.)	Generalized anaphylaxis	Generalized urticaria, rhinitis, asthma, laryngeal edema, and obstruction of the airway; shock; death

reactions occur rapidly following exposure to the allergen. An injection of penicillin, for example, commonly produces signs of anaphylaxis in a susceptible individual in less than a minute. This kind of allergic reaction rarely begins more than an hour after antigenic exposure.

Diagnosis of immediate hypersensitivity is usually made on the basis of the patient's history of anaphylactic-type response to allergens. When there is some uncertainty regarding the history, a skin test can be performed. Allergen can be introduced into the skin in several ways, the safest and easiest method being the prick or scratch test. A drop of allergen solution is applied to an area of skin (usually on the forearm or back) that has been cleaned with alcohol. Then a needle is used to either puncture the skin or abrade 4 to 8 mm of skin surface. This procedure should not produce any bleeding.

Another common method of skin testing is the intradermal test in which 0.03 to 0.05 cc is injected into the upper layers of the skin. Intradermal testing can induce serious systemic reactions in highly allergic individuals, so the prick test should be performed first. A positive reaction is indicated by a wheal and flare reaction occurring between 10 to 20 minutes after injection. An initial irritative flare before 10 minutes has elapsed should be disregarded. Certain substances, such as morphine, iodinated contrast media, and certain extracts of house dust will produce a wheal and flare in a high percentage of normal subjects. Patients with dermatographism will react to any skin test with a wheal and flare. It is therefore essential to include a skin test using a diluent as a negative control. When unfamiliar substances are used, it is a reasonable precaution to test the substance in one or more normal subjects to rule out nonspecific effects of the extract. A positive skin test with the above reservations can be taken as a reasonably certain indication of the presence of IgE antibody.[7]

In the future, measurement of serum IgE antibody by radioimmunoassay (the radioallergosorbent test or RAST) has the potential of being more reliable and convenient than skin testing in some circumstances. It has been shown in a number of allergen systems that serum IgE antibody levels generally correlate with skin test reactivity. Skin testing is often more sensitive than the RAST, given the concentration of allergen extracts customarily used. The skin test, therefore, tends to be positive in a higher percentage of patients without overt disease. Even though commercial laboratories have the capability of measuring IgE antibody to multiple inhalent allergens and a few drugs such as penicillin, skin testing seems likely to remain the mainstay of the diagnosis of immediate hypersensitivity.[8]

Delayed Hypersensitivity (Lymphocyte Mediated)

Although lymphocytes may be observed histologically in many inflammatory states (especially those that are chronic) and are probably essential in the protective immune response to certain infections such as tuberculosis, they also participate in the pathogenesis of certain disease states. A good example of this involvement is allergic contact dermatitis. The antigens that most commonly elicit contact dermatitis include a number of fairly simple molecules: metals, such as nickel and mercury; preservatives, such as methylparaben and formalin; and plant oleoresins, such as those derived from poison ivy. Many of these are incomplete antigens or haptens that must complex to skin protein before activation of lymphocytes can take place.

The allergic reaction is characterized by the appearance of a papulovesicular rash at the site of skin contact. The rash takes 48 to 72 hours to develop fully—hence the term "delayed hypersensitivity." The histologic appearance of contact dermatitis is not significantly different from other forms of dermatitis. Depending on the chronicity of the lesions, the following changes may be seen in varying degrees: intracellular edema, acanthosis spongiosis, parakeratosis, exocytosis, and formation of multilocular bullae.

Vasodilation and extravasation of mononuclear cells may be observed very early in the development of the lesions.[9]

The manifestations of delayed hypersensitivity are probably mediated in part by a number of soluble factors derived from lymphocytes (lymphokines) and monocytes (monokines) elaborated as these cells respond to the antigenic stimulus. Some of these factors have a direct effect on target cells (lymphotoxin). Other factors are chemotactic for neutrophils, eosinophils, and basophils.

The most reliable test for contact dermatitis is the "patch test." The substance to be tested is applied to the skin with an occlusive dressing which is removed after 24 to 72 hours.[9] If a local dermatitis results, this can be taken as evidence of delayed hypersensitivity. The interpretation of patch tests is often less clear than the interpretation of skin tests for IgE mediated reactions. While there are currently many in vitro tests that measure lymphocyte function, none has proven useful in the diagnosis of contact dermatitis.

Reactions analogous to allergic contact dermatitis can occur in other body tissues, although they are less frequent. Examples of these are oral mucous membrane reactions to dental appliances and tissue reactions to various prostheses.

TREATMENT OF GENERALIZED ANAPHYLACTIC REACTIONS

The onset of symptoms and signs of generalized anaphylaxis should be treated quickly. The symptoms can progress rapidly over a period of minutes and result in airway obstruction and shock. Therefore, at the first indication of an anaphylactic reaction—swelling of the throat, difficulty in swallowing, stridor, and generalized urticaria—treatment should be started. The equipment and medication needed for treating generalized anaphylaxis are listed in Table 2.

The treatment consists of the following steps:

1. Make sure the airway is clear. If not, endotracheal intubation or tracheostomy may be necessary.
2. A. Inject 0.3 to 0.5 cc of epinephrine (1:1000) subcutanteously. In a monitored patient, this dose may be repeated every 15 to 20 minutes for several doses. In instances of profound shock, epinephrine (5 to 10 cc of a 1:10,000 dilution) may be administered intravenously.
   B. Administer 20 to 30 mg of diphenhydramine hydrochloride (Benadryl) intravenously. This dosage may be repeated 2 hours after the first administration.
3. Monitor cardiac status since the use of beta-adrenergic agents, especially in the presence of hypoxia, can lead to serious cardiac arrhythmias.
4. A. Set up IV infusion. Sodium chloride can be supplemented with 20 mEq ampules of sodium bicarbonate to correct any associated acidosis. Elevation of the foot of the bed and intravenous saline will correct transient hypotension.
   B. Treat severe hypotension with vasopressors such as dopamine or levarterenol, the dosage of which can be titrated according to the response.

TABLE 2. Equipment and Medication for Treating Anaphylactic Reactions

Equipment
Endotracheal tube pack
Tracheotomy pack
Venous cutdown pack
IV infusion set
Oxygen administration equipment
Sphygmomanometer
Medication
Adrenergic agents: epinephrine (1:1000), dopamine, levarterenol
Antihistamines: diphenhydramine (Benadryl)
Phosphodiesterase inhibitors: aminophylline
Corticosteroids: methylprednisolone, hydrocortisone
Intravenous fluids: normal saline

5. If asthmatic symptoms are present, infuse 250 to 350 mg of aminophylline slowly over a 10 to 15 minute period (adult dose). Follow this with an infusion at a rate of 0.5 to 0.9 mg/kg/hr.
6. Administer 60 to 100 mg of methylprednisolone intravenously. Although the drug is ineffective for treating the symptoms of acute anaphylaxis, it can prevent delayed reactions that sometimes occur 8 to 12 hours after the onset of symptoms.

The patient's response to this course of treatment is usually very rapid, and the acute administration of these agents can frequently be suspended within an hour. Occasionally, however, some of the anaphylactic symptoms recur within 24 hours after the treatment has been suspended. These symptoms are usually less severe and easily managed.

INHALANT ALLERGIES

Allergens

SEASONAL ALLERGENS

Airborn allergens impinge upon permeable membranes of the respiratory tract and conjunctiva, causing the allergic syndromes of asthma, rhinitis, and conjunctivitis. Among the more important airborn allergens are those derived from pollen produced by the flowers of plants that depend on wind for cross-fertilization. Since plants pollinate at regular times throughout the year, it is possible to predict when a person who is allergic to a particular pollen will manifest symptoms. In general, in the northeast United States, trees and grasses pollinate from spring to early summer, while some weeds pollinate throughout the summer months and into the early fall. One of the most important allergens is ragweed pollen, which is distributed widely in the northern United States. It is somewhat less significant in the Northwest and is virtually nonexistent in the deep South. Ragweed begins pollinating in mid-August and persists until the first frost. Mountain cedar, on the other hand, is mainly a problem in the southern states and pollinates from December through February.[10]

NONSEASONAL ALLERGENS

Other important allergens prevalent in the air at all times include house dust, of which the house dust mite (Dermatophagoides) is an important component. Certain people react very strongly to mite allergens, manifesting symptoms similar to those associated with pollens. Animal danders and feathers are also important nonseasonal allergens and are associated with asthma and rhinoconjunctivitis.

Antigens from mold spores straddle the seasonal and nonseasonal categories. Mold spores are present indoors throughout the year but are most prevalent outside in late summer and fall. Spores are liberated into the air through sporulation and tend to be ubiquitous. Since spores have a mean diameter of less than 20 microns (μ), they can penetrate into the lungs very easily. In contrast, pollens tend to be larger than 20 μ in diameter and do not penetrate the lungs as easily.[10]

Manifestations of Inhalant Allergy

ASTHMA

Asthma is the most serious manifestation of inhalant allergy. It presents with a variety of symptoms, the most common being wheezing, tightness in the chest, and shortness of breath. These symptoms may also occur in other chronic pulmonary diseases. The distinctive feature of asthma, however, is the variability of symptoms. It is therefore necessary to have an objective measure for diagnosis, such as spirometry to detect air flow obstruction. The most commonly used spirometric measurement is the one second forced expiration volume (FEV_{25-75}). One confusing aspect of asthma is that in addition to IgE mediated mechanisms, it can be precipitated by a number of other factors that mimic IgE mediated mechanisms. These include viral infections; irritants such as cold air, smoke, and strong odors; aspirin and other prostaglandin inhibitors; beta-adrenergic blocking agents; and psychosomatic factors.

Aspirin Sensitivity

In certain individuals, asthmatic symptoms can be induced by aspirin 1 to 2 hours after ingestion. Such hypersensitivity seems to be related to aspirin but not to salicylate as aspirin sensitive asthmatics can ingest sodium salicylate or methylsalicylate, as well as other salicylate-containing products without ill effect.

The mechanism of aspirin induced asthma has been studied extensively and is probably not mediated by immediate hypersensitivity or any other immunologic reaction. Rather, it appears to be a pharmacologic effect in susceptible individuals and may be related to the action of aspirin on prostaglandin metabolism.

Asthmatics who are sensitive to aspirin also react to drugs such as indomethacin and ibuprofen, which act on prostaglandin metabolism. There have been widespread claims that tartrazine, a yellow dye additive in foods and drugs, will also induce asthma in aspirin sensitive individuals. The mechanism is not known, although it appears that tartrazine does not affect prostaglandin synthesis.[11, 12]

Beta-Adrenergic Blocking Agents

Drugs such as propranolol will produce bronchospasm in a significant number of asthmatics. Adrenergic stimulation produces an increase in cyclic adenosine monophosphate intracellularly, which results in a decrease in mast cell mediator release. Beta-adrenergic stimulation also has a direct effect on reducing bronchial smooth muscle tone. In the perioperative period, the blocking of these beneficial effects with propranolol should be avoided or done with caution in patients known to have asthma.[13]

Psychologic Factors

It appears that stress of any kind will aggravate asthmatic conditions. However, stress seldom brings on serious asthma in a patient who does not already have significant manifestations of the disease.[14]

Viral Infections

Viral infections will frequently lead to a state of bronchial hyperresponsiveness that may persist for a period of many weeks after the acute signs of the viral infection have subsided. Bacterial infections are not usually responsible for acute exacerbation of asthma.[15]

RHINOCONJUNCTIVITIS

While not as severe an allergy syndrome as asthma, rhinoconjunctivitis can be a significant factor in the comfort of a patient during the peak of pollen season. In addition to the basic problems of sneezing, coughing, and nasal congestion, complications such as sinusitis and otitis media can generate extreme discomfort and complicate the management of the patient in the perioperative period.

Perioperative Management of Inhalant Allergies

Several environmental considerations are important in the surgical patient. If a patient's seasonal allergies create a potential problem from excessive coughing and sneezing, elective surgery should be planned for a time of year when the particular allergen is not at its peak prevalence. A number of measures can also be taken in the hospital for patients who have allergic reactions to nonseasonal allergens. These include: eliminating feather pillows, minimizing dust exposure, and replacing or sealing old mattresses that may well be heavily contaminated with dust and mite allergens.

The general principles of the pharmacologic treatment of asthma are given in Chapter 12, Pulmonary Management. Particular consideration should be given to the use of corticosteroids perioperatively. In general, patients who have been maintained on oral corticosteroids for the treatment of asthma to any extent within the year prior to surgery should receive parenteral corticosteroid coverage to treat any absolute or relative hypothalmic-pituitary-adrenal axis insufficiency that may be present.

In addition, patients maintained on inhaled corticosteroids such as beclomethasone dipropionate may experience an exacerbation of asthma when these sprays are withdrawn. A single steroid coverage regimen can serve to prevent both the adrenal insufficiency provoked by the stress of surgery and the possible occurrence of asthma in the patient who has needed oral or inhaled corticosteroids to control the condition in the recent past. See Chapter 5, Endocrinology, for steroid coverage regimens.

Antihistamines are the mainstays in managing rhinoconjunctivitis. Diphenhydramine hydrochloride (Benadryl) is effective but is not desirable because of its sedative effects. The more preferable antihistamines are chlorpheniramine in doses up to 32 mg/day total and tripelennamine at 150 mg/day total. These drugs are effective for the majority of patients with allergic rhinitis and can be given intramuscularly during the perioperative period.

In severe rhinitis, additional forms of treatment are necessary, such as oral or parenteral corticosteroids. However, this type of treatment should be reserved for the most severe reactions. The recent availability of potent topical corticosteroid sprays represents an improvement in the treatment of rhinitis. If used at the onset of rhinitis symptoms, these sprays are effective. Improvements resulting from their use is usually gradual, requiring three to seven days. One particularly effective steroid spray is beclomethasone dipropionate. This agent may also be useful in preventing or retarding the growth of nasal polyps.

Vasoconstrictor sprays effectively provide temporary relief from rhinitis symptoms. Their overuse, however, can lead to rebound, which only aggravates the condition. In general, vasoconstrictor sprays should be avoided in chronic rhinitis.

Another drug, cromolyn sodium, may be useful for treating rhinitis and conjunctivitis as well as asthma. It is used prophylactically for relatively short periods of high intensity antigenic stimulation, such as in the pollen season. Cromolyn sodium is not useful in the treatment of acute exacerbation of rhinitis and conjunctivitis.

Immunotherapy

Immunotherapy or "desensitization" has been in use for more than 50 years and consists of a series of injections of allergen extract. The injections are given over a period of months in gradually increasing doses. The purpose is to make the patient less susceptible to inhaled pollen and other allergens. The efficacy of immunotherapy in rhinitis and to a lesser extent in asthma has been well established in recent years.[16]

The mechanism by which immunotherapy works is not completely clear; however, it does result in the production of IgG or blocking antibody. IgG may have the effect of complexing to the allergen and preventing its attachment onto cell-bound IgE antibody. In addition, immunotherapy results in the reduction of the maximum ability of mast cells to release histamine via antigenic stimulation. When given for more than a year, immunotherapy is associated with a decrease in IgE antibody synthesis which may be related to the induction of antigen specific suppressor T cells.

Currently, there is wide variation in the way immunotherapy is administered with regard to dose of extract and interval between injections. Most commonly, when the dose of extract is being increased, the injections are given at weekly intervals. Following the build-up period, the injections are given as boosters at two to six week intervals. Especially during the build-up period, such injections can result in a systemic anaphylactic reaction if the dose given exceeds the patient's tolerance. A local reaction at the site of the injection is usually seen. Systemic reactions and severe local reactions will require modification of the dosage schedule. The effect of immunotherapy is very gradual. During hospitalization, it is seldom essential that the patient be given injections at the exact planned interval. Injections can usually be postponed for a period of weeks without ill effect, although the dosage schedule will need some modification when resumed.

FOOD ALLERGIES

Patients can be allergic to a number of different kinds of food. The most common are fruits, nuts, fish, shellfish, and peanuts.[17, 18] These reactions are mediated by IgE antibody and produce the symptoms of anaphylaxis within 10 minutes to an hour. The relationship of the acute symptoms and the food intake usually presents with few diagnostic difficulties. It is important to take a history of food allergy and avoid foods in the hospital that contain hidden allergens. This is particularly important with patients who are allergic to soy protein, since soy is an additive found in many foods. Certain individuals who are highly allergic to penicillin may react to trace amounts of the drug found in milk and milk products. Finally, some dyes in foods such as tartrazine (yellow dye #5) can induce an allergic reaction consisting of asthma and urticaria; however, such reactions are fairly unusual and the mechanism is not understood.

It should be recognized that much intolerance to food is not allergic (i.e., IgE mediated). Examples of this include upper gastrointestinal symptoms in response to a variety of foods in patients with a tendency to acid peptic disease or specific gluten (wheat) or milk intolerance (celiac disease and intestinal lactase deficiency, respectively). Certain children with nodular hyperplasia of the small bowel thought to be due to a sensitivity to various foods are now being treated with oral cromolyn sodium.

In recent years, many symptom complexes have been ascribed to food additives. However, many claims lack a firm scientific basis, and reactions that occur more than several hours after the ingestion of food must be treated with some skepticism.

DRUG ALLERGIES

Reactions to drugs can be broadly categorized into two different types:

1. Exaggerated pharmacologic actions that are usually predictable and dose dependent.
2. Aberrant drug actions that are unpredictable and would not be expected on the basis of the agent's known pharmacologic properties.

The first category includes direct toxicity of drugs, overdosage, side effects, and most drug interactions.[19] Interactions between drugs often lead to enhanced or diminished effects by altering the pharmacokinetics of the individual drugs. Thus, one drug may affect the adsorption, distribution in blood or tissues, metabolism, and elimination of the second drug. Some drugs combine with specific host receptors, and the dynamics of target organ sensitivity depend on drug competition or potentiation and the influence of disease on the host's cell membrane receptors. In surgical patients who are being treated with several different medications, there is often concern about the interaction of drugs with analgesics and anesthetic agents. Many of these adverse interactions are predictable; however, with the vast array of different drugs currently utilized, the pharmacologic explanation is easy to overlook and the adverse effect is often mislabeled "allergic." As a result, in many patients who recount so-called "allergic" reactions to drugs, there is often no immunologic basis for hypersensitivity.

The second category of adverse effects to drugs includes the unpredictable aberrant reactions which would not be apparent during conventional toxicologic screening. For example, malignant hyperpyrexia, the inherited disturbance of intracellular calcium transport, occurs in rare individuals (1:15,000) when they are given general anesthetic agents.[20] Malignant hyperpyrexia manifests by hyperthermia, increased muscle tone, hyperventilation, acidosis, and hyperkalemia.[21] Allergic drug reactions would also fit into this category, being defined as those reactions mediated immunologically. In a prospective questionnaire study of 10,000 patients presenting for anesthesia in Britain,[22] an overall frequency of 13.5 percent was obtained for a history of allergies which were identified as allergy to penicillin (6.2%), other antibiotics (0.5%), narcotics (0.5%), iodine (0.4%), zinc oxide plaster (2.2%), and other agents (5%). Although this figure exceeds the true incidence of drug allergy in a surgical population, it indicates the importance of eliciting a detailed history of allergy in patients prior to anesthesia and surgery when many agents may be administered to the unknowing patient.

Immunologic Drug Reactions

Immunologic drug reactions can be subdivided into the four categories outlined in the beginning of this chapter. Type I or IgE mediated anaphylactic reactions are an important cause of fatal reactions to drugs. Type II or cytotoxic reactions include hemolysis, thrombocytopenia, and agranulocytosis. These are due to antibody sticking to the surface of cells which are then hemolyzed by complement activation or destroyed by phagocytosis in the reticuloendothelial system. Type III or immune-complex type reactions occur as the result of antibodies to drugs, usually of the IgG or IgM class. Immune complexes can deposit in various tissues and mediate syndromes such as nephritis and vasculitis. Finally, Type IV or delayed type reactions mediated by lymphocytes can result in contact dermatitis from topical application of drugs on the skin.[9]

A large group of drug reactions remain that defy a simple classification but probably involve immunologic mechanisms. It is essential to appreciate the scope of these reactions so that associations with drug intake are not overlooked.

A wide variety of cutaneous eruptions can be caused by drugs.[23] These include erythematous, papular, vesicular, bullous, and various raised wheal-like eruptions. The most severe generalized skin eruption is exfoliative dermatitis, which can be fatal. Erythema multiforme is a highly variable erythematous, raised macular eruption which can be vesiculobullous and which includes typical iris or target configurations. Erythema nodosum consists of tender subcutaneous lesions that have a predilection for the lower extremities and persist for a number of weeks. Generalized skin rashes can also be associated with systemic manifestations. Stevens-Johnson syndrome is a particularly fulminant bullous form of erythema multiforme with mucous membrane involvement, fever, myalgias, and occasionally sepsis.

Localized skin eruptions associated with drug intake include fixed drug eruptions which are well-demarcated, rounded plaques that tend to relapse at the same site. Photosensitivity dermatitis consists of immediate urticarial erythematous reactions or delayed vesiculobullous reactions, which result from systemic or topical administration of drugs followed by exposure to sunlight.

Drugs can be associated with the occurrence of necrotizing venulitis or arteritis (periarteritis nodosa) with a wide spectrum of cutaneous and systemic manifestations. Serum sickness consists of fever, arthralgias, lymphadenopathy, peripheral neuropathy, and occasionally joint effusions. Cutaneous manifestations include urticaria (mediated by IgE antibody), erythema multiforme, and purpura. Many of the manifestations of serum sickness are believed to be caused by the deposition of immune complexes. Initial sensitization to a drug is followed by the appearance of symptoms within 3 to 12 days. An accelerated serum sickness reaction can occur in two to four days if the patient is already sensitized.

Persistent fever can be the sole manifestation of a drug reaction. Drug fever can also be associated with a variety of skin rashes or the systemic manifestations of vasculitis.

Allergic Reactions to Penicillin

Penicillin allergy is frequently seen and has been studied extensively. Skin testing with penicillin itself is unreliable because penicillin is a poor antigen in that it is monovalent (or haptenic). The introduction of a polyvalent skin test antigen, penicilloyl-polylysine (PPL), has improved the capacity to diagnose immediate hypersensitivity to penicillin.[24, 25] There are, however, metabolic products of penicillin (nonpenicilloyl or "minor" determinants) that can produce severe allergic reactions and current data suggest that most anaphylactic reactions to penicillin are associated with IgE mediated reactions to these minor determinants.[26] Currently, no reliable skin test reagents for detecting them are commercially available. Aged aqueous penicillin preparations contain variable amounts of these minor determinants, and it is useful to test with both PPL and aged penicillin before treating patients with a history of allergic reactions to the drug. A negative reaction to these two skin test preparations reduces the risk of immediate anaphylaxis.

Skin rashes encountered during penicillin therapy are frequently labeled penicillin allergy. While a variety of immunologic responses are seen (IgG, IgM, lymphocyte, and so forth), the relationship of these changes to pathogenesis remains unclear. It should be emphasized that maculopapular and bullous eruptions are *not* associated with an increased risk of anaphylaxis of immediate hypersensitivity. Skin testing is not useful in these situations. Ampicillin commonly causes a mildly pruritic maculopapular eruption appearing 1 to 20 days after the start of therapy. Patients with infectious mononucleosis are particularly prone to react to ampicillin in this way. The mechanism of this rash is unclear.[27]

Since cephalosporins are commonly considered alternatives to penicillin, it should be pointed out that they share with the penicillins a beta-lactam structure and that cross-reactivity has been reported in up to 20 percent of patients. A skin test with cephalosporins prior to administration might single out those individuals who have immediate hypersensitivity.

The extent of cross-reactivity between the various synthetic penicillins and their metabolic degradation products is completely uninvestigated, and it would be wise to assume that extensive cross-reactivity does exist. Skin testing with the specific penicillin derivative that is to be used is appropriate, as long as the physician is aware that a negative test may not be completely reliable. A safe skin testing procedure is as follows:

> A solution containing 1 to 10 mg/ml of the antibiotic is diluted serially 1:10, 1:100, and 1:1000 in normal saline. Prick testing is first done with the 1:1000 dilution and, if no reaction is seen at 20 minutes, a ten-fold greater concentration is used. This procedure is repeated until the most concentrated solution is used. The same process is then repeated using an intradermal test.

Skin tests, in particular the intradermal test, may result in a nonspecific irritative reaction when the more concentrated solutions are used. Irritative reactions can be documented by skin testing in one or more normal subjects.

A patient may have an urgent need to take an antibiotic to which he had anaphylactic sensitivity. If alternative antibiotics are not adequate, it is possible to desensitize the patient safely.[28] The intravenous route is recommended because an allergic reaction is apparent immediately. Briefly, desensitization involves the intravenous infusion of gradually increasing concentrations of penicillin, starting with a concentration of 0.0001 mg/ml in a 50 ml volume over 20 to 30 minutes. Resuscitation equipment and the drugs necessary to treat an anaphylactic reaction must be available. If no adverse reaction occurs, 50 ml volumes of solutions containing penicillin at a concentration of 0.001, 0.01, 0.1, and 1.0 mg/ml are sequentially administered. If no reaction occurs at these concentrations, therapeutic dosages of penicillin can be started. Typical early manifestations of anaphylaxis, which are treated as they occur, include flushing, symptoms of rhinitis and asthma, hives and/or angioedema of the face, tongue, or larynx. The infusion of penicillin is discontinued while the acute manifestations of anaphylaxis are being treated, after which it is cautiously resumed at a slower rate.

Attempts to desensitize patients with a drug allergy that has produced a maculopapular or other nonurticarial eruption are fraught with much uncertainty and the small risk of exfoliative dermatitis. From a practical standpoint, it should be mentioned that a majority of such patients can be given the drug in question without ill effects. This may mean either that the patient has lost his sensitivity or that the reaction was falsely ascribed to the drug in the first place.

Local Anesthetic Hypersensitivity

Adverse reactions to local anesthetics are of great concern to dentists and surgeons, particularly those working in emergency room situations where many patients report that they are allergic to "-caine anesthetics," but seldom know the exact identity of the offending anesthetic. Fortunately for the clinician, very few of these reactions are immunologically mediated. Less than 1 percent represent immediate IgE reactions, and a careful history will serve to give a high index of suspicion for these cases.[29, 30] Adverse reactions include a wide variety of local and systemic symptoms. These vary from local swelling at the injection site to generalized urticaria, angioedema, and a variety of nonspecific systemic symptoms including nausea, central nervous system symptoms, and cardiovascular symptoms. The timing of these reactions is critical in evaluating their etiologies.[31, 32]

The severe allergic reactions are IgE mediated and occur within minutes of administration, leading to local and systemic urticaria/angioedema and hypotension with peripheral vasodilation. Late allergic reactions may occur from 8 to 24 hours after exposure but are usually less serious clinically. Such reactions may lead to excessive local swelling and skin rashes of various sorts, including contact dermatitis from topical preparations. Systemic reactions to local anesthetics can often be attributed to overdosage rather than allergy. Rapid absorption or inadvertent intravenous injection of relatively large quantities of these lipid soluble agents can lead to initial central nervous system excitation and possibly convulsions, followed by central nervous system depression that accounts for the respiratory arrest and coma rarely encountered.

Direct action of the anesthetic agents on the myocardium and peripheral vasculature has been implicated as the cause of vasodilation and hypotension which may also be confused with an allergic response. A transient "vagal response" can occur following an injection of any kind. Thus, patients who claim to be "allergic to local anesthetics" require careful assessment of the nature of the adverse reaction, the identity of the local anesthetic, and the exact time of the reaction relative to the administration of the agent.

There are several chemical classes of local anesthetics. One major group includes esters containing the benzoic acid ring. These agents (Table 3) are structurally and antigenically distinct from the other groups of local anesthetics, which include amides, ketones, and derivatives of phenetidin. Thus, patients with a clear history of allergy to drugs of one group can be safely switched to a structurally different agent. It should be remembered that most local anesthetics contain preservatives. In the case of the amides, Paraben is the usual preservative. Paraben is structurally related to the benzoic acid ester group of local anesthetics and has rarely been implicated in immediate hypersensitivity reactions.[33]

Often in dental practice, local anesthetics are administered with epinephrine which, in combination with the large quantities of epinephrine released by the anxious patient, can cause tachycardia, restlessness, and agitation that may be interpreted as an adverse reaction to the anesthetic.

Skin testing can be useful in patients with a convincing history of an adverse reaction but should only be performed where there are adequate facilities to treat a

TABLE 3. Chemical Classes of Local Anesthetics

Generic Name	*Proprietary Name*
Benzoic Acid Esters	
Procaine hydrochloride	Novocain
Butethamine	Monocaine
Chloroprocaine hydrochloride	Nesacaine
Cocaine	
Meprylcaine hydrochloride	Oracaine
Tetracaine hydrochloride	Pontocaine
Metabutethamine hydrochloride	Unacaine
Isobucaine	Kincaine
Amides	
Dibucaine hydrochloride	Nupercaine
Lidocaine hydrochloride	Xylocaine
Mepivacaine hydrochloride	Carbocaine
Prilocaine hydrochloride	Citanest
Others (available as topical agents)	
Pramoxine	Tronothane
Dyclonine	Dyclone
Phenacaine hydrochloride	Holocaine

severe reaction.[34] A reasonable protocol in each case is to start with prick testing and then proceed to intradermal injection, first using a 1:1000 dilution of the normally available 1 percent solution and then progressing with ten-fold greater concentrations at 20 minute intervals until the 1 percent solution is tested. Finally, a progressive subcutaneous challenge with 0.1 ml, 0.5 ml, and 1 ml of the local anesthetic will demonstrate to the patient and his physician that the drug can be safely administered. If the history suggests a late reaction, it would be wise to observe the skin testing sites 24 hours after testing. There are occasional false positive local reactions to skin testing with undiluted local anesthetic, but in at least two studies, provocative challenge with higher doses failed to demonstrate an allergic response.

In someone with a convincing history of an allergic reaction to a local anesthetic, skin challenge with an agent belonging to another chemical class is warranted, particularly to exclude the possibility of sensitivity to the Paraben preservative. It is helpful to remember how unusual the IgE mediated reactions to local anesthetics are and that even if the patient has a convincing history, there are almost always alternative chemical types of anesthetics available that do not cross-react antigenically.

REACTIONS TO RADIOGRAPHIC CONTRAST MEDIA (RCM)

Contrary to common belief, a history of sensitivity to seafood is not associated with an increased risk of allergic reaction to iodinated contrast media. A history of previous reaction to RCM, however, should be taken seriously. A survey of more than 112,000 contrast media studies yielded about 5 percent adverse reactions with over half being nausea and vomiting. Urticaria and flushing were the next most common reactions, and the risk of a further reaction was 16 to 21 percent in those who had experienced a previous reaction.[35, 36, 37]

The increasing use of iodinated contrast media for radiographic techniques has led to as many as 500 deaths per year in the United States from systemic anaphylaxis which is reported to occur in 2 percent of dye studies in some series. Various mechanisms have been suggested for the pathogenesis of RCM reactions. Some RCM reactions are clearly of nonallergic etiology, although severe adverse reactions are usually immediate in onset and the symptoms resemble allergic disease with rhinitis, wheezing, urticaria, angioedema, and anaphylaxis. There is little proof that these reactions are mediated by IgE antibodies which have only been rarely demonstrated in patients with RCM reactions. Also, reactions can occur in patients who have not been previously exposed to contrast dyes, and even after one reaction, further exposure to the same RCM may not lead to another reaction.

Nonimmunologic mechanisms for RCM reactions have been suggested based on findings of complement activation and histamine release in some individuals.[38] However, not all patients suffering from RCM reactions show changes of complement activity, and reactions occur only in a minority of those individuals in whom there is evidence for complement activation following RCM infusion. Complement activation by RCM has also been demonstrated in vitro. It is thus possible that one mechanism for immediate reactions to RCM is release of histamine from mast cells mediated by the anaphylatoxins C3a and C5a. These can be generated by proteolytic cleavage of C3 and C5 either via the alternative complement pathway or by other nonsequential proteolytic enzymes such as those of the clotting and fibrinolytic pathways.[39] However, conflicting evidence from different studies and the poor correlation between clinical reactions and complement abnormalities suggest that these findings may not be directly related to the pathogenesis of RCM reactions.

Another mechanism of immediate reactions to RCM is direct release of histamine and other mediators from mast cells and platelets. Although changes in histamine do occur after RCM infusions and histamine is released by RCM-challenged basophils in vitro, clinical correlations of RCM reactions with plasma histamine have not been conclusive. Recent evidence suggests that basophils and mast cells release histamine in vitro in response to hyperosmolar solutions of a variety of solutes including RCM and mannitol. Thus, it appears that some individuals are abnormally sensitive to hyperosmolar stimuli which cause the noncytotoxic release of histamine.[40]

Skin testing is not useful in identifying those at risk of severe reactions because of the high incidence of false positive cutaneous reactions. Many radiologists continue to pretest patients by administering intravascular injections of a small dose of dye, but such pretesting tends to give a false sense of security. Since it is not possible to identify which of those patients who have a prior history of RCM reactions will react when rechallenged, various pretreatment regimens have been proposed.

Depending on the severity of the previous reaction and assuming that the dye study is unavoidable, the patient should be pretreated with a glucocorticoid and an antihistamine.[41, 43] For example, 50 mg of prednisone can be administered every 6 hours, starting 18 hours before the study and continuing for 12 hours afterwards. An intravenous infusion should be started prior to the dye study, and an antihistamine (such as diphenhydramine 50 mg) should be administered an hour before the study. By using this simple regimen, the risk of reaction is reduced and, if a reaction does occur, it will be less severe. Acute reactions to RCM are treated as outlined above in Treatment of Generalized Anaphylactic Reactions.

Dye studies should only be undertaken with caution in patients with diabetes, dehydration, or multiple myeloma. In these patients, acute renal failure is a potential hazard following cholecystography, angiography, CT scanning and, in particular, intravenous pyelography.[42] The pathogenesis is unclear but may be due to hyperosmolarity of RCM, causing direct toxicity and hemodynamic changes. RCM has also been shown to precipitate Bence Jones protein, the urinary Tamm Horsfall mucoprotein, and uric acid crystals. These nephrotoxic reactions can usually be prevented by avoiding unnecessary dye studies in high risk groups including older aged patients and by assuring adequate hydration rather than the usual pretest dehydration. Dosage of dyes should be kept to safe limits (0.88 mg iodine/kg) and multiple repeated doses avoided if possible.

REFERENCES

1. Gell, PGH, and Coombs, RRA: *Clinical Aspects of Immunology.* Philadelphia: F.A. Davis Co., 1964.
2. Edelman, GM (ed.): *Cellular Selection and Regulation in the Immune Response.* New York: Raven Press, 1974.
3. Paul, WE: *Lymphocyte biology* in Parker, CW (ed.): *Clinical Immunology.* Philadelphia: W.B. Saunders Co., 1980, pp. 19–48.
4. Ishizaka, K, and Ishizaka, T: *Immunology of IgE mediated hypersensitivity* in Middleton, E, Reed, CE, and Ellis, EF, (eds.): *Allergy Principles and Practice* St. Louis: C.V. Mosby Co., 1978, pp. 52–78.
5. Lewis, RA, Austen, KF, Drazen, JM, et al.: *Slow reacting substances of anaphyaxis: identification of leukotrienes C-1 and D from human and rat sources.* Proc Natl Acad Sci (USA) 77:3710, 1980.
6. Offesen, EA, and Cohen SG: *The eosinophil, eosinophilia and eosinophil-related disorders* in Middleton, E, Reed, CW, and Ellis, EF (eds.): *Allergy Principles and Practice.* St. Louis: C.V. Mosby Co., 1978, pp. 584–632.
7. Booth, BH: *Diagnosis of immediate hypersensitivity* in Patterson, R (ed.): *Allergic Diseases.* Philadelphia: J.B. Lippincott Co., 1972, pp. 63–86.
8. Gleich, GJ, Adolphson, CR, and Yunginger, JW: *The mini-RAST: comparison with other varieties of the radioallergosorbent test for the measurement of immunoglobulin E antibodies.* J Allergy Clin Immunol 65:20, 1980.
9. Fisher, AA: *Contact Dermatitis,* ed. 2. Philadelphia: Lea & Febiger, 1973.
10. Solomon, WR, and Matthews, KP: *Aerobiology and inhalant allergens,* in Middleton, E, Reed, CE, and Ellis, EF (eds.): *Allergy Principles and Practice.* St. Louis: C.V. Mosby Co., 1978, pp. 899–956.
11. Weber, RW, Hoffman, M, and Raine, DA, et al.: *Incidence of bronchoconstriction due to aspirin, azo dyes, non-azo dyes, and preservatives in a population of perennial asthmatics.* J Allergy Clin Immunol 64:32, 1979.
12. Gerber, JS, Payne, NA, Oelz, O, et al.: *Tartrazine and the prostaglandin systems.* J Allergy Clin Immunol 63:289, 1979.
13. Ryo, UY, and Townley, RG: *Comparison of respiratory and cardiovascular effects of isoproterenal, propranolol, and practolol in asthmatics and normal subjects.* J Allergy 57:12, 1976.
14. Graham, DT: *Psychology, behavior and the treatment of asthma.* J Allergy Clin Immunol 60:273, 1977.
15. Minor, TW, Dick, EC, DeMeo, AN, et al.: *Viruses as precipitants of asthmatic attacks in children.* JAMA 227:292, 1974.
16. Norman, PS: *An overview of immunotherapy: implications for the future.* J Allergy Clin Immunol 65:87, 1980.
17. Galant, SP, Bullock, J, and Frick, OL: *An immunologic approach to the diagnosis of food sensitivity.* Clin Allergy 3:363, 1973.

18. Bock, SA, Wai-Ying, L, Remingio, LK, et al.: *Studies of hypersensitivity reactions to foods in infants and children.* J Allergy Clin Immunol 62:327, 1978.

19. Rawlins, MD, and Thompson, JW: *Pathogenesis of adverse drug reactions* in Davies, DM, (ed.): *Texbook of Adverse Drug Reactions.* Oxford: Oxford University Press, 1977, p. 10.

20. Lelstrup, J, Reske-Nielsen, E, Haase, J, et al.: *Malignant hyperthermia in a family: a clinical and serological investigation of 139 members.* Acta Anaesthesiol Scand 18:58, 1974.

21. World Health Organization: *Pharmacogenetics.* World Hlth Org Techn Rep Ser 524, 1973.

22. Dundee, JW, Fee, JPH, McDonald, JR, et al.: *Frequency of atopy and allergy in an anaesthetic patient population.* Br J Anaesth 50:793, 1978.

23. Beerman, H, and Kirshbaum, BA: *Drug eruptions* in Moschella, SL, Pillsbury, DM, and Hurley, HJ (eds.): *Dermatology* Philadelphia: W.B. Saunders Co., 1975, pp. 350–384.

24. Green, GR, Rosenblum, AH, and Sweet, L: *Evaluation of penicillin hypersensitivity: value of clinical history and skin testing with penicilloylpolylysine and penicillin G* J Allergy Clin Immunol 60:339, 1977.

25. Green, GR, and Rosenblum, A: *Report of the penicillin study group—American Academy of Allergy.* J Allergy Clin Immunol 48:331, 1971.

26. Levine, BB: *Immunologic mechanisms of penicillin allergy.* N Engl J Med 275: 1115, 1966.

27. Lund, B, and Bergan, T: *Temporary skin reactions to penicillins during the acute stage of infectious mononucleosis.* Scand J Infect Dis 7:21, 1975.

28. Green, GR, Peters, GA, and Geraci, JE: *Treatment of bacterial endocarditis in patients with penicillin hypersensitivity.* Ann Int Med 67:235, 1967.

29. deShazo, RD, and Nelson, HS: *An approach to the patient with a history of local anesthetic hypersensitivity: experience with 90 patients.* J Allergy Clin Immunol 63:387, 1979.

30. Incaudo, G, Schatz, M, Patterson, R, Rosenberg, M, Yamamato, F, and Hamburger, RN: *Administration of local anesthetics to patients with a history of prior adverse reaction.* J Allergy Clin Immunol 61:339, 1978.

31. Verill, PJ: *Adverse reactions to local anesthetics and vasoconstriction drugs.* Practitioner 214:380, 1975.

32. Meyers, FH, Jawetz, E, and Goldfien, A: *Local Anesthetics* in Meyers, PH (ed.): *Review of Medical Pharmacology.* Los Altos, California: Lange Medical Publications, 1976, p. 220.

33. Nagel, JE, Fuscaldo, JT, and Fireman, P: *Paraben allergy.* JAMA 237:1594, 1977.

34. Goodman, MH: *Cutaneous hypersensitivity to procaine anesthetics. Correlation of hypersensitivity with chemical structure.* J Invest Dermatol 2:53, 1939.

35. Shehadi, WH: *Adverse reactions to intravenously administered contrast media.* Am J Roentgenol 124:145, 1975.

36. Lieberman, P, Siegle, RL, and Taylor, WW, Jr.: *Anaphylactoid reactions to iodinated contrast media.* J Allergy Clin Immunol 62:174, 1978.

37. Ansell, G: *Adverse reactions to contrast agents.* Invest Radiol 5:374, 1970.

38. Arroyave, CM, Schatz, M, and Simon, RA: *Activation of the complement system by radiographic contrast media: studies in vivo and in vitro.* J Allergy Clin Immunol 63:276, 1979.

39. Simon, RA, Schatz, M, Stevenson, DD, et al.: *Radiographic contrast media infusions. Measurement of histamine, complement, fibrin split products and correlation with clinical parameters.* J Allergy Clin Immunol 63:281, 1979.

40. Findlay, SR, Dvorak, AM, Kagey-Sobotka, A, and Lichtenstein, LM. *Hyperosmolar triggering of histamine release from human basophils.* J Clin Invest 1981. In press.

41. Zweiman, B, Mishkin, MM, and Hildreth, EA: *An approach to the performance of contrast studies in contrast material reactive persons.* Ann Intern Med 83:159, 1975.

42. Byrd, L, and Sherman, RL: *Radiocontrast induced acute renal failure.* Medicine 58:270, 1979.

43. Greenberger, PA, Patterson, R, Simon, R, et al.: *Pretreatment of high-risk patients requiring radiographic contrast media studies.* J Allergy Clin Immunol. 67:185, 1981.

Chapter 3

CARDIOLOGY

Deeb N. Salem, M.D., F.A.C.C.,
David Homans, M.D.,
James W. McNally, M.D., and
John S. Banas, Jr., M.D., F.A.C.C.

Cardiac disease accounts for a significant proportion of perioperative complications and management of cardiac problems in the perioperative period is one of the most frequent reasons for medical consultations on surgical patients. In the series by Goldman and associates of 1001 patients undergoing general surgical procedures at the Massachusetts General Hospital, approximately one-third of all postoperative deaths were due to cardiac causes.[1, 2] It is thus imperative that the internist consulting on surgical patients be constantly aware of potential cardiac complications.

The role of the internist providing perioperative care for the cardiac patient involves essentially two main functions: first, to aid the patient and surgeon in assessing the impact of the patient's cardiac disease on surgical risk and second, to prevent, diagnose, and treat cardiac disorders in the perioperative period. Accordingly, the first part of this discussion will focus on risk assessment in cardiac patients and the effect of noncardiac factors on postoperative cardiac morbidity and mortality. The remainder of this chapter will discuss specific cardiac disorders in terms of their risk, diagnosis, and treatment in the surgical patient.

RISK ASSESSMENT IN THE CARDIAC PATIENT

It is clear that multiple factors which can be derived from history, physical, and laboratory data influence the operative risk in the cardiac patient. Given the presence of a certain risk factor in a patient, one can generally derive from the literature a rational assessment of his risk or at least the degree to which his risk is increased. This is an assessment of risk based on a univariate analysis of risk factors. That is, *all other things being equivalent,* what is the modification of risk by this factor? However, clinical situations are rarely so simple. For example: Mr. Jones is over 70 years old; has a remote history of myocardial infarction; and has mild dyspnea on exertion, a few basilar rales, frequent premature atrial contractions on his preoperative electrocardiogram, and some cardiomegaly on his chest x-ray. He is to undergo surgery for aortofemoral bypass. We can all agree that he is at increased risk for surgery on the basis of multiple risk factors, each of which by univariate analysis has been associated with an increased operative risk. But how do we quantify his risk given the presence of multiple factors? Clearly, we would not expect his net risk to be a sum of all the individual risks as the factors are interdependent. The rales and dyspnea on exertion presumably both reflect left ventricular dysfunction as may the premature atrial contractions; all may be the result of the previous infarction. Thus, does the presence of all the factors, each of which separately is associated with increased risk, effect his overall risk? This cannot really be ascertained accurately from data gathered by univariate analysis.

Goldman and associates[1, 2] have attempted to devise a scale for the prediction of perioperative cardiac risk in the individual patient based on a multivariate analysis of multiple potential risk factors occurring in a large group of patients. Though their results are preliminary and must be subjected to further study, this type of approach is likely to yield the most useful type of data for the assessment of surgical risk.

Goldman and his colleagues[1, 2] analyzed data gathered prospectively on 1001 consecutive patients over the age of 40 seen in medical consultation preoperatively at the Massachusetts General Hospital. Minor operations under local anesthesia or uncomplicated endoscopies, as well as transurethral prostatectomies, were excluded. With careful preoperative history, physical examination, and laboratory determinations, they gathered data on the presence of the following variables which might conceivably effect cardiac risk: sex, age, body build, dyspnea, orthopnea, edema, angina, history of myocardial infarction, New York Heart Association Functional Class, Dripps American Society of Anesthesiologists' Class, history of specific arrhythmias, diabetes, hypertension, hyperlipidemia, tobacco use, preoperative blood pressure, jugular venous distention, systolic and diastolic murmurs, important valvular aortic stenosis, S_3 gallop, S_4 gallop, rales, peripheral pulses, electrocardiogram rhythm, QRS axis, P-R interval, voltage, ST segments, T waves, P waves, Q waves, R wave progression, bundle branch block, heart size, pulmonary vasculature and aortic shadow by x-ray, available preoperative laboratory data, signs of chronic liver disease, central nervous system status, known cancer, ability to care for oneself, type of operation, type of anesthesia, emergency or elective procedure, and the training level of the surgeon.

They rigidly define *cardiac* mortality and life-threatening morbidity. A cardiac death was defined as death from arrhythmia or from refractory low cardiac output which was not part of an inexorable downhill course of other disease processes. "Life-threatening" cardiac complications were considered to be: pulmonary edema, myocardial infarction, and ventricular tachycardia. All of these complications had a greater than 25 percent cardiac mortality.

They then identified by discriminant analysis nine factors from among all these variables which had *statistically significant independent* correlation with *cardiac* outcome. No other factors or combination of factors could provide any additional statistically significant increment in the ability to predict outcome. This was true even though nearly every sign, symptom, or electrocardiographic criteria of heart disease had a statistically significant *univariate* correlation with postoperative cardiac outcome. Notable variables which were not associated with a significantly increased risk for cardiac death included: hypertension (past or present, treated or untreated) S_4 gallops, systolic ejection murmur without evidence of significant aortic stenosis by physical examination, abnormal aorta on x-ray, diabetes mellitus, hyperlipidemia, and body build.

Having determined the nine significant predictors of outcome by multivariate analysis, the researchers attempted to weight these factors based on their predictive power. Each risk factor was assigned a point value based on its relative significance as a predictor of cardiac outcome. By summarizing the individual scores, it was possible to assign each patient a total point score. This score defined four categories of patients who had different levels of risk.

Table 1 utilizes the scoring system of Goldman and associates which weights each risk factor in terms of its correlation with cardiac outcome. Note that 28 of the 53 points are potentially alterable. Patients can be assigned a class on the basis of this score. This class has been shown to correlate well with the risk of cardiac death and significant cardiac morbidity as outlined in Table 2.

TABLE 1. Cardiac Risk Factors for Patients Going to Surgery

Criteria	*Finding*	*Points*
History	Age over 70	5
	Myocardial infarction in previous 6 months	10*
Physical examination	Third heart sound or jugular venous distention	11*
	Significant aortic stenosis	3
Electrocardiogram	*Any* rhythm other than Normal sinus	7
	Premature atrial contractions on last preoperative electrocardiogram	7*
	More than 5 premature contractions per minute on *any* previous EKG	7
General status	Po_2 less than 60 mm Hg, Pco_2 greater than 50	
	K^+ less than 3.0 mEq/L, Hco_3 less than 20	
	BUN greater than 50 mg/dl, creatinine greater than 3.0 mg/dl.	
	Abnormal SGOT or signs of chronic liver disease	3*
Operation	Emergency surgery	4*
	Intraperitoneal, thoracic, or major vascular procedure	3
		53

*Risk factors which may be altered by preoperative intervention or delay of surgery.
Adapted from Goldman et al.[1]

TABLE 2. Cardiac Risk Classes for Patients Going to Surgery

Risk Class	*Point Score*	*No or Minor Complications (Percentage)*	*Life-threatening Complications* (Percentage)*	*Cardiac Death (Percentage)*
I	0–5	99	0.7	0.2
II	6–12	93	5	2
III	13–25	86	11	2
IV	> 26	22	22	56

*Myocardial infarction, ventricular tachycardia, pulmonary edema.
Adapted from Goldman et al.[1]

To return to Mr. Jones, he scores 5 points for his age; since his infarction occurred over six months ago, this scores no points. He has dyspnea on exertion and some rales but no jugular venous distention or S_3 gallop and, hence, no points. He scores 7 points for his frequent premature atrial contractions on the preoperative electrocardiogram. He also scores 3 points for an intra-abdominal operation on his aorta. His total score is 15 which places him in Class 3. Within the study, this corresponded to a risk of cardiac death of about 2 percent and risk of life-threatening cardiac complications of about 11 percent. The benefits of surgery can now be weighed against this magnitude of risk. Though the data is less clear on whether we can modify his risk, it makes sense to attempt to minimize these factors. Hence, we may recommend preoperative digitalization because of his cardiomegaly, mild failure, and frequent premature atrial contractions. Taking care not to intravascularly volume deplete him or induce electrolyte abnormalities, we give a diuretic which eliminates his rales. Further, we suggest perioperative monitoring and serial electrocardiograms because of his increased risk for perioperative infarction.

NONCARDIAC FACTORS WHICH AFFECT RISK OF PERIOPERATIVE CARDIAC MORBIDITY/MORTALITY

Age

The occurrence of coronary disease as well as manifestations of other forms of cardiac pathology increase with age. In addition, there is an increased incidence of diseases of other organ systems which may alter mortality either directly or indirectly through effects on the cardiovascular system. It is not surprising then to find an increased surgical mortality with advancing age, regardless of whether or not well defined heart disease is present. Though the increased mortality with age is no doubt a continuous function, the increased risk becomes striking beyond age 70 (Table 3). The combined figure for all series is a mortality of nearly 14 percent for patients over 70. Though few authors have addressed the issue of mortality in patients over 60, it would appear that the

TABLE 3. Effect of Age Greater than 70 Years on Mortality Rates in Surgical Patients (Literature Review)

Author	*Year of Publication*	*Number of Cases*	*Number of Deaths*	*Percentage of Mortality*
Krieger-Lassen[3]	1962	1197	191	15.9
Parsons et al.[4]	1956	146	12	8.2
Nachlas et al.[5]	1961	77	10	14.3
Arkins et al.[6]	1964	605	65	10.8
Goldman et al.[1,2]	1977, 1978	324	16	5.0* cardiac death only
Bosch et al.[9]	1952	159	28	17.0
Owen and Murphy[10]	1952	434	117	27.2
Anglem and Bradford[11]	1953	621	62	10.0
Stewart and Alfano[12]	1954	290	39	13.0
Mithoefer and Mithoefer[13]	1954	240	20	8.3
Limbosch[14]	1956	336	69	20.5
Mitty and Echemeudia[15]	1953	589	70	11.9
		5726	778	13.6

*5% cardiac mortality in patients over 70 in Skinner's series compares with 0.4% mortality for patients less than 70 in their series.

mortality in these patients is only about one-half of that of those over 70 (i.e., about 7%).

Type of Surgery

Intraperitoneal and thoracic surgery have been shown to involve greater risk to the patient with cardiac disease than other surgical procedures (Table 4). Though patient population and institutional factors resulted in a relatively high overall mortality in the series summarized in Table 4,[16] the conclusions regarding relative risks of various procedures are supported by other investigators.[1,17]

TABLE 4. Operative Mortality in Various Types of Surgery in Patients with Heart Disease

Type of Procedure	*Number of Cases*	*Percentage of Mortality*
Transurethral resection of prostate	124	2
Urologic (other than transuretheral resection of prostate)	96	12
Hernia	80	0
Cholecystectomy	48	12
Other intra-abdominal	232	12–30
Thoracic (noncardiac)	36	30

Adapted from Skinner and Pearce[16]

Emergency Operations

Goldman and associates[1,2] found that patients who had emergency procedures were four times more likely to develop a postoperative myocardial infarction or cardiac death. This is reflected as a risk factor in their index (see Table 1). In other older series, emergency surgery resulted in an approximate two-fold increase in mortality compared to elective surgery.[16,18]

The reasons for increased mortality in patients with heart disease undergoing emergency surgery are no doubt myriad and may relate largely to factors associated with the disease for which surgery is being performed. It is not clear whether or not some cases of "emergency surgery" might not benefit from a 24 to 48 hour delay to optimize factors which may have a negative impact on cardiac risk (such as treatment of congestive failure, volume depletion, anemia, hypoxia, arrhythmias, correction of electrolyte and acid-base disturbances, and so forth). At present, one has to consider "emergency surgery" a potentially modifiable risk factor in the cardiac patient. However, the actual decision regarding the timing of surgery in a given case is dependent on an estimation of the risks of delay versus the benefits of optimizing the patient's condition prior to surgery.

Duration of Surgery

Table 5 lists some of the data on the relationship between the duration of surgery and mortality in the cardiac patient. When all operations are considered, the length of procedure directly correlates with increased mortality. However, when the results of *specific types of procedures* are analyzed separately, there is actually a *negative* correlation between length of procedure and mortality though there may be some influence on the incidence of postoperative complications.[6,16,20] Similarly Goldman and associates[1,2] found only an increased risk of perioperative congestive heart failure and *noncardiac* death in procedures lasting over 5 hours, but no effect on the incidence of infarction or *cardiac* death even at this length of procedure.

TABLE 5. Duration of Procedure and Perioperative Mortality or Reinfarction (Literature Review)

		Number of Patients			
Author	*Year of Publication*	*Less than 60 Minutes*	*60 to 120 Minutes*	*120 to 180 Minutes*	*Greater than 180 Minutes*
Arkins et al.[6]	1964	270 (15*)	406 (19.4*)	183 (25*)	146 (32.8*)
Skinner and Pearce[16]	1964	196 (8*)	314 (11*)	130 (17*)	126 (23*)
Tarhan et al.[19]	1972	46 (6.5†)	78 (5.1†)	53 (7.5†)	41 (5†)

*Percentage of mortality
†Percentage of reinfarction

Anesthetic Agents

All general anesthetics depress the mechanical performance of the isolated heart muscle or decrease the cardiac output of experimental heart lung preparations at concentrations which produce surgical anesthesia. With cyclopropane and ether there is a simultaneous increase in sympathetic activity and, hence, the blood pressure tends to be maintained or even increased slightly. Halothane and methoxyflurane do not cause the same increase in sympathetic tone, therefore the systemic blood pressure tends to fall as the level of anesthesia rises. Nitrous oxide is similar to the latter two agents but has less of a myocardial depressant effect. With spinal or epidural anesthesia, hypotension is common because of blockade of sympathetic outflow.[21]

In general, literature on patients with heart disease fails to document any substantial differences in morbidity and mortality among the various general anesthetic agents and between general and spinal anesthesia.[6,19,20,22] However, there are differences between general and local anesthesia. These sorts of comparisons may be treacherous because of differences in patients, underlying illnesses, and the types of surgical procedures being done.

Goldman and associates[1,2] found that among patients who had general anesthesia, the agent used had no effect on the development of cardiac complications. Those who received spinal or epidural anesthesia were no less likely to develop intraoperative hypotension or perioperative cardiac death than those receiving general anesthesia. However, in terms of one cardiac complication, spinal or epidural anesthesia appeared to have an advantage: no patient who received spinal anesthesia developed new or experienced worsened congestive heart failure while new congestive heart failure developed in 4.3 percent of patients receiving general anesthesia and worsened in 22 percent of the patients with preoperative failure. This consequence of general anesthesia is probably due to its direct myocardial depressant effects which are not shared by the spinal anesthetics. Thus, although spinal anesthesia carries a risk of intraoperative hypotension and may not significantly alter cardiac mortality or infarction rate, it has clear advantages over general anesthesia particularly in patients with a history of heart failure.

DATA BASE

It appears that a number of cardiac and noncardiac factors can exert a powerful influence on the risk of postoperative cardiac complications in the surgical patient. The question next arises as to what constitutes an adequate data base from which to assess these cardiac risk factors. The answer must, of course, be individualized according to the presence of certain pre-existing risk factors and the nature of the procedure that the patient is about to undergo. Certainly, the "sicker" the patient and the more extensive the procedure, the greater the importance of defining exactly the degree of cardiac disability. This section presents our general approach to the routinely available diagnostic studies. Their application to specific cardiac disorders will be clarified in the subsequent discussions of those entitles.

History

In addition to a thorough medical evaluation, the following are of particular concern in assessing risk in the cardiac patient: age; presence of risk factors for coronary disease; history of murmur or rheumatic fever; history of hypertension; presence or absence of angina with the determination of its pattern particularly with regard to stability of frequency, duration, nocturia, edema, history of palpitations, presyncope, and syncope; and some assessment of cardiac functional impairment (such as, the New York Heart Association Classification, Table 6). Cardiac medications (if any) should be noted. If the patient has had previous surgery, it is useful to know what cardiovascular complications may have occurred at that time. Finally, the type of procedure and the anesthesia planned should be ascertained.

Physical Examination

In the physical examination, particular attention should be paid to the following: blood pressure with orthostatic variation; presence of rales or pleural fluid; evidence of other lung disease which might effect cardiac function; carotid pulse contour; presence of significant jugular venous distention; abnormalities of cardiac impulse or presence of rhythm disturbances which may have been missed on preoperative electrocardiogram; presence of gallops, murmurs, or rubs; evidence of edema; and evidence of artherosclerotic disease elsewhere.

Laboratory Data

The chest x-ray is useful in assessing cardiac size, presence of failure, and presence of other lung disease. The electrocardiogram should be reviewed for evidence of ischemic changes, conduction or rhythm disturbances, chamber enlargement, and drug or electrolyte effects. In addition to these two laboratory procedures, general laboratory evaluation should be performed to discover alterations which might effect cardiac risk including assessment of hemoglobin and hematocrit, electrolytes (particularly potassium and bicarbonate), BUN and creatinine as evidence of renal function and perfusion, and liver function tests to evaluate hepatic function or congestion. In addition to their value in assessing organ function, the renal and hepatic function tests are useful in the event that

TABLE 6. New York Heart Association Functional Classification

CLASS I	Asymptomatic
CLASS II	Asymptomatic at rest Symptoms with ordinary activity
CLASS III	Asymptomatic at rest Symptoms with minimal activity
CLASS IV	Symptoms at rest

renal or hepatic metabolized cardiac medications are needed in the perioperative period. Though not necessary in all patients, an arterial blood gas study to assess oxygenation or further clarify acid-base disturbances should be obtained where clinically indicated. In addition, there are several noninvasive studies which may be useful in selected patients. Isotope angiocardiography can be utilized to assess left ventricular function and aortic stenosis. Echocardiography may yield information concerning left ventricular function, chamber size, and valvular lesions. The exercise stress test can be used to evaluate functional status and reserve or unusual chest pains which may or may not be due to coronary artery disease.

Cardiac catheterization generally provides the most definitive information as to the presence and severity of cardiac disease. In view of its own complication rate, however, it is usually reserved for situations in which major intervention (frequently cardiac surgery) is being contemplated prior to the noncardiac procedure.

CORONARY ARTERY DISEASE

It is not surprising that patients with coronary artery disease undergoing anesthesia and surgery have an increased risk over the general population. The administration of anesthetics and the performance of operations clearly place increased demands on the myocardium, both directly and through indirect mechanisms. There are demands for increased cardiac output in the perioperative period and simultaneously there are multiple factors which can adversely effect myocardial function and perfusion. Increased demands for cardiac output result from many factors: pain, anxiety, increased metabolic requirements, catecholamine release, hypoxia, hemorrhage, and fever with or without bacteremia or infection. Concomitantly, multiple factors have an adverse impact on myocardial function and perfusion: anesthetics which depress the myocardium, hypoxia, electrolyte and acid-base disturbances, anemia, tachycardia, hypotension, and rapid fluctuations in intravascular volume.

The literature documenting an increased surgical mortality in patients with cardiac disease is summarized in Table 7. The bulk of cardiac disease included represents coronary disease, but particularly in early studies, data from patients with other forms of acquired heart disease were intermixed with data from the majority of patients who had coronary disease. The amount of increased risk varies from 1½ to 4 times that of controls, and in the overall combination of data, surgical mortality in patients with cardiac disease is 3½ times that of controls (10.1% vs. 2.8%).

Angina Pectoris

Patients with angina pectoris, a marker for coronary artery disease, are clearly at increased operative risk (Table 8). The overall mortality derived by combining the series in the literature is almost 9 percent. Most studies do not comment on the stability of anginal pattern. Of these studies only Skinner and Pearce[16] specifically identified patients with unstable angina as a separate group. Though the mortality in this group was not substantially higher, the number of cases was small and we would caution against drawing conclusions from this. Most cardiologists would agree that the risks are proba-

TABLE 7. Effect of Heart Disease on Surgical Mortality (Literature Review)

Author	Year of Publication	Definition of Cardiac Disease	*Cardiac Patients* Number of Cases	Percentage of Mortality	*Controls (If Any)* Number of Cases	Percentage of Mortality
Butler et al.[23]	1930	Acquired heart disease	414	12		
Hickman et al.[24]	1935	Cardiac disease	103	9.7*		
Morrison[25]	1948	Acquired heart disease	701	12	9137	2.8
Hannigan et al.[26]	1951	Old myocardial infarction	58	5.2	260	3.4
Garcia et al.[27]	1952	Acquired heart disease	500	5.0†		
Etsten and Proger[28]	1955	Coronary artery disease	1624	3.4‡	4154	2.0
Lockhead et al.[29]	1954	Coronary artery disease	51	6		
Nachlas et al.[5]	1961	Arteriosclerotic heart disease	200	10.5	6059	3.5
Arkins et al.[6]	1964	Coronary artery disease	1005	22.3§		
Skinner and Pearce[16]	1964	Defineable cardiac disease	766	13‖		
Lewin et al.[31]	1971	Arteriosclerotic coronary vascular disease	43	32.5#	22	23
Sapala et al.[22]	1975	Coronary artery disease	416	5.3		
Goldman et al.[1,2]	1978	Ischemia by hypoxia or EKG	269	4*	732	1*
		Combined Series	*6150*	*10.1*	*20,364*	*2.8*

*Includes "cardiac" death only.
†Very low number of intra-abdominal procedures.
‡Only 60% "major" operations.
§Includes all deaths occurring up to 2 months post-op.
‖Is twice the mortality for similar populations without coronary artery disease in their institution.
#Study of 65 elderly, seriously ill patients.

TABLE 8. Angina: Effect on Perioperative Mortality (Literature Review)

Author	Year of Publication	Definition of Patients	Number of Cases	Percentage of Mortality
Butler et al.[23]	1930	Angina	41	12.2
Morrison[25]	1948	Angina	58	8.6
Dana and Ohlar[32]	1956	Angina	37	16.2
Nachlas et al.[5]	1961	Angina	41	12.2
Lockhead et al.[29]	1954	Angina	21	0
Sapala et al.[22]	1975	Angina	99	5.0
		Angina and old infarct	55	11.0
Skinner and Pearce[16]	1964	Angina	192	11.0
		Unstable angina	20	10.0
Goldman et al.[1,2]	1978	Angina	70	4.0*
		Combined Series	*634*	*8.7*

**Cardiac* mortality only; compares with cardiac mortality of 1.0% in 850 patients in their study who had no angina.

bly higher if angina is unstable (i.e., occurring with increasing duration or with diminishing response to nitroglycerin). Hard data on this question is lacking partly, no doubt, because of a reluctance to allow patients to undergo elective surgery when their anginal pattern is not stable. Nevertheless, it has been demonstrated that patients admitted to hospitals with unstable angina have a 12 month mortality in the range of 15 percent despite the exclusion of infarction during the admission. This is clearly higher than the yearly mortality for all patients with angina. By extrapolating from this data, we recommend that whenever possible noncardiac surgery be delayed in the patient with an unstable anginal pattern for several months until the pattern has stabilized on medical antianginal therapy.

Previous Myocardial Infarction

Patients with previous myocardial infarction have a clearly increased risk of perioperative infarction with extremely high mortality when this event occurs (Tables 9 and 10). The incidence of new perioperative infarction in patients with previous myocardial infarctions is 6 to 7 percent,[19,20,33,34] in contrast to an incidence of 0.1 to 1.5 percent in the overall population. Table 11 indicates the ominous prognostic significance of a perioperative transmural infarction. Combining the data available in the literature yields a figure of 51.6 percent for the mortality of patients with perioperative myocardial infarction.

Although some have suggested that the older literature fails to accurately reflect current risk because of improvement in surgical and anesthetic techniques and the use of perioperative intensive care monitoring, it is noteworthy that Tarhan and associates [19,33] work fails to substantiate this notion. There is no substantial difference in the incidence of perioperative myocardial infarction or the mortality associated with this occurrence in his two large reviews, one done during 1967 and 1968 and the other done during 1974 and 1975.

The timing of previous infarctions prior to surgery appears to have a dramatic effect on the occurrence of new infarcts and on mortality (Table 9, Fig. 1). In large series, approximately one-third of the patients who have had myocardial infarctions in the previous three months who undergo surgery experience a reinfarction with exceedingly high mortality. This figure is reduced to approximately one-sixth in the period of three

TABLE 9. Effect of History of Previous Myocardial Infarctions on Incidence of Perioperative Myocardial Infarction and on Mortality (Literature Review)

		Patients with History of Previous Infarct		*Patients without History of Infarct*
Author	*Year of Publication*	*Percentage of Patients Developing New Infarcts Postoperatively*	*Percentage of Mortality in Patients with New Postoperative Infarcts*	*Percentage Developing Infarct Postoperatively*
Tarhan et al.[19]	1972	6.6	54	0.13 (32,455*)
Steen et al.[33]	1978	6.1	69	
Topkins and Artusio[20]	1964	6.5	70	0.66 (12,054*)
Knapp et al.[34]	1962	6.0	58	0.7 (8557*)
Combined Series		*6.4%*		*0.37*

*Number of control patients in series.

TABLE 10. Influence of Timing of Preoperative Myocardial Infarctions on Surgical Outcome (Literature Review)

Author	*Year of Publication*	*Timing of Previous Myocardial Infarctions Preoperatively*	*Percentage of New Infarcts*	*Percentage of Mortality*
Tarhan et al.[19]	1972	0 to 3 months	37	54 overall
		3 to 6 months	16	
		> 6 months	4.5	
Steen et al.[33]	1978	0 to 3 months	27	69 overall*
		3 to 6 months	11	
		> 6 months	4.5	
Topkins and Artusio[20]	1964	< 6 months	54	70 overall*
		6 months to 2 years	24	
		2 to 3 years	6.0	
		> 3 years	1.0	
Goldman et al.[1,2]	1978	< 6 months	3	22.7*
		> 6 months	3	
Skinner and Pearce[16]	1964	< 3 months		40**
		> 3 months		14**
Dana and Ohler[32]	1956	< 3 months		40**
		> 3 months		10**
Fraser et al.[35]	1967	< 3 months		38**
Etsten and Proger[28]	1955	< 1 month		18**

*Cardiac mortality only.
**Figure for overall mortality without specifying whether new infarct occurred.

TABLE 11. Mortality of Perioperative Myocardial Infarctions (Literature Review)

Author	*Year of Publication*	*Number of Patients with Myocardial Infarctions*	*Number of Deaths*	*Percentage of Mortality*
Arkins et al.[6]	1964	55	38	69
Tarhan et al.[19]	1972	71	43	60*
Goldman et al.[1,2]	1978	18	8	44
Master et al.[36]	1938	35	23	66
Topkins and Artusio[20]	1964	122	52	42
Mauney et al.[37]	1970	30	16	53
Knapp et al.[34]	1962	26	15	58
Wasserman et al.[38]	1955	25	5	20
Sapala[22]	1975	18	10	56
Wroblenski and Ladve[39]	1952	15	6	40
Etsten and Proger[28]	1955	11	2	18
DePeystter et al.[40]	1952	10	7	70
Total		*436*	*225*	*51.6*

*Compares with mortality of 69% in his later series of patients from 1974–1975 (Tarhan[47]).

to six months. Most studies indicate that beyond six months, the risk of reinfarction and mortality levels off at approximately 5 percent, a figure which is higher than that of the general population but comparable to the figure in patients with angina pectoris. The reasons for this are not clear but may relate to improvement in ventricular compliance,

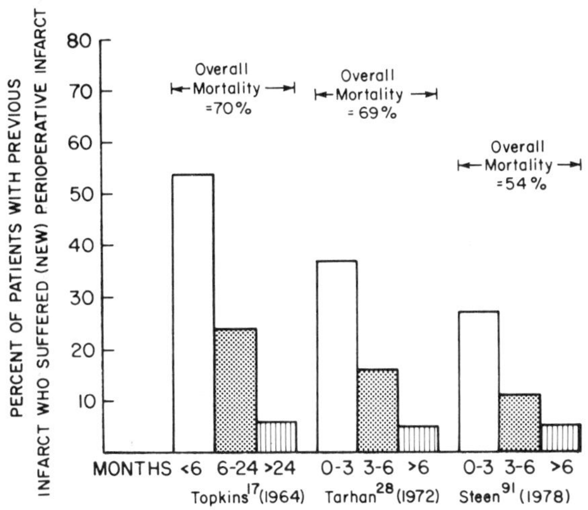

FIGURE 1. Influence of timing of preoperative myocardial infarction on new perioperative infarction and operative mortality. (Number of months indicated on horizontal axis represents the interval between previous infarction and subsequent surgery.)

stabilization of myocardial irritability and perhaps development of collateral circulation. In any event, as a practical principle it appears that the risk of surgery in the first three months following infarction prohibits all but "lifesaving" surgical procedures.

Perioperative Management of the Patient with Coronary Artery Disease

A review of the literature indicates that patients with coronary artery disease probably have a risk of perioperative mortality two to three times that of a similar population without known coronary artery disease. The risk of perioperative infarction in a patient with angina or an old infarct (greater than one year old) is on the order of 5 to 7 percent, and when this complication occurs, it is accompanied by an approximately 50 percent mortality.

In general, elective surgery should be delayed in any patient who has had an infarction in the previous six months. A more conservative approach would be to delay a minimum of one year. Certainly, only "lifesaving" surgery (as discussed above) should be performed in the patient who has had an infarction during the preceding three months.

Though the data are less clear, we would recommend delaying elective surgery several months in the patient with unstable angina. The unstable angina should be treated medically, or if necessary, the coronary anatomy should be studied and coronary artery bypass grafting, if advisable, should be performed.

MEDICATIONS

Unless the patient is hypotensive, the nitrate regimen which successfully controlled angina prior to surgery should, in general, be continued during the perioperative period.

When the order for the patient is NPO either sublingual long acting nitrates or paste preparations for use on the skin may be used. In general, propranolol should be continued in the preoperative and perioperative period when it is being used successfully for control of angina (see below).

CONTROL OF PRECIPITANTS

A vigorous attempt must be made to control those factors which inevitably accompany surgery and which adversely effect the patient with coronary artery disease. These would include hypoxia, acid-base disturbances, hypotension, hypertension, and tachycardia. Fever should be reduced with antipyretics while attempts are being made to elucidate and treat its etiology. Similarly, causes of sinus tachycardia should be vigorously sought and treated. It is especially important to use adequate doses of analgesics and sedatives to avoid the adverse effects of catecholamine discharge on the patient with coronary disease who is in pain, anxious, and sleep deprived. When the patient with known angina experiences an attack under the stress of the preoperative and perioperative period, it is important that he have quick access to the nitroglycerin he would use for a similar attack at home. Too often an inordinate delay occurs in the hospital while the nurse responds, the doctor is notified, electrocardiograms are obtained, and so forth.

In the patient at high risk for perioperative myocardial infarction (the patient with angina or a history or electrocardiographic evidence of an old infarct), we would recommend perioperative monitoring as well as serial electrocardiograms and enzyme determinations. In addition, to avoid missing a substantial number of infarcts, we would recommend extending the serial electrocardiogram observation to five days postoperatively.

ELECTROCARDIOGRAMS

The finding of "nonspecific" ST-T wave changes in a preoperative patient is a common problem. Goldman and associates[1,2] noted that "nonspecific" electrolyte induced or nonclassifiable ST segment changes and flat or inverted T waves were all associated with an increased postoperative cardiac mortality (4 to 8%) by univariate but not by multivariate analysis. It is interesting to note that ischemic appearing ST segment deviations were not associated with either a higher incidence of postoperative myocardial infarction or cardiac deaths in this series. Goldman and associates' findings with respect to the importance of nonspecific or metabolic ST-T wave changes are not surprising in view of data from the Framingham study indicating that these patients have higher cardiac mortality at follow-up. It would thus appear that these patients should be carefully assessed preoperatively for ischemic or valvular heart disease and possible metabolic derangements. Postoperatively, it would be prudent to monitor them for possible postoperative myocardial infarction and other cardiac complications.

Another frequent problem is the finding of electrocardiographic changes consistent with a myocardial infarction of indeterminate age in the asymptomatic preoperative patient. In view of studies documenting the high risk accompanying surgical procedures performed in the first three to six months following a myocardial infarction, this age of the infarction can be crucial. However, these studies have dealt only with surgical procedures following *symptomatic* infarctions. Since patients with symptomatic and asymptomatic infarctions have been found to have similar long term survival rates,[7] the findings concerning the age of the infarction and surgical risk in patients with symptomatic infarcts may well apply to patients with preoperative silent infarctions as well. Obviously, the evaluation of such a patient should begin with a careful assessment of possible ischemic disease and cardiac risk factors. A thorough search for old electrocardiographic tracings may yield important information. If no older tracings can be found and a reasonable likelihood exists that the patient has in fact sustained an unrecognized myocardial infarction at some point in the past, the conservative approach would be to delay elective surgery a minimum of three months. If the need for surgery is more urgent, the risks and benefits of early operation must be carefully analyzed. However, the cardiac risk of early operation under these circumstances must be assumed to be 5 to 10 percent. Techniques such as thallium scanning and vectorcardiography may help identify patients with Q waves due to ischemic disease and higher surgical risk.

There is now good evidence that transmural and subendocardial infarction have the same long term prognosis. It is, therefore, our feeling that a patient sustaining a nontransmural myocardial infarction in the six months preceding surgery should be treated in the same manner as a patient with a transmural infarction.

STRESS TESTING

The role of stress testing as a preoperative screening measure is as yet undefined. At present, its application lies mainly in the diagnosis of chest pain syndromes or the evaluation of arrhythmias in preoperative patients. In view of its higher false positive rate in asymptomatic patients, its use as a routine screen for "silent" coronary artery disease must be questioned, particularly in the absence of firm data that any preoperative intervention is likely to reduce the cardiac surgical mortality in such patients. It should be noted that in one study of 100 patients with occlusive arterial disease of the lower extremities coming to surgery, 50 percent were found to have severe coronary artery disease at cardiac catheterization.[8] However, these patients were, on the whole, readily identified by histories of angina, myocardial infarctions, or abnormal electrocardiograms, and it is uncertain what the contribution of stress testing would have been. Should "prophylactic" coronary artery bypass grafting be shown to be of value, however, routine preoperative exercise testing in high risk individuals may be a more reasonable approach. Certainly, some insight into the functional limitations imposed by cardiac disease can be gained from exercise testing in selected individuals, but there are as yet no studies correlating this type of information with surgical outcome.

Postoperative Myocardial Infarction

In view of the high incidence of "silent" infarcts in the postoperative period,[41] accurate laboratory diagnosis is essential. Unfortunately, tissue trauma during surgery may cause elevations of serum glutamic-oxalacetic transaminase (SGOT), lactic dehydrogenase (LDH), and creatine phosphokinase (CPK), thus confusing the diagnosis. CPK-MB isoenzyme elevation in the postoperative period is specific for myocardial damage, however.[30] Cardiac surgery poses particular problems. Ten of thirty patients undergoing cardiac surgery studied by Pyle and associates[43] demonstrated evidence of CPK-MB band in the serum. Eight of these had electrocardiograms and a postoperative course consistent with myocardial infarction. Two "false positives," however, had undergone valve replacement and had no evidence of infarction. When there is question about postoperative infarction, technetium pyrophosphate scanning may be useful in detecting the presence of infarcted tissues.[44]

Tarhan and associates[19] reviewed the distribution of occurrence of postoperative infarctions over time (Fig. 2). Of note is the fact that the peak occurrence of infarctions was on postoperative day three with nearly 40 percent of the infarctions occurring on days four through six. These data illustrate the importance of following serial studies, such as electrocardiograms and enzymes, for at least five days postoperatively. If this is not done, a significant number of postoperative infarcts will not be detected.

Patients with Previous Coronary Artery Surgery

With large numbers of patients undergoing coronary artery bypass grafting (CABG) annually, it can be expected that many of these patients will be undergoing subsequent noncardiac surgery. The overall mortality from subsequent noncardiac surgery appears to be 1 to 2 percent with myocardial infarction rates of 1 percent and serious perioperative arrhythmias occurring in 4.6 percent (Table 12). Timing of the second procedure does appear to be critical, since in Crawford and associates' series,[48] 75 percent of the deaths occurred in patients undergoing the second procedure within 30 days of the cardiac surgery. However, this higher risk may be secondary to more serious disease (either cardiac or noncardiac) and may not be solely a function of timing. This data compares very favorably with the postoperative course in patients with coronary artery

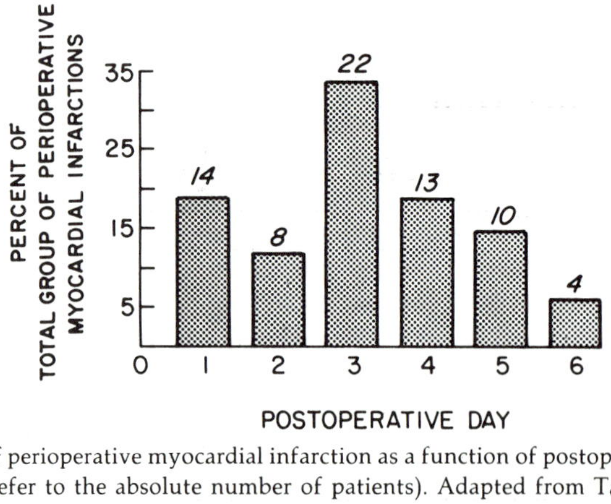

FIGURE 2. Incidence of perioperative myocardial infarction as a function of postoperative day. (Number on the top of each column refer to the absolute number of patients). Adapted from Tarhan et al.[19]

TABLE 12. Noncardiac Surgery Following Coronary Artery Bypass Grafting (Literature Review)

Author	*Year of Publication*	*Number of Patients*	*Percentage of Perioperative Mortality*	*Percentage of Perioperative Myocardial Infarctions*	*Percentage of Serious Perioperative Arrhythmias*
Scher and Tice[45]	1976	20	10	5	15
Edwards et al.[46]	1978	53	3.8	0	9.4
McCollum et al.[47]	1977	60	0	0	11.6
Crawford et al.[48]	1978	358	1.1	1.2	2.9
Total		*491*	*1.2*	*1*	*4.6*

disease previously outlined. Although this suggests a rational for prophylactic CABG in patients undergoing general surgery, there are no prospective randomized studies of this issue. Retrospective studies with small groups of patients suggest that CABG prior to general surgery decreased morbidity and mortality. Bernhard and associates[49] retrospectively analyzed 30 patients with both coronary artery disease and extracranial occlusive disease. Fifteen of these patients had carotid endarterectomy before cardiac surgery and 3 of these (20%) died postoperatively or had cardiac complications. The other 15 patients had both CABG and endarterectomy done during the same anesthesia. There were no deaths in this group and 3 of them had subsequent surgical procedures without cardiac problems. Additional similar series of simultaneous CABG and noncardiac surgery have been reported upon, but results are as yet preliminary and this approach must be viewed with caution. Larger, prospective, randomized, controlled studies will be necessary to clarify this issue.

The relatively low mortality (1 to 2%) for CABG surgery at major centers currently should be emphasized. This contrasts sharply with the higher mortality figures given in the literature for noncardiac surgery in the patient with coronary disease. Though these are obviously very different types of surgery, these data suggest that perhaps the morbidity and mortality of noncardiac surgery in the coronary patient could be reduced by application of techniques of anesthesia and perioperative management originally developed for cardiac surgery.

VALVULAR HEART DISEASE

The management of the surgical patient with valvular heart disease requires that attention be directed not only at the severity and location of the valvular lesion but also at possible complications such as endocarditis, arrhythmias, and congestive heart failure.

Risk Assessment

The risk of perioperative death in patients with clinically significant valvular heart disease appears to be 6 to 14 percent;[1,2,16,25] however, this is highly dependent on the location of the lesion, the degree of valve involvement and the underlying ventricular function. In Goldman and associates' study[1,2] (Table 13), multivariate analysis was used

TABLE 13. Valvular Heart Disease and Operative Risk*

Valve Lesion	*Number of Patients*	*Percentage with Postoperative Myocardial Infarction*	*Percentage of Cardiac Mortality*
Mitral regurgitation	55	9	7
Mitral stenosis	14	7	7
True aortic stenosis	23	0	13
II/VI Systolic murmur without true aortic stenosis	248	2	2
Aortic insufficiency	12	8	8

*Results of study of Goldman and Associates.[1,2]

to exclude the influence of associated cardiac disease. Using this approach, only true aortic stenosis was found to significantly increase surgical mortality.

Aortic Stenosis

The cardiac mortality in patients with aortic stenosis was 13 percent compared to an overall cardiac mortality of only 1.9 percent.[1,2] Similarly, Skinner and Pearce[16] reported an operative mortality of 10 percent in all patients with aortic valve disease and this mortality was increased to 20 percent in patients undergoing intrathoracic or intra-abdominal surgery. However, both Morrison[25] and Skinner and Pearce[16] noted no increment in surgical mortality when patients with aortic and mitral disease were compared to patients having mitral disease only. As can be seen from Table 13, the distinction between true aortic stenosis and a systolic ejection murmur without true stenosis is very important as the perioperative mortality in these conditions is considerably different. Unfortunately, Goldman and coworkers[1,2] could not apply uniform objective criteria when making the diagnosis of aortic stenosis in their report. Given the importance of a correct diagnosis in this case, every effort should be made to document aortic stenosis objectively prior to surgery. Certainly, clinical features such as angina, congestive heart failure, syncope, diminished arterial pulse pressure with slowly rising carotid upstroke, sustained and prominent left ventricular impulse, and diminished intensity of aortic closure may be associated with aortic stenosis and should prompt further study. Aortic valve calcification, left ventricular hypertrophy (LVH), or poststenotic aortic dilation may be found on chest x-ray; and atrial fibrillation, LVH, left anterior fascicle block, AV block, or T wave inversion may be found on routine electrocardiogram. Eddleman and associates[50] found that angina, congestive heart failure, syncope, and LVH on electrocardiograms were not predictive of a systolic aortic valve gradient of greater than 50 mm Hg. In that study, a diminished carotid upstroke, calcified aortic valve, prominent left ventricular thrust, and precordial T wave inversion on electrocardiograms were predictive of such a gradient. Franks and colleagues[51] also had difficulty in correlating symptoms with hemodynamic parameters although they noted that symptoms correlated better with survival than did hemodynamic parameters. It may be that symptoms are more indicative of the ability of the left ventricle to tolerate the hemodynamic burden. On the other hand, hemodynamic parameters, particularly systolic gradient, more accurately reflect the degree of stenosis but yield less information as to its consequences in terms of ventricular function or oxygen supply and demand. Since both valve gradient and cardiac output are used in determination of valve *area,* this last parameter would be expected to be the most "reliable" of the hemodynamic parameters.

Unfortunately, the literature has not attempted to distinguish between these types of diagnostic criteria in assessing aortic stenosis in surgical patients. Until these issues are resolved, it would seem prudent to assume that either prominent symptoms or definite laboratory data place the patient in the "high risk" aortic stenosis group. Certainly, angina and/or congestive heart failure (CHF) may be due to concomitant coronary artery disease and patients with these symptoms must be screened perioperatively.

Mitral Valve Disease

In mitral valve disease, an increased risk of surgery appears to be related primarily to the complications of CHF or atrial fibrillation. Overall mortality rates for all patients with mitral stenosis are reported to be 5 to 7 percent in three studies.[1,16,25] However, when atrial fibrillation was present mortality increased to 18 percent and a significant complication rate of 10 to 18 percent was also noted.[16,25] The surgical mortality associated with atrial fibrillation in these series appears to remain approximately 18 percent whether or not mitral stenosis is present. Thus, it is possible that the arrhythmia rather than the mitral valve lesion is the critical factor. Alternately, atrial fibrillation may simply be a marker for severe cardiac disease, be it ischemic, valvular, or whatever. Certainly the loss of diastolic filling time and the loss of atrial contribution to ventricular filling can have profound hemodynamic consequences in mitral stenosis and these features may also contribute to its powerful impact on perioperative mortality.

A similar relationship exists between CHF and mitral stenosis. Perioperative risk is considerably higher in patients with mitral stenosis and CHF and approximates the mortality of patients with CHF due to other forms of cardiac disease.[16,25]

In summary, patients with mitral stenosis and no complications appear to have a surgical mortality close to 5 percent for major operative procedures, whereas patients with complicated mitral stenosis (i.e., atrial fibrillation or CHF) have a surgical mortality of 15 to 20 percent. Although one might expect an increased frequency of atrial fibrillation postoperatively in patients with mitral stenosis, Goldman and associates[2] were unable to demonstrate this. It is probable that the occurrence of atrial fibrillation is mainly a function of left atrial size[52] and the stress of surgery is not the critical factor.

Other Valvular Lesions

Data for other valvular lesions is quite fragmentary and the overall mortality rates range from 7 to 10 percent in the reported series (see Table 14). It should be noted that CHF

TABLE 14. Valvular Heart Disease and Operative Mortality (Literature Review)

Author	*Year of Publication*	*Percentage of Mortality in Mitral Valve Disease*	*Percentage of Mortality in Aortic Valve Disease*	*Percentage of Mortality in Combined Aortic and Mitral Valve Disease*
Goldman et al.[1,2]	1978	7	13	
Morrison[25]	1948	4.8		4.9
Skinner and Pearce[16]	1964	6	10	6

appears to be a frequent postoperative complication of valvular heart disease occurring in about 20 percent of patients with mitral regurgitation, mitral stenosis, aortic regurgitation, or aortic stenosis.[1,2]

Management of Patients with Valvular Heart Disease

The available data would thus indicate that the surgical risk in the patient with valvular heart disease correlates mainly with the clinical severity of the valvular lesion as manifested by complications such as CHF and arrhythmias. The noteworthy exception to this is true aortic stenosis which should be regarded as a serious surgical risk factor whenever it is detected. As previously mentioned, heavy reliance has been placed on clinical assessment of the nature and severity of valvular disease in the published data. At the present time there is no large scale published body of data using more objective information such as cardiac catheterization, echocardiography, or isotope studies.

If there is a question as to the severity of the valvular lesion, the possible need for more sophisticated perioperative monitoring, or cardiac surgery, appropriate additional studies including echocardiogram, isotope angiocardiogram, fluoroscopy, and/or catheterization should be performed. The question of valve replacement must, of course, be individualized. Certainly, if the noncardiac operation is elective and the patient is found to have tight symptomatic aortic stenosis, valve replacement may be given first consideration. With mitral disease, the physical status of the patient and presence of other complications may help to determine the need for definitive cardiac surgery. If valve replacement is not possible and cardiac compensation is borderline, hemodynamic monitoring with a Swan-Ganz catheter should be considered during the perioperative period. In all cases, the volume status should be carefully monitored and large infusions of fluid avoided if possible. Supraventricular tachyarrhythmias, which may be particularly likely to precipitate hemodynamic deterioration in this group, should be looked for and treated as outlined elsewhere. In patients receiving anticoagulation for valvular heart disease, we use the same approach as that which will be outlined for patients with prosthetic valves. As previously noted, bacterial endocarditis prophylaxis should be provided according to American Heart Association guidelines (see Chap. 8, Infectious Diseases).

Special Situations

MITRAL VALVE PROLAPSE

Mitral valve prolapse is a relatively common disorder that is usually seen as an isolated finding with no other underlying abnormalities. It may occur with a frequency of up to 10 percent in young females. The typical patient with mitral valve prolapse is a woman between 20 and 50 years of age;[53] however, this disorder may occur in males and in people of any age.

There is a growing feeling among physicians involved with patients with mitral valve prolapse that these patients should be subdivided into two groups. The first group contains those patients who have significant underlying disease such as rheumatic heart disease, musculoskeletal disease such as Marfan's syndrome, atrial septal defects, and Turner's syndrome. The patient may have significant cardiovascular impairment and should receive special attention. This would include careful assessment of underlying disease, severity of mitral regurgitation, and extent of arrhythmias. The second group consists of individuals in whom the diagnosis of mitral valve prolapse is made incidentally. This group usually consists of relatively asymptomatic young men and women in whom the diagnosis is made on a routine physical examination or because of some nonspecific symptoms. On auscultation a midsystolic click is often heard and occasionally a late systolic murmur. There is usually no evidence of significant mitral regurgitation. The echocardiogram will often, but not invariably, show evidence of mitral valve prolapse. For this group, it is the feeling of most that little else besides reassurance, and perhaps bacterial endocarditis prophylaxis during dental work, should be recommended.

Supraventricular arrhythmias, ventricular arrhythmias, and bradyarrhythmias have all been implicated in mitral valve prolapse.[54–66] It is not clear whether arrhythmias associated with mitral valve prolapse syndrome have the same high surgical risk as those found in patients with other causes of cardiac arrhythmia (see below). However, in view of reports of sudden death in patients with this syndrome,[61, 64–66] it would seem prudent to recommend propranolol therapy and continuous EKG monitoring in the perioperative period for those patients with high grade ventricular ectopy. Again, it should be emphasized that the risks of complications with mitral valve prolapse seem to be far greater in patients with the "full-blown" syndrome that includes severe arrhythmias, electrocardiographic abnormalities, disabling chest pain, and hemodynamically significant mitral regurgitation. Although some consider endocarditis prophylaxis controversial in the asymptomatic patient with mitral valve prolapse, there is little argument that patients with significant mitral regurgitation and mitral valve prolapse should be given bacterial endocarditis prophylaxis. Since there are a significant number of reported cases of endocarditis in this syndrome,[67–72] it has been our practice to provide endocarditis prophylaxis in all patients after the diagnosis is made.

HYPERTROPHIC CARDIOMYOPATHY

Hypertrophic cardiomyopathy is a general term that includes hypercontractile states such as idiopathic hypertrophic subaortic stenosis (IHSS) and asymmetric septal hypertrophy. These conditions are seen at any age and may include a wide clinical spectrum. Patients with this disorder may be totally asymptomatic, but in the severest form, patients may have incapacitating chest pain, arrhythmias, CHF, and even sudden death. The diagnosis may be suspected from the patient's clinical course, family history, and physical examination; however, it should be confirmed by echocardiography and/or cardiac catheterization. This discussion will focus upon the management of patients with hypertrophic cardiomyopathy in the perioperative period and will assume a familiarity with the physical findings.

Volume depletion perioperatively may result in increased left ventricular outflow tract obstruction and, thus, careful fluid management is mandatory in these patients. This is best accomplished by the preoperative insertion of a Swan-Ganz catheter. During surgery, intra-arterial lines may be useful in the optimal management of severe cardiomyopathy. In patients with IHSS who develop hypotension, care must be used to avoid beta-adrenergic stimulating agents such as isoproterenol and dopamine. Besides volume repletion, the immediate management of significant hypotension in these patients is by use of pure peripheral vasoconstricting agents such as Neo-Synephrine. Because of decreased myocardial compliance in hypertrophic cardiomyopathy, supraventricular tachyarrhythmias may lead to considerable hemodynamic deterioration and require prompt treatment (frequently including electrical cardioversion). Atrial fibrillation has been associated with a significant risk of systemic embolization in IHSS[52] and anticoagulation should be considered. Propranolol is the drug of choice for rate control in this syndrome (see below). Although no firm data are available, it would be reasonable to assume that the perioperative mortality rate in patients with IHSS and atrial fibrillation would be at least as high as in those patients with atrial fibrillation due to other causes and probably higher.

Mention has previously been made of the importance of avoiding inotropic agents in this syndrome as increased outflow obstruction may result. In addition to isoproterenol and dopamine, digitalis preparations are often poorly tolerated. Atrial fibrillation should initially be managed with propranolol to control ventricular rate. If there is no response despite adequate dosage, digitalis may then be considered.

Sudden death has long been recognized as a complication in patients with hypertrophic cardiomyopathy. It has recently been reported that there is a subgroup of patients with "malignant" hypertrophic cardiomyopathy with a high incidence of sudden death.[73,74] In one series of 26 such patients,[73] the majority were young and had frequently been asymptomatic without evidence of outflow obstruction. Most had a family history of asymmetric septal hypertrophy with sudden death. The vast majority had notable murmurs (19 out of a group of 22) and abnormal electrocardiograms (19 of 19). Death was frequently related to exercise and appeared to be related to ventricular ectopy despite the infrequent presence of ectopy on routine electrocardiograms. In view of the fact that 6 patients had been on propranolol at the time of death, this drug cannot be viewed as wholly protective. In a similar series,[74] it was concluded that severe septal thickening (20 mm or more during systole) may help identify the subgroup of patients who are at relatively high risk of sudden death. There also may be some relationship between the degree of electrocardiographic abnormalities and the risk of sudden death. An increased frequency of high grade ventricular ectopy has recently been documented in a series of 100 patients with 19 percent exhibiting ventricular tachycardia.[75] Two of the patients with ventricular tachycardia suffered cardiac arrest in the follow-up period. These patients also had a significantly greater mean septal thickness. Asymptomatic patients with severe outflow obstruction constituted another group at increased risk for high grade ectopy. The import of this data for surgical patients with asymmetrical septal hypertrophy is uncertain. Of concern, however, is the possibility that surgical stress and associated catecholamine release may simulate the metabolic/hemodynamic derangements associated with exercise thereby increasing the risk of malignant ventricular ectopy. At present, it is our practice to treat all symptomatic patients with propranolol or other antiarrhythmics and to consider monitoring and propranolol therapy in asymptomatic patients with significant ectopy, significant obstruction, or family history of sudden death. Endocarditis has also been reported in this syndrome[76] and prophylaxis here is indicated.

PROSTHETIC VALVES

With the increasing frequency of cardiac valvular surgery, a growing number of patients with prosthetic valves will be undergoing general surgery.[77] Katholi and associates[78] have reported their experience in a noncontrolled, retrospective study of 44 operations in 35 patients with prosthetic valves. Twenty-two procedures were considered major and 22 minor. Overall mortality was 6.8 percent and was in all cases related to hemostatic problems. Patients in whom anticoagulants were discontinued one to five days preoperatively had a 5.7 percent mortality and complication rate, whereas patients in whom anticoagulation was continued perioperatively had 11 percent mortality and a 44 percent complication rate. All of the deaths in the group not receiving anticoagulation therapy were related to thromboembolic problems. Tinker and Tarhan[79] reported on 187 patients with prosthetic valves who underwent 180 subsequent noncardiac operations. Anticoagulation therapy was discontinued preoperatively in 87 percent (62 percent had anticoagulation discontinued for one to three days preoperatively). Immediate postoperative thromboembolic complications were rare. However, hemostatic complications were common with a 6 percent incidence of hematoma, 4 percent incidence of "prominent" postoperative bleeding, 2.2 percent incidence of subdural hematoma, and 1.7 percent incidence of bleeding duodenal ulcer. The total hemorrhagic complication rate was 13 percent. It should also be noted that almost all patients with bleeding complications had prothrombin times greater than 20 percent above the normal range.

In the majority of patients in reported series, anticoagulation therapy was resumed one to three days after surgery. Only 1 patient[79] had a thromboembolic complication occur within 2 years following general surgery. However, as previously noted Katholi and associates[78] reported a higher incidence of perioperative thromboembolic episodes with a 6 percent mortality due to such complications. These occurred only in patients with mitral prostheses.

Thus, it appears that anticoagulation therapy should be maintained in the therapeutic range until one to three days prior to surgery and resumed one to three days postoperatively. With this approach there seems to be an unavoidable incidence of hemorrhagic complications that should be considered in deciding upon the need for surgery.

An alternative approach may also be considered. This is to discontinue oral anticoagulation therapy three to five days preoperatively (or reverse it with vitamin K) and substitute full dose heparin by continuous infusion. The infusion can be discontinued six hours preoperatively and reinstituted 12 to 24 hours postoperatively. Oral anticoagulation can then be begun and the heparin infusion discontinued when therapeutic prothrombin times have again been achieved. This has considerable theoretical merit in terms of providing the fullest possible anticoagulation for the longest period of time while still insuring adequate clotting capabilities during the critical immediate perioperative period. A similar approach was used in a prospective study by Katholi and associates [80] in patients with mitral valve prostheses. Only 2 of 26 operations were complicated by hemorrhage, and neither of these bleeding episodes were life threatening. There were no thrombolic complications in this group.

The preoperative evaluation of the patient with prosthetic valves must include evaluation for paravalvular leak and other forms of mechanical dysfunction as well as the underlying myocardial status. Routine preoperative blood tests for bilirubin, lactic dehydrogenase, and reticulocyte count are helpful in detecting occult hemolysis which may indicate valve dysfunction or paravalvular leak. Of course, careful physical examination to detect changes in valve sounds and the appearance of new murmurs is essential. Phonocardiogram, fluoroscopy, echocardiography, and occasionally cardiac catheterization may need to be performed in assessing the patient's valve function, particularly if the screening procedures outlined above disclose significant abnormalities. In view of the high risk and poor prognosis of prosthetic valve endocarditis,[81,82] antibiotic prophylaxis is mandatory in patients with prosthetic valves (see Chap. 8, Infectious Diseases).

CONGENITAL HEART DISEASE

The management of patients with congenital heart lesions must be individualized and related to the specific lesion, the degree of the lesion, and presence or absence of arterial desaturation. In general, subacute bacterial endocarditis prophylaxis will be indicated.

CONGESTIVE HEART FAILURE

Preoperative Congestive Heart Failure

Congestive heart failure may have a profound effect on the perioperative course, and it is essential that careful attention be given to its etiology, severity, and treatment. Preoperative CHF increases surgical risk and the increment in risk appears proportional to the extent of hemodynamic compromise. In Goldman and associates'[1,2] study a variety of signs and symptoms of CHF were correlated with the operative course. When multivariate analysis was performed and the effects of associated cardiac disease eliminated, the only two findings which correlated with operative risk were increased venous pressure (by clinical exam or central venous pressure measurement) and an S_3 gallop. These were associated with an 18 percent and 22 percent incidence of postoperative cardiac death, respectively. A variety of other parameters were associated with increased cardiac mortality by univariate analysis: pulmonary edema (14%), shortness of breath, orthopnea or peripheral edema of cardiac origin (6%), cardiomegaly (5%), and rales (5%). A past history of CHF without evidence of CHF was associated with a cardiac mortality of 4 percent which was not significantly different from the overall cardiac mortality of 1.9 percent for the entire series. In Skinner and Pearce's study of cardiac patients undergoing general surgery,[16] operative mortality was closely associated with preoperative New York Heart Association Class: Class I having 4.3 percent mortality; Class II, 10.6 percent mortality; Class III, 25 percent mortality; and Class IV, 67 percent mortality. Hewson[83] noted that preoperative CHF became worse in 11.4 percent of cases, pneumonia developed in 17 percent, and respiratory insufficiency in 11 percent. Morrison[25] confirmed Goldman and associates' findings with respect to the weak predictive power of cardiomegaly without other evidence of CHF. In Morrison's study, patients with cardiomegaly and coronary artery disease had an operative mortality of 12.7 percent with a complication rate of 3.5 percent. This was little different from the mortality rate of 14.8 percent and the complication rate of 4.3 percent observed in patients with coronary artery disease and no cardiomegaly.

It thus appears that preoperative CHF is associated with an increased cardiac mortality for two reasons. In those patients with severe CHF, as manifested by an S_3 gallop, jugular venous distention, or pulmonary edema, the increment in cardiac mortality appears to be due to the direct effects of hemodynamic compromise. The increased risk in these patients is 15 to 20 percent. Patients in CHF without an S_3 gallop or venous distention appeared to have a surgical mortality that was much smaller (5%) and due primarily to the associated cardiac disease. In the former group with florid CHF, every attempt should be made to correct the hemodynamic derangements prior to surgery. The necessity of surgery should be carefully considered in view of the patient's increased risk. In the group with mild CHF, careful attention should be directed at the associated cardiac disease and its management as the congestive failure itself is likely to be of relatively less consequence.

In patients with acute myocardial infarction, a discrepancy may be present between clinical and hemodynamic findings due to a temporal delay that may occur before the hemodynamic events result in the clinical findings of CHF.[84] Thus, total reliance on clinical features and chest x-ray may at times be misleading. Occasionally, preoperative hemodynamic assessment with Swan-Ganz catheterization may be necessary. However, there is presently no data correlating hemodynamic findings with risk in patients undergoing general surgery.

Postoperative Congestive Heart Failure

The incidence of postoperative CHF is difficult to determine from the available literature, occurrence rates vary from 0.02 percent to 5.8 percent depending on patient population, surgical procedures, and case finding techniques.[1,25,85]

Several factors (chronic obstructive pulmonary disease, emergency surgery, thoracic or major intra-abdominal surgery and valvular heart disease) have been found to increase the risk of developing postoperative CHF.[1,83] Significant worsening of preoperative CHF has been commonly found in patients with preoperative findings of an S_3 gallop (47%), jugular venous distention (35%), or history of pulmonary edema (32%).[1] Overly aggressive fluid administration has been thought to be at least contributory to the pulmonary edema in approximately 50 percent of the cases.[85] The correlation of preoperative New York Association Class with significant postoperative worsening of heart failure was found to be strong in Goldman and associates' study[1] (Class 1, 5%, Class II, 7%, Class III, 18%, Class IV, 31%). However known pre-existing heart disease is present in only 40 to 50 percent of patients developing postoperative CHF.[1,85] The use of propranolol does not appear to contribute to the development of CHF postoperatively! However the direct myocardial depressant effects of general anesthesia may be contributory as 5 percent of cases of perioperative CHF have been found to occur during induction of anesthesia.[85]

The mortality of postoperative pulmonary edema is high; 40 percent die from cardiac causes, 17 percent from noncardiac causes.[1] Juler and associates[86] noted an 87 percent mortality in patients developing pulmonary edema following thoracotomy; this figure is high and may represent a selected patient population. Simple postoperative CHF is associated with a mortality of 15 to 20 percent[1,85] usually from noncardiac causes. Postoperative CHF associated with coronary artery disease has a higher mortality (25 to 79%) than CHF due to other cardiac disease (0 to 17%).[25,85]

The presence of overt CHF is an ominous finding at any point in the perioperative period and necessitates an immediate search for the etiology as well as institution of appropriate therapy. If failure is severe, surgery should be postponed if possible while hemodynamic derangements are corrected. Underlying causes (coronary artery disease, valvular heart disease, cardiomyopathy, arrhythmias, therapeutic noncompliance, metabolic demands for increased cardiac output, hypoxia, and so forth) should be sought and corrected when feasible. Coronary artery disease as an underlying etiology should perhaps be viewed with particular concern. Routine treatment is indicated with digitalis, diuretics, oxygen, and sodium and fluid restriction. Adjunctive measures such as vasodilators, aminophylline, morphine, and phlebotomy may be required in more severe cases. If the underlying pathophysiologic mechanisms cannot be corrected and lifesaving surgery is required, perioperative monitoring with a Swan-Ganz catheter should be considered with meticulous attention given to fluid and electrolyte balance, oxygenation, cardiac arrhythmias, electrocardiographic changes, and the possibility of pulmonary and thromboembolic complications.

Mild CHF constitutes less of a threat, however, diagnostic and therapeutic interventions are usually indicated. In all patients with coronary artery disease, myocardial infarction should be excluded postoperatively and pulmonary toilet may be indicated to reduce the incidence of pneumonia postoperatively.

Although experimental design was suboptimal and numbers were small, two studies have demonstrated some benefit of prophylactic digitalization in preventing postoperative CHF in patients undergoing thoracotomy.[86,87] The data is preliminary, but this approach may be considered in elderly patients with cardiomegaly particularly if atrial rhythm disturbances are present.

CARDIAC RHYTHM DISORDERS

Cardiac arrhythmias are not only the most common of all cardiac disorders, they are also potentially the most lethal. The management of these diverse disorders is of paramount importance in caring for surgical patients. The incidence, as well as the significance of cardiac arrhythmias, is clearly related to the patient population being studied. Evaluation and treatment of arrhythmias occurring in the preoperative patient hinges clearly on the patient's underlying cardiac and metabolic status.

Supraventricular Arrhythmias

Although supraventricular tachyarrhythmias are not as immediately life threatening as the more serious ventricular arrhythmias, at times they may be of great concern. Patients with ischemic, myopathic, or valvular heart disease tend to suffer from both the rapid heart rate as well as the loss of atrial contribution to ventricular filling associated with these arrhythmias. When atrial arrhythmias are associated with very rapid heart rates, even "normal" patients may experience a significant fall in cardiac output. Supraventricular tachyarrhythmias may also be an initial manifestation of serious medical complications such as myocardial infarction, pulmonary embolization, and systemic infection.

Even excluding sinus tachycardia, supraventricular tachyarrhythmias are clearly the most frequent cardiac rhythm disturbances noted in the surgical patient. It should be remembered that there is some degree of overlap between the atrial arrhythmias.

Goldman and associates[1,2] have demonstrated that nearly any preoperative tachyarrhythmia increases operative risk. In their series, the overall mortality was 1.9 percent whereas the overall mortality for any rhythm other than normal sinus rhythm was 18 percent. This increased mortality extends even to patients with premature atrial contractions in whom a postoperative mortality of 8 percent was found. It should be noted that these data were generated from routine preoperative electrocardiograms. Data from patients showing arrhythmias only on 24 hour Holter monitors or other more sophisticated monitoring systems cannot be directly extrapolated to this study. Furthermore, it should be noted that premature atrial contractions resulted in excess cardiac mortality only in elderly patients who are unstable medically or surgically and this excess risk probably does not apply to healthy young patients with occasionally premature atrial contractions. With respect to atrial fibrillation, studies have shown a 13 to 18 percent surgical mortality when this arrhythmia was present on preoperative electrocardiograms (see Table 15) and an increased overall complication rate.[22,88] Patients with atrial fibrillation with rapid ventricular response do particularly poorly.[39] Preoperative atrial flutter has been reported to have as high as a 50 percent surgical risk,[16] but the numbers of patients studied are quite small. Although the effects of treatment on preoperative supraventricular arrhythmias and its relationship to surgical mortality is not well documented, it is considered prudent to have these rhythm disorders optimally treated prior to surgery.

PREOPERATIVE ATRIAL ARRHYTHMIAS

In evaluating the patient with atrial fibrillation or flutter preoperatively, a careful assessment of other cardiac disease is indicated. Certainly, valvular disease should be excluded. A loud S–1, diastolic rumble, vertical axis on EKG, or left atrial enlargement on chest x-ray may be valuable clues to the presence of mitral stenosis. The clinical features of aortic stenosis have been reviewed previously. Other less common structural defects such as atrial septal defect (ASD), IHSS, atrial myxoma, and mitral regurgitation may cause atrial fibrillation and should be excluded. Wolff-Parkinson-White syndrome (WPW) should be considered in view of its unique therapeutic requirements. A cardiac echo is usually indicated to help exclude these conditions as well as to measure left atrial size (see below). Atrial fibrillation with a particularly slow ventricular response and/or a history of bradyarrhythmias may suggest a sick sinus syndrome and the possible need for perioperative pacemaker insertion. Thyrotoxicosis should also be considered particularly since its clinical manifestations may be subtle in the elderly. If the atrial fibrillation is of recent onset, more acute problems should be sought (e.g., pulmonary embolus, infection, metabolic derangements, myocardial ischemia, pericarditis).

Having considered the diagnosis and the treatment of any coexistent cardiac or systemic illness, the question of proper management of atrial fibrillation remains. Given the high perioperative mortality associated with atrial fibrillation and its persistence as a strong prognostic indicator even after multivariate analysis, the question arises as to whether patients would benefit from preoperative cardioversion to normal sinus rhythm. Unfortunately, there are no studies of this approach and it is likely, in any event, that the question should be individualized. Certainly, a patient with longstanding atrial fibrillation and massive left atrial enlargement is unlikely to remain in normal sinus rhythm for a great length of time and the approach would be conservative (i.e., no cardioversion). On the other hand, a patient with the acute onset of atrial fibrillation (particularly if due to some potentially reversible metabolic upset) may benefit from conversion to normal sinus rhythm. This may also be considered in a patient who

TABLE 15. Preoperative Supraventricular Tachyarrhythmia* as Operative Risk Factor (Literature Review)

Author	*Date of Publication*	*Percentage of Surgical Mortality in All Patients in the Series*	*Percentage of Surgical Mortality in Patients without Arrhythmia*	*Percentage of Surgical Mortality in Patients with Arrhythmia*	*Total Number of Operations*
Morrison†[25]	1948	11.6	10	18	701
Skinner and Pearce†[16]	1964	13	7	14	857
Sapala et al.†[22]	1975	5.3	6	2.2	416
Goldman et al.[1,2]	1978	1.9	1	18	1001
Total		*7.7*	*5.5*	*14.5*	*2975*

*Majority of tachyarrhythmias are atrial fibrillation and flutter.
†Only cardiac patients included in series.

because of structural cardiac disease (e.g., aortic stenosis) might be expected to tolerate atrial fibrillation particularly poorly. It should be noted that anticoagulation therapy is usually indicated prior to conversion in order to avoid systemic embolization. This may complicate the surgical course and it is therefore advisable to plan conversion well in advance of scheduled surgery if at all possible. The approach to conversion usually involves digitalization then conversion with quinidine or D.C. current. Cardioversion is thoroughly discussed elsewhere and will not be dealt with in detail here. It would be reasonable to maintain the converted patient on digitalis plus quinidine throughout the perioperative period, although again the data are not conclusive (see below).

When it is not felt appropriate to cardiovert the patient preoperatively, the heart rate must be well controlled with digitalis (and propranolol if necessary). Since rate is an important determinant of cardiac output in atrial fibrillation, propranolol or digitalis given for this determinant should be continued throughout the perioperative period. The question of anticoagulation frequently arises. The well accepted association of atrial fibrillation with systemic embolization in patients with mitral valve disease has been extended in recent studies. These have demonstrated a significant incidence of systemic embolization in atrial fibrillation due to other disorders as well and many cardiologists are broadening their indications for anticoagulation. Anticoagulation during surgical procedures carries a significant morbidity and mortality. Although the incidence of systemic embolization during the perioperative period may, on theoretical grounds, be expected to be significant, available studies in general fail to document this for most types of cardiac disease. Goldman and associates[1,2] mentioned no fatal emboli in their 48 patients with perioperative atrial fibrillation. Morrison[25] noted 3 cases of arterial emboli (2 fatal) in their series of 701 operations on patients with cardiac disease. Assuming that all of these occurred in their subset of 84 patients with preoperative atrial fibrillation, the mortality from this complication at most would be 2.3 percent. The subgroup of 22 patients with rheumatic heart disease and atrial fibrillation had a higher embolism rate however (4.5% mortality and 4.5% morbidity vs. 1.6% mortality and 0% morbidity from arterial emboli in patients with atrial fibrillation and coronary artery disease). Although these data are inconclusive, it would seem reasonable to approach anticoagulation in patients with mitral valve disease and atrial fibrillation in the same manner as outlined above for patients with valvular protheses. In patients with atrial fibrillation due to other types of disease, anticoagulation can probably be stopped three to five days preoperatively and restarted three to five days postoperatively without ill effect.

Certainly patients with atrial fibrillation due to the sick sinus syndrome should be assessed for bradyarrhythmias, and if any questions arise, perioperative pacemaker insertion should be planned. In patients with atrial fibrillation due to WPW or IHSS, digitalis may be contraindicated. Patients with IHSS respond to propranolol and patients with WPW may require treatment with drugs such as quinidine, lidocaine, and procainamide.

Atropine may facilitate AV conduction and its use should be limited in patients with atrial fibrillation. The same is true for other chronotropic agents or anesthetic agents such as cyclopropane which may release endogenous catecholamines. The other preoperative atrial arrhythmias, such as frequent premature atrial contractions (PACs) and multifocal atrial tachycardia, present a rather different problem in that treatment is more likely to be directed at underlying systemic illness.

Frequent PACs are associated with a significant perioperative morbidity and mortality only in elderly patients with underlying systemic illness[1,2] including metabolic derangements, pulmonary disease, infection, myocardial ischemia, and hypotension. Although it might seem likely that PACs would simply be serving as a marker for poor overall medical condition in this situation, the fact that frequent PACs retain their strong prognostic value even after multivariate analysis at least suggests that they are of importance in and of themselves. This may be because they frequently presage more serious rhythm disturbances (atrial flutter or fibrillation), or because they are indicative of a diseased or unstable myocardium which cannot tolerate stress. In any event, major efforts should be aimed at correcting the underlying derangements when approaching preoperative patients with these rhythm disorders. Certainly, the intrinsic cardiac diseases noted in the previous section should also be considered as premature atrial contractions may be present as forerunners of atrial fibrillation in such patients. The data on the value of preoperative digitalization to prevent postoperative atrial fibrillation in these syndromes are reviewed elsewhere. Although inconclusive, these data would at least suggest that elderly patients, patients with known cardiac disease, or patients undergoing thoracotamy may benefit. Unfortunately, the underlying systemic illnesses may predispose to digitalis toxicity which must be watched for.

Multifocal atrial tachycardia usually occurs in the setting of severe pulmonary compromise and may be associated with life threatening ventricular ectopy. It is unlikely to respond to digitalization and pulmonary function is likely to be the major concern. The excess surgical risk associated with all these disorders should of course be considered carefully when assessing the need for surgical intervention under these circumstances.

POSTOPERATIVE ATRIAL ARRHYTHMIAS

Atrial arrhythmias are quite common in the postoperative period. Their incidence often depends on the methodology used for detection. Goldman and associates[1,2] noted an overall incidence of 4 percent in general surgical patients when screening consisted of a routine electrocardiogram performed on the fifth postoperative day or whenever a change occurred in the clinical status of the patient. They identified a number of factors which increased the risk of developing postoperative arrhythmias: age of 70 years or older (10% developed arrhythmia), congestive heart failure (13%), preoperative rales (8%), chronic obstructive pulmonary disease (9%), preoperative nondiagnostic ST-T wave changes (7%), and intra-abdominal thoracic or major vascular procedures (6%). There was a definite relationship between the occurrence of these arrhythmias and medical problems such as cardiac disorders (46%), infections (31%), hypotension (29%), anemia (26%), and hypoxia (20%). The mortality of patients with postoperative arrhythmias was high (49%). As expected, this was not directly due to the arrhythmias themselves but rather to the underlying problem. Most of the arrhythmias reverted to normal sinus rhythm (40% reverted without the use of antiarrhythmic agents). Table 16 summarizes the incidence of postoperative supraventricular arrhythmias in general surgical patients. Atrial flutter and atrial fibrillation compose 70 percent of reported

TABLE 16. Postoperative Arrhythmias in General Surgical Patients (Literature Review)

Author	*Date of Publication*	*Number of Patients*	*Percentage of Patients Developing Arrhythmias*	*Mortality Rate in Those with Arrhythmia*
Goldman et al.[1,2]	1978	916	4	49
Sapala et al.[22]	1975	424	0.7	100
Hewson[83]	1973	616	1.3	85
Rogers et al.[99]	1953	28,000	1	12% (due directly to arrythmia)

postoperative arrhythmias; atrial tachycardia, supraventricular tachycardia, and nodal tachycardia account for another 18 percent of postoperative supraventricular tachyarrhythmias.[89] These arrhythmias most often occur on postoperative days two and three.[101]

POSTOPERATIVE SUPRAVENTRICULAR TACHYARRHYTHMIAS

Management of supraventricular arrhythmias begins with a thorough search for underlying causes. Arterial blood gas analysis and a chest x-ray examination as well as a full 12-lead electrocardiogram must be considered the first steps in determining the management of these rhythm disorders. A thorough search for pulmonary embolism and pulmonary infection is mandatory. In trauma cases both direct myocardial injury and pericarditis may cause atrial arrhythmias. Congestive heart failure, occult valvular heart disease, hypertension, thyrotoxicosis, congenital heart disease, and invasive tumors may all lead to any of these rhythm disturbances.[91] An "uncomplicated" thoracotomy itself may be associated with atrial arrhythmias (Table 17). Digitalis is the most useful therapy for most atrial tachyarrhythmias. However, digitalis excess must always be considered in

TABLE 17. Postoperative Arrhythmias in Thoracotomy Patients (Literature Review)

Author	*Date of Publication*	*Number of Patients*	*Percentage of Patients Developing Arrhythmias*	*Percentage of Mortality Rate in Those with Arrhythmias*
Goldman et al.[1,2]	1978	31	10	
Beck-Nielsen et al.[92]	1973	300	21	3
Mowry and Reynolds[91]	1964	574	3.8	9
Ghosh and Pakrashi[93]	1957	100	16	
Cohen and Pastor[94]	1957	92	16.3	
Cerney[127]	1957	76	20	
Krosnik and Wasserman[95]	1955	82	12.2	20
Massie and Valle[98]	1947	120	9	27
Currens et al.[96]	1943	43	21	20
Baily and Betts[97]	1943	78	10	0
Total		*1496*	*11*	*10*

any patient taking this medication who develops atrial arrhythmias. Certain atrial arrhythmias are highly suggestive of digitalis toxicity. They include atrial tachycardia with conduction block, atrial and ventricular arrhythmias occurring together, and atrial fibrillation with irregular, slow, or "grouped" ventricular response. Serum levels are quite helpful in determining the role of digitalis therapy in the genesis of an arrhythmia, but care must be taken not to rely too heavily on this test.

Electrical countershock is effective in converting atrial flutter, atrial fibrillation, and paroxysmal atrial tachycardia and may be employed on an emergency basis if the patient is experiencing severe hemodynamic impairment or cardiac ischemia from these arrhythmias. Countershock is generally contraindicated in a digitalized patient and should be used only after careful consideration. When countershock is thought to be absolutely necessary in a patient receiving digitalis, the intravenous administration of phenytoin (Dilantin) may prevent postcardioversion ventricular arrhythmias.

Maneuvers, such as carotid sinus massage and the Valsalva maneuver, may be quite helpful in certain atrial arrhythmias. Because of their simplicity, they should be attempted in most instances of supraventricular tachycardia for therapeutic as well as diagnostic purposes (presuming that there is no contraindication, e.g., carotid artery stenosis). Propranolol, quinidine, procainamide, sympathomimetic agents, parasympathomimetic agents, and atrial pacing all have a role in managing these rhythm disorders.

DIGITALIS IN THE PERIOPERATIVE PERIOD

With respect to the often debated question of preoperative digitalization, there seem to be at least four issues: (1) the risk of developing atrial fibrillation in a given patient population, (2) the morbidity/mortality of the arrhythmia, (3) the efficacy of preoperative digitalization in preventing this arrhythmia, and (4) the risk of preoperative digitalization.

The literature cited above does delineate several risk factors for the development of postoperative atrial fibrillation: advanced age, pulmonary resectional surgery, CHF, chronic obstructive pulmonary disease (COPD), major surgery, lung cancer, other operative complications, preoperative pneumonia or arrhythmia, preoperative PACs. It would be reasonable to add a history of atrial fibrillation, significant valvular disease, and generally poor medical condition to this list. The exact estimate of the risk of developing atrial fibrillation is difficult to make, but an estimate of 10 to 15 percent in a patient with several of these factors is not unreasonable. The literature is much less explicit about the increment in mortality which can be attributed solely to the arrhythmia. Most studies imply that the excess mortality is usually attributable to other associated conditions. Despite this, it would seem that the added stress of an arrhythmia and the complications in management that would arise would justify low risk prophylactic measures.

The majority of studies show a reduction in the rate of atrial fibrillation in preoperatively digitalized patients (Table 18). However, the studies by Juler and associates[86] and Tyrus and coworkers[100] show quite the opposite. The study by Juler and coworkers[86] was biased in that the group receiving digitalis was on the average about 10 years older

TABLE 18. Efficacy of Prophylactic Preoperative Digitalization in Preventing Postoperative Supraventricular Tachyarrhythmias

Author	*Year of Publication*	*Total Number of Patients*	*Percentage of Patients Developing Supraventricular Tachyarrhythmias*		*Percentage of Operative Mortality*	
			Digitalis Therapy	*No Digitalis*	*Digitalis Therapy*	*No Digitalis*
Thoracotomy						
Burman[121]	1965	244	3.2	16.4	1.3	7.0
Shields and Ujiki[122]	1968	125	2.7	14.0	4.0	14.0
Juler et al.[86]	1962	563	14.3	2.0	4.1	1.5
Wheat and Burford[123]	1961	439	9.6	16.1	5.0	5.0
Hurt* and Bates[124]	1958	100	9.0	31.0		
Total		*1377*	*9.0*	*11.0*	*3.5*	*4.0*
Aortocoronary Bypass Graft						
Johnson et al.[125]	1976	120	9.0	27.0	5.0	5.0
Tyras et al.[100]	1979	140	27.8	11.4	1.6	0.0
O'Kane et al.[126]	1972	33	0.0	50.0		
Total		*293*	*15.4*	*21.5*	*3.0*	*1.8*

*Quinidine prophylaxis used instead of digitalis.

than the group not receiving digitalis. In view of the profound effect of advanced age on the frequency of postoperative fibrillation, this data must be questioned. The study by Tyrus and coworkers[100] dealt only with patients undergoing CABG surgery in whom propranolol was being tapered. With respect to overall mortality, there seems to be very little difference between the digitalized and the nondigitalized group. Data concerning the risks of preoperative digitalization are scarce. Several studies[10,86,102] have noted increased bradyarrhythmias in digitalized patients. This was especially true in those digitalized rapidly preoperatively; however, there was no analysis to exclude effects of other risk factors. Goldman and associates[2] noted perioperative bradyarrhythmias in 24 percent of digitalized patients although this was of little clinical significance.

In summary, it seems justifiable to recommend preoperative digitalization in a metabolically suitable patient who has several of the above noted risk factors provided that appropriate precautions are taken to avoid digitalis toxicity. It should be noted that patients with WPW or hypertrophic cardiomyopathy usually should *not* be digitalized preoperatively. We do not believe that advanced age in and of itself is a reason for preoperative digitalization; however, patients over 60 years of age undergoing thoracotomy as well as patients undergoing CABG receive preoperative digitalization in many institutions.[89]

It has recently been noted that the administration of quinidine to patients already receiving digitalis raises serum digitalis levels and predisposes to digitalis toxic rhythms.[103] Finally, it is common practice at many institutions to withhold digitalis on the morning of surgery. The evidence supporting the potential benefit for this practice is minimal.

Ventricular Arrhythmias

Ventricular arrhythmias range from the relatively common and usually benign occurrence of an occasional premature ventricular contraction to the lethal condition of ventricular fibrillation.

PREMATURE VENTRICULAR CONTRACTIONS

In their evaluation of operative risks, Goldman and associates[1,2] noted that five premature ventricular contractions per minute on any previous electrocardiogram increased the cardiac mortality from surgery to 14 percent (overall cardiac mortality being 1.9%). However, the clinical significance of spontaneously occurring premature ventricular contractions can best be related to their cause (Table 19).

Premature ventricular contractions (PVCs) occurring in "normal hearts" are far less serious than those occurring in ailing hearts. Isolated instances of PVCs have been reported to occur in 0.5 to 4 percent of routine electrocardiograms taken in asymptomatic individuals.[104,105] Furthermore, 24 hour continuous ambulatory electrocardiogram (Holter) monitoring typically demonstrates one or more ectopic ventricular beats in about 50 percent of a normal young population. Thus, the defining of "high risk populations" is absolutely necessary in the management of PVCs.

PVCs seem to be more serious in older age groups. This probably reflects the greater likelihood that they are manifestations of ischemic heart disease. Relating PVCs to coronary artery disease is usually no problem in a patient who has a clear cut history of angina pectoris or myocardial infarction. However, "occult coronary artery

TABLE 19. Etiologies of Premature Ventricular Beats

Benign idiopathic origin
Underlying myocardial disease
Coronary heart disease
Cardiomyopathy
Infiltrative and metastatic disorders
Ventricular aneurysms
Myocardial contusion
Mitral valve prolapse syndrome (floppy mitral valve)
Metabolic disorders, e.g., hypoxia, electrolyte disorders
Prolonged Q-T interval syndrome
Drugs, e.g., digitalis, phenothiazines, lithium carbonate, tricyclic antidepressants, sympathetic agents, aminophylline, cyclopropane, alcohol, caffeine
Central nervous system disorders
Miscellaneous, e.g., displaced vascular catheters, pulmonary emboli, hypothermia, smoking

disease" causing PVCs may require a careful history and evaluation for risk factors (i.e., family history, hyperlipidemia, diabetes, smoking, and hypertension) as well as diagnostic procedures. Graded exercise testing has become a valuable tool in evaluating isolated premature contractions. Those that disappear with exercise and are not associated with ST segment changes are much less likely to be due to ischemic heart disease. Coronary angiography, which at present is felt to be the final word in clinical diagnosis of coronary artery disease, is usually not performed merely to find the etiology of PVCs. However, radioisotope techniques, such as in exercise thallium studies, result in useful screening tests with greater sensitivity and specificity for ischemic heart disease than exercise testing alone. Within the category of ischemic heart disease, PVCs are felt to be far more serious in the setting of acute ischemia than they are in long standing coronary disease.

Several other underlying cardiac disorders may commonly be associated with PVCs and other forms of ventricular arrhythmias. The floppy mitral valve syndrome (Barlow's, click murmur, or mitral valve prolapse syndrome) is being recognized as a very common cause of ventricular arrhythmias particularly in young females (see Mitral Valve Prolapse, above). The significance of PVCs occurring in the perioperative period in these patients has not been well defined. However, in view of reports of sudden death occurring in patients with the floppy mitral valve syndrome, it is our feeling that propranolol therapy and continuous EKG monitoring should be considered perioperatively in patients with this condition who demonstrate more than just an occasional PVC in their preoperative EKG.

Idiopathic hypertrophic subaortic stenosis (see above) may present with ventricular or supraventricular arrhythmias. Left ventricular aneurysms and cardiomyopathy of many etiologies can also present with ventricular arrhythmias as their first manifestations. Echocardiography and isotope angiocardiography are very useful noninvasive tools in establishing diagnoses.

In 1957 Jervel and Lange-Nielsen[106] reported upon a family with a high incidence of congenital deafness as well as prolonged Q-T intervals. The family members were subject to PVCs and recurrent bouts of syncope. It has now become apparent that the long Q-T interval syndromes are not rare and may occur without deafness.

In the absence of a detectable underlying cause, treatment of sporadically occurring PVCs is not usually indicated. However, treating isolated PVCs should be considered in two situations. The first is when this arrhythmia is causing incapacitating symptoms, such as loss of sleep and severe apprehension. Often these symptoms can be alleviated by counseling and reassurance. A small population of these patients may require pharmacologic therapy. The second situation involves the presence of certain patterns of occurrence associated with more serious ventricular arrhythmias. The occurrence of PVCs with a frequency greater than 12 per minute, paired contractions (two consecutive PVCs), multifocal PVCs, and early PVCs (those occurring on the T wave previous beats) all have been linked to a higher incidence of premature death. Therefore, the occurrence of even a short burst of ventricular tachycardia during a routine electrocardiogram or electrocardiographic monitoring may be grounds for treatment.

INTRAOPERATIVE ARRHYTHMIAS

Intraoperative arrhythmias are common, the vast majority are benign, and their management lies within the province of the anesthesiologists.[107] Of major concern, however, are instances of intraoperative cardiac arrest and the degree to which these can be prevented by preoperative interventions. Reported incidence rates vary from 0.03 percent to 0.12 percent of all operative procedures depending on the study (see Table 20), with mortality rates of 50 to 90 percent in patients sustaining an arrest. Approximately 15 to 36 percent appear due to problems with anesthetic management and these patients are generally from the group of patients who were previously healthy. Another 5 to 25 percent are primarily due to surgical problems (e.g., excessive blood loss), whereas 13 to 22 percent of these deaths are secondary to poor overall condition of the patient prior to surgery. The remainder of the deaths are due to a combination of these factors. Physical status has a marked effect on the incidence of intraoperative arrest: patients judged to be American Society of Anesthesiologists' (ASA) Class I* had a rate of 0/16192 (0%); Class II, 12/12154 (0.1%); Class III, 24/4070 (0.6%); Class IV, 33/720 (4.5%); and Class V, 8/87 (9.1%).[112] In addition, another study demonstrated that the chance of successful resuscitation falls dramatically with increasing ASA Class: Class I, 84 percent resuscitated; Class II, 37 percent; and Class III, 0 percent.[110] Fifty percent of arrests were asystolic, the remainder being due to ventricular fibrillation; there was no difference in the prognosis in the two groups.[110] Of cardiac arrests 12 to 24 percent occur during the induction of anesthesia, approximately 67 percent occur during the surgery itself, and 8 to 22 percent occur during the immediate postoperative period.[108,109]

Review of the available literature indicates that there does not seem to be any clearly identifiable subgroup of patients who appear to be healthy but are, in fact, at increased risk of sudden intraoperative cardiac arrest which the physician can identify preoperatively. Two groups who theoretically might fall within this category would be asymp-

TABLE 20. Intraoperative Cardiac Arrest (Literature Review)

Author	*Year of Publication*	*Patients Experiencing Arrest/Total Patient Population*	*Percentage of Cardiac Arrest*	*Percentage of Mortality of Cardiac Arrest*	*Cause (Percentage)*		
					Anesthesia	*Surgical*	*Underlying Illness*
Taylor et al.[108]	1976	41/?	?	?	22	?	22
McClure et al.[109]	1972	24/ 82,671	0.03	50	?	15	?
Pierce[110]	1966	22/ 18,062	0.1	63	36	5	15
Stephen[111]	1962	164/118,552	0.12	93	15	25	13
Dripps et al.[112]	1961	80/ 33,224	0.2	?	33	?	72
Bomar and Thompson[113]	1960	30/ 68,913	0.04	94	?	?	14

*For a description of ASA classes see Chapter 16.

tomatic patients with significant arrhythmias and patients with anatomically advanced but as yet occult coronary artery disease. It appears from the study of Goldman and associates[1,2] that a routine preoperative electrocardiogram is sufficient to identify the first group, but at present, there is no evidence to support *routine* preoperative screening with Holter monitor, stress testing, or echocardiography in the absence of suggestive data obtained from the history, physical examination, or routine laboratory examinations.

MANAGEMENT OF VENTRICULAR ARRHYTHMIAS

The majority of ventricular arrhythmias fall into the category of isolated PVCs in asymptomatic patients and do not require therapy. However, in critically ill patients, patients with underlying cardiac disorders, and patients with various forms of metabolic abnormalities, ventricular arrhythmias are much less likely to be "innocent." Unfortunately, there is often a tendency to initiate pharmocologic antiarrhythmic therapy without fully assessing the patient and looking for causes of the arrhythmia that might be easily treated. Arrhythmias due to metabolic derangements, however, are often quite refractory to drug therapy.

Hypoxia and electrolyte disturbances are the most common noncardiac causes of treatable ventricular arrhythmias. These conditions are usually associated more with postoperative than preoperative arrhythmias. Arterial blood gas determinations are mandatory in the postoperative patient with ventricular irritability. Simple adjustment of the inspired O_2 fraction may be all that is needed to treat a rhythm abnormality. Decreased serum potassium and/or magnesium levels and increased serum calcium levels may all cause ventricular excitability in an otherwise normal heart. Growing use of potent diuretic agents has greatly increased the incidence of ventricular arrhythmias due to electrolyte disturbances. Patients with diuretic induced hypokalemia and arrhythmia who do not respond to potassium replacement may have hypomagnesemia, and the arrhythmia may resolve following magnesium replacement.[115] Patients with prolonged gastrointestinal disorders requiring nasogastric suction are also quite likely to have electrolyte abnormalities as the cause of their arrhythmia.

Smoking and chronic alcohol and caffeine intake must also be considered as potential sources of ventricular irritability. High anxiety states have been linked to the development of life threatening arrhythmias without any underlying cardiac cause. In these situations, management of the arrhythmia relates to eliminating the precipitating factors and/or the use of sedatives.

In hospitalized patients, an occasionally overlooked source of cardiac arrhythmias is a displaced intravascular line, such as a Swan-Ganz catheter; central venous pressure tubing; pacemaker electrode; or a sheared indwelling peripheral venous catheter embolism. These causes of arrhythmia must be promptly treated by removing or repositioning the mechanical irritant to the ventricle. Hypothermia, whether accidental or medically induced, may cause ventricular fibrillation, usually at a temperature of 28° C or less. A normal rhythm can usually be re-established by rewarming. Postoperatively, pulmonary embolic disease may be responsible for ventricular arrhythmias. Again, the diagnosis and treatment of the underlying disorder and the treatment of hypoxia are the most important factors in the management of the arrhythmia.

Finally, it should be remembered that many drugs themselves may cause ventricular ectopy. These drugs include digitalis, beta-adrenergic stimulating agents (even nose drops), cyclopropane and chloroform anesthetics, phenothiazines, injected radiopaque dyes, aminophylline, lithium carbonate, tricylic antidepressants, and antiarrhythmic agents themselves. Blood levels, particularly of cardiac drugs, may help clarify the issue.

In summary, it is clear that ventricular arrhythmias may be due to a wide variety of etiologies and the current literature does not explicitly define which etiologies are responsible for the increased perioperative risk in patients with ventricular ectopy. Nevertheless, it is reasonable to assume that patients with serious underlying disease and/or high grade ventricular ectopy would be at higher risk in the perioperative period. It is in this group that we would recommend antiarrhythmic therapy in the perioperative period. The drugs routinely used in this country for the treatment of ventricular arrhythmias are described in the Appendix to this chapter. For parenteral therapy, lidocaine is usually considered the drug of first choice. If lidocaine therapy is unsuccessful, procainamide or bretylium should be considered. Quinidine, procainamide, and disopyramide may be used orally with good results. Ventricular arrhythmias related to ischemia, IHSS, and the floppy mitral valve syndrome may respond well to propranolol. If ventricular arrhythmia is felt to be secondary to digitalis excess, diphenylhydantoin therapy should be considered.

The treatment of sustained ventricular tachycardia is cardioversion. If the patient is still conscious during the arrhythmia, intravenous administration of a sedative such as diazepam should be considered. If the patient is unconscious, cardiopulmonary resuscitation maneuvers should be initiated while cardioversion is being prepared. The optimal energy levels for cardioversion and defibrillation have not yet been determined. For ventricular tachycardia, cardioversion should be synchronized (i.e., programmed to discharge simultaneously with the QRS complexes) in order to avoid inadvertent discharge into the repolarization cycle and the chance of inducing ventricular fibrillation. One can start with 50 joules or less for cardioversion, but if a true emergency exists, time should not be wasted and the energy level should be turned up to 200 to 400 joules.

Ventricular fibrillation must be treated immediately with cardioversion. Again, cardiopulmonary resuscitation must also be initiated. The administration of lidocaine to enhance the effectiveness of the cardioversion should be considered if cardioversion initially fails. If cardioversion with lidocaine also fails, other agents such as procainamide and/or bretylium should be tried.

Rarely, recurrent ventricular arrhythmias may be controlled with "overdrive" atrial or ventricular pacing (80 to 120 per minute). Very rarely, emergency surgical procedures such as aneurysmectomy or coronary artery bypass surgery may be lifesaving in refractory ventricular arrhythmias, but the role of such procedures is controversial.

CARDIAC CONDUCTION ABNORMALITIES

With the development of simple, reliable, and safe techniques for both temporary and permanent pacemaker insertion, recognition of the patient with conduction abnormalities has become an important aspect of the care of the perioperative patient. Some of the many causes of cardiac conduction abnormalities are summarized in Table 21.

TABLE 21. Causes of Cardiac Conduction System Abnormalities

Congenital heart block
Coronary artery disease
Collagen disease (i.e., rheumatoid spondylitis, rheumatoid arthritis, scleroderma)
Cardiomyopathy
Amyloidosis
Hemochromatosis
Infiltrative and granulomatous diseases
Valvular heart disease (usually chronic)
Infectious diseases
Trauma
Metabolic disorders
Idiopathic degenerative disorders
Iatrogenic disorders (i.e., following digitalis therapy or cardiac surgery)

First-degree heart block (PR interval prolongation) is usually a benign abnormality and results in no significant clinical impairment. However, digitalis induced first-degree heart block may be a precursor of more serious manifestations of digitalis toxicity.

Second-degree heart block of the Wenckebach (Mobitz type I) variety is most often seen during digitalis intoxication or acute inferior myocardial infarction but may also be seen in "normal" hearts (i.e., patients engaging in long distance running). It may be abolished by vagolytic agents such as atropine. The management of the occasional patient with the Wenkebach form of second-degree heart block must be individualized. Factors such as the patient's age and symptoms must be taken into account before a decision is made regarding pacemaker insertion. Mobitz type II second-degree heart block is a more serious disorder, often being a harbinger of complete heart block and thus usually requiring pacemaker insertion.

Third-degree (complete) heart block is almost always considered to be a serious condition. Vandam and McLemare[115] demonstrated that 5 of 11 patients with third-degree heart block and a history of Stokes-Adams attacks developed cardiac arrest in the perioperative period while 1 of 11 patients with third-degree heart block but no history of syncope had postoperative cardiac arrests. All patients with third-degree heart block should be considered candidates for pacemaker insertion preoperatively.

Data from seven studies (Table 22) with a total of 306 patients document that otherwise uncomplicated bifascicular block does not significantly increase the risk of development of complete heart block in asymptomatic patients during the perioperative period. The addition of a prolonged P-R interval may or may not slightly increase this risk. In these studies there were 2 instances of progression to third-degree heart block perioperatively, and 1 occurred in a patient who had Mobitz type II heart block preoperatively. As a whole, these patients had an increased surgical mortality, but as Goldman

TABLE 22. Preoperative Bilateral Bundle Branch Block as an Operative Risk Factor (Literature Review)

Author	*Date of Publication*	*Number of Patients*	*Number Progressing to Complete Heart Block*	*Percentage of Operative Mortality*
Berg and Kotler[116]	1971	30	0	10
Venkataraman et al.[117]	1975	38	1	10
Pastore et al.[118]	1974	44	1	7
Kunstadt et al.[119]	1973	24	0	8
Rooney et al.[120]	1976	27	0	
Goldman et al.[1,2]	1978	45	0	9
Bellocci et al.[152]	1980	98	0	4.0
Totals		*306*	*2*	*6.7*

and associates[1,2] demonstrated with multivariate analysis, the excess mortality can be attributed to other frequently associated cardiac diseases and not to the conduction abnormality itself. Bellocci and associates[152] noted that prolongation of the H-V interval was a marker for underlying cardiac disease in patients with bilateral bundle branch block.

The designation sick sinus syndrome covers a wide variety of clinical states. It is usually characterized by sinus bradycardia alternating with supraventricular tachycardia. Patients who have a history of syncopal attacks and sinus bradycardia should be considered candidates for preoperative pacemaker insertion. It should also be noted that patients with sick sinus syndrome are often quite sensitive to digitalis preparations.

Management of Patients with Conduction Abnormalities

Before pacemaker insertion some "reversible" causes of conduction disorders should be considered. These include use of digitalis, antiarrhythmic agents such as quinidine or procainamide, sympathetic blocking agents used in the treatment of hypertension, and tricyclic antidepressants. It should be remembered that any monitoring lines that cross the tricuspid valve (e.g., Swan-Ganz catheters) have the potential of producing right bundle branch block. This is usually of no consequence. However, if the patient has a pre-existing left bundle branch block, right heart catheterization may produce complete heart block and ventricular asystole. Our policy is to not insert a Swan-Ganz catheter in any patient with left bundle branch block without considering prior insertion of a temporary transvenous pacing wire.

Patients with asymptomatic conduction disturbances that otherwise would not be candidates for pacemaker insertion may require such intervention when they develop ventricular irritability requiring antiarrhythmic therapy. Potent antiarrhythmic agents theoretically may exacerbate a pre-existing conduction problem and thus promote the development of high-degree AV block.

Currently, we recommend permanent pacemaker insertion or temporary transvenous pacemaker insertion prior to elective surgery for patients with complete heart block or Mobitz type II second-degree heart block and for patients with a history of syncope due to any of the other conduction abnormalities.

In patients with conduction problems in whom transvenous pacing is not indicated, the following protocol is used. Prior to the induction of anesthesia, external pacing electrodes are positioned on the patient's chest with the positive electrode at the second right interspace at the right sternal border and the negative electrode at the apex of the left ventricle. By attaching these wires to an appropriate external pacemaker impulse source, a number of patients (but not all) may be paced if necessary. Syringes containing atropine (2 mg), epinephrine (10 cc of 1:10,000 solution), and an intravenous solution of isoproterenol (2 mg in 500 cc of 5% dextrose in water) should be available for immediate use in the operating room.

Occasionally, patients who are paced ventricularly become hypotensive because of loss of their "atrial kick." Some of these patients may be helped by the adjustment of pacing rates, but a few may require atrioventricular synchronous pacing to maintain an adequate stroke volume as well as heart rate.

Patients with permanent pacemakers pose special problems. Knowledge of the location, type, manufacturer, and age of the pacing unit is of great importance in managing such patients. Demand pacemakers may be temporarily "turned off" by electrical cautery and extreme caution must be taken in keeping cauterization units as far as possible from the pacing site. Patients must be monitored carefully while such devices are being used. A magnet for conversion of the pacemaker to fixed mode should be available for use should the demand pacer be suppressed by the cauterization unit. Although present day pacemakers are said to be "protected" from the effects of defibrillation currents, there is still a threat, and if defibrillation is indicated, initial attempts should be made with the axis of defibrillation perpendicular to the axis of the pacing wire (i.e., if the pacing unit is under the right clavicle and the wire is implanted in the apex of the right ventricle, the paddles should be placed from front to back). The defibrillator paddles should never be placed directly over a pacemaker unit.

Many patients now have rate adjustable ("programmable") permanent pacemakers. These units may be helpful in a critically ill patient who may benefit from an increase in heart rate for the suppression of tachyarrhythmia and/or increase in cardiac output.

Needless to say, any patient with a permanent pacer unit should have his pacemaker function thoroughly evaluated preoperatively. This usually includes accurate measurement of R-R intervals with and without a magnet and measurement of pulse duration and sensing function when applicable.

PROPRANOLOL IN THE PERIOPERATIVE PERIOD

With the widespread use of beta-adrenergic blocking agents in the management of hypertension, coronary artery disease, cardiac arrhythmias, mitral valve prolapse, and hypertrophic cardiomyopathy, increasing concern has been raised about the proper management of these agents in the perioperative period. This discussion will focus on the patient with cardiac disease, as the hypertensive patient is discussed elsewhere (see Chapter 14, Renal Disease and Hypertension).

Theoretical concerns have been raised about the possibility of additive effects of beta-adrenergic blocking agents and general anesthetics with direct myocardial depressant activity. It should be noted that in the patient with good left ventricular function, cardiac performance is not dependent on adrenergic stimulation and this possibility is of less concern. In 1972 Viljoen[128] reported on 5 patients with intraoperative cardiac failure who had previously been on chronic propranolol therapy and suggested its withdrawal 2 weeks prior to surgery. The pharmacologic basis for the two week period is uncertain, and this is very likely far in excess of what is really necessary, as will be discussed later. It should be noted that all of his patients had elevated left ventricular end diastolic pressures (LVEDP) previously and that it was not specified how many, if any, were actually on propranolol at the time of surgery. Additional support has been given to this view by experimental data demonstrating an increase in LVEDP and a decrease in cardiac output in volume-loaded dogs on propranolol who were subjected to cardiopulmonary bypass.[129] A number of other studies, however, have demonstrated no significant differences in the frequency of perioperative hypotension, CHF, bradycardia, or mortality when propranolol was continued until just prior to aortocoronary bypass graft surgery (Table 23). Kopriva and associates[153] noted no significant difference in cardiac output, mean arterial pressure, or stroke volume when patients on chronic propranolol for control of angina pectoris and undergoing coronary artery bypass grafting were compared with similar patients not receiving this medication. Significantly, however, patients with left ventricular "power failure" were excluded from this study. In the only prospective randomized study of this problem, Kirsch and associates[133] found no significant difference in the incidence of postoperative myocardial infarction and hypotension, mortality, or requirement for prolonged intra-aortic balloon support when patients whose propranolol was stopped 48 hours prior to surgery were compared with patients who were given propranolol until one to two hours preoperatively. It should be noted that this study (as well as most propranolol studies) was done in patients undergoing general surgical procedures, but the available results appear to be as in those undergoing cardiac surgery (Table 24). Unfortunately, these latter studies involve small numbers of patients and the indications for propranolol therapy are variable making it difficult to draw firm conclusions.

TABLE 23. Effect of Propranolol on Patients Undergoing Aortocoronary Bypass Graft Surgery

			Percentage of Mortality		*Percentage with Significant Hypertension*	*Significant Bradycardia*
Author	*Year of Publication*	*Timing of Last Dose Pre-operatively*	*without Propranolol*	*with Propranolol*	*with Propranolol*	*with Propranolol*
Kaplan et al.[130]	1975	24 h	6	4	3.1	
Jones et al.[131]	1976	< 24 h	0	0	20	0
		24 to 48 h	0	4.8	10	0
		> 48 h	0	6.5	10	0
Moran et al.[132]	1974	< 48 h	6.6	3.8	15	
Kirsh et al.[133]	1978	< 1 h		0	2.1	
		>48 h		0	3.8	
Carlaps et al.[134]	1974	24 h	0	0	5.5	
Manners and Walters[135]	1979	< or > 16 h	0	0	6.2	
Boudoulas et al.[136]	1978	< or > 10 h		0	0	0

TABLE 24. Effects of Propranolol in Patients Undergoing Elective Noncardiac Surgery

Author	*Year of Publication*	*Mortality with Propranolol*	*Percentage of Patients with Significant Hypotension or Congestive Heart Failure with Propranolol*	*Percentage of Patients with Bradycardia with Propranolol*	*Percentage of Patients with Hypotension or Congestive Heart Failure without Propranolol*
Prys-Roberts et al.[137]	1973	0	0	0	
Kaplan and Dunbar[138]	1976	0	3.2	1.3	9
Goldman et al.[2]	1978		4		6.2

With regard to the pharmacokinetics of propranolol withdrawal, it is now fairly clear that no propranolol (or active metabolites) are detectable in the blood or left atrial tissue 24 to 48 hours after its discontinuation.[139,140] Furthermore, beta-blockade as measured by left atrial sensitivity to norepinephrine or isoproterenol in vitro is also nonexistent at this time interval.[139,140] However, other studies, using noninvasive techniques, have suggested that some beta-blockade persists for 12 to 24 hours following the last dose.[141,142]

Controversy has similarly existed over the danger of abrupt withdrawal of propranolol in the patient with severe angina pectoris. A number of case reports and small series have documented an increased incidence (3.7 to 14%) of unstable angina and myocardial infarctions in patients following abrupt withdrawal of propranolol.[130,131,134,143,145-147] Unfortunately, these are all uncontrolled series in patients undergoing cardiac catheterization or aortocoronary bypass graft surgery. That these patients are frequently unstable, with a significant myocardial infarction rate, whether or not any therapeutic manipulation is undertaken was shown by Myers and associates[146] who found an identical incidence of new ischemic events just prior to and immediately following propranolol withdrawal in patients about to undergo cardiac catheterization. Kirsch and associates,[133] in the one prospective randomized study, noted a similar perioperative myocardial infarction rate in patients whose propranolol was discontinued 48 hours prior to surgery and those who were maintained on propranolol until the time of surgery. Boudoulas and coworkers[136] noted a higher incidence of subendocardial (17 vs. 3%) but not of transmural (10 vs. 10%) myocardial infarction in patients whose propranolol was stopped 24 hours preoperatively when compared with patients in whom it was continued until 4 to 10 hours preoperatively. Unfortunately, this series was retrospective with historical controls. Miller and coworkers[154] in a double-blind crossover study found a 15 percent incidence of death or life-threatening complications and a 10 percent incidence of significant exacerbations of angina following abrupt withdrawal of chronic propranolol. The patients in this study were not receiving long-acting nitrates, thus this figure would be higher than expected in optimally managed patients. It should be noted that the withdrawal complications occurred up to 2 weeks following propranolol withdrawal in this study and might have been avoided if propranolol had been reinstituted shortly after surgery.

In summary, it appears that due to methodological problems in reported series, both the danger of continuing propranolol perioperatively and the danger of abrupt withdrawal may well have been exaggerated. In the absence of a sufficient number of good prospective studies, definitive answers to these pressing questions are not possible at present.[144,148,149] It nevertheless seems that there is no reason to discontinue propranolol in a patient receiving it for control of arrhythmias, mitral valve prolapse, or hypertrophic cardiomyopathy. Similarly, in a patient with significant angina and good left ventricular function, it is probably safer to continue the drug perioperatively. In the patient with severe angina and questionable or poor left ventricular function, the question is particularly difficult and the solution must be individualized. It may be necessary to define the extent of left ventricular dysfunction preoperatively by noninvasive or invasive means. Possible solutions may include the use of "cardiac" type anesthesia to lessen the myocardial depressant effect, pharmacologic ionotropic therapy, mechanical circulatory support, or even aortocoronary bypass grafting prior to the noncardiac procedure. Although it is uncertain that the last procedure will increase myocardial performance, it is likely to reduce the requirement for propranolol. Should propranolol be discontinued preoperatively in order to avoid myocardial depressant activity, 48 hours should be sufficient to assure absence of beta blockade at the time of surgery.

HYPOTENSION

The patient with postoperative hypotension presents a challenge to the internist, surgeon, and anesthesiologist alike, as the cause may lie in any one of these areas (Table 25). The first etiology to be excluded would be intraoperative blood loss or postoperative bleeding. This may be indicated by decreased hematocrit without obvious signs of

TABLE 25. Etiologies of Perioperative Hypotension

Volume depletion
Hemorrhage (operative site, gastrointestinal, iatrogenic)
Untoward effects of medications
Blood products
Anesthetic agents
Analgesics
Antihypertensives
Idiosyncratic reactions
Reflex mechanisms
Pneumothorax
Pulmonary embolism
Cardiac causes (CHF, arrhythmia, tamponade, ischemia, pacemakers)
Sepsis
Endocrine causes (adrenal insufficiency, myxedema)
Metabolic causes (hypoxia, acid/base/electrolyte irregularities)

external bleeding or hemolysis. However, early in the course, the hematocrit may be unchanged. Careful examination of the operative site may give valuable clues as to the occurrence of bleeding and is mandatory. Not to be neglected in critically ill postoperative patients is the possibility of hemorrhage secondary to invasive monitoring devices such as central venous catheters, arterial lines, or support devices such as intra-aortic balloons. Intubated patients are at risk for the development of pneumothorax, particularly if ventilated under positive pressure. The approach to the above problems is usually surgical although the possibility of an underlying hemostatic defect should be considered in all hemorrhagic cases. Certainly gastrointestinal bleeding secondary to stress ulceration should also be kept in mind in the postoperative patient and the approach in this instance may often be conservative with volume replacement, antacids, or cimetidine and Pitressin if necessary (see Chapter 6, Gastroenterology).

Most patients are subjected to a vast array of medications during the perioperative period, introducing the possibility of drug-induced hypotension. Most anesthetic agents have direct depressant effects on the myocardium. Morphine and other analgesics may induce vasodilation and hypotension; blood products may contain antigenic substances and hypotension may accompany transfusion reactions. Anaphylactic reactions to many different drugs may all result in hypotension. In addition, patients may receive a variety of antihypertensive agents or sympatholytic agents as part of their perioperative care. Spinal anesthesia, by interrupting normal reflex mechanisms, may result in hypotension as is well known. Idiosyncratic reactions to rapid infusions of a whole variety of drugs (e.g., phenytoin, lidocaine, procainamide) should be considered in patients receiving these medications. Hypotensive reactions to the acrylic cement used in stabilizing orthopedic prosthetic devices have been well documented.[150,151] Contrast agents may be used perioperatively and these can also induce hypotension.

Reflex mechanisms may play a role in the hypotension occurring following intubation, carotid endarterectomy, and thoracic or peritoneal procedures in which the vagus nerve is stimulated; ocular surgery may have a vagotonic effect and cause hypotension in this manner also.

Pulmonary or fat embolism usually occurs several days postoperatively and, they are less likely causes of immediate postoperative hypotension. Amniotic fluid embolism, however, may be considered in the obstetrical patient with hypotension following cesarean section. Hypotension following cardiac surgery is a particularly complex subject and will not be dealt with in detail here.

Postoperative patients are at high risk for a large number of cardiac disorders which may result in hypotension. Most commonly these include arrhythmias and heart failure (whether due to ischemia, valvular disease, or cardiomyopathy). Also to be considered is the negative inotropic effect of severe electrolyte and acid-base abnormalities and drugs. The possibility of tamponade may be considered, particularly in patients with thoracic procedures who are on anticoagulants, with neoplastic disease known to involve the mediastinum, or with intracardiac monitoring devices. It should be noted that occasional patients are dependent on the atrial contribution to ventricular filling in order to maintain an adequate cardiac output and pacemaker insertion with a ventricular electrode may result in hypotension in these patients.

Sepsis must always be considered in hypotensive patients. Although fever and leukocytosis may be valuable clues to the presence of a serious underlying infection their absence certainly does not exclude septicemia.

In a patient with unrecognized Addison's disease or myxedema, the stress of surgery may precipitate acute crisis with hypotension and/or coma. This may also be the case in patients on replacement doses of steroids or patients who have recently received steroids for other therapeutic purposes. Any patients having recently received steroids should receive supplemental steroid coverage throughout the perioperative period unless their pituitary adrenal axis has previously been demonstrated to be intact. Adrenal hemorrhage with acute adrenal insufficiency may also occur postoperatively (see Chapter 5, Endocrinology).

Severe hypoxia may also result in hypotension. This may be due to aspiration, pneumonia, mechanical difficulties with endotracheal tube positioning or ventilation assisting devices. Pneumothorax as a consequence of positive pressure ventilation or invasive intrathoracic procedures is also to be considered. In addition, the postoperative patient with significant central nervous system depression may fail to ventilate sufficiently.

Evaluation of the hypotensive patient involves the combined expertise of all physicians involved in the operative and postoperative care. Review of the operative procedure itself in terms of possible sites of hemorrhage and the dosage and method of administration of anesthetic agents and other medications are necessary. Routinely obtained laboratory data include complete blood count, coding parameters, chest x-ray, EKG, serum electrolytes, and arterial blood gases. The remainder of the clinical evaluation is usually guided by the findings on physical examination and this initial laboratory data. Treatment is usually aimed at correcting the underlying abnormality and is discussed further in the appropriate chapters. In addition, effort is directed at raising the blood pressure and, hopefully, thereby improving tissue perfusion. In many patients, administration of fluids will suffice, particularly in hypotensive patients. In patients with questionable or marginally compensated cardiac status, a central venous pressure line or Swan-Ganz catheter may be indicated to help monitor the rate of volume repletion. The rate and kind of fluid administered (crystalloid, colloid, or blood products) must of course be individualized. Certainly in profoundly hypotensive patients, the decreased tissue perfusion may itself be a major threat to life and pressor agents are indicated. The choice of agents includes dopamine, dobutamine, and norepinephrine, which have varying ionotropic activity in addition to pressor effects, and other drugs such as metaraminol and phenylephrine which have pure alpha vasoconstrictor activity. The use of such drugs must be tailored to the individual situation and remains a topic of considerable debate. As was previously noted, patients with hypertrophic cardiomyopathy should receive vasoconstrictor agents only.

INTRA-AORTIC BALLOON COUNTERPULSATION

The use of intra-aortic balloon assist devices has been accepted for several years in the treatment of "high risk" patients undergoing cardiac surgery. Recently the use of such devices has been advocated in patients with severe myocardial ischemia and decreased left ventricular function undergoing noncardiac operations.[155] At the present time, there is too little experience to clearly define guidelines for prophylactic balloon insertion. The recent development of percutaneous insertion techniques may lead to futher evaluation of the efficacy of prophylactic counterpulsation in managing high risk cardiac patients undergoing general surgery.

REFERENCES

1. GOLDMAN, L, CALDERA, DL, NUSSBAUM, SR, ET AL.: *Multifactoral index of cardiac risk in noncardiac surgical procedures.* N Engl J Med 297:845, 1977.
2. GOLDMAN, L, CALDERA, DL, SOUTHWICK, FS, ET AL.: *Cardiac risk factors and complications in non-cardiac surgery.* Medicine 57:357, 1978.
3. KRIEGER-LASSEN, HS: *Geriatric problems in surgery.* J Gerontol 17:167, 1962.
4. PARSONS, WH, WHITAKER, HT, AND HINTON, JK: *Major surgery in patients of 70 years of age and over.* Arch Surg 143:845, 1956.
5. NACHLAS, MM, ABRAMS, SJ, AND GOLDBERG, MD: *The influence of arteriosclerotic heart disease on surgical risk.* Am J Surg 101:447, 1961.
6. ARKINS, R, SMESSAERT, AA, AND HICKS, RG: *Mortality and morbidity in surgical patients with coronary artery disease.* JAMA 190:485, 1964.
7. KANNELL, WB, SORLLE, P, AND MCNAMARA, PM: *Prognosis after initial myocardial infarction—the Framingham study.* Am J Cardiol 44:53, 1979.
8. TOMATIS, LA, FLERENS, EE, AND VERBRUGGE, GP: *Evaluation of surgical risk in peripheral vascular disease by coronary arteriography. A series of 100 cases.* Surgery 71:429, 1972.
9. BOSCH, DT, ISLAMI, A, TANCT, R, ET AL.: *Elderly surgical patient. Analysis of 500 consecutive cases of patients 60 years of age or older.* JAMA 64:269, 1952.
10. OWEN, RAC, AND MURPHY, AF: *Surgery in old age.* Br Med J 2:186, 1952.
11. ANGLEM, TJ, AND BRADFORD, ML: *Major surgery in the aged.* N Engl J Med 249:1005, 1953.
12. STEWART, JD, AND ALFANO, GS: *Surgery of the elderly.* JAMA 154:643, 1954.
13. MITHOEFER, J, AND MITHOEFER, JC: *Studies of aged, surgical mortality.* Arch Surg 69:58, 1954.
14. LIMBOSCH, J: *Experiences with more than 1000 elderly surgical patients.* Arch Surg 73:124, 1956.
15. MITTY, WF, AND ECHEMEUDIA, EM: *Misuse of blood transfusions.* Geriatrics 18:368, 1953.
16. SKINNER, JF, AND PEARCE, ML: *Surgical risk in the cardiac patient.* J Chronic Dis 17:57, 1964.
17. THOMPSON, G, KELALIS, P, AND CONNOLLY, D: *Transurethral prostatic resection after myocardial infarction.* JAMA 182:908, 1962.
18. VACANTI, CJ, VANHOUTEN, RJ, AND HILL, RC: *Statistical analysis of relationship of physical status to postoperative mortality in 68,388 cases.* Anesth Analg 49:564, 1970.
19. TARHAN, S, MOFFITT, EA, TAYLOR, WF, ET AL.: *Myocardial infarction after general anesthesia.* JAMA 226:1451, 1972.
20. TOPKINS, MJ, AND ARTUSIO, JF: *Myocardial infarction and surgery: a five year study.* Anesth Analg 43:716, 1964.
21. HILLIS, LD, AND COHN, PF: *Noncardiac surgery in patients with coronary artery disease.* Arch Int Med 138:972, 1978.
22. SAPALA, JA, PONKA, JL, AND DUVERNOY, WF: *Operative and nonoperative risks in the cardiac patient.* J Am Geriatr Soc 23:529, 1975.
23. BUTLER, S, FEENY, N, AND LEVINE, SA: *The patient with heart disease as a surgical risk.* JAMA 95:85, 1930.
24. HICKMAN, J, LIVINGSTONE, H, AND DAVIES, ME: *Surgical and anesthetic risk in cardiac disease.* Arch Surg 31:917, 1935.
25. MORRISON, DR: *The risk of surgery in heart disease.* Surgery 23:561, 1948.
26. HANNIGAN, CW, WROBLEWSKI, F, LEWIS, WH, ET AL.: *Major surgery in patients with healed myocardial infarction.* Am J Med Sci 222:628, 1951.
27. GARCIA, JE, MIDDLETON, SL, AND ANDERSON, AE: *The cardiac patient as a surgical risk.* New Orleans Med Surg J 104:715, 1952.
28. ETSTEN, B, AND PROGER, S: *Operative risk in patients with coronary heart disease.* JAMA 159:845, 1955.

29. Lockhead, RP, Coakley, CS, and Evans, JM: *The risk of major surgery in patients with coronary artery disease.* Am J Med Sci 227:624, 1954.

30. Roberts, R, and Sobel, B: *Elevated plasma MB creatine phosphokinase activity. A specific marker for myocardial infarction in perioperative patients.* Arch Intern Med 136:421, 1976.

31. Lewin, I, Lerner, AG, Green, SH, et al.: *Physical class and physiologic status in prediction of operative mortality in the aged sick.* Am Surg 46:217, 1971.

32. Dana, JB, and Ohler, RL: *Influence of heart disease on surgical risk.* JAMA 162:878, 1956.

33. Steen, PA, Tinker, JH, and Tarhan, S: *Myocardial reinfarction after anesthesia and surgery.* JAMA 239:2566, 1978.

34. Knapp, RB, Topkins, MJ, and Artusio, JF, Jr.: *The cerebrovascular accident and coronary occlusion in anesthesia.* JAMA 182:332, 1962.

35. Fraser, JG, Ramachandran, PR, and Davis, HS: *Anesthesia and recent myocardial infarction.* JAMA 199:318, 1967.

36. Master, AM, Dack, S, and Jaffe, HL: *Postoperative coronary artery occlusion.* JAMA 116:1415, 1938.

37. Mauney, FM, Ebert, PA, and Sabiston, DC: *Postoperative myocardial infarction: a study of predisposing factors, diagnosis and mortality in a high risk group of surgical patients.* Ann Surg 172:497, 1970.

38. Wasserman, F, Beilet, S, and Saichek, RP: *Postoperative myocardial infarction report of 25 cases.* N Engl J Med 252:967, 1955.

39. Wroblenski, F, and Ladve, JS: *Myocardial infarction as a postoperative complication of major surgery.* JAMA 150:121, 1952.

40. DePeystter, FA, Paul, O, and Gilchrist, RK: *Risk of urgent surgery in the presence of myocardial infarction and angina.* Arch Surg 65: 448, 1952.

41. Driscoll, A, Hobika, J, Esten, BE, et al.: *Clinically unrecognized myocardial infarction following surgery.* N Engl J Med 264:633, 1961.

42. Roberts, R, and Sobel, BE: *Elevated plasma in MB creatine phosphokinase activity. A specific marker for myocardial infarction in perioperative patients.* Arch Intern Med 136:421, 1976.

43. Pyle, RB, Blomberg, DJ, Burke, MD, et al.: *CPK-MB isoenzyme use in diagnosis of acute myocardial infarction in the early postoperative period.* J Thorac Cardiovasc Surg 71:884, 1976.

44. Platt, MR, Mills, LJ, Parkey, RW, et al.: *Perioperative myocardial infarction diagnosed by technetium 99m stannous pyrophosphate myocardial scintigrams.* Circulation 54: (6 suppl 3): III24-7, 1976.

45. Scher, KS, and Tice, DA: *Operative risk in patients with previous coronary artery bypass.* Arch Surg 111:807, 1976.

46. Edwards, WH, Mulhern, JL, and Walker, WE: *Vascular reconstructive surgery following myocardial revascularization.* Ann Surg 187:653, 1978.

47. McCollum, CH, Garcia-Rinaldi, R, Graham, JM, et al.: *Myocardial revascularization prior to subsequent major surgery in patients with coronary artery disease.* Surgery 81:302, 1977.

48. Crawford, ES, Morris, GC, Howell, JF, et al.: *Operative risk in patients with previous coronary artery bypass.* Ann Thorac Surg 26:215, 1978.

49. Bernhard, VM, Johnson, WD, and Peterson, JJ: *Carotid artery stenosis—association with surgery for coronary artery disease.* Arch Surg 105:837, 1972.

50. Eddleman, EE, Frommeyer, WB, Lyle, DP, et al.: *Critical analysis of clinical factors in estimating the severity of aortic valve disease.* Am J Cardiol 31:687, 1973.

51. Franks, S, Johnson, A, and Ross, J: *Natural history of valvular aortic stenosis.* Br Heart J 35:41, 1973.

52. Henry, WL, Morganroth, J, Pearlman, AS, et al.: *Relation between echocardiographically determined left atrial size and atrial fibrillation.* Circulation 53:273, 1976.

53. Devereux, RB, Perloff, JK, Reichek, N, et al.: *Mitral valve prolapse.* Circulation 54:4, 1976.

54. DeMaria AN, Amsterdam, EA, Vismara, ND, et al.: *Arrhythmias in the mitral valve prolapse syndrome—prevalance, nature and frequency.* Ann Intern Med 84:656, 1976.

55. Pocock, WA, and Boriow, JB: *Postexercise arrhythmias in the ballooning posterior mitral valve leaflet syndrome.* Am Heart J 80: 740, 1976.

56. Swartz, MH, Telcholz, LE, and Donoso, E: *Mitral valve prolapse—a review of associated arrhythmias.* Am J Med 62:377, 1977.

57. Sloman, G, Wong, M, and Walker, J: *Arrhythmias on exercise in patients with abnormalities of the posterior mitral valve.* Am Heart J 83:312, 1972.

58. Winkle, RA, Lopes, MG, Popp, RL, et al.: *Life threatening arrhythmias in the mitral valve prolapse syndrome.* Am J Med 60: 961, 1976.

59. LeBauer, EJ, Perloff, JK, and Kelleher, TF: *The isolated systolic click with bacterial endocarditis.* Am Heart J 73:534, 1967.

60. Wei, JY, Buckley, BH, Schaeffer, AH, et al.: *Mitral valve prolapse syndrome and recurrent ventricular tachyarrhythmias.* Ann Intern Med 89:6, 1978.

61. Jeresaty, RM: *Sudden death in the mitral valve prolapse-click syndrome.* Am J Cardiol 37:317, 1976.

62. Gooch, AS, Vicencio, F, Maranhoa, V, et al.: *Arrhythmias and left ventricular asynergy in the prolapsing mitral leaflet syndrome.* Am J Cardiol 29:611, 1972.

63. Campbell, RWF, Goldman, MG, Fiddler, GI, et al.: *Ventricular arrhythmias in the syndrome of balloon deformity of the mitral valve. Definition of a possible high risk subgroup.* Br Heart J 38:1053, 1976.

64. Leichtman, D, Nelson, R, Gobel FL, et al.: *Bradycardia with mitral valve prolapse. A potential mechanism of sudden death.* Ann Intern Med 85:453, 1976.

65. Shappell, SD, Marshal, CE, Brown, RE, et al.: *Sudden death and familial occurrences of mid-systolic click, late systolic murmur syndrome.* Circulation 48:1128, 1973.

66. Shappell, SD, and Marchal, LE: *Ballooning posterior leaflet syndrome: syncope and sudden death.* Arch Intern Med 135:664, 1974.

67. Corrigal, D, Bolen, J, Hancock, EW, et al.: *Mitral valve prolapse and infective endocarditis.* Am J Med 63:215, 1977.

68. Barlow, JB, Bosman, CK, Pocock, WA, et al.: *Late systolic murmur and non-ejection clicks (mid-late) systolic clicks. An analysis of 90 patients.* Br Heart J 30:203, 1968.

69. LeBaner, EJ, Pekioff, JK, and Kellher, TF: *The isolated systolic click with bacterial endocarditis.* Am Heart J 73:534, 1967.

70. Stannard, M, and Gable, AJ: *Endocarditis and the mitral valve.* Br Heart J 4:683, 1967.

71. Lackman, AS, Bramwell-Jones, DM, Lahler, TB, et al.: *Infective endocarditis in the ballooning mitral leaflet syndrome.* Br Heart J 37:326, 1975.

72. Davies, MJ, Moore, BD, and Braimbridge, MV: *The floppy mitral valve, study of incidence, pathology, and complications in surgical, necropsy, and forensic material.* Br Heart J 46:468, 1978.

73. Maron, BJ, Roberts, WC, Edwards, J, et al.: *Sudden death in patients with hypertrophic cardiomyopathy: characterization of 26 patients without functional limitation.* Am J Cardiol 41:803, 1978.

74. Maron, BJ, Lipson, LC, and Roberts, WC: *Malignant hypertrophic cardiomyopathy: identification of a subgroup of families with usually frequent premature death.* Am J Cardiol 41: 1733, 1978.

75. Savage, DD, Seides, SF, Maron, BJ, et al.: *Prevalence of arrhythmias during 24 hour electrocardiographic monitoring and exercise testing in patients with obstructive and non-obstructive hypertrophic cardiomyopathy.* Circulation 59:866, 1979.

76. Frank, S, and Braunwald, E: *Idiopathic hypertrophic subaortic stenosis. Clinical analysis of 126 patients with emphasis on the natural history.* Circulation 37:759, 1968.

77. Maille, JG: *Patients with cardiac valve prostheses. Subsequent anesthetic management for non-cardiac surgical procedures.* Can Aneasth Soc J 20:207, 1973.

78. Katholi, RE, Nolan, SD, and McGuire, L: *Living with prosthetic heart valves. Subsequent non-cardiac operations and the risk of thromboembolism and hemorrhage.* Am Heart J 92:162, 1976.

79. Tinker, JH, and Tarhan, S: *Discontinuing anticoagulant therapy in surgical patients with cardiac valve prostheses.* JAMA 239:738, 1978.

80. Katholi, RE, Nolan, SP, and McGuire, LD: *The managements of anticoagulation during noncardiac operations in patients with prosthetic heart valves. A prospective study.* Am Heart J 96:163, 1978.

81. Arnett, EN, and Roberts, WC: *Prosthetic valve endocarditis.* Am J Cardiol 38:281, 1976.

82. Kaplan, EL, Rich, H, Gerson, YW, et al.: *A collaborative study of infective endocarditis in the 70's; emphasis on infections in patients who have undergone cardiovascular surgery.* Circulation 59:327, 1979.
83. Hewson, J: *Cardiopulmonary complications in the surgical patient.* J Maine Med Assoc 64:73, 1973.
84. Forrester, JS, Diamond, G, Chatterjee, K, et al.: *Medical therapy of acute myocardial infarction by application of hemodynamic subsets.* N Engl J Med 295:1356, 1404, 1976.
85. Cooperman, LH, and Price, HL: *Pulmonary edema in the operative and postoperative period: a review of 40 cases.* Ann Surg 172:883, 1970.
86. Juler, GL, Stemmer, EA, and Connolly, JE: *Complications of prophylactic digitalization in thoracic surgery patients.* J Thorac Cardiovasc Surg 58:352, 1962.
87. Wheat, MW, and Burford, HT: *Digitalis in surgery, extension of classical indications.* J Thorac Cardiovasc Surg 41: 163, 1961.
88. Finkbeiner, JA, Wroblewski, F, and LaDoe, JS: *Effect of chronic auricular fibrillation on operative risk.* Am J Med Sci 227:535, 1954.
89. Deutsch, S, and Dalen, JE: *Indications for prophylactic digitalization.* Anesthesiology. 30:648, 1969.
90. Salem, DN: *Disorders of cardiac rhythm.* Orthop Clin North Am 9:715, 1978.
91. Mowry, FM, and Reynolds, EW, Jr.: *Cardiac rhythm disturbances complicating resectional surgery of the lung.* Ann Intern Med 61:688, 1964.
92. Beck-Nielsen, J, Sorensen, HR, and Alstrup, P: *Atrial fibrillation following thoracotomy for non-cardiac diseases in particular cancer of the lung.* Acta Med Scand 193:425, 1973.
93. Ghosh, P, and Pakrashi, BC: *Cardiac dysrhythmias after thoracotomy.* Br Heart J 34:374, 1972.
94. Cohen, MG, and Pastor, BH: *Delayed cardiac arrhythmias following non-cardiac thoracic surgery.* Dis Chest 32:435, 1957.
95. Krosnik, A, and Wasserman, F: *Cardiac arrhythmias in the older age group following thoracic surgery.* Am J Med Sci 230:541, 1955.
96. Currens, JH, White, PD, and Churchill, ED: *Cardiac arrhythmias following thoracic surgery.* New Engl J Med 229:360, 1943.
97. Baily, CC, and Betts, RH: *Cardiac arrhythmias following pneumonectomy.* New Eng J Med 229:356, 1943.
98. Massie, E, and Valle, AR: *Cardiac arrhythmias complicating total pneumonectomy.* Ann Intern Med 26:231, 1947.
99. Rogers, WR, Wroblewski, F, and Ladvefs, G: *Supraventricular tachycardiac complicating surgical procedures.* Circulation 7:192, 1953.
100. Tyras, DH, Stothert, JC, Jr. Kaiser, GC, et al.: *Supraventricular tachyarrhythmias after myocardial revascularization: A randomized trial of prophylactic digitalization.* J Thorac Cardivasc Surg 77:310, 1979.
101. Goldman, L: *Supraventricular tachyarrhythmias in hospitalized adults after surgery.* Chest 73:450, 1978.
102. Vanik, PE, and Davis, HS: *Cardiac arrhythmias during halothane anesthesia.* Anesth Analg 74:299, 1968.
103. Leahey, EB, Jr., Reiffel, JA, Drusin, RE, et al.: *Interaction between quinidine and digoxin.* JAMA 240:533, 1978.
104. Kennedy, HL, and Underhill, SJ: *Frequent or complex ventricular ectopy in apparently healthy subjects: a clinical study of 25 cases.* Am J Cardiol 38:141, 1976.
105. Ruffy, R, and Ziques, DP: *VPCs in the otherwise normal heart.* Prim Cardiol 3:27, 1977.
106. Jervel, A, and Lange-Nielsen, F: *Congenital deaf-mutism, functional heart disease with prolongation of the QT interval and sudden death.* Am Heart J 59:59, 1957.
107. Katz, RI, and Bloger, ST: *Cardiac arrhythmias during anesthesia and operation.* Anesthesiology 33:193, 1970.
108. Taylor, G, Larson, CP, and Drestwich, R: *Unexpected cardiac arrest during anesthesia and surgery.* JAMA 236:27, 1976.
109. McClure, JN, Skardasis, GH, and Brown, JM: *Cardiac arrest in the operating room.* Am Surg 38: 241, 1972.
110. Pierce, JA: *Cardiac arrests and deaths associated with anesthesia.* Anesth analg 45:407, 1966.
111. Stephen, CR: *Cardiac arrest is on the decline.* Ann Surg 155:345, 1962.
112. Dripps, RC, Lamant, A, and Eckenhoff, JE: *The role of anesthesia in surgical mortality.* JAMA 178:261, 1961.

Goldman, Lee, Cardiac Risks & Complications on Non-Cardiac Surgery, Ann. Surg, 198:780, Dec 1983.

113. Bomar, WE, and Thompson, WR: *Preoperative factors in providing of cardiac arrest.* JAMA 172:41, 1960.

114. Dyckner, T, and Webster, PO: *Ventricular extrasystoles and intracellular electrocytes before and after K+ and Mg++ infusions in patients on diuretic treatment.* Am Heart J 97:12, 1979.

115. Vandam, LD, and McLemare, GA, Jr.: *Circulatory arrest in patients with complete heart block during anesthesia and surgery.* Am J Med 47:518, 1957.

116. Berg, GR, and Kotler, MN: *The significance of bilateral bundle branch block in the preoperative patient. A retrospective electrocardiographic and clinical study in 30 patients.* Chest 59:62, 1971.

117. VenKataraman, K, Madias, JE, and Hood, WB, Jr.: *Indications for prophylactic preoperative insertion of pacemakers in patients with right bundle branch block and left anterior hemiblock.* Chest 68:501, 1975.

118. Pastore, JO, Yurchak, PM, and Jans, KM: *The risk of advanced heart block in surgical patients with right bundle branch block and left axis deviation.* Circulation (Suppl) 50:218, 1974.

119. Kunstadt, D, Punja, M, Cagin, N, et al.: *Bifascicular block: a clinical and electrophysiologic study.* Am Heart J 86: 173, 1973.

120. Rooney, SM, Goldiner, PL, and Muss, E: *Relationship of right bundle branch block and marked left axis deviation to complete heart block during general anesthesia.* Anesthesiology 44: 64, 1976.

121. Burman, SO: *Digitalis and thoracic surgery.* J Thorac Cardiovasc Surg 50:875, 1965.

122. Shields, TW, and Ujiki, GT: *Digitalization for prevention of arrhythmias following pulmonary surgery.* Surg Gynecol Obstet 126:743, 1968.

123. Wheat, MW, Jr., and Burford, TH: *Digitalis in surgery: extension of classical indications.* J Thorac Cardiovasc Surg 41:162, 1961.

124. Hurt, RL, and Bates, M: *The value of quinidine in the prevention of cardiac arrhythmias after pulmonary resection.* Thorax 13:39, 1958.

125. Johnson, JW, Dickstein, RA, Fruvehan, CT, et al.: *Prophylactic digitalization for coronary artery bypass surgery.* Circulation 53:819, 1976.

126. O'Kane, H, Geha, A, Bale, A, et al.: *Prophylactic digitalization in aorta coronary bypass patients.* Circulation 45&46 (Supl II):199, 1972.

127. Cerney, CI: *The prophylaxis of cardiac arrhythmias complicating pulmonary surgery.* Scand J Thoracic Surg 34:105, 1957.

128. Viljoen, JF: *Propranolol and cardiac surgery.* Thorac Cardiovasc Surg 64: 826, 1972.

129. Tyerg, GF: *Circulatory effects of propranolol and cardiopulmonary bypass.* J Surg Res 18:181, 1975.

130. Kaplan, JA, Dunbar, RW, Bland, JW, et al.: *Propranolol and cardiac surgery: A problem for the anesthesiologist.* Anesth Analg 59:571, 1975.

131. Jones, EL, Kaplan, JA, Dorney, ER, et al.: *Propranolol therapy in patients undergoing myocardial revascularization.* Am J Cardiol 38:696, 1976.

132. Moran, JM, Mulet, J, Caralps, JM, et al.: *Coronary revascularization in patients receiving propranolol.* Circulation 50 (Supp): 116, 1974.

133. Kirsh, MM, Behreudt, DM, Jackson, AP, et al.: *Myocardial revascularization in patients receiving long term propanolol therapy.* Ann Thorac Surg 25:117, 1978.

134. Carlaps, JM, Mulet, J, Weinice, HR, et al.: *Results of coronary artery surgery in patients receiving propranolol.* J Thorac Cardiovasc Surg 67:526, 1974.

135. Manners, JM, and Walters, FJ: *Beta adrenergic blockade and anesthesia.* Anesthesia 34:3, 1979.

136. Boudoulas, H, Snyder, GL, Lewis, RP, et al.: *Safety and rationale for continuation of propranolol therapy during coronary bypass operation.* Ann Thorac Surg 26:222, 1978.

137. Prys-Roberts, E, Foex, P, Bird, GP, et al.: *Studies of anesthesia with relation to hypertension V: Adrenergic beta receptor blockade.* Br J Anesth 45:671, 1973.

138. Kaplan, JA and Dunbar, RW: *Propranolol and surgical anesthesia.* Anesth Analg 55:1, 1976.

139. Faulkner, SL, Hopkins, JT, and Boerth, RC: *Time required for complete recovery from chronic propranolol therapy.* New Engl Med J 289:607, 1973.

140. Coltart, DJ, Cayen, MN, Stinson, EB, et al.: *Investigation of the safe withdrawal period for propranolol in patients scheduled for open heart surgery.* Br Heart J 37:1228, 1975.

141. Boudoulas, N, Beaver, BM, Kates, RE, et al.: *Pharmaco dynamics of ionotropic and chronotropic responses to oral therapy with propranolol.* Chest 73:146, 1978.

142. Myers, JH, and Horwitz, LD: *Hemodynamic and metabolic response after abrupt withdrawal of longterm propranolol.* Circulation 58:196, 1976.

143. Mizgala, HF, and Coonsell, J: *Acute coronary syndromes following abrupt cessation of oral propranolol therapy.* Can Med Assoc J 114:1123, 1976.

144. *Should propranolol be stopped before surgery?* Med Letter 18:41, 1976.

145. Harrison, DC, and Alderman, EL: *Discontinuation of propranolol therapy-cause of rebound angina pectoris and acute coronary events.* Chest 69:1, 1976.

146. Myers, MG, Freeman, MR, Juna, ZA, et al.: *Propranolol withdrawal in angina pectoris, a prospective study.* Am Heart J 97:298, 1979.

147. Raabe, DS, Meengs, WL, Crary, SL, et al.: *Risk of suddenly discontinuing propranolol therapy before coronary arteriography.* Circulation 52:12, 1975.

148. Shand, DG, and Wood, AJ: *Propranolol withdrawal syndrome—Why?* Circulation 58: 202, 1978.

149. Spitzer, S, Corver, J, and Mason, D: *Withdrawal of cardiac drugs prior to general surgery.* Practical Cardiol 5:121, 1979.

150. *Acrylic cement and the cardiovascular system.* Lancet 3: 1002, 1974.

151. Modig J, et al: *Arterial hypotension and hypoxemia during total hip replacement. The importance of thromboplastic products, fat embolism and acrylic monomers.* Acta Anaesthesiol Scand 19:28, 1975.

152. Bellocci, F, Santarelli, P, DiGennaro, M, et al.: *The risk of cardiac complications in surgical patients with bifascicular block. A clinical and electrophysiologic study in 98 patients.* Chest 77:343, 1980.

153. Kopriva, CS, Brown, AC, and Pappas, G: *Hemodynamics during general anesthesia in patients receiving propranolol.* Anesthesiol 48:28, 1978.

154. Miller, RR, Olson, HG, Amsterdam, EA, et al.: *Propranolol-withdrawal rebound phenomenon. Exacerbation of coronary events after abrupt cessation of antianginal therapy.* N Engl J Med 293:416, 1975.

155. Bonchek, LI, and Olinger, GN: *Intra-aortic balloon counter-pulsation for cardiac support during noncardiac operations.* J Thorac Cardiovasc Surg 78:147, 1979.

APPENDIX: DRUGS USED IN THE TREATMENT OF VENTRICULAR ARRHYTHMIAS

Quinidine

USES

Control of atrial and ventricular extrasystoles
Use in atrial fibrillation and atrial flutter, after digitalization, and when ventricular rate is controlled
Ventricular tachycardia
Wolff-Parkinson-White syndrome

DOSAGE, ADMINISTRATION, AND FATE

Intravenous administration rarely used because of severe hypotensive action
Intramuscular quinidine gluconate, 200 mg every 8 hours; peak effect in 30 to 90 minutes
Oral doses of quindine rapidly and completely absorbed by gastrointestinal tract; maxi-

mal effects in 1 to 3 hours; effects last 6 to 8 hours; quinidine sulfate, 200 mg tablets, every 6 hours; quinidine sulfate, 300 mg tablets every 6 hours; quinidine gluconate, 330 mg tablets every 8 hours
Half-life of quinidine: 7 hours
Therapeutic blood levels, 1 to 5 mcg/ml
Ten to fifteen per cent excreted by kidneys unchanged in 24 hours
Appreciable amount bound to plasma protein
Remainder degraded by liver
Special high dose schedules used in initial conversion of atrial arrhythmias

SIDE EFFECTS AND COMPLICATIONS

Hypotension
Widened QRS normally occurs but is discontinued if widening is greater than 25 percent
Prolongation of P-R interval
Depression of sinoatrial node may lead to nodal or ventricular escape rhythm
Anorexia, nausea, vomiting, diarrhea
Tinnitus, hearing disturbance, visual disturbances, headache, urticaria
Idiosyncratic reactions (vascular collapse)
Thrombocytopenia
Convulsions
Quinidine fever
May cause a rise in digitalis levels, necessitating reduction in digitalis dosage

CONTRAINDICATIONS

Second-degree or third-degree heart block
History of quinidine related thrombocytopenia
Use cautiously in presence of digitalis toxicity and hypotension

Propranolol

USES

Digitalis induced arrhythmias, both ventricular and supraventricular
Atrial flutter and fibrillation: increase degree of atrioventricular block
Paroxysmal atrial tachycardia, nodal tachycardia
Premature atrial contractions, premature nodal contractions
Premature ventricular contractions
Arrhythmias associated with Wolff-Parkinson-White syndrome

DOSAGE, ADMINISTRATION, AND FATE

Intravenous dosage, 0.5 to 1.0 mg given at 2 to 3 minute intervals
Total dose not to exceed 0.1 mg/kg

Onset of action within 3 minutes
Duration of action, 4 to 6 hours
Oral dosage, 10 to 100 mg every 6 hours
Half-life: 6 hours for oral dose
Therapeutic plasma levels, 40 to 85 mcg/ml

SIDE EFFECTS AND COMPLICATIONS

Hypotension
Acute onset of heart failure
Bronchospasm
Hypoglycemia
Nausea, tiredness, visual disturbances, nightmares, insomnia
Mild diarrhea, rashes

CONTRAINDICATIONS

Severe hypotension
Bronchial asthma
Severe congestive heart failure
Presence of atrioventricular block

Diphenylhydantoin

USES

Best results when arrhythmias are transient, as is often seen with anesthesia induction after cardioversion and digitalis toxicity
Generally no effects on atrial arrhythmias other than in digitalis toxicity

DOSAGE, ADMINISTRATION, AND FATE

Intravenous administration must be very slow and drug diluted with normal saline
Usual dosage, 75 to 250 mg over 2 to 5 minutes
Onset of action, within 10 minutes
Oral or intramuscular dosage is a 1 gm loading dose in individual dose, then 300 to 400 mg every day
Therapeutic drug level, 10 to 20 mcg/ml
Half-life: 24 to 36 hours
Parahydroxylated in the liver

SIDE EFFECTS AND COMPLICATIONS

Hypotension
Sinoatrial node depression resulting in bradycardia

Nervousness, ataxia, tremor, nystagmus
Bone marrow depression, megoblastic anemia, lupus-like syndrome, infectious mononucleosis-like syndrome, lymphadenopathy
Transient headache or nausea

CONTRAINDICATIONS

Severe sinus bradycardia
Second-degree or third-degree heart block

Lidocaine

USES

Ventricular arrhythmias
Rarely, if ever, used in atrial arrhythmias but may be useful in pre-excitation syndromes (Wolff-Parkinson-White syndrome)

DOSAGE, ADMINISTRATION, AND FATE

Intravenous dosage: 50 to 100 mg bolus followed by constant drip of 1 to 4 mg/min (20 to 50 mcg/kg/minute)
Rapid onset within 1 to 2 minutes
Metabolized 90 percent in liver
Ten percent excreted unchanged by the kidneys
Half-life: 1½ to 2 hours
Therapeutic plasma levels: 1.4 to 6.0 mcg/ml

SIDE EFFECTS AND COMPLICATIONS

Hypotension
Central nervous system depression, convulsions, muscular twitching, vague visual disturbances, tinnitus, dizziness, sweating, sensations of heat or cold or numbness, discomfort in breathing or swallowing, and slurred speech
Anorexia, nausea, vomiting

CONTRAINDICATIONS

Second-degree or third-degree atrioventricular block

Procainamide

USES

Control of atrial and ventricular extrasystoles
Ventricular tachycardia

Use in atrial flutter and atrial fibrillation after digitalization
Control of arrhythmias in Wolff-Parkinson-White syndrome

DOSAGE, ADMINISTRATION, AND FATE

Intravenous administration in initial bolus of 25 to 100 mg followed by carefully titrated drip of 1 to 4 mg/minute
  Blood pressure should be monitored carefully and patient's electrocardiogram should be continually monitored
Oral doses of procainamide rapidly and almost completely absorbed
  Maximal blood level reached in 1 hour
  Widely distributed and tissue concentration higher than plasma concentrations
Most procainamide excreted unchanged by the kidneys
  Usual dosage, 250 mg to 1 gram every 3 to 4 hours
Half-life: 3 to 4 hours
Therapeutic plasma levels: 4 to 10 mcg/ml

SIDE EFFECTS AND COMPLICATIONS

Idiosyncratic reaction (vascular collapse)
Hypotension
Widening of QRS complex greater than 25 percent
Skin rash
Lupus-like syndrome of agranulocytosis
Cinchonism, tinnitus, headache, nausea, visual disturbances
Nausea, vomiting

CONTRAINDICATIONS

Second-degree or third-degree atrioventricular block
History of lupus-like syndrome
Caution in presence of digitalis toxicity, hypotension

Disopyramide Phosphate

USES

Ventricular arrhythmias

DOSAGE, ADMINISTRATION, AND FATE

Initial loading dose of 300 mg followed by 400 to 800 mg every day in divided doses
Therapeutic effects are usually attained 30 minutes to 3 hours after administration of loading dose

Almost completely absorbed by gastrointestinal tract
Therapeutic plasma levels: 2 to 4 mcg/ml
Plasma half-life: 6.7 hours
Clearance, 80 percent by kidney and 10 percent by bowel

SIDE EFFECTS AND COMPLICATIONS

Hypotension
Heart failure
Heart block
Urinary retention
QRS widening
Atrial tachyarrhythmias in undigitalized patients

CONTRAINDICATIONS

Glaucoma
Benign prostatic hypertrophy
Cardiogenic shock
Pre-existing heart block

Bretylium Tosylate

USES

Acute control of recurrent ventricular tachycardia or ventricular fibrillation which has been resistant to standard antiarrhythmia drugs
It is unclear from available data if bretylium tosylate significantly suppresses premature ventricular contractions
Bretylium tosylate is not a "first line" antiarrhythmic agent. It should be used only when traditional drugs have been ineffective.

DOSAGE, ADMINISTRATION, AND FATE

Oral bretylium tosylate is unavailable
Intravenous undiluted bretylium tosylate (500 mg/10cc ampules)
- For ventricular fibrillation: 5 to 10 mg/kg of body weight by rapid intravenous infusion
- Repeated at 15 to 30 minute intervals until a total of 30 mg/kg of body weight has been given
- Onset of action is rapid—within minutes

Intravenous diluted bretylium tosylate (500 mg/10cc ampule with 40cc of dextrose or sodium chloride solution)

For ventricular tachycardia and premature ventricular contractions: 5 to 10 mg/kg of body weight over a period of 78 minutes
Repeat dose in 1 to 2 hours
Onset of action is 20 minutes to 2 hours
Constant intravenous drip (1 gm bretylium tosylate in 500DSW)
For ventricular tachycardia, ventricular premature contractions: infuse 1 to 2 mg/minute
Intramuscular undiluted bretylium tosylate
For ventricular tachycardia and premature ventricular contractions: 5 to 10 mg/kg of body weight
Dosage may be repeated in 1 to 2 hours
Every 6 to 8 hours for 3 to 5 days
Onset of action 20 minutes to 2 hours
70 to 80 percent is excreted unchanged in the urine within 24 hours
Another 10 percent is excreted over the next 72 hours

SIDE EFFECTS AND COMPLICATIONS

Hypotension is seen in most patients due to adrenergic neuronal blockade
Patient should be kept supine until a tolerance develops
Transient hypertension and aggravation of arrhythmia
Nausea and vomiting is associated with rapid intravenous infusion

CONTRAINDICATIONS AND SPECIAL WARNINGS

Current data contraindicates use of bretylium tosylate in arrhythmias associated with digitalis toxicity
Critical aortic stenosis, pulmonary hypertension, or other conditions with fixed cardiac output

Chapter 4
DERMATOLOGY

Stephanie H. Pincus, M.D.

This chapter will focus on two aspects of dermatologic problems: those common problems likely to be encountered in a surgical patient and those infrequent problems where modification of standard surgical procedures and/or specialized therapy may be necessary. For more extensive information one of the standard dermatologic textbooks[1,2,3] should be consulted.

DERMATOLOGIC DIAGNOSIS

History

Dermatologic diagnosis depends upon an accurate history. Family history, occupational history, drug history, and environmental exposure (e.g., sunlight) may be of particular relevance.

Questions of particular importance include:

1. When did the eruption (or lesion) begin? Have there been exacerbations and remissions?
2. Where did the eruption (or lesion) begin? Were there multiple sites or was the lesion solitary?
3. What did the initial lesions look like? Were they pruritic? Painful?
4. Has the eruption spread? Locally or widely?
5. Has the area (or lesion) been previously treated? By a physician or the patient? What medications have been applied?

6. Are there any other environmental factors? Toxic exposure? Sunlight? Ingested medications? What is the time relation between the suspected environmental factor and the eruption?

Diagnostic Tests

In addition to the standard hematologic, biochemical, and bacteriologic tests, certain specialized diagnostic tests are useful in dermatologic diagnosis. For more detailed descriptions of how to perform these tests a useful source is *A Manual of Dermatologic Therapeutics* by Kenneth A. Arndt.[4]

KOH PREPARATION

Microscopic examination of skin scrapings in the presence of 10 percent potassium hydroxide (KOH) is employed for detection of dermatophyte and yeast infection. If hyphae and/or spores are detected in the keratinous material, the KOH text is regarded as positive. Tinea versicolor is distinguished by many short hyphae and numerous spores. In candidal infections, budding yeast and/or pseudohyphae may be detected. A KOH preparation is indicated in all cases of suspected fungal disease such as scaling eruptions of the scalp, body, groin, intertriginous folds, feet, and jaw. This test is usually available in microbiology laboratories.

FUNGAL CULTURE

When culture of skin, nails, and/or hair is combined with a KOH examination, fungus is identified in a greater percentage of cases. However, fungal cultures rarely provide results in less than two weeks. Fungal culture is indicated in tinea capitis, suspected animal-borne fungus, and in refractory or diagnostically puzzling eruptions.

CYTOLOGIC EXAMINATION (TZANCK TEST)

Cytologic examination of material from bullae and vesicles is utilized in the diagnosis of bullous and viral diseases and depends upon recognition of acantholytic cells or multinucleate giant cells, respectively.

PATCH TESTS

Patch testing involves the application of suspected allergens to the skin in order to ascertain whether the patient is indeed allergic to the material.[5]

SKIN BIOPSIES

The microscopic examination of tissue is an essential aid to diagnosis. Though frequently a biopsy can be deferred until advice can be obtained from a consultant, in certain instances (such as vasculitis) a prompt biopsy is indicated. Small elliptical excisions may be done, however, circular punch biopsies are simpler, leave a minimal scar, and usually do not require the use of sutures. The biopsy site should be selected with care. For most inflammatory processes, nodules or plaques, the center should be selected. When purpuric or vesicular-bullous lesions are biopsied, fresh, nontraumatized lesions should be selected. For most bullous lesions the biopsy should include the edge of the lesion and some adjacent normal skin. A 4 mm punch will usually provide adequate tissue. However, when multiple bacteriologic tests are to be performed, multiple biopsies may be required. Histopathologic interpretation of skin lesions is a difficult task. The specimens may on occasion need to be submitted to pathologists specifically trained in dermatopathology.

CUTANEOUS IMMUNOFLUORESCENCE

There are two types of immunofluorescence available: *direct immunofluorescence,* utilized to detect the presence of immunoglobin and complement in skin and *indirect immunofluorescence,* which identifies the presence of circulating antibodies directed against skin tissue.[6] Direct immunofluorescence is indicated in the diagnosis of bullous disease and may be helpful in systemic lupus erythematosus or vasculitis. Indirect immunofluorescence is indicated in the diagnosis of bullous eruptions such as pemphigus and bullous pemphigoid.

DERMATOLOGIC THERAPEUTICS

In an effort to modify the physical chemical properties of the skin surface, numerous medications and treatments may be applied. In general, when the skin is acutely inflammed, topical steroids are employed to reduce the inflammation and wet dressings are used to remove the exudate and edema fluid. At the other end of the dermatologic spectrum are conditions characterized by "dryness" with scaling and thickening. These conditions are treated by the use of occlusive ointments which retain water within the skin, thus providing additional lubrication.

Wet Dressings

Wet dressings are used in many different acute inflammatory conditions characterized by serous exudate and crusts. These relieve the patient's symptoms and gently debride the lesion regardless of the cause of the acute dermatitis. They are also helpful in superficial erosions and deep ulcers where necrotic and/or infected material must be removed. Wet dressings depend upon evaporative cooling and must be open in order to be effective. Covering wet dressings with plastic causes maceration, retards evaporation, and promotes secondary infection. Burow's solution (aluminum acetate) used in a 1:20 or 1:40 dilution (.01 to .005%) is rarely irritating. However, if Burow's solution is not available or the patient cannot tolerate it, normal saline can be employed. Silver nitrate and potassium permanganate both tend to cause excessive staining. The total duration of wet dressing application should be 20 to 30 minutes and treatments should be repeated three or four times a day. If any additional medications are to be employed, a good time to apply them is immediately after completing a wet dressing treatment.

Occlusive Dressings

In order to increase the penetration of various topical medications, air-tight plastic wrap may be applied to the skin. Occlusion is especially helpful in refractory, inflammatory conditions of the hands and feet. Though occlusion is frequently useful on a short term basis, a potential complication is the development of bacterial or fungal superinfection in the moist occluded areas. This is especially a problem in hair bearing areas where folliculitis may develop. In addition, long term use of occlusion may lead to atrophy and telangiectasis. When large areas of the body surface are covered by occlusive plastic, there may be significant precutaneous absorption of steroids. Usually only creams or gels are covered by occlusive wraps.

Hair Removal

Incisions in hair bearing areas require the removal of hair prior to the procedure. The usual method employed is shaving. Problems include multiple nicks and/or abrasions as well as the discomfort experienced during hair regrowth. For patients with very curly hair where ingrown hairs are a problem (such as pseudofolliculitis barbae) the use of depilatory cream will provide more satisfactory hair removal. A variety of commercially produced agents are available, the most satisfactory of which contain thioglycolate.

TOPICAL MEDICATIONS

Dermatologic vehicles can be characterized by their water content: *Liquids* with or without active ingredients such as aluminum acetate or potassium permanganate are used primarily for wet dressings. *Creams* consist of an emulsion or semisolid suspension of oil in water and are used when eruptions are moist or do not require lubrication. *Gels* which liquify upon contact with skin are especially useful in hair bearing areas. *Ointments* consist of emulsions of water in oil. In general, ointments are more occlusive, retain water, and provide additional lubrication.

Steroids

The mainstays of topical dermatologic treatment are topical steroids (Table 1). Vehicles for topical steroids include: ointments, creams, gels, and liquids. The particular form selected will, of necessity, vary with the particular condition under treatment. A wide variety of topical formulations are available, and the differences between apparently similar products may be slight. The accompanying table divides topical steroids into various groups depending upon their potency. It may be best for the nondermatologist to select one product from each potency group and learn how to work with the particular product.

Certain general principles should be kept in mind when topical agents are employed.[7,8,9]

TABLE 1. Commonly Employed Topical Steroid Preparations

Relative Strength	*Formulation*	*Proprietary Products**
Lowest Potency		
Hydrocortisone 0.25%, .5%, 1.0%	Creams	Hytone
Low Potency		
Triamcinolone acetonide or diacetate .025%	Cream or ointment	Aristocort, Kenalog
Fluocinolone acetonide .01%	Cream or solution	Synalar, Fluonide
Intermediate Potency		
Betamethasone valerate or benzoate .01%	Cream, ointment, or solution	Valisone, Benisone
Triamcinolone acetonide .01%	Cream or ointment	Aristocort, Kenalog
Fluocinolone acetonide .025%	Cream or ointment	Synalar, Fluonide
High Potency		
Fluocinonide .05%	Cream, ointment, or gel	Lidex, Topsyn
Betamethasone dipropionate .05%	Cream, ointment, or solution	Diprosone
Halcinonide 0.1%	Cream, ointment, or solution	Halog

*For informational purposes only; this is not a product endorsement

1. The least potent steroid anticipated to be effective should be employed and given an adequate therapeutic trial.
2. Fluorinated steroids (those other than hydrocortisone) should not be applied to the face or groin.
3. Creams are most effective for acute inflammatory processes, and ointments are more satisfactory for chronic (i.e., dry, scaly) processes. Lotions, solutions, or gels are more appropriate for hairy areas.
4. A severe acute inflammatory process will usually respond to an intermediate strength steroid. A mild to moderate process will usually respond to a low strength steroid. The most potent fluorinated steroids should be reserved until other preparations have been tried.

A word should be said about the tars. These preparations have little therapeutic use except for the coal tar derivatives which are frequently employed for chronic atopic dermatitis, seborrheic dermatitis, psoriasis, and refractory eczematous processes.

Anti-Infective Agents

Topical anti-infective agents may be divided into chemical antiseptics and antibiotics.

ANTISEPTICS

An antiseptic is a substance that will inhibit the growth and development of microorganisms without necessarily destroying them. Chemical antiseptics are widely used in an attempt to reduce the incidence of surgical infections and are frequently applied to minor wounds and skin lesions to reduce possible skin infections. A wide variety of agents has been employed and use is frequently dictated by custom of the particular

TABLE 2. Topical Antiseptic Agents

Agent	*Advantages*	*Disadvantages*
Alcohol (70%)	Effective against gram-negative and gram-positive bacteria	Drying to skin; must remain for 2 minutes for optimal effect
Iodine	Very potent	Irritating; contact sensitivity
Hexachlorophene	Effective against gram-negative bacteria	Can be absorbed; toxic in neonates; repeated application necessary for best effect; contact sensitivity
Iodophors	Effective against gram-negative and gram-positive bacteria. Rarely sensitizing	May be toxic if large doses are applied to broken skin
Chlorhexidine	Effective against gram-negative and gram-positive bacteria	Persists on skin
Organic mercurials (i.e., Merthiolate, mercurochrome)		Contact sensitivity; weak bactericidal action toxic to epidermal cells

hospital (Table 2). There are few objective data, however, the following conclusions appear justified.

1. Normal persons disseminate more than 10^7 particles of skin per day, and when skin is colonized by bacteria these bacteria will also be shed.[10]
2. The dispersal of skin organisms can be reduced by the use of topical antiseptics,[10] such as iodophors or chlorhexidine. Persons carrying large numbers of skin microorganisms may benefit from regular treatment with these agents.
3. Controlled studies have failed to demonstrate significant advantages between various surgical scrub techniques.[11]
4. The use of topical antiseptics may reduce the incidence of infection in contaminated wounds, however, added detergents, irritants, and toxins may damage tissues.[13,14]
5. One should be alert for possible adverse effects of the use of antiseptics such as irritant and allergic contact dermatitis and systemic absorption.

ANTIBIOTICS

An antibiotic is an antiseptic substance produced by a microorganism which has the ability to inhibit the growth of or to kill other microorganisms. Topical antibiotics are widely employed and widely promoted for a variety of indications including treatment of infected burns, surgical incisions, pyoderma, and dermatitis as well as for prophylaxis of similar uninfected conditions. Though clinical experience may appear to validate their use, it must be remembered that the majority of uninfected skin injuries will heal without specific antimicrobial treatment.[15,16] Whether or not topical antibiotics are useful has been the subject of considerable controversy with little objective data. A consensus of the available information supports the following conclusions:

1. Topical antibiotics such as neomycin and/or bacitracin and/or polymyxin may be effective in reducing the number of bacteria at a specific site, but systemic antibiotics more effectively and quickly treat individual lesions as well as reduce the number of bacteria at other sites.[15,16,17]
2. Topical antibiotics are somewhat effective in clean wounds or in prophylaxis of infection at sites of intravenous catheters, however, topical iodophors are even more effective.[14,16]
3. No significant advantages of steroid-antibiotic combination medications have been noted.
4. The use of topical antibiotics, as opposed to chemical antiseptics, may promote the development of resistant bacterial strains.[10]
5. The antibiotics as well as additives within the preparations may be a cause of allergic contact dermatitis. This may interfere with wound healing when an acute inflammatory process develops. If the patient develops a contact dermatitis in response to the antibiotic itself, severe reactions may develop if the antibiotic is administered systemically.[5] Though topical antibiotics such as neomycin, polymyxin, or bacitracin are not commonly used for systemic therapy, gentamicin now available as a topical preparation, is used for life threatening gram-negative infections. The risk of systemic skin reactions from the administration of aminoglycosides to patients allergic to the structurally related neomycin is unknown. Topical antibiotics are a common cause of contact dermatitis as illustrated by the fact that neomycin is one of the ten most common contact allergens in North America.[5]

Thus, it seems in the absence of clearcut advantages for these medications that they should be avoided whenever possible.

Antifungal Agents

A variety of agents are available to treat cutaneous fungal infections due to *Candida* and dermatophytes (Table 3). Since all medications are not effective against both organisms, whenever possible, a specific etiologic diagnosis should be made prior to therapy. If such a distinction cannot be made, either clotrimazole or miconazole should be selected since these agents are effective against both dermatophytes and yeasts. Nystatin is effective only against yeasts. Though many agents may be effective against tinea versicolor, the least expensive is selenium sulfide shampoo applied as a lotion to the entire trunk (including areas without apparent involvement).

Griseofulvin is the only systemic antifungal agent employed in the treatment of dermatophyte infections. For that reason it is discussed here. It is the drug of choice in extensive skin involvement and inflammatory fungal infections. Griseofulvin has a

TABLE 3. Antifungal Agents

	Action Spectrum	*Usage*	*Comments*
Topical Agents			
Clotrimazole	Candida Dermatophyte infection Tinea versicolor	1% cream, 1% solution, 2–3 times a day to affected areas; vaginal tablets, 1 per day	Relatively expensive; equivalent to Nystatine
Miconazole	Candida Dermatophyte infection	2% cream, 2–3 times a day	
Nystatin	Candida	Ointment: cream 100,000 units/gm), 2–3 times a day. Oral suspension, 400–600,000 units, 4 times a day. Tablets: (500–100,000 units), 3 times a day	Powder of limited effectiveness; should not be employed in combination mixtures with antibiotics
Selenium sulfide	Tinea versicolor	Apply shampoo or lotion to entire trunk for 15–30 minutes nightly for 5–7 days	Best method for treating tinea versicolor; if used for long periods of time may be irritating
Systemic Agents			
Amphotericin B	Most systemic fungal infections		See Chapter 8, Infectious Diseases
Griseofulvin	Dermatophyte infection	Tablets: 250–500 mg. microsize or 125 mg. ultramicrosize. Skin: 1 gm/day micronized for 1 month. Hair: 1 gm/day, 3–6 weeks. Nails: 1 gm/day, 6–18 months	Interacts with many drugs including anticoagulants and phenobarbital; headache, gastrointestinal distress at high doses

number of adverse effects such as headache and gastrointestinal intolerance and may be carcinogenic; however, the incidence of life threatening complications is low.

SYSTEMIC MEDICATIONS

Patients requiring systemic medication (other than antihistamines) for dermatologic disease should, whenever possible, be seen by a consultant prior to treatment. It is rare for dermatologic disease to be of such severity that such delays will significantly alter the disease's course. Table 4 lists systemic medications employed by dermatologists. It should be noted that patients who have received long term therapy with prednisone, dapsone, sulfapyridine, or methotrexate should not have the medication abruptly dis-

TABLE 4. Systemic Medications Commonly Employed in Dermatology

	Therapeutic Indication	*Usage*
Antibiotics		
Erythromycin	Acne	250 mg, 1 to 4 times/day
Tetracycline	Acne, rosacea, perioral dermatitis	250 mg, 1 to 4 times/day
Antihistamines		
Diphenhydramine	Pruritus of multiple causes including urticaria, acute and chronic dermatitis, infestations, drug eruptions	50 mg, prn up to q 4 hr
Tripelennamine		50 mg, prn to q 4 hr
Hydroxyzine		10–50 mg, po prn to q 4 hr
Chlorpheniramine		4 mg, po prn to q 4 hr
Cyproheptadine	Cholinergic urticaria	4 mg, po q 4 h
Steroids		
Prednisone*	Acute inflammatory disease of skin; contact dermatitis, severe erythema multiforme, and severe drug eruptions; lupus, dermatomyositis, vasculitis, pemphigus, pemphigoid	30–60 mg, daily for initial therapy; then tapered
Triamcinolone acetonide or triamcinolone hexacetonide	Used in depot form for some unreliable patients with chronic dermatitis	30–60 mg IM
Sulfa and Sulfone Medications		
Dapsone†	Dermatitis herpetiformis, subcorneal pustular dermatosis, refractory inflammatory processes	50–100 mg up to 200 mg/day, many adverse effects, variable hemolytic anemia
Sulfapyridine	Dermatitis herpetiformis, subcorneal pustular dermatosis	500 mg up to 3 gm/day
Miscellaneous		
Psoralens	Psoriasis and pigment disorders (frequently with ultraviolet light	
Methotrexate	Severe psoriasis, pustular psoriasis, psoriatic arthropathy, pityriasis rubra pilaris	Must be individualized; frequently given at 7–10 day intervals

*Contraindicated in psoriasis
†Contraindicated in patients with G6PD deficiency

continued without the expectation that a significant relapse may occur. It should also be noted, in particular, dapsone, sulfapyridine, and methotrexate have a variety of toxic adverse effects which must be monitored.

COMMON SKIN DISEASES

Pre-Existing Diseases

The following diseases are all relatively common and are likely to be found in surgical patients. Frequently they are present when a patient is admitted for a surgical procedure. Preoperative evaluation should include history relative to existing skin disease as well as inspection of the planned operative site. Considerations include: What is the skin disease? How should it be treated? How does the skin condition effect the planned surgery? Few precedents and scientific studies relate to the surgical risks of performing procedures in patients with known cutaneous disease. As always, the benefits of the procedure must be balanced against possible risks.

ACNE

Acne is a common disorder of the pilosebaceous apparatus which frequently presents as papular-pustular lesions on the face, anterior chest, and back. In addition, there may be open and closed comedones ("whiteheads" and "blackheads"). When acne is more severe and inflammatory, there may be large nodular cysts. Contrary to popular beliefs, acne frequently persists into the late 20s and 30s. The diagnosis of *mild* to *moderate* acne is usually readily apparent and many patients will have made an appropriate self diagnosis. Therapy of mild to moderate acne includes use of topical agents such as benzoyl peroxide, vitamin A acid, topical clindamycin, and various sulfur and salicylic acid mixtures. Oral treatment with tetracycline or erythromycin is frequently indicated in moderate acne. The presence of mild to moderate acne should not interfere with any contemplated surgical procedure.

Nodular Cystic Acne

This form of acne may present both diagnostic and therapeutic problems. The presence of large, inflammatory, painful cysts, and nodules on the face, chest, and back plus papulopustular lesions and comedones should lead to the consideration of severe acne as a diagnosis. When few in number, these lesions may be confused with an acute bacterial pyoderma. The absence of "pathogenic organisms" in an apparently purulent cutaneous abscess should be an additional clue. Whenever possible, surgery of areas involved with cystic acne should be avoided because the inflammatory nodules may interfere with proper wound healing and may predispose to bacterial superinfection. However, the presence of cystic acne in one area should not necessarily contraindicate surgery in a distant, uninvolved area. Treatment of cystic acne usually requires a minimum of 6 to 8 weeks of therapy to achieve an adequate therapeutic effect. The mainstay of treatment is tetracycline usually administered at a dose of 250 mg, four times a day. Adjunctive topical therapy may include benzoyl peroxide or vitamin A acid. A patient with severe cystic acne should be referred to a dermatologist for further treatment prior to elective surgery of involved areas.

ACNE ROSACEA

Sometimes known as rosacea, this term is applied to a papulopustular, erythematous, central facial eruption common in middle-aged persons. It is frequently associated with telangiectasia and proliferation of the nasal tissue (rhinophyma). Patients with rosacea will commonly give a history of intermittent flushing and exacerbation by hot liquids, alcohol, and caffeine. Rosacea should not be confused with photosensitivity eruptions, lupus erythematosus, or drug eruptions. Treatment of rosacea includes oral tetracycline and topical agents. Rosacea should be treated to minimize complications such as telangiectasia and rhinophyma, however, in itself it is not a contraindication to surgical treatment.

DERMATITIS

The term dermatitis is used in this chapter to apply to any acute and/or chronic inflammatory process of the skin manifested by erythema, edema, and vesicle formation. If the process is relatively acute, there will be more erythema and edema with serous exudate and crust formation. In more chronic processes, there will be thickening and prominence of the skin markings (lichenification) and increased scaling with less evidence of weeping and oozing. Dermatitis can be classified both on the basis of etiology and the apparent morphology. This leads to categorization such as irritant contact dermatitis, allergic contact dermatitis, atopic dermatitis (classifications based on suspected etiology) as well as lichen simplex chronicus and nummular dermatitis (classifications based on morphologic appearance).

Allergic Contact Dermatitis

Of special relevance to the surgical patient is allergic contact dermatitis. The sudden development of an intensely pruritic vesicular eruption with clearcut demarcation should suggest allergic contact dermatitis. Frequently the allergen will have been applied 24 to 48 hours prior to the development of dermatitis. Common allergens in a hospital setting include: adhesive tape, iodide (not organic iodides such as Betadine), tincture of benzoin, and topical antibiotics, such as neomycin. The history should be reviewed and the eruption examined to see if any correlation with external factors can be identified. Treatment should be initiated with wet dressings when the eruption is acutely inflammed. When less exudation of fluid is present, treatment may be initiated with one of the intermediate strength topical steroids listed in Table 1. The eruption should respond within several days. Failure to respond may indicate either continued exposure to the allergen or improper diagnosis. Allergic contact dermatitis is likely to be a problem of the immediate postoperative period rather than a pre-existing disease. However, if patients give a history of intensely pruritic eruptions previously associated with surgical procedures, the diagnosis of contact dermatitis to a commonly utilized substance should be entertained.

Chronic Dermatitis

In the surgical patient, chronic dermatitis is of importance because such areas tend to be heavily colonized with bacteria. For elective procedures such colonization may increase the risk of postoperative wound infection and/or infection of synthetic materials such as prostheses. Chronic dermatitis is likely to be a long-standing problem which will be evident prior to surgery. It can be treated with one of the intermediate strength steroids listed in Table 1. The eruption should improve within three to seven days. If it does not significantly improve, a more potent steroid may be necessary. Whenever possible, chronic dermatitis should be treated prior to surgery, and every effort should be made to avoid incision in this area.

Seborrheic Dermatitis

Dandruff or seborrheic dermatitis is often a problem in the postoperative patient. A common antecedent is a history of mild scaling controlled by shampoos which were discontinued during hospitalization. Seborrheic dermatitis is recognized by diffuse erythema, scaling, and pruritus involving the entire scalp. There may be associated involvement of the nasolabial fold, eyebrows, and central face. On occasion the eruption may extend to the presternal area and may be accompanied by a moderate amount of yellowish greasy scale. Patients with seborrheic dermatitis will complain of pruritus and/or increased scaling. Patients should be treated with daily or alternate day shampoos with selenium sulfide or zinc pyrithione (Selsun or Head & Shoulders). For patients who have significant pruritus and/or inflammation, the addition of topical steroids may be helpful. For the scalp, a gel or liquid should be selected; for facial seborrhea, 1 percent hydrocortisone cream may be helpful. Seborrheic dermatitis is not a contraindication to surgery. However, the physician should be aware of its frequent appearance in the postoperative patient, and the eruption should not be confused with lupus erythematosus.

FUNGAL INFECTIONS

Cutaneous fungal infections may be divided into dermatophyte infections and yeast infections. Dermatophyte infections are further categorized according to affected area: tinea capitis (scalp), tinea corporis (body), tinea pedis (foot), tinea manum (hand), and onychomycosis (nails). Tinea capitis is relatively uncommon in adult patients. In children it may present as localized areas of alopecia with "broken off" hairs. Because of important epidemiologic considerations, the presence of tinea capitis in a child should lead to consultation. Tinea corporis or cruris is usually manifested by a long standing relatively asymptomatic or mildly pruritic process with characteristic erythematous or brownish, scaling, annular lesions. Tinea pedis is known in the vernacular as "athlete's foot." However, many patients with "athlete's foot" may have nonspecific maceration without dermatophyte fungi. Tinea pedis can be manifested as fine erythema and scaling or interdigital maceration as well as vesicular bullous eruption of the sole. Tinea manum frequently is characterized by mild scaling of the hands, however on occasion a vesicular eruption may be noted. It is rare in the absence of tinea pedis. In all cases, the diagnosis may be confirmed by a KOH examination. Patients with involvement of the skin of the hand or foot may also have a nail infection or onychomycosis. The nails may become thick and/or crumbly, accumulate yellow debris, or develop white discoloration. Fingernail involvement is of more than cosmetic significance since it may impair hand function and be painful. Tinea infections are not a contraindication to surgery since the fungi do not live in body tissue other than the stratum corneum. However, they may be a cause of discomfort in preoperative or postoperative patients. When tinea involves the planned operative site, the area should be treated prior to surgery, since local inflammation and a defective skin barrier may predispose to the development of local bacterial infection. Symptomatic relief of the tinea may be obtained by using one of the topical fungicides (see Table 3). Griseofulvin is indicated in very inflammatory fungal infections and in nail infections. However, because a sizable percentage of patients with nail infections fail to respond, many physicians no longer recommend treatment of onychomycosis.

Tinea Versicolor

Tinea versicolor (ringworm) is a very common cutaneous infection manifested by erythematous or white or brownish, scaling macules on the central trunk. Many patients who are darkly pigmented will notice a loss of pigment in the affected areas. Tinea versicolor is important because it must be differentiated from the other causes of papulosquamous disease such as psoriasis, lichen planus, pityriasis rosea, and secondary syphilis. Tinea versicolor is not a contraindication to surgery since the etiologic agent does not grow in other environments.

Candidal Infections

The yeast *Candida albicans* is a frequent commensal organism of the skin. However, under appropriate circumstances it may be a cause of cutaneous infection (candidiasis). Candida can be responsible for infection of the nail folds (paronychia), intertriginous infection, or oral infection. The diagnosis should be entertained when an area is intensely erythematous and scaling; satellite papules or pustules are frequently noted. Oral infection or thrush is manifest by loosely adherent, white plaques. In all cases, the diagnosis can be confirmed by a KOH preparation. In addition, bacterial and/or fungal culture will provide confirmation within 72 to 96 hours. Patients who have received steroids and/or high dose antibiotics or who are diabetic or debilitated are at risk for developing candidiasis. Once the diagnosis is established, appropriate topical therapy should be initiated (see Table 3). When areas are moist and weeping, an additional drying effect can be provided by the use of compresses. Incisions should not be made through areas of active infection since the organism may be innoculated into deeper tissues. The presence of active candidal infection in one site may increase the risk of candidal infection at a distant site, and procedures involving implantation of inert materials should be deferred.

INFESTATIONS

Infestations with either lice (pediculosis) or scabies may be present when patients are admitted to the hospital.

Lice

Patients with lice will complain of intense pruritus in the affected area. Pediculosis can be subdivided into three classes: pediculosis capitis (scalp), pediculosis pubis (groin), or pediculosis corporis (body). In pediculosis capitis or pubis, the organisms reside in the affected area and deposit eggs (nits) which are attached to the hairs. The nits may be identified as small, oval, gray-white bodies attached to the hairs. Frequently, the eruption consists of excoriations with or without secondary pyoderma. Patients with public lice may in addition have involvement of the eyelashes, beard, or axillary hair. Both pediculosis capitis and pubis should be treated with gamma benzene hexachloride according to the directions in Table 5. To prevent secondary infection of hospital personnel, clothing, bed linens, and towels should be washed in hot water or dry cleaned. In pediculosis corporis, the lice frequently live in the garments rather than on the body and treatment of the clothing is frequently adequate. Good hygiene and clean clothing will frequently treat the primary problem. Pyoderma should be treated as necessary after appropriate treatment with a pesticide. Improvement should be apparent subjectively within 24 to 48 hours. Persistent pruritus should suggest inadequate treatment or another diagnosis.

Scabies

Scabies is an infestation of the superficial skin by the mite *Sarcoptes scabiei.* The mite burrows within the stratum corneum depositing eggs. This may be responsible for the patient's complaint of intense pruritus of the finger webs, groin, forearms, and lower abdomen. Primary lesions themselves may be difficult to identify. Burrows, 5 to 10 mm long, resembling thin, black threads may be seen in the affected areas. However, frequently excoriations and secondary eczematous changes with or without bacterial superinfections may be the sole findings. Whenever possible, a diagnosis may be confirmed

TABLE 5. Treatment of Infestations

	Action Spectrum	*Usage*	*Comments*
Gamma benzene hexachloride (Kwell)	Scabies	Apply to all areas below neck and leave in place for 24 hours	Systemically absorbed. Should not be used in infants, children, pregnant women
	Lice	Head lice: Shampoo, lather leave in place for 5 minutes Pubic lice: Cream, apply to pubic region for 24 hours	Dry cleaning or hot water washing of clothing necessary.
Crotamiton (Eurax)	Scabies	2 applications within 48 hour period.	Alternate therapy for those patients who cannot be treated with gamma benzene hexachloride

by removing the "small, black dot" from the end of a burrow or a vesicle. The black dot is the mite which may be identified under low power with the microscope. All too frequently the diagnosis cannot be confirmed definitively. However, a strong clinical suspicion which includes the presence of affected friends or family members in a characteristic history justifies treatment with gamma benzene hexachloride as described in Table 5. For young children and pregnant women alternative therapies discussed in standard dermatology texts should be employed. In most cases, one treatment with gamma benzene hexachloride should be adequate although, on occasion, retreatment may be necessary one week later. Patients admitted to the hospital with suspected scabies should be treated immediately after arrival in order to minimize possible spreading of the infection. Patients with scabies may be bothered by persistent itching and, especially in patients who have developed nodular lesions, pruritus may persist for two to three weeks. Another problem is the development of secondary eczematous dermatitis due to irritant effects from the scabicide. If necessary, emollients and/or mild steroids may be used.

LICHEN PLANUS

Lichen planus is a relatively common cutaneous disease characterized by multiple, pruritic, shiny, violaceous, flat-topped papules of variable size with fine, white striae or dots (Wickham's striae). The disease is commonest around the wrists and ankles, and lesions of the mucous membranes are frequent. The cause of the disease is unknown, but most cases clear spontaneously within one to two years. The disease is not a contraindication to surgery, however, new lesions may develop at sites of incision (as in psoriasis).

PSORIASIS

Psoriasis is a fairly common cutaneous disease which is recognized by the presence of discrete, erythematous, scaling plaques likely to be distributed over extensor surfaces. The scale is typically thick and silvery, however, the appearance may be modified by prior treatment. Areas of involvement in addition to the elbows and knees frequently include the scalp, genitalia, and glutteal cleft. Cutaneous disease may be manifested by punctate pitting of the nails and/or psoriatic arthritis. Some patients have pruritus. The most common complaint relates to the cosmetic appearance. Psoriasis may be classified according to the extent of involvement. For patients with mild to moderate cutaneous involvement, treatment with sunlight and/or intermediate strength steroids (see Table 1) and emollients is frequently adequate.

Psoriasis is of importance in the surgical patient for several reasons. Psoriatic plaques may be colonized with pathogenic organisms such as *Staphylococcus aureus.* Hence, in certain procedures such as elective joint replacement every effort should be made to treat the psoriatic lesions prior to surgery and thus reduce the risk of postoperative infection. An additional problem relates to the Koebner phenomenon, the development of psoriatic lesions in areas of trauma. Thus, a patient with psoriasis may develop new lesions at the site of a surgical incision. The time course is such that usually the surgical incision is completely healed prior to the development of psoriatic lesions. Psoriasis in intertriginous areas such as the groin may be confused with candidiasis. However, skin scrapings will not reveal fungi and the eruption will not respond to antifungal treatment. Patients who have been treated with antimetabolites (such as methotrexate) or psoralen and ultraviolet light may have little evidence of active disease. However, when their therapy is stopped for surgical procedures they may relapse. This will be manifested by the appearance of plaque-like lesions or by the development of psoriatic erythroderma. Physicians should be alert to the possibility of a recrudescence of psoriasis and appropriate consultative assistance sought. The patients maintained on these treatments are frequently unresponsive to the usual topical medications.

Diseases Developing in Hospitalized Patients

DERMATITIS

Dermatitis may be either a preexisting condition or develop after the patient has been hospitalized. The discussion of dermatitis above covers either eventuality.

DRUG ERUPTIONS

Drug eruptions are commonly seen in a hospitalized population. They can appear as an immediate urticarial eruption shortly after administration or ingestion of the drug. A more common form is an erythematous, maculopapular eruption usually beginning on the head and progressing to the trunk. The palms and soles may be involved. Drug eruptions are characterized by pruritus, and the absence of pruritus should mitigate against the diagnosis of a drug eruption. The morphology is nonspecific; many different drug reactions can be manifested by the same morphologic eruption. A diagnosis of drug eruption should be entertained in any hospitalized patient with a pruritic, maculopapular eruption. Sulfonamide (in combination with trimethoprim), erythromycin, gentamicin, cephalosporins, and quinidine are agents which may be likely to cause drug eruptions. In addition, blood and blood products are frequent causes of eruptions with a cutaneous appearance similar to that of drug eruptions. An eruption can suddenly develop in a patient who has previously tolerated an agent or in a patient who has received long-standing therapy with a medication. Treatment should be initiated with antihistamines (see Table 4) and a mild to intermediate strength topical steroid cream. For patients with a severe drug eruption such as a bullous drug eruption, systemic steroids will be necessary. The commonly employed dose is 60 mg of prednisone tapering to none over ten to fourteen days.

ERYTHEMA MULTIFORME

Erythema multiforme is a cutaneous hypersensitivity reaction characterized by erythematous macules and papules that have a target or iris appearance. These lesions have a purpuric center and an outer, erythematous ring. Some lesions may have a pale periphery and appear similar to urticaria. Typically, the extremities are the most common sites of involvement. In more severe forms, the central area develops into a vesicle or bulla. Severe erythema multiforme (known as Stevens-Johnson syndrome) is characterized by extensive bullae of the skin; ulceration of the mucous membranes of the mouth, eyes, and genitalia; and systemic signs of fever and malaise. Some patients may have only mucosal lesions or relatively few skin lesions. Frequently, the cause is unknown, however, antecedent herpes infection is not unusual. In the hospitalized patient hypersensitivity to a drug (such as penicillin, sulfonamides, or phenytoin) is the most common cause of erythema multiforme. There is considerable variation in the severity of the disease. In mild cases, symptomatic treatment with antihistamines and topical steroids is adequate. In more severe cases, systemic steroids (prednisone, 60 mg daily) are indicated. Once no new lesions are noted, the steroids can be reduced over a 10 to 14 day period. Adjunctive topical care includes wet dressings or tub baths to remove crusts. Careful observation is necessary since superinfection of the widespread erosions is frequent. It is important to search for a cause, since drug induced erythema multiforme will recur when the patient receives the medication again. Patients with severe erythema multiforme should be seen by a dermatologist, and whenever possible a skin biopsy (for routine and immunofluorescence studies) should be obtained prior to therapy.

VIRAL INFECTIONS

Herpes Simplex

Commonly known as cold sores or fever blisters, herpes simplex presents as a recurrent vesicular eruption around the mouth or nares. The virus appears to dwell in the skin or nerve endings and may reappear after appropriate stimulation. Stimuli include: sunlight, emotion, fever, or viral infections such as upper respiratory infections. The sudden appearance of a vesicular, crusted eruption around the mouth or nares following surgery is consistent with a diagnosis of herpes simplex. The diagnosis can be confirmed with cytologic examination if clinical examination is not adequate. Recognition of herpes simplex in the surgical patient is important for several reasons. Firstly, the lesions may be mistakenly identified as the effects of the anesthetic and/or intubation procedure. In addition, they may become secondarily infected with bacteria. Finally, they may represent a hazard to nursing and medical personnel via innoculation. Relief may be obtained with topical compresses. Sometimes herpes simplex may involve other areas of the body and present as a recurrent, vesicular eruption precipitated by trauma or other stimuli. Lesions may be sexually transmitted and appear as grouped vesicles on an erythematous base located on the penis or vulva. The question of whether vaginal delivery is contraindicated in pregnant patients with active genital herpes is controversial and appropriate consultation should be sought several weeks before the anticipated date of delivery. The presence of recurrent, multiple, small, superficial erosions on male genitalia should suggest a diagnosis of herpes simplex. This diagnosis is the most important in distinguishing it from primary syphilis. On occasion, low dose topical steroids are used to decrease accompanying inflammation.

Herpes Zoster

Herpes zoster (shingles) is a frequent manifestation of the reactivation of the varicella virus. It usually presents with premonitory pain or tenderness in a dermatomal area. Within several days, the patient will notice grouped vesicles on an erythematous base. Over the next few days, the lesions will crust and be sloughed. Patients with herpes zoster have a history of prior chicken pox. Herpes zoster can be identified on the basis of the clinical appearance, however, on occasion it may be necessary to confirm the diagnosis by cytologic examination. When a Tzanck test is done, multinuclear giant cells will be seen. Diagnosis of herpes zoster is important for several reasons. Firstly, patients with unusual pain may indeed have herpes zoster. A patient who develops a cutaneous eruption in an area of such pain should be strongly suspected of having herpes zoster. Many patients will have one to two dozen lesions outside of the original dermatome, however, the presence of multiple lesions (more than 25 outside the original dermatome) may be associated with defective immunity. Herpes zoster lesions also can become secondarily infected with bacteria. Treatment consists of symptomatic relief with compresses employing Burow's solution, pain medications as necessary, and local steroids during the healing phase. It is important to provide for adequate pain relief since the development of postherpetic neuralgia may be related to this problem.

SYSTEMIC DISEASE WITH CUTANEOUS MANIFESTATIONS

Entire textbooks have been written on this topic, illustrating the multiple acquired and hereditary conditions falling under this heading. The cutaneous manifestations may vary from a small seemingly insignificant lesion (such as pigmented macules in Peutz-Jeghers syndrome) to an extensive process involving all body tissues (such as pseudoxanthoma elasticum). This chapter will not cover this topic, and when skin findings raise the question of an associated systemic disease one of the standard textbooks should be consulted. However, genetic biochemical disorders may present special problems in wound healing in selected instances.

Ehlers-Danlos Syndrome

Ehlers-Danlos syndrome is a hereditary, generalized defect of connective tissue associated with fragile skin and blood vessels, cutaneous hyperelasticity, and joint hyperextensibility. The degree of these abnormalities and the hereditary pattern varies with the particular subtype. Specific enzymatic defects leading to defective collagen production have been identified in four of the seven variants of the syndrome. Of importance to surgeons is that the fragile skin of these patients is easily torn. Healing occurs slowly and the scars tend to be wide and gaping ("fish-mouth"). Pseudotumors may form in the scars. Sutures do not hold well in the friable tissue and pressure dressings and adhesive strips may be helpful. One variant (type 4) is associated with severe vascular fragility and should be considered in patients with unexplained cardiovascular and gastrointestinal hemorrhage.

Epidermolysis Bullosa

Epidermolysis bullosa is an hereditary disease associated with frequent blister formation of the skin and mucous membranes. It is divided into subtypes depending upon the hereditary pattern and severity; some variants are associated with severe scarring and esophageal stricture formation. Surgery is occasionally indicated for correction of strictures and scars. Meticulous technique is necessary since minimal pressure and/or new trauma may induce new blisters and lead to further scar formation.

MAJOR ACQUIRED DERMATOLOGIC DISEASES

Bullous Disease

The category bullous disease includes the acquired diseases pemphigus vulgaris, dermatitis herpetiformis, and bullous pemphigoid. The blisters result from cleavage within the skin, and the conditions are distinguished by the level of the split (intraepidermal or subepidermal), the histologic appearance of the infiltrate, and the immunofluorescent findings. Pemphigus vulgaris, a disease of older patients, frequently presents with large, denuded areas which are easily colonized by bacteria. The superficial, flaccid blisters resulting from intraepidermal cleavage and acantholysis (separation of cells) rupture easily. Patients with controlled pemphigus should be maintained on their therapy throughout the operative period since failure to do so may lead to a severe exacerbation.

Bullous pemphigoid, a subepidermal disease, is manifest by multiple, large, tense bullae frequently on an inflammatory base, which typically arise after an eczematous prodromal eruption. The disease tends to require chronic steroid therapy, but remissions are not uncommon. Dermatitis herpetiformis, another supepidermal bullous disease is characterized clinically by recurrent, intensely pruritic urticarial, erythematous, papulovesicular or bullous lessions and may be associated with a gluten-sensitive enteropathy. Histologically, localized microabscesses of eosinophils and neutrophils accumulate within the dermal papillae leading to blister formation. Patients with subepidermal bullous disease should be maintained on prednisone (bullous pemphigoid) or dapsone or sulfapyridine (dermatitis herpetiformis). Patients on dapsone or sulfapyridine may have a compensated hemolytic anemia and methemoglobinemia which should be evaluated prior to surgery.

Mycosis Fungoides

Mycosis fungoides is a T-cell infiltrate of the skin, notorious for its long pruritic course. Patients frequently live 10 to 20 years after diagnosis so the presence of mycosis fungoides is not a contraindication to operative intervention. A variety of treatments are employed including topical steroids, electron beam therapy, topical nitrogen mustard, and chemotherapy. In the latter case, the physician supervising the chemotherapy should be contacted prior to treatment to ascertain marrow reserves and expected complications.

REFERENCES

1. Rook, A, Wilkinson, DS, and Ebling, FJG: *Textbook of Dermatology,* ed. 3. Oxford: Blackwell Scientific Publications, 1979.
2. Fitzpatrick, TB, Eisen, AZ, Wolff, K, et al.: *Dermatology in General Medicine,* ed. 2. New York: McGraw Hill Inc., 1979.
3. Moschella, S, Pillsbury, DM, and Hurley, HJ: *Dermatology.* Philadelphia: W.B. Saunders Co., 1975.
4. Arndt, KA: *Manual of Dermatologic Therapeutics,* ed. 2. Boston: Little, Brown & Co., 1978.
5. Fisher, A: *Contact Dermatitis,* ed. 2. Philadelphia: Lea & Febiger, 1973.
6. Jablonska, S, Beutner, EH, Beno, M, et al.: *Uses of immunofluorescence tests of skin and sera.* Arch Dermatol 111:371, 1975.
7. Munro, DD: *The effect of percutaneously absorbed steroids on hypothalamic—pituitary—adrenal function after intensive use in in-patients.* Br J Dermatol 94 (suppl. 12): 67, 1976.
8. Maibach, HI, and Stoughton, RB: *Topical steroids* in *Symposium on steroid therapy.* Med Clin North Am 57:1253, 1973.
9. Sneddon, IB: *Atrophy of the skin: The clinical problems.* Br J Dermatol 94 (suppl. 12): 121, 1976.
10. Noble, WC: *Dispersal of skin microorganisms.* Br J Dermatol 93:477, 1975.
11. Galle, PC, Homesly, HD, and Rhyne, AL: *Reassessment of the surgical scrub.* Surg Gynecol Obstet 147:215, 1978.
12. Edlich, RF, Custer, J, Madden, J, et al.: *Studies in the management of the contaminated wound. III. Assessment of the effectiveness of irrigation with antiseptic agents.* Am J Surg 118:21, 1969.
13. Custer, J, Edlich, RF, Prusak, M, et al.: *Studies in the management of the contaminated wound. V. An assessment of the effectiveness of pHisoHex and Betadine surgical scrub solutions.* Am J Surg 121:572, 1971.
14. Gilmore, OJA, Reed, C, and Strokon, A: *A study of the effect of povidone-iodine on wound healing.* Postgrad Med J 53:122, 1977.
15. Leyden, JJ, and Kligman, AM: *The case for topical antibiotics.* Prog Dermatol 10:13, 1976.
16. Rasmussen, JE: *The case against topical antibiotics.* Prog Dermatol 11:1, 1977.
17. Rasmussen, JE: *Criticism of "the case for topical antibiotics."* Prog Dermatol 11:5, 1977.
18. Stoughton, RB: *Perspectives in topical glucocorticosteroid therapy.* Prog Dermatol 9:7, 1975.

Chapter 5
ENDOCRINOLOGY

Mark E. Molitch, M.D.

Endocrinologic diseases usually do not create serious problems for patients who need surgical procedures when the diagnoses are known. It is in the patient who is first found, for example, to be hyperthyroid, diabetic, or adrenally insufficient intraoperatively or postoperatively that life-threatening situations arise. Since diabetes, hyperthyroidism and hypothyroidism, hypercalcemia, and other endocrine dysfunctions occur rather frequently in the population, problems associated with their management may often be found when treating surgical patients. In the following discussion, the diseases of each endocrine organ system are discussed separately, but it must be remembered that multiple endocrine organ excess (multiple endocrine adenomatosis) and deficiency (autoimmune endocrine insufficiencies) states may occur together; the presence of one may be a clue to the presence of others.

PANCREAS

Diabetes Mellitus

Diabetes mellitus has been estimated to affect 2 to 5 percent of the population in the United States, with about 50 percent of these cases being undiagnosed and not on any form of therapy.[1] Because of this high prevalence in the population, diabetes would be expected to make up a similar proportion in any surgical practice, especially in older individuals. Surgical illness commonly punctuates the life of a diabetic; sometimes trauma or a surgical procedure brings out the presence of diabetes for the first time. Despite the greater difficulties in management of metabolic disturbance in the diabetic patient, in most large series the overall mortality rate for diabetics undergoing a variety of surgical procedures is about 2 percent, a figure that is not higher than that for nondiabetics.[2,3] In the large series of 667 diabetic patients reported upon by Galloway and Shuman,[2] 29 percent of the deaths were due to cardiovascular causes and 16 percent were due to staphylococcal septicemia.

Diabetic patients appear to be older physiologically than they actually are chronologically, suggesting that they age more rapidly. In fact, Steinke[4] has suggested that in thinking about such patients the duration of the diabetes should be added to the chronologic age of the patient to get a rough approximation of the patients' cardiovascular and renal status. The possibility that cardiac function might be more compromised than expected should promote caution in the administration of large amounts of fluids intraoperatively and postoperatively. Careful cardiac monitoring during surgery and in the recovery room may also be important. The presence of renal insufficiency will influence not only the amount of intravenous fluids that can be given but also the rate of excretion of various medications, so that alterations in drug dosage amounts and intervals are needed (see Chapter 14, Renal Disease and Hypertension).

PREOPERATIVE EVALUATION

Besides the usual careful history and physical examination, preoperative evaluation of the diabetic should focus on certain specific problems. In the history specific attention should be paid to the following: (1) Is the patient a ketosis prone or a "brittle" diabetic (subject to wide swings from hypoglycemia to hyperglycemia)? (2) Precisely what kind of therapy is being used to control the diabetes—diet, oral hypoglycemic agents (Table 1), or insulin (Table 2) with exact data as to type, dosage, and timing of administration? (3) How well controlled has the diabetes been, especially in the few days prior to admission—has the patient had polyuria, polydipsia, nausea, vomiting, fatigue, blurring of vision, or marked glycosuria or ketonuria on home urine testing? (4) Has the patient had any of the chronic complications of diabetes, particularly nephropathy, neuropathy, peripheral vascular disease, or cardiac disease? (5) Is the patient taking medications which influence surgical outcome such as propranolol (Inderal), diuretics, other antihypertensive agents, or digitalis?

On physical examination, attention should be directed particularly to organ systems

TABLE 1. Oral Hypoglycemic Agents

Generic Name	*Trade Name*	*Available Form (mg)*	*Average Daily Dose (mg)*	*Duration of Action (Hours)*
Tolbutamide	Orinase	500	500–1000	6–12
Acetohexamide	Dymelor	250 500	250–1000	12–24
Tolazamide	Tolinase	100 250	100–500	16–24
Chlorpropamide	Diabinese	100 250	100–500	24–36

TABLE 2. Types of Insulin Preparations

Type	*Onset (Hours)*	*Peak (Hours)*	*Duration (Hours)*	*Modifier*
Regular (CZI)	1	2–4	5–7	None
NPH	3–4	5–20	24–28	Protamine
Protamine zinc	4–6	14–24	36+	Protamine
Semilente	1	2–4	5–7	Zinc
Lente	3–4	6–20	24–28	Zinc
Ultralente	4–6	18–24	36+	Zinc

that can be affected by diabetes and that may influence the patient's management. Does the patient have evidence of hypertension, retinopathy, neuropathy, cardiac disease, or peripheral vascular disease? Recently it has been found that patients with diabetes may develop congestive heart failure due to a cardiomyopathy that appears to be related to diffuse small vessel disease rather than to disease of the larger coronary arteries.[5] Thus, a patient may develop heart failure in the absence of known heart or vascular disease and caution must always be used in administering fluids to such patients.

The presence of autonomic neuropathy should also be ascertained. There may be bladder neuropathy which can lead to difficulty in voiding postoperatively. Neuropathic bladders are also prone to infection when catheterized so this should be avoided. Vagal neuropathy may lead to delayed gastric emptying (gastroparesis diabeticorum);[6] if this is present a nasogastric tube should be placed preoperatively to empty the stomach of food which may be present from supper the night before. Autonomic neuropathy can also result in esophageal motility dysfunction[7] and intestinal dysfunction leading to both increased and decreased transit times with the production of diarrhea and even steatorrhea due to bacterial overgrowth in some patients.[8,9] It is conceivable that decreased intestinal motility combined with gastroparesis might give the clinical impression of an ileus so that this altered intestinal physiology must be kept in mind when a patient presents with a possible intrabdominal process. Another source of confusion can be the abdominal pain associated with a diabetic radicular neuropathy; electromyography in such circumstances is usually diagnostic and may prevent the carrying out of invasive procedures and even laparotomy.[10]

Of great importance is the detection of a cardiac autonomic neuropathy[11] since patients with this appear to be at high risk for the development of sudden cardiorespiratory arrest in the intraoperative and postoperative (recovery room) periods and for pneumonias.[12] Most patients with cardiac autonomic neuropathy have symptoms and signs of orthostatic hypotension, a mild resting tachycardia, and evidence of peripheral neuropathy and other autonomic neuropathies such as nocturnal diarrhea and sweating.[12] Although the 8 patients with cardiac arrest associated with cardiac autonomic neuropathy described by Page and Watkins[12] were not being monitored so that the exact precipitating arrhythmia is not known, patients were usually found apneic and pulseless.

Upon resuscitation their heart rhythm stabilized quickly, but they often required prolonged mechanical ventilation, suggesting that an impairment of respiratory reflexes might be primary.

Cardiac autonomic neuropathy can be easily diagnosed preoperatively at the bedside using an electrocardiogram. One method employs the calculation of the ratio of the longest R-R interval to the shortest R-R interval following the Valsalva maneuver. A normal response is greater than 1.21, a borderline response is 1.11 to 1.20, and an abnormal response is less than 1.11.[13] Figure 1 illustrates the lack of response to the Valsalva maneuver seen in an insulin dependent diabetic (studied by Dr. William Cobb in our division) who also had peripheral neuropathy, gastroparesis diabeticorum, and an abnormal CO_2-ventilatory response curve; she also had no change in heart rate in response to standing. Ewing and colleagues[14] have found that the response to standing can be useful in this regard. They found that measuring the ratio of the R-R interval at 15 beats after standing to the R-R interval at 30 beats after standing was reproducible and could distinguish young normals (ratio of 1.03 or greater) from diabetics with autonomic neuropathy (ratio of 1.03 or less). Older nondiabetics, however, occasionally have a ratio of less than 1.03. Because of the ease of performing these two maneuvers (Valsalva and standing) and because of the importance of detecting cardiac autonomic neuropathy in the perioperative setting, calculation of this ratio should become routine in the preoperative evaluation of all diabetics. In addition to the immediate risk in the perioperative period, long term follow-up of patients with cardiac autonomic neuropathy has revealed the strikingly high mortality rate of 50 percent within 2½ years.[15] The causes of death in this group included renal failure (6 patients), cerebrovascular accident (2 patients), hypoglycemia (1 patient), and "sudden death" (1 patient). This generally poor prognosis should promote caution in the decision to perform elective surgery in such patients.

Finally, a relatively rare form of neuropathy has been termed diabetic neuropathic cachexia by Ellenberg.[16] These patients develop anorexia with profound weight loss, painful peripheral neuropathy, depression, and impotence. The syndrome is reversible with spontaneous recovery in about one year. These patients all appear to be harboring an occult malignancy and, indeed, evaluation for this is needed in each patient. However, before exploratory laparotomy is performed in a diabetic with unexplained weight loss, it is important to recall this syndrome to avoid unnecessary surgery. Recently, this syndrome has been found to be responsive to therapy with amitriptyline and perphenazine.[17] Apathetic thyrotoxicosis (see below) should also be excluded, of course, in older patients with unexplained weight loss.

In addition to the standard laboratory tests, daily fasting blood sugars (FBS) should be obtained as well as a midafternoon glucose. Urinary glucose testing four times a day using the double voiding method (on awakening, before lunch, before supper, and at bedtime) should be performed. The electrolytes give a clue to the presence of metabolic acidosis by a widening of the "anion gap" (see Chap. 15, Fluid, Electrolyte, and Acid-Base Disorders). If the gap is widened in a diabetic, the serum bicarbonate is lowered and the arterial pH is decreased; this usually is due to one or more of the following: (1) ketones in ketoacidosis, (2) lactate in lactic acidosis, and (3) increased phosphate and sulfate in the face of renal insufficiency. Since severe trauma can precipitate any one or

CONTROL

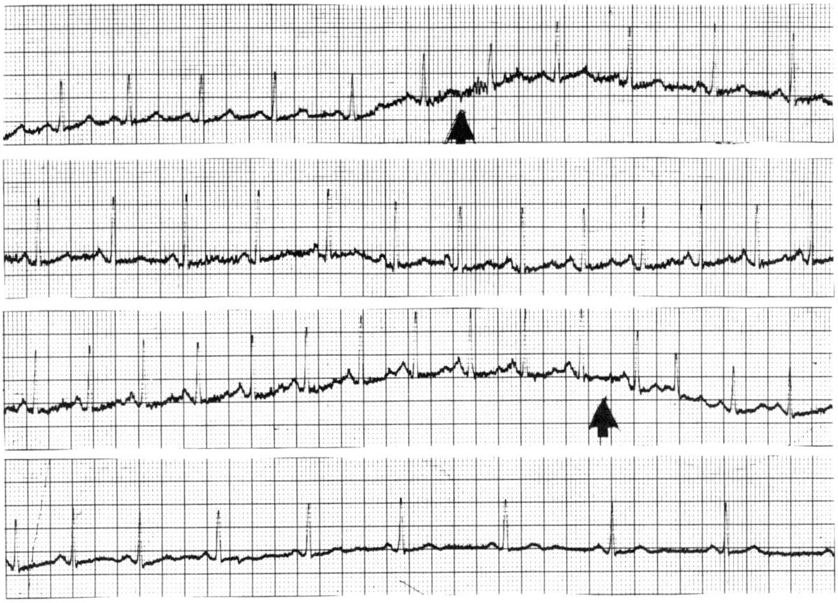

DIABETIC

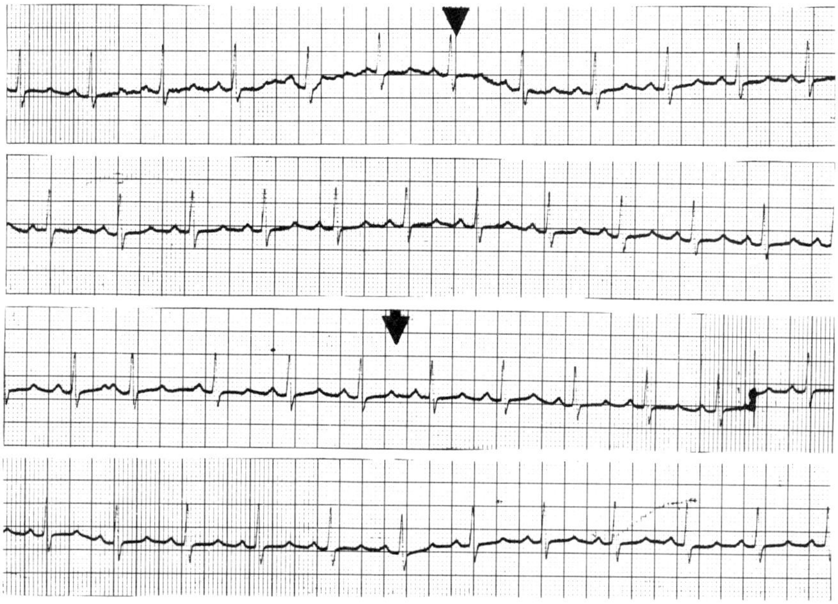

FIGURE 1. Comparison of heart rate responses to Valsalva maneuver (onset and offset noted by arrows) in normal person and patient with diabetic cardiac autonomic neuropathy. Note the lack of variation in heart rate in diabetic patient.

all of these, and since the therapy is different for each, it is important to determine which disorder is present. Serum or plasma ketones can be measured easily at the bedside. A clotted or anticoagulated blood specimen should be centrifuged and a drop of serum or plasma can be added to a crushed Acetest tablet (normally used for urine ketone testing). If the color reaction reads "large," then the serum or plasma is serially diluted with water to give samples at 1:1, 1:2, 1:4, 1:8, and 1:16 dilutions, and a drop of each of these is added to a crushed Acetest tablet. If ketones are found in greater than 1:2 dilution of plasma, ketoacidosis is present. If ketones are not present in significant amounts, and the BUN and creatinine are not significantly elevated, the patient most likely is in lactic acidosis (see Chap. 15, Fluid, Electrolyte, and Acid-Base Disorders). The nitroprusside reagent in the Acetest tablet, however, reacts only with acetoacetate and not β-hydroxybutyrate. In states of severe ketoacidosis or ketoacidosis combined with lactic acidosis[18] the redox reaction

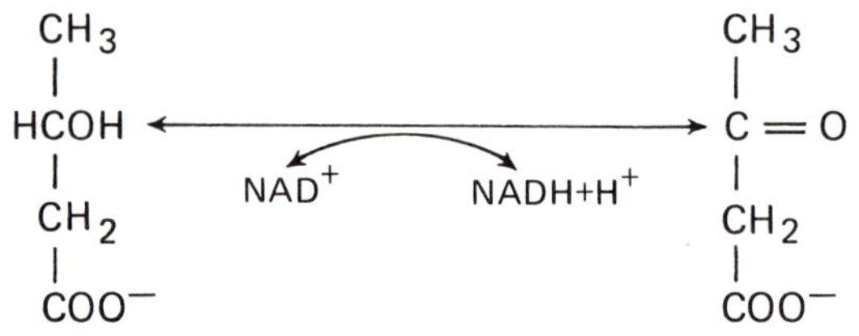

β−hydroxybutyrate Acetoacetate

may be shifted toward β-hydroxybutyrate so that the Acetest reading will give a falsely lowered "ketone" reading associated with a widened anion gap. Paradoxically as the pH is raised during therapy, this reaction shifts back toward acetoacetate with an increase in measured "ketones" by the nitroprusside method but the decreasing anion gap will indicate that the sum of acetoacetate and β-hydroxybutyrate is really decreasing. It is important to remember that all three of the above types of acidosis can coexist in the same patient. An example might be a diabetic patient with multiple fractures secondary to falling down the steps who was not found for several hours or days. The stress of such trauma together with lack of insulin can precipitate ketoacidosis in an otherwise stable patient; the polyuria combined with the lack of fluid intake could lead to dehydration and hypotension with resultant lactic acidosis and/or acute tubular necrosis.

It has become apparent in the past few years that diabetics are prone to develop acute renal failure following the administration of the iodinated contrast agents used in intravenous pyelography, arteriography, and computerized tomographic scanning (CT scan). Diabetics who have early onset disease (onset under 40 years of age) with a serum creatinine over 2 mg/dl and who have other evidence of vascular disease appear to be particularly at risk for this complication. In one series[19] 22 of 29 (76%) diabetic patients with a creatinine greater than 2 mg/dl developed acute renal failure following intravenous pyelography and in 9 this was irreversible. Patients undergoing studies utilizing these contrast agents should be kept well hydrated, although there is no conclusive evidence supporting a protective effect on hydration. Therefore, renal function must be checked serially for a few days following such procedures to detect any deterioration of function.

PREOPERATIVE AND INTRAOPERATIVE MANAGEMENT

Diabetic Treated with Diet Alone

This type of patient is usually fairly stable and is not ketosis prone. Blood sugars usually range between 100 and 250 mg/dl. When such a patient undergoes an elective surgical procedure, we usually do not recommend the routine use of insulin and prefer to continue to manage this patient with diet alone.

Occasionally patients who ordinarily do not require insulin will manifest blood sugars in the 300 to 600 mg/dl range. This is especially true if they suffer trauma or infection, either of which creates a state of insulin "resistance," partly attributable to the elevated levels of catecholamines, glucagon, cortisol, and growth hormone that occur with various forms of stress. These elevated "counter-regulatory" hormones result in increased proteolysis, lipolysis, and gluconeogenesis[20,21] and the elevated catecholamines may suppress any residual insulin secretion.[22] Such patients then require insulin on a short term basis to lower the blood glucose before, during, and immediately after surgery. (For the treatment of severe hyperglycemia, ketoacidosis, or hyperosmolar coma see below). Table 2 shows the different types of the commonly used insulin preparations. It is always preferable to stabilize a patient for several hours or for a few days before surgery when possible. If several days are available, the patient can be started on 10 to 15 units (U) of lente or NPH insulin once a day in the morning and the fasting and late afternoon blood glucose checked to assess the adequacy of control. Optimally, blood glucose should be in the range of 100 to 250 mg/dl. On the day of surgery, one half of the dose of lente or NPH insulin should be given preoperatively and an infusion of 5 percent dextrose in water begun to replace the carbohydrate content of breakfast. Surgery should be carried out in the morning if possible, so that meals can be given later in the day. We advocate giving this small dose of insulin preoperatively since it is known that the stress of both anesthesia and surgery serves to raise blood sugar in the normal individual,[23–25] and even more so in the diabetic who is relatively insulin deficient. In the uncontrolled diabetic who already has accelerated glycogenolysis and gluconeogenesis, the additional stress of anesthesia and surgery can precipitate ketoacidosis or hyperosmolar coma if no insulin is present to at least partially control the lipolysis, glycogenolysis, and gluconeogenesis. Although some anesthesiologists fear the development of hypoglycemia with this regimen, in practice we have found that this is not a problem and this has been the experience of other groups who report upon large series of cases.[2,3]

Often there is little time available for stabilization of the patient prior to emergency surgery. Under these circumstances, even a few hours can be helpful in replacing any fluid and electrolyte deficiencies that may be present as well as lowering blood glucose below 300 mg/dl. Only regular (crystalline) insulin should be used. This can be given subcutaneously in a dose of 5 to 20 U every 4 to 6 hours depending on the blood sugar. However, we believe that constant intravenous infusion of insulin is generally superior. In this approach, 50 U of regular insulin is added to 500 ml of normal saline (Table 3). Of this solution, 60 ml is drained through the needle prior to beginning the infusion to saturate all the insulin binding sites on the plastic administration set. Then 60 ml (6 U) is infused rapidly (over 5 to 10 minutes) to obtain a loading dose. Thereafter, insulin can

TABLE 3. Method of Continuous Intravenous Insulin Infusion

1. Regular insulin 50 U in 500 ml of normal saline. No albumin needed.
2. Let 60–80 ml of this mixture run out to saturate the binding sites on tubing.
3. Infuse 60 ml (6 U) rapidly (5–10 minutes) to achieve a loading dose.
4. Then infuse at rate of 10–60 ml (1–6 U)/hour.
5. Infuse via a constant infusion pump (e.g., IVAC) piggybacked into the IV tubing or into a separate IV site via a pediatric drip infusion set to insure constant flow.
6. Double the rate of infusion if response not adequate (e.g., about 100 mg/dl fall in glucose per hour when treating ketoacidosis).
7. When blood glucose is less than 250 mg/dl, either:
   (a) adjust infusion rate to 1–2 U/hr and start 5% dextrose at 100–200 cc/hr to maintain glucose in this range.
   (b) stop infusion, start 5% dextrose at 100–200 cc/hr, check blood glucose every 4–6 hours, and give 5–10 U of regular insulin subcutaneously every 4–6 hours. *Do not omit a dose of insulin;* give a smaller dose for lower blood sugars.
8. Fluids, potassium, bicarbonate, and so forth may be given in standard fashion.
9. Strict flow sheets should be kept.

be infused at 10 to 40 ml (1 to 4 U) per hour using an infusion pump depending on the blood glucose. With very high blood glucose levels seen in ketoacidosis or hyperosmolar coma (see below), 6 to 10 U per hour should be infused. Once the blood glucose level falls below 250 mg/dl, the infusion rate should be reduced to 1 to 2 U per hour and 5 percent glucose should be infused at the rate of about 100 ml per hour. The blood glucose will need to be checked every few hours to assess the need for adjusting either the insulin or glucose administration rate. Alternatively, when the blood glucose level falls below 250 mg/dl the insulin infusion can be stopped and regular insulin can be administered subcutaneously in 5 to 10 U amounts every 4 to 6 hours. Although 5 to 25 percent of insulin is absorbed to the glass and plastic when insulin is given by intravenous infusion, enough gets into the patient to be effective and it is not necessary to add albumin to the bottle.

With patients who look like they will need insulin for only a short time in the perioperative period, it may be prudent to give them one of the new, highly purified insulins (Novo, Nordisk, and Lilly Iletin II) to avoid antibody formation and possible insulin resistance or allergy should they need insulin again in the future.

Diabetic Treated with Oral Hypoglycemic Agents

At present, the only oral hypoglycemic agents available in the United States are the sulfonylurea derivatives listed in Table 1. These drugs act by facilitating insulin-mediated glucose uptake in peripheral tissues.[26] Recently the biguanide phenformin was removed from the market in the United States because of its association with the development of lactic acidosis in some patients. It has no place in the therapy of patients in the perioperative period because of this tendency to facilitate the development of lactic acidosis. Should patients be admitted for emergency surgery while taking phenformin, lactic acidosis should be watched for with extra care by frequent measurement of the "anion gap" (see above).

If the patient being treated with oral agents is under reasonable control (FBS less than 150 mg/dl, 2 hour postprandial blood sugar [PPBS] less than 200 mg/dl), then these agents should be continued until the day before surgery and then withheld the day of surgery. Because of the long half-life of Diabinese (chlorpropamide), the drug should be omitted the day prior to surgery as well if the patient's blood glucoses are generally under 200 mg/dl. If the glucose becomes elevated postoperatively, this can be treated with supplemental doses of regular insulin (see below). If the patient's glucose levels are in the 300 to 500 mg/dl range, it is preferable to bring these down into the 150 to 250 mg/dl range with the use of insulin (see above).

Diabetic Treated with Insulin

Most diabetics receiving insulin will be on a regimen consisting of an intermediate-acting insulin such as lente or NPH given once or twice a day, often with additional short-acting insulin such as semilente or regular insulin given with the intermediate-acting insulin. If the blood glucose levels of this patient are generally less than 250 mg/dl, one-half the usual daily dose of insulin should be given on the morning of surgery together with an infusion of 5 percent dextrose equivalent to the usual breakfast carbohydrate load (i.e., about 1000 to 1500 ml of 5 percent glucose). If the blood glucose is significantly higher than this, supplemental regular insulin 5 to 10 U subcutaneously every 4 to 6 hours can be used to bring it down prior to surgery. The morning of surgery, one-half of the required daily insulin dose can be given as NPH or lente. If emergency surgery must be performed shortly after the administration of a large dose of insulin, the blood glucose must be monitored carefully to avoid hypoglycemia.

The Undiagnosed Diabetic

In Galloway and Shumway's series of 667 operations in diabetics, about 20 percent were performed in patients first diagnosed as having diabetes in the perioperative period.[2] These patients should be considered as diabetics treated with diet alone and treatment should follow the guidelines established for that group discussed above, which includes provision for the occurrence of high blood glucose levels.

The Diabetic in Ketoacidosis

The stress of severe trauma or infection will often trigger the development of ketoacidosis in a diabetic who has otherwise been reasonably well controlled. The accumulation of ketoacids leads to a severe acidosis and patients may show rapid deep respiration (Kussmaul's respiration) in an attempt to compensate. The massive osmotic diuresis that occurs due to the glycosuria leads to severe dehydration and total body potassium, phosphate, and sodium depletion.[27]

As outlined above, the laboratory data will show hyperglycemia, a depressed bicarbonate with an increased anion gap, ketones present in the blood at greater than 1:2 dilution, and a low pH with a low P_{CO_2}. The serum sodium concentration is usually decreased due to a shift of water from the intracellular compartment to the extracellular fluid along the osmotic gradient. Roscoe and coworkers have calculated that there should be a drop in serum sodium of 1.35 to 1.6 mEq/L for every 100 mg/dl rise in the blood glucose. In the absence of hyperlipidemia, a deviation from this expected value should suggest a disproportionate loss in free water compared to sodium as the ketoacidosis developed.

In ketoacidosis, the serum amylase is substantially elevated in about 60 percent of cases[29] and can be a source of confusion. Although abdominal pain is found in about 50 percent of patients with ketoacidosis, there is no correlation between the pain and the presence of an elevated amylase: the patients clinically do not have pancreatitis, and lipase levels are normal.[29] The amylase/creatinine clearance ratio is also elevated.[30] Recently Warshaw and associates[31] found that the amylase elevation is usually due to an increase in the salivary amylase isoenzyme. Although pancreatitis can precipitate ketoacidosis in a diabetic, it is now clear that this is rare and this possibility can be excluded by measuring the lipase as well as the amylase. In addition to amylase, serum glutamic-oxaloacetic transaminase (SGOT), serum glutamic pyruvic transaminase (SGPT), lactic dehydrogenase (LDH), and creatine phosphokinase (CPK), and creatinine are often found to be artifactually elevated in diabetic ketoacidosis due to interference in the measurements by the elevated acetoacetate levels.[32–34] Because of this, invasive maneuvers to investigate the cause of these elevations (e.g., liver biopsy, intravenous pyelography) should be delayed until several days after resolution of the ketoacidosis. However, creatinine may be measured accurately by a manual method, thereby allowing the assessment of coexisting renal disease.[34]

Detailed discussions of the pathophysiology and management of diabetic ketoacidosis are available[35–38] and only a brief guide can be given here (Table 4). These patients usually have an overall fluid deficit of 5 to 10 L of a composition that approximates 0.5 N saline. They also have deficits of 100 to 200 mEq of potassium. If the patient is hypotensive, 1 to 2 L of normal saline is infused over about 1 to 3 hours, and the rest of the fluid should be 0.5 N saline. About one-third of the estimated fluid deficit should be corrected in the first 8 hours, one-third over the next 16 hours, and the final third over the next 24 hours. In the older patient, one must watch for signs of congestive heart failure and a central venous pressure (CVP) line may often be helpful. Although the initial potassium may be elevated because of the acidosis, it gradually falls as intravenous fluids and insulin therapy are given. After it has been established that there is a good urinary output and as soon as plasma potassium levels are below 4.5 mEq/L, 20 to 40 mEq/L of potassium should be given.

The use of bicarbonate therapy in diabetic ketoacidosis has been controversial. Because respiration[39] and myocardial function[40] are depressed when blood pH is less than 7.10 we prefer to raise the pH to 7.10 to 7.20 with a small amount of bicarbonate

TABLE 4. Management of the Patient in Ketoacidosis

1. Measure blood glucose, BUN, electrolytes, ketones, pH, Po_2, Pco_2.
2. Replace fluid deficits initially with normal saline and later half-normal saline.
3. Replace potassium deficits as potassium chloride, 20–40 mEq/L once urine output is achieved.
4. Give small amounts of bicarbonate (50–100 mEq) only when pH is less than 7.10 to raise pH above 7.10.
5. Give regular insulin 6 U/hr by constant intravenous infusion (See Table 3).
6. Give 5% dextrose when glucose is less than 250 mg/dl.
7. When glucose is less than 250 mg/dl, decrease infusion rate to 1–2 U/hr or give 5–10 U regular insulin SQ every 4–6 hr.
8. Start NPH or lente insulin in a.m. when patient is stable, afebrile, and eating.

(1 to 2 ampules of 50 mEq each) intravenously if the initial pH is less than 7.10. Over time, the acidosis will resolve spontaneously as insulin therapy halts lipolysis, the ketoacids are metabolized, and bicarbonate is regenerated in the kidney.

Insulin therapy can be given either as repetitive subcutaneous or intramuscular injections of 50 to 100 U every 2 to 4 hours or by intravenous infusion. We prefer the intravenous infusion method because of its reliability, its ease of use, the relatively linear rate of fall of the glucose (Fig. 2), and the ability to stop administration abruptly should hypoglycemia occur. A loading dose of 6 U and an infusion of 6 U per hour as noted

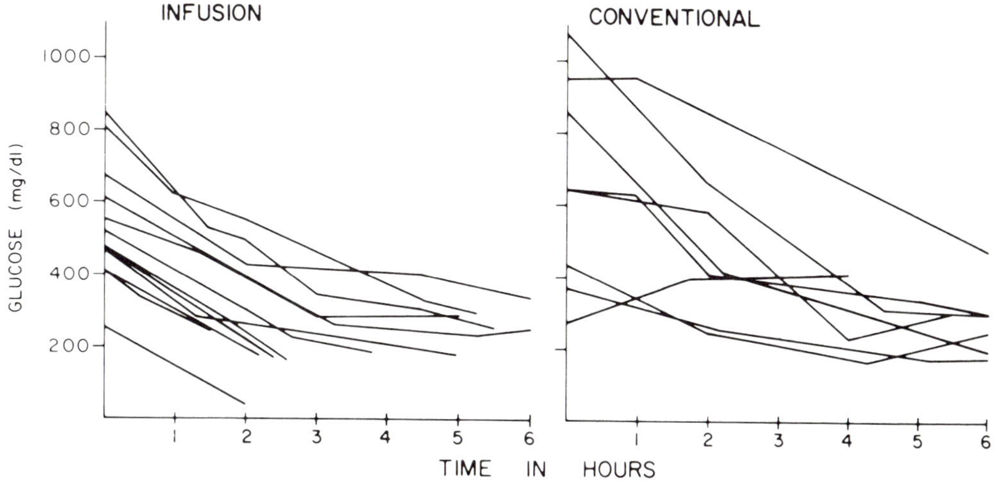

FIGURE 2. Individual patterns of glucose level fall in patients receiving low-dose infusion and conventional insulin therapy for diabetic ketoacidosis. (From Heber, D, Molitch, ME, and Sperling, MA: Low-dose continuous insulin therapy for diabetic ketoacidosis. Arch Intern Med 137:1377, 1977. Copyright 1977, American Medical Association.)

above has proved to be quite successful.[41] When the blood glucose drops below 250 mg/dl, the infusion can be reduced to 1 to 2 U per hour and an infusion of dextrose 5 percent in water or dextrose 5 percent in 0.5N saline at about 100 cc per hour is begun. Alternatively, regular insulin 5 to 10 U subcutaneously every 4 to 6 hours can also be begun at this point. Some insulin must be given at the end of the higher dose infusion to allow continued resolution of the ketoacidosis, because in the absence of insulin the factors that initially precipitated the ketoacidosis will put the patient right back into ketoacidosis.

To lessen the likelihood of cardiac arrhythmias during anesthesia, surgery should be postponed as long as possible until the ketoacidosis is at least stabilized and partially resolved. Preferably, the pH should have risen to at least 7.25, hypokalemia been prevented, and fluid deficits partially corrected. Blood glucose, electrolytes, and arterial blood gases should be checked every 1 to 2 hours for the first 4 hours and then every 2 to 4 hours for the next 4 to 8 hours, depending upon the clinical state of the patient. If surgery cannot be delayed by even 1 to 2 hours, then aggressive insulin, fluid, and electrolyte therapy should be continued into the operating room and through surgery. Close cooperation between the surgeon, anesthesiologist, and internist is vital in the management of these critically ill patients.

Hyperglycemic Hyperosmolar Nonketotic Coma

This state is characterized by extreme hyperglycemia with glucose levels in the 700 to 2000 mg/dl range unaccompanied by ketoacidosis.[42] Trauma or infection in the older adult-onset diabetic will usually lead to this state as opposed to ketoacidosis. Why some patients go into ketoacidosis and others into hyperosmolar coma is not clear. The hyperglycemia together with severe dehydration due to the persistent glycosuria leads to the hyperosmolar state.

Because these patients often have coexisting diseases, careful evaluation for cardiopulmonary and renal disease is very important. It is necessary to rule out a hypotension-related myocardial infarction or acute tubular necrosis before instituting surgery and vigorous potassium and fluid therapy. The electrolytes and arterial blood gases of these patients may point to a coexistent lactic acidosis due to hypotension. The BUN is usually elevated out of proportion to the creatinine, reflecting the state of dehydration. Serum ketones may be present but only in a dilution of 1:2 or less.

Therapy in this state is primarily directed at the severe dehydration (Table 5). If the patient is hypotensive, the first fluids given should be normal saline until the blood pressure is normal. Thereafter, half normal saline should be given. Replacement of the fluid deficits is similar to that in ketoacidosis in that about one-third should be replaced in the first 8 hours, one-third in the next 16 hours, and the final third in the following 24 hours. Since these patients are often elderly a central venous pressure (CVP) line may be helpful. If lactic acidosis appears to be present, bicarbonate therapy may be needed to keep the pH above 7.20 to 7.25. Usually with correction of the hypotension, resolution of the acidosis will not be difficult. Because some of these patients are prone to thromboembolic events and because of the hyperosmolar state, the administration of colloid solutions such as dextrans is not recommended. As in ketoacidosis, potassium replace-

TABLE 5. Management of the Patient in Hyperosmolar Nonketotic Coma

1. Measure blood glucose, BUN, electrolytes, ketones, pH, Po_2, Pco_2.
2. Vigorously replace fluid deficits with normal saline initially and half-normal saline later.
3. Replace potassium deficits as potassium chloride, 20–40 mEq/L once urine output is achieved.
4. Give regular insulin 2–6 U/hr by constant intravenous infusion (see Table 3).
5. Give 5% dextrose when glucose is less than 250 mg/dl.
6. When glucose is less than 250 mg/dl, decrease infusion rate to 1–2 U/hr or give 5–10 U regular insulin SQ every 4–6 hr.
7. Observe for need for daily insulin therapy. If needed, start NPH or lente insulin when patient is stable, afebrile, and eating.

ment should be given in 20 to 40 mEq/L amounts depending on the serum electrolyte concentrations which should be measured every 2 to 4 hours in the acute phase.

Insulin therapy for patients with hyperosmolar coma varies a bit from that for ketoacidosis. The blood glucose will usually fall 200 to 400 mg/dl just from rehydration. If insulin is given subcutaneously or intramuscularly, it should be in small 10 to 20 U doses every 2 to 4 hours depending on the rate of fall of the glucose. We have used the constant insulin infusion method outlined above for ketoacidosis with considerable success for this state also with doses of 4 to 6 U per hour. Again it is always preferable to stabilize a patient for several hours before surgery. Anesthesia in the face of hypovolemia may lead to a worsening of hypotension; adequate fluid replacement before surgery is essential. When the blood glucose falls below 250 mg/dl, 5 percent dextrose should be added to the intravenous fluids at a rate of about 50 to 100 cc per hour. The insulin infusion can then be reduced to about 1 U per hour. Alternatively, regular insulin can be given every 4 to 6 hours in 5 to 10 U amounts depending on the blood glucose. Once hypovolemia is largely corrected and the blood sugar is below 300 to 400 mg/dl, emergency surgery can proceed, although it is better to wait until the patient has stabilized for a few days if possible.

POSTOPERATIVE MANAGEMENT

Diet Controlled Diabetic

If the diet controlled diabetic has been under fair control before surgery, we prefer to keep this patient on diet therapy alone in the immediate postoperative period if the blood glucoses remain below about 300 mg/dl. There usually is not sufficient glycosuria to cause significant polyuria. When the glucoses are persistently above 300 mg/dl insulin therapy may be necessary (see below). In the patient with a benign postoperative course, the blood glucose probably needs to be checked only twice a day for the first few days and then daily thereafter.

Diabetic on Oral Hypoglycemic Agents

If the patient is eating postoperatively, we usually restart these patients on their oral agents the day following surgery. Often these patients will require insulin for persistent hyperglycemia only for a few days following surgery and then later can be switched back to their oral agents.

Insulin Requiring Diabetic

As mentioned previously, these patients should usually receive about one-half their daily dose of insulin preoperatively. In this type of patient as well as in the patient treated with diet or oral hypoglycemic agents who becomes moderately hyperglycemic following surgery, regular insulin should be given every 4 to 6 hours depending upon the results of blood glucose testing which should be obtained every 4 to 6 hours.

We are strongly opposed to giving insulin based on a *urinary* glucose sliding scale system for the following reasons: (1) The renal threshold for spilling glucose is highly variable in different individuals ranging from 130 mg/dl to over 300 mg/dl so that 4+ glucose in one patient could reflect a blood sugar of 200 mg/dl while in another 400 mg/dl. (2) Unless the urinary measurement is from a catheterized or doubly-voided specimen it may reflect the blood glucose from hours before. (3) Postoperatively, patients may have difficulty voiding for several hours so that an accurate assessment of urinary glucose can be difficult to make. This may be especially true in the diabetic with a neurogenic bladder. Urinary catheters should be avoided in diabetics because of the possible predisposition to urinary tract infections. (4) Since urine specimens are difficult to obtain at exact times, the covering insulin may be given too frequently or too infrequently. (5) A urine glucose of 4+ indicates a concentration of 2 percent or *greater*, so that it may reflect a blood glucose of 250 mg/dl or anywhere higher (e.g., 1000 mg/dl). The insulin dose that might be satisfactory for 250 mg/dl probably will not be satisfactory for 1000 mg/dl. For all of these reasons, we recommend obtaining a blood glucose value every 4 to 6 hours postoperatively until the morning following surgery and giving regular insulin every 4 to 6 hours depending on the blood glucose obtained. If the patient is stable, then the usual dose of insulin or the oral hypoglycemic agent can be reinstituted in the morning.

Patients who are unstable postoperatively can be continued on the above regimen of glucose measurement every 4 to 6 hours and regular insulin subcutaneously. Alternatively, insulin can be given by constant intravenous infusion at 1 to 2 U per hour along with intravenous glucose, and the rates of infusion of each can be varied depending on the blood glucose measurements. In patients with infection and trauma, the insulin requirements may vary greatly depending on the degrees of resolution or exacerbation of these complications. The frequent measurement of the glucose and the giving of frequent doses of short-acting insulin to such patients will insure that adequate insulin levels are maintained to prevent severe hyperglycemia while at the same time avoiding hypoglycemia. We have seen 2 patients in the past two years who required more than 100 U per hour of regular insulin given by intravenous infusion, when septic, with much smaller doses needed when the infection resolved.

Nutritional requirements of severely ill patients, both diabetic and nondiabetic, are often overlooked because of the concern with other aspects of patient care. If such patients cannot be fed by mouth within 24 to 48 hours following surgery, they should be given amino acids intravenously to help prevent protein breakdown[43] as well as vitamin supplements. If patients cannot eat after 5 to 6 days, then consideration should be given to providing adequate protein and calories by nasogastric tube or via total parenteral nutrition (see Chapter 16, Nutrition). Diabetics who are managed in this way, receiving a continuous caloric intake either enterally or parenterally, can be treated with regular insulin subcutaneously every 6 hours by intravenous infusion if they are unstable or with NPH or lente insulin every 12 hours with or without added regular or semilente insulin if they are stable. It is important that calories be given at a constant rate in these diabetics to avoid hypoglycemia or hyperglycemia.

Hypoglycemia

Patients will occasionally develop hypoglycemia in the postoperative period. Usually this occurs in a diabetic who has received a dose of insulin that is excessive for the amount of nutrient supplied. Uncommonly, a patient with severe underlying liver disease may get hypoglycemic when receiving a grossly inadequate caloric intake since glycogen stores may become depleted within 48 hours and the liver disease may prevent gluconeogenesis.

A more frequent occurrence of hypoglycemia is in the patient who is receiving total parenteral nutrition (TPN) which is stopped suddenly rather than tapered off gradually. The prolonged high glucose and amino acid loads stimulate endogenous insulin release with resultant high insulin levels. If the TPN is stopped suddenly, these high insulin levels may cause hypoglycemia. Therapy for this includes the resumption of a high caloric intake with gradual tapering down of this intake over a few days. Other rare causes of hypoglycemia include (1) an insulinoma being present, (2) errors in insulin dosage, (3) the wrong patient getting an insulin dose, and (4) the patient surreptitiously self-administering insulin. The differential diagnosis between these disorders employs a wide variety of tests including fasting, stimulation tests, and the measurement of the connecting or C-peptide as well as insulin levels. Details of these tests are beyond the scope of this discussion and are available elsewhere.[44–47]

A pre-existing diagnosis of "reactive hypoglycemia" in a patient usually implies a modest degree of hypoglycemia (40 to 50 mg/dl) occurring 2 to 4 hours after a meal.[48] This usually does not produce any problems for patients undergoing surgical procedures. A proportion of patients carrying this diagnosis, however, have been found to have anxiety neurosis[49, 50] and this needs to be taken into consideration in the overall management of the patient.

THYROID

The major thyroid disorders that should be considered in the patient undergoing surgery are hyperthyroidism and hypothyroidism. Whether the patient has Hashimoto's thyroiditis, a simple goiter, or a nodular goiter is relatively unimportant except that a goiter may cause mechanical difficulties if the surgeon is operating in the neck area. Goiters may also cause upper airway obstruction[51] and difficulty with intubation. The discovery of a goiter in a patient with previously undiagnosed thyroid disease makes it mandatory that the functional state of the thyroid be assessed preoperatively. When hyperthyroidism is suspected, a total thyroxine (T_4), an assessment of thyroid hormone protein binding (e.g., T_3 resin uptake), and a total triiodothyronine (T_3, performed by radioimmunoassay) should be obtained. Conversely, when hypothyroidism is suspected, a T_4, a T_3 resin uptake, a free T_4 (measuring unbound T_4), and a thyroid stimulating hormone (TSH) level should be obtained (Table 6). A detailed discussion of thyroid function testing is available.[52] Because of the danger of precipitating thyroid storm in a hyperthyroid patient by a surgical procedure (see below) or myxedema coma in a hypothyroid patient by anesthesia or analgesics, it is necessary to have at least the T_4 and T_3 resin uptake available before surgery.

Hyperthyroidism

In hyperthyroidism, the T_4, the T_3 resin uptake, and the T_3 will all be elevated except in some rare forms of hyperthyroidism in which the T_3 alone or the T_4 alone may be elevated. Clinically, the signs and symptoms of hyperthyroidism may be divided into two categories: adrenergic hyperthyroidism, characterized by nervousness, anxiety, restlessness, tremor, tachycardia, and perspiration and nonadrenergic hyperthyroidism, characterized by weight loss, myopathy, exophthalmos, and dermopathy. The beta-receptor blocker propranolol has proven to be extremely useful in the management of hyperthyroidism, especially in the emergency treatment of this disorder.

The major manifestations of hyperthyroidism that are of concern in the perioperative period are the effects on cardiac function. Many of these effects are mediated by adrenergic mechanisms. However, thyroid hormones also appear to exert direct effects on the heart with resultant increased rate and contractility.[53–54] It is important to separate out these effects because of the recent tendency to use beta-blocking agents alone in the therapy of hyperthyroidism. It is also necessary to lower thyroid hormone levels to reduce these direct effects. The high output heart failure that is occasionally

TABLE 6. Normal Values of Commonly Used Thyroid Function Tests*

T_4 (thyroxine)	5–13 μg/dl (radioimmunoassay)
	4–11 μg/dl (competitive protein binding assay)
T_3 (triiodothyronine)	70–170 ng/dl (radioimmunoassay)
T_3 Resin Uptake	25–35%
Free T_4	0.8–2.4 ng/dl (dialysis)
TSH (thyroid stimulating hormone)	less than 8 μU/ml
^{131}I Uptake (24 hrs)	5–30%

*Values may vary depending on laboratory.

seen in severe cases is usually the result of hyperthyroidism plus additional, underlying cardiovascular disease, but some patients may develop heart failure without any other disease.[53–55] Cardiac manifestations must be corrected prior to any surgery.

In addition to cardiac effects, hyperthyroidism may be associated with a profound catabolic state with weight loss and loss of lean body mass associated with an elevation of basal metabolic rate. In the presence of this catabolic state, elective surgery should be deferred for several weeks to months while the hyperthyroid state is corrected and lean body mass is restored. Beta-blocking agents alone are not effective in reducing the metabolic rate or allowing weight gain,[56] although some nitrogen retention does occur;[57] antithyroid drugs are necessary to correct the catabolic state.

Several other findings associated with hyperthyroidism may be of importance in the differential diagnosis, especially in the patient with undiagnosed disease. Such patients may have an anemia with a hematocrit of 27 to 30 mm/dl, anisocytosis and hypochromic on peripheral smear, a normal bone marrow, and a defective utilization of iron—all of these findings return to normal with treatment of the hyperthyroidism.[58] Furthermore, about 3 percent of patients with Graves' disease may have pernicious anemia.[59] About 10 percent of patients with hyperthyroidism may have a mild granulocytopenia with a relative lymphocytosis before any therapy, but platelets and clotting are normal.[60] Splenomegaly and lymphadenopathy also occur in 5 to 10 percent of hyperthyroid patients.[60] Also, it should be noted that patients with hyperthyroidism may have increased intestinal motility with diarrhea, nausea, and vomiting and may even present with acute abdominal symptoms which subside with therapy of the hyperthyroidism.[61] Finally, about 20 percent of hyperthyroid patients have hypercalcemia[62] that is responsive to antithyroid therapy and this may further confuse the picture. It should be remembered that many older hyperthyroid patients may lack many of the usual symptoms of hyperthyroidism and they may appear apathetic,[63] but they still may have the cardiac and catabolic manifestations of the disease.

Recently it has been found that even in regions where iodine is not deficient, iodine administration (e.g., used as an expectorant) can induce the development of hyperthyroidism in patients with nontoxic goiters,[64] a phenomenon referred to as the Jodbasedow phenomenon. Of great practical importance, have been the reports of hyperthyroidism[65] and even thyroid storm[66] occurring in initially euthyroid individuals with goiters following the administration of iodinated contrast media used in roentgenographic procedures. Clearly, any patient with a toxic or nontoxic goiter must be observed carefully for the occurrence of hyperthyroidism following such procedures. Although it has not become standard therapy, it may be useful to take the precautionary step of blocking iodine uptake into the gland in patients (especially in known hyperthyroid patients) utilizing thionamide drugs prior to the procedure and for several weeks following the procedure.

MANAGEMENT OF THE CONTROLLED HYPERTHYROID STATE

Elective surgery should be deferred until the functional state of the patient's thyroid is clarified and the hyperthyroidism is brought under control. If cardiac disease, marked weight loss, or myopathy are present then it is preferable to wait for several months before proceeding with surgery, if possible, to allow the catabolic damage to tissues to be repaired. Most such patients are treated with methimazole or propylthiouracil (PTU) to render them euthyroid and occasionally adjunctive agents such as propranolol or iodides are also used (Table 7).

It is not necessary to wait for a remission of the disease or to use definitive ablative therapy such as ^{131}I or thyroidectomy before proceeding with surgery as long as the patient is euthyroid. If the patient is taking PTU or methimazole, these drugs should be continued through the day prior to surgery. If iodinated contrast media are used in diagnostic procedures prior to surgery, it might be prudent to double or triple the dose of the medication before and for several days after the procedure to prevent the stimulation of new thyroid hormone formation, but it is uncertain whether this is necessary. Unfortunately there is no parenteral preparation of these drugs, so that if the patient is to have nothing by mouth for several days following surgery, they cannot be given. Usually this will not result in any sudden exacerbation of the hyperthyroidism, but it is advisable that these drugs be resumed as soon as the patient is able to take oral medications. If necessary, these drugs can be crushed and given by nasogastric tube to unconscious patients. If the patient is euthyroid and in addition to a thionamide is taking propranolol, the latter drug can be stopped prior to surgery and does not routinely have to be resumed postoperatively.

MANAGEMENT OF THE UNCONTROLLED HYPERTHYROID PATIENT NEEDING EMERGENCY SURGERY

An attempt must be made to lower thyroid hormone levels and reduce adrenergic "overactivity" rapidly in the untreated hyperthyroid patient prior to needed urgent or emergency surgery because of the known ability of surgery to precipitate thyroid storm in such patients.[67] In this setting PTU would appear to be more advantageous than methimazole because of its ability to inhibit the conversion of T_4 to T_3 in addition to inhibiting hormone synthesis.[68] It should be given in high doses with an initial dose of 600 to 1000 mg and subsequent doses of 150 to 200 mg every 4 to 6 hours until surgery (if it is to be performed within 72 hours). One to two hours following the initial PTU dose, saturated solution of potassium iodide (SSKI) 2 to 5 drops every 8 hours orally or NaI 0.5 to 1 g intravenously every 8 hours should be given to block thyroid hormone release.[60] Dexamethasone, 2 mg every 6 hours for four doses, can also be given to decrease hormonal release and peripheral conversion of T_4 to T_3.[69] Finally, propranolol, 20 to 80 mg orally every 4 to 6 hours, should be administered to reduce adrenergic "overactivity."[70] Thyroid storm has occurred in patients treated with propranolol alone, so it should always be used in conjunction with other agents.[71] Lithium carbonate, 300 mg every 6 to 8 hours, can be used in place of iodide to inhibit thyroid hormone release[72] if the patient is hypersensitive to iodides. With this regimen, T_3 levels can be halved and clinical improvement (largely due to the propranolol) is seen in 24 to 48 hours. If emergency surgery must be performed within a few hours, the above regimen should be carried out but intravenous propranolol (1 to 10 mg) may be necessary, using cardiac monitoring. In the patient with high output heart failure, intravenous rapid digitalization may also prove beneficial (see Chap 3, Cardiology).

TABLE 7. Drugs Useful in the Treatment of Hyperthyroidism

Name	*Mode of Action*	*Usual Dose*	*Side Effects*	*Indication*
Propylthiouracil (PTU)	Inhibition of thyroid hormone synthesis. Decreased conversion of T_4 to T_3	50–150 mg q 8h po	Rash, fever, agranulocytosis lupus-like syndrome	All hyperthyroidism
Methimazole	Inhibition of thyroid syndrome synthesis	5–20 mg q 8h po	Rash, fever, agranulocytosis lupus-like syndrome	All hyperthyroidism
Propranolol	Decreases adrenergic signs and symptoms by beta blockade. Decreased conversion of T_4 to T_3	10–80 mg q 6h po 1–10 mg q 6h IV	Bronchospasm, congestive heart failure	Thyroid storm, symptomatic relief of adrenergic symptoms
Iodide SSKI NaI	Inhibits thyroidal hormone release	1–2 drops (50–100 mg) q 8h po 1 gm. q 8h IV	Sialadenitis, rash, conjunctivitis	Thyroid storm adjunctive to other agents in severe hyperthyroidism
Glucocorticosteroids (dexamethasone)	Inhibits thyroidal hormone release and decreases conversion of T_4 to T_3	2 mg q 6h × 4 (effects last 7 days)	None in this short time period	Thyroid storm, adjunctive to other agents in severe hyperthyroidism
Lithium carbonate	Inhibits thyroidal hormone release	600–1500 μg/day po in divided doses	Nausea, vomiting, anorexia, stupor, tremor, ataxia. (Dangerous in salt-depleted state)	Adjunctive to other agents
Reserpine	Decreases adrenergic signs and symptoms by depleting catecholamines, sedation	1–5 mg q 4–6h IM	Sedation, postural hypotension	Thyroid storm
Guanethidine	Decreases adrenergic signs and symptoms by depleting catecholamines	1–2 mg/kg/day in divided doses po	Postural hypotension, diarrhea	Thyroid storm
Phenobarbital	Sedation, increases T_4 catabolism.	30–60 mg q 6–8h po	Sedation	Thyroid storm

Intraoperatively, intravenous propranolol can be administered judiciously to help control tachyarrhythmias in the partially treated patient. Ether anesthesia should be avoided since it results in an acute increase in serum T_4 because of a redistribution from tissues into blood.[73] Postoperatively intravenous propranolol, 1 to 10 mg every 6 hours, plus NaI, 0.5 to 1 gm every 8 hours, should be continued. Administration of PTU should be restarted as soon as the patient can take oral medication in doses of 100 to 200 mg every 6 to 8 hours with subsequent reduction to the normal maintenance dose of 100 to 300 mg per day. Intravenous propranolol and iodide should be changed to the oral forms along with resumption of the PTU. The propranolol should be adjusted to keep the heart rate in the range of 60 to 90 beats per minute and the SSKI can be reduced to 1 to 2 drops every 8 hours for 1 to 2 weeks and then discontinued.

MANAGEMENT OF THYROID STORM (TABLE 8)

Even with modern diagnostic and therapeutic techniques, occasionally a patient's hyperthyroidism will first be detected with the onset of thyroid storm in the immediate postoperative period. Since the mortality for this entity varies between 20 and 50 percent,[74] it is important to recognize it clinically before laboratory confirmation can be obtained. It almost always occurs in an untreated or only partially treated patient so that preoperative recognition and therapy of hyperthyroidism should prevent most cases.

Fever is invariably present and is progressive. The fever of thyroid storm usually begins a few hours following surgery; fever starting 12 to 24 hours postoperatively is more likely to be due to other causes (e.g., atelectasis, pneumonia).[67] A tachycardia out

TABLE 8. Management of Thyroid Storm

1. Clinical Findings: Fever, tachycardia, restlessness, stupor, diarrhea, vomiting

2. Laboratory Findings: Elevated T_4, T_3, T_3 resin uptake, free T_4

3. Drug Therapy
   - A. Propylthiouracil 600–800 mg po stat then 150–200 mg q 4–6h
   - B. SSKI, 2–5 drops q 8h po or NaI 0.5–1.0 gm IV q8h (starting 1–2 hrs after propylthiouracil)
   - C. Dexamethasone, 2 mg q 6h × 4 doses
   - D. Propranolol, 20–80 mg q 4h po or 1–10 mg IV q 4h
     - 1. If severe bronchospasm give instead: Reserpine, 1–5 mg IM q 4–6h, or Guanethidine 1 mg/kg of body weight po q 12h
   - E. If iodide toxicity: Use lithium carbonate, 300 mg q 6–8 h. Checking lithium levels before each dose
   - F. Phenobarbital, 30–60 mg q 6–8h

4. Supportive Therapy
   - A. Fluids
   - B. Calories
   - C. Oxygen
   - D. Vitamins: Vitamin B complex, thiamine, vitamin C
   - E. Antipyretic: Cooling blanket, iced gavage, aspirin (acetominophen)
   - F. Digitalis if necessary

5. Treat any underlying illness

of proportion to the fever is present; atrial fibrillation with a rapid ventricular response poorly controlled by digitalis may be present, especially in older patients.[75] Heart block, congestive failure, and acute pulmonary edema may complicate the picture.[75] Although the blood pressure is usually normal, showing an increased pulse pressure, shock may ensue with prolonged duration.[75,76] The mental status is frequently altered, ranging from extreme restlessness and nervousness to confusion, psychosis, seizures, and coma.[75,76] Severe diarrhea, nausea, vomiting, abdominal pain, and jaundice may also be present.[75,76] If the patient has a large goiter, exophthalmos, or a known history of hyperthyroidism, the diagnosis of thyroid storm may not be difficult. However, in a patient without these obvious findings, postoperatively it may be difficult to establish the diagnosis of thyroid storm on the basis of the above clinical manifestations. Unfortunately, the clinical assessment is the only tool available under these circumstances, since the necessity for speed in therapy precludes waiting for laboratory confirmation. Nonetheless, blood should be obtained for serum T_3, T_4, T_3 resin uptake, and free T_4 measurements before commencing therapy.

The drug therapy for thyroid storm is the same as that outlined in the previous section for the uncontrolled hyperthyroid patient and will include high dose PTU, iodides, dexamethasone, and propranolol. If it is at all possible, the PTU should be administered orally or by nasogastric tube 1 to 2 hours prior to iodides. In the event that abdominal surgery and/or a postoperative ileus precludes the administration of PTU, it must be omitted since there is no parenteral preparation. In the event that propranolol cannot be used (severe bronchospasm), reserpine, 1 to 5 mg intramuscularly every 4 to 6 hours, or guanethidine, 1 mg/kg of body weight orally every 12 hours, can be given.[77,78] Unlike propranolol, these agents have a delay of several hours before their effects are apparent clinically. It is possible that metoprolol or other cardioselective beta-blocking agents may prove beneficial in patients with bronchospasm but experience in their use in hyperthyroidism is limited. After steroids are given in the first 24 hours, many authorities recommend continuation until the severe toxic state has resolved but there is no real proof that this is efficacious.[75]

In addition to high dose PTU, iodides, steroids, and propranolol, these patients require considerable supportive care and should be managed in an intensive care unit with constant cardiac monitoring. In this setting, intravenous propranolol (1 to 10 mg over 5 to 10 minutes) may be necessary to control tachyarrhythmias. When heart failure is present, digitalization and diuretics may also be helpful. Because of the excessive sweating and fever, insensible fluid losses are often great and careful fluid and electrolyte repletion is necessary. Glucose should be provided to meet immediate caloric needs, and if the patient is unable to eat for more than 24 hours, amino acid supplements should be employed to achieve nitrogen balance and total parenteral nutrition should be considered because of the excessive caloric requirements of the hyperthyroid state. Thiamine, vitamin B complex, and vitamin C should be provided in liberal amounts since subclinical deficits may be present.[75] The body temperature should be reduced using a cooling blanket and iced saline gavage (if the patient is permitted anything by mouth). The use of salicylates is controversial. Larsen[79] has shown that salicylates result in a displacement of T_3 and T_4 from binding protein, resulting in substantial increases in the free hormone concentration in blood. In addition, aspirin is also known to be calorigenic itself.[80] Although acetaminophen might therefore be theoretically the more desirable antipyretic, no untoward effects from the use of aspirin have been reported,[81] and either acetaminophen or aspirin would appear satisfactory in this regard. Sedation is often indicated for extreme restlessness, and because of their effects in lowering thyroid hormones by increasing their catabolism, the barbiturates appear to be the drugs of choice.[82] Phenobarbital, 30 to 60 mg every 6 to 8 hours, has been employed for this purpose. When reserpine is used as the "antiadrenergic" agent, its sedating effect obviates the use of other agents. Oxygen should also be administered to help support the increased oxygen demands of the hyperthyroid tissues. Finally, if surgery itself is not the underlying cause, a precipitating illness such as infection must always be looked for and treated.

MANAGEMENT OF THE PATIENT UNDERGOING THYROIDECTOMY

Indications for thyroidectomy for hyperthyroidism vary from clinic to clinic and will not be dealt with here. Thyroidectomy in the hyperthyroid patient is a purely elective procedure, and all patients should be rendered euthyroid with PTU or methimazole for several weeks before surgery. If there is significant weight loss or cardiac disease, a longer period of up to several months may be necessary to bring the patient to the optimal state of health prior to surgery. For 1 to 2 weeks prior to surgery, iodide (SSKI, 2 drops, 3 times a day) or propranolol (20 to 40 mg, four times a day) should be added to reduce the vascularity and friability of the gland.[83,84] If thyroidectomy is indicated in a patient who has an adverse reaction to both thionamides, surgery can usually be performed safely using propranolol alone.[83,85,86] It should be remembered, however, that propranolol alone will not reverse the altered metabolic rate or the direct effects of thyroid hormones on the heart[54,56] and also that thyroid storm has been precipitated by surgery in patients prepared with just propranolol.[71] Such patients, therefore, should be monitored closely for the development of storm postoperatively. It is felt that the intraoperative manipulation of the gland may result in a release of thyroid hormones when the gland is not properly prepared and that this surge of hormones may be responsible for the postoperative worsening.[82]

In centers with significant experience with thyroidectomies, the postoperative complications of subtotal thyroidectomy for Graves' disease and other conditions range from 0.2 to 9 percent.[87,88] Bleeding, occasionally requiring reoperation or tracheostomy, occurs in 0.3 to 2 percent of cases, and recurrent nerve paralysis occurs in 0.5 to 0.8 percent.[87,88] Hypocalcemia occurs in up to 23 percent of patients following subtotal thyroidectomy for Graves' disease, in 28 percent of patients following total thyroidectomy for thyroid cancer, but in only 1.5 percent of patients following subtotal thyroidectomy for other diseases.[89] The hypocalcemia usually occurs 24 to 36 hours following surgery and is transient in 75 to 80 percent of patients. This transient hypocalcemia has been attributed to several causes, including: (1) hyperthyroid osteodystrophy with a decrease in bone resorption following thyroidectomy, (2) a release of thyrocalcitonin, and (3) parathyroid damage.[89] It is not clear which of these mechanisms is operative and the mechanism may vary from patient to patient. Permanent hypocalcemia is due to hypoparathyroidism caused by inadvertent parathyroidectomy and/or interference with the parathyroid blood supply either at surgery or by late scar formation.[89,90] In some centers, parathyroid autotransplantation to the sternocleidomastoid muscle is routinely performed to prevent late hypoparathyroidism.[90] Postoperative hypocalcemia is not usually symptomatic and, therefore, does not need to be treated unless the patient develops cramping, paresthesias, positive Trousseau's or Chvostek's signs, or Q-T interval prolongation on electrocardiogram. Acutely, calcium gluconate 10 percent can be administered intravenously in 10 ml amounts every 2 to 4 hours should such indications develop. If hypocalcemia persists longer than 72 hours, calcium carbonate (Os-Cal) can be added (4 tablets contain 1 gm elemental calcium). If, after several days, this is not successful in maintaining a normal serum calcium, vitamin D can be added (see below) for the chronic management of hypoparathyroidism.

Overall, the most common complications of thyroidectomy for hyperthyroidism are hypothyroidism and recurrent hyperthyroidism. Recurrent or persistent hyperthyroidism occurs in 4 to 8 percent of patients treated with subtotal thyroidectomy; interestingly, a recurrence may not appear for several years.[91,92] Hypothyroidism is related both to the amount of tissue remaining and the degree of fibrosis and lymphocytic infiltration of the gland.[91,92] Although hypothyroidism usually occurs within the first few months following surgery, long term follow-up studies have shown that it may also be a later complication. In one series of 43 children treated by subtotal thyroidectomy, 58 percent developed hypothyroidism.[93] Postoperative hypothyroidism is treated as any other hypothyroidism with the caveat that the remnant of thyroid tissue may still be autonomous and, therefore, a smaller dose of thyroxine may be needed for adequate replacement. Occasionally postoperative hypothyroidism is only transient and thyroid hormone values return to normal by 6 months following surgery.[94] Clearly the patient whose hyperthyroidism has been treated with surgery must be followed closely and indefinitely for the development of hypothyroidism or hyperthyroidism so that these complications can be treated promptly should they occur.

Hypothyroidism

The clinical presentation of patients with hypothyroidism usually will include symptoms and signs of dry skin, coarsened hair, constipation, sluggishness, modest weight gain, increased sleeping, bradycardia, mental slowing, and periorbital edema. However, it has become apparent that many patients do not manifest many of these symptoms and only a high index of suspicion will point toward the diagnosis. Laboratory testing in patients who are not severely ill should include a T_4 and a T_3 resin uptake, values of both of which will be low, and a TSH which will be high. A T_3 and a free T_4 may be helpful under certain circumstances (see below).

Although mildly to moderately hypothyroid patients do not fair worse with surgery than euthyroid patients,[95] there is considerable evidence that hypothyroidism adversely affects a number of body systems, so that optimally it is preferable to make a patient euthyroid first before an elective procedure. On the other hand, emergency surgery in a hypothyroid patient does not carry the risks that are inherent in not treating the hyperthyroid patient.

The cardiac effects of hypothyroidism are prominent. In severe myxedema the myocardium is fibrotic, edematous, and has a loss of striations. Myocardial contractility is impaired in hypothyroidism. Crowley and associates[96] have shown excellent correlation between systolic time intervals and thyroid hormone levels in hypothyroid individuals with a return to normal of cardiac function with thyroxine therapy. In addition to impaired myocardial contractility, bradycardia is seen due to the direct effects of thyroid hormone deficiency on the sinoatrial node.[97] The impaired contractility and bradycardia result in decreased cardiac output and stroke volume. Blood volume is decreased and is accompanied by a normal to increased peripheral resistance.[97] In severe hypothyroidism, pericardial effusions are common, being documented by echocardiography in 9 of 14 patients in one series.[96] The pericardial effusions are high in protein, as are the ascites, pleural effusions, and joint effusions also seen in hypothyroidism.[98] Although serious cardiac impairment does not usually occur with these pericardial effusions due to their slow development, tamponade does rarely occur.[97] A chest x-ray often reveals cardiomegaly with a globular configuration suggestive of pericardial effusion. The electrocardiogram characteristically shows generalized low voltage with T wave flattening, bradycardia, and occasionally right bundle-branch block. These changes revert to normal with thyroid replacement.[97]

Patients with long-standing myxedema appear to have an increased amount of coronary artery disease as shown by autopsy studies,[99] although this may be partly related to the hypertension seen in many of these patients.[100] Although the decreased metabolic requirements of the hypothyroid state usually protect the individual from going on to infarction, it should be remembered that such a patient with coronary artery disease must be started on thyroid hormone replacement extremely cautiously. Similarly, the increased metabolic requirements induced by the stress of surgery or infection may be a problem for the hypothyroid patient with compromised coronary arteries. Nitroglycerin use has occasionally produced hypotension and syncope in hypothyroid patients with angina due to their decreased blood volume.

In hypothyroidism the serum enzymes SGOT, LDH, and CPK are often elevated into the ranges seen in myocardial infarction, and the SGPT remains normal.[97] Isoenzyme analysis of the CPK elevation reveals the MM isoenzyme, reflecting skeletal muscle component, to be elevated, with the cardiac MB band being normal.[101] Therefore, CPK isoenzyme analysis may be essential in excluding a myocardial infarction in the hypothyroid patient who develops chest pain. If this type of analysis is not available then it would be important to have values for preoperative or prestress enzymes as a baseline.

Respiratory function is also impaired in hypothyroidism. Pulmonary function tests reveal significant decreases in diffusing capacity and maximal breathing capacity.[102] Alveolar hypoventilation also occurs to a varying degree owing to a markedly depressed hypoxic ventilatory drive in all hypothyroid patients and a depressed hypercapnic drive in severely hypothyroid patients; occasionally this may result in respiratory failure.[103] It is well known that drug metabolism is considerably slowed in patients with hypothyroidism.[104] All sedating drugs, especially narcotic analgesics, must be used in small doses and with great caution in such patients not only because of the excess sedation but also because of the additive suppressive effects they may have on respiration. Myxedema coma can be precipitated by the injudicious use of morphine or other analgesics for postoperative pain.

A variety of mechanisms may lead to impaired consciousness in the patient with severe hypothyroidism. As noted, the most common of these are (1) the impaired metabolism of administered sedatives, (2) depressed hypoxic and hypercapnic ventilatory drives leading to carbon dioxide retention with hypoxia, and (3) decreased cardiac output with an increase in cerebrovascular resistance[105] leading to decreased cerebral perfusion. Hyponatremia, occasionally severe enough to cause mental impairment, may also occur in hypothyroidism although the mechanism is not clear.[106,107] Since postoperative hyponatremia is commonly seen in euthyroid patients, special care is needed postoperatively to restrict free water intake in hypothyroid patients to avoid this complication. It should also be remembered that hypothyroidism may be secondary to hypopituitarism and that adrenal insufficiency may also be present. The hypotension, hypothermia, and coma seen in severe myxedema may also occur in hypopituitarism[108] and both steroids and thyroid hormone may be necessary in therapy (see below).

Hematologic abnormalities may also be found in patients with hypothyroidism. Bruising and excessive bleeding have been found in some patients, with defective platelet adhesiveness found in 12 of 16 patients, a prolonged bleeding time in 4 of 16, and an abnormal partial thromboplastin time (PTT) in 5 of 16 patients in one series.[109] It is uncertain how often these changes result in a clinically significant bleeding diathesis that would impede surgery. The total circulating red cell mass and plasma volume are decreased in hypothyroidism resulting in a normal or low hematocrit.[110] Erythropoiesis is diminished and an anemia due to folate,[111] vitamin B_{12}, or iron deficiencies[112] can be seen in association with hypothyroidism. Optimally these deficiencies should be corrected before surgery or at least treated in the perioperative period so as to allow the marrow to replace blood loss and to correct leukopenia or thrombocytopenia if they are present.

Other potentially important findings in the hypothyroid patient needing surgery relate to the skin and gastrointestinal tract. The dermal layer of the skin is infiltrated with a mixture of mucopolysaccharides associated with a decrease in collagen synthesis and degradation.[113] It has been suggested that myxedematous tissues hold sutures less well than normal tissues, but there is no firm data to support or refute this concept. Gastrointestinal motility is usually slowed, resulting in constipation and distention. Rarely, patients with myxedema will appear to have a paralytic ileus which has led to unnecessary surgery in the past.[114]

EUTHYROID SICK SYNDROME

As noted earlier, laboratory evaluation in hypothyroidism will show a low T_4, a low T_3 resin uptake, and a high TSH. Additionally the nonprotein bound or free T_4 will be low and T_3 levels are low to normal. It is of importance to distinguish the state of hypothyroidism biochemically from the "euthyroid sick syndrome," in which the laboratory values may initially appear to suggest hypothyroidism but the patient is relatively euthyroid. In this syndrome, severe acute stresses such as infection and surgery result in a decrease in serum T_3 levels by decreasing the peripheral deiodination of T_4 to T_3.[115] This effect lasts for several days and low T_3 levels are seen in many chronic disease states, such as malignancy, renal failure, infection, and pulmonary and hepatic diseases.[116,117] A similar fall in T_3 is seen with fasting and hypocaloric intake associated with weight loss.[118] We have shown that in septic patients some of the fall in T_3 is due to the stress of the infection but part is due to the decreased caloric intake of these sick patients.[119] These low serum T_3 levels are reflected in similarly low tissue T_3 levels.[120] In addition to these low T_3 levels, total T_4 levels are normal to low due to accelerated metabolism of T_4,[121] a decrease in thyroidal T_4 release,[122] and a decrease in thyroxine binding prealbumin (TBPA) and occasionally in thyroxine binding globulin (TBG).[123] Importantly, in this syndrome the free T_4 level is normal to slightly elevated and the TSH levels are normal;[120,123] it is necessary, therefore, to check the free T_4 and TSH levels in these patients. We have even seen patients with this syndrome who also had low free T_4 levels but normal TSH levels, so that a low free T_4 level is no guarantee of hypothyroidism. It is still unclear as to whether these patients are truly euthyroid or hypothyroid (which may be a compensatory mechanism to reduce body metabolism in the face of stress), since it is difficult to assess the usual parameters of tissue function related to thyroid status (i.e., cholesterol and CPK levels and basal metabolic rate) in these ill patients.[124] A special case is the patient with head trauma and coma who may have low T_4, T_3, free T_4, and TSH measurements.[125] It is uncertain whether these patients represent the euthyroid sick syndrome or have true hypothalamic hypothyroidism, since their TSH response to thyrotropin-releasing hormone (TRH) is actually exaggerated.

The euthyroid sick syndrome is very common, occurring in 37 percent of 70 patients admitted to an acute medical ward in a city hospital.[126] Patients preoperatively and postoperatively may often be found to have this syndrome, with low T_3 and low to normal T_4 and T_3 resin uptake values. Under these circumstances it is necessary to obtain values for a free T_4 and a TSH to separate euthyroid sick from hypothyroid patients. Clinically, these patients are usually quite ill, and it may not be possible to assess the thyroid state accurately by examination. The hardest distinction is in the severely ill, comatose patient in whom a low T_4 value is obtained with the other studies pending. Since it is important to begin treatment of myxedema coma with thyroid hormone rapidly (see below), it is probably better to err by giving thyroxine to a euthyroid sick patient (if the thyroid is normal, the only result will be a shutting off of TSH and thyroid hormone synthesis) than to possibly withhold thyroxine from a patient with myxedema coma. Therefore, if the T_4 value is very low and the clinical suspicion is high for hypothyroidism, I recommend obtaining the free T_4 and TSH measurements and starting either low dose levothyroxine for the routine patient or higher dose levothyroxine (0.1 mg daily) for the patient with possible myxedema coma, continuing such therapy until the results of these laboratory tests are obtained.

MANAGEMENT OF THE HYPOTHYROID PATIENT UNDERGOING ELECTIVE SURGERY

When possible, surgery should be deferred in hypothyroid patients until the hypothyroidism has been corrected. Therapy should be carried out using levothyroxine exclusively. It was formerly thought that T_3 was primarily secreted by the thyroid and that thyroid medication containing T_3 was necessary for proper hormone replacement. It is now clear that 70 to 80 percent of circulating T_3 is derived from the peripheral deiodination of T_4,[117] and normal T_4 and T_3 levels have been found with pure levothyroxine therapy in doses of 0.1 to 0.20 mg daily.[127] In fact, therapy with T_4 and T_3 combinations[128] and dessicated thyroid U.S.P.[129] have both been found to result in a greater incidence of hyperthyroid side effects, resulting in normal T_4 levels but usually elevated T_3 levels,[129] than therapy with levothyroxine. Switching patients to levothyroxine corrects this imbalance. Because of its long half-life of 7 days, levothyroxine results in sustained even levels of both T_4 and T_3, but T_3 preparations (Cytomel) and T_4 and T_3 combinations result in markedly fluctuating T_3 levels due to the short half-life (24 hours) of T_3[130] and so they should not be used routinely.

In patients below the age of 40, therapy is usually begun with doses between 0.05 and 0.1 mg of levothyroxine, increasing the dosage at 2 to 4 week intervals until full replacement dosage is reached. In the older patient, some degree of coronary artery disease is presumed and therapy is begun at 0.025 to 0.05 mg daily with increasing increments usually at 4 week intervals. Crowley and associates[96] have shown that a significant improvement in cardiovascular dynamics occurs with doses of 0.075 to 0.1 mg daily of levothyroxine. The dosage is gradually increased until the TSH level is normal and the T_4 and T_3 levels are normal.

The patient with advanced coronary artery disease and angina pectoris presents a special problem. In these patients thyroxine is started at very low doses—0.0125 mg every day or even every other day. The increment should be similarly small, at intervals of 4 to 8 weeks. Should increased angina occur, the medication is halted for a few days and therapy is reinstituted at the preceding lower dose. Often long-acting nitrates and propranolol may be helpful while instituting therapy in such patients. Paine and associates[101] have found that myxedematous patients whose angina pectoris is severe enough to warrant coronary bypass surgery tolerate cardiac catheterization and surgery reasonably well, and thyroid hormone therapy can be initiated safely the first postoperative day. Under these circumstances, the decision to start thyroid hormone preoperatively is an exceedingly difficult one at best. On the basis of our own experience, I would favor starting levothyroxine, 0.0125 mg every other day, and if angina worsened at all then surgery should proceed forthwith. However, the report of Paine and associates[101] suggests that perhaps coronary artery surgery should proceed first. Such decisions must be individualized for each patient with combined consultation of cardiologist, endocrinologist, and cardiac surgeon. Even after surgery, patients with angina pectoris may often benefit by thyroid hormone therapy that results in their being slightly under replaced.

Levothyroxine is 79.9 percent absorbed in the fasting state and 59.6 percent absorbed when taken with meals.[131] Because of this, when patients are unable to take medications orally we usually recommend giving about half to two-thirds of the usual dose intravenously. Since the usual replacement dose is about 0.15 mg, this corresponds to 0.1 mg of levothyroxine intravenously once a day. If the patient is to have nothing by mouth for only 2 to 3 days, then such parenteral therapy is not necessary because of the long half-life of the drug.

In hypothyroidism due to pituitary insufficiency, there is a high likelihood that the hypothalamic-pituitary-adrenal axis will be impaired as well. When the hypothyroidism is due to Hashimoto's thyroiditis a concomitant autoimmune adrenal insufficiency (Schmidt's syndrome) occurs infrequently.[132] Because of these two possibilities, if the clinical situation warrants it, a limited investigation of adrenal function should be done before starting thyroid replacement because thyroid hormone replacement might exacerbate adrenal insufficiency. Obtaining a basal morning cortisol level plus a cortisol value from a sample obtained 30 to 60 minutes following the intravenous or intramuscular administration of synthetic 1–24 ACTH (Cortrosyn) will suffice. Then therapy with glucocorticoids (see below) should be begun along with levothyroxine.

MANAGEMENT OF THE HYPOTHYROID PATIENT NEEDING EMERGENCY SURGERY

As noted in the preceding sections, such patients appear to tolerate surgery satisfactorily without thyroid hormone replacement although certain precautions need to be taken. Levothyroxine should be started as soon as possible orally or intravenously in the same doses as suggested above. Glucocorticoids should be given (see below) because of the possibility of coexistent adrenal insufficiency. Great caution should be exerted in the administration of sedatives and analgesics preoperatively and postoperatively because of their slow metabolism. Because of the prolonged effects of these drugs and anesthesia and because of the depressed hypoxic and ventilatory drives of these patients, they may need to be intubated and ventilated with a respirator for a prolonged period. As mentioned earlier, the hyponatremia often seen postoperatively may be exaggerated in these patients because of their impaired ability to clear free water. Consequently, their water intake should be restricted. Because of the volume contraction normally seen in hypothyroidism, the vasodilation that may occur with anesthesia and morphine may result in hypotension that will respond to fluids. However, care must be exercised so that when the effects of these agents wear off the impaired myocardial contractility doesn't result in the patient going into pulmonary edema. Finally, a postoperative ileus might be prolonged in patients with hypothyroidism.

MANAGEMENT OF MYXEDEMA COMA

Myxedema coma is a true medical emergency with a 20 percent mortality even when treated properly.[133] On surgical services, it is usually seen in a patient in whom hypothyroidism had not been recognized and who had become comatose as a result of hyponatremia, excessive sedation, infection, hypoxia, hypoglycemia, or CO_2 narcosis. Clinical features suggestive of myxedema coma include hypothermia ($<36°C$), bradycardia, delayed return of or absent deep tendon reflexes, impaired consciousness, evidence of a goiter or a thyroidectomy scar, exophthalmos, periorbital edema, coarse dry skin, and alopecia.[133–136] Appropriate blood tests should be performed to evaluate the possibilities of hyponatremia, hypoglycemia, hypoxia, and hypercapnia. Full thyroid function studies should be obtained, including a free T_4 and TSH to help to differentiate the euthyroid sick syndrome from myxedema, although therapy must proceed before the results can be obtained.

Therapy for myxedema coma consists of general supportive care with the correction of metabolic abnormalities and thyroid hormone administration. Supportive care consists of the rapid correction of hyponatremia (see Chapter 15, Fluid, Electrolyte and

TABLE 9. Management of Myxedema Coma

1. Clinical Findings: Hypothermia, bradycardia, obtundation (thyroidectomy scar; exophthalmos, occasionally)

2. Laboratory Findings: Low T_4, T_3 resin uptake, T_3, and free T_4 levels. Elevated TSH (unless hypopituitary). Frequently, low Po_2, high Pco_2, low Na, low glucose

3. Hormone Therapy
   A. Levothyroxine, 500 μg IV stat then 50 μg IV daily
   B. Hydrocortisone, 100 mg IV q 8h

4. Supportive Therapy
   A. Correction of hypoxia and hypercapnia. Intubation and mechanical ventilation if necessary
   B. Correction of hypoglycemia
   C. Correction of hyponatremia if sodium <120 mEq/L with 3% NaCl and furosemide
   D. Correction of hypotension with colloid
   E. Treatment of any underlying infection
   F. Nasogastric suction
   G. Bladder catheterization
   H. Avoid rapid warming
   I. Avoid pressors if possible
   J. Pericardiocentesis if signs of tamponade

Acid-Base Disorders), the administration of glucose and other intravenous fluids, respiratory management (including intubation and mechanical ventilation if necessary), and appropriate antibiotics if infection is present. External warming should not be performed because it may result in peripheral vasodilation and hypotension. However, central warming via heated air or oxygen may be useful.[137] Hypotension should be managed with fluids or whole blood, utilizing a CVP line. Pressors should be avoided if possible because myxedematous patients appear to be more sensitive to ventricular arrhythmias.[133] Rarely, the pericardial effusion present in such patients will lead to tamponade and will require tapping. A paralytic ileus may require nasogastric suction and urinary retention may require catheterization.[134] There is some controversy regarding the adequacy of the hypothalamic-pituitary-adrenal response in myxedema coma, but most authors advocate giving steroids for the first 24 to 48 hours of therapy after a basal cortisol level is obtained.[133,134] Hydrocortisone, 100 mg intravenously every 8 hours, will be sufficient.

As opposed to the usual hypothyroid patient who initially should receive small doses of thyroid hormone, large doses are given to patients in myxedema coma. An intravenous dose of 0.5 mg of levothyroxine is usually recommended initially and results in repletion of the total thyroxine pool.[133–136] The long half-life of thyroxine obviates giving additional drug for a few days,[133,136] although Menendez and Rivlin[135] recommend giving an additional 0.05 mg intravenously daily. This dose results in a rise in T_4 to the low normal range and a decrease in TSH by 39 percent with 24 hours.[138] The peak metabolic effects of this dose do not occur for about 10 days, but some improvement is usually seen by 6 to 12 hours and clear-cut improvement (increased body temperature, improved mental status) should be seen within 24 hours.[133] Many of these patients will have a decrease in conversion of the T_4 to T_3 as might be expected because of their severe illnesses.[130] Unfortunately, only T_4 is routinely available for intravenous injection; T_3 can be given only orally or via nasogastric tube. A parenteral preparation of T_3 can be made by dissolving the sodium salt of T_3 in a few drops of 0.1 N NaOH. This is then diluted with 5 ml of sterile saline containing 1 percent albumin and sterilized using a Millipore filter.[133,136] Twenty-five μg are then given intravenously every 8 to 12 hours. Because of its more rapid effects, T_3 might appear to be the drug of choice, but much more experience has been obtained using T_4 and the results with T_4 appear satisfactory. The intravenous route is much to be preferred since the ileus commonly seen with this condition may significantly delay and decrease intestinal absorption. Administration of T_4 is also favored as large doses of T_3 may promote arrhythmias should the diagnosis of myxedema coma prove erroneous (in actual practice this is not infrequent) while T_4, even in large doses, appears to be well tolerated.[136] Because of its ready availability in parenteral form, its documented efficacy, and the lack of ill effects when the condition is misdiagnosed, T_4 would appear to be the preparation of choice.

ADRENALS

The most common adrenal hormonal disorder that affects patients having surgical procedures is iatrogenic adrenal insufficiency from glucocorticosteroid therapy. Such patients are easy to manage. Fortunately, spontaneous Cushing's syndrome, Addison's disease, hyperaldosteronism, and hypoaldosteronism are quite rare.

Adrenal Insufficiency (Addison's Disease)

The symptoms of chronic adrenal insufficiency are relatively nonspecific and include weakness, fatigue, lethargy, apathy, confusion, anorexia, weight loss, nausea, constipation alternating with diarrhea, hyperpigmentation (especially of scars, skin creases, and mucosal surfaces), hypotension, and amenorrhea. Occasionally, the gastrointestinal features may predominate and the abdominal pain that may occur may simulate an acute abdomen.[139,140] Any form of stress can convert this clinical situation into one of acute adrenal insufficiency or adrenal crisis, which is manifested by hypotension and shock that is poorly responsive to pressors. Such stresses would include surgical procedures, infection, invasive diagnostic procedures, and anesthesia. Unexplained hypotension in a patient should always raise the possibility of adrenal insufficiency.

The clinical background of the patient is important in arriving at a diagnosis. Autoimmune and tuberculous adrenalitis are by far the most common causes of adrenal insufficiency,[140] and autoimmune adrenalitis is often associated with other endocrine insufficiencies, especially that of the thyroid.[141] However, metastases to the adrenals, especially from lung and breast cancer,[142] adrenal venography,[143] histoplasmosis, sarcoidosis, irradiation,[140] and amyloidosis have all been documented to cause adrenal insufficiency as well. Acute adrenal insufficiency may develop in any of these settings when the patient is stressed. Of great importance is the occurrence of adrenal hemorrhage in patients in the perioperative period. This usually presents as an acute adrenal crisis that is manifested by fever, abdominal or flank pain, vomiting, confusion, and hypotension.[144–146] Spontaneous adrenal hemorrhage has been reported in the postoperative period up to 33 days following surgery[144] and should be considered in cases of unexplained rapid deterioration postoperatively. Adrenal hemorrhage has also been found with anticoagulant therapy,[147] severe burns, meningococcemia (Waterhouse-Friderichsen syndrome) and other septic states, and cardiovascular collapse.[145]

Laboratory features of adrenal insufficiency include hyperkalemia due to aldosterone deficiency, hyponatremia due to an inability to clear free water by the kidney, azotemia, eosinophilia, and a lymphocytosis.[148] If the signs, symptoms, and laboratory data base suggest adrenal insufficiency, then diagnostic procedures and therapy should be carried out quickly and simultaneously.

DIAGNOSTIC PROCEDURES

Not only is it important to establish a diagnosis of adrenal insufficiency, it is also important to distinguish between primary adrenal dysfunction and secondary dysfunction due to hypopituitarism. The method that will yield the most information in the shortest time is outlined in Table 10. Blood for cortisol and ACTH levels is obtained. The latter should be drawn into a heparinized tube (green top) and stored on ice immediately. Both values will be low in hypothalamic/pituitary disease but the ACTH will be elevated in primary adrenal insufficiency; these two values alone may be sufficient to discriminate between these two disorders.[148] After these basal samples are obtained, dexamethasone, 4 mg, and ACTH (Cortrosyn) (1 ampule = 25μg) are given intravenously. A second cortisol level is obtained 1 hour later. (The dexamethasone does not interfere with the cortisol assay or the adrenal's response to ACTH.)

The minimum values for cortisol in the Cortrosyn stimulation test that are accepted as normal are a basal cortisol of greater than 5 μg/dl and an increment of over 7 μg/dl, with the actual level reached over 18 μg/dl.[140, 149] In a stressed patient, the basal cortisol levels would be expected to be much higher than 5 μg/dl and ordinarily the

TABLE 10. Diagnostic Protocol in Adrenal Insufficiency

1. Clinical Presentation: Hyperpigmentation, apathy, lethargy, weight loss, nausea, diarrhea, abdominal pain, hypotension, fever
2. Draw blood for cortisol (serum) and ACTH (heparinized on ice) electrolytes, BUN, creatinine
3. Give dexamethasone, 4 mg IV
4. Administer Cortrosyn (synthetic ACTH), 1 ampule (0.25 μg), IM or IV
5. Draw blood for cortisol evaluation 1 hour after administration of Cortosyn
6. Administer hydrocortisone, 100 mg IM or IV q8h for 24 hours and then taper down
7. Administer 1-3 L of D_5 saline over first 24 hours to correct fluid deficit
8. If Cortrosyn stimulation test substantiates hypoadrenalism, further detailed testing should be carried out when patient is stable

response is close to a doubling of the basal value. In patients with disease secondary to ACTH deficiency, a subnormal but definite response is seen, and in patients with primary adrenal disease, little or no response is seen. The Cortrosyn stimulation test should be regarded as a screening test only. An abnormal test requires confirmation using more prolonged testing with ACTH stimulation and dynamic tests of the entire hypothalamic-pituitary-adrenal axis such as hypoglycemic stimulation and metyrapone testing. Details of such tests are available.[139,140,148] However, it is important to carry out this brief, simple diagnostic Cortrosyn stimulation test when a patient is thought to be in adrenal insufficiency so that prolonged steroid administration can be avoided in the case of diagnostic error. The ready availability of ACTH assays in commercial laboratories now makes this once difficult to obtain measurement easily available.

TREATMENT OF KNOWN ADRENOCORTICAL INSUFFICIENCY

The average glucocorticoid maintenance dosages for an adult are: cortisol (hydrocortisone), 20 mg in the morning and 10 mg in the evening; cortisone acetate, 25 mg in the morning and 12.5 mg in the evening; and prednisone, 2.5 to 5 mg in the morning and 2.5 mg in the evening. Patients with primary adrenal insufficiency usually also require a mineralocorticoid and the usual dose is 0.05 to 0.15 mg per day of fludrocortisone (Florinef) as an oral preparation or 2.5 to 5 mg per day of deoxycorticosterone acetate (DOCA) subcutaneously or intramuscularly. Since normal individuals secrete 100 to 300 mg of cortisol in 24 hours in the face of severe stress,[139] we recommend giving 300 mg per day on the day of surgery or in the face of severe stress such as overwhelming infection. Assuming that the stress resolves over a few days, the dose can be decreased by 50 percent every 1 to 2 days (Table 11). In the typical patient undergoing elective surgery, we normally recommend giving 50 to 100 mg of hydrocortisone sodium succi-

TABLE 11. Glucocorticoid Therapy for Surgery in Adrenal Insufficiency

1. Hydrocortisone, 100 mg IM the night prior to surgery
2. Hydrocortisone, 100 mg IM in AM on call to operating room
3. Hydrocortisone, 100 mg IV over course of surgery
4. Hydrocortisone, 100 mg IM or IV evening of surgery
5. Postoperative day (POD) 1: Hydrocortisone, 50–100 mg* IM or IV q 8h
6. POD 2: Hydrocortisone, 25–50 mg IM or IV q 8h
7. POD 3: Hydrocortisone, 25 mg IM, IV, or po q 12h
   Fludrocortisone (Florinef), 0.1 mg daily
8. POD 4: Hydrocortisone, 20 mg in AM, 10 mg in PM
   Fludrocortisone, 0.05–0.1 mg daily

*For major procedures, unstable course, or supervening infection the higher dosage figures should be used with slower tapering off.

nate (Solu-Cortef) on the night before surgery to cover the psychologic stress of the impending procedure. On the day of surgery, we recommend giving 100 mg of hydrocortisone intramuscularly in the morning, 100 mg of hydrocortisone as an intravenous drip in dextrose in saline during the surgery itself, and finally 100 mg intramuscularly in the late evening.[139] On the first postoperative day, 50 mg of hydrocortisone intramuscularly every 8 hours is given; on the second postoperative day, 25 mg intramuscularly every 8 hours is given; on the third postoperative day, 25 mg intramuscularly or orally every 12 hours is given; and then maintenance dosage is resumed. If the postoperative course is not smooth or if infection supervenes, then the rate of tapering should be slower. Hydrocortisone in large doses has enough mineralocorticoid activity that additional therapy with Florinef or deoxycorticosterone acetate is not necessary until the dose of hydrocortisone is 100 mg or less per day.

With more minor acute stresses, such as a pneumoencephalogram or a dental extraction, 50 to 100 mg of hydrocortisone before and after the procedure will usually suffice. If the stress is more prolonged, as with a myocardial infarction, a pneumonia, or metastatic cancer, two to three times the usual maintenance dose should be given for the stressful period. We have had the experience of 2 patients who had bilateral adrenalectomies for palliation of metastatic breast cancer who developed signs and symptoms of adrenal insufficiency on prednisone, 7.5 mg daily, but who did well on 15 mg daily. Mineralocorticoid replacement does not usually have to be increased with stress, but patients should be given a liberal amount of salt in their diet. With all of the above suggestions, it is better to give a bit too much glucocorticoid transiently than too little to allow the patient to meet the stress adequately. On the other hand, the known effects of high doses of glucocorticoids may combat the response to infection (see below) so that it is wise not to give too much for too long. The above guidelines have stood the test of time[139] and patients usually do well with this type of coverage.

TREATMENT OF ACUTE ADRENAL INSUFFICIENCY

The patient who develops acute adrenal insufficiency usually has had some acute stressful process like surgery that has precipitated this event. If the process is not obvious, an underlying illness (e.g., infection, myocardial infarction, occult malignancy) must be looked for and treated. In the hospitalized patient, adrenal hemorrhage due to anticoagulation, infection, or the postoperative state must be suspected (see above). These patients are acutely ill with up to 20 percent dehydration[139] and hypotension being the usual manifestations. Unexplained hypotension in the postoperative period should always raise the possibility of adrenal insufficiency.

Therapy should consist of the administration of 1 to 3 L physiologic saline with glucose (D5NS) to correct the sodium deficit and hypoglycemia and steroids. As mentioned above, diagnosis and therapy can proceed simultaneously by performing a Cortrosyn stimulation test and administering dexamethasone (see Table 10). Hydrocortisone, 100 mg is then given intravenously or intramuscularly every 8 hours (if the patient is not hypotensive) until the acute event has resolved and the dose is then tapered as mentioned above.[150]

Cushing's Syndrome

This syndrome of excess cortisol secretion may be due to (1) bilateral adrenal hyperplasia secondary to excess pituitary ACTH secretion or to ectopic ACTH secretion by a nonendocrine neoplasm (e.g., oat cell of lung, thymus, islet cell), (2) an adrenal adenoma, (3) an adrenal carcinoma, or (4) the administration of exogenous corticosteroids. The clinical manifestations of Cushing's syndrome are familiar to most clinicians and these manifestations as well as the detailed testing needed to differentiate which type is present can be found in many reviews.[139,151–153]

Certain of the clinical features of this syndrome bear importantly upon the patient's ability to tolerate major surgical procedures. Hypertension is present in about 80 percent of patients.[139] Although only some of the patients present with a hypokalemic alkalosis (especially those with the ectopic ACTH syndrome) we have found that treatment of the hypertension with a thiazide diuretic usually results in marked hypokalemia. Glucose intolerance occurs in about 90 percent of patients with Cushing's syndrome but only 20 percent develop overt diabetes.[139] In the perioperative period, the stress of the procedure combined with these other effects might necessitate the use of insulin for control of hyperglycemia in some patients.

The marked catabolic effects of the hypercortisolism results in muscle wasting, osteoporosis, and thinning of skin. At surgery, the tissues are often found to have poor tensile strength, tear easily, retain sutures poorly, heal slowly, and become infected.[139,154] Healing may also be slowed due to steroid induced zinc deficiency.[155] Finally, the psychologic changes of depression, emotional lability, and even psychosis may be important factors in managing these patients.[156]

Because of all of these adverse effects of excess corticosteroids, it is preferable to defer elective surgery for several weeks to months following correction of the hypercortisolism. Although this correction is normally done with surgery or pituitary irradiation, it should be remembered that there are several pharmacologic agents that are capable of reducing ACTH secretion (cyproheptadine, bromocriptine) and cortisol secretion (metyrapone, mitotane, aminoglutethimide) in many patients.[157] In a patient who has not had major catabolic effects and who has normal tissues, there is no problem with proceeding with surgery immediately. Emergency surgery requires no special precautions in the patient with Cushing's syndrome provided the glucose, electrolytes, and blood pressure are in order. Although theoretically such patients might not be able to increase their steroid secretion adequately in the face of stress, this has generally not been a problem and steroid supplementation is not usually employed.

In the patient who undergoes unilateral adrenalectomy for an adrenal adenoma or carcinoma, the opposite normal gland is usually atrophied. Therefore, such a patient should receive full steroid coverage intraoperatively and postoperatively as outlined above. Liddle[139] advocates giving about twice the maintenance dose for about two weeks to such patients, gradually tapering down to 20 mg of hydrocortisone in the morning and 10 mg in the afternoon after about 2 months. Then the evening dose should be dropped for about six months, allowing ACTH stimulation and the other gland to recover. The patient should then be tested (see below) to see if return of function is complete. In the patient undergoing bilateral adrenalectomy, full maintenance glucocorticoid and mineralocorticoid therapy is necessary as well as full intraoperative and postoperative steroid coverage. When a patient with Cushing's disease undergoes hypophysectomy, full steroid coverage is also needed and the patient should be placed on maintenance steroids. Patients who undergo selective resection of an ACTH secreting adenoma may have suppression of their pituitaries for months;[158] their steroid dosage should be tapered as described above for adrenal adenomas. As in the patient who undergoes unilateral adrenalectomy for an adenoma, patients who undergo bilateral adrenalectomy or hypophysectomy should also initially be tapered to twice maintenance dose for a few weeks since their bodies had gotten used to high glucocorticoid levels. This dose can then be tapered to maintenance levels over the next several weeks.

Exogenous Glucocorticoid Therapy

High doses of steroids are commonly used for a variety of neoplastic and inflammatory conditions. Patients receiving these drugs may become very cushingoid and the tissue effects resemble those described above for endogenous Cushing's syndrome; this subject has been well described in the literature.[159,160] Interestingly, certain side effects appear to be much more common with steroid administration, such as benign intracranial hypertension (pseudotumor cerebri), glaucoma, posterior subcapsular cataract, pancreatitis, aseptic necrosis of bone, and panniculitis.[161] Many of the side effects of high dose steroids may be avoided or decreased by using an alternate day regimen.[161]

One of the major side effects of high dose daily steroid therapy is suppression of the hypothalamic-pituitary-adrenal axis, so that after therapy is stopped the patient will be unable to respond to stress with an adequate outpouring of glucocorticoids. This suppression clearly occurs within 10 days, and there is evidence that there may be suppression as early as 3 days after beginning such therapy.[161] Suppression of this axis may last for up to a year.[162] All patients who have had high dose steroid therapy within the previous year should be considered to have partial adrenal insufficiency and should receive high dose steroids during surgery, as outlined in Table 11.

Withdrawing a patient from steroid therapy can be very difficult. Often the underlying inflammatory condition dictates that the withdrawal be slow so as to prevent a flare-up. Usually these patients can be gradually switched to an alternate day regimen to lessen side effects and also to lessen suppression of the hypothalamic-pituitary-adrenal axis. Alternate day therapy may not be effective in controlling giant cell arteritis, polymyositis, severe rheumatoid arthritis, and some complications of systemic lupus erythematosus (nephritis, thrombocytopenia, central nervous system involvement).[160] Occasionally, the underlying conditions for which the steroids have been given are excised (e.g., a colon involved by ulcerative colitis or a rejected kidney). Under these circumstances, the steroids can usually be tapered to close to maintenance doses rapidly and further tapering is limited by the development of the "steroid-withdrawal syndrome" which consists of lethargy, arthralgias, headaches, anorexia, myalgias, nausea, vomiting, and skin desquamation. Byyny[163] has suggested a useful protocol to follow in the presence of this syndrome: (1) The patient is first switched to a single dose of 20 mg of the short-acting hydrocortisone in the morning, with no afternoon dose. (2) This dose is then reduced by 2.5 mg per day every one to two weeks until a dose of 10 mg is reached. (3) When the patient has been taking 10 mg daily for several weeks, the 8 AM cortisol level is checked monthly, and when this level reaches 10 μg/dl some degree of restoration of function can be assumed. Although Byyny[163] provides no data in support of this method, it appears to be sound and useful. However, it would be prudent to check the response of the hypothalamic-pituitary-adrenal axis to stress through pyrogen[160] or insulin-induced hypoglycemic stimulation once steroids are withdrawn when such testing is practical. Patients withdrawn in such a manner are still considered to be at risk for developing adrenal insufficiency with surgery and other major stresses for up to one year following cessation of steroids, and steroid administration during such stresses is necessary. Whenever there is any doubt about the adequacy of the adrenal response, regardless of the mode of steroid administration, steroid coverage should be given for any major stress.

Congenital Adrenal Hyperplasia

Patients with congenital adrenal hyperplasia are always deficient in glucocorticoids and may be deficient in mineralocorticoids, depending upon the specific enzymatic deficiency involved. This can usually be determined by the type of medications they are receiving. However, many of the patients who have 21-hydroxylase deficiency (the most common variety) may only be mildly mineralocorticoid deficient and require exogenous saline or mineralocorticoids when they are salt deprived or are placed in a salt-depleting environment.[164] All patients with these syndromes will require full steroid coverage as if they were completely adrenally insufficient (see Table 11) with appropriate tapering postoperatively. Additionally, at least 1 L of physiologic saline should be administered daily, and the electrolytes should be monitored carefully to avoid hyperkalemia. When the dose of exogenous hydrocortisone is reduced to below 75 to 100 mg per day, additional mineralocorticoid may be necessary. Maintenance steroid doses for these conditions are slightly higher than for routine Addison's disease patients in order to shut off ACTH and androgen secretion. Brook and associates[165] have found the best daily maintenance doses to be 25 mg of hydrocortisone or 6 mg of prednisone per square meter of body surface area.

Hyperaldosteronism

Patients with primary hyperaldosteronism usually have moderate hypertension and present with a hypokalemic alkalosis. The diagnostic maneuvers necessary (1) to establish a diagnosis of hyperaldosteronism, (2) to distinguish the various types of hyperaldosteronism, and (3) to localize the site of the tumor have been well reviewed.[166,167] Once the diagnosis has been made, it is important to correct the electrolyte abnormalities to prevent the intraoperative and postoperative development of arrhythmias (see Chap. 3, Cardiology). Additionally, the hypokalemia may contribute to mild glucose intolerance and to hypokalemic nephropathy in which the kidneys may not be able to concentrate properly. The hypokalemia may be responsive only to very high doses of potassium supplementation (40 to 120 mEq/day) because of the kaliuresis, and spironolactone in high doses (100 to 400 mg/day) may be helpful in treating both the hypertension and the hypokalemia. Great caution must be exercised if both spironolactone and potassium are given together to avoid sudden life-threatening hyperkalemia. In a patient who is to have elective surgery for removal of an aldosterone producing adenoma (as opposed to bilateral hyperplasia), spironolactone should be given for several weeks to normalize the blood pressure, potassium, and blood volume. If this is not done, the patient may develop hypotension and hyperkalemia from postoperative hypoaldosteronism because of suppression of the renin-angiotensin-aldosterone system. Exogenous mineralocorticoid and saline may be necessary under these circumstances.[168]

Hypoaldosteronism

Many older diabetics who have modest renal insufficiency (BUN 25 to 60 mg/dl) and hypertension have hyperkalemia due to hyporeninemic hypoaldosteronism. Although this group makes up the bulk of the patients, the syndrome also occurs in nondiabetics and diabetics without renal insufficiency.[169] Rarely, the hyperkalemia in this syndrome can be life-threatening with varying degrees of heart block reported. When the hyperkalemia becomes severe, normotensive patients may need to be treated with a mineralocorticoid, and hypertensive patients may need a kaliuretic diuretic, a mineralocorticoid, or both together. The therapeutic regimen has to be adjusted individually for each patient.

Pheochromocytomas

Pheochromocytomas have been found in up to 0.1 percent of hypertensive patients in some series,[170] and malignant pheochromocytomas make up between 1 and 10 percent of these patients.[170,171] The clinical features and diagnostic tests have been well described,[170–172] but certain features of pheochromocytomas are worth reemphasizing. Many patients do not have paroxysmal hypertension associated with headaches and flushing, but rather have sustained hypertension. Some patients may have episodes of hypertension that are very infrequent, and therefore they may be operated upon for other reasons and the first suspicion of the pheochromocytoma may occur with a blood pressure rise during the induction of anesthesia or at surgery. Failure to recognize this possibility may result in death of the patient.[173] On the other hand, extra-adrenal tumors may provoke paroxysmal symptoms after particular activities. For example, an intrathoracic tumor pressing against the esophagus resulted in attacks upon swallowing in one patient, and in another woman a tumor in the organ of Zuckerkandl caused attacks during sexual intercourse, particularly at orgasm.[171] Importantly, pheochromocytomas have extra-adrenal locations in 10 to 20 percent of patients with a large percentage being in the organ of Zuckerkandl at the bifurcation of the aorta.[174] An interesting variant can occur in the bladder wall and is usually associated with micturition induced symptoms of palpitations, fatigue, headache, sweating, and anxiety. These lesions can be seen at cystoscopy.[175]

In addition to the usual symptoms commonly associated with pheochromocytomas, patients occasionally have recurrent abdominal pain and frequently suffer weight loss. Rarely, the catecholamine induced decrease in peristalsis can mimic an ileus with progressive abdominal distention and an ischemic enterocolitis can also occur. Occasionally, extremity pain may occur from catecholamine induced vasoconstriction and ischemia. Shock may occur in predominantly epinephrine secreting tumors or after hemorrhage into a tumor.[170] Some patients develop a "catecholamine cardiomyopathy" with resultant congestive heart failure even when they are not hypertensive.[176] Clearly, caution is needed in the administration of fluids to such patients.

Other pathologic conditions may be associated with pheochromocytomas and these should be looked for. The excessive catecholamines suppress insulin release, and varying degrees of glucose intolerance may occur.[176] Cholelithiasis occurs in up to 30 percent of patients with paroxysmal hypertension and in about 10 percent of patients with sustained hypertension.[170]

Medullary carcinoma of the thyroid occurs in many patients with familial pheochromocytomas, an association known as multiple endocrine adenomatosis type II or Sipple's syndrome. In screening programs carried out in kindreds with this syndrome, a precursor form of both diseases (i.e., C-cell and medullary hyperplasia) can be found in patients detected early.[177] Bilateral pheochromocytomas are more common in the familial variety. Coexistent hyperparathyroidism may also occur in these patients although occasionally hypercalcemia occurs in patients with pheochromocytomas without hyperparathyroidism and the hypercalcemia disappears with adrenalectomy.[178] Among kindreds with Sipple's syndrome, many also have a marfanoid habitus and multiple mucosal neuromas. Some of these patients have diffuse ganglioneuromatosis extending throughout the gastrointestional tract from tongue to rectum and may have clinical problems ranging from constipation to megacolon requiring surgery.[179] Cutaneous neurofibromatosis (von Recklinghausen's disease) occurs in about 5 percent of patients with pheochromocytomas, and pheochromocytomas occur in about 1 percent of patients with neurofibromatosis.[170]

PREOPERATIVE MANAGEMENT

Although the hypertensive crisis induced by surgery and/or anesthesia is the problem most feared in these patients, it should also be remembered that these patients are quite prone to both ventricular and supraventricular ectopy and tachyarrhythmias. Reversible electrocardiographic changes suggestive of an acute myocardial infarction have been seen in rare patients.[170] Occasionally, the hypertensive attacks result in a bradycardia instead of a tachycardia due to the vagal response to the elevated pressure.[170] Nodal escape and AV dissociation have been noted during both bradycardia and tachycardia.[170]

Because of the high likelihood of precipitating a hypertensive crisis or an arrhythmia by anesthesia, surgery, or arteriography, it is important to have patients well blocked with alpha-adrenergic (and occasionally beta-adrenergic) blocking agents prior to such procedures. Manger and Gifford[170] and Zelch and coworkers[180] have reported that in patients that have tumors that are difficult to localize by arteriography or in whom the biochemical parameters are not conclusive, arteriography without or with only partial adrenergic blockade may be useful as a provocative test for both diagnosis and localization. These authors suggest that an increase in blood pressure of greater than

20 to 40 mm Hg over baseline with the injection of contrast material is very suggestive of a pheochromocytoma and at that point they will give intravenous phentolamine to lower the pressure. We have found that constant electrocardiographic and blood pressure monitoring utilizing a radial artery cannula and transducer during the procedure is essential and have found that nitroprusside is useful in the rapid correction of the blood pressure rise. Either agent should be in solution and on standby for immediate infusion into the patient (see Table 12). Similarly, propranolol should be available for intravenous injection for arrhythmias. Rarely phentolamine can cause a marked sustained hypotension in such patients and therefore norepinephrine should also be available for rapid intravenous infusion. If alpha blockade is complete, then norepinephrine infusion may not be successful in raising the blood pressure; in this situation angiotensin II infusion has been successful in restoring the blood pressure.[170] For these reasons we and others have come to prefer nitroprusside to phentolamine.

Surgical removal of the pheochromocytoma should take precedence over all but the most emergent surgical conditions. Indeed, some patients with an accelerating frequency and severity of hypertensive crises are medical emergencies themselves. The hypertensive crisis itself may be treated with phentolamine, nitroprusside, and propranolol (for

TABLE 12. Drugs Used in the Management of Pheochromocytomas

Hypertensive Emergencies

1. Phentolamine (Regitine)
    - a. Given in 1–5 mg boluses IV at 1 mg/min
    - b. Low-dose IV drip: 10 μg/ml (5 mg in 500 ml D5W)
    - c. High-dose IV drip: 80 μg/ml (40 mg in 500 ml D5W)
2. Nitroprusside (Nipride): Light-sensitive, shield with aluminum foil; stable in solution for only 4 hrs
    - a. Low-dose IV drip: 100 μg/ml (50 mg in 500 ml D5W)
    - b. High-dose IV drip: 500 μg/ml (250 mg in 500 ml D5W)
3. Norepinephrine (Levophed): For phentolamine induced hypotension
    - a. Low-dose IV drip: 4 μg/ml (4 ml in 1000 ml D5W)
    - b. High-dose IV drip: 64 μg/ml (64 ml in 1000 ml D5W)

Arrhythmias

1. Lidocaine (Xylocaine)
    - a. Given in 50–100 mg boluses IV at 25–50 mg/min
    - b. IV drip: 1 mg/ml (1 gm in 1000 ml D5W)
2. Propranolol (Inderal)
    Given in 0.25–5 mg boluses at maximum rate of 1 mg/min

Chronic Management

1. Phenoxybenzamine (Dibenzyline): 10 mg capsules
    Usual dose: 10–20 mg 3–4 times a day
2. Phentolamine (Regitine): 50 mg tablets
    Usual dose: 50–100 mg every 4–6 hours
3. Propranolol (Inderal): 10, 40, 80 mg tablets
    Usual dose: 10–40 mg every 6 hours
    N.B.—only to be used after alpha blockade achieved
4. Alphamethyltyrosine: 250 mg tablets
    Usual dose: 250–1000 mg every 6 hours

arrhythmias) as discussed earlier. Because the hypertension is mediated by alpha-adrenergic mechanisms, propranolol, a beta blocker, should never be used without prior alpha blockade (or nitroprusside) because a worsening of the hypertension may result.

While the patient is being evaluated and prepared for surgery the longer acting alpha blocker phenoxybenzamine (Dibenzyline) should be used in a dose of about 10 to 20 mg orally two to four times daily with meals to control the hypertension. Side effects include nasal congestion, sedation, nausea, vomiting, and orthostatic hypotension, which may be dose-limiting. Phentolamine (Regitine) can be added in 25 to 50 mg doses four to six times a day orally (duration only 2 to 4 hours) to help control the blood pressure but is even more likely to cause nausea, vomiting, diarrhea, and abdominal cramping. A combination of these drugs at lower dosage may be successful in controlling blood pressure with lessened side effects.[170] In practice, the dose of phenoxybenzamine is started low, for example, 20 to 30 mg daily in three or four doses and is increased by 10 to 20 mg a day until control of the blood pressure is effected. Should side effects intervene, then the phentolamine can be added. If blood pressure control can only be achieved at the expense of orthostatic hypotension, then the patient must be kept at bed rest. Should treatment with alpha-adrenergic blocking agents not result in satisfactory lowering of the blood pressure, the recently released drug alphamethyltyrosine (Demser), a substance which interferes with catecholamine synthesis, may prove useful in doses of 1 to 4 gm daily in divided doses.[279]

If arrhythmias or tachycardia are a problem, propranolol can be added after alpha blockade has been achieved in doses of 10 to 40 mg four times a day. Although most centers do not add propranolol routinely, ReMine and associates[181] have found that the routine preoperative use of propranolol decreased cardiac arrhythmias during surgery. The myocardial irritability due to the high catecholamine levels dictates caution in the administration of digitalis preparations.[170] In addition to controlling the blood pressure, the use of alpha blockers for several days preoperatively will allow the contracted plasma volume to re-expand; this will largely prevent the hypotension that may occur following resection of the pheochromocytoma.[182] A minimum of three days of blockade is usually required for normalization of blood pressure and plasma volume (with a reduction of hematocrit of about 5%).[182,183] Engelman[176] maintains that the plasma volume is not altered in patients with pheochromocytomas and that the hypotension seen following tumor removal is related to a functional autonomic insufficiency with vasodilation; however, the proper therapy in this situation is still volume expansion.

OPERATIVE MANAGEMENT

Most experienced physicians taking care of these patients advocate preoperative alpha blockade but there is considerable controversy as to the desirability of continuing alpha blockers into surgery. As discussed above, such blockade should allow the induction of anesthesia and surgery to proceed without problems. However, complete blockade may prevent a diagnostic rise in blood pressure when the surgeon manipulates tissue that may be the tumor. Similarly, a fall in blood pressure following tumor resection is desirable to show that there are no other tumors or that the tumor is not bilateral.[170] Therefore, to allow the surgeon this diagnostic help, I would recommend stopping the phenoxybenzamine after the morning dose the day before surgery. The 24 hour half-life of the drug[170] means there will be incomplete alpha blockade at the time of surgery.

All patients should have constant electrocardiographic monitoring, arterial blood pressure monitoring using an indwelling radial artery catheter and transducer, and a central venous pressure line to help assess volume. Intravenous solutions of phentolamine, nitroprusside, norepinephrine, and lidocaine should be attached to the intravenous lines using stopcocks so that they can be administered quickly.[184] Propranolol should also be readily available for intravenous injection. Premedication can be achieved with diazepam or droperidol.[170,185] Morphine can cause a release of catecholamines and atropine may aggravate the tachycardia that may be present and therefore they should not be used.[170] Both phenothiazines[170] and thiopental[183] have been associated with hypotension, so care must be exercised when these agents are used.

Intubation may cause a severe hypertensive crisis. To avoid such hypertensive reactions, Manger and Gifford[170] advocate giving a small, nondepolarizing dose of *d*-tubocurarine, followed by a small dose of thiopental, and then a small amount of the general anesthetic and succinylcholine (Anectine) to facilitate intubation. Muscle relaxation is maintained with *d*-tubocurarine. Currently, the anesthetic agent of choice appears to be enflurane (Ethrane) which affords good muscular relaxation and has little of the myocardial sensitization to catecholamines that is seen with halothane and especially cyclopropane plus nitrous oxide.[170,185] Enflurane also produces some degree of peripheral vasodilatation which may be useful.[185] Innovar (fentanyl plus droperidol) and nitrous oxide/oxygen have also been used successfully[181,185] (see also Chapter 17, Anesthesiology).

Intraoperative hypertensive episodes can be controlled with nitroprusside as a 0.25 mg intravenous bolus followed by an infusion (see Table 12) or by phentolamine as a 1 to 5 mg bolus (1 mg/ml) followed by an infusion. Arrhythmias usually appear during the hypertensive episode and disappear as the blood pressure is lowered.[170] Should the arrhythmia persist, intravenous boluses of lidocaine (50 to 100 mg) or propranolol (0.1 to 2.5 mg) are indicated. Although either agent will be useful for ventricular arrhythmias, propranolol is the agent of choice for supraventricular arrhythmias.[170] Hypotension intraoperatively or postoperatively is due either to (1) excessive alpha blockade, in which case norepinephrine infusion is necessary, or (2) hypovolemia due to hemorrhage or vasodilatation following tumor removal, in which case volume expansion is the proper therapy and not administration of pressors.

POSTOPERATIVE MANAGEMENT

Alpha and beta blocking agents should not be needed postoperatively unless all of the tumor was not removed or if hypertension persists. Occasionally, fluid administration for intraoperative hypotension is too vigorous and when normal autonomic reflexes return the patient may become hypertensive due to volume overload; this responds to furosemide.[176] Finally, persistent hypertension postoperatively may be due to inadvertent renal artery ligation at surgery[176] or to the development of nephrosclerosis secondary to the catecholamine induced hypertension. More commonly, hypotension occurs and is due to blood loss or vasodilation as noted above, and responds to volume replace ment with blood. If bilateral adrenalectomy is performed, steroid coverage will be needed as outlined in Table 11. Urinary measurements of vanillylmandelic acid (VMA), catecholamines, and metanephrines should be performed in all patients to check for residual tissue several days postoperatively. In patients with malignant disease in whom all of the tissue cannot be resected or in patients who are too poor risks for surgery, longterm therapy with phenoxybenzamine or alphamethyltyrosine can be used.[170]

Other Emergency Surgery

Rarely, some pheochromocytoma patients will need other surgery before their pheochromocytomas can be resected. Under these circumstances, full alpha blockade should be carried through surgery. The anesthetic considerations mentioned above are applicable and hypertensive episodes and arrhythmias can be controlled with nitroprusside, phentolamine, and propranolol, as discussed. Clearly such patients are at high risk and every effort should be made to treat the patient conservatively until the pheochromocytoma can be removed.

DISORDERS OF CALCIUM, PHOSPHORUS, MAGNESIUM, AND BONE

Calcium

Because of variations in methodology, each hospital laboratory should establish its own range of normal calcium values. The usual normal range is about 8.8 to 10.5 mg/dl.[186–188] Approximately 47 percent of calcium in serum is present in the unbound or ionized form and appears to be the physiologically active component; about 40 percent of the total calcium is bound to protein (mainly albumin), and about 13 percent is complexed with organic anions.[188] The total serum calcium may alter when the amount of proteins in the blood alters, but under these circumstances the unbound calcium usually remains unchanged. Many formulas have been devised to "correct" the measured total serum calcium in states of altered protein concentrations, but none of these formulas hold true in all situations. The most common abnormality in "sick" patients and in the postoperative period is that of hypocalcemia due to hypoalbuminemia. Ladenson and colleagues[188] have found that in this particular situation the algorithm devised by Payne and associates[189] is very accurate. According to this equation, the corrected serum calcium (Ca_c) equals the measured serum calcium (Ca_s) minus 0.989 times the measured serum albumin +4.0 (i.e., $Ca_c = Ca_s - 0.989\,[Alb] + 4.0$).

HYPERCALCEMIA

A wide variety of conditions may be associated with hypercalcemia and hypercalcemia itself is very common, being present in 0.1 to 0.6 percent of the population.[186,190] A careful investigation of hypercalcemia should always be performed. The great majority of patients will be found to have hyperparathyroidism. Whenever possible, the patient scheduled for surgery who is found to be hypercalcemic should be fully evaluated before surgery. Because many such patients will prove to have malignancy or hyperthyroidism as the cause of the hypercalcemia, it is important to establish these diagnoses preoperatively. Only a brief discussion of the evaluation of hypercalcemic patients can be presented here but detailed discussions are available in the literature.[191–193]

Table 13 lists the known causes of hypercalcemia. This list can be broken down into those causes in which parathyroid hormone (PTH) is elevated (i.e., primary hyperparathyroidism and malignancies producing PTH [ectopic PTH production]) and those in which PTH is suppressed (i.e., all others). Accordingly, after discontinuing any thiazide medication, a PTH measurement (readily available from many commercial laboratories) is the first step in evaluating the hypercalcemic patient. With the knowledge that PTH induces a renal loss of phosphate and bicarbonate, Palmer and associates[194] have nicely devised a "poor man's" PTH assessment utilizing the serum chloride and phosphate measurements. In their hands, the chloride/phosphate ratio was greater than 33 in 96 percent of patients with hyperparathyroidism and less than 30 in 92 percent of patients with hypercalcemia due to other causes. The zone between 30 and 33 was indeterminant. We have found this ratio to be exceedingly helpful.

In the high PTH, high Cl/PO_4 group, the major differentiation is between primary hyperparathyroidism and ectopic PTH secretion. Although the PTH levels are often not as high in the ectopic PTH patients,[195] in the individual patient neither PTH level nor other biochemical parameters are able to distinguish between these two entities. Because of the high proportion of malignancies associated with hypercalcemia that are squamous cell carcinomas of the lung; hypernephromas; squamous cell carcinomas of the head, neck, and esophagus; and tumors of the female genital tract[195–197] we routinely obtain a chest x-ray, intravenous pyelogram (IVP), barium swallow, and formal otolaryngologic consultation and examination and perform a careful pelvic examination in all older patients in whom malignancy is a distinct possibility. It should be remembered, however, that both primary hyperparathyroidism and malignancy can coexist in the same patient.[198] Although thiazide diuretics are frequently associated with hypercalcemia, many patients who become hypercalcemic on thiazide will show

TABLE 13. Etiologies of Hypercalcemia

Common	*Uncommon*
Hyperparathyroidism	Sarcoidosis
Malignancies (solid) with osseous metastases	Diuretic phase of acute tubular necrosis
Malignancies (solid) without osseous metastases	Immobilization (in adolescent and in patients with Paget's disease)
Secreting parathormone	Addison's disease
Secreting prostaglandin E_2	Myxedema
Secreting ?	Vitamin A toxicity
Hyperthyriodism	Leukemia/lymphoma
Thiazide diuretics	Other granulomatous diseases (tuberculosis, coccidioidomycosis, berylliosis, blastomycosis)
Multiple myeloma	Milk-alkali syndrome
Vitamin D toxicity	Idiopathic etiology (associated with supravalvular aortic stenosis in childhood)
Estrogen (androgen) therapy of breast cancer	

persistent hypercalcemia off the medication and will eventually be found to have hyperparathyroidism.

In the low PTH, low Cl/PO_4 group the most common causes are hyperthyroidism,[62] malignancies not secreting PTH,[199] malignancies with osseous metastases, multiple myeloma, and sarcoidosis. Although it is uncommon, it is important to remember that estrogen (or androgen or tamoxifen) therapy of breast cancer patients can induce a striking rise in serum calcium levels in 24 to 48 hours.[200]

EFFECTS OF HYPERCALCEMIA

Calcium is important in regulating the excitation-contraction coupling that occurs in cardiac and noncardiac muscle. Hypercalcemia results in a decrease in myocardial automaticity, a shortening of ventricular systole, and an increase in myocardial contractility.[201] Electrocardiographic findings include P-Q and QRS prolongation with ST shortening and an overall shortened Q-T interval.[201,202] The decreased conduction velocity and shortened refractory period are said to predispose to arrhythmias[201] but significant problems are not seen with the degrees of hypercalcemia usually seen clinically.[203] If the serum calcium is acutely raised by the intravenous infusion of calcium, however, bradycardia, heart block, sinus arrest, and premature ventricular contracting may occur.[204,205] Although chronic hypercalcemia does not appear to cause arrhythmias, it has been associated with varying degrees of heart block.[206,207] Hypercalcemia can potentate the effect of digitalis preparations on cardiac contractility,[203] and caution is needed in administering these preparations to hypercalcemic patients to avoid digitalis toxicity.

Increasing degrees of hypercalcemia can progressively affect mental function. With calcium levels below 16 mg/dl the most common findings are personality changes, characterized by depression, loss of initiative, and irritability, and memory impairment. When calcium levels increase above 16 mg/dl, it is more common to see acute organic psychoses characterized by disorientation, confusion, paranoid ideation, and hallucinations. Finally, calcium levels above 19 mg/dl are usually associated with somnolence and coma. These changes are almost always completely reversible with a reduction of calcium to normal levels.[208]

Other depressant effects of hypercalcemia on the nervous system include impaired reflexes, constipation, and even a partial ileus.[209] Hypercalcemia can further confuse the picture of a patient with an apparent intra-abdominal process in that it can cause anorexia, nausea, vomiting, and generalized abdominal pain.[209] Acute pancreatitis occurs in association with both parathyroid[210] and nonparathyroid[211] hypercalcemia.

Hypercalcemia has several effects on kidney function. Both hypercalcemia and elevated PTH levels independently and additively reduce the glomerular filtration rate (GFR) and hypercalcemia can reduce renal blood flow. The latter effect may be due to a vasconstrictive effect of calcium on the renal arterioles. Hypercalcemia also effects tubular function, inhibiting NaCl reabsorption in the thick ascending limb of the loop of Henle, the distal convoluted tubule, and the collecting duct which results in NaCl loss and dehydration with an attendant kaliuresis and hyperuricemia. In the collecting duct, hypercalcemia interferes with the action of vasopressin (ADH) by a variety of mechanisms leading to a state of nephrogenic diabetes insipidus.[212] Usually these changes are reversible when the calcium is lowered, but the defects in renal concentrating ability and renal insufficiency may not recover in patients with longstanding hypercalcemia in whom calcium may be deposited in the renal parenchma (nephrocalcinosis). Finally, the hypertension that is seen in up to 50 percent of patients with hypercalcemia resolves in a variable percentage of patients when the hypercalcemia is corrected.[209,213]

These aspects of hypercalcemia are important to remember in the patient going to surgery. Since most patients with hypercalcemia will be moderately dehydrated, NaCl and water administration will be necessary for rehydration. Free water requirements may be greater than what would ordinarily be expected because of the inability of the kidney to concentrate. Finally digitalis administration must be done cautiously should it be needed to avoid toxicity.

Effects of Hyperparathyroidism

In addition to the effects of hypercalcemia described above that may be important in the surgical patient, there are some selected aspects of hyperparathyroidism that may bear on the patient going to surgery. In the series of Mallette and associates,[187] of 57 cases of primary hyperparathyroidism, one-third had significant weight loss and 16 percent had documented peptic ulcer disease. Of these patients, 42 percent complained of weakness and 14 of 16 of these patients who had detailed testing showed a neuropathic myopathy that was predominantly proximal and resolved with parathyroidectomy.[214] A moderate normochromic, normocytic anemia (hematocrit 23 to 33%) that is not due to iron, folate or vitamin B_{12} deficiency or to blood loss has been found in 5 to 21 percent of patients.[187,215] The sedimentation rate was found to be elevated in 48 percent, the uric acid was elevated in 62 percent of patients, and the alkaline phosphatase was elevated in 30 percent of patients.[187] Hypomagnesemia was found in 14 percent and a moderate hyperchloremic acidosis (due to the decrease in bicarbonate reabsorption caused by the PTH and hypophosphatemia) was found in 24 percent of patients in the same series.[187]

Patients with hyperparathyroidism often have other family members who have hyperparathyroidism; most familial cases have hyperplasia of all glands instead of solitary adenomas.[216] Such patients with familial disease are at increased risk to be part of the multiple endocrine adenomatosis syndromes (type I: parathyroid, pituitary, pancreas; type II: parathyroid, medullary carcinoma of the thyroid, and pheochromocytomas) although such an association can exist without the disease being familial.[216] Patients who are found to have hyperplasia should have screening for other gland involvement as part of the multiple endocrine adenomatosis syndromes and family members should also be screened. The yield in such screenings shows that over 50 percent of family members may be affected.[216] Another interesting association that has recently been found is that in one series of 89 patients with primary hyperparathyroidism, 30 percent had a history of external irradiation to the head and neck in childhood for benign diseases.[217] Of these 27 patients, 4 had coexistent thyroid carcinomas. In hyperparathyroid patients, therefore, a history of any childhood or early adulthood irradiation should be elicited and the thyroid and salivary glands of such patients should be carefully examined.

Therapy of Hypercalcemia (Table 14)

When possible, it is best to establish the etiology of the hypercalcemia as quickly as possible. If the calcium level is lower than 15 mg/dl, there usually is no severe alteration of mental or cardiac function but renal impairment may well occur. For this reason, it is advisable to bring down the calcium level to less than 12 mg/dl preoperatively. Calcium levels below 12 mg/dl do not appear to cause significant dehydration or cardiac problems and, therefore, no additional therapy other than attention to perioperative fluid status is needed. Bed rest and dehydration both tend to worsen hypercalcemia so early postoperative mobilization and adequate hydration are paramount.

In the severely hypercalcemic patient (calcium greater than 14 mg/dl or in the obtunded patient) the first step in emergency therapy is adequate rehydration. The most frequently used and rapidly effective method of reducing the calcium level employs a saline diuresis utilizing intravenous saline and furosemide (Lasix).[218] A central venous pressure line should be used so that it is possible to ensure that intravascular volume

TABLE 14. Treatment of Hypercalcemia

Method	*Dose*	*Efficacy*	*Mechanism*	*Side Effects*
1. Saline and furosemide	4–10 L/24 hrs 40–80 mg q 1–2h IV	>90% in 12–24 hrs	↑Ca excretion	↓K^+, ↓Mg^+, congestive heart failure, dehydration
2. Mithramycin	25 μg/kg of body weight IV	>90% in 24–48 hrs	Inhibits bone resorption	Thrombocytopenia, hepatic and renal failure
3. Glucocorticoid	30–60 mg prednisone	Myeloma, sarcoid, vitamin D and A toxicity, Addison's disease	↓Ca absorption	Cushing's syndrome
4. Calcitonin	1–2 MRC units/kg of body weight q 6–8h IM	75%	Inhibit bone resorption	Hypersensitivity: test with 0.5 U intradermally
5. Phosphate, IV	500 ml over 8h of 0.1M solution of 0.081M Na_2HPO_4 and 0.019M KH_2PO_4	>90%	Ca deposition in tissues	Death, hypotension, renal failure
6. Phosphate, oral	5–10 ml of Fleet Phospho-Soda tid		Inhibits bone resorption	Diarrhea
7. Indomethacin	25–50 mg q 8h	In tumors secreting prostaglandin E	Decrease prostaglandin E synthesis	GI upset

is kept on the "full" side and it is preferable to put the patient in an intensive care unit. With this method, 40 to 80 mg intravenous furosemide is given every 1 to 4 hours to promote a diuresis of greater than 200 ml/hour once initial volume depletion has been corrected. Plasma electrolytes and urine sodium and potassium are measured every 2 to 4 hours and urinary losses are replaced intravenously. Urinary magnesium losses can be very high with this method and if renal function is not severely impaired, 10 to 15 mg of magnesium should be given as magnesium sulfate intramuscularly every 2 to 4 hours during the course of the diuresis. Evaluation of serum magnesium levels in the middle and at the end of the diuresis is needed, and careful clinical monitoring is necessary to avoid precipitating congestive heart failure or dehydration.

Mithramycin is the next agent of choice if saline plus furosemide are not successful. It is given in a dose of 25 μg/kg of body weight, and reductions of calcium (to normal in 80 to 90% of patients) are obtained in 24 to 48 hours.[219] Mithramycin works by inhibiting bone resorption and the effects usually last for up to a week, at which time the dose can be repeated.[192] Rarely, side effects of thrombocytopenia and renal insufficiency are seen and we have seen one case of marked, transient transaminase rise due to this drug.

Glucocorticoids are specifically indicated in hypercalcemia due to vitamin D intoxication, adrenal insufficiency, and sarcoidosis and result in decreased intestinal calcium absorption. The hypercalcemias associated with multiple myeloma, lymphoma, and estrogen/androgen therapy of breast cancer are also amenable to treatment with steroids in doses of 30 to 60 mg daily of prednisone.[192]

Thyrocalcitonin therapy may be useful in the rare patient who does not respond to diuresis, mithramycin, or steroids. It is effective in about 75 percent of patients but usually results in a decrease in the serum calcium of only 2 to 4 mg/dl.[220] Intravenous phosphate therapy is highly effective in treating hypercalcemia but it is associated with a relatively high incidence of ectopic calcification, hypotension, renal insufficiency, and sudden death. For these reasons, it should be used only after all other methods have failed. Should it be needed, 50 mM of phosphate should be given over 6 to 8 hours. This solution can be made up by adding 81 mM of Na_2HPO_4 and 19 mM of KH_2PO_4 to 1000 ml of 5 percent dextrose in water; 500 ml of this solution are then given over 6 to 8 hours.[192]

Oral phosphate may be useful in the chronic management of hypercalcemia which is not amenable to specific therapy, in particular the hypercalcemia of malignancy. It works by both inhibiting bone resorption and binding dietary calcium in the gut.[221] The dose is 1 to 3 gm of elemental phosphorus daily (Table 15). Finally, indomethacin 25 to 50 mg every 8 hours may be useful in those patients with malignancies whose hypercalcemia is mediated by prostaglandin E.[199]

HYPOCALCEMIA

True hypocalcemia (when corrected for any decrease in binding proteins (see above) usually is due to hypoparathyroidism or to insufficient quantities of the active form of vitamin D,-1,25$(OH)_2$D. The most common form of hypoparathyroidism is surgical. Permanent hypoparathyroidism occurs in 3 to 15 percent of patients operated on for

TABLE 15. Oral Phosphate Preparations*

Name	Dose to Provide 1.0 gm Elemental Phosphorus	Cation (mEq) Na	K
Phospho-Soda	6.2 ml	57	
Neutra-Phos	300 ml or 4 capsules	28.5	28.5
Neutra-Phos-K	300 ml or 4 capsules		57
K-Phos	8 tablets		29.4
K-Phos Neutral	4 tablets	48	8.3
Hyper Phos K	6 tablets		57
Phos-tabs	6 tablets		52
Uro-KP-Neutral	6 tablets	36.9	21.8

*After Rude and Singer[222]

hyperparathyroidism[187,209] and in about 1 percent of patients operated on for thyroid disease (see above). A transient hypocalcemia often occurs after parathyroidectomy for hyperparathyroidism with the nadir at 48 to 72 hours following surgery. In most patients, this is usually due to the "hungry" bones taking up calcium and phosphate, leading to a fall in both serum calcium and phosphate. When the hypocalcemia is due to hypoparathyroidism, the phosphate level usually rises. Postparathyroidectomy patients may develop a hyperchloremic acidosis due either to a release of hydrogen ions from bone during remineralization or to an alteration in renal bicarbonate reabsorption secondary to the hypophosphatemia attendant upon remineralization.[187] Hypomagnesemia may also occur due to the remineralization of bone[187] and this may further impair PTH action (see below). A transient reversible decrease in creatinine clearance over the first three postoperative weeks has also been described.[187]

Hypomagnesemia results in decreased PTH secretion and a decreased response of target organs (bone and kidney) to the actions of the PTH. Under these circumstances, magnesium replacement results in a return to normal calcium levels.[222] In pancreatitis, hypocalcemia is accompanied by inadequate PTH secretion for uncertain reasons.[223] Other less common causes of hypoparathyroidism include irradiation of the parathyroids, infiltration with hemochromatosis or metastatic cancer, dysembryogenesis (along with an absent thymus and altered T-lymphocytes—the Di George syndrome), autoimmune disease (often in association with other autoimmune endocrine insufficiencies such as Addison's disease and Hashimoto's thyroiditis), a defective PTH molecule, and a decreased tissue responsiveness to PTH (pseudohypoparathyroidism).[224]

Recent studies have shown that for vitamin D_3 to be active in the body it must initially be hydroxylated in the 25 position in the liver to $25(OH)D_3$ and then further hydroxylated in the 1 position in the kidney (a process enhanced by hypophosphatemia and PTH) to $1,25(OH)_2D_3$.[225,226] The effects of this activated $1,25(OH)_2D_3$ are primarily to increase calcium mobilization from bone and intestinal transport of calcium and phosphorus. Hepatic and renal disease may alter the production of these more active metabolites and thereby contribute to disordered calcium regulation. Many of the inherited vitamin D deficiencies have been found to be due to defects in these activation steps of vitamin D. In patients with alterations of vitamin D metabolism (exclusive of renal insufficiency which is much more complex), the serum calcium level is not markedly reduced and the phosphorus level may be low. In malabsorption states in which both the fat soluble vitamin D and calcium (and possibly magnesium) are absorbed poorly, more marked degrees of hypocalcemia may occur. Although the serum calcium levels are not markedly reduced in these states, bone does not mineralize properly and osteomalacia may occur.

Effects of Hypocalcemia

Although hypocalcemia does not usually produce arrhythmias, it can depress myocardial contractility and prolongs systole.[201] Clinically, however, acute hypocalcemia does not appear to exert significant hemodynamic effects. Electrocardiographic findings of hypocalcemia include a prolonged Q-T interval due to ST segment prolongation with a normal T wave. The Q-T prolongation is proportional to the degree of hypocalcemia. The Q-T interval should be corrected for rate (Q-T_C) by the formula:

$$\text{Q-T}_C = \text{Q-T}/\sqrt{\text{R-R interval}}$$

with the normal range being 0.35 to 0.44 second in adults.[201] Hypocalcemia may reduce the effects of digitalis on the heart, and rapid correction of hypocalcemia in a digitalized patient may bring out digitalis toxicity.

The other major clinical manifestations of hypocalcemia are neurologic. Heightened muscle contraction can cause cramps, carpopedal spasm, and even tetany. Chvostek's sign, a contraction of the eyelid muscles elicited by tapping on the facial nerve in front of the ear, is usually positive with significant hypocalcemia, although it may also be positive in some normal people. Trousseau's sign, carpal spasm elicited by impairing blood return by inflating a blood pressure cuff on the arm at a level to impede venous return for 3 to 5 minutes, is also usually positive in patients with significant hypocalcemia and is rarely positive in normals. Sensory paresthesias in the hands and feet and periorally may occur. Other less common problems include seizures, choreiform movements, parkinsonian-like rigidity, anxiety, agitation, delirium, cataracts, raised intracranial pressure, calcifications of the basal ganglia and choroid plexus, and a variety of electroencephalographic (EEG) abnormalities.[227–229] These neurologic changes are usually seen in states of both idiopathic and postsurgical hypoparathyroidism. In patients with hypoparathyroidism, phenothiazines may cause an acute dystonic syndrome and these medications should be avoided in such patients.[230] Chronic mucocutaneous moniliasis occurs commonly in idiopathic and rarely in postsurgical hypoparathyroidism.

Therapy of Hypocalcemia

Postoperative hypocalcemia need only be treated if it is symptomatic, that is, causing paresthesias, cramping, or tetany, although many physicians would treat a patient manifesting positive Trousseau's or Chvostek's signs. In acute situations, calcium gluconate can be given as an intravenous infusion of 15 to 20 mg/kg of body weight of calcium (the 10% solution contains 9 mg/ml of elemental calcium) over 4 to 6 hours and can be

TABLE 16. Calcium Supplement Preparations

Generic Name	*Trade Name*	*Calcium Content*	*Route*
Calcium carbonate	Os-Cal Titralac	250 mg/tablet 168 mg/tablet	oral oral
Calcium glubionate	Neo-Calglucon	115 mg/5cc	oral
Calcium lactate		80 mg/650 mg tablet	oral
Calcium gluconate 10%		9 mg/ml	intravenous
Calcium gluceptate		18 mg/ml	intravenous

repeated at 4 to 6 hour intervals.[229] Alternatively 10 to 20 ml of 10 percent calcium gluconate can be given over 10 minutes intravenously and repeated every 4 to 6 hours. The aim of this therapy should be the correction of symptoms and not a specific serum calcium level. If symptomatic hypocalcemia requiring intravenous therapy persists into the second postoperative week, oral calcium supplements can be given (Table 16). We prefer calcium carbonate because of the low cost and small number of tablets but many patients feel better with calcium glubionate. Some preparations cause bloating, cramping, and diarrhea in individual patients, and it is often necessary to switch from one preparation to another. The usual dose is 1 to 3 gm of calcium daily.

Patients with permanent hypoparathyroidism usually need supplemental vitamin D to maintain a normal serum calcium (Table 17). The usual dose of vitamin D_3 (cholecalciferol) or vitamin D_2 (ergocalciferol) is 50,000 to 100,000 IU (1.25 to 2.50 mg) per day but dosage requirements may fluctuate and the individual patient may be hypocalcemic or hypercalcemic on the same dose at different times.[231] There is a delay of several days to weeks until the onset of action and several weeks until the effects wear off. These delays are due to the necessary activation of vitamine D to 1,25 $(OH)_2D$ and the solubility of vitamin D in fat. Dihydrotachysterol (DHT) has been found to be much

TABLE 17. Vitamin D Preparations*

Name	*Usual Dose (in hypoparathyroidism)*	*Time to Restore Normocalcemia*	*Persistence after Stopping Drug*
Cholecalciferol (vitamin D_3)	50–100,000 IU	4–8 weeks	6–18 weeks
Ergocalciferol (vitamin D_2)	50–100,000 IU	4–8 weeks	6–18 weeks
Dihydrotachysterol (DHT)	0.25–1.25 mg	1–2 weeks	1–3 weeks
25 OHD_3	50–200 μg	2–4 weeks	4–12 weeks
$1,25(OH)_2D_3$	0.5–2.5μg	3–7 days	3–7 days
$1\alpha OHD_3$	0.5–3μg	1–8 weeks	6–14 days

*Modified from Parfitt[234]

more effective than ergocalciferol and cholecalciferol in the treatment of the hypocalcemia of hypoparathyroidism and renal insufficiency.[232] The recent discoveries of the metabolic changes necessary to activate cholecalciferol suggest that the steric configuration of DHT obviates the 1 alpha hydroxylation step in the kidney that is partially regulated by PTH.[233] An additional advantage to DHT is that its effects begin in 1 to 2 weeks and persist for only 1 to 3 weeks following cessation.[232] The usual dose is 0.25 to 1 mg daily. Parfitt[234] has recently shown that purified 25(OH)D_3, which only needs 1 alpha hydroxylation, is intermediate between ergocalciferol and DHT in latency of action and persistence of effects. Although doses of 50 to 200 μg of 25 (OH)D_3 provided clear cut advantages over ergocalciferol with regard to the stability of serum calcium levels, no advantage was found in comparison with DHT.[234]

The final metabolic product 1,25$(OH)_2D_3$ has also been shown to be very effective in the treatment of the hypocalcemia of hypoparathyroidism. Normocalcemia may be achieved 3 to 7 days after beginning therapy with 0.5 to 2.5 μg daily and the calcium levels remain quite stable.[233,235] The effects persist for only a few days and hypercalcemia is readily reversible should it occur.[233,235] Similar dose and activity characteristics have been reported for the 1αOHD_3 analog in hypoparathyroidism.[236,237] Both 1,25$(OH)_2D_3$ and 1αOHD_3 offer significant advantages over the other preparations in the rapidity of onset and offset of action. For these reasons, it would be prudent to make initial dosage adjustments as an inpatient. After the initial adjustment, periodic calcium measurements will still be needed to avoid late hypocalcemia or hypercalcemia.

In the long term management of hypoparathyroidism, both calcium supplements in the range of 1 to 3 gm per day and a vitamin D preparation are usually needed. Porter and associates,[238] however, have recently shown that hypoparathyroid patients can be successfully treated with a thiazide-type diuretic (in this case chlorthalidone, 50 mg daily) and salt-restriction, without vitamin D, and with variable calcium supplementation. They found that this form of therapy prevented the hypercalciuria sometimes seen with vitamin D therapy and was successful in maintaining normocalcemia. This may be an effective approach in some patients.

Phosphorus

The normal range of serum inorganic phosphate in adults is 2.7 to 4.5 mg/dl (1.3 to 2.3 mM/L);[239] children have higher levels. Modest hypophosphatemia (1.0 to 2.5 mg/dl) may be seen in association with starvation, hyperparathyroidism, glucose administration, malabsorption, vitamin D deficiency, respiratory alkalosis, vomiting, hemodialysis and renal tubular disease.[239,240] Severe hypophosphatemia (less than 1.0 mg/dl) may be seen in association with alcoholism and especially with alcohol withdrawal; insulin therapy in diabetic ketoacidosis; phosphate binding antacids; total parenteral nutrition without phosphate supplementation; severe, prolonged respiratory alkalosis; and the diuretic recovery phase sometimes seen after extensive third degree burns.[239,240] Severe hypophosphatemia is also occasionally seen in patients 2 to 3 days postoperatively who are maintained on dextrose and saline.[241]

Severe hypophosphatemia can give rise to a variety of clinical syndromes which may be of major importance in the surgical patient. Erythrocyte metabolism becomes altered with deficits in adenosine triphosphate (ATP) and 2,3 diphosphoglycerate (2,3 DPG); the consequent shift in the oxygen-hemoglobin dissociation curve results in a decreased ability of the blood to release oxygen to tissues.[242] The low levels of ATP also make the erythrocytes less deformable and a hemolytic anemia may occur.[243] The low intracellular ATP due to hypophosphatemia in phagocytes may lead to decreased chemotaxis, phagocytosis, and bactericidal activity, thus rendering patients more susceptible to infections.[244] Although platelet structure and function has been shown to be abnormal in hypophosphatemia, no clinical evidence of a bleeding diathesis has yet been shown.[239]

Severe hypophosphatemia has been associated with a metabolic encephalopathy consisting of irritability, paresthesias, dysarthria, confusion, seizures, stupor, and coma; the pathophysiology is uncertain, however.[239] Similar degrees of hypophosphatemia have been associated with osteomalacia and muscle weakness.[239,245] Recently, acute respiratory failure has been seen as a result of severe weakness due to hypophosphatemia.[246] Hypophosphatemia has also been shown to decrease myocardial contractility significantly.[247] Obviously lactic acidosis, infection, decreased consciousness, respiratory failure, and congestive heart failure all occur not infrequently postoperatively, and there are multifactorial causes for these complications. It is important, therefore, to exclude hypophosphatemia, which occurs commonly in this setting, as a potential contributing factor.

Hypophosphatemia can be corrected using any of the preparations listed in Table 15 or simply by providing milk which contains 1 gm of phosphorus and 1 gm of calcium per quart.[248] An initial daily dose of 0.08 to 0.16 mM/kg of body weight of phosphate (2.5 to 5.0 mg/kg of body weight of phosphorus) has been recommended.[249] In severe hypophosphatemia resulting in coma, seizures, or severe hemolysis, intravenous phosphate can be used (see Table 14). The parenteral dose is similar to the oral dose and is given every 6 hours.[249] The serum phosphate, calcium, potassium, and ECG should be monitored closely, and oral phosphate should be substituted as soon as possible to avoid metastatic calcification and hypotension.

Magnesium

The normal blood magnesium levels are 1.53 to 1.99 mEq/L.[250] Hypermagnesemia occurs primarily in patients with renal insufficiency who are treated with magnesium containing antacids. Conditions which are associated with magnesium depletion include poorly controlled diabetes mellitus and diabetic ketoacidosis,[250] alcoholism, congestive heart failure, diuretic usage, malabsorption, extensive bowel resection, prolonged parenteral fluid therapy, the diuretic phase of acute tubular necrosis, hypoparathyroidism, hyperaldosteronism, acute pancreatitis,[251] and gentamycin therapy.[252] Magnesium depletion can occur while the serum magnesium remains normal; therefore, when the serum magnesium is low, marked depletion has already taken place.[251]

Clinically, magnesium depletion may be manifested by signs of neuromuscular irritability, such as lethargy, weakness, tremors, athetoid movements, cramping, mental irritability, seizures, stupor, and coma.[251] Anorexia, nausea, and vomiting may occur. As mentioned earlier, hypomagnesemia can give rise to hypocalcemia. Magnesium deficiency has been found to cause both atrial and ventricular tachyarrhythmias, especially when digitalis is also being administered and appears to make the heart more vulnerable to digitalis toxicity.[251]

If severe central nervous system symptoms or cardiac irritability can be accurately attributed to magnesium depletion, therapy with parenteral magnesium sulfate is warranted. A dose of 10 to 15 ml of 10 percent magnesium sulfate should be given intravenously over 15 minutes followed by 500 ml of 2 percent magnesium sulfate intravenously over 6 hours. If arrhythmias recur, a second 500 ml bottle can be given over the next 18 hours.[251] Alternatively 1 gm may be given IM every 4 to 6 hours. If the injection has been too rapid, flushing, sweating, and heat may occur. With therapy, magnesium levels should be checked 1 to 2 times daily and the patellar reflexes should be tested before each dose. With magnesium levels above 5.5 mEq/L, hypotension may occur, and with levels above 6 mEq/L, deep tendon reflexes disappear. At toxic levels (above 10 mEq/L) P-R prolongation and QRS widening are seen on electrocardiography, and respiratory depression and cardiac arrest may occur.[251]

As with hypophosphatemia, the clinical syndromes (cardiac and central nervous system) seen with hypomagnesemia are nonspecific. It is important to remember, however, that in the postoperative setting with prolonged intravenous fluid therapy, hypomagnesemia may well occur and can cause these syndromes. Once hypomagnesemia is found in the setting of central nervous system disturbance or arrhythmias, therapy is specific.

Metabolic Bone Disease

In general, bone disease does not affect the immediate management of the surgical patient. Paget's disease of bone can give rise to significant hypercalciuria and hypercalcemia when a patient is immobilized for several days.[253] Rarely, these patients may also develop high output cardiac failure due to increased blood flow in the affected bones.[253] It is necessary to exercise care in the movement of patients with osteoporosis and other osteopenias to avoid fractures.

From the opposite viewpoint, gastrointestinal surgery may have significant late effects on calcium metabolism and bone. Varying degrees of osteomalacia were seen on iliac crest bone biopsies in 44 percent of patients who had undergone a partial gastrectomy or a vagotomy and pyloroplasty 3 to 9 years earlier for nonmalignant disease.[254] The most severe degrees of osteomalacia were seen in women who had undergone a Polya-type partial gastrectomy. Osteomalacia has also been seen on bone biopsy in 36 percent of patients who had varying degrees of small bowel resection.[255] In both of these studies, no combination of biochemical or radiographic studies was able to predict the histology correctly. Since such patients respond to vitamin D supplementation, it may be advisable to treat all patients undergoing partial gastrectomy and intestinal resection with vitamin D. No prospective studies have documented the efficacy of such therapy, however.

PITUITARY

Anterior Pituitary

Both secreting and nonsecreting pituitary tumors can cause hypopituitarism by either compressing the normal tissue or by interruption of the hypothalamic-pituitary portal vessels through which flow the controlling releasing hormones. Varying degrees of hypopituitarism may also be seen with hypothalamic disease (tumors, infiltrative disease such as sarcoidosis and eosinophilic granuloma), infarcts, vascular insufficiency, the empty-sella syndrome, pituitary surgery and irradiation, head trauma, and hemochromatosis. However, most cases are idiopathic. The hormones are usually lost in the order of (1) gonadotropins, (2) growth hormone, (3) TSH, (4) adrenocorticotropic hormone (ACTH) and (5) prolactin.[256]

In adults, many cases of hypopituitarism without tumors occur after postpartum hemorrhage (Sheehan's syndrome), although pituitary apoplexy unassociated with pregnancy is not uncommon and we see 1 or 2 instances of the latter each year. Pituitary apoplexy is usually associated with severe headache, visual disturbance, and often with decreased consciousness and vascular collapse. The cerebrospinal fluid is hemorrhagic. A high index of suspicion is needed to recognize these cases. Such patients need full doses of corticosteroids (see Table 11) and may need surgical decompression.[257]

Patients with hypopituitarism should be tested thoroughly to determine which hormones are deficient, and then appropriate replacement therapy with thyroxine, corticosteroids, and sex steroids is begun. The patient with known hypopituitarism should be treated as someone with combined adrenal and thyroid insufficiency (see above). Some patients with only borderline ACTH reserve deficiency may not need steroid replacement on a daily basis but should receive full steroid coverage for surgery (see Table 11). When there is insufficient time before surgery to permit detailed testing, the patient with suspected but unproven hypopituitarism should be assumed to be ACTH deficient and thereby adrenally insufficient and receive full steroid coverage. Any patient with an enlarged sella turcica on x-ray who has not been fully evaluated should be assumed to have hypopituitarism and should be covered with steroids when undergoing emergency surgery. Following surgery, the steroid dosage should be tapered as outlined and a maintenance dose of 30 mg of hydrocortisone or 5 to 7.5 mg of prednisone should be administered for a few weeks until recovery is complete. Then the patient should be admitted and taken off steroids for 48 to 72 hours for retesting to determine whether there is ACTH deficiency and to establish a need for lifelong steroid therapy. We have performed such testing in over 50 patients who have had transsphenoidal adenomectomies for prolactin secreting adenomas and have found that a daily dose of 5 to 7.5 mg of prednisone for 4 to 8 weeks does not result in suppression of the hypothalamic-pituitary-adrenal axis.[258] Although it is desirable to correct hypothyroidism secondary to TSH deficiency prior to surgery, this is not of crucial importance (see p. 000). T_4, T_3, T_3 resin uptake, and TSH values should be obtained prior to surgery, however. Deficiencies of gonadotropins, prolactin, and growth hormone do not appreciably affect the course of surgery in adults.

Of the hormonal oversecretion states seen with pituitary tumors, Cushing's disease has already been discussed. Although prolactin is the most common hormone secreted by tumors, this is not usually of any concern with respect to a patient's ability to tolerate surgery. TSH secreting tumors are very rare, and the mild hyperthyroidism that may ensue can be treated in the emergency situation like routine hyperthyroidism, although definitive therapy would be aimed at the pituitary tumor.

Acromegalic patients do have certain characteristics that bear upon their ability to tolerate surgery and their perioperative care. About 50 percent have impaired glucose tolerance, and 10 percent have overt diabetes mellitus.[256] Varying degrees of hypopituitarism are found in about 40 to 50 percent.[259] Hypertension is common in acromegalics, being present in 23 percent in one series.[260] Although cardiomegaly, arrhythmias, congestive heart failure, and coronary artery disease are seen in acromegaly, it is not clear that these cardiac disorders occur with increased frequently in acromegaly.[260] Therefore, cardiac disease should be looked for and managed in routine fashion in all acromegalics going to surgery but no extraordinary measures need be taken.

Posterior Pituitary

Diabetes insipidus (DI) may be classified into central and nephrogenic varieties. Central DI is due to varying degrees of deficiency of the secretion of vasopressin or antidiuretic hormone (ADH). While most cases of acquired central DI are idiopathic, structural lesions of the hypothalamus and pituitary stalk must be excluded. Such lesions include brain tumors (especially craniopharyngiomas), metastatic cancer (especially breast), leukemia, eosinophilic granuloma, sarcoidosis, meningitis, encephalitis, vascular infarcts, and trauma (accidental or neurosurgical).[261] Central DI is occasionally seen following transsphenoidal pituitary surgery, and it is usually transient, lasting from a few hours to several weeks, although we have seen a few patients in whom it lasted for several months.

Nephrogenic DI may be inherited (very rarely) or may be due to a number of conditions in which a disturbance of the urinary concentrating mechanisms causes an inability to concentrate the urine that is unresponsive to endogenous or exogenous antidiuretic hormones. Such conditions include renal insufficiency, sickle cell anemia, hypokalemia, hypercalcemia, and the use of lithium carbonate, demeclocycline (Declomycin), and the anesthetic agent methoxyflurane (Penthrane).[262] Usually, the first three conditions only produce an inability to concentrate fully but do not cause symptomatic polyuria whereas the drugs mentioned may give rise to symptomatic polyuria.

Mild chronic central DI is often managed with oral pharmacologic agents which act to either increase the secretion of ADH or enhance the sensitivity of the collecting duct to ADH. Such agents include chlorpropamide, carbamazepine and clofibrate. Thiazide diuretics are also often used to enhance water and sodium resorption proximally.[263] Patients chronically controlled on such medications can usually be managed in the perioperative period by discontinuing such medications and matching input to the previous 6 to 8 hour output plus insensible loss. Since the output is mostly free water, the input should be dextrose 5 percent in water. The amount of saline per day is not different than that for any postoperative patient. In the fluctuating perioperative and immediately postoperative period, the patient should be weighed on the same scale twice daily and the serum osmolality (or serum sodium if osmolality measurements are not available) measured twice daily. A specific gravity should be performed on each urine and careful input and output records maintained. Once the patient is able to drink, fluids are taken according to thirst and the oral medication taken before surgery may be resumed.

Patients who are taking Pitressin tannate in oil (PTO), lysine vasopressin (LVP) nasal spray, or the new synthetic agent 1-desamino-8-D-arginine vasopressin (dDAVP) should be continued on their standard dose perioperatively and postoperatively. Because they will be receiving a fixed amount of antidiuretic hormone, intravenous water overloading can cause a dilutional hyponatremia. These patients also need to have their weights, serum osmolalities, serum sodiums, and urine specific gravities determined twice daily until their course becomes stable. Patients usually receive dDAVP by blowing through the oral end of a piece of plastic, the other end of which is inserted in the nose, a device known as a Rhinyle. Unconscious patients can be administered dDAVP intranasally by pushing air quickly through the oral end of the Rhinyle with a syringe.[264] Alternatively, the antidiuretic preparation can be discontinued postoperatively and the urine output matched with dextrose 5 percent in water as discussed above.

It is important to recognize the new development of diabetes insipidus in postoperative patients, especially in neurosurgical patients.[265] The first occurrence is the development of polyuria of up to 400 to 500 ml per hour. This may be of sudden onset, usually within 24 to 48 hours postoperatively. The differential diagnosis at this point includes glycosuria from diabetes mellitus which may be precipitated by high dose steroids (easily diagnosed by measuring urinary glucose), osmotic diuresis from mannitol (high urinary specific gravity), the diuretic phase of acute tubular necrosis (prior history and measurements of renal function), diuretic administration (medium to high urinary sodium), and nephrogenic diabetes insipidus. The urine specific gravity will be low and the serum sodium and osmolality will be high in both central and nephrogenic diabetes insipidus.

A protocol developed by Miller and colleagues[266] is very useful in recognizing mild degrees of central DI and separating this from nephrogenic DI and primary polydipsia (Table 18). Since the number of conditions that cause nephrogenic DI is quite small and should be clear from the patient's course, it is actually relatively easy to arrive at a clinical diagnosis of central DI. The dehydration testing and protocol as outlined in Table 18 will only confirm what may be clinically evident.

The management of acute and often transient DI in such patients is similar to what was outlined above. In the initial stages, patients should have their weights and serum osmolalities (and/or sodiums) evaluated twice daily, specific gravities determined on all urines, and careful input and output records maintained. The output can be matched with oral fluids and dextrose 5 percent in water, allowing for insensible losses additionally. If urine volumes become very large (over 4,000 cc), it is usually difficult to keep up with fluids and an antidiuretic preparation should be used. Aqueous vasopressin 5 to 10 IU can be given intramuscularly or subcutaneously with repeat doses every 4 to 8 hours as needed. This preparation is in short supply. Overall, the best preparation and the easiest to use is dDAVP in doses of 2.5 to 10 μg intranasally every 12 hours.[264] It can

TABLE 18. Protocol for Assessing Diabetes Insipidus (DI)*

Procedure

1. Weigh patient at beginning of test (usually 6 P.M. if mild polyuria or 7 A.M. if severe polyuria)
2. Complete fluid deprivation for 14 hours (usually overnight) or until 3–5% of body weight is lost
3. Measure urine specific gravities hourly beginning at 6 A.M. or when 3–5% of body weight lost (save specimens for osmolality measurements)
4. When specific gravities constant for two or preferably three consecutive specimens, obtain serum for osmolality
5. After serum and last urine specimens obtained, administer 5 U of aqueous vasopressin (Pitressin) SQ or 5 μg of dDAVP intranasally
6. Measure hourly urine specific gravities and osmolalities for next 2 hours.

Interpretation

1. At end of dehydration period in normal individuals, plasma osmolality averages 289.7 mOsm/kg of body weight and urinary osmolality is greater than 866 mOsm/kg of body weight
2. In patients with various illnesses, varying degrees of DI, and primary polydipsia, urinary osmolality may not reach 866 mOsm/kg of body weight
3. Only patients with central DI will have a rise in urinary osmolality of greater than 9% in response to vasopressin
4. Patients with nephrogenic DI may have a significant rise in urinary osmolality, but this is usually small and not to a level greater than plasma osmolality

*After Miller et al.[266]

be administered to unconscious patients as indicated above. An intravenous preparation may soon become available in this country. Lysine vasopressin nasal spray (50 IU/ml) can be given as 1 to 2 sprays every 4 to 6 hours also; each spray contains about 2 IU.[265] Neither intranasal preparations should be used for several weeks following transsphenoidal hypophysectomy until the nasal mucosa has healed. Finally, Pitressin Tannate in Oil can be given in doses of 2.5 to 5 IU by deep intramuscular injection for effects that last 24 to 48 hours. It is important to warm and agitate the vial of PTO thoroughly to resuspend any precipitate to obtain full activity. If patients are conscious and taking fluids orally, they should be allowed to drink according to thirst. In the first several days of therapy, the effect of each dose of antidiuretic preparation should be allowed to wear off for a short period before administering the next dose to see if the DI is persistent. Over these first several days, the dose and interval between doses can be adjusted. At home, the patient should also try letting the effects of a dose run out periodically to determine if therapy is still needed.

Thiazide diuretics are the only useful drugs in treating familial nephrogenic diabetes insipidus. The vasopressin resistant states due to demeclocycline, lithium, and methoxyflurane are usually reversible upon stopping the drug. However, in the immediate postoperative period, patients receiving methoxyflurane anesthesia should have their urine output and renal function monitored carefully to watch for both DI and renal insufficiency. Patients with hypercalcemic, hypokalemic, and sickle cell nephropathy may get into trouble with postoperative hypernatremia if not enough free water is given since they cannot concentrate properly. All patients with renal concentrating defects need to have weights, urine specific gravities, electrolytes, BUN, creatinine, and input and output measured daily in an effort to avoid problems before they arise.

OBESITY

Obesity only begins to affect overall mortality rates when weight exceeds 120 percent of the average body weight for a given height.[267] Massively obese patients at surgery often present with a problem of sheer bulk, with the surgeon having to reach over and around layers of fat. Postoperatively these increased layers of fat predispose toward wound dehiscence. In addition to these mechanical factors, obese individuals have an increased likelihood of having hypertension, diabetes mellitus, hypertriglyceridemia, and coronary artery disease (when one of the first three are present). The hypertension, diabetes, and hypertriglyceridemia are often reversible with weight loss.[267] The individual problems of diabetes and hypertension and their interaction with surgery are discussed elsewhere (see Diabetes Mellitus above and Chapter 13, Renal Disease and Hypertension).

Obese patients who are greater than 120 percent overweight have two to three times the general incidence of cholesterol gallstones.[268] Liver function tests are abnormal in some obese patients,[269–271] but only the SGOT and SGPT could be correlated with the degree of fat infiltration seen by biopsy in one study.[269] In this same study, periportal fibrosis and inflammation were also seen in some patients. Clearly, liver function tests should be performed preoperatively to avoid confusion when abnormal test results are found postoperatively.

The major source of perioperative morbidity that may be directly linked to obesity is respiratory impairment which takes three forms. The first form appears to be directly due to increased chest wall and abdominal fat and consists of a reduction in lung and chest wall compliance. This results in the closure of small peripheral lung units, an increased energy cost of breathing with decreased respiratory muscle efficiency, hypoventilation of dependent lobes, and a reduction in vital capacity and functional residual capacity.[272,273] In an ambulatory setting, these patients do not retain carbon dioxide,[272,274] but they may be slightly hypoxic, especially when supine.[274] After abdominal surgery, massively obese patients have a further reduction in PaO_2 with the nadir appearing on the second postoperative day.[274]

A much smaller group of massively obese patients have hypoventilation, hypercapnea, hypoxia, somnolence, and markedly reduced lung compliance—a constellation of findings that has been referred to as the Pickwickian syndrome.[272] Further testing reveals these patients to have blunted O_2 and CO_2 response curves.[275] The prognosis in patients with Pickwickian syndrome is exceedingly poor,[276] but considerable improvement can be achieved if significant weight loss occurs.[272] Finally, some patients with obesity develop upper airway obstruction when asleep (or given sedation) and become hypoxic and even apneic.[277,278]

From the foregoing it can be seen that many patients with moderate to massive obesity may have varying degrees of respiratory insufficiency, especially following thoracic or abdominal surgery. Every effort should be made to encourage deep breathing (incentive spirometers) and coughing in such patients. Preoperative arterial blood gases should be obtained since significant hypoxia or hypercapnea will signal that severe postoperative respiratory problems may occur. Sedation should be employed with extreme caution. If there is a history of periodic awakening with sleep disturbance, upper airway obstruction should be suspected, and such patients may need prolonged postoperative intubation (see Chapter 12, Pulmonary Diseases). Finally, it should be remembered that patients with massive obesity are prone to thrombophlebitis and pulmonary embolism.[276] In addition to these respiratory problems, obese patients may have an increased susceptibility to anesthetic toxicity as a result of altered anesthetic biotransformation. The increased bulk of adipose tissue allows for continued biotransformation of methoxyflurane and enflurane, resulting in elevated serum levels of inorganic fluoride and potential nephrotoxicity.[271]

REFERENCES

1. Williams, RH, and Porte, D, Jr.: *The pancreas,* in Williams, RH (ed.): *Textbook of Endocrinology,* ed. 4. Philadelphia: W.B. Saunders Co., 1974, p. 502.
2. Galloway, JA, and Shuman, CR: *Diabetes and surgery.* Am J Med 34:177, 1963.
3. Wheelock, FC, Jr, and Marble, A: *Surgery and diabetes,* in Marble, A, White, P, Bradley, RF, et al. (eds.): *Joslin's Diabetes Mellitus,* ed. 11. Philadelphia: Lea & Febiger, 1971, p. 599.
4. Steinke, J: *Management of diabetes in the surgical patient.* Med Clin North Am 55:939, 1971.
5. Hamby, RI, Zoneraich, S, and Sherman, L: *Diabetic cardiomyopathy.* JAMA 229:1749, 1974.
6. Zitomer, BR, Gramm, HF, and Kozak, GP: *Gastric neuropathy in diabetes mellitus; clinical and radiologic observations.* Metabolism 17:199, 1968.
7. Hollis, JB, Castell, DO, and Braddom, RL: *Esophageal function in diabetes mellitus and its relation to peripheral neuropathy.* Gastroenterology 73:1098, 1977.
8. Goldstein, F, Wirts, W, and Kowlessar, OD: *Diabetic diarrhea and steatorrhea.* Ann Intern Med 72:215, 1970.
9. Ellenberg, M: *Diabetic neuropathy; clinical aspects.* Metabolism 25:1627, 1976.
10. Longstreth, GF, and Newcomer, AD: *Abdominal pain caused by diabetic radiculopathy.* Ann Intern Med 86:166, 1977.
11. Page, MM, and Watkins, PJ: *The heart in diabetes: autonomic neuropathy and cardiomyopathy.* Clinics in Endocrinol Metab 6:377, 1977.
12. Page, MM, and Watkins, PJ: *Cardiorespiratory arrest and diabetic autonomic neuropathy.* Lancet 1:14, 1978.
13. Fraser, DM, Campbell, IW, Ewing, DJ, et al.: *Peripheral and autonomic nerve function in newly diagnosed diabetes mellitus.* Diabetes 36:546, 1977.
14. Ewing, DJ, Campbell, IW, Murray, A, et al.: *Immediate heart-rate response to standing; simple test for autonomic neuropathy in diabetes.* Br Med J 1:145, 1978.
15. Ewing, DJ, Campbell, IW, and Clarke, BF: *Mortality in diabetic autonomic neuropathy.* Lancet 1:601, 1976.
16. Ellenberg, M: *Diabetic neuropathic cachexia.* Diabetes 23:418, 1974.
17. Gade, GN, Hofeldt, FD, and Treece, GL: *Diabetic neuropathic cachexia. Beneficial response to combination therapy with amitriptyline and fluphenazine.* JAMA 243:1160, 1980.
18. Marliss, EB, Ohman, JL, Jr, Aoki, TT, et al.: *Altered redox state obscuring ketoacidosis in diabetic patients with lactic acidosis.* N Engl J Med 283:978, 1970.
19. Harkonen, S, and Kjellstrand, CM: *Exacerbation of diabetic renal failure following intravenous pyelography.* Am J Med 3:939, 1977.
20. Beisel, WR: *Magnitude of the host nutritional responses to infection.* Am J Clin Nutr 30:1236, 1977.
21. Long, CL: *Energy balance and carbohydrate metabolism in infection and sepsis.* Am J Clin Nutr 30:1301, 1977.
22. Wilmore, DW: *Carbohydrate metabolism in trauma.* Clin Endocrinol Metab 5:731, 1976.
23. Clarke, RSJ: *The hyperglycaemic response to different types of surgery and anaesthesia.* Br J Anaesth 42:45, 1970.
24. Giddings, A: *The control of plasma glucose in the surgical patients.* Br J Surg 61:787, 1974.

25. Schweizer, O, and Howland, WS: *Some metabolic changes associated with anesthesia and operation.* Surg Clin North Am 49:223, 1969.
26. Shen, SW, and Bressler, R: *Clinical pharmacology of oral antidiabetic agents.* N Engl J Med 296: 493, 787, 1977.
27. Gennari, FJ, and Kassirer, JP: *Osmotic diuresis.* N Engl J Med 291:714, 1974.
28. Roscoe, JM, Halperin, ML, Rolleston, FS, et al.: *Hyperglycemia-induced hyponatremia: metabolic considerations in calculation of serum sodium depression.* Can Med Assoc J 112:452, 1975.
29. Knight, AH, Williams, DN, Ellis, G, et al.: *Significance of hyperamylasemia and abdominal pain in diabetic ketoacidosis.* Br Med J 3:128, 1973.
30. Levine, RI, Glauser, FL, and Berk, JD: *Enhancement of the amylase-creatinine clearance ratio in disorders other than acute pancreatitis.* N Engl J Med 292:329, 1975.
31. Warshaw, AL, Feller, ER, and Lee, KH: *On the cause of raised serum amylase in diabetic ketoacidosis.* Lancet 1:929, 1977.
32. Chen, JC, Marsters, R, and Wieland, RG: *Diabetic ketosis. Interpretation of elevated serum glutamic acid-oxaloacetic transaminase (SGOT) by multi-channel chemical analysis.* Diabetes 19:730, 1970.
33. Knight, AH, Williams, DN, Spooner, RJ, et al.: *Serum enzyme changes in diabetic ketoacidosis.* Diabetes 23:126, 1974.
34. Molitch, ME, Rodman, E, Dubinsky, E, et al.: *Spurious serum creatinine elevations in ketoacidosis.* Ann Intern Med 93:280, 1980.
35. Winegrad, AI, and Clements, RS, Jr: *Diabetic ketoacidosis.* Med Clin North Am 55:899, 1971.
36. Matz, R: *Diabetic coma. Guidelines in therapy.* NY State J Med 74:642, 1974.
37. Alberti, KGMM, and Hockaday, TDR: *Diabetic coma; a reappraisal after five years.* Clin Endocrinol Metab 6:421, 1977.
38. Kreisberg, RA: *Diabetic ketoacidosis: new concepts and trends in pathogenesis and treatment.* Ann Intern Med 88:681, 1978.
39. Kety, SS, Polis, BD, Nadler, CS, et al.: *The blood flow and oxygen consumption of the human brain in diabetic acidosis and coma.* J Clin Invest 27:500, 1948.
40. Thrower, WB, Darby, TD, and Aldinger, EE: *Acid-base derangements and myocardial contractility.* Arch Surg 82:76, 1961.
41. Heber, D, Molitch, ME, and Sperling, MA: *Low-dose continuous insulin therapy for diabetic ketoacidosis.* Arch Intern Med 137:1377, 1977.
42. Arieff, AI, and Carroll, HJ: *Nonketotic hyperosmolar coma with hyperglycemia; clinical features, pathophysiology, renal function, acid-base balance, plasma-cerebrospinal fluid equilibrium and the effects of therapy in 37 cases.* Medicine 51:73, 1972.
43. Blackburn, GL, Flatt, JP, Clowes, GHA, Jr, et al.: *Protein sparing therapy during starvation with sepsis or trauma.* Ann Surg 177:588, 1973.
44. Schein, PS, DeLellis, RA, Kahn, CR, et al.: *Islet cell tumors: current concepts and management.* Ann Intern Med 79:239, 1973.
45. Stefanini, P, Carboni, M, Patrassi, N, et al.: *Beta-islet cell tumors of the pancreas: results of a study of 1,067 cases.* Surgery 75:597, 1974.
46. Service, FJ, Dale, AJD, Elveback, LR, et al.: *Insulinomas. Clinical and diagnostic features of 60 consecutive cases.* Mayo Clin Proc 51:417, 1976.
47. Horwitz, DL, Kuzuya, H, and Rubenstein, AH: *Circulating serum C-peptide. A brief review of diagnostic implications.* N Engl J Med 295:207, 1976.
48. Hofeldt, FD: *Reactive hypoglycemia.* Metabolism 24:1193, 1975.
49. Anthony, D, Dippe, S, Hofeldt, FD, et al.: *Personality disorder and reactive hypoglycemia. A quantitative study.* Diabetes 22:664, 1973.
50. Ford, CU, Bray, GA, and Swerdloff, RS: *A psychiatric study of patients referred with a diagnosis of hypoglycemia.* Am J Psychiatry 133:290, 1976.

51. Jauregui, R, Lilker, ES, and Bayley, A: *Upper airway obstruction in euthyroid goiter.* JAMA 238:2163, 1977.

52. Fisher, DA: *Advances in the laboratory diagnosis of thyroid disease.* J. Pediatrics 82:1, 187, 1973.

53. Levey, GS: *The heart and hyperthyroidism. Use of beta-adrenergic blocking drugs.* Med Clin North Am 59:1193, 1975.

54. Skelton, CL, and Sonnenblick, EH: *Hyperthyroidism: cardiovascular system,* in Werner, SC, and Ingbar, SH (eds.): *The Thyroid,* ed 4. New York: Harper and Row, 1978, p. 688.

55. Sandler, G, and Wilson, GM: *Nature and prognosis of heart disease in thyrotoxicosis.* Q J Med 28:347, 1959.

56. Mazzaferri, EL, Reynolds, JC, Young, RL, et al.: *Propranolol as primary therapy for thyrotoxicosis. Results of a long-term prospective study.* Arch Intern Med 136:50, 1976.

57. Georges, LP, Santangelo, RP, Mackin, JF, et al.: *Metabolic effects of propranolol in thyrotoxicosis. I. Nitrogen, calcium, and hydroxyproline.* Metabolism 24:11, 1975.

58. Rivlin, RS, and Wagner, HN, Jr.: *Anemia in hyperthyroidism.* Ann Intern Med 70:507, 1969.

59. Herbert, V: *Hyperthyroidism: blood,* in Werner, SC, and Ingbar, SH (eds.): *The Thyroid,* ed. 4. New York: Harper and Row, 1978, p. 773.

60. Ingbar, SH, and Woeber, KA: *The thyroid gland,* in Williams, RH, (ed.): *Textbook of Endocrinology,* ed. 5. Philadelphia: W.B. Saunders Co., 1974, p. 95.

61. Palmer, HM, and Beardwell, CG: *Hyperthyroidism presenting with acute abdominal symptoms.* Practitioner 212:239, 1974.

62. Burman, KD, Monchik, JM, Earll, JM, et al.: *Ionized and total serum calcium and parathyroid hormone in hyperthyroidism.* Ann Intern Med 84:668, 1976.

63. Davis, PJ, and Davis, FB: *Hyperthyroidism in patients over the age of 60 years.* Medicine 53:161, 1974.

64. Vagenakis, AG, Wang, CA, Burger, A, et al.: *Iodide-induced thyrotoxicosis in Boston.* N Engl J Med 287:523, 1972.

65. Blum, M, Weinberg, U, Shenkman, L, et al.: *Hyperthyroidism after iodinated contrast medium.* N Engl J Med 291:24, 1974.

66. Blum, M, Kranjac, T, Park, CM, et al.: *Thyroid storm after cardiac angiography with iodinated contrast medium.* JAMA 235:2324, 1976.

67. Nelson, NC, and Becker, WF: *Thyroid crisis. Diagnosis and treatment.* Ann Surg 170:263, 1969.

68. Braverman, LE: *Therapeutic considerations in thyrotoxicosis.* Clin Endocrinol Metabol 7:221, 1978.

69. Williams, DE, Chopra, IJ, Orgiazzi, J, et al.: *Acute effects of corticosteroids on thyroid activity in Graves' Disease.* J Clin Endocrinol Metab 41:354, 1975.

70. Grossman, W, Robin, NI, Johnson, LW, et al.: *Effects of beta blockade on the peripheral manifestations of thyrotoxicosis.* Ann Intern Med 74:875, 1971.

71. Eriksson, M, Rubenfeld, S, Garber, AJ, et al.: *Propranolol does not prevent thyroid storm.* N Engl J Med 296:263, 1977.

72. Temple, R, Berman, M, Carlson, HE, et al.: *The use of lithium in Graves' Disease.* Mayo Clin Proc 47:872, 1972.

73. Fore, W, and Wynn, J: *Rapid redistribution of serum thyroxine during ether anesthesia.* J Clin Endocrinol Metab 26:821, 1966.

74. Mackin, JF, Canary, JJ, and Pittman, CS: *Thyroid storm and its management.* N Engl J Med 291:1396, 1974.

75. Ingbar, SH: *Thyroid storm,* in Werner, SC, and Inbar, SH (eds.): *The Thyroid,* ed 4. New York: Harper and Row, 1978, p. 800.

76. Rosenberg, IN: *Thyroid storm.* Pharmacol Ther C 1:423, 1976.

77. Dillon, PT, Baba, J, Meloni, CR, et al.: *Reserpine in thyrotoxic crises.* N Engl J Med 283:1020, 1970.

78. Mazzaferri, EL, and Skillman, TG: *Thyroid storm.* Arch Intern Med 124:684, 1969.

79. Larsen, PR: *Salicylate-induced increases in free triiodothyronine in human serum.* J Clin Invest 51:1125, 1975.

80. Hoch, FR: *Synergism between calorigenic effects: L-thyroxine and 2,4 dinitrophenol or sodium salicylate in euthyroid rats.* Endocrinology 76:335, 1965.

81. Newmark, SR, Himathongkam, T, and Shane, JM: *Hyperthyroid crisis.* JAMA 230:592, 1974 and 233:508, 1975 (correspondence).

82. Cavalieri, RR, Sung, LC, and Becker, CE: *Effects of phenobarbital on thyroxine and triiodothyronine kinetics in Graves disease.* J Clin Endocrinol Metab 37:308, 1973.

83. Zouszein, J, Santangelo, RP, Mackin, JF, et al.: *Propranolol therapy in thyrotoxicosis. A review of 84 patients undergoing surgery.* Am J Med 66:411, 1979.

84. Thomas, CG, Jr: *Surgery of the thyroid.* Med Clin North Am 59:1247, 1975.

85. Caswell, HT, Marks, AD, and Channick, BJ: *Propranolol for the preoperative preparation of patients with thyrotoxicosis.* Surg Gynecol Obstet 146:908, 1978.

86. Toft, AD, Irvine, WJ, Sinclair, I, et al.: *Thyroid function after surgical treatment of thyrotoxicosis. A report of 100 cases treated with propranolol before operation.* N Engl J Med 298:643, 1978.

87. Feind, CR: *Hyperthyroidism: surgery,* in Werner, SC, and Ingbar, SH (eds.): *The Thyroid,* ed. 4. New York: Harper and Row, 1978, p. 822.

88. Foster, RS, Jr: *Morbidity and mortality after thyroidectomy.* Surg Gynecol Obstet 146:423, 1978.

89. Burnett, HF, Mabry, CD, and Westbrook, KC: *Hypocalcemia after thyroidectomy: mechanisms and management.* South Med J 70:1045, 1977.

90. Gann, DS, and Raone, JF: *Delayed hypocalcemia after thyroidectomy for Graves' disease is prevented by parathyroid autotransplantation.* Ann Surg 190:508, 1979.

91. Green, M, and Wilson, GM: *Thyrotoxicosis treated by surgery or iodine-131 with special reference to development of hypothyroidism.* Br Med J 1:1005, 1964.

92. Hedley, AJ, Flemming, CJ, Chesters, MI, et al.: *Surgical treatment of thyrotoxicosis.* Br Med J 1:519, 1970.

93. Wesley, JR, Buckingham, BA, Gahr, JA, et al.: *Surgical treatment of hyperthyroidism in children.* Surg Gynecol Obstet 145:343, 1977.

94. Toft, AD, Irvine, WJ, McIntosh, D, et al.: *Temporary hypothyroidism after surgical treatment of thyrotoxicosis.* Lancet 2:817, 1976.

95. Weinberg, AD, Brennan, MD, Marsh, HM, et al.: *Anesthetic and post-operative risks in hypothyroid patients.* Program of the 56th Meeting of the American Thyroid Association. San Diego, 1980, p. 8.

96. Crowley, WF, Jr, Ridgway, EC, Bough, EW, et al.: *Noninvasive evaluation of cardiac function in hypothyroidism.* N Engl J Med 296:1, 1977.

97. Skelton, CL, and Sonnenblick, EH: *Hypothyroidism: cardiovascular system,* in Werner, SC, and Ingbar, SH (eds.): *The Thyroid,* ed. 4. New York: Harper and Row, 1978, p. 861.

98. Sachdev, Y, and Hall, R: *Effusions into body cavities in hypothyroidism.* Lancet 1:564, 1975.

99. Vanhaelst, L, Neve, P, Chailly, P, et al.: *Coronary artery disease in hypothyroidism.* Lancet 2:800, 1967.

100. Steinberg, AD: *Myxedema and coronary artery disease—a comparative autopsy study.* Ann Intern Med 68:338, 1968.

101. Goldman, J, Matz, R, Mortimer, R, et al.: *High elevations of creatine phosphokinase in hypothyroidism. An isoenzyme analysis.* JAMA 237:325, 1977.

102. Turino, GM: *Hypothyroidism: respiratory system,* in Werner, SC, and Ingbar, SH (eds.): *The Thyroid,* ed 4. New York: Harper and Row, 1978, p. 857.

103. Zwillich, CW, Pierson, DJ, Hofeldt, FD, et al.: *Ventilatory control in myxedema and hypothyroidism.* N Engl J Med 292:662, 1975.

104. Eichelbaum, M, Bodem, G, Gugler, R, et al.: *Influence of thyroid status on plasma half-life of antipyrine in man.* N Engl J Med 290:1040, 1974.

105. O'Brien, MD, and Harris, PWR: *Cerebral-cortex perfusion rates in myxedema.* Lancet 1:1170, 1968.

106. DiScala, VA, and McKinney, MJ: *Effects of myxedema on the renal diluting and concentrating mechanism.* Am J Med 50:325, 1971.

107. DeRubertis, FR, Jr., Michelis, MF, Bloom, ME, et al.: *Impaired water excretion in myxedema.* Am J Med 51:41, 1971.

108. Royce, PC: *Severely impaired consciousness in myxedema—a review.* Am J Med Sci 261:46, 1971.

109. Edson, JR, Fecher, DR, and Doc, RP: *Low platelet adhesiveness and other hemostatic abnormalities in hypothyroidism.* Ann Intern Med 82:342, 1975.

110. DAS, KC, MUKHERJEE, M, SARKAR, TK, ET AL.: *Erythropoiesis and erythropoietin in hypo– and hyperthyroidism.* J Clin Endocrinol Metab 41:211, 1975.

111. HINES, JD, HALSTED, CH, GRIGGS, RC, ET AL.: *Megaloblastic anemia secondary to folate deficiency associated with hypothyroidism.* Ann Intern Med 68:792, 1968.

112. HORTON, L, COBURN, RJ, ENGLAND, JM, ET AL.: *The haematology of hypothyroidism.* Q J Med 45:101, 1976.

113. FREEDBERG, IM: *Hypothyroidism: skin,* in WERNER, SC, AND INGBAR, SH (eds.): *The Thyroid,* ed. 4. New York: Harper and Row, 1978, p. 851.

114. JAVITT, NB: *Hypothyroidism: gastrointestinal tract,* in WERNER, SC, AND INGBAR, SH (eds.): *The Thyroid,* ed. 4. New York: Harper and Row, 1978, p. 869.

115. BRANDT, MR, KEHLET, H, SKOVSTED, L, ET AL.: *Rapid decrease in plasma-triiodothyronine during surgery and epidural analgesia independent of afferent neurogenic stimuli and of cortisol.* Lancet 2:1333, 1976.

116. CAVALIERI, RR, AND RAPOPORT, B: *Impaired peripheral conversion of thyroxine to triiodothyronine.* Ann Rev Med 28:57, 1977.

117. SCHIMMEL, M, AND UTIGER, RD: *Thyroidal and peripheral production of thyroid hormones.* Ann Intern Med 87:760, 1977.

118. MOLITCH, ME, SPILER, IJ, MODELL, E, ET AL.: *Suppression of hypothalamic-pituitary thyroid axis during prolonged protein supplemented semi-starvation.* Int J Obesity 2:389, 1978.

119. RICHMAND, D, MOLITCH, ME, AND O'DONNELL, TF: *Altered thyroid hormone levels in bacterial sepsis: the role of nutritional adequacy.* Metabolism 29:936, 1980.

120. SULLIVAN, PRC, BOLLINGER, JA, AND REICHLIN, S: *Selective deficiency of tissue triiodothyronine; a proposed mechanism of elevated free thyroxine in the euthyroid sick.* J Clin Invest 52:83, 1973.

121. DERUBERTIS, FR, AND KOSCH, PC: *Accelerated host metabolism of L-thyroxine during acute infection: role of the leukocyte and peripheral leukocytosis.* J Clin Endocrinol Metab 40:589, 1975.

122. WARTOFSKY, L: *The response of the thyroid gland and thyroid hormone metabolism to infectious disease.* Horm Res 5:112, 1974.

123. LUTZ, JH, GREGERMAN, RJ, SPAULDING, SW, ET AL.: *Thyroxine binding proteins, free thyroxine and thyroxine turnover interrelationships during acute infectious illness in man.* J Clin Endocrinol Metab 35:230, 1972.

124. UTIGER, RD: *Decreased extrathyroidal triiado thyroxine production in nonthyroidal illness: benefit or harm?* Am J Med 69:807, 1980.

125. RUDMAN, D, FLEISCHER, AS, KUTNER, MH, ET AL.: *Suprahypophyseal hypogonadism and hypothyroidism during prolonged coma after head trauma.* J Clin Endocrinol Metab 45:747, 1977.

126. WILSON, H, SILVERMAN, V, BOYD, AE, III, ET AL.: *Are patients with low serum triiodothyronine (T3) really euthyroid?* Clin Res 26:792A, 1978.

127. STOCK, JM, SURKS, MI, AND OPPENHEIMER, JH: *Replacement dosage of l-thyroxine in hypothyroidism. A reevaluation.* N Engl J Med 290:529, 1974.

128. SMITH, RN, TAYLOR, SA, AND MASSEY, JC: *Controlled clinical trial of combined triiodothyronine and thyroxine in the treatment of hypothyroidism.* Br Med J 4:145, 1970.

129. JACKSON, IMD, AND COBB, WE: *Why does anyone still use dessicated thyroid USP?* Am J Med 64:284, 1978.

130. SABERI, M, AND UTIGER, RD: *Serum thyroid hormone and thyrotropin concentrations during thyroxine and triiodothyronine therapy.* J Clin Endocrinol Metab 39:923, 1974.

131. WENZEL, KW, AND KIRSCHSIEPER, HE: *Aspects of the absorption of oral l-thyroxine in normal man.* Metabolism 26:1, 1977.

132. CARPENTER, CCJ, SOLOMON, N, AND SILVERBERG, SG: *Schmidt's syndrome (thyroid and adrenal insufficiency); a review of the literature and a report of fifteen new cases, including ten instances of coexistent diabetes mellitus.* Medicine 43:153, 1964.

133. NICOLOFF, JF: *Myxedema coma.* Pharmacol Ther C 1:161, 1976.

134. BLUM, M: *Myxedema coma.* Am J Med Sci 264:432, 1972.

135. MENENDEZ, CE, AND RIVLIN, RS: *Thyrotoxic crisis and myxedema coma.* Med Clin North Am 57:1463, 1973.

136. WERNER, SC: *Myxedema coma,* in WERNER, SC, AND INGBAR, SH (eds.): *The Thyroid,* ed 4. New York: Harper and Row, 1978, p. 971.

137. REULER, JB: *Hypothermia; pathophysiology, clinical settings and management.* Ann Intern Med 89:519, 1978.

138. RIDGWAY, EC, MCCAMMON, JA, BENOTTI, J, ET AL.: *Acute metabolic responses in myxedema to large doses of intravenous l-thyroxine.* Ann Intern Med 77:549, 1972.

139. LIDDLE, GW: *The adrenal cortex,* in WILLIAMS, RH (ed.): *Textbook of Endocrinology,* ed. 5. Philadelphia: W.B. Saunders Co., 1976, p. 233.

140. IRVINE, WJ, AND BARNES, EW: *Adrenocortical insufficiency.* Clin Endocrinol Metabol 1:549, 1972.

141. APPEL, GB, AND HOLUB, DA: *The syndrome of multiple endocrine gland insufficiency.* Am J Med 61:129, 1976.

142. HILL, GJ, II, AND WHEELER, HB: *Adrenal insufficiency due to metastatic carcinoma of the lung.* Cancer 18:1467, 1965.

143. EAGAN, RT, AND PAGE, MI: *Adrenal insufficiency following bilateral adrenal venography.* JAMA 215:115, 1971.

144. CLARK, OH: *Postoperative adrenal hemorrhage.* Ann Surg 182:124, 1975.

145. XARLI, VP, STEELE, AA, DAVIS, PJ, ET AL.: *Adrenal hemorrhage in the adult.* Medicine 57:211, 1978.

146. ALFORD, WC, JR, MEADOR, CK, MIHALEVICH, J, ET AL.: *Acute adrenal insufficiency following cardiac surgical procedures.* J Thorac Cardiovasc Surg 78:489, 1979.

147. PORTNAY, GI, VAGENAKIS, AG, BRAVERMAN, LE, ET AL.: *Anticoagulant therapy and acute adrenal insufficiency.* Ann Intern Med 81:115, 1974.

148. WEST, CD, AND DOLMEN, LI: *Plasma ACTH radioimmunoassays in the diagnosis of pituitary-adrenal dysfunction.* Ann NY Acad Sci 297:205, 1977.

149. SPECKART, PF, NICOLOFF, JT, AND BETHUNE, JE: *Screening for adrenocortical insufficiency with cosyntropin (synthetic ACTH).* Arch Intern Med 128:761, 1971.

150. HIMATHONGKAM, T, NEWMARK, SR, GREENFIELD, M, ET AL.: *Acute adrenal insufficiency.* JAMA 230:1317, 1974.

151. GOLD, EM: *The Cushing syndromes: changing views of diagnosis and treatment.* Ann Intern Med 90:829, 1979.

152. EDDY, RL, JONES, AL, GILLILAND, PF, ET AL.: *Cushing's syndrome: a prospective study of diagnostic methods.* Am J Med 55:621, 1973.

153. MOLITCH, ME: *ACTH-secreting adenomas,* in POST, KD, JACKSON, IMD, AND REICHLIN, S (eds.): *The Pituitary Adenoma.* New York: Plenum Press, 1980, p. 118.

154. OXLUND, H, FOGDESTAM, I, AND VIIDIK, A: *The influence of cortisol on wound healing of the skin and distant connective tissue response.* Surg Gynecol Obstet 148:876, 1979.

155. FLYNN, A, STRAIN, WH, PORIES, WJ, ET AL.: *Zinc deficiency with altered adrenocortical function and its relation to delayed healing.* Lancet 1:789, 1973.

156. REGESTEIN, QR, ROSE, LI, AND WILLIAMS, GH: *Psychopathology in Cushing's syndrome.* Arch Intern Med 130:114, 1972.

157. MOLITCH, ME: *Medical therapy of pituitary tumors,* in POST, KD, JACKSON, IMD, AND REICHLIN, S, (eds.): *The Pituitary Adenoma.* Plenum Press, New York, 1980, p. 323.

158. SALASSA, RM, LAWS, ER, JR., CARPENTER, PC, ET AL.: *Transsphenoidal removal of pituitary microadenoma in Cushing's disease.* Mayo Clin Proc 53:24, 1978.

159. DAVID, DS, GRIECO, MH, AND CUSHMAN, P, JR: *Adrenal glucocorticoids after twenty years. A review of their clinically relevant consequences.* J Chron Dis 22:637, 1970.

160. MELBY, JC: *Clinical pharmacology of systemic corticosteroids.* Ann Rev Pharmacol Toxicol 17:511, 1977.

161. AXELROD, L: *Glucocorticoid therapy.* Medicine 55:39, 1976.

162. GRABER, AL, NEY, RL, NICHOLSON, WE, ET AL.: *Natural history of pituitary-adrenal recovery following long term suppression with corticosteroids.* J Clin Endocrinol Metab 25:11, 1965.

163. BYYNY, RL: *Withdrawal from glucocorticoid therapy.* N Engl J Med 295:30, 1976.

164. ROOT, AW, BONGIOVANNI, AM, AND EBERLEIN, WR: *The adrenogenital syndrome,* in CHRISTY, NP (ed.): *The Human Adrenal Cortex.* New York: Harper and Row, 1971, p. 427.

165. BROOK, CGD, ZACHMAN, M, PRADER, A, ET AL.: *Experience with long-term therapy in congenital adrenal hyperplasia.* J Pediatrics 85:12, 1974.

166. McGuffin, WL, Jr., and Gunnells, JC, Jr.: *Primary aldosteronism.* Urol Clin North Am 4:227, 1971.

167. Weinberger, MH, Grim, CE, Hollifield, JW, et al.: *Primary aldosteronism.* Ann Intern Med 90:386, 1979.

168. Spark, R, and Eisenberg, H: *Medical aspects of adrenal surgery.* Urol Clin North Am 3:433, 1976.

169. Perez, GO, Lespier, L, Jacobi, J, et al.: *Hyporeninemia and hypoaldosteronism in diabetes mellitus.* Arch Intern Med 137:852, 1977.

170. Manger, WM, and Gifford, RW, Jr.: *Pheochromocytoma.* New York: Springer-Verlag, 1977.

171. Melmon, KL: *The Adrenals. Part II: Catecholamines and the adrenal medulla,* in Williams, RH (ed.): *Textbook of Endocrinology.* Philadelphia: W.B. Saunders Co., 1974, p. 283.

172. Freier, DT, Eckhauser, FE, and Harrison, TS: *Pheochromocytoma. A persistently problematic and still potentially lethal disease.* Arch Surg 115:788, 1980.

173. Cross, DA, and Meyer, JS: *Postoperative deaths due to unsuspected pheochromocytoma.* South Med J 70:1320, 1977.

174. Melicow, MM: *One hundred cases of pheochromocytoma (107 tumors) at the Columbia-Presbyterian Medical Center, 1926–1976. A clinicopathological analysis.* Cancer 40:1987, 1977.

175. Raper, AJ, Jessee, EF, Texter, JH, Jr., et al.: *Pheochromocytoma of the urinary bladder: a broad clinical spectrum.* Am J Cardiol 40:820, 1977.

176. Engelman, K: *Phaeochromoctyoma.* Clin Endocrinol Metabol 6:769, 1977.

177. Graze, K, Spiler, IJ, Tashjian, AH, Jr, et al.: *Natural history of familial medullary thyroid carcinomas.* N Engl J Med 299:980, 1978.

178. Kukreja, SC, Hargis, GK, Rosenthal, IM, et al.: *Pheochromocytoma causing excessive parathyroid hormone production and hypercalcemia.* Ann Intern Med 79:838, 1973.

179. Carney, JA, Go, VLW, Sizemore, GW, et al.: *Alimentary tract ganglioneuromatosis.* N Engl J Med 295:1287, 1976.

180. Zelch, JV, Meaney, TF, and Belhobek, GH: *Radiologic approach to the patient with suspected pheochromocytoma.* Radiology 111:279, 1974.

181. ReMine, WH, Chong, GC, Van Heerden, JA, et al.: *Current management of pheochromocytoma.* Ann Surg 179:740, 1974.

182. Gittes, RF, and Mahoney, EM: *Pheochromocytoma.* Urol Clin North Am 4:239, 1977.

183. Ross, EJ, Prichard, BNC, Kaufman, L, et al.: *Preoperative and operative management of patients with pheochromocytoma.* Br Med J 1:191, 1967.

184. Pertsemlidis, D, Gitlow, SE, Siegel, WC, et al.: *Pheochromocytoma: 1. Specificity of laboratory diagnostic tests. 2. Safeguards during operative removal.* Ann Surg 169:376, 1969.

185. Stephen, CR: *Anesthesia for adrenal surgery.* Urol Clin North Am 4:319, 1977.

186. Boonstra, CE, and Jackson, CE: *Serum calcium survey for hyperparathyroidism. Results in 50,000 clinic patients.* Am J Clin Path 55:523, 1971.

187. Mallette, LE, Bilezikian, JP, Heath, DA, et al.: *Primary hyperparathyroidism: clinical and biochemical features.* Medicine 53:127, 1974.

188. Ladenson, JH, Lewis, JW, and Boyd, JC: *Failure of total calcium corrected for protein, albumin and pH to correctly assess free calcium state.* J Clin Endocrinol Metab 46:986, 1978.

189. Payne, RB, Little, AJ, Williams, RB, et al.: *Interpretation of serum calcium in patients with abnormal serum proteins.* Br Med J 4:643, 1973.

190. Christensson, T, Hellstrom, K, and Wengle, B: *Hypercalcemia and primary hyperparathyroidism.* Arch Intern Med 137:1138, 1977.

191. Rasmussen, H: *Parathyroid hormone, calcitonin and the calciferols,* in Williams, RH (ed.): *Textbook of Endocrinology.* Philadelphia: W.B. Saunders Co., 1974, p. 660.

192. Schneider, AB, and Sherwood, LM: *Calcium homeostasis and the pathogenesis and management of hypercalcemic disorders.* Metabolism 23:925, 1974.

193. Purnell, DC, Scholz, DA, and Smith, LH: *Diagnosis of primary hyperparathyroidism.* Med Clin North Am 57:543, 1977.

194. Palmer, FJ, Nelson, JC, and Bacchus, H: *The chloride-phosphate ratio in hypercalcemia.* Ann Intern Med 80:200, 1974.

195. Skrabanck, P, McPartlin, J, and Powell, D: *Tumor hypercalcemia and "ectopic hyperparathyroidism."* Medicine 59:262, 1980.

196. Singer, FR, Sharp, CF, Jr., and Rude, RK: *Pathogenesis of hypercalcemia in malignancy.* Mineral Electrolyte Metab 2:161, 1979.

197. Stephens, RL, Hansen, HH, and Muggia, FM: *Hypercalcemia in epidermoid tumors of the head and neck and esophagus.* Cancer 31:1487, 1973.

198. Drezner, MK, and Lebovitz, HE: *Primary hyperparathyroidism in paraneoplastic hypercalcemia.* Lancet 1:1004, 1978.

199. Fisken, RA, Heath, DA, Somers, S, et al.: *Hypercalcaemia in hospital patients. Clinical and diagnostic aspects.* Lancet 1:202, 1981.

200. Swaroop, S, and Krant, MJ: *Rapid estrogen-induced hypercalcemia.* JAMA 223:913, 1973.

201. Wenger, NK, and Herndon, EG, Jr: *Endocrine and metabolic disorders,* in Hurst, JW, Logue, RB, Schlaut, RC, et al. (eds.): *The Heart, Arteries and Veins,* ed. 3. New York: McGraw Hill Book Co., 1974, p. 1478.

202. Nierenberg, D, and Rausil, BJ: *Q-aTc interval as a clinical indicator of hypercalcemia.* Am J Cardiol 44:263, 1979.

203. Bronsky, D, Dubin, A, Waldstein, SS, et al.: *Calcium and the electrocardiogram. II. The electrocardiographic manifestations of hyperparathyroidism and of marked hypercalcemia from various other etiologies.* Am J Cardiol 7:833, 1961.

204. Berliner, K: *The effect of calcium injections on the human heart.* Am J Med Sci 191:117, 1936.

205. Clark, NE: *The action of calcium on the human electrocardiogram.* Am Heart J 22:367, 1941.

206. Crum, WD, and Till, HJ: *Hyperparathyroidism with Wenckebach's phenomenon.* Am J Cardiol 6:838, 1960.

207. Ginsberg, H, and Schwartz, KV: *Hypercalcemia and complete heart block.* Ann Intern Med 79:903, 1973.

208. Petersen, P: *Psychiatric disorders in primary hyperparathyroidism.* J Clin Endocrinol Metab 28:1491, 1968.

209. Paloyan, E, Lawrence, AM, and Straus, FH: *Hyperparathyroidism.* New York: Grune and Stratton, 1974.

210. Ludwig, GD, and Chaykin, L: *Pancreatitis associated with primary hyperparathyroidism.* Med Clin North Am 50:1403, 1966.

211. Gafter, U, Mandel, EM, Har-Zahav, L, et al.: *Acute pancreatitis secondary to hypercalcemia. Occurrence in a patient with breast carcinoma.* JAMA 235:2004, 1976.

212. Benabe, JE, and Martinez-Maldonado, M: *Hypercalcemic nephropathy.* Arch Intern Med 138:777, 1978.

213. Christensson, T, Hellstrom, K, and Wengle, B: *Blood pressure in subjects with hypercalcemia and primary hyperparathyroidism detected in a health screening programme.* Eur J Clin Invest 7:109, 1977.

214. Patten, BM, Bilezikian, JP, Mallette, LE, et al.: *Neuromuscular disease in primary hyperparathyroidism.* Ann Intern Med 80:182, 1974.

215. Boxer, M, Ellman, L, Geller, R, et al.: *Anemia in primary hyperparathyroidism.* Arch Intern Med 137:588, 1977.

216. Marx, SJ, Spiegel, AM, Brown, EM, et al.: *Family studies in patients with primary parathyroid hyperplasia.* Am J Med 62:698, 1977.

217. Prinz, RA, Paloyan, E, Lawrence, AM, et al.: *Radiation-associated hyperparathyroidism; a new syndrome?* Surgery 82:296, 1977.

218. Suki, WN, Yium, JJ, Von Minden, M, et al.: *Acute treatment of hypercalcemia with furosemide.* N Engl J Med 283:836, 1970.

219. Perlia, CP, Gubisch, NJ, Wolter, J, et al.: *Mithramycin treatment of hypercalcemia.* Cancer 25:389, 1970.

220. Silva, OL, and Becker, KL: *Salmon calcitonin in the treatment of hypercalcemia.* Arch Intern Med 132:337, 1973.

221. Deftos, LJ, and Neer, R: *Medical management of the hypercalcemia of malignancy.* Ann Rev Med 25:323, 1974.

222. Rude, RK, Oldham, SB, and Singer, FR: *Functional hypoparathyroidism and parathyroid hormone end-organ resistance in human magnesium deficiency.* Clin Endocrinol 5:209, 1976.

223. Robertson, GM, Jr., Moore, EW, Switz, DM, et al.: *Inadequate parathyroid response in acute pancreatitis.* N Engl J Med 294:512, 1976.

224. Nusynowitz, ML, Frame, B, and Kolb, FO: *The spectrum of the hypoparathyroid states; a classification based on physiologic principles.* Medicine 55:105, 1976.

225. Haussler, MR, and McCain, TA: *Basic and clinical concepts related to vitamin D metabolism and action.* N Engl J Med 297:974, 1977.

226. Habener, JF, and Mahaffey, JE: *Osteomalacia and disorders of vitamin D metabolism.* Ann Rev Med 29:327, 1978.

227. Fonseca, OA, and Calverley, JR: *Neurological manifestations of hypoparathyroidism.* Arch Intern Med 120:202, 1967.

228. Dimich, A, Bedrossian, PB, and Wallach, S: *Hypoparathyroidism. Clinical observations in 34 patients.* Arch Intern Med 120:449, 1967.

229. Schneider, AB, and Sherwood, LM:*Pathogenesis and management of hypoparathyroidism and other hypocalcemic disorders.* Metabolism 24:871, 1975.

230. Schaaf, M, and Payne, CA: *Dystonic reactions to prochlorperazine in hypoparathyroidism.* N Engl J Med 275:991, 1966.

231. Avioli, LV: *The therapeutic approach to hypoparathyroidism.* Am J Med 57:34, 1974.

232. Harrison, HE, Lifshitz, F, and Blizzard, RM: *Comparison between crystalline dihydrotachysterol and calciferol in patients requiring pharmacologic vitamin D therapy.* N Engl J Med 276:894, 1967.

233. Neer, RM, Holick, MF, DeLuca, HF, et al.: *Effects of 1α-hydroxy-Vitamin D_3 and 1,25 dihydroxy-vitamin D_3 on calcium and phosphorus metabolism in hypoparathyroidism.* Metabolism 24:1403, 1975.

234. Parfitt, AM: *Adult hypoparathyroidism. Treatment with calcifediol.* Arch Intern Med 138:874, 1978.

235. Rosen, JF, Fleischman, AR, Finberg, L, et al.: *1,25 Dihydroxycholecalciferol: its use in the long-term management of idiopathic hypoparathyroidism in children.* J Clin Endocrinol Metab 45:457, 1977.

236. Lewin, IG, Paapoulos, SE, and O'Riordan, JLH: *1α-hydroxy vitamin D_3 in the long-term management of hypoparathyroidism and pseudohypoparathyroidism.* Clin Endocrinol 7(suppl.):203s, 1977.

237. Heyburn, PJ, and Peacock, M: *The management of hypoparathyroidism with 1α-hydroxy vitamin D_3.* Clin Endocrinol 7(suppl.):209s, 1977.

238. Porter, RH, Cox, BG, Heaney, D, et al.: *Treatment of hypoparathyroid patients with chlorthalidone.* N Engl J Med 298:577, 1978.

239. Knochel, JP: *The pathophysiology and clinical characteristics of severe hypophosphatemia.* Arch Intern Med 137:203, 1977.

240. Fitzgerald, F: *Clinical hypophosphatemia.* Ann Rev Med 29:177, 1978.

241. Guillou, PJ, Morgan, DB, and Hill, GL: *Hypophosphatemia: a complication of "innocuous dextrose-saline."* Lancet 2:710, 1976.

242. Travis, SF, Sugerman, HJ, Ruberg, RL, et al.: *Alterations of red-cell glycolytic intermediates and oxygen transport as a consequence of hypophosphatemia in patients receiving intravenous hyperalimentation.* N Engl J Med 285:763, 1971.

243. Territo, MC, and Tanaka, KR: *Hypophosphatemia in chronic alcoholism.* Arch Intern Med 134:445, 1974.

244. Craddock, PR, Yawata, Y, Van Santen, L, et al.: *Acquired phagocyte dysfunction. A complication of the hypophosphatemia of parenteral hyperalimentation.* N Engl J Med 290:1403, 1974.

245. Baker, LRI, Ackrill, P, Cattell, WR, et al.: *Iatrogenic osteomalacia and myopathy due to phosphate depletion.* Br Med J 3:150, 1974.

246. Newman, JH, Neff, TA, and Ziporin, P: *Acute respiratory failure associated with hypophosphatemia.* N Engl J Med 296:1101, 1977.

247. O'Connor, LR, Wheeler, WS, and Bethune, JE: *Effect of hypophosphatemia on myocardial performance in man.* N Engl J Med 297:901, 1977.

248. Rude, RK, and Singer, FR: *When dietary phosphate is not enough.* Drug Therapy, August:114, 1976.

249. Lentz, RD, Brown, DM, and Kjellstrand, CM: *Treatment of severe hypophosphatemia.* Ann Intern Med 89:941, 1978.

250. Jackson, CE, and Meier, DW: *Routine serum magnesium analysis. Correlation with clinical state in 5100 patients.* Ann Intern Med 69:743, 1968.

251. Iseri, LT, Freed, J, and Bures, AR: *Magnesium deficiency and cardiac disorders.* Am J Med 58:837, 1975.

252. Bar, RS, Wilson, HE, and Mazzaferri, EL: *Hypomagnesemic hypocalcemia secondary to renal magnesium wasting. A possible consequence of high-dose gentamycin therapy.* Ann Intern Med 82:646, 1975.

253. Singer, FR: *Treatment of Paget's disease of bone.* Postgrad Med 57:117, 1975.

254. Garrick, R, Ireland, AW, and Rosen, S: *Bone abnormalities after gastric surgery. A prospective histologic study.* Ann Intern Med 75:221, 1975.

255. Compston, JE, Horton, LWL, Ayers, AB, et al.: *Osteomalacia after small-intestinal resection.* Lancet 1:9, 1978.

256. Daughaday, WH: *The adenohypophysis,* in Williams, RH (ed.): *Textbook of Endocrinology,* ed. 5. Philadelphia: W.B. Saunders Co., 1974, p. 31.

257. Zervas, NT, and Mendelson, G: *Treatment of acute haemorrhage of pituitary tumors.* Lancet 1:604, 1975.

258. Post, KD, Biller, BJ, Adelman, LS, et al.: *Results of selective transsphenoidal adenomectomy in women with galactorrhea-amenorrhea.* JAMA 242:158, 1979.

259. Goldfine, ID, and Lawrence, AM: *Hypopituitarism in acromegaly.* Arch Intern Med 130:720, 1972.

260. McGuffin, WL, Sherman, BM, Roth, J, et al.: *Acromegaly and cardiovascular disorders. A prospective study.* Ann Intern Med 81:11, 1974.

261. Martin, JB, Reichlin, S, and Brown, GM: *Clinical Neuroendocrinology.* Contemp Neurol Ser Vol 14, 1977.

262. Singer, I, and Forrest, JN, Jr.: *Drug-induced states of nephrogenic diabetes insipidus.* Kidney Int 10:82, 1976.

263. Moses, AM, and Miller, M: *Drug-induced dilutional hyponatremia.* N Engl J Med 291:1234, 1974.

264. Cobb, WE, Spare, S, and Reichlin, S: *Neurogenic diabetes insipidus: management with dDAVP (1-desamino-8-D-arginine vassopressin).* Ann Intern Med 88:183, 1978.

265. Shucart, WA, and Jackson, I: *Management of diabetes insipidus in neurosurgical patients.* J Neurosurg 44:65, 1976.

266. Miller, M, Dalakos, T, Moses, AM, et al.: *Recognition of partial defects in antidiuretic hormone secretion.* Ann Intern Med 73:721, 1970.

267. Bray, GH: *The Obese Patient.* Philadelphia: W.B. Saunders Co., 1976.

268. Freeman, JB, Meyer, PD, Printen, KJ, et al.: *Analysis of gall bladder bile in morbid obesity.* Am J Surg 129:163, 1975.

269. Danowski, TS, Fisher, ER, Gregorio, RM, et al.: *Correlates of fatty liver in morbid obesity.* Obesity/Bariatric Med. 4:232, 1975.

270. Bray, GA, Dahms, WT, Greenway, FL, et al.: *Evaluation of the obese patient. 2. Clinical findings.* JAMA 235:2008, 1976.

271. Vaughan, RW, Gardolfi, AJ, and Bentley, JB: *Biochemical consideration of morbid obesity.* Life Sci 26:2215, 1980.

272. Rochester, DF, and Euson, Y: *Current concepts in the pathogenesis of the obesity hypoventilation syndrome.* Am J Med 57:402, 1974.

273. Vaughan, RW, and Conahan, TJ, III: *Cardiopulmonary consequences of morbid obesity.* Life Sci 26:2119, 1980.

274. Vaughn, RW, Engelhardt, RC, and Wise, L: *Postoperative hypoxemia in obese patients.* Ann Surg 180:877, 1976.

275. Zwillich, CW, Sutton, FD, and Pierson, DJ: *Decreased hypoxic ventilatory drive in the obesity-hypoventilation syndrome.* Am J Med 59:343, 1975.

276. Miller, A, and Granada, M: *In-hospital mortality in the pickwickian syndrome.* Am J Med 56:144, 1974.

277. Walsh, RE, Michaelson, ED, Harkleroad, LE, et al.: *Upper airway obstruction in obese patients with sleep disturbance and somnolence.* Ann Intern Med 76:185, 1972.

278. Kryger, M, Quesney, LF, Holder, D, et al.: *The sleep deprivation syndrome of the obese patient. A problem of periodic nocturnal upper airway obstruction.* Am J Med 56:530, 1974.

279. Engleman, K, Horwitz, D, Jéquier, E, et al.: *Biochemical and pharmacologic effects of α-methyltyrosine in man.* J Clin Invest 47:577, 1968.

Chapter 6

GASTROENTEROLOGY

Daniel S. Matloff, M.D., and
Marshall M. Kaplan, M.D.

Problems related to dysfunction of the gastrointestinal system and the liver are common in the patient requiring surgery. Some, such as postoperative ileus, are predictable consequences of intra-abdominal surgery and are rarely serious. Others, such as acute upper gastrointestinal bleeding and pancreatitis may be life threatening if not recognized and treated promptly. This chapter discusses the diagnosis and treatment of gastrointestinal and hepatobiliary disorders commonly seen in the perioperative period. It will not attempt to cover long term consequences of abdominal surgery such as the postgastrectomy syndrome.

JAUNDICE AND LIVER DYSFUNCTION

The majority of surgical procedures, whether carried out under general or local anesthesia, affect liver function adversely. Most postoperative changes in liver function are minor and subclinical, resolve spontaneously, and are correlated in a general way with the duration and extent of the operation. Jaundice, that is, the accumulation of bilirubin in tissues, usually implies more serious postoperative impairment of liver function. It has been estimated that approximately 1 percent of all postoperative patients develop clinically significant jaundice (bilirubin greater than 2 mg/dl) if their surgery is performed under general anesthesia.[1] With some operations, such as portal-systemic shunts or prolonged cardiovascular surgery, the incidence of postoperative jaundice is much higher.

Postoperative hepatic dysfunction can be divided into six main groups:

1. Mild, transient disturbances of liver function. These are clinically unimportant and are recognized by minor changes in liver function tests.

2. Jaundice due to pigment overload. This may occur after multiple blood transfusions or as a result of the resorption of large hematomas.
3. Jaundice secondary to hepatic hypoxia. This occurs in seriously ill postoperative patients with hypotension, hypoxia, and heart failure.
4. Jaundice secondary to hepatitis or hepatocellular disease. Hepatitis may be caused by viral infection or adverse reactions to drugs. Occasionally jaundice develops in postoperative patients who have unrecognized liver disease, such as cirrhosis.
5. Jaundice secondary to extrahepatic biliary obstruction.
6. Combinations of the above. These are usually the most serious and difficult to diagnose and treat.

Many different factors may work in concert to contribute to the development of jaundice, particularly in elderly patients with cardiovascular, renal, pulmonary, or hematopoietic functional impairment. Prolonged hypoxia, hypertension, and cardiac failure—all of which may occur during or immediately after major surgical procedures —can initiate multisystem organ failure, including jaundice. A consultant must approach patients who develop postoperative jaundice or liver failure in a practical and orderly way to make an accurate diagnosis. Most cases of postoperative jaundice will subside spontaneously if the underlying disorders can be corrected. Only rarely does the development of postoperative jaundice necessitate invasive testing, repeat surgery, or specific pharmacologic treatment.

Liver Function Tests

Judicious use of liver function tests is needed to elucidate the type, severity, and prognosis of postoperative hepatic dysfunction. A battery of liver function tests should be ordered at one time. If used alone, each test lacks specificity and sensitivity. A comprehensive battery of serum tests should include: serum glutamic-oxaloacetic transaminase (SGOT, also known as AST), serum glutamic-pyruvic transaminase (SGPT, also known as ALT), alkaline phosphatase, bilirubin, albumin, and prothrombin time. A more complete list of tests is given in Table 1. It is rare that all of these need to be ordered. Although most clinicians are familiar with these tests, several points deserve emphasis.

TABLE 1. Useful Liver Function Tests

Serum glutamic-oxaloacetic transaminase (SGOT)
Serum glutamic-pyruvic transaminase (SGPT)
Gamma-glutamyl transpeptidase (GGTP)
Alkaline phosphatase
5′-Nucleotidase
Bilirubin
Prothrombin time
Albumin
Total protein
Hepatitis B surface antigen (HB_SAg)
Hepatitis B surface antibody (HB_SAb)

TRANSAMINASES (AMINOTRANSFERASES)

The transaminases (aminotransferases) are serum enzymes that reflect hepatocyte damage and/or necrosis. Postoperative elevations of transaminase levels of up to two times normal in the absence of other liver function test abnormalities are common and rarely are of concern. Whereas an elevated serum glutamic-oxaloacetic transaminase may originate from the liver or heart and skeletal muscle, an elevated serum glutamic-pyruvic transaminase is usually specific for liver damage. Significant elevations of transaminases above normal are consistent with hepatocellular damage. However, the degree of elevation of the transaminases is rarely of prognostic value.

GAMMA-GLUTAMYL TRANSPEPTIDASE

Gamma-glutamyl transpeptidase (GGTP) is an enzyme that is elevated in a wide variety of hepatobiliary diseases. Marked elevations are seen most often in cholestatic disorders, both intrahepatic and extrahepatic. The GGTP may be used to confirm hepatic origin of an elevated alkaline phosphatase since it is not increased in other disorders such as those involving bone. Other methods for documenting the origin of an elevated alkaline phosphatase are given below. GGTP may also be used as a marker for alcoholic liver disease.[2]

ALKALINE PHOSPHATASE

Although alkaline phosphatase has many sources in the body, most serum elevations occur in patients with liver or bone disorders. If the cause of an elevated serum alkaline phosphatase is unclear, it may be fractionated accurately by electrophoresis. If this test is not available, there are alternative methods. The 5′-nucleotidase level parallels the alkaline phosphatase elevation in 85 percent of patients with hepatobiliary disease and is rarely elevated in bone disorders. The GGTP determination is equally reliable.

An occurrence that may cause undue concern in the postoperative period is the finding of an isolated elevated alkaline phosphatase in a patient without obvious liver disease. The alkaline phosphatase may be up to three times normal with further tests indicating that it is of liver origin. Before subjecting a patient to extensive and expensive testing, consider the entire setting. An alkaline phosphatase elevation in this range may be a consequence of the operation alone and may be nonspecific and clinically unimportant.[3] Pursue the work-up only if the clinical setting suggests potentially serious hepatobiliary disease.

PROTHROMBIN AND ALBUMIN

The prothrombin time and serum albumin concentration test the biosynthetic capacity of the liver. Vitamin K resistant hypoprothrombinemia implies a serious diminution of functioning liver mass. However, before one assumes that serious liver disease is present, a patient should always be given parenteral vitamin K; an adequate dose is 5 to 10 mg.

If the prothrombin time returns to normal within 24 hours, the prolongation was due to vitamin K deficiency rather than to intrinsic liver disease. If the prothrombin time remains abnormal, hematologic consultation should be obtained prior to any surgical procedure. A low serum albumin is not as specific for liver disease. It may occur as a consequence of poor nutrition, chronic disease with associated diminished albumin synthesis, and urinary and gastrointestinal loss.

BILIRUBIN

The presence of clinically detectable jaundice indicates a serum bilirubin of at least 2 mg/dl. If the serum bilirubin concentration is elevated, it is helpful to fractionate bilirubin into unconjugated (indirect) and conjugated (direct) forms to separate prehepatic causes of jaundice, such as hemolysis or hematoma resorption, from hepatocellular or extrahepatic etiologies. With prehepatic causes of jaundice, the unconjugated (indirect) bilirubin fraction is elevated and the direct fraction is normal. This is also true in Gilbert's syndrome, a benign condition in which the indirect bilirubin is slightly increased.

Tests for Viral Hepatitis

Sensitive serological tests have been developed over the past decade that have greatly increased our ability to accurately diagnose viral hepatitis. Hepatitis A (short incubation) is caused by a RNA virus. It is now possible to detect hepatitis A antibody in the serum with sensitive immunologic techniques.[4] Surveys have shown that about 25 to 30 percent of healthy adults in the United States are anti-HA positive; that is, they have recovered from hepatitis A and are now immune to it. Hepatitis A is not a common postoperative problem, and there is no known chronic carrier state for the hepatitis A virus.

The presence of hepatitis B surface antigen (HB_sAg, formerly called Australia antigen and HAA) can be determined readily by radioimmunoassay. This test is an excellent screen for hepatitis B (formerly called serum hepatitis). Hepatitis B is caused by a DNA virus. The presence of antibody to surface antigen (anti-HB_s) can also be measured and is indicative of previous exposure to hepatitis B virus; its presence implies immunity to this disease. Because of our ability to screen blood donors for the presence of markers of the hepatitis B virus, hepatitis B is now a rare cause of post-transfusion hepatitis. In fact, the availability of accurate and sensitive tests for hepatitis A and B have allowed us to document a new type of post-transfusion hepatitis called, for lack of a better term, non-A, non-B hepatitis. This is now the most common cause of post-transfusion hepatitis. Several different viruses, in fact, may prove to be responsible for this entity. To date, there are no serologic tests available to diagnose non-A, non-B hepatitis. There are asymptomatic chronic carriers of the non-A, non-B hepatitis virus. The same is true for hepatitis B.

Preoperative Considerations

It is helpful to obtain a complete set of liver function tests in patients scheduled for major surgery. Suggested tests include the transaminases, alkaline phosphatase, bilirubin, albumin, and prothrombin time. Less crucial, but often helpful, is screening for HB_sAg. With these tests, it is possible to identify patients with unsuspected liver diseases such as early or anicteric viral hepatitis, alcoholic liver disease, or postnecrotic cirrhosis. In addition, it is useful to have baseline values in case the postoperative course is not smooth and liver function tests are abnormal.

Surgery in the Patient with Pre-Existing Liver Disease

One important consideration in the preoperative evaluation of a patient is the risk of general anesthesia with pre-existing liver disease. Unfortunately, there are little hard data on this subject. The older literature suggests that there is between a 14 and 21 percent combined morbidity and mortality rate in patients with viral hepatitis who undergo surgery.[5] Complications include infection, pulmonary embolus, and hepatic encephalopathy. Patients with drug hepatitis, on the other hand, appear not to have an increased incidence of serious complications from surgery.[5] Most of these data are from patients operated upon because of unexplained jaundice during the 1950s and early 1960s. Many of these patients had very severe viral hepatitis that was not at that time recognized preoperatively because tests such as serum transaminases were not widely available. With the liver function tests available today plus other more definitive procedures such as percutaneous needle biopsy of the liver, it should be possible to distinguish between acute viral hepatitis and cholestatic disorders. Despite the absence of hard data, most experts recommend that patients with acute viral hepatitis not undergo elective surgery until liver function tests have returned to normal. The findings of nonspecific portal tract inflammation (triaditis) on liver biopsy in asymptomatic patients with minimal liver function test abnormalities is no reason to delay urgent surgery. If there is an acute surgical emergency, surgery should, of course, be performed even if a patient has acute viral hepatitis. These patients will require vigilant postoperative follow-up and appropriate precautions concerning handling of used needles and stool to prevent infecting the hospital staff. With modern anesthesia, most of these patients will tolerate surgery well.

With any acute or chronic hepatitis, regardless of etiology, there is a risk of exacerbation of the disease from the surgical insult with possible development of liver failure. There are no data on the frequency of this complication. In general, the worse the liver disease, the higher the risk. Certain liver diseases, such as alcoholic hepatitis, carry a particularly high risk for postoperative hepatic decompensation. Patients with the clinical picture of acute alcoholic hepatitis should be treated with rest and nutritional therapy in the hospital until fever resolves and bilirubin and white blood cell count fall toward normal. These patients often require six weeks or more of hospitalization and abstinence from alcohol before elective surgery should be considered. In addition, percutaneous liver biopsy should be done prior to surgery. If there is still active liver cell necrosis and Mallory's bodies are present, it is best to wait for further improvement and repeat the liver biopsy if there is any question about continued activity of the alcoholic hepatitis.

There is more information about the risks of surgery in patients with cirrhosis. In general, patients with well-compensated inactive cirrhosis tolerate anesthesia well and there are few complications. Lindenmuth and Eisenberg showed that the complication rate of surgery varied directly with the degree of impairment of liver function in males with active alcoholic cirrhosis.[6] They stressed the importance of deferring elective surgery in patients with active alcoholic liver disease until nutritional deficiencies were corrected and abstinence from alcohol had led to an improvement in and stabilization of liver function tests. Similarly, surgery should be delayed, if possible, in patients with apparently compensated cirrhosis whose liver function tests deteriorate markedly in response to an acute episode such as an upper gastrointestinal hemorrhage.

Child's criteria (Table 2) correlate well with survival in patients with cirrhosis who undergo portal-systemic shunts and can be used as a rough guide to predict response to other types of surgery.[7,8] Regardless of the cause of cirrhosis, patients with decompensated cirrhosis, Child's class B and C, do poorly after surgery and may develop liver failure (see below). Patients in Child's class A tolerate surgery relatively well. However, any patient with cirrhosis or chronic active liver disease has an increased risk of developing postoperative hepatic decompensation. Accordingly, the indications for elective surgery in these patients should be stringently met. For minor procedures, local anesthesia should be used whenever possible. Patients being treated with corticosteroids for chronic active hepatitis should have their dosages increased during the intraoperative and postoperative period. If azathioprine is being used, it should be continued during this time. (See Chapter 5, Endocrinology.)

Liver Disease and Anesthetic Agents

All general and spinal anesthetic agents lower splanchnic blood flow. In normal patients this effect is not harmful. However, in patients whose liver function is already compromised, further damage may occur, particularly if hypotension or hypoxia are present. Cyclopropane and ether, both now largely abandoned in favor of newer compounds, have not been demonstrated to be hepatotoxic despite marked effects on splanchnic circulation.[9] Halothane and enflurane affect liver blood flow least yet have been implicated as occasional hepatotoxins. Despite these theoretical considerations, the type of anesthetic agent appears to have a minor impact on the outcome of surgery in cirrhotic patients. The most likely determinant of morbidity and mortality, in fact, relates to the patient's pre-existing liver disease. Zimmerman recently has reviewed the effect of anesthetic agents on the liver.[10] Anesthetic hepatotoxicity will be discussed below.

In patients with compensated, inactive cirrhosis, premedication agents and intravenous induction agents may be given with complete safety. There is no evidence that

Table 2. Clinical and Laboratory Classification of Cirrhosis According to Functional Reserve*

	Class A	*Class B*	*Class C*
Serum bilirubin	< 2	2–3	> 3
Serum albumin	> 3.5	3.0–3.5	< 3.0
Ascites	None	Easily controlled	Poorly controlled
Neurologic disorder	None	Minimal	Advanced
Nutrition	Excellent	Good	Poor, wasting
Risk of perioperative mortality	Low	Moderate	High

*Modified from Child.[8]

nitrous oxide or intravenous barbiturates cause hepatic injury. In decompensated cirrhosis, however, any sedative or narcotic may precipitate or aggravate hepatic encephalopathy.

Postoperative Jaundice

Clinically significant liver disease after surgery is often heralded by the development of jaundice. Three distinct pathophysiologic mechanisms may cause jaundice in the postoperative patient: (1) increased pigment load to the liver, (2) impaired hepatocellular function, and (3) extrahepatic obstruction (Table 3). Impaired hepatocellular function is clearly the most common cause. However, many different factors may work together to contribute to the development of jaundice. For example, in the elderly patient with pre-existing cardiovascular disease, intraoperative or postoperative hypotension, hypoxia, or cardiac failure may initiate multisystem organ failure with accompanying jaundice. In order to diagnose the cause of jaundice in the postoperative patient, the following factors should be assessed: (1)prior history of alcohol abuse or hepatitis exposure, (2)preoperative liver function, (3)type of anesthesia used and reaction (if any) to previous anesthetics, (4)duration between surgery and onset of liver dysfunction, (5)type and duration of surgery and operative findings, (6)evidence of hypotension or anoxia during or after surgery, (7)number of blood transfusions, (8)postoperative medications, and (9)evidence of hemolysis, heart failure, or sepsis.

INTERVAL BETWEEN SURGERY AND JAUNDICE

The timing between surgery and the development of jaundice is the most critical factor in making an accurate diagnosis (Table 4). For example, jaundice that develops within

TABLE 3. Causes of Postoperative Jaundice

I. Increased pigment load
   - A. Multiple blood transfusions
   - B. Resorption of large hematomas
   - C. Hemolytic anemia

II. Hepatocellular dysfunction
   - A. Hepatitis-like picture
     1. Hypotension, anorexia, heart failure
     2. Anesthetic hepatotoxicity
     3. Viral hepatitis
     4. Drug hepatitis
   - B. Cholestatic picture
     1. Benign postoperative intrahepatic cholestasis
     2. Drug induced cholestasis
     3. Sepsis

III. Postoperative cholecystitis

IV. Postoperative pancreatitis

V. Common bile duct obstruction

VI. Miscellaneous
   - A. Gilbert's syndrome
   - B. Dubin-Johnson syndrome
   - C. Total parenteral nutrition

TABLE 4. Interval between Surgery and Jaundice

Cause	*Timing of Jaundice after Surgery*	*Associated Findings*	*Typical Pattern of Liver Function Tests*
Normal individual			Total bilirubin, up to 1.0 mg/dl. Alkaline phosphatase, normal. SGOT, 10–40 units, normal.
Benign postoperative cholestasis	2–10 days	Hypotension, prolonged surgical procedure, hemorrhage, sepsis, advanced age	Bilirubin variably elevated as high as 50 mg/dl. Alkaline phosphatase strikingly elevated (may suggest obstructive process). Transaminases only slightly elevated, seldom greater than 200 units
Anesthetic hepatitis	7–10 days	Fever, eosinophilia, previous exposure to halogenated anesthetic	Bilirubin variably elevated, as high as 50 mg/dl. Alkaline phosphatase elevated, seldom greater than 3 times normal. Transaminases markedly elevated, ranging from several hundred to several thousand
Viral hepatitis	Late, weeks to months	Malaise, anorexia, HB_sAg*, elevated cytomegalovirus* or Epstein-Barr virus titers*	
Hypotension	Early, usually 1–5 days	Acute tubular necrosis, heart failure, shock, hypoxemia	
Drug hepatitis	Variable	Fever, chills, rash, eosinophilia	Similar to above but transaminases seldom greater than 500 units
Hematoma	Early	Unexplained drop in hematocrit, large ecchymoses, swelling of affected limb	Isolated elevation of bilirubin (1-8 mg/dl)with normal alkaline phosphatase and transaminases
Hemolysis	Variable	Unexplained drop in hematocrit, elevated reticulocyte count	
Postoperative cholecystitis	1–2 weeks	Fever, abdominal pain, right upper quadrant mass, leukocytosis; usually no past history of gallstones	Similar to benign postoperative cholestasis but with less striking elevations of bilirubin and alkaline phosphatase

*Uncommon causes of post-transfusion hepatitis

one to three days of surgery should suggest causes such as prolonged hypotension during or after surgery or brisk hemolysis. The jaundice caused by anesthetic related hepatitis rarely develops before the seventh postoperative day and is usually heralded by the development of fever. Drug-induced hepatitis or cholestasis is often related to the institution of a new therapeutic agent but indeed may be noted weeks to months after starting a new medication. Viral hepatitis from transfused blood, on the other hand, would not be seen for at least several weeks or, more often, several months following surgery. Often serial liver function tests and careful clinical observation are needed before the correct diagnosis can be made.

INCREASED PIGMENT LOAD

A normal liver conjugates and excretes into the bile between 250 and 300 mg of bilirubin daily, mostly from destruction of senescent red blood cells by the reticuloendothelial system. Each 50 ml of blood generates 250 mg of bilirubin. Bilirubin loads six to ten times this amount can be handled by the normal liver without the development of jaundice. Red blood cell transfusions contribute significantly to this bilirubin load. Approximately 10 percent of transfused erythrocytes are hemolyzed within 24 hours of transfusion. Thus, the average 500 ml unit of banked blood leads to the production of 250 mg of bilirubin. With multiple unit transfusions, the functional reserve of the liver for conjugation and excretion of bilirubin can be overwhelmed. This will result in jaundice with the greatest increase in the unconjugated bilirubin fraction. The presence of preexisting liver disease, of course, would greatly lower the hepatic functional reserve.

By a similar mechanism, resorption of large hematomas or extravascular pools of blood may result in jaundice. In these situations, the bilirubin loads may be even higher and be present over longer periods of time. Hypoxemia, hypotension, and sepsis all inhibit bilirubin metabolism and excretion and will increase the serum bilirubin even further in this situation. Both unconjugated and conjugated bilirubin fractions will be elevated. Since conjugated bilirubin may be excreted by the kidney, particularly if its concentration is increased in serum, any renal impairment will aggravate the degree and duration of jaundice. With acute anuric renal failure complicating the picture, the serum bilirubin may reach levels of 60 mg/dl or higher. Fortunately, elevations of the serum bilirubin in this range are not harmful. The treatment of this type of postoperative jaundice is conservative. The liver will take care of itself if the underlying disorders are corrected.

Hemolytic anemia is a rare cause of postoperative jaundice. Patients with chronic hemolytic states, such as sickle cell anemia or thalassemia, may develop more brisk hemolysis after the stress of surgery. Patients with undiagnosed glucose-6-phosphate dehydrogenase (G-6-PD) deficiency may be given medications such as sulfonamides, chloramphenicol, nitrofurantoin, and aspirin, which induce hemolysis. Alternatively, autoimmune mechanisms and Coombs' positivity have been associated with hemolysis induced by other drugs, including penicillin, the cephalosporins, methyldopa, phenacetin, quinidine, and the sulfonylureas. If hemolysis is the cause of the jaundice, the bilirubin will be mostly unconjugated and associated with a falling hematocrit, elevated reticulocyte counts, a very much elevated lactate dehydrogenase, and normal transaminase and alkaline phosphatase levels (see Chapter 8, Infectious Diseases).

IMPAIRED HEPATOCELLULAR FUNCTION

By far the majority of cases of postoperative jaundice reflect direct hepatocyte injury from various etiologies, such as hypotension, hypoxia, anesthesia, drugs, and sepsis.

From a clinical point of view, the syndrome of postoperative jaundice can be manifested as prominent hepatocellular damage, a cholestatic (obstructive) picture, or, most commonly, a combination of the two. For example, with hepatocellular damage, a prototype of which is halothane hepatitis, one sees predominantly elevation of serum transaminase levels with a smaller elevation of the alkaline phosphatase level. The magnitude of the bilirubin elevation may be quite variable and usually reflects the degree of hepatocellular damage. In the cholestatic picture, frequently seen after the administration of certain medications such as phenothiazines, there is a marked elevation of the bilirubin or alkaline phosphatase level with only a modest elevation of transaminase level.

Impaired Hepatic Perfusion and Jaundice

Hypotension and anoxia are two frequently coexisting conditions associated with abnormal liver function in the postoperative period. They probably account for a majority of cases of postoperative jaundice. The liver is exceedingly sensitive to a reduction in perfusion and oxygenation. Patients with this type of hepatic injury may have strikingly elevated transaminase levels with marked elevation of bilirubin. Jaundice typically occurs between 1 and 5 days after surgery and peaks between 7 and 18 days. The liver is remarkably resilient to the changes and will recover completely after transient hypotensive or anoxic episodes.[11] Commonly, however, the insult to the liver is a prolonged one, either initiated or complicated by other conditions—renal failure, myocardial failure, and sepsis—all of which prolong and worsen the jaundice. Although deep jaundice will often alarm the attending physicians, it is rare for this type of liver dysfunction to be a critical, life-threatening problem. The other problems such as heart failure and renal failure are usually more immediately life threatening and will require close attention and treatment.

Congestive Heart Failure

A less catastrophic cause of impaired hepatic perfusion is congestive heart failure. Both right-sided and left-sided heart failure can result in jaundice. In some instances, patients with isolated left-sided failure can present with a picture difficult to distinguish from acute viral hepatitis because of strikingly elevated transaminase levels. A liver biopsy is sometimes needed to recognize this type of liver disease. The biopsy will show marked centrilobular necrosis without evidence of acute or chronic hepatitis.[12]

Anesthesia Related Liver Disease

Anesthesia related hepatotoxicity is an increasingly recognized, albeit rare, problem that occurs in approximately one in ten thousand patients who receive the halogenated anesthetics, halothane and methoxyflurane (Penthrane), for the first time.[13] Hepatotoxicity has recently been reported following enflurane administration but these case reports have been challenged.[13,14] The incidence of this type of liver dysfunction increases after multiple exposures to these agents. The exact pathophysiology of liver damage is not completely understood. In many patients, there appears to be a hypersensitivity phenomenon, while in others there may be a metabolic conversion of the anesthetic to a hepatotoxin.[16,17]

Unexplained postoperative fever, occurring anywhere from 1 to 11 days after surgery (typically the second or third postoperative day) is the most constant clinical feature of this entity. Unfortunately, fever in this period is common and may be due to numerous other causes. The fever is more important if it is accompanied by right upper quadrant pain and malaise, although these are not constant features of anesthetic-induced hepatitis. Serum transaminase levels rise early and often dramatically in halothane hepatitis. Jaundice does not develop until after transaminase levels are elevated, usually 7 to 10 days postoperatively. The alkaline phosphatase level may be variably elevated. Anicteric cases of halothane hepatitis have been observed. Although the leukocyte count is usually normal, both the percentage of eosinophils and the total eosinophil count are usually elevated.

The clinical spectrum of this disease ranges from transient unexplained fever to fulminant hepatic failure and death. Indeed, icteric cases carry up to a 20 percent mortality rate. With massive hepatic necrosis, the finding of a rapidly decreasing liver size is a poor prognostic sign. A liver biopsy usually does not distinguish the lesion of halothane hepatitis from acute viral hepatitis, but is useful in gauging the severity of the disease. However, the rapid onset of fever, transaminase elevation, and jaundice after anesthesia along with the eosinophilia, usually allow one to differentiate between halothane hepatitis and viral hepatitis. The development of hepatic encephalopathy and vitamin K resistant hypoprothrombinemia are poor prognostic signs for survival. Other than general supportive measures, there is no specific treatment for halothane hepatitis. Although there is no convincing evidence that corticosteroids are of benefit, some experts believe they are helpful.[18]

In situations where multiple anesthetic agents are needed, the slightest suspicion of hepatitis after the first use of a halogenated anesthetic should be an absolute contraindication to repeated use of any halogenated agent. The data suggest that once a patient has developed halothane hepatitis, subsequent use of a halogenated anesthetic in this same patient will invariably cause an even more severe, possibly fatal hepatitis. Despite the severity of the initial histologic damage, the lesion often will heal completely with only minimal abnormalities on follow-up biopsy.[19] There is no evidence that patients with underlying liver disease, such as Laennec's cirrhosis, have an increased incidence of adverse reactions to these anesthetic agents.

Most anesthesiologists are likely to see only one case of halothane hepatitis within a lifetime. Halothane and other halogenated anesthetics are safe, acceptable agents. However, they can, in rare instances, be hepatotoxic substances in man with a mechanism of liver damage most likely to be metabolically and immunologically determined.

Viral Hepatitis

Postoperative viral hepatitis is not a common problem in the immediate postoperative period. Transfusions of blood and blood products certainly can transmit viral hepatitis, but generally the incubation period is six weeks to six months following transfusion. In rare cases, the incubation period has been as short as two to three weeks.[20] Several outbreaks of type B hepatitis have been traced to chronic carriers of hepatitis B surface antigen (HB_sAg) among medical and paramedical personnel.[21] Because there are no known chronic carrier states for hepatitis A, it is not a common cause of postoperative hepatitis. With screening of all red blood cell transfusions for HB_sAg by sensitive tests, most cases of post-transfusion hepatitis are felt to be secondary to an as yet unidentified viral agent (or agents), called non-A, non-B. The incubation period, infectivity, and need for gamma globulin prophylaxis are unknown in patients with non-A, non-B hepatitis.

Other relatively uncommon causes of viral hepatitis in postoperative patients are infectious mononucleosis and cytomegalovirus.[22] Both of these typically occur three to eight weeks after an episode of extracorporeal circulation. Tests to measure Epstein-Barr virus, the presumptive cause of mononucleosis, and cytomegalovirus are available. For mononucleosis, the Monospot test and heterophile antibody tests are both convenient and highly accurate.

Drug Hepatitis

Drug-induced hepatic dysfunction, ranging from minimally elevated serum transaminase levels to acute hepatitis, may occur in the postoperative period. Many drugs commonly used in surgical patients including aspirin, diphenylhydantoin, phenothiazines, erythromycin estolate, methyldopa, and quinidine have been implicated in the development of either a hepatitis-like picture, cholestasis, or both (Table 5). Essentially, any drug may cause allergic hepatitis, although the incidence is usually very low.[23]

TABLE 5. Drugs That Have Caused Hepatitis or Liver Damage

Anabolic and Contraceptive Steroids	Anticonvulsants
C-17 Alkylated anabolic steroids	Diphenylhydantoin
Oral contraceptives	Phenobarbital*
Analgesics	Antihypertensive Agents
Aspirin	Methyldopa
Acetaminophen	Anti-inflammatory Agents
Anesthetics	Phenylbutazone
Halothane	Gold*
Methoxyflurane	Indomethacin*
Enflurane*	Probenecid*
Antiarrhythmics	Antimetabolites
Quinidine	Methotrexate
Procainamide*	Azathioprine*
Antibiotics	Antithyroid Agents
Erythromycin estolate	Propylthiouracil
Tetracycline	Methimazole
Rifampin	Psychotropic Agents
Isoniazid	Chlorpromazine
Sulfonamides	Thioridazine
Penicillin and semisynthetic penicillins*	Prochlorperazine*
Nitrofurantoin	
Carbenicillin*	

*Either very rare causes or causal relationship disputed

Frequently, patients with drug hepatitis become ill abruptly, with symptoms and signs of hypersensitivity, such as chills, fever, rash, pruritus, and arthralgias. The eosinophil count is often elevated. With a cholestatic type of drug hepatitis, such as that associated with phenothiazines, the clinical manifestations are often minimal, other than jaundice or itching. The key to diagnosing this complication is a careful review of the patient's medical record with temporal comparison to results of liver function tests. Discontinuation of all potentially implicated drugs is the simple and effective treatment of this complication.

Benign Postoperative Jaundice

The term benign postoperative intrahepatic cholestasis has been used to describe a cholestatic picture that occurs in the postoperative period.[24,25] Typically, lengthy and extensive surgical procedures have been performed with multiple complications, including hemorrhage, hypotension, hypoxia, sepsis, cardiac decompensation, and renal failure. As already discussed, any of these factors individually is reason enough for postoperative jaundice to develop. Marked hyperbilirubinemia, with peak bilirubin levels of 10 to 40 mg/dl, have been noted between 2 and 10 days after surgery with this syndrome. The alkaline phosphatase level is usually elevated and found to be of hepatic origin. Transaminase levels, however, are rarely in the range of acute hepatitis and are seldom more than five times normal.

The diagnosis can often be made from the clinical picture alone. If the diagnosis is in doubt, a liver biopsy is helpful. It will reveal only cholestatic changes, with few or no signs of liver cell necrosis and inflammation. This type of jaundice clears completely if other medical problems can be corrected or avoided. Often, however, multiorgan failure is present in these acutely ill patients and their prognosis is grave. One must be careful to distinguish postoperative cholestasis from extrahepatic biliary obstruction. In an occasional patient with known cholelithiasis or with an unusually complicated course, the possibility of extrahepatic obstruction may require further diagnostic tests. Both thin needle transhepatic cholangiography and endoscopic retrograde cholangiography are feasible in these acutely ill patients and should be used before undertaking surgery. In benign postoperative intrahepatic cholestasis, both of these tests will demonstrate normal-sized bile ducts with free flow of contrast material into the duodenum.

EXTRAHEPATIC OBSTRUCTION

The common bile duct may be damaged by extensive trauma, such as occurs in automobile accidents, or in complicated biliary tract surgery. Causes of postoperative bile duct obstruction include complete transection from trauma, accidental ligature, and transient edema from manipulation, injury, or surrounding inflammatory processes. Following gallbladder and common duct explorations, occasional patients develop obstructive jaundice because of retained common duct stones that escaped detection during initial ductal exploration.[26] The advent of ultrasonography, thin needle transhepatic cholangiography, and endoscopic retrograde cholangiography has simplified the diagnosis in these patients. The increasing use of T-tube basket extraction of stones and endoscopic papillotomy has decreased the frequency of repeat operations in patients with retained common duct stones.[27]

Postoperative Acute Cholecystitis

Acute cholecystitis is an uncommon but increasingly recognized postoperative problem that may present with jaundice.[28,29] Most patients with this complication, up to 80 percent, have no previous history of biliary disease. Typically, these patients present within two weeks of major surgery with unexplained fever associated with either right upper quadrant or epigastric pain. In about one-half of cases, a palpable mass, the boggy, edematous, inflamed gallbladder, is noted in the right upper quadrant. The leukocyte count is usually markedly elevated with a left shift. Unlike anesthetic-induced liver disease, an entity which may present clinically in a similar fashion, liver function tests show only slight elevations of bilirubin and alkaline phosphatase levels, with the transaminases being normal or minimally elevated.

Gallbladder echography may be useful, but often the diagnosis can be made only at laparotomy. This is one of the few causes of postoperative jaundice where early surgical intervention is needed if the diagnosis appears likely. The mortality of this entity, even with surgery, is between 20 and 47 percent and is almost always secondary to infection, cholangitis, or multiple hepatic abscesses. Indeed, many patients develop gangrene or perforation of the gallbladder. Since only 50 percent of these patients are shown to harbor gallstones, other theories, such as inspissated bile or decreased gallbladder blood flow have been implicated to explain the cholecystitis. Unaccountably, in the two large series of such patients reported upon, there was a high percentage of antecedent orthopedic operations, 45 percent in one series and 30 percent in another.

Postoperative Pancreatitis

Another uncommon etiology for postoperative jaundice is the development of acute pancreatitis following abdominal surgery and, even rarer, following surgery of areas remote from the pancreas. Approximately 30 percent of patients with postoperative pancreatitis develop jaundice due to blockage of the bile duct as it courses through the head of the pancreas.[30] Midepigastric pain, often radiating to the back, associated with nausea and vomiting, are common symptoms.

The laboratory diagnosis of this problem still rests in elevated levels of amylase and lipase in the serum. Both tests should be obtained since amylase may be elevated from many nonpancreatic problems and is relatively short-lived in the serum. Warshaw has suggested that the amylase to creatinine clearance ratio, C_{amy}/C_{cr} is a sensitive and specific test for acute pancreatitis.[31] However, elevated ratios may occur in patients with burns, diabetic acidosis, renal failure, and after cardiac surgery.[32,33] In addition, the normal limits of the C_{amy}/C_{cr} ratio must be determined in each individual laboratory because the values depend upon the specific amylase assay used.[34] We have not found the C_{amy}/C_{cr} ratio to be as useful as the serum amylase in our institution in the diagnosis of acute pancreatitis.

Treatment consists of usual measures for acute pancreatitis: nasogastric suction, intravenous fluid administration, and narcotic analgesics. The use of anticholinergic drugs and antibiotics is controversial and is not advised, but cimetidine, the new histamine H_2 blocker, may be beneficial. In patients with known chronic pancreatitis, there is not an increased risk of pancreatic insufficiency or diabetes mellitus following general surgery.

Inherited Disorders of Bilirubin Metabolism

Three unusual causes of jaundice, Gilbert's syndrome, Rotor's syndrome, and the Dubin-Johnson syndrome are occasionally diagnosed after a surgical procedure, often minor in nature. Gilbert's syndrome is a benign inherited condition in which patients have a slightly elevated unconjugated bilirubin level, seldom greater than 3.0 mg/dl.[35] The direct bilirubin is normal, as are all other liver function tests. Liver biopsy shows normal histology. There is a diminished capacity of the liver to clear bilirubin from the blood, with a reduced amount of the hepatic conjugation enzyme, glucuronyl transferase. Hemolysis can give a similar picture but can be readily diagnosed in most cases.

The Dubin-Johnson and Rotor's syndromes, characterized by elevation of unconjugated and conjugated bilirubin, are caused by defects in the hepatic excretion of organic anions into the bile.[36] The characteristic liver biopsy finding in Dubin-Johnson syndrome is the presence of a melanin-like pigment. It is absent in Rotor's syndrome. Oral cholecystography fails to visualize the gallbladder in Dubin-Johnson syndrome. The important point to remember in both of these syndromes is that fasting, physical strain, and mild infections often cause the bilirubin level to increase further and become clinically evident. The bilirubin level returns to its original slightly elevated level with resumption of feeding or control of infection. These syndromes require no treatment.

Total Parenteral Nutrition and Liver Dysfunction

The addition of total parenteral nutrition (TPN) to the preoperative and postoperative management of malnourished, acutely ill surgical patients has evolved dramatically over the past five years. Hepatomegaly, due to fatty infiltration, with nonspecific periportal inflammation and minor elevation of transaminases, are frequently seen in patients on TPN.[37] Whether the high glucose load, general malnourished state, or other medications cause these findings is difficult to ascertain. Pediatric patients, particularly premature infants, have been described who develop a syndrome of intrahepatic cholestasis that has been completely reversible with cessation of total parenteral nutrition.[38] Jaundice has been reported rarely in adults as a complication of total parenteral nutrition. This difference is presumably a reflection of more mature excretory function in mature livers. The addition of intravenous fat emulsions in most patients receiving total parenteral nutrition has made mild hepatic dysfunction even rarer than previously noted, possibly secondary to correction of essential fatty acid deficiency. The development of severe hepatic dysfunction or jaundice in a patient receiving TPN should prompt an extensive search for etiologies other than the nutrition itself.

Hepatic Encephalopathy

Postoperative hepatic encephalopathy, recognized by disturbances of mental function, neurologic abnormalities, and characteristic laboratory findings, is seen most often in patients with chronic parenchymal liver disease associated with portal-systemic shunting. Specific precipitating events are often responsible for the development of encephalopathy (Table 6). Hepatic encephalopathy may also occur in acute hepatic failure, a rare complication of viral hepatitis and halothane hepatitis.

The precise pathogenetic mechanisms for hepatic encephalopathy remain to be elucidated. A multifactorial etiology is likely. Various toxins, such as ammonia, mercaptans, and fatty acids, along with altered amino acid profiles, have been proposed to explain the deranged neurosynaptic transmission, altered neuronal membrane function, and impaired brain energy metabolism seen in these patients.[39]

The accepted form of treatment of hepatic encephalopathy is based on three goals: (1) recognition and treatment of precipitating events, (2) reduction of exogenous and endogenous nitrogenous compounds by dietary protein restriction, bowel cleansing, and use of neomycin or lactulose, and (3) administration of adequate calories and vitamins (Table 7). Treatment is frequently successful in exacerbations of chronic liver disease, but in encephalopathy complicating fulminant hepatic failure, where no precipitating event is present, mortality approaches 80 percent.[40] In this subset of patients with encephalopathy, various support systems such as exchange transfusions and extracorporeal liver perfusion have been tried. None of these measures have been shown to improve survival.

The amino acids in TPN solutions do not appear to exacerbate hepatic encephalopathy. Correction of the altered serum amino acid profile by the parenteral administration of an amino acid solution containing a greater than normal concentration of branched-chain aliphatic amino acids and a low concentration of aromatic amino acids has been used experimentally to treat hepatic encephalopathy.[41]

DIGESTIVE TRACT

Unlike the development of postoperative hepatic dysfunction, which often is clinically silent aside from jaundice, postoperative derangements of digestive tract function may be dramatically obvious. In this situation, the physician's role is not only to restore normal physiologic mechanisms, but, equally important, provide symptomatic relief.

TABLE 6. Precipitating Events in Hepatic Encephalopathy

Gastrointestinal bleeding
Drugs: Sedatives, tranquilizers, analgesics, diuretics
Excess dietary protein
Infection
Metabolic alkalosis
Hypokalemia
Azotemia
Constipation

TABLE 7. Treatment of Hepatic Encephalopathy

Accepted Forms of Treatment

1. Identification and Treatment of Precipitating Events
2. Dietary Protein Restriction
   - A. No protein initially
   - B. Increase by 10–20 gm of protein per day every 2–5 days with improvement
   - C. Total dietary protein tolerated often approximately 60 gm/day
3. Bowel Cleansing
   - A. Purgatives, enemas, stool softeners
   - B. Neomycin
     - (1) Oral dose: 2–4 gm/day in divided doses
     - (2) Rectal dose: 1% solution once or twice daily
   - C. Lactulose
     - (1) Oral dose: 50–150 ml/day in divided doses, enough to cause 2–3 soft stools/day
     - (2) Rectal dose: 300 ml in 700 ml of water by enema
     - (3) May have additive effect with neomycin
4. Provision of Adequate Calories
   - A. Carbohydrate source, 1,600–2,000 calories/day
   - B. Multivitamins
   - C. Potassium replacement if necessary

Experimental or Unproven Forms of Treatment

1. Amino Acid Administration: High concentration of branched chain and low concentration of aromatic amino acids
2. Ketoanalogues of Amino Acids
3. L-dopa
4. Bromocriptine
5. Colon Bypass
6. Corticosteroids
7. Biological Support Systems
   - A. Exchange transfusion
   - B. Plasmapheresis
   - C. Cross-circulation
   - D. Extracorporeal liver perfusion
   - E. Total body washout

This section discusses the pathophysiology and management of common postoperative gastrointestinal problems, namely gastrointestinal bleeding, vomiting, diarrhea, constipation, gas, and paralytic ileus.

Gastrointestinal Bleeding

Whether manifested by a slow ooze or a torrential gush, postoperative gastrointestinal bleeding can be a serious postsurgical problem having a mortality rate of 8 to 10 percent.[42] In the face of common postoperative factors such as respiratory failure, renal failure, jaundice, hypotension, peritonitis, and sepsis, both the incidence and mortality of bleeding are increased significantly.[43] The approach to these patients, after initial stabilization of hemodynamic parameters, is an aggressive diagnostic search for the source of bleeding. Only after the site is identified can specific, intelligent treatment be initiated.

Patients with significant gastrointestinal bleeding in the postoperative period may have several different presentations. The clinician must first distinguish between an upper and lower gastrointestinal bleeding. Both hematemesis (vomiting of bright red blood) and coffee-ground vomitus usually imply a site of bleeding above the ligament of Treitz, although more distal small bowel sites have been seen with these symptoms on rare occasions. The absence of either of these signs does not always preclude an upper gastrointestinal source of bleeding. An actively bleeding duodenal ulcer is not always associated with reflux of blood into the stomach. Such factors as marked duodenal bulb edema, pyloric scarring from previous ulcer disease, or simply a competent pyloric sphincter may prevent reflux of blood into the stomach. Melena (dark, guaiac-positive stools) most often indicates bleeding from above the ileocecal valve but occasionally is seen from lesions in the right colon. Hematochezia (bright red rectal bleeding) is less specific. Both lesions distal to the ileocecal valve and massive bleeding from the duodenum or stomach may present in this way.

The more common causes of postoperative gastrointestinal hemorrhage are listed in Table 8. Detailed discussion of each cause is beyond the scope of this chapter and readers are referred to more general gastroenterology texts for further descriptions. Several of the more common causes, however, deserve additional comment. Specific plans of management will be limited to these more common postoperative problems.

TABLE 8. Common Causes of Postoperative Gastrointestinal Bleeding

I. Upper Gastrointestinal Bleeding
- A. Inflammatory causes
  1. Stress erosions and ulcer
  2. Gastritis/duodenitis
  3. Duodenal ulcer
  4. Gastric ulcer
  5. Esophagitis
- B. Mechanical causes
  1. Mallory-Weiss syndrome
  2. Suture line following gastroduodenal surgery
  3. Hematobilia following trauma or procedure
- C. Vascular causes
  1. Esophageal or gastric varices
  2. Aortoduodenal fistula
  3. Mesenteric vascular occlusion
  4. Vascular malformation
- D. Systemic causes
  1. Uremia
  2. Blood dyscrasias
- E. Neoplasms
  1. Carcinoma
  2. Polyps

II. Lower Gastrointestinal Bleeding
- A. Inflammatory causes
  1. Diverticulitis
  2. Inflammatory bowel disease
  3. Enterocolitis: radiation, toxic, bacterial
- B. Mechanical causes
  1. Diverticulosis
- C. Vascular causes
  1. Ischemic bowel disease
  2. Aortointestinal fistula
  3. Aortic aneurysm
  4. Hemorrhoids
  5. Vascular malformations (angiodysplasia)
- D. Systemic causes
  1. Uremia
  2. Blood dyscrasias
- E. Neoplasms
  1. Carcinoma
  2. Polyps
- F. Anomalies
  1. Meckel's diverticulum

ACUTE STRESS EROSIONS AND ULCERS

Acute stress erosions of the stomach and duodenum, unrelated to previous peptic ulcer disease, are common in acutely ill, traumatized, and postoperative patients. Endoscopic studies have demonstrated a 90 to 100 percent incidence of stress erosions in such patients.[44] The vast majority of these cases, of course, are clinically silent. Pathologically, superficial mucosal necrosis (erosion) is seen within 24 hours of the insult. By 48 hours, these same areas may show extension into the muscularis mucosa (ulceration). Various stages of the same disease, ranging from patchy areas of mild gastritis to multiple deep ulcerations, may be seen simultaneously in any individual patient. These lesions typically develop in the more proximal portions of the stomach (fundus and body) and, occasionally, spread distally to involve the antrum. Isolated antral disease is distinctly unusual.

The overall incidence of stress erosion and ulceration in the postoperative period is unknown. However, several risk factors for bleeding from these lesions have been identified. These risk factors, all common in surgical patients, are: (1) respiratory failure, (2) sepsis, (3) peritonitis, (4) burns, (5) trauma, (6) hypotension, (7) renal failure, (8) jaundice, and (9) surgery itself. Hastings and associates recently demonstrated that the risk of bleeding correlated directly with the number of such factors.[45] With one factor, the incidence of bleeding is 9 percent, with two factors the incidence is 20 percent, and with three or more factors, the incidence of bleeding is 40 percent. The loss of blood from this syndrome, usually painless, may range from guaiac-positive stools to brisk hematemesis. Even with aggressive medical and surgical management, the development of massive bleeding is associated with a 30 percent mortality.[46]

The mechanisms that lead to this pathologic spectrum of lesions and occasional bleeding are poorly understood. Considerable experimental data suggest that some intraluminal acid is needed for acute stress erosions and ulcerations to develop.[47] In experimental animals, the complete buffering of acid prevents such lesions from developing. Other factors thought to play a role in the pathogenesis include: (1) altered mucosal microcirculation, (2) acute energy deprivation of mucosal cells, and (3) mucosal injury from refluxed duodenal fluid containing bile acids and lysolecithin.

With the above discussion in mind, an approach to both prophylaxis and treatment of this syndrome can be formulated. Since acid is a sine qua non in the pathogenesis of these lesions and since high risk patients clearly have been identified, prevention of acute gastrointestinal bleeding might be expected with neutralization of gastric acid. Hastings and coworkers demonstrated in a randomized, controlled trial the effectiveness of liquid antacid in significantly reducing the occurrence of acute gastrointestinal hemorrhage in critically-ill patients.[45] Between 30 and 60 ml of antacid was instilled by nasogastric tube hourly to maintain the gastric pH above 3.5 when it was tested 60 minutes later. Whereas 24.5 percent of nontreated patients bled, only 3.9 percent of antacid-treated patients had gastrointestinal hemorrhage. Both groups were comparable in age, sex, and number of risk factors. A similar study of antacid prophylaxis in patients with major burns of the skin reached the same conclusion.[48] Controlled trials using the H_2 receptor antagonist cimetidine, both alone and in combination with antacids, currently are being conducted.

Cimetidine has been shown more effective in preventing acute gastrointestinal bleeding in patients with hepatic failure compared to low dose antacids.[49] However, hourly administration of antacid is more effective than cimetidine in preventing stress ulceration in intensive care unit patients.[76]

In summary, acute stress erosion and ulceration, leading to gastrointestinal bleeding, is a common problem in a well-defined subset of postoperative patients. In these patients we strongly recommend prophylactic gastric acid neutralization with either hourly antacids, or a combination of antacid plus cimetidine. If cimetidine is used, the amount of antacid can be reduced. The goal of treatment should be to prevent bleeding by keeping the gastric pH above 3.5 and, preferably, closer to 7. In those patients who need nasogastric tubes for other purposes, the tube serves as a convenient device to sample gastric acidity. We do not recommend, however, prolonged nasogastric intubation simply to check the pH.

Reactivation of Chronic Peptic Ulcer Disease

Hemorrhage is a frequent complication of peptic ulcer disease, occurring in 15 to 20 percent of patients some time after diagnosis of their ulcer.[50] The incidence of rebleeding from either duodenal or gastric ulcer is between 30 and 50 percent, indicating that one bleeding episode increases the likelihood of a second. Although well-controlled, endoscopically verified studies are lacking, clinical experience suggests that the incidence of both initial bleeding and rebleeding increases significantly following nonulcer surgery of any type. The exact precipitating factors are unknown, although hypotension, stress, anxiety, and drugs all have been implicated. The vast majority of patients with bleeding peptic ulcers stop bleeding with medical management (see below). However, emergency surgery due to refractory bleeding carries a 7 to 28 percent mortality rate.[51] We recommend that patients with previously documented peptic ulcer disease, with or without a previous history of bleeding, be placed on prophylactic acid neutralization. In these patients, an adequate program would include either cimetidine or liquid antacids (see below).

INITIAL MANAGEMENT

Depending upon the rapidity of bleeding, the initial step in treatment is restoration of fluid volume by appropriate replacement with blood and plasma expanders. Normal saline is useful until blood is available. Particular care must be taken to prevent overexpansion of intravascular volume, particularly in elderly patients with underlying heart disease. With brisk bleeding, central venous pressure, urinary output, and the electrocardiogram need initial measurement and careful monitoring.

A nasogastric tube should be passed both to facilitate diagnosis and begin specific treatment, even if the patient has hematochezia. Gastric contents are aspirated and, if found to contain blood, an upper gastrointestinal source of bleeding may be definitely diagnosed. It must be stressed that a negative nasogastric aspirate does not rule out upper gastrointestinal tract bleeding. Lavage of bloody gastric contents is performed for two purposes. First, clinical experience shows that removal of bloody stomach contents increases the likelihood of spontaneous cessation of bleeding. In addition, upper gastrointestinal endoscopy, the next step in evaluation of most such patients, is most satisfactorily performed in a clean, blood-free stomach. Due to the presence of large clots, appropriate lavage in most cases of brisk bleeding requires a large orogastric tube. Lavage is recommended with either normal saline or tap water.

ENDOSCOPY

Upper Gastrointestinal Endsocopy

The advent and rapid technical refinement of fiberoptic panendoscopy in the past 15 years has revolutionized the diagnosis of bleeding lesions, improving both the rapidity and accuracy of diagnosis. We suggest that endoscopy be used as the initial diagnostic step in most cases when an upper gastrointestinal source of bleeding is suspected or questioned.

Endoscopy may be performed safely and quickly with minimal sedation (often diazepam) in the vast majority of acutely ill postoperative patients. The esophagus, stomach, duodenal bulb, and most of the descending duodenum can be easily visualized in most patients. Absolute contraindications include: (1) an uncooperative patient, (2) recent myocardial infarction, (3) severe pulmonary disease in the absence of endotracheal intubation, (4) marked hypotension from blood loss, (5) a probable perforated viscus, and (6) a patient who has just had gastric surgery. In the last instance, there is danger of disrupting the suture line and perforating the stomach. The patient who has just undergone abdominal surgery should be approached cautiously for the same reason. He should be adequately sedated to prevent retching and sudden increases in intra-abdominal pressure. With brisk hemorrhage, unaltered by gastric lavage, endoscopic visualization may prove to be impossible or, at best, inadequate for diagnostic purposes due to obscuration of lesions by large clots and pools of blood. However, in bleeders who have ceased bleeding or who are bleeding slowly, upper gastrointestinal panendoscopy will locate the bleeding site in 70 to 90 percent of cases, depending on the expertise of the individual endoscopist.[52] Therapeutic endoscopy, using techniques such as electrosurgical coagulation and laser photocoagulation to stop bleeding, is still in the experimental stage.

Several points about the timing of endoscopy in relation to the onset of bleeding need to be emphasized. In general, a patient should be studied as soon after the initial bleeding episode as possible. However, it is imperative to stabilize the patient's blood pressure with intravenous fluids and transfuse with blood as necessary to return the hematocrit towards baseline value. An electrocardiogram needs to be obtained in every acutely ill patient to exclude any coexistent myocardial ischemia. Unless gastric lavage through a large-bore orogastric tube becomes clear of blood or pink tinge, endoscopy will be technically difficult, if not impossible. This maneuver should be started early in the management of a brisk bleeder and not as an afterthought when the endoscopist arrives on the scene. With less active bleeders, a large nasogastric tube may suffice for adequate cleansing lavage. Finally, if endoscopy is contemplated within a six hour period, food and particularly antacids should be withheld to insure a better view of the mucosa.

The causes of upper gastrointestinal bleeding determined by endoscopy in any particular series will vary widely according to patient population. In postoperative patients, stress erosions and ulcerations, along with peptic ulcer disease, prove to be the most common cause of upper gastrointestinal hemorrhage. A common postoperative bleeding site, usually after gastroduodenal surgery, is the suture line. Other lesions of increased incidence include Mallory-Weiss tears, drug-induced gastritis, and esophagitis (frequently associated with nasogastric intubation). Gastroesophageal varices may bleed in cirrhotic patients after surgery. The role of gastroesophageal reflux and coexistent esophagitis in the pathogenesis of variceal hemorrhage is controversial.[53]

Colonoscopy

Although proctosigmoidoscopy should be done, colonoscopy usually has no role in the evaluation of acute lower gastrointestinal bleeding. Large amounts of blood and clots prevent adequate mucosal visualization. With intermittent rectal bleeding, however, colonoscopy is valuable. A recent study demonstrated that routine proctosigmoidoscopy and single contrast barium enema studies miss a large percentage of bleeding lesions.[54] Colonoscopy yielded an additional diagnosis in 32.9 percent of patients with intermittent rectal bleeding and only diverticula seen on barium enema and in 20 percent of anemic patients with occult blood in the stool and negative barium studies, proctosigmoidoscopies, and upper gastrointestinal endoscopy results.

BARIUM STUDIES

The use of barium contrast studies, either upper gastrointestinal series or barium enema, should be discouraged in acutely ill patients with massive bleeding for several reasons. First, in upper gastrointestinal bleeding, patients may bleed extensively from superficial lesions (tears and erosions) which are undetectable by most x-ray techniques. Second, the mere demonstration of a lesion by barium techniques does not mean that the lesion is the bleeding site. Indeed, in 20 to 50 percent of bleeding patients with known demonstrable esophageal varices, another lesion is the source of hemorrhage.[55] Third, with massive bleeding, angiography is often the only way to make a diagnosis (see below). Filling the gastrointestinal tract with barium prevents adequate blood vessel demonstration for many hours at least and may delay diagnosis and definitive treatment. The use of water soluble contrast agents, such as Gastrografin, to avoid this problem is of no benefit. In addition, the water soluble contrast agents are very hypertonic and may aggravate an already compromised vascular volume by causing massive outpouring of fluid into the gut.

With lower gastrointestinal bleeding, if the bleeding is not acute, barium enema may be of some use. Lesions such as polyps, colonic neoplasms, diverticular disease, ischemic colitis, and inflammatory bowel disease may be visualized, particularly if air contrast technique is used. Of course, a thorough rectal examination and proctosigmoidoscopy, either with a standard rigid scope or the newer flexible sigmoidoscope, should be the initial evaluation of such patients. If large clots or active bleeding are noted, selective angiography is the most useful diagnostic and potentially therapeutic test.

ANGIOGRAPHY

With active gastrointestinal bleeding, defined as a rate exceeding 0.5 ml per minute, contrast material may be seen to extravasate into the intestinal lumen with angiography.[56] At times, this extravasation can be dramatic and will identify the bleeding site. Additionally, structural lesions, such as arteriovenous malformations, may be noted. These lesions frequently cause intermittent bleeding but any single episode may be acute.

In acute upper gastrointestinal hemorrhage, the celiac axis is catheterized from a femoral approach and injected first, followed by selective injections of the left gastric and gastroduodenal arteries. If no bleeding site is identified, the superior mesenteric artery is injected to inspect the proximal small intestine. In the case of suspected lower gastrointestinal hemorrhage, the superior mesenteric artery is first catheterized, followed by the inferior mesenteric artery. Frequently, with massive hemorrhage, a simple midstream aortogram will demonstrate the bleeding site. Demonstration of bleeding (extravasation) from esophageal varices is seldom seen from the venous phase of a left gastric artery injection, although the varices themselves will usually be visualized.

The value of arteriography rests not only in its diagnostic value for acute bleeding but, increasingly, in therapy. Selective intra-arterial infusion of Pitressin, a potent vasoconstricting agent, has been used with varying degrees of success in upper gastrointestinal hemorrhage.[57] In general, the more superficial lesions, such as gastritis, duodenitis, and Mallory-Weiss tears, respond better to this therapy than do frank ulcerations. Pitressin infusion into the superior mesenteric artery has proven to be an effective treatment for diverticular bleeding in the colon.[58] In addition, for bleeding gastroesophageal varices, superior mesenteric artery infusion has been beneficial, at least temporarily, in many acutely ill patients. However, a recent report suggests that equally good control occurs with intravenous administration of Pitressin.[59] Most commonly, between 0.1 and 0.4 U per minute are infused. If bleeding is controlled, the infusion rate is decreased by 0.1 U per minute at 12 to 24 hour intervals. Complications include the development of angina pectoris in patients with coronary artery disease, intestinal ischemia with pre-existing mesenteric insufficiency, and bowel necrosis in the hyperviscosity syndromes.

In addition to vasoconstrictor treatment, selective embolization of bleeding arterial vessels with various materials, such as Gelfoam and autologous clot, have been employed by some investigators with at least temporary success. For better control of variceal hemorrhage, transhepatic portal vein catheterization and selective embolization of the coronary and short gastric veins has been advocated recently. The long-term efficacy and risk-benefit ratio of such treatment remains to be determined.[60]

Once a definitive diagnosis has been made by any of the above means, appropriate treatment may be initiated and tailored for the individual patient. In the vast majority of patients with either upper or lower gastrointestinal bleeding, medical management will be sufficient. Less commonly, angiographic techniques will be necessary to stop the hemorrhage. Only rarely, with massive bleeding, uncontrollable by less invasive techniques, will surgical intervention be necessary.

ANTACIDS AND CIMETIDINE

In the large group of postoperative patients with gastrointestinal bleeding secondary to inflammatory lesions (stress ulceration, esophagitis, gastritis, duodenitis, and peptic ulcer) or mechanical lesions (Mallory-Weiss syndrome and hiatus hernia), acid neutralization is the cornerstone of treatment. As alluded to above, this goal can be accomplished with either antacids, cimetidine, or both.

Depending upon the severity of bleeding, the appropriate frequency of antacid therapy is variable, ranging from half-hourly (often 30 to 90 ml per dose) to four times per day. Tablet antacids are not recommended in this situation. In patients with brisk bleeding and a nasogastric tube already in place, the pH should be measured periodically and the antacid dose titrated accordingly just prior to the next scheduled dose to keep it above pH 4.0. In patients without nasogastric tubes and with less bleeding, we do not recommend intubation of the stomach simply to check gastric pH. The intubation itself may promote bleeding through the development of gastric erosions or esophagitis.

Not all liquid antacid preparations have equally potent neutralizing capacity. The volume of antacid necessary to provide 140 mEq of neutralizing capacity (a dose shown effective in duodenal ulcer disease when given one and three hours after meals and at bedtime) may range from 16 to 350 ml (Table 9).[61] Since all antacids have some predictable side effects, including diarrhea, constipation, phosphorus depletion, cation absorption, and alkalosis, the lowest effective volume is desirable. In some patients, doses two to four times the usual sufficient dose will be needed for adequate gastric neutralization.

Cimetidine, a histamine H_2-antagonist, is a potent inhibitor of gastric acid secretion. The appropriate initial dose is 300 mg with meals and at bedtime, either orally or by intravenous infusion. When given intravenously, the drug may be given either by slow bolus injection over 1 to 2 minutes or by infusion over 15 to 20 minutes. In some patients it may be necessary to increase the dosage to a maximum of 2400 mg per day. The usefulness of cimetidine in the treatment of gastrointestinal bleeding is being evaluated in several large prospective studies. Little is known about the long-term effects of this agent, but other than mental confusion (particularly in the elderly), the drug appears safe. Since cimetidine is relatively free of side effects and well-tolerated by most patients, we advocate its use initially in most patients with upper gastrointestinal bleeding from inflammatory lesions. When anacidity cannot be achieved with cimetidine alone, concomitant administration of antacid is indicated. Although anticholinergic drugs may contribute to lowering gastric acid secretion, they are not usually recommended in the immediate postoperative period. However, anticholinergics will enhance the acid lowering effect of cimetidine.[62] Their usage should be considered in the individual whose gastric acid secretion, measured by nasogastric aspiration, does not fall adequately in response to cimetidine alone.

TABLE 9. Potency and Characteristics of Selected Liquid Antacids

Antacid	*Components*	*Neutralizing Capacity (mEq/15 ml)**	*Comments*
Mixtures Containing Aluminum Hydroxide and Magnesium Hydroxide			
Mylanta-II	Aluminum and magnesium hydroxides, simethicone	62	Aluminum hydroxide and magnesium hydroxide mixtures may produce diarrhea, phosphorus depletion, hypermagnesemia (in renal insufficiency) and increased fluid retention
Aludrox	Aluminum hydroxide gel, magnesium hydroxide	42	
Maalox	Aluminum and magnesium hydroxide gel	39	
Di-Gel	Aluminum and magnesium hydroxides, simethicone	38	
Mylanta	Aluminum and magnesium hydroxides, simethicone	36	
Wingel	Aluminum and magnesium hydroxides, hexitol stabilized	34	
Single Entity			
Titralac	Calcium carbonate	58	Produces "acid rebound"; milk-alkali syndrome occasionally results
Basaljel	Aluminum carbonate	50	May cause constipation and phosphorus depletion
Milk of magnesia	Magnesium hydroxide	35	Diarrhea limits acceptability
Riopan	Magaldrate	33	Low sodium content
Amphogel	Aluminum hydroxide gel	29	May cause constipation and phosphorus depletion
Phosphaljel	Aluminum phosphate	6	see above
Other Mixtures			
Ducon	Aluminum and magnesium hydroxides, calcium carbonate	105	Calcium-containing (see above)
Camalox	Aluminum and magnesium hydroxides, calcium carbonate	54	Calcium-containing (see above)
Gelusil	Magnesium trisilicate, aluminum hydroxide gel	20	Silicate kidney stones reported

*Milliequivalents of antacid is defined by the mEq of hydrochloric acid required to keep an antacid suspension at pH 3.0 for two hours in vitro.[61]

Vomiting

Nausea and vomiting are frequent problems both during and after surgery. Many specific causes for these problems can be identified. Drugs, such as general anesthetics, opiates, and digitalis, may act centrally on receptors in the medulla (vomiting center) and fourth ventricle floor (chemoreceptor trigger zone) as well as through other less well defined reflex arcs. With gastrointestinal surgery or manipulation, peristaltic coordination is temporarily altered, leading to gastric atony or, more commonly, adynamic ileus. With premature resumption of oral feedings, vomiting frequently occurs. Central nervous system lesions associated with increased intracranial pressure are occasionally associated with projectile vomiting. Prolonged total parenteral nutrition has been associated with a syndrome of food intolerance, manifested by vomiting, when oral feeding is restarted. The mechanism of this is poorly understood. Finally, an intra-abdominal catastrophe, such as intestinal obstruction, peritonitis, pancreatitis, or cholecystitis may be heralded by vomiting.

Besides patient discomfort, complications of postoperative vomiting include: (1) aspiration pneumonia, (2) Mallory-Weiss syndrome with extensive gastrointestinal hemorrhage, (3) esophageal perforation with mediastinitis (Boerhaave's syndrome), (4) electrolyte and acid-base disturbances, and (5) wound dehiscence or delayed healing. Treatment includes removal of any obvious precipitating causes, awareness of potential complications, and antiemetic drugs. The most commonly used antiemetics in these situations are prochlorperazine, chlorpromazine, and haloperidol. Constant aspiration of gastric secretions and air via a nasogastric tube may be necessary if there is prolonged gastric atony. Metoclopramide, an investigational drug, is currently being evaluated in patients with postoperative gastric atony. It stimulates gastric motility in normal individuals.[63] In practice, antiemetics often prove to be more effective in prophylaxis than in treatment.

Diarrhea

Although more quantitative definitions have been proposed, diarrhea may be regarded as a significant increase from baseline stool volume. The postoperative period offers numerous predisposing factors for the development of diarrhea. Most often the diarrhea is self-limited with a readily identifiable cause. Depending upon the type of surgery performed, diarrhea in this setting may occasionally reflect significant pathology and make diagnosis and therapy difficult, for example, in abdominal vascular surgery where intestinal blood flow may be compromised. Diarrhea in the postoperative period is, on rare occasions, massive enough to become life threatening. The common causes of postoperative diarrhea are listed in Table 10. Several of the most common causes of diarrhea will be discussed in detail.

TABLE 10. Causes of Postoperative Diarrhea

1. Drugs: Antibiotics, antacids, digitalis, laxatives (including surreptitious abuse), antihypertensive agents, chemotherapeutic agents
2. Antibiotic-Associated Colitis (Pseudomembranous Colitis)
3. Ischemic Bowel Disease
4. Infection: Viral infection, salmonellosis, shigellosis, infection with *Escherichia coli,* giardiasis, amebiasis
5. Fecal Impaction
6. Excessive Bile Salts in Colon: Choleretic diarrhea
7. Inflammatory Bowel Disease
8. Postvagotomy
9. Blind Loop Syndrome/Bacterial Overgrowth
10. Unmasking of Celiac Sprue
11. Unmasking of Lactase Deficiency
12. Radiation Enteritis
13. Tumors of the Bowel
14. Endocrine Tumors

If severe, difficult to control diarrhea develops postoperatively, several orderly diagnostic studies should be obtained. A proctosigmoidoscopy, without cleansing enemas, should be performed. This test can be done quickly at the bedside even in acutely ill patients. The mucosa can be inspected for ulcerations, pseudomembranes, friability, or tumors. A normal mucosa rules out several of the more serious causes of diarrhea, including antibiotic-associated colitis. In addition, direct fresh stool smears may be taken for microscopic exam and occult blood testing. Finally, if bleeding is present, the site of bleeding may be identified or localized. A stool culture should be obtained to look for shigellosis and salmonellosis; stool for ova and parasites should also be sent to the laboratory. A smear for stool leukocytes should be made. The finding of polymorphonuclear leukocytes suggests either inflammatory bowel disease or invasive infection, such as caused by Shigella or Salmonella. If surreptitious laxative abuse is present, alkalinization of the stool with sodium hydroxide will cause a purple color if a phenolphthalein derivative is being ingested. In most cases, barium enema studies should be reserved until these studies are completed.

There is no simple formula for the management of postoperative diarrhea and each patient should be treated on an individual basis. For instance, if a patient who hourly has been taking magnesium-containing antacids develops diarrhea, the best approach is discontinuation of the antacids and observation. If diarrhea does not subside within 24 hours, the above tests would be indicated. Similarly, the use of antidiarrheal agents such as diphenoxylate with atropine (Lomotil), loperamide, and opiates needs to be individualized. In most cases, they can be used with excellent symptomatic relief. In others, for example, with acute infectious diarrhea or inflammatory bowel disease, there is a risk that they may prolong the diarrhea or produce toxic dilatation of the colon—toxic megacolon.

ANTIBIOTICS

Surgical patients frequently receive antibiotics. Antibiotics are probably the single most common cause of postoperative diarrhea.[64] Fortunately, the vast majority of such patients are troubled only by frequent, loose stools without any significant discomfort, caused by an altered colonic bacterial flora. Discontinuation of the antibiotic or, if necessary, changing to a different antibiotic usually will result in prompt resolution.

A much more serious but less common antibiotic-associated diarrheal state is pseudomembranous colitis.[65] This complication usually occurs in patients without any serious underlying gastrointestinal disease. The diarrhea is almost always accompanied by fever and patients frequently have leukocytosis. Less commonly, hematochezia, abdominal tenderness, and volume depletion are noted. Although lincomycin and clindamycin have been implicated in many cases, virtually any antibiotic may be the cause. Individual cases of pseudomembranous diarrhea due to ampicillin, amoxicillin, penicillin G, cephalosporins, tetracycline, chloramphenicol, and trimethoprim–sulfamethoxazole, have been reported. Sigmoidoscopy is diagnostic and shows numerous yellowish-white plaques or even a contiguous membrane on boggy edematous, erythematous base. The plaques represent the pseudomembranes which can be definitely identified with biopsy.

Recent studies have increased our understanding of the etiology, pathophysiology, and treatment of pseudomembranous colitis (also termed antibiotic-associated colitis).

Using both hamster and human experimental models, several independent investigators have demonstrated high concentrations of *Clostridium difficile* and its cytopathic toxin in stools of patients with this disease.[66,67] In certain individuals, the selective influence of antimicrobial therapy enables this resistant cytotoxigenic strain to proliferate and elaborate toxin. The *C. difficile* strain is sensitive to vancomycin and pseudomembranous colitis responds well to oral vancomycin, 125 mg every 6 hours.[68] In addition, the implicated antibiotic must be discontinued immediately. With relatively mild diarrhea, antidiarrheal agents such as diphenoxylate may be used. In more severe cases, uncontrolled with the above measures, corticosteroids or cholestyramine may be tried. In the past, colectomy or diverting ileostomy has been needed in some desperately ill patients. It is doubtful if surgical intervention will be necessary now that the cause and effective medical treatment has been found.

ISCHEMIC COLITIS

Segmental ischemic disease of the colon, ischemic colitis, often presents with grossly bloody diarrhea associated with varible degrees of nonspecific abdominal pain. Most patients are over age 50 and typically have evidence of atherosclerotic disease. Following certain types of surgery, such as aortoiliac reconstruction or abdominoperineal resection, the incidence of colonic ischemia may approach 2 percent.[69] There is also evidence suggesting an association with oral contraceptive agents.[70]

Particularly susceptible areas of involvement are the so-called "watershed" areas between two adjacent arterial supplies. These are the splenic flexure area (between the superior mesenteric and inferior mesenteric arteries) and the rectosigmoid area (between the inferior mesenteric and internal iliac arteries). However, any area of the colon may be affected. Diagnosis rests on a strong clinical suspicion, negative stool cultures, and typical barium enema findings showing the characteristic picture of intramural hemorrhage and edema. These findings include "thumbprinting" (often seen on plain film), tubular narrowing, ulcerations, and sacculations. With bowel rest, intravenous fluids, and antibiotics, the vast majority of such patients improve spontaneously with complete resolution of symptoms. Follow-up barium enema often shows a residual stricture which, depending on the degree of lumen compromise, may necessitate a future operation for resection. In the rare patient, bowel infarction develops and surgery is required.

FECAL IMPACTION

A paradoxical consequence of a large fecal impaction is uncontrollable passage of liquid stool around the impaction, simulating diarrhea. This problem can occur in patients inactive for long periods of time who continue to eat, such as elderly postoperative patients or orthopedic patients of any age. Abdominal examination often reveals a large mass which may be recognized on plain film. Treatment consists of removal or disruption of the fecal mass, either directly with a gloved finger or employing a sigmoidoscope. Enema treatment with saline or mineral oil may also be necessary for complete disimpaction.

STRUCTURAL GASTROINTESTINAL CHANGES

With ileal resection or disease, bile salt resorption is interrupted. Due to the functional reserve of the liver and the enterohepatic circulation, there is no alteration noted in bowel function with limited ileal removal. However, with more extensive ileal dysfunction, diarrhea may develop by one of several mechanisms. If bile salts pass into the colon, they directly stimulate colonic secretion and, hence, diarrhea. Cholestyramine, a nonabsorbable binding resin, is effective treatment for this type of diarrhea. When ileal malabsorption is even greater (more than 100 cm removed or diseased), steatorrhea develops due to insufficient luminal concentration of bile salts. Again, the colon becomes a secretory organ. In this case, it is due to hydroxy-fatty acids, which are produced by the action of bacteria on malabsorbed dietary triglycerides. A low fat diet or medium chain triglycerides may be necessary to treat this type of diarrhea.

There are several other situations leading to diarrhea due to gastrointestinal structural alteration from surgery. Clinically important diarrhea occurs in approximately 5 percent of patients who undergo vagotomy for ulcer disease. Treatment with cholestyramine, 4 gm three times a day, or aluminum hydroxide gel, 1 oz, one hour following meals, recently have been shown to be useful.[71] Blind loop syndrome, caused by bacterial overgrowth and consequent malabsorption, may be seen in certain situations. These include (1) long blind loops of bowel resulting from various types of abdominal surgery, (2) Crohn's disease with partial bowel obstruction and dilatation proximal to a diseased segment of bowel, and (3) patients with diseased bowel motility such as occurs in scleroderma. Broad spectrum antibiotics, such as tetracycline, are used to reduce or eliminate the bacterial overgrowth. Rarely, both celiac sprue and lactase deficiency may be "unmasked" by gastric surgery and present as intractable, chronic diarrhea weeks or months later. Appropriate basic treatment involves a gluten-free diet and avoidance of lactose containing foods, respectively.

RADIATION ENTERITIS

Radiation injury to the small bowel and colon is an increasingly recognized cause of diarrhea in patients undergoing radiotherapy for lymphoma and carcinoma of pelvic, retroperitoneal, and intra-abdominal structures.[72] Most such patients have had a total of at least 4,000 rads of radiation and often have received simultaneous chemotherapy. Symptoms may develop early, that is, during or immediately after treatment, or late, that is, months to many years after treatment. Diagnosis may be made by finding characteristic sigmoidoscopic and x-ray changes. These lesions may be similar to those found in inflammatory bowel disease, and include ulcerations, fistulas, and, at later stages, stenotic areas. Treatment is difficult and often unsatisfactory. In the acute phase, if the diarrhea is incapacitating, the patient is given nothing by mouth, stool volume is monitored, and electrolytes and water are given parenterally. There is no evidence that corticosteroids help although inhibitors of prostaglandin synthesis, including aspirin, may provide some symptomatic relief. Diphenoxylate, loperamide, and opiates may be given for similar purposes.

Inflammatory Bowel Disease

When patients with inflammatory bowel disease require nonbowel related surgery, there is a risk of flare-up of the underlying disease with the development or exacerbation of diarrhea. This complication is unrelated to the type of inflammatory bowel disease (either ulcerative colitis or Crohn's disease) or the preoperative activity of the disease. The incidence of this complication is unknown. When other causes of diarrhea have been excluded, treatment with corticosteroids is often required. Depending upon the clinical setting, the equivalent of 40 to 80 mg of prednisone is usually necessary initially. With less severe disease, sulfasalazine, 2 to 4 gm per day, may suffice.

Constipation

Constipation is a common problem in bedridden postoperative patients. However, proper management of this problem is seldom difficult. The causes of constipation are myriad and can be broadly categorized into the following groups: (1) drug-induced, (2) metabolic-induced, (3) neurogenic, and (4) structural disorders. Several specific causes are common in the postsurgical period (Table 11). With mild cases of constipation, not associated with either intestinal obstruction or ileus, treatment consists of resumption of normal dietary and physical activity, discontinuation of any medications known to predispose to constipation, and mild laxative administration.

A traditional classification of laxatives consists of five categories: (1) osmotically active agents, (2) mucosal irritants, (3) lubricants, (4) bulk increasing agents, and (5) stool softeners. Recent studies on laxative action have suggested, however, that effective

TABLE 11. Common Causes of Postoperative Constipation

1. *Medications*	3. *Mechanical Obstruction*
Analgesics	Tumors
Anesthetic agents	Strictures
Antacids (aluminum and calcium)	Diverticulitis
Anticholinergics	Ischemic colitis
Anticonvulsants	Radiation colitis
Antidepressants	Fecal impaction
Anti-parkinsonism agents	
Hypotensive agents	4. *Pseudo-Obstruction*
Iron preparations	
Muscle paralyzers	5. *Anal Disorders*
Opiates	Fissures
Psychotropic agents	Perirectal abscesses
	Hemorrhoids
2. *Metabolic Disorders*	
Hypokalemia	6. *Irritable Bowel Syndrome*
Uremia	
Acidosis	
Diabetes	
Hypocalcemia	
Hypomagnesemia	
Infection	

laxatives function by altering intestinal fluid and electrolyte transport, resulting in increased fecal water excretion.[73] Combinations of active ion secretion, altered intestinal motility, increased mucosal permeability, and mucosal damage all contribute to altered fluid and electrolyte movement. A surfeit of laxative preparations are on the market. We recommend bulk agents in most postoperative patients with judicious addition of mineral oil or milk of magnesia if bulk agents alone are not potent enough.

Gas, Postoperative Ileus, Obstruction, and Pseudo-Obstruction

Transabdominal surgery of any type has a profound inhibitory effect on gastrointestinal motility. Its cause is poorly understood. Investigations in experimental animals have demonstrated that even with sham operations (transient clamping of a renal pedicle), normal bowel motility is lost and not restored for at least 72 hours.[74] These observations are compatible with the clinical observation of a three to four day hiatus between simple abdominal surgery (e.g., uncomplicated appendectomy) and return of bowel sounds or, more importantly, the ability of a patient to pass gas per rectum. Nasogastric suction during this period will usually prevent bowel distension and its attendant discomfort. Certainly, a plain abdominal film at this time may show dilated loops of small and large bowel with air fluid levels compatible with obstruction. With more extensive bowel manipulation or resection, resumption of normal function is even further delayed.

Occasionally, these postoperative changes are acutely exaggerated or markedly prolonged, particularly in seriously ill patients having undergone extensive surgery. In this situation, patients may present with symptoms and signs of intestinal obstruction. It is imperative to distinguish between a true mechanical obstruction and a prolonged ileus causing a transient acute pseudo-obstruction. Abdominal plain films are often inconclusive helping to make this distinction. Mechanical obstruction is said to show little or no gas in the distal colon and rectum, whereas both ileus and pseudo-obstruction usually do.

Barium studies are often necessary for proper diagnosis. A careful barium enema should always be done before upper G.I. series. This is done to avoid inspissation of barium in the colon if an obstructing colonic lesion is present. Only after the colon has been thoroughly examined and found not obstructed should a barium meal be given. There is no evidence that a barium concretion can occur in the small bowel. Water soluble contrast agents are not useful in diagnosing small bowel obstruction. They are hyperosmolar, cause a secretion of water into the intestinal lumen, and usually become too dilute to give accurate information by the time most obstructing lesions are encountered. With pseudo-obstruction, no obstruction will be seen.

With few exceptions, the treatment of mechanical obstruction is surgical. Treatment of pseudo-obstruction, occasionally called Ogilvie's syndrome, is not surgical but is directed at treatment of any underlying associated problem such as infection, congestive heart failure, chronic renal failure, chronic pancreatitis, hypokalemia, or hypocalcemia.[75] Symptomatic relief is provided by decompression with gastric or intestinal intubation. In very rare patients, who continue to develop progressive bowel dilatation despite intubation and correction of underlying conditions, a decompressive cecostomy is necessary. When a prolonged ileus prevents enteral feeding, consideration should be given to providing calories parenterally within three to five days following surgery (see Chapter 16, Nutrition).

REFERENCES

1. LaMont, JT, and Isselbacher, KJ: *Current concepts of postoperative hepatic dysfunction.* Conn Med 39:461, 1975.
2. Rosalki, SB, and Rau, D: *Serum gamma-glutamyl transpeptidase activity in alcoholism.* Clin Chim Acta 39:41, 1972.
3. Brensilver, HJ, and Kaplan, MM: *Significance of elevated liver alkaline phosphatase in serum.* Gastroenterology 68:1556, 1975.
4. Purcell, RIT, Wong, DC, Moritsugu, Y, et al.: *A microtiter solid-phase radioimmunoassay for hepatitis A antigen and antibody.* J Immunol 116:349, 1976.
5. Harville, DD, and Summerskill, WHJ: *Surgery in acute hepatitis.* JAMA 184:257, 1963.
6. Lindenmuth, WW, and Eisenberg, MN: *The surgical risk in cirrhosis of the liver.* Arch Surg 86:235, 1963.
7. Kanel, GC, Kaplan, MM, Zawacki, JK, et al.: *Survival in patients with postnecrotic cirrhosis and Laennec's cirrhosis undergoing therapeutic portacaval shunt.* Gastroenterology 73:679, 1977.
8. Child, CG: *The liver and portal hypertension,* In Child, CG (ed.): *Major Problems in Clinical Surgery.* Vol. 1. Philadelphia: WB Saunders Co., 1964, pp. 1–83.
9. Peters, RL, Edmondson, HA, Reynolds, TB, et al.: *Hepatic necrosis associated with halothane anesthesia.* Am J Med 47:748, 1969.
10. Zimmerman, HJ: *Anesthetic agents,* in Zimmerman, HJ: *Hepatotoxicity.* New York: Appleton-Century-Crofts, 1978, pp. 370–394.
11. Nunes, G, Blaisdell, FW, and Margaretten, W: *Mechanism of hepatic dysfunction following shock and trauma.* Arch Surg 100:546, 1970.
12. Cohen, JC, and Kaplan, MM: *Left-sided heart failure presenting as hepatitis.* Gastroenterology 74:583, 1978.
13. Sherlock, S: *Halothane hepatitis.* Gut 12:324, 1971.
14. Van der Reis, L, Askin, SJ, Frecker, GN, et al.: *Hepatic necrosis after enflurane anesthesia.* JAMA 227:76, 1974.
15. Higgins, WL: Correspondence. JAMA 228:158, 1974.
16. Klatskin, G, and Smith, DP: *Halothane-induced hepatitis,* in Gerok, W, and Sickinger, K (eds.): *Drugs and the Liver.* Stuttgart: T.K. Schattauer-Verlag, 1975, pp. 289–296.
17. Uehleke, H, and Werner, T: *A comparative study on the irreversible binding of labeled halothane, trichlorofluoromethane, chloroform, and carbon tetrachloride to hepatic protein and lipids in vitro and in vivo.* Arch Toxicol 34:289, 1975.
18. Klatskin, G: *Toxic and drug-induced hepatitis,* in Schiff, L (ed.): *Diseases of the Liver.* Philadelphia: J.B. Lippincott, 1975, p. 638.
19. Miller, DJ, Dwyer, J, and Klatskin, G: *Halothane hepatitis: benign resolution of a severe lesion.* Ann Intern Med 89:212, 1978.
20. Senior, JR: *Post-transfusion hepatitis.* Gastroenterology 49:315, 1965.
21. Snydman, DR, Hindman, SH, Wineland, MD, et al.: *Nosocomial viral hepatitis B.* Ann Intern Med 85:573, 1976.
22. Stern, H: *Cytomegalovirus and EB virus infection of the liver.* Br Med Bull 28:180, 1972.
23. Zimmerman, HJ: *Hepatotoxicity.* New York: Appleton-Century-Crofts, 1979.
24. Schmid, M, Hefti, ML, Galtiker, R, et al.: *Benign postoperative intrahepatic cholestasis.* N Engl J Med 272:545, 1965.
25. Kantrowitz, PA, Jones, WA, Greenberger, NJ, et al.: *Severe postoperative hyperbilirubinemia simulating obstructive jaundice.* N Engl J Med 276:591, 1967.
26. Hall, RC, Sahiyalah, P, Kim, SK, et al.: *Failure of operative cholangiography to prevent retained common duct stones.* Am J Surg 125:51, 1973.
27. Zimmon, DS: *Endoscopic management of biliary calculi.* Hosp Pract 13:103, 1978.
28. Howard, RJ, and Delaney, JP: *Postoperative cholecystitis.* Am J Dig Dis 17:213, 1972.

29. Ottinger, LW: *Acute cholecystitis as a postoperative complication.* Ann Surg 184:162, 1976.

30. Weinstein, BR, Korn, RJ, and Zimmerman, HJ: *Obstructive jaundice as a complication of pancreatitis.* Ann Intern Med 58:245, 1963.

31. Warshaw, AL, and Fuller, AF: *Specificity of increased renal clearance of amylase in diagnosis of acute pancreatitis.* N Engl J Med 292:325, 1975.

32. Levine, RL, Glauser, FL, and Berk, JE: *Enhancement of the amylase-creatinine clearance ratio in disorders other than acute pancreatitis.* N Engl J Med 292:329, 1975.

33. Traverso, LW, Ferrari, BT, Buckberg, GD, et al.: *Elevated postoperative renal clearance of amylase without pancreatitis after cardiopulmonary bypass.* Am J Surg 133:298, 1977.

34. Levitt, MD, Johnson, SG, Ellis, CJ, et al.: *Influence of amylase assay technique on renal clearance of amylase-creatinine ratio.* Gastroenterology 72:1260, 1977.

35. Powell, LW, Hemingway, E, Billing, GH, et al.: *Idiopathic unconjugated hyperbilirubinemia (Gilbert's syndrome).* N Engl J Med 227:1108, 1967.

36. Butt, HR, Anderson, VE, Fovik, WT, et al.: *Studies of chronic idiopathic jaundice (Dubin-Johnson syndrome).* Gastroenterology 51:619, 1966.

37. Sheldon, GF, Petersen, SR, and Sanders, R: *Hepatic dysfunction during hyperalimentation.* Arch Surg 113:504, 1978.

38. Bernstein, J, Chang, CH, Brough, AJ, et al.: *Conjugated hyperbilirubinemia in infancy associated with parenteral alimentation.* J Pediatr 90:361, 1977.

39. Zieve, L, and Nicoloff, DM: *Pathogenesis of hepatic coma.* Ann Rev Med 26:143, 1975.

40. Hoyumpa, AM, Desmond, PV, Avant, GR, et al.: *Hepatic encephalopathy.* Gastroenterology 76:184, 1979.

41. Fischer, JE, Rosen, HM, Ebeid, AM, et al.: *The effect of normalization of plasma amino acids on hepatic encephalopathy in man.* Surgery 80:77, 1976.

42. Yajko, RD, Norton, LW, and Eiseman, B: *Current management of upper gastrointestinal bleeding.* Ann Surg 181:-474, 1974.

43. Skillman, JJ, Bushnell, LS, Goldman, H, et al.: *Respiratory failure, hypotension, sepsis, and jaundice: a clinical syndrome associated with lethal hemorrhage from acute stress ulceration of the stomach.* Am J Surg 117:523, 1969.

44. Lucas, CE, Sugawa, C, Riddle, J, et al.: *Natural history and surgical dilemma of "stress" gastric bleeding.* Arch Surg 102:266, 1971.

45. Hastings, PR, Skillman, JJ, Bushnell, LS, et al.: *Antacid titration in the prevention of acute gastrointestinal bleeding.* E Engl J Med 298:1041, 1978.

46. Wilson, WS, Gadacz, T, Olcott, C, et al.: *Superficial gastric erosions.* Am J Surg 126:133, 1973.

47. Moody, FG, and Aldrete, JS: *Hydrogen permeability of canine gastric secretory epithelium during formation of acute superficial erosions.* Surgery 70:154, 1971.

48. McAlhany, JC, Jr, Czaja, AJ, and Pruitt, BA, Jr.: *Antacid control of complications from acute gastroduodenal disease after burns.* J Trauma 16:645, 1976.

49. MacDougall, BRD, Bailey, RJ, and Williams, R: *H_2-receptor antagonists and antacids in the prevention of acute gastrointestinal hemorrhage in fulminant hepatic failure: two controlled trials.* Lancet 1:617, 1977.

50. Walker, CO: *Complications of peptic ulcer disease and indications for surgery,* in Sleisenger, M, and Fordtran, J (eds.): *Gastrointestinal Disease,* Philadelphia: WB Saunders Co., 1978, pp. 914–946.

51. Allen, R, and Dykes, P: *A study of the factors influencing mortality rates from gastrointestinal hemorrhage.* Q J Med 180:533, 1976.

52. Morris, DW, Levine, GM, Soloway, RD, et al.: *Prospective, randomized study of diagnosis and outcome in acute upper gastrointestinal bleeding: endoscopy versus conventional radiography.* Am J Dig Dis 20:1103, 1975.

53. Eckardt, VF, and Grace, ND: *Gastroesophageal reflux and bleeding esophageal varices.* Gastroenterology 76:39, 1979.

54. Tedesco, FJ, Waye, JD, Raskin, JB, et al.: *Colonoscopic evaluation of rectal bleeding.* Ann Intern Med 89:907, 1978.

55. McCray, RS, Martin, F, Amir-Ahmadi, H, et al.: *Erroneous diagnosis of hemorrhage from esophageal varices.* Am J Dig Dis 14:755, 1969.

56. Baum, S, Nusbaum, M, Clearfield, HR, et al.: *Angiography in the diagnosis of gastrointestinal bleeding.* Arch Intern Med 119:16, 1967.
57. Conn, HO, Ramsby, GR, Storer, EH, et al.: *Intra-arterial vasopressin in the treatment of upper gastrointestinal hemorrhage: a prospective, controlled clinical trial.* Gastroenterology 68:211, 1975.
58. Athansoulis, CA, Baum, S, and Rosch, J: *Mesenteric arterial infusions of vasopressin for hemorrhage from colonic diverticulosis.* Am J Surg 129:212, 1975.
59. Johnson, WC, Widrich, WC, Ansell, JE, et al.: *Control of bleeding varices by vasopressin: a prospective randomized study.* Ann Surg 186:369, 1977.
60. Viamonte, M, Jr., Pereiras, R, Russell, E, et al.: *Transhepatic obliteration of gastroesophageal varices: results in acute and non-acute bleeders.* Am J Roentgenol 129:237, 1977.
61. Fordtran, JS, Morawshi, SG, Richardson, CT: *In vivo and in vitro evaluation of liquid antacids.* N Engl J Med 288:923, 1973.
62. Feldman, M, Richardson, CT, Peterson, WL, et al.: *Effect of low-dose propantheline on food-stimulated gastric acid secretion.* N Engl J Med 297:1427, 1977.
63. Pinder, RM, Brogden, RN, Sawyer, PR, et al.: *Metoclopramide: a review of its pharmacological properties and clinical use.* Drugs 12:81, 1976.
64. Keighley, MR, Burdon, DW, Alexander-Williams, J, et al.: *Diarrhoea and pseudomembranous colitis after gastrointestinal operations. A prospective study.* Lancet 2:1165, 1978.
65. Tedesco, FJ, Barton, RW, and Alpers, DH: *Clindamycin-associated colitis—a prospective study.* Ann Intern Med 81:429, 1974.
66. Bartlett, JG, Onderdonk, AB, Cisneros, RL, et al.: *Clindamycin-associated colitis due to a toxin-producing species of Clostridium in hamsters.* J Infect Dis 136:701, 1977.
67. George, WL, Sutter, VL, Goldstein, EJC, et al.: *Aetiology of antimicrobial-agent-associated colitis.* Lancet 1:802, 1978.
68. Keighley, MRB, Burdon, DW, Arabi, Y, et al.: *Randomized controlled trial of vancomycin for pseudomembranous colitis and postoperative diarrhea.* Lancet 2:1667, 1978.
69. Ottinger, LW, Darling, RC, Nathan, MJ, et al.: *Left colon ischemia complicating aorto-iliac reconstruction.* Arch Surg 105:841, 1972.
70. Cotton, PB, and Thomas, ML: *Ischaemic colitis and the contraceptive pill.* Br Med J 3:27, 1971.
71. Allan, JG, and Russell, RI: *Cholestyramine in treatment of postvagotomy diarrhoea—double-blind controlled trial.* Br Med J 1:674, 1977.
72. DeCosse, JJ, Rhodes, RS, Wentz, WB, et al.: *The natural history and management of radiation-induced injury of the gastrointestinal tract.* Ann Surg 170:369, 1969.
73. Binder, HJ, and Donowitz, M: *A new look at laxative action.* Gastroenterology 69:1001, 1975.
74. Woods, JH, Erickson, LW, Condon, RE, et al.: *Postoperative ileus: a colonic problem?* Surgery 84:527, 1978.
75. Faulk, DL, Anuras, S, and Christensen, J: *Chronic intestinal pseudo-obstruction.* Gastroenterology 74:922, 1978.
76. Priebe, HJ, Skillman, JJ, Bushnell, LS, et al.: *Antacid versus cimetidine in preventing acute gastrointestinal bleeding. A randomized trial in 75 critically ill patients.* N Engl J Med 302:426, 1980.

Chapter 7
HEMATOLOGY

Rita A. Blanchard, M.D., Bruce Furie, M.D., and
Robert S. Schwartz, M.D.

PREOPERATIVE EVALUATION OF THE SURGICAL PATIENT

History and Physical Examination

A well-conducted medical history can yield much information related to an underlying hematologic disorder. For example, the potential for a hemostatic complication may be recognized by learning that the patient had unusual bleeding associated with prior surgery or dentistry. Moreover, a history of *uncomplicated* surgery or trauma weighs against the possibility of an otherwise clinically silent hemorrhagic disorder, especially of the hereditary variety. A clinical history of spontaneous bruising, epistaxis, or mucosal bleeding requires detailed evaluation, as does a family history of bleeding.

The preoperative history should always include inquiries about drugs. Patients may not perceive words like "drugs" or "medication" in the same way as physicians, especially in relation to compounds such as aspirin or cough syrups. However, the use of these and many other widely employed agents inhibits platelet function, which in turn can be associated with intraoperative or postoperative bleeding. Specific questions can often evoke information that may be missed by merely asking the patient, "Do you take drugs?" Table 1 lists medications that interfere with platelet function. Drug-induced inhibition of blood coagulation is another potential cause of abnormal hemostasis. Procainamide,[1] chlorpromazine,[2,3] penicillin, streptomycin, and isoniazid[4] have been implicated in this phenomenon. Still other drugs are associated with the development of idiosyncratic thrombocytopenia, anemia, or neutropenia

TABLE 1. Drugs Affecting Platelet Function

In Vivo	*Lesser Effect or in Vitro Effect*
Aspirin and aspirin containing compounds	Antihistamines
Atromid and Atromid S(clofibrate)	Beta blockers
Dextran	Chloroquine and hydroxychloroquine
Dipyridamole	Chlorpromazine
Glyceryl guaiacolate	Ethanol
Indomethacin	Furosemide
Meclofenamic acid	General anesthetics
Methylxanthines (aminophylline, theophylline, papaverine)	Imipramine
Penicillin (high dose) and carbenicillin	Nitrofurantoin
Phenylbutazone	Phentolamine and other alpha blockers
Prostacyclin	Serotonin antagonists
Prostaglandin E_1	
Sulfinpyrazone	
Tolmetin sodium	

(Table 2). A history of treatment with warfarin is obviously important. Occasionally, however, this information is not obtained and the operative complications under such circumstances can be predicted. The addition of new medications to the regimen of the patient on chronic warfarin therapy may also precipitate a bleeding episode by potentiating the effect of the anticoagulant (Table 3). Self-poisoning with warfarin, a rare manifestation of a psychiatric disturbance, can present as massive gastrointestinal bleeding.

The physical examination may disclose evidence of underlying hematologic disease or of a disease with hematologic complications, such as cirrhosis of the liver. Petechiae or ecchymoses are associated with quantitative or qualitative platelet defects, whereas purpura in the absence of ecchymoses is generally associated with coagulopathy. Splenomegaly, commonly an incidental finding, may be a clue to the diagnosis of a variety of disorders, hematologic and otherwise (Table 4). To some extent, the size of the spleen influences the diagnostic considerations. The etiology of splenomegaly should be ascertained insofar as possible in advance of the surgical procedure. We have, for instance, encountered patients with isolated splenomegaly and minimal disturbance of liver function who, at surgery, were found to have severe portal cirrhosis. Hemorrhagic complications in these cases were severe.

Laboratory Evaluation

The routine preoperative evaluation includes a series of laboratory screening tests related to the identification of latent hematologic disease. The extent of this evaluation is controversial. It is influenced by the nature of the surgical procedure anticipated and the availability of certain diagnostic tests. With the advent of automated cell counting techniques, the complete blood count is routinely performed on all hospitalized patients. The complete blood count includes the *hemoglobin, hematocrit,* and *white blood cell* count. Also included are the measurements of the volume (mean corpuscular volume or MCV), hemoglobin content (mean corpuscular hemoglobin or MCH), and hemoglobin concen-

TABLE 2. Drugs Associated with Idiosyncratic Reactions

A. Drugs Associated with Thrombocytopenia

Acetaminophen	Flucytosine
Acetazolamide	Furosemide
Acetylsalicylic acid	Heparin
Allyliospropylacetylurea (Sedormid)	Hydrochlorothiazide
Alpha-methyldopa	Hydroxychloroquine
Amphotericin B	Isoniazid
Ampicillin	Miconazole
Antazoline	Nitrofurantoin
Carbamazepine	Novobiocin
Carbenicillin	Oxyphenbutazone
Centulun	Para-aminosalicylic acid (PAS)
Cephalothin	Penicillin
Chloroquine	Phenylbutazone
Chlorothiazide	Phenytoin
Chlorpropamide	Quinidine
Chlorthalidone	Quinine
Clopamide	Rifampin
Desipramine	Stibophen
Diazoxide	Sulfonamides
Digitoxin	Tolbutamide

B. Drugs Associated with Neutropenia

Acetanilid	Mepazine
Acetazolamide	Methicilline
Alpha-methyldopa	Methimazole
Aminopyrine	Novobiocin
Amphenidone	Oxyphenbutazone
Ampicillin	Penicillin
Carbenicillin	Perphenazine
Carbimazole	Phenacetin
Cephalothin	Phenindione
Chloramphenicol	Phenytoin
Chlorothiazide	Procainamide
Chlorpromazine	Prochlorperazine
Chlorpropamide	Promazine hydrochloride
Chlorthalidone	Propylthiouracil
Cimetidine	Sulfaguanidine
Dinitrophenol	Sulfamethoxypyridazine
Dipyrone	Sulfanilamide
Ethacrynic acid	Sulfazosulfapyridine
Flucytosine	Thioridazine
Gold salts	Thiouracil
Hydrochlorothiazide	Tolbutamide
Ibuprofen	Triflupromazine hydrochloride
Imipramine	Trimethadione

TABLE 2. *Continued*

C. Drugs Associated with Anemia

1. Aplastic Anemia

Acetazolamide	Methimazole
Amphotericin B	Organic arsenicals
Aspirin	Oxyphenbutazone
Azathioprine	Penicillin
Benzene	Perchlorate
Carbamazepine	Phenacetin
Carbimazole	Phenylbutazone
Carbon tetrachloride	Phenytoin
Carbutamide	Primidone
Chloramphenicol	Promazine
Chlordane	Pyrimethamine
Chlordiazepoxide	Quinacrine
Chlorpheniramine	Streptomycin
Chlorpromazine	Sulfamethoxypyridazine
Chlorpropamide	Sulfisoxazole
Colchicine	Sulfonamides
DDT	Tetracyclines
Dinitrophenol	Thiocyanate
Gold salts	Thiosemicarbazone
Indomethacin	Thiouracil
Mephenytoin	Thorotrast
Meprobamate	Tolbutamide
Mercury	Triflupromazine hydrochloride
Methicillin	Trimethadione
Miconazole	Tripelennamine

2. Hemolytic Anemia

Acetanilid-phenacetin	Levodopa
Alpha-methyldopa	Mefenamic acid
Amphotericin B	Para-aminosalicylic acid
Arsine	Pamaquin
Cephalexin	Penicillin
Cephaloridine	Quinidine
Cephalothin	Quinine
Chlorate	Salicylazosulfapyridine
Chlorpromazine	Stibophen
Copper	Sulfadiazine
Diaminodiphenylsulfone	Sulfonamides

tration (mean corpuscular hemoglobin concentration or MCHC) of the red cell. In toto, these laboratory tests provide considerable information concerning the hematologic status of the patient. First, is the patient anemic? Anemia should be suspected in men when the hemoglobin is below 14 gm/dl and the hematocrit is below 42 ml/dl. In women the lower limits of accepted normal values for the hemoglobin and hematocrit are 12 gm/dl and 36 ml/dl, respectively. The often ignored red cell indices (MCV, MCH, and MCHC) offer the first clue to the etiology or classification of an anemia. The normal range of the MCV is 85 to 98 μm^3. Values above the normal range indicate macrocytosis,

TABLE 3. Effect of Drugs on Warfarin Response

Medications which Potentiate the Effect of Warfarin	
Acetaminophen	Indomethacin
Acetohexamide	Isoniazid
Allopurinol	Mefenamic acid
Androgenic and anabolic steroids	Methimazole
Alpha-methyldopa	Methotrexate
Antibiotics which disrupt intestinal flora: tetracyclines, streptomycin, erythromycin, kanamycin, nalidixic acid, neomycin	Methylphenidate
Cephaloridine	Nalidixic acid
Chloramphenicol	Nortriptyline
Chlorpromazine	Oxyphenbutazone
Chlorpropamide	Para-aminosalicylic acid
Chloral hydrate	Paromomycin
Cimetidine	Phenylbutazone
Clofibrate	Phenytoin
Diazoxide	Phenyramidol
Disulfiram	Propylthiouracil
Ethacrynic acid	Quinidine
Glucagon	Salicylate
Guanethidine	Sulfinpyrazone
	Sulfonamides
	Thyroid hormone
	Tolbutamide
Medications which Depress the Effect of Warfarin	
Antipyrine	Glutethimide
Barbiturates	Griseofulvin
Carbamazepine	Haloperidol
Chlorthalidone	Oral contraceptives
Cholestyramine	Phenobarbital
Digitalis	Prednisone
Ethanol	All vitamin preparations containing vitamin K
Ethchlorvynol	

while those below normal indicate microcytosis. The range for the MCH is 28 to 32 pg and for the MCHC 28 to 32 gm/dl. Low values indicate hypochromia of the red cells. Is the white blood cell count normal? The normal white count ranges from 4,000 to 10,000 mm^3 in Caucasian adults.[5] In the black population, white blood cell counts as low as 2,000/mm^3 may be in the normal range.[6]

Examination of the peripheral blood smear is also an essential and routine aspect of the preoperative laboratory evaluation. Specific attention is paid to the presence of immature myeloid cells, abnormal red cell morphology, eosinophilia, monocytosis, neutropenia, lymphocytosis, and evidence of thrombocytopenia.

The extent of the preoperative hemostasis evaluation is less well defined and depends upon the nature of the surgical procedure. Since latent congenital and acquired hemostatic defects can seriously compromise the perioperative and postoperative course, these defects should be identified before the operation. A prothrombin time and a partial thromboplastin time should be obtained to evaluate the extrinsic and intrinsic pathways

TABLE 4. Causes of Splenomegaly

Infectious	*Hematologic and Neoplastic*
Brucellosis (acute)	Acute leukemias
Cytomegalovirus infection	Chronic granulocytic leukemia
Histoplasmosis	Chronic hemolytic anemia, e.g., hereditary spherocytosis
Infectious mononucleosis	Chronic lymphocytic leukemia
Kala-azar	Essential thrombocythemia
Leishmaniasis	Hodgkin's Disease
Malaria	Lymphoma
Rocky Mountain spotted fever	Macroglobulinemia
Schistosomiasis	Metastases to spleen
Subacute bacterial endocarditis	Myelofibrosis-agnogenic myeloid metaplasia
Syphilis	Polycythemia rubra vera
Toxoplasmosis	Thalassemia
Tuberculosis	
Viral hepatitis	
Autoimmune	*Miscellaneous*
Chronic autoimmune hemolytic anemia	Acromegaly
Rheumatoid arthritis	Amyloidosis
Systemic lupus erythematosus	Gaucher's disease
	Hyperthyroidism
	Portal hypertension
	"Pseudolymphoma" secondary to Dilantin therapy
	Regional enteritis
	Sea-blue histiocyte syndrome
	Splenic cysts

of blood coagulation. In addition, a platelet count below the normal range (150,000 to 350,000 mm^3) must be evaluated preoperatively. A bleeding time is sufficient to identify patients with qualitative defects of platelet function. Other coagulation studies, including the thrombin time, fibrinogen level, fibrin split products, and platelet function studies, are not recommended in the routine preoperative screening. Table 5 summarizes the routine preoperative laboratory screening useful in identifying latent hematologic disorders. If results of the history, physical examination, and laboratory screening are negative, the patient may proceed to surgery without further evaluation.

ANEMIA

In the United States, there is only one important cause of iron deficiency: bleeding. Anemia due to iron deficiency is generally hypochromic and microcytic, but in mild cases these changes are absent or minimal. The diagnosis is established in classical cases by a low serum iron and a high iron binding capacity. Determination of serum ferritin or a bone marrow stained for iron which assesses marrow storage iron can be valuable in subtle cases, especially when the distinction between the anemia of bleeding and the anemia of chronic disease is difficult. The importance of recognizing iron deficiency

TABLE 5. Laboratory Procedures in Routine Preoperative Screen for Hematologic Disorders

Hemoglobin
Hematocrit
Red cell indices (MCV, MCH, MCHC)
White blood cell count
Examination of peripheral smear
Platelet count
Prothrombin time
Partial thromboplastin time
Bleeding time

before elective surgery, especially in the patient who does not have an obvious source of blood loss, cannot be overemphasized. Identification and treatment of the cause of the blood loss, which is usually in the gastrointestinal tract, prior to the stress of surgery may prevent postoperative hemorrhage from the lesion. Therapy of the iron deficiency should be undertaken with oral preparations of the simple ferrous salts—such as ferrous sulfate, 325 mg, three times daily. Iron therapy is preferable to transfusions, because it is virtually risk free and far less expensive.

Some patients with mild anemia and microcythemia may not have iron deficiency, but a benign form of thalassemia, a condition which should not interfere with surgery. As a rule of thumb, these patients may be identified using the MCV and red cell count.[93] If the MCV divided by the red cell count is less than 13, the diagnosis of β-thalassemia trait is likely. Hemoglobin electrophoresis will confirm the diagnosis. If, however, this value is greater than 13, iron deficiency should be suspected. Other forms of anemia characterized by microcythemia include lead poisoning and the sideroblastic anemias. Both types of anemia require intensive hematologic evaluation for adequate diagnosis.

The anemia of chronic disease or chronic inflammation is common in hospitalized patients and is often a diagnostic problem. This type of anemia can complicate chronic infection, rheumatoid arthritis, various malignancies, collagen-vascular disorders, fractures, and severe tissue injury.[7] Chronic renal failure and hypothyroidism may be overlooked causes of this form of anemia. Laboratory features include decreased serum iron, a decreased serum iron binding capacity, a high serum ferritin, and an elevated erythrocyte sedimentation rate. The anemia may respond to treatment of the underlying primary disorder. However, in the context of anticipated surgery, these patients should be transfused preoperatively to an adequate level (a hematocrit of 25ml/dl for patients less than 40 years, 30 ml/dl for those greater than 40 years).

The common macrocytic anemias are associated with deficiencies of either vitamin B_{12} or folic acid. These forms of anemia are characterized by hypersegmentation of the nuclear lobes of the neutrophil and megaloblastic changes in the bone marrow. Wound healing is impaired in these deficiency states. Recognition of either of these deficiencies should lead to specific diagnosis and therapy prior to surgery. Malabsorption of B_{12} and folate is associated with a variety of diseases involving the small intestine.[8] Folic acid deficiency in the United States is almost always associated with some other medical condition, such as alcoholism or pregnancy.

Occasionally, malabsorption syndromes that cause nutritional deficiencies may be associated with surgery of the gastrointestinal tract. Iron deficiency is often a complication of gastrectomy.[9] Postgastrectomy anemia may also be due to vitamin B_{12} deficiency or, less commonly, folate deficiency. Deficiencies of both iron and B_{12} may also occur in this situation.[10] Removal of major portions of the jejunum or ileum can lead to malabsorption of folate and vitamin B_{12}, respectively. In addition, intestinal bacteria overgrowth, either in a surgically created blind loop or in diverticula of the small intestine, can lead to vitamin B_{12} deficiency.

ERYTHROCYTOSIS

True erythrocytosis is an increase in the circulating red cell mass in a patient with a normal or increased plasma volume. This possibility should be considered when the hematocrit is over 50 ml/dl in the normally hydrated patient. Most patients have true erythrocytosis when the hematocrit exceeds 60 ml/dl. Regardless of its etiology, erythrocytosis can increase blood viscosity; as a result, circulatory stasis and increased cardiac effort to maintain cardiac output may result.

When erythrocytosis is recognized, an underlying disease should be sought. Erythrocytosis secondary to hypoxia and pulmonary disease or a left-to-right shunt as part of a cardiac malformation will surely influence the surgical approach. Erythrocytosis has many causes (Table 6), but cases can be classified into three groups. The commonest cause is *reactive*, this erythrocytosis is secondary to a decreased blood oxygen saturation. In this type of erythrocytosis, the Pa_{O_2} is usually low, but there are also rare cases in which tissue hypoxemia rather than arterial unsaturation accounts for the erythrocytosis (cobalt ingestion, hemoglobins with high oxygen affinity).

The second group consists of patients with the myeloproliferative disorder polycythemia rubra vera. These patients may be distinguished from those in the first group because they have an increase in the blood of all three cell lines (white cell and platelet as well as red cell) and splenomegaly is usual. In addition, the Pa_{O_2} is normal. Surgery in patients with polycythemia rubra vera will be discussed below.

The third kind of true erythrocytosis can be a difficult diagnostic problem. In this heterogeneous group are patients whose erythrocytosis is secondary to an elevated erythropoietin, usually due to abnormal secretion of this hormone. Generally, this situation occurs in association with certain tumors, malignant or benign, such as hypernephroma, liver cell carcinoma, and uterine fibroma (Table 6 I & H). Balcerzak and Bromberg give a comprehensive review of this topic.[11]

There is one additional type of erythrocytosis: stress erythrocytosis or Gaisböck's syndrome. Patients with this condition are often overweight, high-strung, hypertensive, and prone to thromboembolic complications, but they do not have a true increase in red cell mass. Instead, their plasma volume is decreased. When the hypertension is con-

TABLE 6. Causes of Erythrocytosis

1. Polycythemia rubra vera: Myeloproliferative disorder characterized by an increase in all three cell lines, splenomegaly, and normal Pao_2

2. Secondary polycythemia
   - A. High altitude
   - B. Chronic obstructive lung disease
   - C. Pickwickian syndrome
   - D. Cardiovascular anomalies with right-to-left shunt
   - E. Postural hypoxemia
   - F. Hemoglobinopathy with high oxygen affinity
   - G. Heavy smoking
   - H. Tumors
     1. Renal carcinoma
     2. Hepatoma
     3. Cerebellar hemangioblastoma
     4. Uterine fibroid
     5. Adrenal cortical hyperplasia or adenoma
     6. Ovarian carcinoma
   - I. Renal involvement
     1. Cysts
     2. Hydronephrosis
     3. Bartter's syndrome
     4. Renal transplant
   - J. Cobalt therapy
   - K. Familial etiology

3. Stress erythrocytosis (Gaisböck's syndrome)

trolled, the plasma volume and hematocrit are often restored to normal. It is important to recognize and treat these patients prior to surgery.[12]

NEUTROPENIA

A total granulocyte count of less than $1000/mm^3$ should lead to cancellation of surgery except in unusual circumstances. There are grave risks of infectious complications when the granulocyte count is less than $500/mm^3$, and these risks must be balanced by the indications for surgery. Granulocytopenia may occur transiently in acute viral infections, in which case there is usually a lymphocytosis. There are also *normal* individuals among certain population groups (black Americans, black Africans, and Yemenite Jews) who have consistently lower neutrophil counts than Caucasians, but counts below $800/mm^3$ are rare.[6] Agranulocytosis or neutropenia may be due to congenital or acquired defects in myeloid maturation in the bone marrow or to accelerated clearance of white cells from the circulation, problems that require full hematologic evaluation. In favorable cases, such as those related to drug or viral-induced neutropenia, the disorder is reversible and surgery can be reconsidered after recovery.

Emergency surgery in severely neutropenic patients can be performed provided certain principles are followed. Septicemia should be recognized and appropriate treatment started prior to surgery. Infection in a closed space will often not produce a typical walled-off abscess and pus when there is severe neutropenia. Oral and rectal areas are particularly prone to invasion by common bacterial commensals in such cases. Prophylactic antibiotics are of minimal value, with the exception of trimethoprim-sulfamethoxazole for prolonged neutropenia, gut sterilization prior to colonic surgery, penicillin for emergency oral surgery, and ampicillin and gentamicin for cystoscopy. Operative intervention should be minimal and rely mainly on diversion and drainage procedures (see discussion of surgical management of acute leukemia below). The use of granulocyte transfusions is discussed in the section on Transfusion Therapy below.

GRANULOCYTOSIS

Granulocytosis can be defined as a persistent granulocyte count above 10,000/mm.[3] Apart from the usual, well known causes of granulocytosis, granulocytosis is also seen in pregnancy, following splenectomy, and as a side effect of certain drugs, such as corticosteroids, lithium, and epinephrine. If none of these causes are evident, then elective surgery should be postponed and a search for an underlying myeloproliferative disease, occult abscess, malignancy, or inflammatory disease should be undertaken. Leukocyte counts up to 100,000/mm^3 should not interfere with *emergency* surgery although the cause of the leukocytosis may.

LYMPHOCYTOSIS

The commonest cause of lymphocytosis in adults (lymphocyte count greater than 4,000/mm^3) is acute viral infection. Infectious mononucleosis, viral hepatitis, and cytomegalovirus infection are characterized by lymphocytosis, especially with atypical lymphocytes, splenomegaly, and abnormal liver function tests. Heterophile antibodies, hepatitis associated antigen, cytomegalovirus in the urine, or acute-convalescent sera for CMV complement fixing antibodies can diagnose these disorders. Elective surgery should be postponed in these cases, especially during acute viral hepatitis, because of the high risk of postoperative complications.[13]

Occasionally, complications of viral illnesses require emergency surgery. For example, splenic rupture occurs in 1 or 2 cases of infectious mononucleosis per thousand. This usually occurs 10 to 21 days after the onset of illness and is heralded by abdominal pain —an unusual finding in uncomplicated cases of infectious mononucleosis. Other more unusual causes of lymphocytosis include occult or apathetic hyperthyroidism and toxoplasmosis. In the patient with persistent lymphocytosis in whom heterophil, hepatitis antigen, and CMV antibodies are not found, a lymphoproliferative disorder, such as chronic lymphocytic leukemia, should be considered. The bone marrow is usually diagnostic; a predominance in the blood of monoclonal lymphocytes of the B cell type often helps in early diagnosis.

In addition to the white cell disorders mentioned above, other abnormalities include monocytosis, eosinophilia, and leukocytosis. These in themselves will not complicate surgery, but the underlying condition (e.g., amebic abscess) may give rise to unanticipated surgical problems. Therefore, such laboratory findings should be a signal to cancel all but urgent surgery.

HEMOSTATIC DISORDERS

It is important to recognize that some hemorrhagic disorders are clinically *latent,* with bleeding manifestations that declare themselves only after trauma or surgery. Other conditions, such as certain instances of circulating anticoagulants, are associated with grossly abnormal coagulation tests, but there is no bleeding even after major surgery. Therefore, laboratory tests should be used as guides; *they are not infallible.* There is still no substitute for a careful history and physical examination and individual analysis of each patient's problem. For a more extensive review see Bowie and Owen.[14]

Thrombocytopenia

The risk of hemorrhage in thrombocytopenia is related to the extent of the decrease in circulating platelets. There is little risk when the platelet count exceeds 100,000/mm^3; by contrast, a platelet count of less than 20,000/mm^3 is often associated with bleeding complications.[15] With platelet counts between 50,000 to 100,000/mm^3, the hemorrhagic tendency is variable and related to the nature of the surgical procedure, the surgical technique, and other factors, such as fever, infection, and metabolic disturbances. It seems reasonable to attribute operative bleeding to the thrombocytopenia in such marginal cases unless, of course, another more obvious cause can be identified.

Thrombocytopenia due to increased platelet destruction is usually characterized by the presence of large, dense platelets in the blood smear and increased numbers of megakaryocytes in the bone marrow. This form of thrombocytopenia may be seen in patients with idiopathic (autoimmune) thrombocytopenic purpura, systemic lupus erythematosus, and some drug-induced thrombocytopenias. Therapy should be directed at the primary disease before surgery, since these patients do not respond adequately to platelet transfusions. Thrombocytopenia associated with decreased platelet production is characterized by small platelets in the blood smear. Such thrombocytopenia is often associated with serious hematologic disorders, such as aplastic anemia or leukemia. In some cases, however, thrombocytopenia is self-limited or drug-induced, and surgery may be postponed until the condition is corrected. In refractory cases or in emergency situations, the patient should be transfused with platelets prior to surgery. As a rule of thumb, a single unit of random donor platelets will raise the platelet count by 5,000/mm^3. The platelet count should be maintained in excess of 50,000/mm^3 intraoperatively and postoperatively for at least four or five days. The half-life of infused platelets is about two to three days.

Platelet Dysfunction

The bleeding time, barring severe thrombocytopenia, is a screening test for disorders of platelet function. With the Ivy method, a wound is made in the forearm maintained at a venous pressure of 40 mm Hg. A template is used to make a wound 1 by 9 mm in the volar aspect of the forearm. The bleeding time is usually 4 to 9 minutes.

Aspirin

An abnormal bleeding time must be evaluated. Aspirin increases the bleeding time in most persons, and this effect may be marked in about 10 percent of the population.[16] A single aspirin tablet may interfere with platelet function for as long as seven days. Therefore, aspirin and the other compounds listed in Table 1 must be strictly avoided within a week of surgery. The discovery of an abnormal bleeding time should be an indication for studies of platelet aggregation and platelet adhesiveness. Although the results of these tests do not correlate well with some hemorrhagic disorders, these procedures may allow identification and diagnosis of patients with qualitative platelet disorders.

These diagnoses have therapeutic implications. Thrombocytopathies, characterized by prolongation of the bleeding time, abnormal platelet adhesiveness, and abnormal platelet aggregation studies may be managed using platelet transfusions. For patients with modestly abnormal laboratory results and no history of bleeding, surgery may be performed without platelet transfusion. In the event of postoperative hemorrhage, platelet transfusions can be administered. A prolonged bleeding time, abnormal platelet adhesiveness, abnormal platelet aggregation and a low Factor VIII activity characterize von Willebrand's disease. Management of these patients, described in detail below, is directed at elevating the Factor VIII activity and the von Willebrand's protein by infusion of fresh frozen plasma or cyroprecipitate 12 to 24 hours prior to surgery. Platelet transfusions are not useful because the abnormalities of platelet function are secondary to the disturbance of a plasma protein, the von Willebrand's protein.

THROMBOCYTOSIS. Thrombocytosis is defined as a platelet count above 350,000/mm.[3] Conditions known to be associated with thrombocytosis are malignancy, iron deficiency anemia, chronic inflammatory diseases (rheumatoid arthritis or collagen vascular disease), and the postsplenectomy state. By itself, thrombocytosis associated with these conditions does not appear to increase operative morbidity with respect to bleeding or thrombosis and therefore requires no treatment.

The treatment of thrombocytosis in association with a myeloproliferative disorder such as polycythemia vera, primary thrombocythemia, chronic granulocytic leukemia, or agnogenic myeloid metaplasia is a more difficult matter. Many of these patients have platelet counts in excess of 1,000,000/mm^3 and may have either thrombotic or hemorrhagic manifestations. Therefore, the thrombocytosis in these patients should be treated in advance of elective surgery.

In patients requiring emergency surgery, the treatment must be individualized. The age of the patient, the type of surgery, the patient's past history of bleeding or thrombotic episodes, and the bleeding time must all be taken into account in addition to the absolute level of the platelet count. For example, a young patient with a myeloproliferative disorder who has no past history of bleeding or thrombotic episodes and who is to undergo an appendectomy with a normal bleeding time and a platelet count of 1,000,000/mm^3 probably has little increased risk and would therefore require no therapy. With increasing age, abnormal bleeding time, history of thrombotic or bleeding episodes, surgery that carries a greater thrombotic risk (i.e., prostatectomy or splenectomy), and very high platelet counts, surgical risk increases and emergency therapeutic measures are necessary. Many patients with myeloproliferative disorders may, in fact, come to surgery because of thrombotic episodes. Thrombosis in these disorders tends to involve the large vessels, such as the mesenteric artery, the splenic artery or vein, and the heptatic vein.

Emergency therapy should be directed at decreasing both bone marrow production of platelets and the circulating platelet count. The most effective immediate method of rapidly reducing the quantity of circulating platelets is by plateletphoresis. If plateletphoresis is used without suppressing bone marrow platelet production, there will be a rapid rebound in platelet count generally in 24 to 72 hrs. Therefore, this therapy is often given in conjunction with chemotherapy in patients with myeloproliferative disorders. If repeated plateletpheresis were undesirable or unavailable, mechlorethamine hydrochloride (nitrogen mustard), 0.4 mg/kg of body weight, given intravenously will diminish platelet production over five to eight days. More commonly, alkylating agents (Myleran, chlorambucil) or ^{32}P are used but often take four to six weeks before the platelet count is altered.

In the bleeding patient with abnormal platelet function studies, platelet transfusions should be given in the face of a qualitative and quantitative platelet disorder. Although monitoring of the platelet count in this situation is of no value, the clinical response to transfusion can be predicted by titration of the bleeding time.

Coagulopathies

The fluid phase of blood coagulation is generally assessed by the prothrombin time (PT) and activated partial thromboplastin time (PTT). Because of the different reagents and procedures currently in use, there are no absolute values for either the prothrombin time or the PTT. The test results must be related to the normal range of values for that laboratory. In general, most normal prothrombin times are about 12 seconds. The patient's prothrombin time is compared to that obtained with normal plasma. A prothrombin time that is longer than two seconds over that of the control is considered abnormal. A prolonged partial thromboplastin time or prothrombin time is not a specific finding. The nature of the hemostatic defect that causes the abnormality must be identified. It should be appreciated, however, that the yield of this evaluation may be low when the partial thromboplastin time and prothrombin time are only modestly prolonged.

First, the distinction between the presence of a circulating inhibitor of blood coagulation and a deficiency of one or more of the components of the blood coagulation cascade must be made. Clotting studies are performed on an incubated mixture of normal plasma and the patient's plasma. If the normal plasma does not correct the abnormality in the patient's plasma, an anticoagulant is present in the patient's plasma. Circulating anticoagulants may be associated with systemic lupus erythematosus, pregnancy, malignant disorders,[3] or certain medications such as procainamide[1] and chlorpromazine.[2] Many of these anticoagulants are not associated with a bleeding tendency.[4] In these cases, antibodies may be directed against proteins in the contact phase of blood coagulation that may not participate in hemostasis in vivo. In a low percentage of cases, however, circulating anticoagulants may be associated with a hemorrhagic diathesis.

Unfortunately, it is not possible to predict from the routine laboratory results which patients with circulating anticoagulants will have major bleeding complications. The potential risks of serious bleeding must be weighed against the indications for surgery. Clearly, if the clotting studies are only modestly prolonged or if those studies can be corrected in vitro by the addition of small amounts of normal plasma, surgery may be done at less risk.

For example, a patient has a prolonged partial thromboplastin time and a normal prothrombin time. A test for a circulating anticoagulant is positive. This result suggests an inhibitor directed against a component of the intrinsic pathway. Will the infusion of fresh frozen plasma into the patient during surgery correct the abnormal PTT? To answer this question preoperatively during the laboratory evaluation, mixtures of normal and patient plasmas are prepared in ratios which simulate those that could be obtained in vivo by plasma infusion. If one part of normal plasma to three parts of patient plasma yields a mixture with a normal PTT, it may be anticipated that infusion of 4 units of plasma (1000 ml) into a 75 kg man (plasma volume 3000 ml) will also correct the PTT.

If the PTT remains significantly prolonged, the risk of hemorrhage during surgery must be weighed against the benefits of surgery. A recent history of uncomplicated surgery or trauma is reassuring if the operation is required. Similarly, the diagnosis of a circulating anticoagulant in a disorder in which such an anticoagulant does not often lead to a bleeding tendency (e.g., lupus erythematosus, some types of multiple myeloma) can be helpful. Intensive plasmaphoresis may decrease the concentration of high titer circulating anticoagulants, especially of the IgM class. However, this modality is not often helpful.

The development of intraoperative bleeding can pose serious management problems. Fresh frozen plasma should always be employed first. However, this modality may not be successful in patients with high inhibitor titers. For this reason, plasma exchange transfusion may prove useful. Some centers have gained experience in the use of the activated form of the Factor IX concentrates. However, this therapy is usually not readily available and must be considered experimental. Even standard Factor IX containing concentrates may be associated with an increase in thromboembolic complications in the surgical patient[17] and with hepatitis.

The deficiency states are usually easily identified by direct assay of components of the extrinsic or intrinsic pathway (Table 7). The exception is Factor XIII deficiency, a rare disorder which can be either congenital or acquired. In this disorder, a history of bleeding may be obtained in which significant bleeding from a wound is considerably delayed. The PT and PTT are normal. However, the patient's plasma clot is soluble in 5M urea. The common isolated congenital deficiencies, in order of frequency, include Factor VIII, Factor IX, and Factor XI deficiency. Decreased activities of any of the coagulation protein activities may, however, be observed. The magnitude of the deficiency correlates with the degree of prolongation of the partial thromboplastin time or the prothrombin time, but the clinical significance of the deficiency depends upon which clotting protein activity is decreased. For example, although a deficiency of Factor XII, high molecular weight kininogen or prekallikrein is associated with a markedly prolonged partial thromboplastin time, hemorrhage, even under the stress of surgery, does not occur. Deficiency of Factor XI is also uncommonly associated with an important bleeding tendency except in severe homozygous states.

TABLE 7. Identification of Hereditary Blood Coagulation Factor Deficiencies

	Prothrombin Time	*Partial Thromboplastin Time*	*Thrombin Time*	*Bleeding Time*	*Tendency to Bleed*	*Inheritance*
Factor VIII deficiency	N	P	N	N	Yes	X-linked
Factor IX deficiency	N	P	N	N	Yes	X-linked
Factor X deficiency	P	P	N	N	Yes	Autosomal
Factor XI deficiency	N	P	N	N	Variable	Autosomal
Factor XII deficiency	N	P	N	N	No	Autosomal
Factor VII deficiency	P	N	N	N	Yes	Autosomal
Prothrombin deficiency	P	P	N	N	Yes	Autosomal
Factor V deficiency	P	P	N	Maybe P	Yes	Autosomal
von Willebrand's disease	N	P	N	P	Yes	Autosomal
Afibrino genemia	P	P	P	Maybe P	Variable	Autosomal
Dysfibrino genemia	P	P	P	Maybe P	Variable	Autosomal

N = normal,
P = prolonged

Deficiency states involving more than one coagulation protein usually suggest an acquired coagulation disorder, such as vitamin K deficiency or liver disease. Vitamin K is necessary for the production of biologically active prothrombin, Factor X, Factor IX, and Factor VII. Deficiency of vitamin K, as in malnutrition, celiac disease, or prolonged broad spectrum antibiotic therapy, will lead initially to a prolongation in the prothrombin time and then in the partial thromboplastin time. Vitamin K antagonists, such as sodium warfarin (Coumadin), produce the same result. The coagulation abnormalities can be reversed, usually within 6 to 12 hours, by parenteral administration of vitamin K_1, 10 to 15 mg, given over 15 minutes. Because intramuscular injection of vitamin K may lead to local hematoma formation and oral vitamin K may be variably absorbed, careful intravenous administration is often the method of choice. The package insert of the drug warns, however, that this route of administration may be associated with anaphylactic reactions. By contrast, vitamin K is useless in the management of *isolated* deficiencies of coagulation proteins, such as hemophilia. It is also of no value in intravascular coagulation, which may be confused with vitamin K deficiency (see below). Since all the vitamin K-dependent factors are synthesized in the liver, severe liver disease may mimic vitamin K deficiency with low levels of Factors IX, X, VII, and prothrombin and a prolonged prothrombin time. It is often difficult to differentiate these syndromes initially. However, the correction of the coagulation tests by vitamin K administration strongly suggests severe liver disease as the etiology. If the patient is bleeding, fresh frozen plasma should be administered. Factor IX concentrates rich in the vitamin K-dependent blood coagulation proteins should be avoided, since they may cause thrombosis and intravascular coagulation in patients with severe liver disease.[18]

Acquired Factor IX deficiency may be associated with nephrotic syndrome and marked proteinuria.[19] Acquired Factor X deficiency may be associated with primary amyloidosis; patients with this disorder are refractory to replacement therapy.[20] A variety of coagulation protein abnormalities may be observed in chronic disseminated intravascular coagulation. Specific therapy for the hemostatic disorders is described below.

THROMBOSIS: PREVENTION AND RISK. Thrombophlebitis and pulmonary embolus are important causes of morbidity and mortality in the postsurgical patient. (For details on the diagnosis and management of thrombophlebitis and pulmonary embolism see Chapter 12, Pulmonary Diseases). A variety of anticoagulant and antiplatelet drugs have been advocated to prevent these complications. The results of several large cooperative, randomized studies of the use of mini-doses of heparin have indicated that this therapy markedly decreases the occurrence of death due to pulmonary emboli.[21] The recommended regimen is 5,000 U of heparin by subcutaneous injection every 12 hours for 5 days. The initial dose is administered six hours prior to surgery. Intraoperative and postoperative bleeding complications from this therapy may be slightly increased, but these problems are usually easily managed. This treatment plan has been advocated by some for all types of major surgical procedures except orthopedic procedures involving hip replacement. For the latter, this form of prophylaxis appears ineffective. Instead, aspirin or aspirin and dextrans are suggested.[22] Other experts in this field believe that use of small doses of heparin should be reserved for those patients with a high risk of thromboembolic diseases.

Some of the general risk factors for developing a thrombotic complication include age (older patients), heart failure, obesity, prior thromboembolic disorders, particular types of surgery (e.g., prostatic, gynecologic), and venous disease. Patients with prosthetic heart valves[23] or who have atrial fibrillation or subacute bacterial endocarditis have an increased incidence of arterial emboli. Certain other conditions may predispose to thrombosis including homocystinuria, systemic lupus erythematosus, nephrotic syndrome, and certain hyperlipidemias. There are also a certain number of chronic primary hematologic diseases associated with a thrombotic tendency: essential thrombocythemia, polycythemia vera, sickle cell anemia, and paroxysmal nocturnal hemoglobinuria. The surgical management of these disorders is discussed in this chapter under their individual headings. Several rare primary coagulation disorders are also associated with an increased risk of thromboembolism either as the primary or a predominant clinical manifestation: congenital dysfibrinogenemia,[24] antithrombin III deficiency,[25] and plasminogen deficiency. With the exception of congenital dysfibrinogenemia, these disorders all have a normal coagulation screen and require special assays for detection. Patients have also been described with elevated levels of Factor VIII[26, 27] or Factor V[28] where there appears to be a predisposition to thrombosis.

Unfortunately, none of the routine screening tests is useful in predicting the hypercoagulable state, although there are several specialized tests whose results are correlated with increased risk or presence of thromboembolism.[29]

POSTOPERATIVE HEMATOLOGIC COMPLICATIONS

Anemia

In the patient with normal preoperative hematologic values, a rapidly falling hemoglobin in the immediate postoperative period is generally due to blood loss or, rarely, hemolysis. Postoperative anemia may also in part be dilutional due to expansion of the blood volume by transfusion of colloid or crystalloid. Apart from the obvious causes, the importance of repeated phlebotomy for laboratory tests as a cause of postoperative anemia cannot be overemphasized.

The otherwise healthy patient responds to acute blood loss rapidly by releasing reticulocytes into the circulation. This reaction requires an adequate supply of marrow iron and a normal bone marrow. Any disorder of marrow structure such as tumor invasion, prior irradiation, or fibrosis will limit the capacity of the marrow to produce red cells. Azotemia, inflammation, or a poor nutritional state will also blunt the erythroid response to blood loss. Even the inflammatory effects of surgery may impair the hematopoietic response to anemia. In the normovolemic patient with an adequate nutritional status and no postoperative complications, anemia does not seem to impair wound healing. Therefore, it is wise to avoid transfusion and its attendant risks in such patients unless there are clinical indications for transfusion. Oral iron supplementation, however, may be given in the form of simple ferrous salts to the menstruating woman or the patient suspected to have low iron stores before surgery.

If blood loss is excluded, the rapid development of anemia should suggest hemolysis. Increased red cell destruction occurs in many conditions including hypersplenism, severe liver disease, disseminated intravascular coagulation, septicemias, and drug-related hemolysis. It is characterized by a normochromic, normocytic, or macrocytic anemia, with reticulocytosis and often spherocytosis. In uncomplicated cases, there is erythroid hyperplasia of the bone marrow. Hemolysis that is primarily extravascular (i.e., due to increased phagocytosis of red cells by the reticuloendothelial system) is also characterized by elevation of the indirect bilirubin and an increased excretion of urine urobilinogen. Intravascular hemolysis may lead initially to a fall in the serum haptoglobin and to the appearance of free plasma hemoglobin. The formation of methemalbumin and an elevation of the indirect bilirubin follows these events. If hemolysis is intravascular, hemoglobinuria and an eventual increase in urine hemosiderin occurs. These tests are not always abnormal or positive, especially when hemolysis is extravascular (reticuloendothelial), and the only manifestation may be a persistent anemia with an elevated reticulocyte count. The findings depend on the extent of the hemolysis, liver function (ability to clear unconjugated bilirubin), and the chronicity of the process.

Chronic infections may lead to bone marrow depression and slightly increased red cell destruction, but there are some infections in which marked hemolysis occurs. Infection of the postoperative patient with *Aspergillus*,[30] pneumococcus, *Escherichia coli*, *Hemophilus influenzae*, *Neisseria meningitidis*, *Salmonella*, *Streptococcus*,[31] and clostridia species[32] may cause such a picture. Clostridia may lead to a clinical syndrome of overwhelming intravascular hemolysis with hemoglobinuria, shock, and renal and hepatic failure. The hemolysis subsides with control of the underlying infectious process.

Medication-induced hemolytic anemias may evolve postoperatively via two different mechanisms. In the first category is the patient with a hereditary red cell enzyme deficiency or unstable hemoglobin who may develop rapid and severe hemolysis induced by certain medications. The second category consists of idiosyncratic drug-induced hemolytic anemias, which may occur through a variety of immune mechanisms. Perhaps the most important of the red cell enzyme deficiencies is deficiency of the hexosemonophosphate shunt enzyme, glucose-6-phosphate dehydrogenase (G-6-PD). Deficiency of this enzyme is sex-linked and occurs almost exclusively in males. The two most important variants are GdA, which is found in about 10 percent of American blacks, and Gd Mediterranean, which is found in Caucasians of Mediterranean ancestry. Patients with either form develop hemolysis when given oxidant drugs (Table 8). Patients with deficiency of G-6-PD may also hemolyze within a few days after onset of an infection,[33] especially with infectious hepatitis.[34] In the GdA-variant G-6-PD activity in young cells is normal but declines rapidly as the erythrocytes age. Consequently, hemolysis is limited to older red cells and the severity of the anemia is limited. The Mediterranean variant has low enzymatic levels in all red cells and can lead to severe and potentially fatal hemolysis. The diagnosis is made by the presence of Heinz bodies in red cells and by direct assay for G-6-PD. In patients with a past history of episodic or drug-induced hemolysis, an enzyme screen should be ordered prior to surgery.

Oxidant drugs can also precipitate a rare form of hemolytic anemia in which unstable hemoglobins form due to increased quantities of methemoglobin. Patients with this disorder may have pre-existing anemia, reticulocytosis, and splenomegaly. The hemoglobin electrophoretic pattern is usually normal, but the unstable hemoglobins may be identified by heat denaturation and isopropanol stability.

Drugs may also induce hemolytic anemia in otherwise normal postoperative patients by idiosyncratic immune mechanisms. In the "innocent bystander" reaction, an immune complex consisting of drug and antibody is adsorbed onto the red cell and the cell is lysed by complement-mediated mechanisms. The prototype drug for this mecha-

TABLE 8. Drugs Known to Cause Hemolysis in GC-6-PD Deficiency

Acetanilid	Potassium menaphthosulfate
Aspirin (mild hemolysis)	Primaquine
Chloramphenicol	Probenecid
Chloroquine (mild hemolysis)	Quinacrine
Dapsone	Quinidine
Furazolidone	Quinine
Menazodine	Quinocide
Methylene blue	Salicylazosulfapyridine
Nalidixic acid	Solapsone
Naphthalene	Sulfacetamide
Neoarsphenamine	Sulfamethoxypyridazine
Nitrofurantoin	Sulfanilamide
Nitrofurazone	Sulfapyridine
Pamaquin	Sulfisoxazole
Phenacetin	

nism is quinidine. Phenacetin, sulfonamides, isoniazid, indomethacin, and chlorpromazine can also produce hemolytic anemia by this mechanism. The direct antiglobulin test (Coombs) usually reveals complement components and immunoglobulin on the cell. In suspected cases, the drug should be stopped immediately.

In the second type of immune hemolysis, the drug is adsorbed onto the red cell membrane and forms a hapten, which together with the cell membrane induces antibody formation. The antibody in turn causes destruction of red cells that display the haptenic moiety. Penicillin in large doses and some cephalosporins can induce this form of hemolysis. The Coombs test is usually strongly positive, with IgG and occasionally complement on the red cells.

Finally, alpha-methyldopa produces a hemolytic anemia of gradual onset, usually over a period of months, with a positive direct Coombs due to an IgG coating of the cells. The presence of the drug is not required for hemolysis. About 1 percent of patients taking the drug for at least three months have laboratory evidence of hemolysis.[35] Hemolysis may take some time to abate once the drug is stopped and the Coombs test may remain positive for one month to two years. Drugs causing hemolytic anemia are listed in Table 2 and a more complete listing is found in a review by Garratty and Pete.[35]

Hemolytic anemia with red cell fragmentation may occur in patients who have had intracardiac surgery involving placement of prostheses. Although some evidence of hemolysis was present in the majority of patients in one large series,[36] only 5 percent had hemoglobin less than 10.5 gm/dl irrespective of iron therapy. Serum lactic dehydrogenase (LDH) and reticulocyte count elevations correlate well with the eventual development of anemia[37] and so should be monitored in all patients with cardiac prosthesis. Severe anemia may require reoperation; with milder forms, chronic oral iron therapy should be given.

Anemias associated with bone marrow depression are generally slow to develop and characterized by normochromic, normocytic red cells and by a decreased or inappropriately low reticulocyte count. In assessing whether there is a true reticulocytosis, we correct for the degree of anemia by multiplying the reticulocyte percentage by a ratio of the patient's hematocrit (or hemoglobin) to an average normal value. If this corrected reticulocyte percentage is the same as or below normal, it suggests that bone marrow suppression is a least partly responsible for the anemia.

Drug induced suppression of the bone marrow should be suspected if reticulocytopenia, anemia, and decreased erythroid precursors in the bone marrow coexist in the patient who is not seiously ill. If the index of suspicion is sufficiently high, the drug should be discontinued and an appropriate substitute found. If reticulocytosis begins within 10 days to 2 weeks, this is suggestive although not diagnostic of a drug-induced idiosyncratic reaction.

Chloramphenicol predictably causes a brief, reversible bone marrow suppression in most patients. This is accompanied by an increase in the serum iron, reticulocytopenia, and nuclear vacuolization of the erythroid cells in the bone marrow. The effect is directly related to the amount of drug and the length of exposure to the drug. This predictable reversible effect can not, however, be distinguished from idiosyncratic chloramphenicol-induced irreversible aplastic anemia whose incidence is about 1 in 25,000[94] in chloramphenicol treated patients. It is prudent to recommend that this drug be used only for certain serious illness where there is no effective alternative antimicrobial agent.

White Blood Cell Disorders

Severe neutropenia is an uncommon complication of surgery. Neutropenia may often accompany septicemia or fulminant infections and should resolve with appropriate treatment. When granulocytopenia occurs postoperatively in a previously healthy patient without severe infection or nutritional deficiency, drugs should always be suspected (see Table 2). Two basic mechanisms of drug-induced idiosyncratic agranulocytosis are known. One, associated with leukoagglutinins and a rapid onset, may develop soon after ingestion of a small amount of drug in a patient who has been sensitized by its prior administration. The classical example is aminopyrine, but similar cases of immune agranulocytosis have been ascribed to dipyrone, phenylbutazone, sulfonamides, chlorpropamide, chlorpromazine, and mercurial diuretics.[38] The second variety of agranulocytosis occurs several weeks after initiation of continuous treatment and is generally due to interference with granulocyte production in the bone marrow. Characteristic drugs in this class are thionamide antithyroid medications (propylthiouracil, methimazole, and carbimazole), phenothiazines (chlorpromazine, promazine, thioridazine, and prochlorperazine), phenylbutazone and oxyphenbutazone, phenytoin, certain antibiotics (cephalothin, sulfonamides, carbenicillin, ampicillin), cardiovascular agents (quinidine and procainamide), oral hypoglycemics drugs (chlorpropamide and tolbutamide), thiazide diuretics (chlorothiazide) and antihistamines (Pyribenzamine and cimetidine) (See Table 2).

When drug-induced agranulocytosis occurs, the suspected agent should be discontinued and the patient observed. Early recovery is usually heralded by a transient increase in absolute monocyte count, then by monocytosis.

In those patients in whom severe granulocytopenia develops, infection in closed spaces will often not lead to walled-off abscesses and pus. Indeed, pyelonephritis may not be associated with pyuria. The oral and rectal mucosa are particularly susceptible to invasion. Because of the increased susceptibility to infection, manipulations which might introduce bacteria should be kept to a minimum. If the use of intravenous catheters is necessary, the site should be examined daily for signs of infection and changed frequently. Surveillance cultures of the throat, sputum, urine, intravenous sites, and rectum are useful in helping to plan antibiotic therapy if fever develops. The role of isolation and gut sterilization in the prevention of infection in the neutropenic patient is controversial. We use oral trimethoprim–sulfamethoxazole if prolonged neutropenia is expected and gut sterilization only with colonic surgery.

If fever or hypotension without evidence of hypovolemia or blood loss occurs in the neutropenic patient, infection should be suspected. Treatment with cephalosporin and aminoglycoside antibiotics, with the addition of carbenicillin or ticarcillin if a colonic or rectal source is suspected, should be instituted. As soon as the infecting organism is identified and its antibiotic susceptibility known, antibiotic therapy should be adjusted accordingly. If fever and neutropenia persist, we recommend a full course of antibiotics even if cultures are negative. Treatment of *drug-induced* neutropenia with granulocyte transfusion is, for the majority of cases, unwarranted because there is usually rapid recovery once the causative drug is stopped. White cell transfusions should be reserved for the patient with overt sepsis in whom a prolonged period of agranulocytosis is expected, that is, when the bone marrow contains no granulocyte precursors (see section on Transfusion Therapy, below).

Postoperative granulocytosis in the range of 10,000 to 16,000 cells/μl is usual for the first 36 to 48 hours. If, however, granulocytosis persists for more than a week, an underlying cause should be sought. The most common causes are occult infection, bleeding, hematoma formation, or tissue necrosis. Corticosteroids and other drugs such as epinephrine and lithium may also cause leukocytosis. In addition, metabolic disorders such as azotemia, acidosis, anoxia, and hepatic necrosis can cause granulocytosis. Splenectomy predictably leads to a chronic increase in the granulocytes and platelets. If eosinophilia predominates postoperatively, a drug reaction or allergic disorder should be suspected.

Postoperative lymphocytosis may relate to viral infection. The postperfusion syndrome that occurs after cardiopulmonary bypass or multiple transfusions is caused by cytomegalovirus.[39,40] In addition to lymphocytosis, this syndrome is characterized by transient hepatosplenomegaly, abnormal liver function, and a negative heterophile test. The diagnosis is confirmed by a rise in the complement fixing antibodies to cytomegalovirus. No treatment is necessary.

Thrombocytosis

Postoperative thrombocytosis following surgery is not uncommon. Usually the thrombocytosis (defined as a platelet count in excess of 350,000 cells/μl) is modest and part of the acute phase reaction associated with inflammation. Occasionally persistent blood loss, hemolysis, or leukocytosis may be associated with thrombocytosis. This laboratory finding is of no clinical consequence and requires no therapy.

The spleen is the primary organ involved in the clearance of platelets from the blood. Normally, platelet production by the marrow is balanced by platelet destruction within the spleen, yielding a constant level of circulating platelets. Thrombocytosis characteristically occurs immediately after splenectomy, peaking between the third and fifth postoperative day. Typically, the platelet count reaches 600,000 to 800,000 cells/μl but may rise in excess of 1,000,000 before reequilibrating at a level below 500,000. Although thrombocytosis can be associated with a thrombotic tendency, there is no evidence that the transient thrombocytosis observed after splenectomy carries a risk directly related to the magnitude of thrombocytosis. In otherwise healthy patients without myeloproliferative disorders, postsplenectomy thrombocytosis does not require antiplatelet therapy.

Postoperative Bleeding

Postoperative hemorrhagic complications are among the most serious surgical management problems directly related to hematology. Bleeding from the surgical wound may be due to either acquired or congential defects in hemostasis or to problems of surgical technique. The distinction between a hemostatic defect and problem of surgical technique may be both difficult and important. The diagnosis of hemorrhage related to surgical technique is a diagnosis of exclusion. Abnormalities of hemostasis should be considered before a decision is made to re-explore the surgical site. As might be suspected, surgery in the hemorrhaging patient with an acquired disorder such as intravascular coagulation can have fatal consequences and must be avoided.

In an urgent situation, several facts should be rapidly established: Has this patient ever had a hemorrhagic syndrome or any abnormalities of preoperative testing? Has this patient been treated with drugs capable of aggravating a bleeding tendency? This information should have been obtained, of course, during the preoperative evaluation. Next, firsthand information must be obtained from the surgeon and anesthesiologist. If the problem is noted during the operation, the consultant should be present in the operating room. He should obtain a clear image of its magnitude and should note personally the nature of the surgery, any technical difficulties, unusual complications, and the number of units of blood or blood products that have been given. A coagulation screen (prothrombin time, partial thromboplastin time, thrombin time, fibrinogen level, platelet count, and bleeding time) should be obtained. Since hemolytic transfusion reaction can cause intravascular coagulation (see below), the consultant should request a review of the transfused blood. The site of bleeding is often an important clue to the etiology of bleeding. If the patient is bleeding from all mucosal surfaces, venepuncture sites, as well as the surgical wound, disseminated intravascular coagulation should be suspected. Bleeding from drains within the wound is more likely to represent a surgical problem or a congenital deficiency of a particular clotting protein.

If the preoperative coagulation evaluation has been normal, any underlying hemostatic defect must have been acquired intraoperatively. Nevertheless, the possibility of laboratory error should be borne in mind before exclusion of a congenital hemorrhagic disease. Coagulation studies should be performed as rapidly as possible. Blood should always be obtained by venipuncture. Although central venous lines or arterial lines are enticing, these lines are often anticoagulated with heparin. Despite vigorous flushing, heparin bound to the walls of the tubing may contaminate blood samples and artifactually alter the coagulation studies. Coagulation studies of immediate interest include the prothrombin time, partial thromboplastin time, bleeding time, thrombin time, and platelet count. If available, quantitation of the fibrin split products and the fibrinogen level are also helpful. If heparin has been used intraoperatively, the conversion of fibrin to fibrinogen may still be assessed by ordering a Reptilase time. It will not be affected by heparin but will be sensitive to a low fibrinogen level and fibrin split products.

DISSEMINATED INTRAVASCULAR COAGULATION

Disseminated intravascular coagulation (DIC) is a complex hemorrhagic syndrome in which the normal regulatory mechanisms of hemostasis which localize and control clot and platelet plug formation are overwhelmed by activation of the plasma coagulant proteins. Severe intravascular coagulation is often fatal and is characterized clinically by marked ecchymoses and purpura (purpura fulminans), spontaneous bleeding from venepuncture sites, hematuria, mucosal bleeding (gastrointestinal, vaginal, oral, nasal), and wound hemorrhage. Occasionally, thrombotic manifestations can also be observed, for example, on the distal appendages.

In less serious cases, disseminated intravascular coagulation may be manifested by bleeding in the surgical wound alone or only by abnormalities of in vivo laboratory studies. These laboratory tests are useful in defining the presence and magnitude of intravascular coagulation. The pathophysiology of intravascular coagulation is reasonably well understood and the characteristic abnormalities of the tests reflect this pathophysiology. Intravascular coagulation is associated with the activation, consumption, and depletion of the plasma components of the coagulation system. Therefore, the prothrombin time and partial thromboplastin time are prolonged and the plasma fibrinogen concentration is reduced. This syndrome is also associated with the activation of the fibrinolytic pathways which also contributes to the depletion of the fibrinogen. This does not automatically mean that the fibrinogen level will be below normal, since many surgical patients start with an elevated fibrinogen level preoperatively. However, invariably the fibrinogen level will drop compared to the preoperative value if disseminated intravascular consumption is present. The action of plasmin on fibrinogen yields fibrin degradation products, which can be detected in increased concentration in the plasma. The fibrin degradation products are helpful in documenting the existence of increased fibrinolysis although low levels of split products (< 40 μg/ml) may occur with routine surgery. The fibrin split products can be measured directly. Alternatively, a prolongation of the thrombin time correlates with an elevation of fibrin split products in excess of 60 μg/ml. However, other causes of a prolonged thrombin time, including circulating heparin, low fibrinogen levels, or dysfibrinogenemia, must be first excluded. Consumption of platelets yields thrombocytopenia, another classic laboratory manifestation of intravascular coagulation. Lastly, fragmented red cells may be observed in the peripheral blood smear of about 30 percent of patients with intravascular coagulation. These fragmented cells are the result of microangiopathic changes in the vasculature caused by fibrin deposition.

In summary, the minimum diagnostic criteria for disseminated intravascular coagulation include: (1) a coagulation disorder manifested by a prolonged prothrombin and partial thromboplastin time, (2) thrombocytopenia or abrupt drop in platelet count with adequate megakaryocytes in the marrow, and (3) abnormal fibrinolytic screening studies (e.g., prolonged thrombin time, elevated fibrin split products).

The treatment of intravascular coagulation is controversial. Therapeutic options have included heparin, fibrinogen, fresh frozen plasma, ϵ-aminocaproic acid, and exchange transfusion. One salient guiding principle, however, is not controversial: *specific therapy should be directed at the underlying cause of the disseminated intravascular coagulation.* As a practical matter, DIC is *always* secondary to some underlying disturbance (Table 9). Intravascular coagulation secondary to sepsis and endotoxemia must be treated aggressively with the appropriate parenteral antibiotics. Intravascular coagulation due to a placental abruption or a retained dead fetus must be managed by delivery of the fetus.

In head injury with brain tissue destruction, defibrination commonly occurs acutely and returns toward normal after several hours. This is a critical period for the potentially

TABLE 9. Disorders Associated with Diffuse Intravascular Coagulation

1. Obstetric complications
   a. Septic abortion
   b. Abruptio placentae
   c. Amniotic fluid embolism
   d. Retained dead fetus
   e. Hypertonic saline abortion
   f. Hydatidiform mole
   g. Abdominal pregnancy
   h. Toxemia of pregnancy
2. Infections
   a. Viral (disseminated herpes, influenza A)
   b. Rickettsial (Rocky Mountain spotted fever)
   c. Bacterial: meningococcemia and other gram negative organisms, pneumococcal septicemia, rarely staphlococcal or streptococcal infections
   d. Protozoa: Falciparum malaria
3. Malignancy
   a. Metastatic carcinoma (prostate, pancreas, lung)
   b. Leukemia (acute promyelocytic)
4. Tissue damage
   a. Brain tissue destruction
   b. Massive trauma, crush injury
   c. Heatstroke
   d. Burns with infection
5. Hemolytic transfusion reaction
6. Acute systemic vasculitis
7. Extracorporeal circulation
8. Arterial aneurysms
9. Giant hemangiomas
10. Cardiac arrest
11. Snakebite
12. Hypothermia
13. Anaphylaxis
14. Acute pancreatitis

salvageable patient with brain injury where maintenance of adequate hemostasis is of prime import. Thus Goodnight and associates[41] have stressed the need to screen all such patients for DIC. While awaiting the results of the laboratory tests, cryoprecipitate (12 U), fresh frozen plasma (2 to 4 U), and platelet concentrates should be administered.

We recommend that management of DIC be treated in a rational, practical manner. Patients should be given blood components with three goals in mind: (1) maintenance of oxygen carrying ability, (2) maintenance of blood pressure and intravascular volume, (3) repletion of blood coagulation proteins and platelets. Packed red blood cells, fresh frozen plasma, and platelets should be transfused in sufficient quantities to partially or completely correct these deficiency states. "Feeding of the fire" by plasma or platelet transfusion has been overemphasized and, in our opinion, this consideration is clinically unimportant. The degree of anemia and the extent of coagulopathy should be monitored regularly by determining the prothrombin time, the partial thromboplastin time, the fibrinogen level, the fibrin split products, and the platelet count.

Occasionally, thrombotic complications of intravascular coagulation predominate.[42]

Purpura fulminans, gangrene of the distal appendages, and acute renal failure are the hallmarks of this clinical syndrome. In this situation, systemic anticoagulation with heparin is indicated, despite concomittant hemorrhage, to minimize ischemia and infarction due to large and small vessel occlusion. Other therapeutic agents are widely used in the treatment of intravascular coagulation, but clinical evidence to support their continued use is lacking. Specifically, ϵ-aminocaproic acid carries significant risk of promoting systemic thrombosis. Therefore, it should be avoided. Fibrinogen concentrates have also been employed to correct hypofibrinogenemic states. However, these concentrates were prepared commercially from over 400 U of plasma and carried a high risk of transmission of post-transfusion hepatitis. They have been withdrawn from the market. If specific fibrinogen therapy is indicated, cryoprecipitate should be used.

THROMBOCYTOPENIA

Postoperative thrombocytopenia is uncommon, since thrombocytosis is the general response to surgery. However in the absence of a platelet functional defect, abnormal bleeding is generally not encountered if the platelet count is above 100,000/μl. Postoperative thrombocytopenia may occur if the patient has had transfusion of large quantities of platelet-poor packed cells without platelet replacement. Operations involving extracorporeal perfusion are regularly associated with thrombocytopenia and perhaps platelet dysfunction.[43] Presumably platelets are damaged and form microaggregates in the perfusion apparatus. As with the development of any cytopenia, drugs should be suspected as a cause of thrombocytopenia (Table 2). Thrombocytopenia is also one of the hallmarks of disseminated intravascular coagulation. Marrow depression due to inflammation and rapid clearance of IgG-coated platelets in septicemia also cause thrombocytopenia.[44] A rare cause of immune thrombocytopenia, post-transfusion purpura, occurs five to six days after platelet or blood transfusion. This can be severe and persist for several weeks. Therapy with exchange transfusion[45] or intensive plasmaphoresis[46] has been successful in several cases.

PLATELET DYSFUNCTION

Bleeding in the postoperative period may be due to an acquired abnormality in platelet function. This is reflected in a prolongation of the bleeding time. Platelet dysfunction is most commonly secondary to the treatment of the patient with a medication (Table 1). Abnormalities of platelet function as well as a reduction in the platelet count may also accompany cardiopulmonary bypass.[43] Therefore, even if the platelet count is in the normal range, the bypass patient with bleeding and a prolonged bleeding time in the absence of other coagulation abnormalities should receive platelet transfusions.

The patient with significant renal dysfunction often requires invasive procedures or major surgery. Uremia is commonly associated with a hemorrhagic tendency characterized by a prolonged bleeding time and platelet dysfunction. Clinical response of the bleeding, uremic patient to either dialysis or platelet transfusion may be disappointing. A recent report suggests that improvement in hemostasis may be achieved in the uremic patient with severe bleeding by the infusion of cyroprecipitate.[47]

COAGULOPATHIES

Given a normal preoperative coagulation screen (prothrombin time and PTT), an isolated acquired coagulation abnormality with bleeding in the postoperative period is unusual. However, occasionally a mild hemophilia with factor levels in the 20 to 30 percent range will be missed by the routine screening tests. With extensive surgery and plasma dilution with crystalloid, the level of the deficient factor may fall below a critical point and bleeding ensues. Once the possibility that the patient may have a congenital coagulation disorder is considered, the diagnosis is relatively straightforward. Treatment of the hemophiliac is discussed later in this chapter.

Borderline preoperative liver dysfunction or acquired perioperative hepatic injury may result in multiple abnormalities in coagulation and bleeding. Initially there is a prolongation of the prothrombin time due to a decrease in the vitamin K dependent blood clotting proteins. With more severe disease deficiencies in Factor V and fibrinogen also occur. This may be difficult to distinguish from intravascular coagulation. Treatment is with fresh frozen plasma and platelet concentrates if thrombocytopenia is present.

More subtle is the development of vitamin K deficiency in the postoperative patient who is on broad spectrum antibiotic therapy or who is eating a marginal diet. This results in a gradual prolongation of the prothrombin time. The development of vitamin K deficiency can be prevented and treated in this group with small (1 to 2 mg) subcutaneous doses of vitamin K.

BLEEDING WITH ANTITHROMBOTIC THERAPY

Bleeding is the major complication of antithrombotic therapy. The risk of bleeding during standard heparin therapy may be minimized by (1) giving the heparin by continuous infusion, (2) daily monitoring of an in vitro test such as the PTT, (3) avoiding aspirin and other drugs that interfere with platelet function, and (4) avoiding intravascular injections and invasive procedures such as paracentesis, arterial puncture, lumbar puncture, thoracocentesis, and vascular cut downs. Even if these directives are followed, hemorrhagic complications occur.[48]

In the case of uncontrolled hemorrhage, the most rapid means of reversing the effect of heparin is by protamine sulfate neutralization. Protamine is strongly basic protein which binds to heparin and inactivates it. In fact, 1 mg of protamine sulfate neutralizes approximately 100 U of heparin. The half-life of intravenous heparin is 60 minutes; 30 minutes after a dose of intravenous heparin, only about 0.5 mg of protamine is required to antagonize each 100 U injected. One may calculate the dose of protamine needed if the time of administration of the intravenous bolus of heparin is known. With continuous infusion of heparin, the heparin level is generally between 0.2 to 0.3 U/ml (PTT 1.5 to 2 times control) and the neutralizing dose can be calculated from an estimation of the patient's plasma volume and the time the heparin was discontinued. With subcutaneous injection of heparin, the protamine should be given in a dose to neutralize approximately 50 percent of the last heparin dose. In all cases, care should be taken to administer the protamine sulfate slowly over a 10 to 30 minute period to avoid a hypotensive response. Seldom should a single dose of more than 50 mg of protamine have to be used. Treatment with protamine may, however, have to be repeated when counteracting the effect of subcutaneous heparin since protamine is cleared from the blood more quickly than heparin.

One cause of bleeding during heparin therapy is heparin-associated thrombocytopenia. This complication probably occurs in about 5 percent of the patients on heparin anywhere from 2 to 14 days after the initiation of therapy. It is more frequent with the beef lung preparations.[49] Occasionally, this thrombocytopenia is associated with a syndrome of multiple arterial emboli,[50] a complication that has significant morbidity and mortality. Since there is no way to predict which patients will develop thrombocytopenia, all patients on heparin therapy should have their platelet counts monitored frequently. If thrombocytopenia develops, an immediate search should be made for an underlying cause such as sepsis or drugs other than heparin. If heparin induced thrombocytopenia is suspected, the heparin should be discontinued immediately and oral anticoagulants begun. Dextran may be used to achieve anticoagulation for the first several days until the effect of oral anticoagulants is in the therapeutic range.

Anticoagulation with oral anticoagulants, the vitamin K antagonists, is also associated with an increased risk of bleeding. This can be minimized by adjusting the dose so that the patient's prothrombin time is in the therapeutic range, by avoiding unnecessary invasive procedures, and by avoiding the many drugs which interact pharmacologically with the warfarin-like anticoagulants (Table 3).

Patients who bleed during oral anticoagulant therapy when their prothrombin time is in therapeutic range generally have an underlying anatomic lesion or additional risk factor. Bleeding may occur at sites of recent surgery or trauma. With excessive anticoagulation, bleeding may occur in unusual locations: the retroperitoneal space, the corpus luteum, the gut wall, the pancreas, the joints, and the adrenals. Bleeding into this last site is associated with a high mortality. Intracerebral hemorrhage can occasionally occur, especially if the patient is hypertensive or has had a recent cerebral infarct.

If major bleeding occurs during oral anticoagulant therapy, the therapy should be discontinued and either vitamin K or fresh frozen plasma or both should be given. Treatment with vitamin K alone (5 to 10 mg) given either subcutaneously or by *slow* intravenous infusion should reverse the anticoagulant effect in six to twelve hours in patients with normal hepatic function. Large doses of vitamin K (25 mg) render the patient refractory to treatment with warfarin-like anticoagulants for as much as two weeks. Small doses of vitamin K (1 to 2 mg) or omitting several days of anticoagulant therapy might be used to control minor bleeding when the prothrombin time is beyond the therapeutic range. For further details on bleeding with antithrombotic therapy see the review by Kelton and Hirsh.[51]

Thrombolytic Therapy

Streptokinase and urokinase are two agents used for treatment of massive pulmonary emboli, submassive emboli with shock, extensive deep vein thrombosis (streptokinase only) and arteriovenous-cannula occlusion. These agents are effective only for thrombi having occurred within the last 10 days. One of the contraindications to thrombolytic therapy is a recent surgical procedure, including thoracentesis, paracentesis, invasive biopsy, and intra-arterial diagnostic procedure. Therapy is evaluated by the thrombin time. For further details see the review by Bell and Meeks[52] and the results of the National Institutes of Health conference.[53]

SURGICAL MANAGEMENT OF PATIENTS WITH HEMATOLOGIC DISORDERS

Disorders of the Red Cell and Heme Metabolism

SICKLE CELL ANEMIA

Sickle cell anemia is a disease associated with a hereditary abnormality of hemoglobin structure. Deoxyhemoglobin polymerizes and precipitates intracellularly, causing a chronic hemolytic anemia and painful vascular occlusive crises due to stasis and ischemia. Leukocytosis and thrombosis is common during a crisis, which is usually characterized by increased hemolysis and painful infarcts. Due to repeated splenic infarcts, the spleen is usually small and atrophic. The complications of sickle cell disease are many and include an increased incidence of infection (especially pneumococcal pneumonia and salmonellal osteomyelitis), gallstones and cholecystitis, cerebral vascular accidents, serum hepatitis in those who have had multiple transfusions, hematuria and renal infarcts, priapism, chronic ankle ulcers, and narcotic addiction.

The typical vaso-occlusive crisis is accompanied by pain, tachycardia, leukocytosis, and sometimes by fever and ileus. It is often difficult to distinguish such a crisis from an acute surgical abdomen. Initial treatment should be conservative and aimed at reversing those factors which lead to sickling, that is, acidosis, dehydration, and hypoxemia. Thus, the patient should receive oxygen and vigorous rehydration with alkalinization. Transfusion of packed red cells may be required. Infection is often a cause of sickle crisis and it must be excluded in every patient. Analgesics should be administered to relieve the pain. Persistent symptoms, shaking chills, leukocytosis of greater than 30,000/mm^3 and pain that differs from the patient's usual "crisis" pain are indications that the episode may be more than a vaso-occlusive crisis. A low or normal leukocyte alkaline phosphatase (LAP) would argue for a vaso-occlusive crisis; a high LAP is not helpful in distinguishing infection from crisis. Left upper quadrant pain may be due to splenic infarction or left lower lobe pneumonia. Right upper quadrant pain with fever and jaundice may indicate vaso-occlusive crisis, acute cholecystitis or liver abscess. The presence of radio-opaque stones in the right upper quandrant is not diagnostic of cholecystitis because many patients with chronic hemolytic anemia have asymptomatic gallstones. Appendicitis must be suspected when there is persistent localized right lower quadrant tenderness.

Patients with sickle cell anemia develop certain complications that often require elective surgery, such as aseptic necrosis of the hip and cholecystitis. Preoperative measures must be taken to prevent the development of intraoperative and postoperative vaso-occlusive crisis. A general method that involves exchange transfusion and hypertransfusion therapy is often employed. The goal of this treatment is to replace greater than 75 percent of the patient's red cells by transfused normal erythrocytes. Four to six weeks before surgery, 1 or 2 U of whole blood are removed from the patient and replaced with 2 to 4 U of packed normal red blood cells. With repeated infusion of packed red cells, the hemoglobin is raised from the usual 6 to 8 gm/dl to greater than 12 gm/dl. At these hemoglobin levels, production of red cells containing the abnormal sickle hemoglobin will cease and the reticulocyte count will approach zero. Continued infusion of packed red cells once or twice weekly will replace circulating red cells whose in vivo survival is diminished. The success of replacement can be evaluated by quantitative hemoglobin electrophoresis. Hypertransfusion therapy may be continued for several weeks postoperatively and then discontinued.

These procedures may be undertaken rapidly in the face of emergency surgery, and aggressive exchange transfusion may prove useful in such instances. Careful anesthesia and maintenance of a well-oxygenated state are mandatory, as is meticulous fluid balance. Sickle cell cardiomyopathy may lead to heart failure, so the cardiac status must be carefully monitored. Angiography before and during surgery must be done cautiously because hypertonic contrast media may induce sickling in partially deoxygenated red cells.[54] Since hyposthenuria is characteristic of both sickle cell disease and sickle cell trait,[55] assessment of urine flow and specific gravity may be misleading. If large volumes of intravenous fluids are used, they should contain sodium and potassium. As with all chronic hemolytic states, patients with sickle cell disease should take 1 mg of supplemental folic acid daily. Because these patients are functionally asplenic, they should also receive penumococcal vaccine several weeks before surgery to prevent overwhelming pneumococcal sepsis.

Surgery in the patient with sickle cell trait is a more difficult question. In the past, it was assumed that the risk of anesthesia is not increased in these patients. This is probably the case in uncomplicated surgery, but when severe hypoxia is anticipated intraoperatively or when total vascular occlusion is required, exchange transfusion may be warranted.[56]

CHRONIC HEMOLYTIC DISEASE

There is an increased incidence of cholelithiasis in patients with chronic hemolytic disease because of the increased load of bile pigment. Transfusion in these patients often does not achieve the desired increment in blood counts, either because of immune destruction of transfused cells or hypersplenism, or both. Patients receiving chronic corticosteroid therapy for immune hemolytic anemias should be treated preoperatively with an increased steroid dose in a manner analogous to patients with adrenal insufficiency (see Chapter 5, Endocrinology). In addition, surgery may stress an already hyperactive marrow, and supplementation with folic acid is therefore recommended preoperatively and postoperatively.

If a patient with hereditary spherocytosis or autoimmune hemolytic anemia has had previous attacks of cholelithiasis or if gallstones are present, combining splenectomy and cholecystectomy should be considered. Similarly, in the patient with chronic hemolytic disease in whom a cholecystectomy is indicated, a combined cholecystectomy-splenectomy should be considered if the spleen is still present. After splenectomy certain hematologic changes occur, such as an occasional nucleated red cell, pitted and bizarre shaped erythrocytes, Howell-Jolly bodies, and increased leukocyte and platelet counts. Although there seems to be no added risk of deep venous thrombosis associated with postsplenectomy thrombocytosis, early mobilization, the wearing of stockings, and leg exercises are recommended. Prophylactic subcutaneous heparin may be considered.

THALASSEMIA

Until a decade ago, only rare patients with homozygous thalassemia (thalassemia major or Cooley's anemia) survived into their late teens and twenties. With more aggressive transfusion regimens and chelation therapy for the inevitable iron overload, more of these patients now come to surgical attention as adults than previously. Although aggressive transfusion therapy may help prevent hypersplenism, splenectomy is indicated if the transfusion requirements increase remarkably or if clinically significant thrombocytopenia develops due to hypersplenism. In addition, a very large spleen may cause discomfort, early satiety, or urinary frequency due to compression of the bladder. The patient should be prepared for splenectomy by transfusion to a hemoglobin of approximately 8 to 10 gm/dl. The operation is generally safe and postoperatively transfusion requirements may decrease.[57] Serious postoperative infection may be averted by giving prophylactic penicillin, 250 mg daily, after splenectomy and by follow-up immunization with pneumococcal vaccine. As with other patients with hemolytic anemia, postoperative leukocytosis and thrombocytosis is common. In addition there will be many more nucleated red cells and pitted and bizarre shaped erythrocytes than prior to splenectomy.

Striking intra-abdominal lymphadenopathy due to extramedullary erythropoietic tissue may occur in thalassemia major.[58] As with other patients with chronic hemolysis, patients with thalassemia may also develop gallstones; one study reported an incidence of about 25 percent.[59] Extrabiliary obstruction due to lymph nodes containing extramedullary erythropoietic tissue may cause obstructive jaundice as well as cholelithiasis.[58] Other complications of thalassemia major include diabetes, cardiomyopathy, and hypopituitarism from iron overload. Hypopituitarism is so common in patients with long-standing disease that all patients should have a full evaluation of pituitary function. If this has not been performed and the patient needs emergency surgery, steroid coverage should be given (see Chapter 5, Endocrinology).

POLYCYTHEMIA RUBRA VERA

Polycythemia rubra vera is a myeloproliferative disorder characterized by an increased red cell mass, thrombocytosis, leukocytosis, and splenomegaly. Abnormal platelet function is often present in polycythemia vera and may cause a bleeding tendency. Patients with this disease may therefore require platelet transfusion before surgery, despite the presence of normal numbers of circulating platelets. Other patients may have a thrombotic tendency, especially when thrombocytosis is marked.

The risk of surgery in polycythemia rubra vera can be considerable.[60,61] Wasserman found that more than 75 percent of the patients with *uncontrolled* polycythemia rubra vera who underwent surgery developed hemorrhagic or thrombotic complications and one-third died as a result.[61] Therefore, phlebotomy with removal of 350 to 500 ml of blood every other day until the hematocrit is 45 ml/dl is recommended in patients with polycythemia rubra vera before elective surgery. Control of both the platelet count and the red cell mass with chemotherapy should be attempted before elective surgery in patients with platelet counts over one million. Caution should be utilized in prescribing aspirin, heparin, or vitamin K antagonists (e.g., warfarin). Patients with enlarged livers and hepatic extramedullary hematopoiesis may be especially sensitive to warfarin.

Splenectomy is often considered in the later phase of polycythemia rubra vera. The usual indications relate to recurrent splenic infarction, hypersplenism with thrombocytopenia and leukopenia, portal hypertension from splenomegaly with varices, or pain and dysphagia due to splenomegaly. The best candidates for splenectomy seem to be those with adequate marrow function and low or normal platelet counts. Platelet counts may rise dramatically following splenectomy, with ensuing thrombotic or hemorrhagic complications. Antiplatelet drugs, such as aspirin or dipyridamole, may prove useful if the platelet count exceeds one million.

PORPHYRIAS

The porphyrias are a group of rare disorders, primarily congenital, of disturbed heme synthesis characterized by greatly increased formation, accumulation, and excretion of porphyrins and/or porphyrin precursors. Congenital erythropoietic porphyria and erythropoietic protoporphyria are rare disorders characterized by dermal sensitivity to light leading to skin lesions and, in erythropoietic porphyria, hemolytic anemia. Porphyrea cutanea tarda begins late in life and is often associated with liver disease and alcoholism. It is aggravated by alcohol and estrogens; phlebotomy often improves both the biochemical and symptomatic manifestations.

The most important disorder of this group in terms of surgical management is acute intermittent porphyria (AIP). This disease is inherited as an autosomal dominant trait, so there is often a family history. Although the basic abnormality in heme synthesis persists throughout life, attacks are intermittent and may not appear until later in life.[62] The commonest clinical picture is that of acute abdominal pain, constipation, vomiting, and abdominal distension secondary to autonomic neuropathy. In severe attacks there are tachycardia, postural hypotension, slight fever, and leukocytosis. Thus, it may be difficult to distinguish acute intermittent porphyrea from a surgical abdomen. Family history, previous attacks with or without negative exploratory laparotomy, and the association of attacks with certain drugs (Table 10) should raise suspicion of AIP. AIP is easily screened for using the Watson-Schwartz test for urobilinogen. A normal color of the urine should not be taken as evidence against AIP, even though in a typical attack the urine is often brownish. Quantitation of delta amino levulinic and porphobilinogen excretion will confirm the diagnosis.

If surgery is indicated, cyclopropane induction, with ether or ketamine anesthesia is recommended.[63] Postoperatively and in the treatment of the acute attack, high carbohydrate and protein intake have been recommended.[62] Hyponatremia and hypomagnesmia with inappropriate secretion of antidiuretic hormone[64] have also been reported during acute attacks and free water intake may need to be restricted.

TABLE 10. Drugs Potentially Dangerous for Individuals with Acute Intermittent Porphyria

Alcohol	Methyl chloride
Ally barbiturates	Methyprylon
Aminopyrine	Pentobarbital
Arsenic	Phensuximide
Cyclobarbital	Phenobarbital
Ergot preparations	Phenytoin
Glutethimide	Progesterone
Griseofulvin	Pyrazinamide
Hexachlorobenzene	Sedormid (Apronalide)
Lead	Sodium thiopental
Megimide	Sulfonal
Meprobamate	Sulfonamides
Mephenytoin	Tolbutamide
Methsuximide	Trional

PAROXYSMAL NOCTURNAL HEMOGLOBINURIA

Paroxysmal nocturnal hemoglobinuria (PNH) is a rare disease in which red cells as well as the platelets and granulocytes are abnormally sensitive to the lytic actions of serum complement. The diagnosis of PNH depends on the demonstration of complement sensitive red cells, either with the Ham test or the sucrose lysis test. There is also abnormal hematopoiesis with deficient and defective production of all three bone marrow elements. The clinical manifestations of PNH are varied. Most commonly there is chronic hemolysis with persistent hemosiderinuria and concomittent iron deficiency. Classically, but occuring in less than 25 percent of the patients, there is acute hemolysis with hemoglobinuria occuring primarily at night. In addition, these patients may develop cytopenias of any hematopoietic line. The patients are also prone to thromboses, especially of the hepatic vein, portal vein, splenic vein, and the intracerebral venous system. These complications are especially likely to occur during abdominal surgery. In addition, patients with PNH may present with severe abdominal or back pain mimicking an acute abdomen, most often prior to an episode of hemolysis.[65] There may be tenderness with rebound and diminished bowel sounds, rarely with marked guarding. Since these attacks are often recurrent, it is helpful to ask the patient whether the present pain differs from that of other attacks in order to exclude other causes of abdominal pain. These patients may also have esophageal spasm with retrosternal fullness and difficulty in swallowing.

White Blood Cell Disorders

ACUTE LEUKEMIA

The surgical management of the patient with acute leukemia is tempered by the prognosis and the hematologic status of the patient. Acute lymphocytic leukemia in children has an excellent chance of a lengthy remission or even cure. By contrast, acute myelogenous leukemia is invariably fatal. The average patient with this disease lives for about 18 months, although an increasing proportion may survive more than three years. The decision for *elective* surgery in these two forms of leukemia may, therefore, be different. The child with acute lymphocytic leukemia in complete remission should, in the absence of complications, be managed like any other patient. But unnecessary hospitalization for the adult with acute myelogenous leukemia, even if in full remission, should be avoided.

Patients with either form of acute leukemia may develop indications for urgent surgical procedures. Diagnostic lung biopsy and drainage of abscesses are probably the most common. Of course, surgery may be required as treatment for disorders unrelated and incidental to leukemia. Patients in complete remission usually have a few unique surgical problems. If these patients are on maintenance chemotherapy protocols, consideration may be given to postponement of chemotherapy until several weeks postoperatively in order to minimize the infectious and hemorrhagic complications of bone marrow suppression. Furthermore, wound healing will proceed more rapidly in the absence of cytotoxic therapy.

Surgery in patients with untreated or partially treated leukemia or acute leukemia in relapse has a high operative risk. These patients are very susceptible to infection because of low granulocyte counts and should be treated like patients with neutropenia with regard to surveillance cultures, monitoring of intravenous lines, and avoidance of unnecessary intravenous or urinary catheters. If the total granulocyte count is below $500/mm^3$, infection as a result of surgery may have fatal consequences.[66] Granulocyte transfusions may offer temporary support of the severely leukopenic patient. If granulocyte transfusions are administered, they should be continued for at least four days and each transfusion should contain at least 10^{10} cells.[67]

Thrombocytopenia, another hallmark of acute leukemia, will predictably lead to hemorrhagic complications during surgery. Platelets should be transfused preoperatively, and the platelet count maintained in excess of 80,000 to $100,000/mm^3$ for at least three or four days after the operation. Although postoperative bleeding is most often secondary to thrombocytopenia, intravascular coagulation or defective synthesis of blood coagulation factors due to therapy (e.g., L-asparaginase) may also cause a hemorrhagic syndrome. Because the risk of fatal complications is so high in the acute leukemia patient, the potential benefits and risks of surgery must be weighed carefully in each individual case. Invariably, the least complicated surgical procedure is usually chosen, if surgical therapy is indicated. For example, perirectal abscesses are treated by drainage and not by excision. Mild gastrointestinal bleeding is common during the period of thrombocytopenia and should not be evaluated unless it causes frank melena or hematochezia and is unresponsive to platelet transfusion up to platelet count of $50,000/mm.^3$ Similarly, acute abdominal pain may arise from hemorrhage into the wall of the gut or the abdominal wall or a retroperitoneal hematoma. Bowel and stomach infiltrates may occur in acute leukemia and they are often portals of entry for infection by intestinal bacteria; nodular leukemic lesions, though uncommon, may lead to intussuception and obstruction.[68,69] Treatment in these cases is conservative decompression and antileukemic therapy. In addition, a syndrome of pseudoacute abdomen (Table 11) has been described both in acute lymphoblastic leukemia and acute myeloblastic leukemia. These patients had signs and symptoms suggesting intestinal obstruction with perfora-

TABLE 11. Hematologic Conditions Which May Mimic an Acute Surgical Abdomen

Sickle cell crisis
Splenic infarct in patient with large spleen
Porphyria
Bleeding into the gut wall in congenital coagulation disorder
Paroxysmal nocturnal hemoglobinuria
Acute leukemia

tion and peritonitis, but at operation or autopsy no perforation was demonstrated.[69] While these considerations obscure the diagnosis of an acute abdomen, new techniques, particularly fiberoptic bronchoscopy with biopsy, have been useful diagnostically in patients with hematologic malignancy, fever, and pulmonary infiltrates of unknown etiology. With platelet transfusions, complications were minimal.[70]

Patients with acute leukemia, and especially those on cytolytic therapy, may require allopurinol before and after the operative procedure. An adequate urine flow must be maintained to prevent uric acid nephropathy. Hypocalcemia, hypomagnesemia, and lactic acidosis are sometimes complications of leukemia or aggressive cytolytic therapy. No intramuscular injections should be given and no enemas or rectal temperatures should be ordered. Peripheral intravenous lines should be inspected and changed frequently.

Prophylactic intravenous antibiotic therapy is unwarranted. However, oral trimethoprim–sulfamethoxazole (320 mg trimethoprim and 1600 mg sulfamethoxazole daily, i.e., 2 tablets twice daily) has been shown to significantly reduce the number of bacteremic episodes and febrile days in the hospitalized granulocytopenic patient.[71,72] Furthermore, this regimen is well tolerated and easily administered. With fever in excess of 38.5°C, broad spectrum antibiotics, generally a cephalosporin and aminoglycoside with or without carbenicillin or ticarcillin, are recommended after appropriate diagnostic tests. This treatment should be maintained until culture results are available and more specific antibiotic therapy can be chosen. With negative cultures but a fever that is responsive to therapy, a full course of therapy is indicated.

CHRONIC LYMPHOCYTIC LEUKEMIA

Chronic lymphocytic leukemia (CLL) is a common form of leukemia seen usually in patients over 60 years of age. The early stages of the disease may manifest only a peripheral blood lymphocytosis. These patients, in general, present no increased surgical risk. Hypogammaglobulinemia, anemia, and thrombocytopenia complicate the later stages of CLL. For these reasons, infection and bleeding are common complications of surgery. Splenectomy can be useful in patients resistant to chemotherapy, in patients with immune thrombocytopenia or hemolytic anemia, or in patients with pancytopenia. Hemorrhage from the splenic bed and infection are the most common postoperative complications.[73,74]

CHRONIC GRANULOCYTIC LEUKEMIA

The natural course of chronic granulocytic leukemia is characterized by a chronic phase, usually lasting from one to four years. The inevitable metamorphosis to acute "blast" crisis of the disease is invariably fatal. During the chronic phase, the white blood cell count can usually be controlled by a variety of chemotherapeutic agents. Patients whose disease is controlled present little increased surgical risk. However, some patients are susceptible to hemorrhagic complications due to a thrombocytopathy, a feature of the myeloproliferative disorders. High granulocyte counts (100,000/mm^3) may also predispose to hemorrhagic complications. Efforts should be made to lower the white blood cell count to below 50,000 before elective surgery. If emergency surgery is indicated when the white blood count is in excess of 150,000/mm^3, leukophoresis should be considered.

Splenectomy has been considered as a therapeutic procedure in chronic myelogenous leukemia to relieve pain due to the immense spleen or to manage the thrombocytopenia or anemia that may result from splenomegaly. When the disease is poorly controlled and advanced,[75] splenectomy carries a high operative and postoperative mortality of about 25 percent. However when splenectomy is done during clinical remission of the disease, the risk is considerably reduced in terms of both morbidity and mortality, and splenectomy may even have a beneficial effect on prognosis.[76]

PLASMA CELL DYSCRASIAS AND DYSPROTEINEMIAS

The plasma cell dyscrasias are malignant neoplasms that arise from lymphocytes and are generally associated with a monoclonal immunoglobin in the blood. The commonest neoplasms of this type are multiple myeloma and Waldenström's macroglobulinemia. These disorders are to be distinguished from idiopathic monoclonal gammopathy (so called benign monoclonal gammopathy). Osteoporosis, osteolytic lesions, and pathologic fractures are the hallmarks of multiple myeloma; by contrast, bony complications are very rare in macroglobulinemia.

Patients with multiple myeloma may develop pathologic fractures or spinal cord compression from a plasmacytoma. Internal surgical fixation of long bone fractures and artificial hip prostheses may reduce pain and allow ambulation. Radiotherapy to areas of spinal cord compression may prevent the need for decompressive laminectomy. Hypercalcemia, infection (especially with *Streptococcus pneumoniae* and *Hemophilus influenzae*), and impaired renal function frequently complicate surgery; immobilization following surgical procedures may cause or exaggerate hypercalcemia. A high fluid intake, diuretics, and corticosteroids can control hypercalcemia, but in refractory cases, treatment with mithramycin may prove necessary. Dehydration induced by diagnostic or surgical procedures may cause azotemia and acute renal failure, therefore, adequate hydration must be maintained, especially when performing radiologic procedures requiring the injection

Brown, General Surgery in Adult Hemophiliacs, Surgery 99:154, Feb 1986.

of hypertonic contrast media.[78] In general, intravenous pyelography and other procedures requiring the injection of intravenous contrast media are *contraindicated* in patients with multiple myeloma.

Hemostatic abnormalities in the dysproteinemias may cause significant problems at surgery. Perkins and associates[79] reported bleeding as a complication in 15 percent of patients with IgG myeloma and in over 38 percent with IgA myeloma or macroglobulinemia. The hyperviscosity syndrome, generally seen only when plasma viscosity is 3 to 4 times normal, may cause recurrent bleeding from mucous membranes, persistent oozing after minor surgery, or hemorrhages and distended retinal veins in the optic fundi. A prolonged bleeding time and abnormal platelet adherence may also occur secondary to functional abnormalities of platelets. Inhibitors of blood coagulation, particularly of fibrin monomer aggregation, can lead to a prolonged thrombin time and are also common.[79] The treatment for clinically apparent hyperviscosity syndrome remains plasmaphoresis. This therapy may also aid the patient with platelet abnormalities and coagulation inhibitors. However, in some patients plasmaphoresis may initially aggravate the reduced clotting factor levels. Clinical remission of the disease induced by chemotherapy with reduction in the monoclonal protein will also improve both laboratory and hemorrhagic manifestations.

Platelet Disorders

IDIOPATHIC THROMBOCYTOPENIC PURPURA

Idiopathic thrombocytopenic purpura is an autoimmune disease characterized by the production of antiplatelet antibodies. Although about 75 percent of patients are responsive to medical management including steroid and immunosuppressive therapy, at least half ultimately require splenectomy.[80] The usual indications for splenectomy include (1) patients who are refractory to medical management, (2) patients who may be steroid-responsive but who are also steroid-dependent.

Before surgery, the platelet count may be below 50,000 to 75,000/mm.^{3} Often it may be as low as 5,000 to 10,000/mm.^{3} Preoperative treatment with prednisone, 80 mg daily, may be useful in increasing the platelet count. It must be remembered that patients on chronic steroid therapy will require continued and perhaps increased steroid therapy intraoperatively and postoperatively (see Chapter 5, Endocrinology). The preoperative transfusion of platelets accomplishes little to elevate the platelet count since these platelets are rapidly cleared. Intraoperatively, the clamping of the splenic artery will often lead to a rapid increase in the platelet count. Bleeding ceases intraoperatively and the postoperative course is without undue complication. Occasionally, the platelet count may not rise due to decreased bone marrow synthesis of platelets. In such cases, platelet transfusions may prove useful. During surgery a careful search for accessory spleens should be conducted. These splenuli may be associated with the failure of splenectomy to correct the disorder. Postoperative thrombocytosis is not of concern.

On the third to seventh postoperative day, the platelet count may peak between 500,000 to 800,000/mm.^{3} No specific therapy is indicated.

CONGENITAL PLATELET DISORDERS

Qualitative congenital platelet disorders are rare. They include the Bernard-Soulier syndrome, Glanzmann's thrombasthenia, platelet storage pool disease, and the thrombocytopathies. All are characterized by a prolonged bleeding time. There is often a history of susceptibility to bruising, epistaxis, and prolonged bleeding after dental procedures. Unlike von Willebrand's disease, the Factor VIII levels are normal. Treatment prior to elective or emergency surgery includes platelet transfusions. Aspirin and other prostaglandin inhibitors are contraindicated (Table 1). A complete discussion of diagnosis and management of these disorders is found in Weiss[81] and Lusher and Barnhart.[82]

Congenital Coagulation Disorders

Patients with congenital coagulation disorders such as hemophilia can usually undergo surgical procedures without undue risk. However, these patients should be managed by physicians experienced in the treatment of these diseases and in institutions in which adequate laboratory facilities are available. Occasionally, however, hemophiliacs require emergency procedures. Therefore, an approach to management of these patients is described here.

HEMOPHILIA A—FACTOR VIII DEFICIENCY

Hemophilia A is a sex-linked hereditary disorder characterized by a deficiency of plasma Factor VIII. In order to decrease the hemorrhagic tendency during surgery, replacement therapy is used to increase the Factor VIII level to concentrations above 30 to 60 percent of the concentration of Factor VIII in normal plasma. At these levels, the partial thromboplastin time is normal and the Factor VIII level is measured by direct assay of Factor VIII.

It must be emphasized that elective surgery can be safely performed only in those hemophiliacs who attain adequate concentrations of Factor VIII in their blood after Factor VIII transfusion. Patients with inducible or high titer Factor VIII inhibitors are not surgical candidates. A careful history and a review of the medical records are thus essential. In addition, inhibitors that have been previously undiagnosed must be identified. A Factor VIII inhibitor assay is required in every patient with classic hemophilia prior to surgery. As standard practice, we also perform a Factor VIII infusion study. A day prior to surgery, a measured dose of Factor VIII is administered intravenously, and plasma Factor VIII levels are measured at timed intervals. The plasma levels of Factor VIII and the biologic half-disappearance rate of Factor VIII achieved may be assessed prior to surgery. Several types of blood components may be infused to obtain satisfactory Factor VIII levels. Fresh frozen plasma contains Factor VIII. However, because of the problems of fluid overload, the amount of plasma that can be infused is limited to about 6 U (1500 ml) daily. This amount of plasma represents about 1500 U of Factor VIII (a unit of Factor VIII is defined as the amount of Factor VIII in 1 ml of normal plasma). This represents a relatively small amount of Factor VIII. The average 70 kg person (assuming 40 ml plasma/kg of body weight) has a plasma volume of 2800 ml. Three units of plasma (750 U of Factor VIII) will raise the in vivo Factor VIII level to about 25 percent of normal. Since the plasma half-life of Factor VIII is about eight hours, infusion of 3 U of plasma every eight hours will not result in sufficient levels of Factor VIII to permit major surgery.

For these reasons, Factor VIII concentrates are usually employed. Cryoprecipitate is prepared in local blood banks and is rich in Factor VIII. A unit of cryoprecipitate contains far less plasma protein than does a unit of plasma but both have roughly equivalent Factor VIII activity. Although cryoprecipitate can be successfully employed in the management of hemophilia A, the intermediate purity Factor VIII concentrates are currently the agents of choice.[83–85] These preparations are available commercially, have a prolonged shelf life, and are standardized for Factor VIII activity.[86] Thus, the plasma Factor VIII level in the patient may be estimated given the amount of Factor VIII infused. It is important, however, that plasma Factor VIII levels be monitored in the coagulation laboratory. Often the levels achieved in vivo are below those expected due to rapid clearance of Factor VIII. The amount of Factor VIII should be adjusted accordingly.

For example, a 70 kg man with severe Factor VIII deficiency requires surgery. The preinfusion level of Factor VIII is less than 1 percent. Tests for a circulating anticoagulant (anti-Factor VIII antibody) are negative. The patient is given 2000 units of Factor VIII concentrate which, by calculation, should give a Factor VIII level of 80 percent initially and 40 percent at 8 hours. Blood samples are taken at various time intervals and the half-life determined. At 15 minutes following infusion, the Factor VIII level is 70 percent; at one hour, it is 53 percent, at three hours 42 percent, and at five hours, it has dropped to 25 percent. The biologic half-life in this patient is three hours. Therefore, he requires 2000 U of Factor VIII every three hours to maintain at least a 40 percent Factor VIII level.

The level of Factor VIII achieved and the duration for which such levels need be maintained depends upon the type of surgery performed and the complications of surgery. Intraoperatively we maintain the Factor VIII level in excess of 50 percent. Factor VIII infusions are continued for three to five days postoperatively at a level of 30 to 50 percent before therapy is tapered off. With major surgery and especially orthopedic procedures and major dental surgery, Factor VIII levels of at least 40 to 50 percent should be maintained for ten days to two weeks. Preinfusion levels of Factor VIII should be monitored daily. A significant decrease in the Factor VIII levels should raise the suspicion that an antibody to Factor VIII may have developed. A test for an inhibitor should be performed.

Although severe hemophilia A and B generally present with spontaneous bleeding into joints or muscles, spontaneous bleeding into psoas muscle or into the gut wall is not uncommon. This may mimic an acute surgical abdomen. These patients should be treated conservatively with infusion therapy and carefully monitored unless signs of overt peritonitis or sepsis are present.

Complications of Factor VIII therapy include (1) a risk of anti-Factor VIII antibody formation, (2) hepatitis, (3) hemolysis from donor anti-A or anti-B antibodies in patients with blood type A or B, and (4) allergic reactions.[87]

HEMOPHILIA B—FACTOR IX DEFICIENCY

Hemophilia B is a sex-linked hereditary disorder characterized by a deficiency of plasma Factor IX. The therapeutic strategy for managing afflicted patients during and after surgery is parallel to that described for Factor VIII deficiency. However, several facts should be stated explicitly. First, cryoprecipitate does not contain Factor IX and should not be used to treat hemophilia B. Second, Factor IX is a smaller molecule than Factor VIII and it is equally distributed intravascularly and extravascularly. Thus, twice the calculated amount of Factor IX is given as a loading dose to account for loss into the extravascular pool. Last, large quantities of intermediate purity Factor IX concentrates have been associated with intravascular coagulation and thrombotic disease.[88] Therefore, this material must be used in moderation.

FACTOR XI DEFICIENCY

Factor XI deficiency, an autosomal recessive disorder, is a common cause of a prolonged partial thromboplastin time but is not associated with a spontaneous hemorrhagic syndrome. In contrast to patients with hemophilia A and B, most patients with Factor XI deficiency have a latent, previously undiagnosed, disorder. Fortunately, the bleeding tendency is mild. Bleeding may be observed following surgical procedures or trauma, but its clinical significance is variable. For instance, many patients with even the severe form of the disorder (Factor XI level below 5% of the normal level) have a history of successful surgery without untoward bleeding.

The therapeutic dilemma may be clearly stated: Should a patient with Factor XI deficiency who has small hemorrhagic risk be subjected to the small hepatitis risk of prophylactic plasma infusion? Since the answer is not known, we currently use the following guidelines: If the Factor XI level is less than 5 to 10 percent, plasma infusions are administered immediately following surgery with the objective of raising the Factor XI level above 30 percent. Because the half-life of Factor XI disappearance is long (24 hours), infusions may be given on a daily schedule. If the Factor XI level in a patient is between 10 to 30 percent, we prefer to initiate surgery without prior plasma transfusion. If excessive bleeding occurs intraoperatively or postoperatively, fresh frozen plasma is administered without delay. Patients with Factor XI levels in excess of 30 percent do not require special consideration during surgery.

VON WILLEBRAND'S DISEASE

The most common hereditary hemorrhagic disorder is von Willebrand's disease. It is manifested clinically by mucosal bleeding and purpura. In the laboratory, it is characterized by a prolonged bleeding time, a prolonged partial thromboplastin time, a low Factor VIII, and a decreased platelet adhesiveness. The abnormal hemostatic function is due to a deficiency of the von Willebrand's protein in the plasma. The therapeutic strategy prior to surgery is to increase the plasma level of this protein by replacement therapy.

Cryoprecipitate and fresh frozen plasma are good sources of von Willebrand's protein. Factor VIII concentrates are not.[89] Infusion of a single unit of fresh frozen plasma or cryoprecipitate is associated with a pronounced increase in the Factor VIII level within 12 hours, but the von Willebrand's protein level is not significantly changed. If the bleeding time is prolonged so as to represent a significant surgical risk, cryoprecipitate should be administered in large quantity (10 U every 12 hours) to attempt to normalize the bleeding time and increase the level of von Willebrand's protein.

TRANSFUSION THERAPY

Whole Blood and Red Cells

ACUTE BLOOD LOSS

The patient with acute blood loss suffers both from hypovolemia and anemia. Since in rapid hemorrhage both red cells and plasma are lost, the systolic blood pressure and pulse are more reliable guides to the amount of blood loss than the hematocrit. If the systolic pressure is below 100 mm Hg in a hemorrhagic patient, the blood volume is probably diminished by about a third.[90] An orthostatic drop in the blood pressure is also indicative of substantial blood loss. Blood samples should be drawn for typing and cross-matching and crystalloid started immediately. When there is frank hemorrhage and the physician deems that immediate transfusion is necessary, Type O Rh negative blood with low anti-A and anti-B antibody titers may be administered. Properly typed and cross-matched blood should be substituted as soon as possible. Either whole blood or a combination of packed red cells and crystalloid or colloid (albumin or plasma) may be given. If large volumes of blood are administered, consideration should be given to warming the blood and to the dilution of platelets and coagulation factors which occur with massive transfusion. This last complication may be overcome by infusion of platelet concentrates, fresh frozen plasma, and cryoprecipitate after 10 to 14 U or by using fresh whole blood every third or fourth unit. Another risk with massive transfusion of stored blood is lowering of the ionized calcium by complex formation with the citrate anticoagulant. This may be avoided by slowly infusing 10 ml of 10 percent calcium gluconate with every 4 to 5 U of blood transfused.

CHRONIC BLOOD LOSS

The optimal level for transfusion in patients with chronic anemia has not been defined. Practically, this depends on the age, and general condition of the patient as well as the contemplated surgical procedure. For elective surgery, preoperative anemia should be thoroughly evaluated and treatment of the primary cause undertaken, for example, oral iron therapy in iron deficiency anemia, rather than transfusion. For those patients in whom the cause of the anemia is not readily reversible, transfusion therapy is indicated. A sufficient quantity of packed red blood cells to raise the hemoglobin level to 10 to 11 gm/dl is normally administered. The transfusion of frozen washed red cells is reserved for those patients who have demonstrated febrile transfusion reactions in the past, or patients with rare blood types in whom autologous transfusion is necessary.

COMPLICATIONS OF TRANSFUSIONS

Short term complications of transfusion include circulatory overload, air embolism, and transfusion reactions. Hypervolemia can be avoided by the use of packed red cells and by transfusing patients with chronic anemia slowly. Elderly patients and patients with cardiovascular disease should also be transfused at a slow rate.

Transfusion reactions are usually immediate and have multiple causes: (1) hemolysis of transfused red cells, (2) allergic reaction to transfused red cells, leukocytes, or platelet antigens, (3) allergic reaction to infused plasma, and (4) bacterial contamination of transfused blood products. These reactions are accompanied by a variety of clinical symptoms including chills, fever, urticaria, dyspnea, nausea and vomiting, back pain, chest tightness, tachycardia, bronchospasm, angioneurotic edema, hypotension, anaphylaxis, and shock. If a transfusion reaction is suspected, the transfusion must be stopped *immediately.* The blood typing and cross-matching should be repeated, and a Coombs' test done on the patient's red cells. The serum of both the donor and the patient should be tested for blood group antibodies. If sepsis is suspected, cultures of the donor blood and that of the patient should be done. Blood should be drawn carefully and tested for free hemoglobin or methemalbumin. A urine sample should be examined for free hemoglobin. The presence of free hemoglobin in the serum or urine indicates a hemolytic transfusion reaction. The complications of hemolytic transfusion reaction may include shock, renal failure, and bleeding due to disseminated intravascular coagulation.[91,92,95]

Some patients, especially those who have had multiple transfusions or multiparous women, become sensitized to leukocytes or platelet antigens and will develop febrile transfusion reactions. These patients should be treated with frozen washed red blood cells. Also, patients who develop urticaria, pruritus, bronchospasm, angioneurotic edema, or anaphylaxis during transfusion should be infused with frozen washed red blood cells.

The primary long-term complication of blood transfusion is the transmission of disease: hepatitis, malaria, cytomegalovirus, and toxoplasmosis. The risk of hepatitis can be lessened but not eliminated by screening donors for hepatitis surface antigen and by using volunteer donors. Other long-term complications of transfusion include iron overload in patients receiving chronic transfusion therapy, sensitization to minor blood group antigen, and HL-A antigen sensitization in the prospective transplant recipient.

Platelet Transfusion

Thrombocytopenia carries a high risk of intraoperative and postoperative bleeding. Since the introduction of routine platelet transfusion over a decade ago, required surgery may be performed at little increased morbidity and mortality in patients with thrombocytopenia. The indications for platelet therapy have been discussed extensively in previous sections. As a rule, the administration of random donor platelets to the recipient leads to development of antiplatelet antibodies in the recipient. After multiple transfusions, these antibodies render the recipient refractory to platelet infusions. For these reasons, platelet infusions should be reserved for patients with clear indications. Intraoperative and postoperative platelet counts should be maintained above 50,000/mm.[3] A single unit of random donor platelets will raise the platelet count by about 5,000/mm.[3] In patients with splenomegaly, immune thrombocytopenia, or prior platelet transfusions, this rule does not hold. Transfusion reactions may be controlled with administration of an antihistamine 30 minutes prior to transfusion. Transfused platelet survival in these patients may be improved by using platelet transfusions from HL-A matched related donors.

Granulocyte Transfusions

Granulocyte transfusions are indicated only in special circumstances and are regarded by some as an experimental therapeutic modality. The circumstances are: when the absolute granulocyte count is less than 500/mm^3, the bone marrow is devoid of myeloid precursors, and the patient has evidence of infection. If granulocyte transfusions are administered, they should be continued for at least four days providing that the patient is still neutropenic. Each transfusion should contain at least 10^{10} cells. Granulocyte transfusions are routinely associated with febrile transfusion reactions. These reactions may be anticipated and controlled by giving the patient an antihistamine such as diphenydramine (25 to 50 mg intravenously) 30 minutes prior to transfusion. When a febrile transfusion reaction occurs, it may be controlled by giving an antihistamine (50 mg intravenously) or morphine (3 mg intravenously). Since the consequences of surgery in this patient population are grave, these patients are not surgical candidates. At present, granulocytic transfusion should be necessary only *rarely* in the management of the surgical patient.

REFERENCES

1. Davis, S, Furie, BC, Griffin, JH, et al.: *Circulating inhibitors of blood coagulation associated with procainamide-induced lupus erythematosus.* Am J Hematol 4:401, 1978.
2. Zucker, S, Zarrabi, MH, Romano, G, et al.: *IgM inhibitors of the contact activation phase of coagulation in chlorpromazine-treated patients.* Br J Haematol 40:774, 1978.
3. Zarrabi, MH, Zucker, S, Miller, F, et al.: *Immunologic and coagulation disorders in chlorpromazine-treated patients.* Ann Intern Med 91:194, 1979.
4. Shapiro, S, and Huttin, M: *Acquired inhibitors to the blood coagulation factors.* Semin Thromb Hemostras 1:336, 1975.
5. Zacharski, LR, Elveback, LR, and Linman, JW: *Leukocyte counts in healthy adults.* Am J Clin Pathol 56:148, 1971.
6. Shaper, AG, and Lewis, P: *Genetic neutropenia in people of african origin.* Lancet 2:1021, 1971.
7. Cartwright, GE: *The anemia of chronic disorders.* Semin Hematol 3:351, 1966.
8. Rosenberg, IH: *Absorption and malabsorption of folates.* Clin Haematol 5:589, 1976.
9. Tovey, FI, and Clark, CG: *Anaemia after partial gastrectomy: a neglected curable condition.* Lancet 1:956, 1980.
10. Bradley, EL, and Issacs, J: *Postresectional anemia.* Arch Surg 111:844, 1976.
11. Balcerzak, SP, and Bromberg, PA: *Secondary polycythemia.* Semin Haematol 12:353, 1975.
12. Weinreb, NJ, and Shih, CF: *Spurious polycythemia.* Semin Haematol 12:397, 1975.
13. Hareville, DD, and Summerskill, WHJ: *Surgery in acute hepatitis: causes and effects.* JAMA 184:257, 1963.
14. Bowie, EJ, and Owen, CA: *The significance of abnormal preoperative hemostatic tests.* Prog Hemost Thromb 5:179, 1980.
15. Gados, LA, Freireich, EJ, and Mantel, N: *The quantitative relation between platelet count and hemorrhage in patients with acute leukemia.* N Engl J Med 266:905, 1962.

16. Mielke, CH, Kaneshiro, MM, Weiner, JM, et al.: *The standardized normal Ivy bleeding time and its prolongation by aspirin.* Blood 34:204, 1969.

17. *Thromboembolic complications of Factor IX complex.* FDA Drug Bulletin 10:25, 1980.

18. Bick, RL, Adams, T, and Radeck, K: *Surgical hemostasis with Factor IX containing concentrates.* JAMA 229:163, 1974.

19. Handley, DA, and Lawrence, JR: *Factor IX deficiency in the nephrotic syndrome.* Lancet 1:1079, 1967.

20. Furie, B, Greene, E, and Furie, BC: *Syndrome of acquired Factor X deficiency and systemic amyloidosis.* New Engl J Med 297:81, 1977.

21. Thomas, DP: *Heparin in the prophylaxis and treatment of venous thromboembolism.* Semin Haematol 15:1, 1978.

22. Harris, WH, Saltzman, EW, Athanasoulis, C, et al.: *Comparison of warfarin, low molecular weight dextran, aspirin, and subcutaneous heparin in prevention of venous thromboembolism following total hip replacement.* J Bone Joint Surg 56A:1152, 1974.

23. Berger, S, and Salzmann, EW: *The thromboembolic complications of prosthetic devices.* Prog Hemost Thromb 2:273, 1977.

24. Egeberg, O: *Inherited fibrinogen abnormality causing thrombophila.* Thromb Diath Haemorrh 17:176, 1967.

25. Marciniak, E, Farley, CH, and DeSimone, PA: *Familial thrombosis due to antithrombin III deficiency.* Blood 43:219, 1974.

26. Kosik, KS, and Furie, B: *Thrombotic stroke associated with elevated plasma factor VIII.* Ann Neurol 8:435, 1980.

27. Penick, GD, Dejanov, II, Reddick, RL, et al.: *Predisposition to intravascular coagulation.* Thromb Diath Haemorrh 21 (Suppl.):543, 1966.

28. Gaston, LW: *Studies on a family with an elevated level of Factor V (proaccelerin) and a tendency to thrombosis.* J Pediatr 68:367, 1966.

29. Hirsh, J: *Hypercoagulability.* Semin Haematol 14:409, 1977.

30. Robboy, SJ, Salisbury, K, Ragsdale, B, et al.: *Mechanism of aspergillos-induced microangiopathic hemolytic anemia.* Arch Intern Med 128:790, 1971.

31. Dacie, JV: *Secondary or symptomatic hemolytic anemias: III. Miscellaneous conditions,* in Dacie, JV (ed.): *The Hemolytic Anemias III.* New York: Grune & Straton, 1967, pp. 908–922.

32. Suzuki, A, Yamada, A, and Maruyama, H: *A case of acute hemolytic anemia due to clostridium perfrigens septicemia.* Jap J Clin Hematol 13:850, 1972.

33. Beutler, E: *Glucose 6-phosphate dehydrogenase deficiency and nonspherocytic congenital hemolytic anemia.* Semin Haematol 2:91, 1965.

34. Phillips, SM, and Silvers, NP: *Glucose 6-phosphate dehydrogenase deficiency, infectious hepatitis, and renal failure.* Ann Intern Med 20:99, 1969.

35. Garatty, G, and Pete, LD: *Drug-induced hemolytic anemia.* Am J Med 58:398, 1975.

36. Crexells, C, Aerichide, N, Bonny, Y, et al.: *Factors influencing hemolysis in valve prosthesis.* Am Heart J 84:161, 1972.

37. Santinga, JT, Flora, JD, Batsakis, J, et al.: *Hemolysis in patients with cloth-covered aortic valve prosthesis. Changing severity of hemolysis and prediction of anemia.* Am J Cardiol 34:533, 1974.

38. Pisciotta, AV: *Immune and toxic mechanisms in drug-induced agranulocytosis.* Semin Haematol 10:279, 1973.

39. Lang, DT, Scolnick, EM, and Willerson, JT: *Association of cytomegalovirus infection with the post-perfusion syndrome.* N Engl J. Med 778:1147, 1968.

40. Prince, AM, Szmuness, W, Millan, SJ, et al.: *A serologic study of cytomegalovirus infection associated with blood transfusions.* N Engl J Med 284:1125, 1971.

41. Goodnight, SH, Kenoyer, O, Rapaport, SI, et al.: *Defibrination after brain tissue destruction.* N Engl J Med 290:1043, 1974.

42. Sack, GH, Jr, Levin, J, and Bell, WR: *Trousseau's syndrome and other manifestations of disseminated intravascular coagulopathy in patients with neoplasms: clinical, pathophysiologic, and therapeutic features.* Medicine 56:1, 1977.

43. Harker, LA, Malpass, TW, Branson, HE, et al.: *Mechanism of abnormal bleeding in patients undergoing cardiopulmonary bypass.* Blood 56:824, 1980.

44. Kelton, JG, Neame, PB, Gauldie, J, et al.: *Elevated platelet-associated IgG in the thrombocytopenia of septicemia.* N Engl J Med 300:760, 1979.

45. Shulman, NR, Aster, RH, Leiter, A, et al.: *Immunoreactions involving platelets V. Post transfusion purpura due to a complement-fixing antibody against a genetically-controlled platelet antigen.* J Clin Invest 40:1597, 1961.

46. Abramson, N, Eisenberg, PD, and Aster, RH: *Post-transfusion purpura: immunologic aspects and therapy.* N Engl J Med 291:1163, 1974.

47. Janson, DA, Jubelirer, SJ, Weinstein, MJ, et al.: *Treatment of the bleeding tendency in uremia with cryoprecipitate.* N Engl J Med 303:1318, 1980.

48. Walker, AM, and Hershel, J: *Predictors of bleeding during heparin therapy.* JAMA 244:1209, 1980.

49. Cines, DB, Kaywin, P, Bina, M, et al.: *Heparin-associated thrombocytopenia.* N Engl J Med 303:788, 1980.

50. Bell, WR, Tomasulo, PA, Alving, BM, et al.: *Thrombocytopenia occurring during the administration of heparin: a prospective study in 52 patients.* Ann Intern Med 85:155, 1976.

51. Kelton, JG, and Hirsh, J: *Bleeding associated with antithrombotic therapy.* Semin Haematol 17:259, 1980.

52. Bell, WR, and Meeks, AG: *Guidelines for the use of thrombolytic agents.* N Engl J Med 301:1266, 1979.

53. *Thrombolytic therapy in thrombosis: a National Institutes of Health concensus development conference.* Ann Intern Med 93:141, 1980.

54. Stockman, JA, Migro, DO, Miskin, MM, et al.: *Occlusion of large cerebral vessels in sickle cell anemia.* N Engl J Med 287:846, 1972.

55. Bucklew, VM, and Someren, A: *Renal manifestations of sickle cell disease.* Arch Intern Med 133:660, 1974.

56. Atlas, SA: *The sickle cell trait and surgical complications: a matched pair analysis.* JAMA 229:1078, 1974.

57. Modell, B: *Total management of thalessemia major.* Arch Dis Child 52:489, 1977.

58. Craig, RP, Bate, CM, and Humpries, G: *Some surgical aspects of homozygous beta-thalessemia.* Br J Surg 64:277, 1977.

59. Deucy, KW, Grossman, L, and Canale, VC: *Cholelithiasis in thalessemia major.* Radiology 96:385, 1970.

60. Rigby, PG, and Leavell, BS: *Polycythemia vera: A review of fifty cases with emphasis on risk of surgery.* Arch Intern Med 106:622, 1960.

61. Wasserman, LR, and Gilbert, HS: *Surgical bleeding in polycythemia vera.* Ann NY Acad Sci 15:122, 1964.

62. Taddeini, L, and Watson, CJ: *The clinical porphrias.* Semin Haematol 5:345, 1968.

63. Rizk, SF, Jacobson, JH, and Silvay, G: *Ketamine as an induction agent for acute intermittent porphyria.* Anesthesiology 46:305, 1977.

64. Nielson, B, and Thorn, NA: *Transient excess urinary excretion of antidiuretic material in acute intermittent porphyria with hyponatremia and hypomagnessemia.* Am J Med 38:345, 1965.

65. Lee, BCD: *Paroxysmal nocturnal haemoglobinuria presenting as acute abdominal emergency.* Br J Radiol 46:467, 1963.

66. Chang, H, Rodriquez, V, Narboni, G, et al.: *Causes of death in adults with acute leukemia.* Am J Med 55:259, 1976.

67. Graw, RG, Jr., Herzig, G, Perry, S, et al.: *Normal granulocyte transfusion therapy: treatment of septicemia due to gram-negative bacteria.* N Engl J Med 287:367, 1972.

68. Haimov, M, Freedman, S, Khilnani, MT, et al.: *Intussusception in acute lymphoblastic leukemia.* Mt Sinai J Med 34:484, 1967.

69. Prolla, JC, and Kirsner, JB: *The gastrointestinal lesions and complications of the leukemias.* Ann Intern Med 61:1084, 1964.

70. Pennington, JE, and Feldman, NT: *Pulmonary infiltrates and fever in patient with hematologic malignancy.* Am J Med 62:581, 1977.

71. Schimpff, SC: *Infection prevention during profound granulocytopenia.* Ann Intern Med 93:358, 1980.

72. Gurwith, MJ, Brunton, JC, Lank, BA, et al.: *A prospective controlled investigation of prophylactic trimethoprim/sulfamethoxazole in hospitalized granulocytopenic patients.* Am J Med 66:248, 1979.

73. Yam, LT, and Crosby, WH: *Early splenectomy in lymphoproliferative disorders.* Arch Intern Med 133:270, 1974.

74. Adler, S, Stutzman, L, Sokai, JE, et al.: *Splenectomy for hematologic depression in lymphocytic leukemia and lymphoma.* Cancer 35:521, 1975.

75. Strumia, MM, Strumia, PV, and Bassert, D: *Splenectomy in leukemia: Hematologic and clinical effects on 34 patients and review of 299 published cases.* Cancer Res 26:519, 1966.

76. Spiers, ASD, Baikie, AG, Galton, DAG, et al.: *Chronic granulocytic leukaemia: effect of elective splenectomy on the course of disease.* Br Med J 1:175, 1975.

77. Spiers, AS, Baikie, AG, Galton, DA, et al.: *Splenectomy for complications of chronic granulocytic leukaemia.* Lancet 2:627, 1975.

78. Myers, GH, and Witten, DM: *Acute renal failure after excretory urography in multiple myeloma.* Am J Roent 113:583, 1971.

79. Perkins, HA, MacKenzie, MR, and Fudenberg, HH: *Hemostatic defects in dysproteinemias.* Blood 5:695, 1970.

80. Karpatkin, S: *Autoimmune thrombocytopenic purpura.* Blood 56:329, 1980.

81. Weiss, NJ: *Congenital disorders of platelet function.* Semin Haematol 17:228, 1980.

82. Lusher, JM, and Barnhart, MI: *Congenital disorders affecting platelets.* Semin Thromb Hemostas 4:123, 1977.

83. Jones, P: *Developments and problems in the management of hemophilia.* Semin Haematol 14:375, 1977.

84. Rizza, CR: *The management of patients with coagulation factor deficiencies,* in Biggs, R (ed.): *Human Blood Coagulation, Hemostasis and Thrombosis.* Oxford: Blackwell Scientific, 1976, pp. 365–398.

85. Krieger, JN, Hilgartner, MW, Redo, FS: *Surgery in patients with congenital disorders of blood coagulation.* Ann Surg 185:290, 1977.

86. Nilsson, IM, and Hedner, U: *Characteristics of various factor VIII concentrates used in treatment of hemophilia A.* Br J Haematol 371:543, 1977.

87. Eyster, ME, Bowman, HS, and Haverstick, JN: *Adverse reactions to factor VIII infusions.* Ann Intern Med 87:248, 1977.

88. Kasper, C: *Postoperative thrombosis in hemophilia B.* N Engl J Med 289:160, 1973.

89. Green, D, and Dotter, EV: *Failure of AHF concentrate to control bleeding in von Willebrand's disease.* Am J Med 60:357, 1976.

90. Blackburn, EK: *Indications for blood transfusion.* Practitioner. 195:174, 1965.

91. Rock, RC, Bove, JR, Nemerson, Y: *Heparin treatment of intravascular coagulation accompanying hemolytic transfusion reactions.* Transfusion 9:57, 1969.

92. Goldfinger, D: *Acute hemolytic transfusion reactions—a fresh look at pathogenesis and considerations regarding therapy.* Transfusion 17:85, 1977.

93. England, JM, and Fraser, PM: *Differentiation of iron deficiency from thalassaemia trait by routine blood count.* Lancet 1:449, 1973.

94. Smick, K, Condit, PK, Proctor, et al.: *Fatal aplastic anemia: an epidemiological study of its relationship to the drug chloramphenicol.* J Chronic Dis 17:899, 1964.

95. Greenwalt, TJ: *Pathogenesis and management of hemolytic transfusion reactions.* Semin Haematol 18:84, 1981.

Chapter 8

INFECTIOUS DISEASES

Ted Butler, M.D., Francis P. Tally, M.D., and Sherwood L. Gorbach, M.D.

Infectious diseases have a major impact on the surgical patient. They may present as clinical syndromes requiring operative intervention for cure or as complications in the postoperative period. Many of the classical infections that plagued patients undergoing surgery in the past are now rare, but change has not occurred without exacting a toll: antibiotic use over the past 30 years has caused a profound change in the epidemiology of nosocomial infections. The formerly prevalent gram-positive cocci have given way to gram-negative bacilli which often colonize surgical wounds and can lead to devastating infections. In addition, modern medical care has promoted violation of man's natural defenses on several fronts: (1) the insertion of prosthetic devices and, (2) immunosuppression induced by steroids and cytotoxic chemotherapy, and (3) widespread use of antimicrobial agents that alter the normal flora. It is not uncommon for a patient to be compromised by all of these factors simultaneously.

Recent studies have documented a decreasing rate of surgical wound infections from 1975 to 1978. Table 1 lists data obtained in a national nosocomial infection study sponsored by the Center for Disease Control.[1] During this period, 40,925 surgical wounds were reported. Surgical wound infection rates decreased in all categories of hospitals, with the largest decrease being reported by university hospitals. Intermediate decreases were experienced in municipal, community teaching, and federal hospitals, and the smallest decrease in community hospitals. Infection rates by service showed a drop of 15 percent on surgical wards and 17 percent on gynecologic services, but there was a 26 percent increase on obstetric services. While these trends generally are encouraging, there still remains a high incidence of postoperative surgical infections with considerable morbidity for the individual patient and a staggering economic toll for society. The cost of nosocomial infections was estimated to be four billion dollars in

TABLE 1. Surgical Wound Infection Rates*: National Nosocomial Infections Study, 1975 to 1978

Service	*1975*	*1976*	*1977*	*1978*
Surgery	170.1	110.8	150.2	144.6
Obstetrics	75.2	85.5	100.1	95.1
Gynecology	125.7	106.3	110.5	104.4
All services**	86.0	80.8	76.1	72.1

*Rates are per 10,000 patients discharged.
**Includes medical and pediatric services.

1978, brought about by the need for more prolonged hospitalization and the use of pharmacologic agents to eradicate the infections.

This chapter will review the infections most likely to be encountered in the surgical patient, both in the preoperative and postoperative periods. Recent developments in the evolving bacteriology and the changing susceptibility patterns of the pathogens have been taken into account in recommending antimicrobial therapy. Many areas remain highly controversial. As is characteristic of most controversies, there is a paucity of data to settle the issues at present. Recognizing the imperfect state of the art, we have attempted to provide guidelines to the diagnostic evaluation of infections in the surgical patient and have set down principles for the rational selection of antimicrobial agents.

PULMONARY INFECTIONS

Infections of the lower respiratory tract are a major cause of fever in surgical patients. Pulmonary infections of interest to the surgeon fall into two categories: (1) those infections requiring drainage to effect a cure such as empyema and, occasionally, lung abscess and (2) pneumonia which occurs in the postoperative patient. The bacteriology of pulmonary infections in these settings ranges from penicillin-sensitive organisms, such as *Streptococcus pneumoniae* and anaerobic bacteria, to highly resistant gram-negative bacilli including *Klebsiella* and *Pseudomonas aeruginosa*. Selection of appropriate antimicrobial therapy is determined by anticipating the pathogens on the basis of the clinical presentation and epidemiology. In general, patients with community-acquired infection have penicillin-susceptible organisms while patients with nosocomial pneumonia have multiple-antibiotic resistant bacteria. In this section we will briefly outline the pulmonary infections requiring surgical intervention and present a diagnostic and therapeutic approach to postoperative pneumonias.

Pulmonary Abscess

Pulmonary abscess is usually considered a medical disease unless there is an obstructing lesion which prevents adequate tracheobronchial drainage. The predisposing cause of lung abscess is aspiration of oropharyngeal contents resulting from impaired consciousness. There is usually a three to four week period of cough, fever, and weight loss. The pathogens involved in lung abscess are anaerobic bacteria in over 90 percent of cases.[2] The aerobic bacteria occasionally encountered as single pathogens in this disease are *Staphylococcus aureus* and *Klebsiella;* these organisms can cause a solitary lung abscess and the patient's condition usually follows a rapid downhill course, often leading to death. Multiple pulmonary abscesses suggest a blood-borne embolic source, either from right-sided endocarditis (usually with *S. aureus*) or from pelvic sepsis (usually involving anaerobes).

In the pediatric and teenage population, *Streptococcus pyogenes* and *S. aureus* are important pathogens in lung abscesses. *Streptococcus pyogenes* infections usually present with a fulminating bronchopneumonia that forms abscesses in two to three days and rapidly spreads to the pleural space. Staphylococcal abscesses may develop during the course of a fulminant pneumonia or may be embolic.

The treatment of pulmonary abscess requires selection of appropriate antimicrobial agents (Table 2) and good tracheobronchial toilet. The antimicrobial agents should be continued until there is radiologic stability, either a residual scar or complete healing; the duration of antibiotic therapy, usually given orally, is 6 to 12 weeks. Surgical intervention is only required when there is an obstructing lesion in the tracheobronchial tree, that is, a foreign body or tumor. On rare occasions, bleeding from vessels traversing an abscess cavity may dictate a surgical approach.

Empyema

The incidence of empyema has been decreasing since the introduction of antimicrobial agents; for example, there were 3.18 cases of empyema per 1000 admissions at the Boston City Hospital in 1935 and 1.85 per 1000 in 1972.[3] In the preantibiotic era, most cases were community-acquired while hospital-acquired empyema accounted for approximately 60 percent of the total cases in the 1970s. At present, 75 percent of community-acquired empyema in adults is caused by anaerobic bacteria, often mixed with aerobes. The pleural space infection is associated with pneumonitis or lung abscess in the adjacent parenchyma.[4] The remaining cases are caused by classic aerobic pathogens: pneumococci, group A streptococci, and staphylococci. These organisms are more frequently encountered as the pathogen in children and young adults.

Hospital-acquired empyema is associated with a wide spectrum of bacteria including aerobic gram-positive cocci, anaerobic bacteria, and gram-negative bacilli. Studies from Boston City Hospital document that *S. aureus* and antibiotic-resistant gram-negative bacilli, such as *Klebsiella, Escherichia coli,* and *Proteus,* are the dominant pathogens.[3] These organisms may be isolated individually or as part of a mixed infection. Since there is uncertainty about the pathogen in either community-acquired or hospital-acquired empyema, it is imperative to perform a diagnostic thoracocentesis before treatment to identify the infecting organisms. The pleural fluid should be submitted for gram stain, cell count, protein and sugar determinations, pH measurements, and aerobic and anaerobic culture.

The treatment of empyema is two-fold: selection of appropriate antibiotics (Table

TABLE 2. Therapy of Pulmonary Infections

		*Antimicrobial Therapy**	
Type of Infection	*Expected Pathogens*	*Primary*	*Secondary*
Pulmonary abscess or necrotizing pneumonitis	Anaerobic bacteria (oral flora): *Bacteroides melaninogenicus, Fusobacterium nucleatum,* Anaerobic cocci	Penicillin G	Clindamycin Erythromycin Chloramphenicol
	Staphylococcus aureus	Nafcillin *or* oxacillin	Cephalothin *or* vancomycin
	Aerobic gram-negative bacilli: *Escherichia coli* Klebsiella	Cephalosporins *or* ampicillin + aminoglycoside	Chloramphenicol and/or aminoglycoside
Empyema	Anaerobic bacteria Oral flora Bowel flora	Penicillin G Clindamycin Chloramphenicol Ticarcillin Carbenicillin Cefoxitin *or* Metronidazole	± Aminoglycoside
	Staphylococcus aureus	Nafcillin *or* oxacillin	
	Aerobic gram-negative bacilli	Cephalosporins *or* ampicillin + aminoglycoside	
Pneumonia	*Streptococcus pneumoniae*	Penicillin G	Erythromycin
	Staphylococcus aureus	Nafcillin *or* oxacillin	Cephalosporins
	Hemophilus influenzae	Ampicillin	Cefamandole
	Aerobic gram-negative bacilli	Cephalosporins *or* ampicillin + aminoglycoside	Cefoxitin, Cefamandole
	Pseudomonas aeruginosa	Aminoglycoside + carbenicillin *or* ticarcillin	

*See section on antibiotics in this chapter for advantages, disadvantages, and dosages of various agents.

2) and adequate drainage of the pleural space. Initial antibiotic selection should cover the possible pathogens, based on gram stain of the pleural fluid and the epidemiologic setting. Subsequent antibiotic therapy is dictated by the results of the culture and susceptibility testing. Drainage of the pleural cavity occasionally may be accomplished by repeated needle aspirations, especially with pneumococci, streptococci, or staphylococci, in the early phases of the disease process. Most cases in the current era, however, are more chronic in nature, associated with anaerobes ensconced in thick pus.

Such infections require prompt insertion of a chest tube under negative pressure. This approach is preferred to needle aspiration because empyema is frequently multiloculated and a large chest tube is useful to break down the loculations. Unless proper drainage is established, the patient will have a septic course with entrapment of the lung by a thick pleural peel, causing extensive loss of pulmonary function. This complication usually requires a thoracotomy and decortication which is a formidable procedure.

Although empyema usually arises from a pulmonary infection, a small percentage of cases are caused by suppurative disease below the diaphragm. The importance of recognizing this condition is that a different set of pathogens may be involved in the abdominal cases, particularly *Bacteroides fragilis* and clostridia. This clinical situation requires appropriate antibiotic therapy and adequate drainage of the intra-abdominal and pleural spaces.

Pneumonia

Pneumonia is the third most frequent postoperative infectious complication, behind infections of the urinary tract and wound. Pneumonia, however, is associated with a higher morbidity and mortality than the other two. This results from the virulent organisms which are encountered in postoperative pneumonia. *S. aureus* and aerobic gram-negative bacilli such as *E. coli, Klebsiella,* and *Pseudomonas aeruginosa* are the frequent pathogens in nosocomial pneumonia in surgical patients. These gram-negative bacteria are resistant to multiple antibiotics. The specific type of pathogen varies from one hospital to another and indeed among different intensive care units in the same hospital. Unusual organisms such as *Serratia marcescens, Acinetobacter calcoaceticus, Pseudomonas cepacia,* and *Proteus rettgeri* account for selected outbreaks of infection. Thus, the epidemiology is important in predicting the type of pathogen in a specific area. Another factor is the use of prophylactic antibiotics which predisposes to infections with organisms multiply resistant to antibiotics. Thus, postoperative pneumonia in patients receiving cephalothin as prophylaxis is usually caused by *Enterobacter* or *P. aeruginosa,* organisms that are resistant to this drug.

Establishing the diagnosis of pneumonia in the postoperative patient is difficult. Many patients have fever and pulmonary infiltrates from atelectasis. In addition, a positive sputum culture for gram-negative rods may only represent colonization of the oropharynx. The diagnosis of pneumonia in the postoperative patient should be based on a constellation of findings, including:

1. Fever
2. Rales and/or dullness on percussion; cough may not be present, depending on level of consciousness or type of surgery
3. X-ray signs of pulmonary infiltrate
4. Purulent sputum
5. Leukocytosis

Three or more of the above findings should be present to sustain the diagnosis of pneumonia. To establish the etiologic agent, an adequate specimen for microbiological analysis must be obtained. The available specimens include coughed sputum or secretions from the lower respiratory tract obtained by nasotracheal suctioning, endotracheal tube aspirates, fiberoptic bronchoscopy, or transtracheal aspiration (TTA). The last method is preferred for isolating the infecting pathogen without contamination by oropharyngeal contents. Unfortunately, TTA is contraindicated in many postoperative patients because of the presence of clotting disorders, hypoxia ($Po_2 \leq$ 50 torr), or an endotracheal tube. When coughed sputum or nasotracheal or endotracheal aspirates are the only specimens available, their validity should be based on the number of squamous epithelial cells (SEC) present in the gram stain. If there are less than 10 SEC per high-power field, the results of the culture closely resemble that obtained with transtracheal aspirates. Larger numbers of SEC indicate contamination from the upper airway.[5]

When the reliability of the specimen is suspect, it is necessary to design antibiotic therapy for all cultured pathogens, especially in seriously ill patients. Sputum cultures in patients with hospital-acquired pneumonia have been compared to those of specimens simultaneously obtained by TTA. When *S. aureus,* coliforms, or pseudomonads were cultured from the TTA specimen, they were virtually always present in the expectorated sputum. The converse was not true, however. In 50 percent of patients with these organisms in the sputum, they could not be recovered from the lower respiratory tract by TTA.[6]

Postoperative pneumonia usually results from aspiration of oropharyngeal contents, and the infecting flora has certain unique features in this setting. Hospitalized patients with underlying diseases rapidly acquire facultative gram-negative bacteria and staphylococci in their oropharynx.[7,8] Changes in this flora are further accentuated by the use of antimicrobial agents. The respiratory equipment used to support the patient also predisposes to the acquisition of resistant bacteria. Thus, a surgical patient with serious illness who has received antimicrobial agents is likely to have coliforms, *Pseudomonas,* or *S. aureus* as the cause of their pneumonia.

The treatment of postoperative pneumonia should be designed initially to cover all possible pathogens (see Table 2) and then tailored to reflect results of the culture. This strategy usually requires therapy with two antibiotics at the onset, particularly when aerobic gram-negative bacilli are present. One of the newer cephalosporins, cefazolin, cefamandole or cefoxitin, may be adequate to cover a broad range of pathogens, including oral anaerobes, gram-positive cocci, and coliforms. An aminoglycoside is used for resistant gram-negative bacilli, especially *P. aeruginosa.* Carbenicillin or ticarcillin is often administered with the aminoglycoside, but there is no compelling evidence that demonstrates improved outcome with such therapy in postoperative surgical patients. Deep nasotracheal suction, endotracheal intubation, or fiberoptic bronchoscopy may be instrumental in clearing the airways so that adequate tracheobronchial toilet is facilitated.

MEDIASTINAL, PROSTHETIC VALVE, AND VASCULAR GRAFT INFECTIONS

Acute Mediastinitis

Acute mediastinitis was an uncommon infection even before the advent of antimicrobial therapy. The proximate causes of nontraumatic mediastinitis in that era were breakdown of caseous tuberculous nodes and extension of infection from a peritonsillar abscess or Ludwig's angina.[9,10] The microbiology reflected the pathogens recovered from upper and lower respiratory disease at that time: hemolytic streptococci, staphylococci, pneumococci, and the tubercle bacillus. The control of tuberculosis, improved dental care, and the liberal use of antibiotics for upper respiratory infections have all contributed to the rarity with which such infections now occur.

Since mediastinitis is encountered infrequently, the diagnosis and management are unfamiliar to many physicians. The symptoms and signs of acute mediastinal infection are fever, dysphagia, chest pain, and respiratory distress, which are manifest to varying degrees by all patients. Leukocytosis is usually present, unless the patient is cachectic or overwhelmingly ill. X-rays of the chest and/or upper neck reveal mediastinal widening, abnormal extra-luminal gas collections, or an associated pleural reaction. Special studies, such as an esophagogram or upper extremity venography, may show encroachment upon the lumen or displacement of vital structures, but these studies are not required for diagnosis or management in most cases.

Recent reports have called attention to mediastinitis arising from odontogenic or deep cervical suppuration.[11] Anaerobic bacteria are often recovered in such situations, since they are the pathogens in the majority of space infections of the head and neck.[12,13] Their infrequent recovery in bygone days reflected a lack of awareness of their virulence and the lack of availability of anaerobic culturing techniques. The pathogenesis of such infections involves dissection of untreated or undrained purulence from the cervical region to the superior mediastinum.

Another route for infection to reach the mediastinum is via esophageal rupture or tears, which not only allows the indigenous microflora to gain access but often causes them to be accompanied by gastric acid, increasing the inflammatory reaction. The eponym Boerhaave's syndrome has been applied to an often lethal scenario of postemetic rupture of the distal esophagus, followed by mediastinitis and empyema. The Dutch physician Hermann Boerhaave witnessed this sequence in 1724 in the Grand Admiral of the fleet who was said to have overindulged in food and drink and then induced vomiting with an emetic.[14] Uniformly fatal if unrecognized, prompt treatment reduces the mortality to less than 50 percent.[15] Perforation of the cervical esophagus is usually due to instrumentation and is not accompanied by extravasation of gastric contents. However, infection often ensues and can culminate in life-threatening mediastinitis.[16] Blunt trauma can also disrupt the esophagus; attention may be drawn away from the mediastinum to an associated intraperitoneal or pulmonary injury, only to be focused on mediastinitis when feeding is resumed.

The principles of management of these infections should include: (1) prompt recognition, (2) aggressive surgical drainage, (3) appropriate cultures of purulent material, and (4) parenteral antimicrobial therapy. Drainage of an involved mediastinum and pleural space should be employed. If an esophageal tear is demonstrated by a contrast exam, immediate repair is indicated. Aerobic and anaerobic cultures should be performed and antimicrobial therapy is adjusted according to culture results and susceptibility studies. Empiric antibiotic therapy, prior to the availability of culture results, should include either penicillin, a cephalosporin, or clindamycin. An aminoglycoside is added when gram-negative organisms are suspected, such as in chronically ill, hospitalized patients.

The duration of therapy is dictated by the clinical response of the patient and a steady decrease in the output from the drainage tubes.

Postoperative Mediastinitis and Sternal Osteomyelitis

The most common form of mediastinal infection encountered in clinical practice today is related to median sternotomy for cardiac surgery. The incidence of this postoperative complication in different centers has ranged from 1 to 5 percent.[17–20] In one large study, the incidence was higher for patients undergoing coronary revascularization (2.5%) than in those having valvular surgery (1.4%). The pathogenesis of the disease is unclear. Routine cultures of the operative field, pump reservoir, or valvular prostheses have revealed a high (71%) rate of bacterial contamination, mostly with diphtheroids and *Staphylococcus epidermidis.* However, in this particular study of 66 patients, none of the infections were due to the recovered organisms[21] perhaps due to cephalosporin administration perioperatively. Some reports have claimed that respiratory infections due to the responsible pathogen preceded mediastinal infection. It is likely that undetected bacteremia from a pulmonary source, an arterial or venous cannula, or urinary catheters in the immediate postoperative period leads to seeding of the mediastinum, only to erupt into mediastinitis days to weeks later. Risk factors for the development of this complication have included in some, but not all series, prolonged cardiopulmonary bypass, reoperation for bleeding, or low cardiac output postoperatively. However, these factors may simply be reflections of a "sicker" group of patients with compromised host defenses rather than independent risk factors.

Because of the seriousness of this complication, most surgeons employ perioperative prophylactic antibiotics. However, a controlled study of antibiotic prophylaxis (penicillin and methicillin or cephalothin) in 904 myocardial revascularization procedures failed to demonstrate any significant difference in the incidence of chest wound infections postoperatively (1.1% treated versus 1.8% untreated). Those in the untreated group usually had infections due to *S. aureus,* while 80 percent of the infections in the prophylaxis group were coliform-associated infections.[20] This is not surprising since streptomycin prophylaxis administered to patients undergoing cardiac surgery has been associated with an increased rate of colonization by gram-negative bacteria and a 50 percent increase in the rate of acquisition of streptomycin-resistant gram-negative bacilli.[22]

The symptoms and signs of mediastinal infections have been fairly uniform in the reported series, with fever, leukocytosis, serous or seropurulent wound drainage, and dehiscence of the sternal fracture site being the major clues to the presence of this complication.[17,20] Routine roentgenograms of the sternum have been unhelpful. Tomography and ^{67}Ga scans have been confirmatory in patients with sternal osteomyelitis,[23] but their predictive value awaits further studies since many patients with a recent sternotomy would be expected to have focal uptake of gallium or radiographic abnormalities. Our own experience with 20 patients with mediastinitis and/or sternal osteomyelitis has been similar. Our cases could be divided into early ($\leq$ 4 weeks postoperative) and late ($>$ 4 weeks). The early cases were more common (70%) and tended to be fulminant with fever in most patients and bacteremia in greater than 40 percent of cases. They were usually due to gram-negative bacilli resistant to antimicrobials used as perioperative prophylaxis. Late cases were usually due to staphylococci (four of six). These patients were often afebrile, and had drainage from the operative site as the hallmark of infection.

Management should include re-exploration of the operative wound with debridement and drainage of all infected areas. This often necessitates reopening the sternal wound and curettage of obviously infected bone. Some authors advocate continuous mediastinal irrigation with dilute povidone-iodine or antibiotic solutions, but there are no data which allow evaluation of its effectiveness.[24] The mainstay of therapy, along with drainage and debridement, is systemic antimicrobial therapy, usually for three or more weeks. It can be predicted that most early infections will be caused by gram-negative bacilli resistant to the agent employed as prophylaxis. In such cases, aminoglycoside administration is usually warranted. The decision is best individualized, depending upon the resistance patterns of nosocomial isolates at a particular institution.

Prosthetic Valve Endocarditis

Infection is an uncommon but serious complication of cardiac prosthetic valve insertion. The incidence of this complication increases with the length of follow-up, but at three years postoperatively, it is approximately 2 percent.[25] Relatively distinct clinical syndromes of "early" and "late" prosthetic valve endocarditis have been described. Early cases, defined as those occurring within 60 days postoperatively, are caused by, in order of frequency, *S. epidermidis*, gram-negative bacilli, *S. aureus*, and miscellaneous pathogens including fungi and streptococci.[25] The pathogens in late cases are reminiscent of infections on natural valves, with streptococci causing the majority of cases. However, there remains a disproportionately high frequency of *S. epidermidis*, gram-negative bacilli, and fungi even in the late cases. Primarily because of the different microbiology, the pathogenesis of early infections is presumed to be intraoperative and perioperative (undetected bacteremia) contamination of the prosthesis; late infections arise secondary to bacteremia known to follow various activities such as dental manipulation or tooth brushing.

The symptoms of prosthetic infection do not differ substantially, whether late or early. Fever is virtually always present. Prominent among symptoms is congestive heart failure due to valve dehiscence and paraprosthetic regurgitation. An elevated white blood cell count is seen in 50 percent of patients, and sustained bacteremia is the rule. The dilemma of prosthetic valve endocarditis lies not so much in awareness of the diagnosis as in management. The reported mortality of early prosthetic valve endocarditis is over 70 percent and of late endocarditis is 45 percent.[25] Both the status of the host and the virulence of the infecting organism contribute to the high mortality.

The appropriate management of the patient with prosthetic valve endocarditis is continuing to evolve. One recurrent theme in recent reports is the emphasis on early surgery to improve the outcome. This is undisputed with fungal infections and major valve dysfunction, as the mortality in these situations approaches 100 percent. While some evidence is available to recommend operative replacement of the valve in early cases due to *S. aureus* and gram-negative bacilli, there are insufficient data to justify a dogmatic approach. Most authorities would recommend a trial of antibiotic therapy for late prosthetic valve endocarditis due to relatively avirulent organisms. The specific antibiotics are dictated by the in vitro sensitivity of the pathogen recovered. Parenteral therapy with a bactericidal antibiotic or combination should be given for four or more weeks. A recent report has demonstrated that rifampin therapy improves bactericidal titers and probably the cure rate in patients with *S. epidermidis* prosthetic valve endocarditis.[26]

Prophylactic antibiotics are recommended during the placement of prosthetic cardiac valves.[27] There is no prospective randomized study which unequivocally demonstrates their efficacy, but available data demonstrate an unacceptable incidence of infections due to susceptible pathogens in patients not receiving such chemoprophylaxis. Two studies have shown that short-term preoperative prophylaxis with cephalothin is as effective as more prolonged prophylaxis.[28, 29] Hence, most authorities recommend a cephalosporin be given preoperatively and for 48 hours after surgery for implantation of cardiac valves. If the operation is prolonged, intraoperative administration of antibiotics should be considered since unacceptably low serum levels of antibiotics have been found during cardiopulmonary bypass.[30]

Vascular Graft Infections

Graft infections are a grave complication of reconstructive vascular surgery. Most surgical groups report the incidence of this complication as 1 to 5 percent.[31–33] Intra-abdominal prostheses are less likely to become infected than more distally positioned grafts. As is the case with prosthetic valve infections, there are early and late graft infections. It is presumed that early infections represent operative or perioperative contamination of the prosthesis; late cases represent lodgement of bacteria due to occult bacteremia with subsequent invasion or a late recrudescence of an operatively contaminated graft. Experimental evidence indicates grafts become less susceptible to infection as a pseudointima forms;[34] this is concordant with the observation that most infections become manifest within 60 days of surgery.

The clinical signs of infection include local inflammation or drainage, thrombosis, hemorrhage, and sepsis. Infected aortoiliac prostheses commonly present with hemorrhage into the peritoneal cavity or gastrointestinal tract, even in the absence of other signs of infection. Aortofemoral or iliofemoral infections, however, are most often recognized because of drainage or cellulitis in the area of the inguinal surgical wound.[35] Hemorrhage is felt to be inevitable if the suture line at the graft site becomes involved.

The microbiology of these infections is dependent upon the nature of antimicrobial prophylaxis and the site in question. Staphylococci, both coagulase-positive and coagulase-negative strains, are the most frequent pathogens in aortofemoral and femoral-popliteal bypasses, while gram-negative bacilli are next in frequency. In aortoiliac operations, gram-negative bacilli are the most frequent pathogens.[35] If anti-staphylococcal prophylaxis is employed (a frequent and justifiable practice), gram-negative bacilli are more frequently encountered.

Recognition of infection is ordinarily not difficult, especially when infection occurs in the groin. Arteriographic examination, often an indispensable tool in management, may disclose an unsuspected false aneurysm. Echography or CT scan may be useful in individual cases. Blood cultures should always be obtained. Some authorities have advocated cultures of arterial blood distal to the prosthesis, but the advantage of this practice remains unproven. Drainage from the wound should be gram-stained and cultured, as should any excised material; in the absence of bacteremia these sources may be the only opportunity to recognize the responsible pathogen.

Management of an infected prosthesis is vexing. Szilagyi and associates have graded infections according to their depth: Grade I—only dermis is involved; Grade II—subcutaneous involvement but no invasion of the implant; and Grade III—the prosthesis is infected.[31] In their experience, infections not involving the prostheses responded to relatively conservative measures and all healed promptly. Conversely, those which involved the prosthesis were extremely difficult to eradicate.

The cardinal principle of removing a foreign body at an infected site usually applies, and surgical removal is the "conservative" approach in this setting, while nonoperative management often invites disaster. If the graft is thrombosed, and therefore useless, or if hemorrhage due to suture line involvement has occurred, there is no quarrel with prompt removal. The more difficult problem is a patient with a functioning but infected graft, in whom efforts are directed at local wound care along with systemic antibiotics. Although failure of this approach is not universal, it is frequent enough to be viewed with scepticism. If graft removal would produce ischemia that threatens the integrity of a limb or other tissue, a two-stage procedure is adopted: (1) placement of an alternative bypass proximally and distally away from the infected area (e.g., an axillofemoral bypass to circumvent an aortofemoral groin infection), and (2) subsequent removal of the infected prosthesis. Antimicrobial therapy for these infections is guided by the sensitivities of the responsible pathogen. If *S. aureus* is responsible, a semisynthetic penicillin (nafcillin or oxacillin) should be given; if gram-negative bacilli are isolated, a cephalosporin or an aminoglycoside is warranted. The drugs should be given intravenously at high doses for at least 4 weeks. The proper duration of therapy is unsettled.

A dogmatic approach to infected grafts should not be adopted as salvage has been documented without removing the graft. Operative debridement of infected tissues around the graft, parenteral antimicrobial therapy, and, in some cases, local instillation of antibiotic solutions have been employed in such cases.[36, 37] Szilagi and coworkers present three criteria to be fulfilled when this approach is to be considered: (1) the periprosthetic infection is lingering and of low virulence, (2) the anastomotic lines are not involved, and (3) there is no evidence of bacterial colonization of the pseudointima.

Dialysis Access Infections

Bacteremic infections in patients undergoing hemodialysis for acute or chronic renal failure frequently arise from the vascular access site. In patients with chronic renal failure, the vascular site is the most likely source of sepsis, while in patients with acute renal failure, pneumonia and intra-abdominal abscesses are more frequently incriminated.[38] *S. aureus* is the responsible pathogen in 70 percent of infections, followed by streptococci and gram-negative bacilli. Recently, fungal infection of access devices has been observed.[39] The frequency of staphylococcal infections and bacteremia no doubt reflects the virulence of this organism and its frequent carriage in patients undergoing chronic dialysis. In one study, 62 percent of patients with chronic renal failure undergoing dialysis carried *S. aureus* in their nose, throat, or skin, compared to a carriage rate of 21 percent in a group of nondialyzed chronic renal failure patients.[40]

This complication presents with fever and chills and may be accompanied by evident inflammation or drainage at the access site. Local signs are more frequent in staphylococcal infections (50%) than in nonstaphylococcal ones (23%).[41] These local signs are more frequent in external shunts than in internal heterograft or native arteriovenous fistula-associated infections.

Antimicrobial therapy of gram-negative associated infections is guided by the antibiotic susceptibilities of the responsible pathogen. Vancomycin has been extremely useful in staphylococcal infections. It is bactericidal, resistance is almost nonexistent, and the pharmacokinetics in patients with renal failure usually allow once-weekly administration.[42, 43] If available, monitoring of serum levels is helpful to avoid excessive or insufficient levels of antibiotic. The duration of therapy should be four to six weeks.

It is controversial whether or not to remove the access device that has led to sepsis. If there is extensive local inflammation, pseudo-aneurysm or abscess formation, hemorrhage, or recurrent thrombosis, most authorities would suggest removal. If these signs are absent and sepsis is quickly controlled by antimicrobial therapy, salvage has been reported, and dialysis through the device can be continued.[41]

INTRA-ABDOMINAL INFECTIONS

Intra-abdominal sepsis following perforation of the gastrointestinal tract provides a challenge to surgical and medical management. Recent studies have called attention to the frequent occurrence of mixed infections in the abdomen involving both aerobic and anaerobic organisms. Knowledge of the normal flora of the gastrointestinal tract allows an accurate prediction of the infecting flora.

The microflora of the normal upper gastrointestinal tract from the stomach to the midileum is comprised of sparse numbers of facultative gram-positive organisms derived from the oropharynx. This situation is altered by anatomic abnormalities (Billroth II gastrectomy, small bowel diverticula, strictures) or pathologic changes (achlorhydria, scleroderma, diabetic autonomic neuropathy); overgrowth of small bowel flora is the consequence of these conditions. Perforation of the upper gastrointestinal tract in a previously healthy individual is associated with a relatively small inoculum and a low risk of infection, while the opposite holds for patients with various disease states.

The large bowel, on the other hand, harbors a luxuriant flora comprised predominantly of anaerobic bacteria.[44] The concentration of organisms in colonic contents approximates 10^{12}/ml, with anaerobes at least three logs more prevalent than aerobes. *Bacteroides,* for example, outnumber *E. coli* by 1000-fold. The lower ileum is a transitional zone containing modest numbers of microorganisms ($\sim 10^8$/ml).

Perforation of the colon releases a large number of bacteria into the peritoneal cavity and its surrounding tissues with a great risk of intra-abdominal sepsis. Common clinical settings which predispose to contamination by colonic flora include perforation of the appendix, diverticulitis, penetrating or blunt abdominal trauma, leakage through intestinal anastomoses, and colon cancer.[45]

Successful therapy of intra-abdominal infections involves judicious surgical intervention with resection of necrotic tissue and drainage of abscesses. The operative approach may be ultimately decisive, but it should be emphasized that surgical treatment alone may be inadequate. Antibiotics prevent spread of infection to adjacent tissues and the bloodstream. They also suppress bacterial growth in the operative site, allowing host defenses to accomplish healing. Intra-abdominal sepsis appears to be a synergistic process in which multiple species of aerobic and anaerobic bacteria act in concert to produce the disease. Our bacteriologic study of 67 patients with peritonitis or intra-abdominal abscess formation is illustrative (Table 3). An average of 5 microbes were isolated from each infected site, 2 aerobic and 3 anaerobic bacteria.[46] Anaerobic bacteria were involved in 63 of 67 cases (94%), being mixed with aerobic organisms in 53 cases (79%). The commonly isolated aerobic or facultative bacteria were *E. coli, Klebsiella, Streptococcus, Proteus,* and *Pseudomonas.* The most common anaerobic bacterium, found in 80 percent of patients, was *B. fragilis,* followed in frequency by various clostridia and anaerobic cocci, particularly *Peptostreptococcus.* Not only did *B. fragilis* emerge as the dominant anaerobic pathogen in intra-abdominal abscess, it was also the most common cause of bacteremia associated with this condition. This is of particular therapeutic importance as *B. fragilis* is resistant to many antimicrobial agents.[47]

Appropriate antimicrobial therapy should be directed at both the aerobic and anaerobic components of a mixed infection. Support for this view is provided by data from an animal model which simulated intra-abdominal sepsis.[48] A gelatin capsule containing cecal contents was inserted into the peritoneal cavity of rats. The gelatin capsule quickly dissolved, releasing the fecal material into the abdomen. A biphasic disease was produced; acute peritonitis occurred during the first five days with an attendant mortality of 43 percent; the second phase, 7 to 14 days following challenge, was characterized by the development of intra-abdominal abscesses in all surviving animals. The predominant organisms during the acute peritonitis phase were *E. coli* and enterococci, with *E. coli*

TABLE 3. Bacteriology of Intra-abdominal Sepsis (67 Patients)

Anaerobic Bacteria	*Number of Patients*	*Aerobic and Facultative Bacteria*	*Number of Patients*
Bacteroides fragilis	54	*Escherichia coli*	44
Bacteroides melaninogenicus	12	*Proteus*	15
Bacteroides species	7	*Klebsiella* species	13
Fusobacterium	14	*Pseudomonas aeruginosa*	10
Peptostreptococcus	18	*Enterobacter*	9
Peptococcus	11	*Staphylococcus epidermidis*	18
Veillonella	2	*Staphylococcus aureus*	3
Anaerobic gram-positive non-sporulating rods	24	Enterococcus	10
Clostridia	43	*Streptococcus* (other than above)	7

Modified from Gorbach.[46]

bacteremia existing in 90 percent of the animals. In the later abscess stage, *B. fragilis* and *Fusobacterium varium* were the predominant isolates.[48, 49]

The efficacy of various antimicrobial agents, singly or in combination, was examined in this model. Gentamicin, which has activity limited to the coliforms, reduced the acute mortality to 4 percent, but 98 percent of survivors developed abscesses. Clindamycin, a drug with excellent activity against most anaerobic bacteria, failed to alter the early mortality rate but reduced abscess formation to 5 percent. The combination of gentamicin and clindamycin significantly reduced both mortality and abscess formation.[50] The implications of these studies are that coliforms are responsible for early mortality associated with peritonitis and septicemia and that anaerobes are responsible for the late stage abscess formation. It is evident that therapy should be directed against both groups of organisms.

A randomized, prospective study conducted in the trauma unit of Cook County Hospital lends support to this therapeutic concept.[51] A group of 100 patients with abdominal trauma which resulted in perforation of the small or large intestine as proven at laparotomy were studied. These patients were previously healthy and had not received prior antibiotics. The traumatic event had occurred within 12 hours of surgical exploration. The selection of antibiotics was randomized to one of two regimens: cephalothin plus kanamycin or clindamycin plus kanamycin. Kanamycin provided activity against the coliforms in both groups. The major comparison was cephalothin, an antibiotic with relatively poor activity against anaerobic bacteria, particularly *B. fragilis,* versus clindamycin, a drug with excellent activity against most anaerobic pathogens.

Detailed bacteriologic studies of the infected wounds showed that the clindamycin regimen reduced the isolation rate of anaerobes when compared to that of patients receiving cephalothin. Of greater interest was the evaluation of clinical efficacy based on the incidence of the two dreaded complications of bowel perforation: intra-abdominal abscess formation and septicemia (Table 4). There were 14 patients with these complications in the cephalothin group compared to 5 in the clindamycin group. The reason for this difference became more apparent when analyzing for episodes associated with anaerobes: anaerobes were involved in 11 septic complications in the cephalothin group but in only 1 in the clindamycin group. Furthermore, in 6 patients who received cephalothin, *Bacteroides* bacteremia developed. These patients were subsequently treated

TABLE 4. Bacteriology of Complications Associated with Abdominal Trauma

Microorganisms	*Number of Patients Receiving Cephalothin and Kanamycin*	*Number of Patients Receiving Clindamycin and Kanamycin*
Aerobes only	3	4
Mixed	6	0
Anaerobes only	5	1
Total	*14*	*5*

Modified from Thadepalli et al.[51]

successfully with clindamycin. The one failure in the clindamycin group was due to a clostridial bacteremia that required chloramphenicol for ultimate cure. These clostridia were shown to be resistant in vitro to clindamycin. The results of this study indicate that maximum reduction of the suppurative complications of bowel perforation is achieved with antibiotic therapy directed at both the aerobic and anaerobic components of the mixed infection.

The selection of appropriate antimicrobial therapy in intra-abdominal sepsis is influenced by the frequent isolation of *B. fragilis* in this clinical setting (> 80%) and by the resistance of this organism to many commonly employed antibiotics. Accepted antibiotic therapy has included the combinations of clindamycin plus an aminoglycoside or chloramphenicol with or without an aminoglycoside. Recent studies have demonstrated that other agents such as ticarcillin, cefoxitin, and metronidazole are efficacious in the therapy of intra-abdominal sepsis. Several antibiotics have poor activity against *B. fragilis,* including penicillin G, tetracycline, cephalosporins (except cefoxitin), and the aminoglycosides.

Many investigators have used combinations of clindamycin and an aminoglycoside in the therapy of intra-abdominal infections with encouraging results. Bartlett and coworkers[52] reported cure in 51 of 75 patients with intra-abdominal sepsis using clindamycin 600 mg intravenously three to four times daily, and gentamicin, 1.5 to 2 mg/kg of body weight intravenously every eight hours. Swenson and Lorber achieved good responses in 51 of 64 patients with intra-abdominal abscess using slightly lower doses of clindamycin (300 to 450 mg intravenously every 6 to 8 hours) and either gentamicin or kanamycin.[53]

Of all the available drugs, chloramphenicol has the broadest spectrum of activity against anaerobes. Chow and Guze[54] reported 27 percent mortality using this agent in treating 48 patients with *Bacteroides* bacteremia, as compared to 21 percent mortality in 42 patients treated with clindamycin. In a recent prospective study, randomized comparison of clindamycin, ticarcillin, and chloramphenicol in combination with gentamicin in the treatment of intra-abdominal sepsis yielded a similar response: 33 of 42 patients (79%) treated with clindamycin, 35 of 39 (90%) treated with ticarcillin, and 43 of 53 (81%) treated with chloramphenicol were cured. The major complication in the chloramphenicol group was hematologic suppression.[55]

However, chloramphenicol failures have been reported. Thadepalli and coworkers[56] described 10 patients with infections with anaerobic bacteria who failed to respond to chloramphenicol; all of the failures subsequently responded to clindamycin. In an animal model of intra-abdominal sepsis, Louie and coworkers[57] noted that chloramphenicol failed to prevent abscesses in 59 percent of the animals. An explanation of these failures may be found in the evidence that *B. fragilis* can inactivate chloramphenicol by two mechanisms: (1) by reduction of the nitro group on the benzene ring and (2) by acetylation of the hydroxyl group on the side chain.

Metronidazole's profound bactericidal activity against anaerobic bacteria has prompted several studies of its efficacy in anaerobic infections. Eykyn and Phillips investigated the use of metronidazole in 50 patients, 36 with intra-abdominal infections, and 6 with pelvic infections. A favorable response was observed in 20 of 24 patients treated with metronidazole alone and in 20 of 26 patients treated with a combination of metronidazole and either gentamicin or ampicillin.[58] Two recent studies have reported that metronidazole or clindamycin, when combined with tobramycin, are equally efficacious in the treatment of serious mixed aerobic-anaerobic infections in the abdomen[212] or female palvis.[213]

Carbenicillin or ticarcillin, either alone or in combination with an aminoglycoside, have been used to treat intra-abdominal sepsis. It should be noted that in vitro susceptibility tests show that carbenicillin is no more active than penicillin G against *B. fragilis* and that 10 to 20 percent of strains are highly resistant. The prospective, randomized trial by Harding and associates[55] demonstrated that ticarcillin was equal to clindamycin or chloramphenicol when combined with an aminoglycoside. The major toxicity with ticarcillin was hypokalemia.

Cephalosporins are widely used in surgical infections. Several studies have shown that cephalothin, cefazolin, and cefamandole have variable activity in vitro against *B. fragilis* with many strains being resistant. Thus, these drugs are not appropriate therapy for intra-abdominal sepsis.

Cefoxitin, a newly-introduced cephamycin, is active against 95 percent of *B. fragilis* strains at the readily achievable concentration of 32 μg/ml. Louie and coworkers[50] evaluated cefoxitin in the animal model of intra-abdominal sepsis; its efficacy was equivalent to that of clindamycin and gentamicin and was superior to that of four cephalosporins. Uncontrolled clinical studies have also demonstrated excellent results with cefoxitin in intra-abdominal infections.[59, 60] In a prospective, randomized study we have demonstrated that cefoxitin, alone or in combination with an aminoglycoside, is equally efficacious as clindamycin plus an aminoglycoside in the treatment of serious anaerobic infections including intra-abdominal infections.[61] Similar results have been obtained in a randomized study in Baltimore.[62]

The choice of appropriate antimicrobial therapy for intra-abdominal infections should be based on comparative studies judging efficacy and safety of the various combinations (Table 5). Based upon the currently available information from clinical and experimental studies of the treatment of mixed aerobic-anaerobic infection, we feel

TABLE 5. Alternative Antibiotic Combinations for Intra-abdominal Sepsis*

Clindamycin or		
Chloramphenicol or		
Carbenicillin or	plus an	Aminoglycoside
Ticarcillin or		
Metronidazole		
	or	
Cefoxitin	alone or with an	Aminoglycoside

*Doses are indicated in section on antimicrobial agents.

Cainzos, Prospective Randomized Controlled Study of Prophylaxis with Cefamandole in High Risk Patients Undergoing Operations upon the Biliary Tract, S.G.O, 160: 27, Jan 1985.

clindamycin and an aminoglycoside or cefoxitin (with an aminoglycoside if cefoxitin-resistant aerobes are suspected or recovered) are the best regimens. If a patient fails to respond to the selected therapy, then alternative agents should be administered. The reasons for failure may include infection with a resistant pathogen or failure to achieve adequate surgical drainage.

Biliary Tract Infections

Biliary tract infections ensue when there is prior bacterial colonization. Bile from a normal biliary tree is usually sterile. However, bacterial colonization of the bile occurs in a diseased biliary tract, especially with cholelithiasis and obstruction. It is presumed, because of the resemblance to the enteric flora, that infecting bacteria reach the biliary tree by ascending from the gut. To convert asymptomatic bactibilia into infection requires another perturbation of host defenses, most commonly impaction of a stone in the cystic or common duct. Obstruction interferes with biliary emptying and vascular supply, providing an opportunity for rapid proliferation of the bacteria present.

The types of infection encountered in the biliary tract include acute cholecystitis, ascending cholangitis, empyema of the gall bladder, and emphysematous cholecystitis. Gall bladder perforation or gangrene are rare in acute cholecystitis but common in emphysematous cholecystitis. Ascending cholangitis is often accompanied by bacteremia and septic shock; this condition also predisposes to multiple small liver abscesses. Empyema of the gall bladder frequently culminates in perforation, either into the peritoneal cavity or a hollow viscus or may spread to the liver causing abscess formation.

Patients with acute cholecystitis have positive bile cultures in 70 percent of cases; when there is common duct obstruction by stones this increases to 90 percent.[63] Acute cholecystitis and ascending cholangitis are usually associated with a single aerobic pathogen such as *E. coli, Klebsiella,* or enterococci. However, emphysematous cholecystitis and gall bladder empyema are most often mixed aerobic-anaerobic infections. Recent bacteriologic studies from Denmark, Japan, and the United States have revealed that anaerobic bacteria may play a more prominent role in biliary tract sepsis than previously thought.[64–66] In one series in which 68 percent of the patients had positive bile cultures, 39 percent yielded potential anaerobic pathogens (Table 6). *B. fragilis* was the most common anaerobic isolate, followed in frequency by *Clostridium perfringens.* Anaerobic bactibilia is encountered more frequently among elderly patients and in patients with severe symptoms, prior biliary-intestinal anastomosis or other complex biliary surgeries, or ductal obstruction.[67] Another unexpected finding has been the isolation of *Pseudomonas* in 5 to 10 percent of primary bile cultures.

Recognition of biliary infection is usually not problematic. Patients with acute cholecystitis present with right upper quadrant pain and ordinarily have fever. Oral cholecystrograms fail to visualize the gallbladder. Intravenous cholecystography may be helpful in excluding common duct obstruction if the bilirubin is below 3.5 mg/dl. Echography has been employed recently to visualize gall bladder stones and exclude common duct dilatation.[68,69] In experienced hands, this procedure is very accurate. Plain films of the abdomen show extra-intestinal, right upper quadrant gas in emphysematous

Nagar, Excretion of Antibiotics by the Biliary Tree, S.G+O, 158: 601, 1984.

TABLE 6. Bacteriology of Biliary Sepsis (371 Patients)*

	Percentage of Positive Cultures (253 patients)
Aerobic pathogens alone	60
Anaerobic pathogens alone	1
Mixed aerobic-anaerobic pathogens	39

Aerobes	*Percentage of Patients with This Isolate/Total Aerobic Isolates*	*Anaerobes*	*Percentage of Patients with This Isolate/Total Anaerobic Isolates*
Escherichia coli	24	*Bacteroides fragilis*	38
Group D streptococci	19	*Clostridium perfringens*	32
Klebsiella	17	*Bacteroides* species	7
Pseudomonas aeruginosa	8	*Clostridium* species	7
Viridans streptococci	7	*Fusobacterium*	5
Enterobacter	3	Anaerobic cocci	3
Proteus mirabilis	3	Nonsporulating gram-positive bacilli	8
Staphylococcus epidermidis	3		
Proteus morganii	2		
Citrobacter	2		
Corynebacterium	2		
Miscellaneous	10		

*Adapted from Bourgault and coworkers[67] and England and Rosenblatt.[66]

cholecystitis. Perforation of the gall bladder is suggested by the development of diffuse peritoneal signs, but not infrequently such signs fail to develop and perforation is found at the time of surgery.

Selection of appropriate antimicrobial therapy in biliary tract sepsis depends on the clinical setting and on achievable drug levels in the bile. In acute cholecystitis and cholangitis without signs of septic shock, therapy directed only at the aerobic pathogens is sufficient. If shock is present or there is evidence of empyema, gangrene, or emphysematous cholecystitis, broad coverage directed at aerobic and anaerobic pathogens should be administered. In the absence of biliary obstruction, chloramphenicol, the aminopenicillins and antipseudomonal penicillins, cephalosporins, clindamycin, tetracycline, and gentamicin reach therapeutic levels in the bile for many of the usual pathogens. A cephalosporin is the best agent if the patient is not gravely ill. However, enterococci are uniformly resistant. Since *Klebsiella* are common in infected bile, ampicillin or carbenicillin alone, to which most *Klebsiella* are resistant, is risky. Most physicians would combine ampicillin with an aminoglycoside for the gravely ill patient. Many *B. fragilis* isolates will be resistant to this combination, and if there are factors which suggest anaerobic bactibilia could be present, we would include a drug effective against this pathogen. Penetration into bile is greatly impared with biliary obstruction, and the therapeutic margin of most drugs is attenuated. Since hepatic-vein bacteremia is proportional to common duct pressure in an experimental model,[70] and antimicrobials reach the infected site so poorly when obstructed, surgical drainage is mandatory to effect a cure when the common duct is obstructed.

In the postoperative patient with continued biliary sepsis despite antibiotic therapy, there may be unrecognized obstruction or abscess formation. They should be searched for with appropriate radiographic or sonographic studies. Alternatively, the presence of a resistant pathogen should be suspected. Appropriate management should include cultures of blood and bile, search for obstruction or an abscess, and adjustment of antibiotic therapy to cover potential resistant pathogens while culture results are pending.

Pyogenic Liver Abscess

Despite advances in surgical technique and antibiotic therapy, liver abscess remains a serious infection with a high mortality. The disease occurs most often in older patients with underlying disorders. Diagnosis may be delayed, many cases being discovered at autopsy. Pyogenic infection of the liver occurs as a discrete abscess or as multiple microabscesses. Clinical settings predisposing to liver abscess include biliary tract disease, abdominal trauma with bowel perforation, appendicitis, hematoma of the liver, and pyelophlebitis of the portal veins. Microabscesses are associated with septicemia, although ascending cholangitis is probably a more common cause.[71,72]

The bacteriology of liver abscess has remained in a confused state for many years. Most reports document the presence of coliforms, facultative streptococci, and staphylococci, the latter being found in cases of septicemia. "Sterile pus" has often been reported in liver abscess; this probably represents anaerobic infection. Recent studies by Sabbaj and coworkers and Altemeier have utilized anaerobic techniques to study liver abscesses. Approximately 50 to 75 percent of their cases were involved with fastidious anaerobes, the most common being *B. fragilis*, anaerobic streptococci, fusobacteria, and clostridia. The majority of cases were coinfected with coliforms and facultative streptococci.[73,74]

The clinical presentation of liver abscess may be obvious on history and physical examination, or may be occult, presenting as a "fever-of-unknown-origin." There are four clinical features which, taken together, suggest liver abscess: First, pain in the right upper quadrant of the abdomen. The pain may be referred to the right shoulder or scapula due to irritation of the diaphragm. Second, fever which may be accompanied by drenching night sweats. Third, vomiting and loss of appetite. Fourth, malaise with weight loss. Other symptoms associated with liver abscess include chills, basilar rales on the right side, diarrhea, jaundice, and cough. Laboratory clues to the presence of a liver abscess are an elevated alkaline phosphatase and a progressive decline in serum albumin. Other laboratory abnormalities may include leukocytosis with a left shift, elevated sedimentation rate, anemia, and elevated liver enzymes including serum glutamic-oxaloacetic transaminase (SGOT), serum glutamic-pyruvic transaminase (SGPT), and lactic dehydrogenase (LDH). The diagnosis of liver abscess is suggested by the presence of a right pleural effusion or an elevated right hemidiaphragm on chest x-ray.

Once a liver abscess is suspected, a number of noninvasive procedures aid in defining the lesion. Plain films of the abdomen should be examined for extra-intestinal gas, an air fluid level over the liver, or gas in the biliary tree. Radionuclide liver scans are very helpful in locating liver abscess. Occasionally, a scan may be negative with a proven abscess, so if clinical suspicion is high, alternative diagnostic procedures should be performed. Ultrasound is another method for detecting intrahepatic abscesses. However, it is only 50 percent accurate. The diagnostic workup for liver abscess has been facilitated by the development of computed tomography (CT). This technique can define even small lesions and can also clearly outline dilated biliary radicles. The CT scan has reduced the need for selective hepatic artery angiography. However, this latter procedure is highly accurate in the detection of lesions greater than 1 cm in diameter and may be needed when a CT scanner is not available.

Large, discrete liver abscesses should be appropriately drained by operative intervention, however, microabscesses cannot be approached in this manner. An underlying cause should be sought in all cases. These include intra-abdominal abscesses, distant sites of persistent bacteremia, and portal vein septic thrombophlebitis. Obstruction of the biliary tract must be ruled out since this will result in persistent bacterial seeding due to ascending cholangitis.

Appropriate antibiotic treatment of liver abscess should include agents for aerobic and anaerobic components of the infection. Coliforms can be treated with an aminoglycoside, while coverage for anaerobic bacteria should include an agent active against *B. fragilis.* Antimicrobial agents with proven activity against *B. fragilis* include cefoxitin, chloramphenicol, clindamycin, metronidazole, and ticarcillin (see discussion on intra-abdominal abscesses above). In patients with shock associated with the abscess, an aminoglycoside should also be included with these agents.

Amebic Liver Abscess

It is important to differentiate a pyogenic liver abscess from an amebic abscess since the chemotherapy and operative approach may be entirely different. Patients with amebic liver abscess tend to have an enlarged, tender liver. Approximately 75 percent have abnormalities in the right chest either noted on physical examination or by chest x-ray. As a general rule, the amebic abscess is associated with less fever and toxicity, a lower white blood cell count, and a more chronic course.[75] However, these findings may be absent in an individual patient. Amebic serology is extremely useful to substantiate the clinical impression. Aspiration of abscess pus may be required for diagnosis in difficult cases. The amebic abscess is filled with reddish-brown material that on microscopic examination has few cellular elements. Trophozoites of Entamoeba histolytica are difficult to identify in pus unless the material is aspirated from the abscess wall. On the other hand, the pus from a pyogenic abscess is yellow or green; polymorphonuclear leukocytes and bacteria can be observed on microscopic examination, and in about one-third of cases there is a distinctly foul odor.

The "therapeutic response" is anathema to most surgeons, but there is some merit to this test in patients with amebic liver abscess. The response to appropriate treatment usually occurs within 2 to 3 days and is often very dramatic with a decrease in pain, toxicity, and size of the liver.

Needle aspiration of an amebic liver abscess is not required either for therapy or diagnosis in the majority of cases. However, the following situations may indicate the need for aspiration: (1) a large abscess which, because of its large volume of fluid, may reabsorb with great difficulty even with adequate chemotherapy, (2) a left lobe abscess that may rupture into the pericardium with catastrophic results (left lobe abscesses should be given a higher priority for drainage), (3) the diagnosis in doubt and the patient's clinical condition requiring rapid decisions, and (4) lack of response to initial therapy (to verify the diagnosis and examine the possibility of bacterial superinfection). It should be mentioned that the major risk of needle aspiration is infection introduced by the procedure.

Several drugs are available for treating amebic liver abscess.[76] One regimen involves metronidazole at a dose of 750 mg by mouth three times a day for ten days. Alternative therapy is intramuscular administration of emetine or dehydroemetine, a less toxic analog, in doses of 1 to 1.5 mg/kg of body weight for 10 days. Some authorities suggest that chloroquine can be used alone or be added to emetine in doses of 1 gm per day for two days and 500 mg daily for three weeks.[75]

Few studies have been performed comparing these regimens. Current evidence suggests that any of the three drugs can be employed alone with excellent results. Metronidazole is less toxic than the other agents and can be given by mouth. However, there have been several treatment failures with this drug. The requirement for oral metronidazole therapy may be difficult in patients who are vomiting or who are extremely ill. The emetine preparations have higher toxicity and must be administered parenterally. If there has been a treatment failure on one regimen, the patient should be restudied by needle aspiration and should have a course of one of the alternate drugs.

Spontaneous Peritonitis

Spontaneous peritonitis is an uncommon condition that is seen mainly in patients with Laennec's cirrhosis with ascites. The pathogenesis probably relates to a septicemia that is metastatically spread to the fluid in the peritoneal cavity. A similar syndrome has been reported in children with nephrotic syndrome.[77,78] Peritoneal dialysis for the treatment of acute renal failure also is associated with peritonitis caused by direct introduction of microorganisms.

The disease is differentiated from peritonitis associated with bowel contamination by the following observations:

1. There is usually a single microorganism seen on gram stain of ascitic fluid and grown on subsequent culture in spontaneous peritonitis. Sheets of polymorphonuclear leukocytes are seen on the stained slide. On the other hand, patients with bowel contamination have multiple organisms associated with their infection, and the polymorphonuclear leukocytes, while abundant, do not have this "wall-to-wall" appearance.
2. The protein content of the ascitic fluid is generally low, often 1 to 2 gm/dl, whereas bowel perforation is associated with a protein concentration of 3.5 gm/dl or higher.
3. There is no anatomic evidence of perforation of the bowel in such patients.

Coliforms, particularly *E. coli* and *Klebsiella,* are found in 70 percent of cases of spontaneous peritonitis. Streptococci such as enterococci and nonclassified streptococci and pneumococci are the second most frequent group of pathogens. Pneumococci have been associated with this syndrome in nephrotic children. Anaerobic bactiascites is distinctly uncommon.

Spontaneous peritonitis in the alcoholic with ascites is associated with a high mortality. Therefore, there should be a high index of suspicion of this infection in these patients. Any patient with ascites presenting with fever or abdominal pain should have a diagnostic peritoneal tap for gram stain and culture. Initial therapy should cover all possible pathogens; subsequent therapy can be tailored to the results of culture. Ampicillin or a cephalosporin plus an aminoglycoside are usually adequate. Surgical drainage is not indicated in the spontaneous form since bowel perforation is not present.

Pseudomembranous Colitis

Recognized since the 1890s, pseudomembranous colitis (PMC) has been associated with gastrointestinal surgery, staphylococcal enterocolitis, high risk newborns, and antibiotics. Many antimicrobial agents have been implicated, including clindamycin, ampicillin, tetracycline, chloramphenicol, cephalothin, erythromycin, and metronidazole. Overwhelming evidence now indicates that PMC and certain cases of antibiotic-associated diarrhea are caused by a cytolytic toxin produced by the anaerobic bacterium *Clostridium difficile.*[79] This organism has been isolated from the feces of most patients with antibiotic-associated PMC utilizing selective culture media, but it is encountered only rarely in the fecal flora of healthy patients. The strains of *C. difficile* isolated from humans with PMC produce the cytotoxin in vitro; the organism or the pure toxin reproduce the disease in hamsters, from which the toxin and organism can be recovered thereby fulfilling Koch's postulates.

The toxin of *C. difficile* is identified in the feces by a tissue culture assay, and its activity is neutralized by gas gangrene antitoxin or *Clostridium sordellii* antitoxin. Fecal specimens from 98 of 102 patients with confirmed PMC contained this cytotoxin.[80] The toxin has not been found in healthy adults; it is present in only 2 percent of patients on antibiotics who are not having diarrhea and in 2 percent of patients with gastrointestinal diseases not related to antimicrobial agents.

The diagnosis of PMC is established by a typical appearance of the colonic mucosa by sigmoidoscopy: there is a cobblestone, ulcerative often hemorrhagic epithelium which is covered by a grey-white, patchy membrane. The clinical presentations range from mild symptomatology with loose stools to severe colitis with toxic megacolon. Fortunately, the latter condition is not frequently encountered, usually occurring in patients with unrecognized PMC who are given opiates such as diphenoxylate or paregoric. Clindamycin cephalosporins and ampicillin have been the antimicrobial agents most frequently incriminated. Antibiotic-associated diarrhea usually begins four to ten days after antimicrobial therapy is initiated but can occur up to three weeks after treatment is discontinued. The incidence of antibiotic-associated diarrhea seems to correlate with increasing patient age but can occur with either oral or parenteral administration of the drugs. Although most patients have a self-limited course, more prolonged diarrhea with marked electrolyte abnormalities, hypoalbuminemia, and even death have occurred.

Therapy for antibiotic-associated diarrhea and PMC initially involves stopping the putative antimicrobial agent and giving supportive fluid and electrolyte replacement. In many instances of mild disease, the diarrhea subsides after these measures. Patients with severe diarrhea or with prolonged symptoms should be administered specific antibiotics directed at *C. difficile.* Vancomycin, 250 mg every six hours by mouth, has been effective in suppressing the diarrhea in 95 percent of patients.[81] However, 14 percent of the patients may be expected to relapse when vancomycin is discontinued. Another antimicrobial agent used to treat PMC is bacitracin. Anecdotal reports indicate that some patients respond to cholestyramine therapy, but the results have been disappointing in others. This agent works by binding the toxin produced by *C. difficile.*[82]

OBSTETRIC AND GYNECOLOGIC INFECTIONS

Postoperative infections in the obstetric and gynecologic patient present either as pelvic abscesses or peritonitis, both of which may be life-threatening. The infections may appear acutely or with a delayed and undulating course. Recent studies have added to our knowledge of the bacteriology of these infections which forms the basis for the selection of antimicrobial therapy.

The microorganisms which predominate in infections of the female pelvis are usually derived from the indigenous vaginal microflora. Quantitative cultures indicate that the total bacterial populations number from 10^8 to 10^9 organisms per milliliter of secretions of the endocervix and vagina. At each site, anaerobes outnumber aerobes by a factor of 10:1.[83] The predominant anaerobic bacteria are *Bacteroides* species, peptococci, peptostreptococci, lactobacilli, and eubacteria. *B. fragilis* is found in only about 3 to 10 percent of healthy women. The predominant aerobic bacteria are *Corynebacterium, Streptococcus,* and *Staphylococcus epidermidis.* Coliforms particularly *E. coli,* are found in 20 to 30 percent of healthy women. There are differences in the types of bacteria in the vaginal flora depending on the time of the menstrual cycle, pregnancy, prior antibiotic administration, and following gynecologic surgery.

In the past, infections of the female pelvis have been synonymous with a few bacteria: the aerobes *Neisseria gonorrhoeae* and streptococci, and the anaerobic streptococci and *C. perfringens.* The modern era of bacteriology has revealed a far more complex picture. Multiple organisms, both facultative and anaerobic, have been implicated and current evidence favors obligate anaerobes as the predominant pathogens in most of the serious infections of the female pelvis. Even milder conditions such as salpingitis may be associated with anaerobes, particularly anaerobic streptococci. In early postoperative cellulitis, *S. pyogenes* and *C. perfringens* are the prime pathogens. In suppurative postoperative disease occurring later in the postoperative period in which there is tissue necrosis and abscess formation, anaerobic microorganisms including *B. fragilis* and the newly recognized species *Bacteroides bivius* and *Bacteroides disiens* are important pathogens. The types of infections that occur in these postoperative patients include pelvic and adnexal abscesses, puerperal sepsis, endometritis, pyometra, amnionitis, suppurative pelvic thrombophlebitis, and cutaneous wound infections.

Pelvic Abscess

Two-thirds of the cases of pelvic abscess are associated with anaerobic-aerobic flora. The number of microbial species per patient ranges from 1 to 12 pathogens with an average being 5 organisms.[84] The aerobic and facultative microflora consists of *E. coli, Klebsiella, Proteus,* and *Streptococcus* while the anaerobic microorganisms include *B. fragilis, B. bivius, B. disiens,* anaerobic streptococci, *Bacteroides melaninogenicus,* and clostridia. Rarely, *P. aeruginosa, S. aureus,* and *Candida* are isolated. There is a high incidence of positive blood culture results in females with suppurative pelvic disease. The most common bloodstream invaders are *Bacteroides,* anaerobic streptococci, *E. coli, Klebsiella,* and clostridia. More than one species of bacterium can often be isolated from a single blood culture if anaerobic and aerobic media are employed.

Posthysterectomy Infections

Infectious complications of hysterectomy complicate 17 to 51 percent of the procedures and are especially common in premenopausal women undergoing vaginal procedures. Of the 64 postoperative pelvic infections studied by Hall and associates, 98 percent were associated with anaerobes.[85] The bacteriology is similar to that ennumerated above in pelvic abscess. Infections in the postoperative patient present as a vaginal cuff abscess, pelvic cellulitis, adnexal abscesses or pelvic thrombophlebitis.

Endomyometritis

The incidence of postpartum endometritis in Sweet and Ledger's prospective study of 2691 deliveries was 3.8 percent.[86] However, this figure is substantially increased to 12 to 27 percent in patients undergoing cesarean section or who have had intrauterine fetal monitoring. Detailed studies by Gibbs and associates[87] and more recently by Ledger's group showed a remarkable similarity between the flora of the infected and noninfected uterus with a mixed flora in 37 percent of those with endometritis and in 53 percent of the uninfected controls. Therapy of postpartum or postcesarean section endometritis should include an antibiotic or combination directed towards the anaerobes and aerobes. A dreaded complication associated with pyoendometritis is bacteremia with septic pulmonary emboli.

Infection following abortion, therapeutic or criminal, usually involves a mixture of microorganisms derived from the vaginal flora and has been known to have a higher frequency of bacteremia than other pelvic infections. Rotheram and Shick noted bacteremia in 61 percent (34 of 56) of patients with septic abortion.[88] Two or three bacterial isolates were recovered from one-half of the blood cultures, indicating the mixed nature of the infection. The anaerobic pathogens include *B. fragilis, B. melaninogenicus, Fusobacterium,* and anaerobic cocci. *C. perfringens* was seen on only two occasions in this study.

Since the most serious form of postabortal sepsis is due to *C. perfringens,* it has received considerable notoriety. The sequence of events is similar to gas gangrene in other sites, although hemolytic anemia and renal failure are more frequent in gas gangrene of the myometrium. The incidence of postabortal *C. perfringens* infections is reported to be 1 in 800 cases in the United States and 1 in 300 cases in Chile. When the complete syndrome occurs, reported mortality is 21 to 85 percent. The major dilemma with bacteriologic isolation of clostridia is differentiating colonization or mild infection from the life-threatening cases caused by massive release of alpha toxin. With gangrene of the uterus, an aggressive surgical approach is necessary in order to prevent the high mortality. In patients with colonization or with *C. perfringens* as one component of a mixed infection, the infection can be managed as are other postpartum pelvic infections. Although antitoxin and hyperbaric oxygen have been recommended for clostridial myonecrosis, these two forms of therapy have unproven merit and are often unavailable. Therefore, aggressive surgical therapy coupled with appropriate antimicrobial agents may be life saving. With pure clostridial infections, penicillin G remains the drug of choice. If the pathogen is felt to be a major component of a mixed infection, then penicillin is often added to the combination used to cover the other components of mixed infections.

S. pyogenes has been a classical cause of childbed fever. This organism has recently been reported in infections related to intrauterine devices and may occasionally be seen in association with pelvic surgery. Treatment of choice is high dose penicillin G, 5 million units intravenously every 4 hours. Surgery is usually not indicated unless necrotic tissue requires debridement.

The importance of treating both the mixed anaerobic-aerobic flora of obstetric and gynecologic infections has been shown by Ledger's group in patients with postoperative endometritis. Two-hundred patients with postcesarean endomyometritis at the Los Angeles County Hospital were randomized to receive either clindamycin plus gentamicin or penicillin plus gentamicin. The major difference in these regimens is the lack of activity of penicillin against the *Bacteroides* and other anaerobic bacteria which are known to be involved in pelvic infections. Each treatment group was evenly matched for clinical status, types of infection, and predisposing features. There was a significant difference in clinical outcome (Table 7); the combination of clindamycin and gentamicin was

TABLE 7. Comparison of Therapy with Clindamycin and Gentamicin versus Penicillin and Gentamicin in Endomyometritis

	Clindamycin and Gentamicin	*Penicillin and Gentamicin*
Number of patients	100	100
No response, third antibiotic	5	29
Wound infections	8	16
Prolonged febrile course	2	12
Median fever index (degree-hours)	77	91

Modified from diZerega and coworkers.[89]

superior to penicillin plus gentamicin considering favorable therapeutic response, incidence of serious postoperative complication, fever index and number of days hospitalized.[89] These data confirm previous clinical observations that optimal therapy is achieved in the treatment of suppurative disease of the female pelvis when antimicrobial therapy is directed at both the aerobic and anaerobic component rather than just at the aerobic organisms.

Several antibiotic regimes employing two drugs have been suggested. Six agents are now available which have been shown to be active against the anaerobic component including clindamycin, chloramphenicol, carbenicillin, ticarcillin, cefoxitin, and metronidazole. These agents are usually combined with an aminoglycoside such as gentamicin, tobramycin, or amikacin to cover the aerobic gram-negative organisms.

Septic Thromboembolism

Septic pulmonary emboli emanating from septic thrombophlebitis are seen occasionally in infected postpartum or postabortal patients and more rarely in patients with other septic disease of the female pelvis. The high incidence of postpartum or postabortal embolization is in part due to the presence of numerous dilated pelvic veins. This syndrome may go unrecognized, and the patients may present with occult pulmonary infiltrates, or the syndrome may be associated with fulminant pelvic infection.[90] Septic pulmonary emboli should be seriously considered in patients with postpartum or postabortal sepsis who are clinically not responding to therapy. A high index of suspicion for this complication should be maintained because heparin therapy may be life saving. Once instituted, heparin therapy should be continued until all signs of sepsis have cleared, usually 1 to 3 weeks. There is no need to institute a prolonged course of oral anticoagulants since the risk of late embolization is low. In rare instances, there may be continued embolization despite adequate anticoagulation and surgical removal of the septic pelvic veins may be required. However, this procedure is difficult and should be undertaken only in dire circumstances.

Pelvic Tuberculosis and Actinomycosis

With chronic infections of the female pelvis, two microorganisms should be seriously considered, *Mycobacterium tuberculosis* and actinomyces. In the pre-antibiotic era, pelvic infection caused by tuberculosis was frequently seen. Fortunately, it has become a rare clinical entity in the industrialized societies. Patients with chronic draining sinuses should be cultured for acid-fast bacilli and, if positive, therapy with two antituberculous drugs should be initiated. Although the incidence of pelvic tuberculosis has been decreasing, the incidence of pelvic actinomycosis has been increasing. Following the introduction of intrauterine contraceptive devices (IUD), there has been a number of reports documenting the association of pelvic actinomycosis with use of IUDs.[91–93] This infection can be diagnosed by finding sulfur granules in the purulent material or seeing the typical clusters of bacteria on gram stain. The organism may be cultured, if good anaerobic techniques are employed and the culture plates are kept for 10 days. Therefore, the laboratory should be alerted to the possible presence of the organisms. Recognition of this disease is important, because it is amenable to antimicrobial therapy with penicillin G, clindamycin, or tetracycline.

GENITOURINARY TRACT INFECTIONS

Urinary tract infections include a spectrum of clinical entities ranging from asymptomatic bacteriuria to pyelonephritis with bacteremia and are among the most frequent bacterial infections to afflict patients. The common denominator in these situations is the presence of significant bacteriuria, commonly accepted as greater than 100,000 organisms/ml. Women are especially prone to bacterial invasion of the normally sterile bladder due to their short urethras.

Acute Symptomatic Urinary Tract Infection

The pathogenesis of urinary tract infection involves an ascending route whereby bacteria reach the upper regions of the excretory system by avoiding the normal defense mechanisms.[94] The ability of clinicians to distinguish between an infection restricted to the bladder and one which has ascended to the kidney is limited. Using bladder wash-out techniques, it has been demonstrated that "upper tract symptoms" (flank pain, chills, and costovertebral area tenderness) are not infrequent in patients with bladder bacteriuria; conversely, such symptoms are not invariably present in upper tract infections.[95,96] High fever, shaking chills, severe nausea, and vomiting are highly suggestive of renal parenchymal infection. Bacteremia is almost invariably associated with upper tract involvement. Frequency, dysuria, and suprapubic discomfort are common to both types of infection and, hence, do not aid in discriminating the site of infection.

The pathogens involved in acute urinary tract infections in the non-hospitalized patient are relatively predictable. *E. coli* accounts for the vast majority of episodes, while other enteric bacteria, such as *Klebsiella, Enterobacter, Proteus,* and enterococci are occasionally recovered. *Staphlococcus saprophyticus, S. aureus* and *S. epidermidis* are less commonly isolated.

Proper bacteriologic diagnosis involves the collection of a midstream sample of urine which is promptly cultured or refrigerated if culture cannot be carried out immediately. Concurrently, microscopic examination of the urinary sediment for the presence of leukocytes should be performed. If pyuria of a significant degree is present (≥ 10 white blood cells/high power field) treatment can be begun while culture results are pending, especially when the patient is acutely symptomatic. A recent report described the utility of quantitative urinalysis to diagnose the presence of infection. Male patients with $\geq 10^4$ WBC/ml uncentrifuged urine were usually found to have infection with $\geq 10^5$ bacteria/ml.[97] It is not known if this holds true for female patients. An extremely useful, but often neglected, adjunctive examination is gram stain of the unspun urine. When bacteria are visualized, it indicates significant bacteriuria ($\geq 10^5$ colonies/ml); in addition, the morphologic and tinctorial properties of the responsible organism are revealed immediately. Enteric bacilli all appear as gram-negative rods. Gram-positive cocci suggest the presence of enterococci or staphylococci.

On the basis of low toxicity, efficacy, and cost, sulfonamides, ampicillin, and tetracyclines are the agents of choice in treatment. Since all of these drugs achieve extremely high urine levels, successful treatment is usual in bladder infections, irrespective of the antimicrobial susceptibility of the responsible pathogen. If the patient has had frequent or relapsing infections, antibiotic-resistant organisms should be suspected and a broader spectrum agent, such as a cephalosporin or trimethoprim-sulfamethoxazole should be chosen.

When pyelonephritis seems likely on clinical grounds (because of high fever or severe toxicity), the patient should be hospitalized and parenteral antibiotics given, especially when there is accompanying nausea and vomiting. Certain underlying conditions lower the threshhold for hospitalization, such as, diabetes, advanced age, and pregnancy. A first episode of urinary infection should be treated with ampicillin or a cephalosporin, but if there is a history of a relapsing or recently treated urinary infection, aminoglycosides are indicated until culture results are available. A gram stain of unspun urine is especially useful in this situation for the presence of gram-positive cocci would dictate the use of nafcillin and gentamicin as coverage for *S. aureus* or enterococcus.[98] The clinical response of the patient with acute pyelonephritis is often sluggish, and it is not uncommon for fever to persist for 48 to 72 hours after treatment has commenced. If fever persists beyond this period or if the patient is otherwise not improving, obstruction should be considered, and appropriate radiologic investigation carried out.

Although it is common practice to treat urinary infections for 7 to 10 days, the optimal length of therapy has not been established. Single dose therapy with kanamycin (500 mg intramuscularly), sulfisoxazole (1 to 2 gm), or trimethoprim-sulfamethoxazole (2 to 4 tablets) has been reported to cure 90 to 95 percent of episodes of bacterial cystitis in females.[99,100] Other studies have shown that three days of treatment with the above agents were equivalent to 10 days of amoxicillin for treating cystitis.[101] In another investigation, a single dose of 3 gm of amoxicillin cured all women with infection confined to the bladder.[102] The problem in clinical practice is how to determine, prior to therapy, which patient has bladder infection only; for them, a shorter course of therapy would be appropriate, while those with upper tract infection would suffer a high failure rate with single dose therapy.

A significant advance in the ability to detect upper tract infection was the discovery that patients with renal infections had antibody-coated bacteria in the urine which could be detected by immunofluorescence, while those with cystitis ordinarily did not.[103,104] This technique has become the method in therapeutic trials of determining the response of patients with cystitis or pyelonephritis to various forms of therapy. The test is imperfect, with false-positive and false-negative results having been noted,[105,106] thereby limiting its predictive value. Also, the test remains largely unavailable to the majority of physicians caring for patients with urinary tract infection. We would recommend that the duration of therapy be dictated by the severity of the illness. In patients with clinical findings of pyelonephritis, we would recommend 10 to 14 days of therapy; in very ill patients, parenteral antibiotics should be given until they respond, and oral therapy can complete the course. Milder cases of presumptive cystitis can be managed with 1 to 3 days of antimicrobial drugs.

Infections Associated with Catheter Use

A frequent problem in hospitalized patients is urinary tract infection associated with an indwelling catheter. The best way to approach this problem is to prevent the acquisition of bacteriuria by using indwelling catheters sparingly. The indications for use of an indwelling catheter are the requirement for rapid, serial determinations of urinary output, the presence of obstruction, and a threat to the integrity of the perineal skin or contiguous wounds from incontinence. Incontinence can be managed in a male patient by a condom catheter, at least for a short period.

The risk of colonizing the urinary tract with bacteria can be correlated to the length of time the catheter is in place.[107] The risk of bacteriuria is greater for elderly, critically ill, and female patients.[108] Disconnecting the catheter system is another factor which predisposes to contamination. The single most important advance in the prevention of infection in the catheterized patient has been the development of the closed urinary drainage system. Though introduced as early as 1928, this technique has not been widely accepted until recently when it became apparent that catheter associated infections were a major cause of nosocomial morbidity.

Since bacteriuria associated with bladder catheterization usually is clinically silent, the infectious process often makes itself known by the abrupt development of fever and gram-negative bacteremia, sometimes with endotoxic shock. In patients with catheter-associated bacteriuria, there is a correlation between the site of infection, as determined by immunofluorescent antibody coating, and the duration of catheterization.[109] During the first three days of catheterization, lower tract colonization was the rule and upper tract infection was uncommon. Beyond this initial three-day period, one-third of the patients had antibody-coated bacteria, indicating upper tract invasion. When a catheterized patient develops fever, the urinary tract should always be suspect. A urinalysis reveals heavy pyuria, and a gram stain of unspun urine shows the morphology of the pathogen. The urine to be examined and cultured should *not* be obtained from the drainage bag since uninhibited bacterial growth occurs there; rather, a freshly aspirated specimen from the drainage tubing, obtained with aseptic technique, should be used. Bacteriuria in an asymptomatic catheterized patient is not an indication for treatment but should forewarn the physician to discontinue or change the catheter.

When symptoms are present, treatment must be initiated prior to identification and sensitivity testing of the pathogen. Many of the nosocomial pathogens are drug-resistant so broad spectrum antibiotics are recommended initially, and these can be modified as sensitivity reports become available. If the patient has not received prior antibiotic therapy and is not terribly ill, a cephalosporin alone may be adequate therapy. However, sick patients, especially those having received antibiotics in the recent past, should receive an aminoglycoside. It is often difficult to eradicate infection with the catheter in situ, though control of the systemic signs can be achieved. One practice which should be abandoned is culturing the tip of the catheter, which has poor predictive value and wastes laboratory resources.[110]

The high frequency of associated infection has caused many workers to seek ways of preventing them with various regimens of chemoprophylaxis. Systemic antimicrobial therapy can decrease the incidence of acquisition of bacteriuria in the first several days of therapy, but its effect is transient and resistant pathogens frequently emerge.[111] Irrigation of the bladder with solutions of neomycin and polymixin through a triple lumen catheter has been widely used, but a well controlled study has demonstrated its lack of efficacy and even a potential danger from this practice. Unirrigated and irrigated patients in the study both acquired infection at a daily rate of 5 percent, but the irrigated group developed bacteria that were resistant to the antibiotics employed and there was a trend toward resistance to many antimicrobial agents.[112] Methenamine mandelate has been used to forestall urinary tract colonization in chronically catheterized patients. Since the antibacterial metabolite of this drug is formaldehyde, an agent which does not have the problem of emerging drug resistance, this approach is theoretically attractive. However, it was unable to prevent infection when administered with 4 gms of ascorbic acid daily to patients with spinal cord injury and indwelling catheters.[113] There has been a suggestion that higher daily doses of 8 to 12 gm could be effective, but the efficacy and toxicity of such regimens remains unproven. In summary, the best method of prevention appears to be avoiding catheters when possible, discontinuing them as soon as feasible, and maintaining the integrity of the closed drainage system in those patients who require long-term catheterization.

Prostatitis and Epididymitis

While women suffer the burden of urinary tract infections, men develop infection of the prostate gland. The genesis of such infections is antecedent or concurrent infection of the bladder. Not all symptoms that arise from an inflamed prostate gland are due to infection. Meares has defined a nonseptic syndrome of "prostatosis," which may be more common than bacterial prostatitis.[114] Such patients have variable degrees of perineal and low back discomfort and most have complaints of urgency or frequency. The common denominator is the inability to recover microbial pathogens, including aerobic and anaerobic organisms, gonococci, or mycoplasma. The pathogenesis and natural history of prostatosis remain unknown. Therapy with prostatic massage or anticholinergics benefits some patients.

Acute bacterial prostatitis is an acute febrile illness with chills, perineal pain, and urinary urgency and frequency. The gland is swollen, warm, and exquisitely tender. The expressed prostatic secretions and the bladder urine ordinarily grow the responsible pathogen. Therapy is directed at the usual urinary pathogens; ampicillin, cephalosporins, and aminoglycosides are all useful. The selection of the proper drug, prior to the availability of sensitivity tests, should be based upon a gram stain of the urine.

Chronic prostatitis is a therapeutically vexing illness. The chief barrier to eradication of the responsible organism is the inability of drugs to penetrate the milieu of the prostate.[115] Elegant studies by Stamey and Meares in dogs have characterized the nature of this penetration constraint. They and others have found that few drugs are likely to achieve therapeutic levels in prostatic fluid. Doxycycline and trimethoprim-sulfamethoxazole appear to be the best available agents.[116, 117] The symptoms of this chronic disorder are indolent, consisting of irritative voiding symptoms, such as frequency, nocturia, and dysuria. The prostate gland is usually unremarkable to palpation. Diagnosis is based on quantitative cultures of the prostatic secretions elicited by prostatic massage, compared to urine voided before and after massage. The colony counts in the prostatic fluid should be several logs higher than in the urine specimens obtained both before and after massage.[115] Treatment is recommended for at least 4 to 6 weeks. Bacteriologic and clinical response is the rule, but long-term cures, even with one of the best available agents, are elusive. For example, only 6 of 18 patients studied by Drach were free of infection 3 months after a course of 28 days of trimethoprim-sulfamethoxazole.[118]

Epididymitis is a readily appreciable inflammatory process associated with swelling, tenderness, and warmth of the affected organ. Theories of pathogenesis have abounded, but recent studies have finally shed some light on the microbial pathogens involved. In young, sexually active men the responsible pathogens were those that caused urethritis: *Neisseria gonorrhoeae, Chlamydia trachomatis* and *Ureaplasma urealyticum.*[119,120] In men over 45 years of age, coliforms and *Pseudomonas* were responsible. The younger group should receive tetracycline for optimal treatment, unless gonococci are found, in which case ampicillin *or* tetracycline could be given. Gram-negative bacilli found in the older patients requires treatment based upon antibiotic susceptibility testing.

Emphysematous Pyelonephritis and Renal Abscesses

Two entities which deserve separate attention are emphysematous pyelonephritis and renal abscess. Emphysematous pyelonephritis is an uncommon, severe, necrotizing form of parenchymal renal infection which has a predilection to affect diabetic patients. The patients are extremely ill, and gas is seen to extend from the perinephric space through the retroperitoneum to the flank, where it is apparent as palpable crepitus. The hallmark is radiographically visible gas in the kidney or adjacent structures.[121] The responsible pathogens are aerobic gram-negative rods, such as *E. coli, Klebsiella, Proteus,* and *Pseudomonas.* In a recent review of the literature, the mortality was found to be 40 percent. Those patients treated only with antibiotics had a higher mortality (70%); surgical therapy, with nephrectomy and/or drainage of the affected tissues, appeared to offer a better chance for survival with a mortality of only 33 percent.[122]

Renal abscess can occur as cortical abscess ("renal carbuncle") or as a perinephric abscess with extension to the adjacent fascial planes. The presentation of either form is similar—fever, chills, and unilateral flank pain being the predominant symptoms.[123]

Cortical abscesses are less commonly encountered. They can rupture through the parenchyma into the pelvis, discharging their contents into the urinary tract, thereby drawing attention to this site, or they can penetrate into the perinephric space so that both cortical and perinephric suppuration are present. At one time the pathogeneses of cortical and perinephric abscess were similar: hematogenous spread was the route of entry and *S. aureus* was the usual pathogen. Recent reports note that intrarenal abscess and perinephric abscess are more often caused by enteric gram-negative bacteria which gain admission through an ascending urinary tract infection.[124, 125]

The treatment of a renal carbuncle traditionally has been surgical drainage and systemic antimicrobial therapy directed at the pathogen, usually *S. aureus.* A report of antibiotic therapy alone, in lesions which had the angiographic characteristics of abscesses, illustrated that this approach can be successful.[126] This has the disadvantage of not yielding material for culture, unless blood cultures are positive. But since staphylococci are so frequently responsible, empiric therapy is justified and surgery can be employed later if the patient fails to respond. Another approach is to localize and percutaneously drain the abscess with echographic guidance.[127]

Since the bacteriology of perinephric abscesses is more complex and empiric antibiotic therapy to cover the putative pathogens would not be without risk, operative drainage should be considered in the first instance. This affords the surgeon a better opportunity to assess how best to drain the area. In those patients in whom the suppurative process is extensive, nephrectomy can then be carried out.

SKIN AND SOFT TISSUE INFECTIONS

Burn Wounds

The major cause of death in the severely burned patient is sepsis,[128] and the burn wound is the usual portal of entry. Before the introduction of topical antimicrobial therapy, burn wound sepsis accounted for three-fourths of deaths in such patients. It is notable that 50 percent of these deaths occurred without spread of the organisms beyond the wound. The role of antimicrobial therapy, while important, should not be overemphasized, for its role is adjunctive. Equally important is removal of nonviable tissue, maintenance of a physical environment that reduces the likelihood of bacterial contamination, and measures to increase host resistance by supplying adequate caloric intake and restoring normal physiology insofar as possible.

Second degree burns are best managed by application of topical antimicrobial agents to minimize contamination. Deeper burns should be debrided and closed primarily with autologous skin grafts. Burns which exceed 25 percent of the body surface cannot be managed in one stage, since too great an area of donor surface is exposed. Topical antibiotics assume a larger role in this setting.

The selection of antimicrobial agents is based on the predicted bacteriology of burn wound sepsis. Early colonization of the wound is predominantly by gram-positive organisms such as *S. pyogenes* and *S. aureus.* By the third day, gram-negative organisms, including *Pseudomonas* and Enterobacteriaceae, usually predominate. Microorganisms invade the burn wound well beneath the surface by the fifth day in concentrations exceeding 100,000/gm of tissue. Septicemia is most frequently due to *S. aureus* or *Pseudomonas.* More recently, burn centers have reported an increasing incidence of candidal sepsis.[129] Invasion by this fungus usually follows alteration of the "normal" bacterial flora secondary to topical and systemic antimicrobial therapy.

Topical antimicrobials have been a major factor responsible for decreased mortality due to burn wound sepsis.[130] Ideally, the topical agents should control the bacteria normally found in burn wounds, have relatively little local and systemic toxicity, and facilitate eschar separation. An ideal agent has not been discovered, but effective agents are currently available that approximate these goals. Sulfamylon (10% mafenide acetate cream) penetrates deeper tissues in effective concentrations and is active against most common organisms. Its main disadvantages are local discomfort and pain upon application, an inhibitory effect on epithelialization, and acid-base disturbances due to inhibition of carbonic anhydrase. Silver nitrate solution (0.5%) is effective in reducing bacterial colonization but requires that an occlusive dressing saturated with solution be kept in contact with the wound. Absorption of this hyptonic solution not infrequently leads to electrolyte disturbances. The solution stains everything dark brown on contact. Active silver penetrates poorly into the wound since it precipitates as silver chloride upon contact with body fluids. Silver sulfadiazine cream (1%) effectively controls the burn wound flora. Unlike silver nitrate, the silver salt is stable and tissue penetration is better. Major side effects appear to be rare, and bacterial resistance has not been observed. The use of topical aminoglycoside creams should be discouraged, as resistant bacteria rapidly emerge, depriving the physician of a major drug in his therapeutic armamentarium. In the absence of comparative data on efficacy, preference for one of the topical agents depends on the experience of the treating physician.

Parenteral penicillin is frequently given in the first few days after a major burn to prevent a catastrophic infection with Group A *Streptococcus*. Parenteral prophylaxis against other pathogens should be avoided, since, predictably, a resistant flora will emerge.

The burn wound eschar presents a barrier to passage of antimicrobial agents, moving from either direction. Parenteral antibiotics do not reach the surface flora, and therefore their use should be reserved for infections that invade adjacent soft tissues or the bloodstream. On the other hand, topical antimicrobials reduce the flora of the burn wound, thereby promoting wound healing, facilitating graft "takes," and reducing the risk of bacteremia.

Therapy for presumed or proven systemic infection with parenteral antibiotics often is required at some point in the management of a serious burn. Since the wounds are always colonized with bacteria, the decision to initiate parenteral treatment for systemic infection must be based on clinical signs, which are often expressed as subtle changes in the patient's course. The experienced physician has a high degree of suspicion and will commence therapy upon minimal symptomatology.

Cellulitis, Erysipelas, and Other Pyodermas

The classification of infections of the integument and adjacent tissues can be based upon the pathogens responsible or the depth and degree of involvement. Fortunately, there is some degree of overlap so that clinical assessment allows a reasonable approximation of the potential pathogens and permits initiation of antimicrobial therapy prior to the availability of culture results.

Cellulitis is most often due to hemolytic streptococci, usually Group A but occasionally Group B or C. The involved area is red, warm, and tender. Fever need not be present. The disease can be lingering or explosive. A rapidly advancing margin of redness and prominent signs of system toxicity (high fever, chills, and tachycardia) call for urgent therapy with hospitalization of the patient, elevation (if a limb is involved), and high-dose parenteral penicillin. Postoperative wound infections that occur early (< 48 hrs) after surgery and progress rapidly should be presumed to be due to a Group A *Streptococcus pyogenes* until proven otherwise. More indolent cellulitis is sometimes seen in the lower extremities, complicating minor trauma, venous ulcers, or lymphedema, or in the upper extremities after mastectomy. Oral therapy and elevation of the affected limb is usually sufficient, but lower limb infections are often resistant to such therapy, perhaps due to poor compliance in elevation of the limb. A brief hospitalization with enforced elevation may then be required. *S. aureus* is sometimes the cause of cellulitis, especially in cases where there is an obvious break in the skin. Because of the lack of differentiating clinical features between streptococcal or staphylococcal cellulitis, it is reasonable to utilize an antistaphylococcal penicillin in place of or with penicillin G in the therapy of severe, rapidly progressive cellulitis. Very rarely, gram-negative bacteria cause cellulitis. This possibility should be considered if there is a contiguous operative wound or if there is compromise of host defenses by cytotoxic chemotherapy, renal failure, or extensive tissue damage. Cellulitis after injuries in fresh water can be due to *Aeromonas hydrophila*, and gentamicin should be included in the initial antimicrobial regimen for severe infections. Less severe infections can be treated with tetracycline.[131,132] Cat bites can initiate a rapidly progressive cellulitis due to *Pasteurella multocida*. High-dose penicillin is the treatment of choice.[133]

Erysipelas is a superficial cellulitis with a bright red, tender, edematous character. There is early lymphatic involvement which can impart a *peau d'orange* appearance. It most frequently occurs at the extremes of age. The extremities or face, especially the cheeks and bridge of the nose, are commonly involved. Group A streptococci are the usual cause, although staphylococci are occasionally isolated.[134]

Other pyodermas encountered in surgical patients include ecthyma gangrenosum, furuncles, and carbuncles. Ecthyma is a "punched-out" necrotic lesion that begins as a violaceous nodule. In recent years, *Pseudomonas* has gained notoriety as the most common etiologic agent—usually as a consequence of bacteremia in a compromised host.[135] Such lesions, however, can result from streptococcal or staphylococcal infection.

Furuncles are staphylococcal infections in areas of hair follicles. Carbuncles are deep and indurated lesions, usually due to staphylococci associated with draining sinuses. The therapy of such infections includes application of moist heat which will promote spontaneous drainage. If fever or secondary cellulitis are present, antistaphylococcal antibiotics should also be given. Carbuncles usually require antibiotic therapy in addition to incision and drainage.

GAS GANGRENE AND CLOSTRIDIAL CELLULITIS

C. perfringens has earned a well-deserved notoriety in soft tissue infections. Although specific syndromes are now recognized, it should be noted that isolation of these organisms is not synonymous with infection since most isolates from wounds represent colonization.[136]

When infection is present it assumes one of two forms: (1) clostridial cellulitis or (2) clostridial myonecrosis. Clostridial cellulitis and fasciitis can erupt rapidly, spreading through tissue planes with abundant gas formation and severe systemic toxicity. Recognition of this form of clostridial infection is important, both to initiate proper antimicrobial therapy and to avoid radical surgery to remove muscle which is not necrotic in this disease. Fasciotomy and drainage of tissue planes is sometimes useful, but the mainstay of therapy is high-dose penicillin and supportive measures.[137] The diagnosis should be made on clinical grounds, and by examination of exudate obtained by needle aspiration of involved tissue; this material should demonstrate abundant leukocytes and gram-positive rods. Clostridial myonecrosis (gas gangrene) is a destructive infection of muscle with tissue crepitation and systemic toxicity. There is severe local pain and the overlying skin becomes magenta-colored. Hemorrhagic bullae often develop. Tissue exudate shows abundant gram-positive rods but a paucity of leukocytes. The patient may display a paradoxical lucidity, which often presages severe toxicity with delirium and coma. Ultimately, the diagnosis is based on operative inspection of involved muscle, which is initially pale and non-contractile, but eventually becomes black and friable. Wide surgical excision of nonviable tissue is essential, and high-dose penicillin should be given. Antitoxin administration is controversial, but may be useful in overwhelming clostridial toxemia accompanied by severe intravascular hemolysis. The role of hyperbaric oxygen is unproven and this modality is generally unavailable.

These severe clostridial infections usually occur in patients with extensive soft tissue damage, that is, traumatic wounds, ischemia, or hypotension, or following intestinal resection. Rarely, nontraumatic myonecrosis occurs which involves silent bacteremia from an occult colonic lesion, with seeding of a specific muscle group. The course then proceeds with the typical virulence of clostridial gas gangrene. Recognition may be difficult at first, due to the absence of a predisposing cause, but the diagnosis soon becomes all too obvious.[138] Treatment is the same as for traumatic clostridial myonecrosis.

MISCELLANEOUS SOFT TISSUE INFECTIONS

Necrotizing Fasciitis

An especially virulent form of soft tissue infection is necrotizing fasciitis. The elderly and diabetics have a predilection for the condition. Drug addicts may also develop such infections at the site of injection.[139] Pathologically, there is extensive dissection of infection and necrosis of fascia. Previously, necrotizing fasciitis was called "streptococcal gangrene," as Group A beta-hemolytic streptococci were frequently recovered from infected tissue.[140] This clinical entity can still be associated with streptococci or *S. aureus* alone, but it is recognized that a diverse group of organisms can be isolated from such lesions, including coliforms and anaerobes. Necrotizing fasciitis originating from an area with a lush polymicrobic flora, such as the perineum or oropharynx, will more likely be caused by a combination of aerobic and anaerobic bacteria. It can arise from a seemingly trivial wound.

The disease has a rapid onset with severe systemic toxicity. The affected skin is painful, reddened, and perhaps bullous. Gas may be present. A tissue aspirate reveals abundant polymorphs and gram-positive cocci (streptococcal or staphylococcal) and/or gram-negative bacilli. Therapy should include incision of tissue, drainage of fascial planes, and excision of necrotic fascia combined with antimicrobial agents directed at the responsible pathogens.

TABLE 8. Selected Features of Soft Tissue Infections*

	Clostridial Cellulitis	*Clostridial Myonecrosis*	*Synergistic Necrotizing Cellulitis*	*Crepitant Cellulitis*	*Necrotizing Fasciitis*	*Anaerobic Streptococcal Myositis*
Predisposing conditions	Trauma Surgery	Trauma Surgery	Diabetes Vascular disease	Diabetes Vascular disease	Diabetes Old age	Local Trauma
Gas	Abundant	Moderate	Moderate	Abundant	Variable	Minimal
Pain	Mild	Severe	Moderate	Mild	Moderate or severe	Late but severe
Toxemia	Marked	Severe	Marked	Minimal	Marked	Marked
Exudate	Polymorphonuclear leukocytes Large gram(+) bacilli	Rare Polymorphonuclear leukocytes Large gram(+) bacilli	Polymorphonuclear leukoeytes Gram(+) cocci or rods and/or gram(−) bacilli	Polymorphonuclear leukocytes Gram(+) cocci or rods and/or gram(−) bacilli	Polymorphonuclear leukocytes Gram(+) cocci and/or gram (−) bacilli	Polymorphonuclear leukocytes Gram(+) cocci
Etiology	Clostridia	Clostridia	Facultative or anaerobic streptococci Facultative or anaerobic gram(−) bacilli Clostridia	Facultative or anaerobic streptococci Facultative or anaerobic gram(−) bacilli Clostridia	Facultative or anaerobic streptococci Facultative or anaerobic gram(−) bacilli *Staphylococcus aureus*	Facultative or anaerobic streptococci *Staphylococcus aureus*
Therapy	Penicillin Incision and drainage	Penicillin Excision of necrotic tissue	Guided by gram stain and culture Excision of necrotic tissue	Guided by gram stain and culture Local debridement	Guided by gram stain and culture Incision and drainage	Penicillin and/or nafcillin Excision of necrotic muscle

*Adapted from: Barza,[147] Flora,[148] and Swartz.[134]

Synergistic Necrotizing Cellulitis

This polymicrobic infection is similar to clostridial myonecrosis in that there is widespread destruction of fascia and muscle, severe systemic toxicity, and an associated high mortality. Most patients have diabetes or vascular insufficiency. There is high fever and exquisite tenderness. The overlying skin may be deceptively unremarkable. The predominant isolates are aerobic gram-negative bacilli, anaerobic cocci, and *Bacteroides* species. Blood cultures are positive in 40 percent of patients.[141] Therapy should be directed at a mixed aerobic-anaerobic flora and aggressive surgical debridement of affected tissues carried out.

Nonclostridial Crepitant Cellulitis

This process can be distinguished from necrotizing fasciitis and synergistic cellulitis by its more gradual onset and minimal systemic toxicity. It is usually a polymicrobic infection with coliforms, *Bacteroides,* and peptostreptococci. Typical patients are those with a lower extremity infection complicating diabetes and vascular disease. Tissue gas is abundant and may remain localized or dissect to adjacent tissues. The overlying skin shows little change and there is minimal pain. Surgical therapy consists of local debridement and drainage. Antibiotics should be given to cover a mixed infection.[137]

Anaerobic Streptococcal Myositis

Anaerobic streptococcal myositis shows muscle necrosis, but the onset is gradual and systemic toxicity is not marked. Nonetheless, severe local pain is present. As originally described, anaerobic streptococci were recovered in most cases, but *S. aureus* and facultative streptococci have also been isolated.[142] A tissue aspirate should reveal abundant leukocytes and gram-positive cocci. Gas formation may be minimal. Necrotic muscle should be excised; antimicrobial therapy is guided by smears and cultures of the affected tissue.

Progressive Bacterial Synergistic Gangrene (of Meleney)

This disease occurs on the abdominal wall, related to an operative wound or colostomy or ileostomy. It begins as a tender, reddened area which ulcerates to produce a necrotic ulcer with a halo of gangrenous skin and an outer zone of violaceous pigmentation. If untreated, the lesion progresses slowly but relentlessly. Systemic signs are absent or minimal but the lesion is painful. It is termed "synergistic" because two organisms are characteristically involved; a microaerophillic or anaerobic *Streptococcus* and *S. aureus.*[143] Debridement and systemic antimicrobial therapy are necessary for cure.

Atypical Organisms and Soft Tissue Infections

The increasing use of immunosuppressive drugs and the impairment of host defenses due to malnutrition in postoperative patients have fostered infections due to atypical organisms. The clues are a progressive skin or soft tissue lesion from which "conventional" pathogens cannot be cultured or that fails to respond to ordinary antibiotics. In such cases, an unusual organism, such as a fungus (e.g., Phycomycetes)[144,145] or atypical mycobacteria[146] can be responsible. Diagnosis is best made by biopsy or excision of involved tissue which should be examined histologically and cultured for fungi and mycobacteria. Treatment can then be logically approached. This may include surgery, antituberculous therapy, or antifungal therapy.

CENTRAL NERVOUS SYSTEM INFECTIONS

It is important to recognize and promptly treat infections occurring in patients after neurosurgical procedures or head trauma as they can quickly lead to a devastating outcome. Besides the risk of central nervous system infection, such patients can develop sepsis at other sites, including pneumonia, urinary tract infection, and catheter-associated bacteremia. However, infections in the central nervous system are the utmost concern.

Noninfectious Causes of Fever

Similar to other postoperative patients, neurosurgical patients may develop noninfectious fever due to atelectasis, sterile phlebitis, or drugs. However, these patients are subject to special situations which give rise to fever. Meningismus, cerebrospinal fluid (CSF) pleocytosis, and high fever have been seen after posterior fossa surgery, often accompanied by a depressed CSF glucose concentration.[149] This aseptic meningitis appears to respond to judicious use of steroids. Differentiation from bacterial meningitis can be difficult initially, but cultures of the CSF should be positive in bacterial meningitis. Another special circumstance is aseptic meningitis after pneumoencephalography, which subsides with no specific therapy.

A clinical situation in which fever is often of noninfectious origin is subdural or intracranial hematomas. Hypoglycorrhachia has also been noted after subdural hematomas.[150] This can represent a perplexing problem to the clinician faced with cerebrospinal fluid findings that include polymorphonuclear leukocytes and a low glucose. An appropriate history (e.g., head trauma or anticoagulation) and adjunctive studies such as echoencephalography, radionuclide brain scanning or CT scanning assist in discriminating pyogenic infection from these other situations. In equivocal situations, empiric therapy for meningitis should be given and subsequently discontinued if cultures remain negative.

Arachnoiditis is a rare clinical event that can follow intrathecal administration of contrast agents.[151] The diagnosis usually is not difficult because of the temporal association with the procedure. This aseptic inflammatory process is accompanied by high fever, headache, pronounced CSF pleocytosis, and low CSF glucose—mimicking a bacterial infection. Another rare occurrence is true pyogenic meningitis after a lumbar puncture.[152] We have seen two cases due to streptococci in our unit in recent years. The pathophysiology of this complication may be an example of "locus minoris resistentiae," that is, a dural puncture before or during a bacteremia that culminates in bacterial contamination of the CSF and subsequent infection. There is experimental support for this scenario.[153] Faced with a patient who manifests signs of an inflammatory process affecting the meninges after lumbar puncture, with or without the prior use of contrast material, CSF examination is mandatory. If no bacteria are visualized on gram stain, empiric antibiotic therapy may be withheld, unless the patient is desperately ill. Steroids have been employed with apparent success in arachnoiditis, though the natural history of this process is unknown and spontaneous recovery is the rule.

Infections after Head Trauma

Trauma to the central nervous system with the development of a CSF leak is an important predisposing cause for the development of bacterial meningitis. The frequency of meningitis appears to be greater with CSF otorrhea than with rhinorrhea at some units.[154] If a fracture of the middle fossa is seen, the likelihood of otogenic meningitis occurring is increased. The absolute incidence of meningitis after this type of injury is 5 to 10 percent in the first week after a dural tear. The pneumococcus accounts for the vast majority of cases of post-traumatic bacterial meningitis,[155] with *Hemophilus influenzae, Neisseria meningitidis* and other pathogens occurring infrequently. Meningitis due to a cryptic CSF leak months after head trauma is possible, and in patients with more than one episode of pneumococcal meningitis, a leak should be assiduously sought.[156] The management of the patient with suspected post-traumatic meningitis should include rapid examination of the CSF for evidence of infection. Therapy is begun on the basis of the gram stain. High-dose penicillin or ampicillin should be given unless nondiplococcal pathogens are visualized on the gram stain or it is negative. If organisms suggestive of *S. aureus* are seen, nafcillin or oxacillin should be given, while gram-negative rods would indicate that chloramphenicol or an aminoglycoside should be administered.

Because of the frequency with which this sequelae follows dural leaks and the predictable bacteriology of this complication, it is common practice to administer prophylactic penicillin to prevent infection. Data indicate that this practice can significantly reduce the frequency of meningitis with post-traumatic CSF rhinorrhea.[154] However, failures with such regimens have been seen, and one can expect the selection of a more resistant flora that might cause disease. In addition, when diagnosed and treated promptly, the outcome of post-traumatic meningitis is favorable. Hence, many do not recommend prophylaxis but urge vigilant observation and aggressive diagnosis and therapy if it is suspected and found. The surgical approach to dural tears is observation initially, followed by operative repair if there is a persistent leak and if recurrent or late meningitis occurs.

Infections after penetrating head trauma are quite different. In this situation, a variable flora is introduced, often an assortment of aerobic and anaerobic bacteria, reflecting that on the scalp, face, or the penetrating instrument. In addition, there is often necrosis of brain tissue with hematoma formation, which provides an excellent substrate for polymicrobial virulence. In this situation, broad spectrum antibiotics, such as an antistaphylococcal penicillin and chloramphenicol should be given, with antimicrobial modifications guided by the pathogens recovered in culture and their susceptibility patterns. Surgical intervention is ordinarily critical in these situations to remove devitalized tissue and drain pus. Subdural empyema can occur after head trauma or spontaneously, arising from chronic sinusitis. It has recently been emphasized as a process with aerobic (streptococci and staphylococci) and anaerobic (*Bacteroides* and anaerobic cocci) components and which requires prompt drainage and appropriate antibiotic therapy.[157]

Infections after Surgery

In contrast to the bacteriology of meningeal infections acquired after head trauma with a CSF leak, the infections occurring after craniotomy more frequently involve hospital acquired gram-negative bacilli. A representative series from Montreal found that 19 (82%) of 23 cases of meningitis after neurosurgical procedures were due to such organisms as *Enterobacter, Klebsiella, Serratia, Pseudomonas,* and *E. coli.*[158] No doubt contributing to this prevalence of gram-negative infections is the use of prophylactic antibiotics and invasive monitoring devices such as bladder catheters, arterial and venous cannulae, and ventricular drainage. The mortality of this type of infection is high; in the Montreal series it was over 50 percent. On occasion, infection is limited to the operative wound itself, and a subgaleal collection of pus develops. This complication has a lesser morbidity, and it can be managed with drainage and antimicrobial agents, most often an aminoglycoside, given systemically.

If infection develops within the central nervous system, therapy is problematic as the drugs which often are most active against the responsible pathogens penetrate the meninges poorly. If the offending agent is sensitive to chloramphenicol, this would be the drug of choice. This is frequently not the case, and gentamicin, tobramycin, or amikacin must be employed. If *P. aeruginosa* is responsible, carbenicillin or ticarcillin should be coadministered, as they penetrate reasonably well and the combination often exerts synergistic bactericidal activity. Intrathecal or intraventricular instillation of an aminoglycoside in addition to systemic therapy has been employed successfully to treat gram-negative meningitis. Although the proper place of this therapy is still being investigated, we would endorse the use of intralumbar therapy for the very ill patient at the time of diagnosis, and recommend it should be added to systemic therapy if there isn't prompt sterilization of the CSF and clinical improvement in moderately ill patients. Intralumbar therapy, unfortunately, does not always lead to adequate ventricular levels of antibiotic,[159,160] and ventriculitis can persist. Ventricular administration has been advocated in these circumstances and this can be accomplished easily if a ventricular drainage system is in use. However, intraventricular therapy in neonatal gram-negative meningitis has been associated with a higher mortality.[161] It is uncertain if this finding can be applied to the postoperative patient. Since no adequate data exist to define whether all patients with gram-negative meningitis should receive intralumbar or intraventricular therapy, we feel it is best to individualize this decision, based upon determination of the minimal inhibitory concentration (MIC) and minimal bactericidal concentration (MBC) of the organism involved, the antimicrobial level achieved in the CSF, and the clinical response of the patient.

Shunt-Associated Infections

The development of ventriculoatrial and ventriculoperitoneal shunts created a new ecologic niche for infection. The incidence of this complication per surgical procedure (placements and revisions) was 13 percent in one large series, and 20% of the shunts became infected at some time.[162] This complication is less frequently seen now. The clinical presentation of the patients can be acute or subacute. Virtually all patients are febrile, but symptoms specifically referable to the central nervous system are often absent. The patient may only complain of malaise, anorexia, and fatigue. If a ventriculoatrial shunt is in place, most patients will have positive blood cultures for the infecting organism. The single most helpful diagnostic test is aspiration of fluid from the shunt, which will show evidence of a pleocytosis. The fluid will virtually always grow a pathogen if infection is present, even in the absence of an inflammatory CSF reaction. The bacteriology has proven to be uniform from different institutions, with *S. epidermidis* the most frequent pathogen.[162–164] Other pathogens of low virulence have been seen, such as *Propionibacteriaceae*,[165,166] while *S. aureus*, and gram-negative bacilli are occasionally seen.

Therapy of these infections should include systemic therapy with an antibiotic to which the organism is susceptible and which penetrates the meninges, usually nafcillin, oxacillin, or chloramphenicol. Prior to the availability of susceptibility studies, we would employ one of the above agents guided by a gram stain of the aspirated CSF. Administration of the antibiotic directly into the shunt has been utilized to achieve higher levels of antibiotic at the infected site.[167] Some authors have reported cures with antibiotic therapy alone,[167] but most feel that complete removal of the shunt and replacement with a new one is the most certain way of eradicating infection and we recommend this approach unless there are technical reasons that preclude its possibility. Rifampin has considerable activity against staphylococci and excellent penetration into the CSF. It has been successfully employed with other antibiotics in the therapy of *S. epidermidis* prosthetic heart valve endocarditis[26] and we have used it to treat CSF-shunt infections. It should not be used alone because of the possibility of selecting a resistant organism. Its proper role in treatment of these infections is uncertain at this time, but as adjunctive antimicrobial therapy, it should be considered if the organism is sensitive.

An occasional extra-central nervous system complication of infected ventriculoatrial shunts is diffuse glomerulonephritis. This has been found to be associated with hypocomplementemia, circulating immune complexes, and bacterial antigens within the renal glomerulus.[168,169] It responds to treatment of the underlying infection.

Brain Abscess and Epidural Abscess

Brain abscesses which arise spontaneously, that is, not after surgery or penetrating trauma, are usually of otic or paranasal sinus origin[170] or are due to covert dental sepsis.[171] As such, they are often polymicrobic mixtures of aerobic and anaerobic bacteria derived from these sites. The chief clinical features are headache and signs of a focal central nervous system (CNS) lesion. Management includes administration of antimicrobial agents, the use of corticosteroids to reduce edema, and judicious surgical drainage. High-dose penicillin and chloramphenicol are recommended initially, except after surgery or trauma, in which case penicillin-resistant staphylococci may be present and nafcillin or oxacillin should be substituted for or added to penicillin. Metronidazole has potent antianaerobic activity and penetrates into the CNS very well. There have been favorable reports from Europe of its use in abscesses due to anaerobic bacteria.[172]

Treatment is ordinarily given for 4 to 6 weeks. Computerized tomography is the most helpful technique in diagnosis and localization of abscesses[173] and is useful in assessing response to therapy.

Management of the patient with focal suppurative disease of the brain, "bacterial cerebritis," entirely with antibiotics and without surgical drainage has been successful in some patients.[174] Rarely, even when upon computerized tomography the process has the hallmarks of abscess formation (i.e., ring enhancement or doughnut lesion) antimicrobial therapy alone has been curative.[175] The timing of neurosurgical intervention is best individualized but is often dictated by the response of the "mass effect" of the abscess to antibiotics and corticosteroids.

A spinal epidural abscess should always be considered in patients with back pain and fever, especially if local tenderness is elicited upon palpation of the vertebral column. The presentation can be either acute or chronic; it is important to recognize the acute presentation immediately, since progression to paraparesis can occur within hours. Not all patients have abnormal neurologic signs and we have seen cases with minimal cellular reaction in the CSF. The responsible pathogen is most often *S. aureus*.[176,177] If suspected, the CSF should be examined promptly, and if there is evidence of an inflammatory process, myelography should be carried out at once. If cord compression is found, the patient should undergo emergency laminectomy and drainage. An antistaphylococcal penicillin can be begun at the time of diagnosis and the regimen modified on the basis of gram stains and cultures of the recovered material.

BACTEREMIA

Surgical patients may develop bacteremia either as part of the underlying disease or as a postoperative complication. Hospitalized patients are particularly at high risk of contracting bacteremia because of intravascular lines, including those for intravenous infusions, arterial monitoring devices, and hyperalimentation.

Bacterial infection of the bloodstream is associated with significant mortality despite the introduction of potent antimicrobial agents.[178] Recent reports still show mortality figures of approximately 25 to 50 percent, the major determinant in mortality being the underlying disease.[179] Thus, leukemia is associated with a high mortality regardless of the antibiotic treatment, whereas bacteremia in an otherwise healthy patient undergoing urinary tract manipulation has a favorable prognosis. Although antibiotics administered prophylactically do not prevent septicemia in a susceptible host, there is evidence that these drugs act to contain underlying infection and to prevent relapse once bacteremia has occurred. The choice of appropriate antimicrobial therapy does produce a significant decline in mortality.

Septic shock is characterized by circulatory insufficiency and inadequate tissue perfusion. Previous reports have emphasized the importance of gram-negative bacteria in septic shock, but this is an oversimplification since gram-positive bacteremia can fully reproduce the hemodynamic complications associated with this syndrome.[180] Despite this potential of gram-positive organisms, septic shock is seen in a small percentage of gram-positive bacteremias, whereas it is encountered in 40 percent of patients with gram-negative bacteremias.[181]

An historical analysis of bacteremia in surgical patients at the Boston City Hospital has revealed a decrease in the gram-positive organisms and an increase in the gram-negative bacilli (coliforms and *Pseudomonas*). This shift seemed to reflect the use of antimicrobial agents and changes in the hospital environment.[178]

Coliform bacteria are the most common organisms causing gram-negative bacteremia and septic shock. In a report from UCLA describing 651 patients with gram-negative bacteremia, *E. coli, Klebsiella, Enterobacter, Serratia,* and *Proteus* accounted for 467 (72%) of the cases. *Pseudomonas* and the obligate anaerobe, *Bacteroides,* were the other major pathogens.[179] In some hospitals *B. fragilis* is second in frequency to *E. coli* as the cause of gram-negative bacteremia in a general surgical unit. This has important therapeutic implications, because certain empiric treatments, for example, a penicillin or cephalosporin combined with an aminoglycoside, may be inadequate for this organism.

The portal of entry of gram-negative bacteria in the series by DuPont and Spink was the urinary tract in 45 percent, gastrointestinal tract in 8 percent, skin and soft tissues in 8 percent, respiratory tract in 7 percent, biliary tract in 7 percent, and indeterminate in 12 percent.[182]

Among the gram-positive cocci, *S. aureus* is the most frequent cause of bacteremia in the postoperative patient, while the pneumococcus and Group A *Streptococcus* are uncommon. *S. epidermidis* and *Propionibacterium acnes* are occasionally encountered in bacteremia, particularly in patients with intravascular or intracranial foreign bodies.

Fungi are most unwelcome in the bloodstream. They occur principally in patients receiving hyperalimentation or broad spectrum antibiotic coverage. The major isolates are yeasts such as *Candida, Torulopsis,* and *Rhodotorula.* The usual presentation of the patient with fungemia is fever which is often associated with shaking chills. If related to an intravascular catheter, its removal often aborts the infection and further therapy is not required. Harbingers of trouble after removal of the catheter are persistent fever and toxicity which may be accompanied by positive blood cultures.

Candidemia has been associated with seeding of the retina and vitreous humor of the eye. In these cases, which are usually related to intravenous hyperalimentation, the initial event of fungemia may escape detection; even when there has been a positive blood culture, a delay of several weeks may ensue between the culture and the eye findings. In the interim, the patient is usually asymptomatic, the first awareness being difficulty with vision. Because of the potential to produce blindness, it is important that all patients with positive blood cultures for *Candida* be monitored by frequent fundoscopic examination for two months after their septic episode. Such metastatic infections of the eye require parenteral therapy with amphotericin B.

The choice of antimicrobial agents to treat suspected bacteremia depends upon the underlying condition of the patient, the source of the bacteremia, and the anticipated bacteriology. Empiric regimes consist of various combinations that provide a broad spectrum of activity. A more rational approach, however, selects antibiotics on the basis of the actual or suspected focus of infection. When cultures and sensitivity tests become available, this drug regime can be adusted. Table 9 lists the antimicrobial agents suggested for bacteremia associated with various clinical situations. Treatment of fungal invasion of the bloodstream requires amphotericin B.

Combination antimicrobial therapy has three advantages: (1) it ensures an effective

TABLE 9. Potential Microorganisms and Antibiotic Therapy in Bacteremia

Site of Infection	*Type*	*Suspected Pathogens*	*Recommended Antibiotics**
Intra-abdominal	Peritonitis	*Bacteroides* (esp. *B. fragilis*) Anaerobic cocci Coliforms *Clostridium*	Clind & Am Chlor & Am Cefox ± Am Carb & Am Mt & Am
		Pneumococcus (spontaneous peritonitis)	Pen
	Liver Abscess	*Bacteroides* (esp. *B. fragilis*) Anaerobic cocci Coliforms Group D *Streptococcus*	Clind & Am Chlor & Am Amp & Am
	Biliary Tract: Cholecystitis or Ascending cholangitis	*Escherichia coli* *Klebsiella* *Clostridium* *Bacteroides fragilis* *Enterococcus*	Ceph ± Am Amp & Am ± Clind
Female genital tract	Septic abortion Salpingitis Pelvic abscess	*Bacteroides fragilis* Anaerobic cocci Coliforms	Cefox ± Am Carb ± Am Clind & Am Chlor & Am Mt & Am
	Postsurgical	*Neisseria gonorrhoeae*	Pen
Urinary tract	Pyelonephritis Renal carbuncle Perinephric abscess	Coliforms *Enterococcus* *Staphylococcus aureus*	Ceph ± Am Amp & Am Naf & Am
Lower respiratory tract	Pneumonia Necrotizing pneumonitis	*Streptococcus pneumoniae* *Staphylococcus aureus* *Klebsiella pneumoniae* Anaerobic cocci *Bacteroides*	Pen (pneumococcus or anaerobes) Clind ± Am Cefox Naf ± Am
	Aspiration pneumonia and lung abscess	*Fusobacterium* *Bacteroides* Anaerobic cocci *Staphylococcus*	Pen Clind
	Hospital-acquired pneumonia	Coliforms *Staphylococcus aureus*	Carb & Am Naf & Am Cefox & Am
Mediastinum	Community-acquired	*Staphylococcus aureus* *Bacteroides* Anaerobic cocci	Cefox ± Am Clind & Am
	Poststernotomy	Coliforms *Staphylococcus aureus*	Ceph & Am Carb & Am

TABLE 9. *Continued*

Site of Infection	*Type*	*Suspected Pathogens*	*Recommended Antibiotics**
Skin and soft tissue	Erysipelas	Group A *Streptococcus* *Staphylococcus aureus*	Pen ± Naf
	Burns	Group A *Streptococcus* *Staphylococcus aureus* *Pseudomonas*	Naf & Am Ceph & Am
	Necrotizing infection: Decubitus ulcer Diabetic foot ulcer Traumatic cellulitis	*Bacteroides* *Staphylococcus aureus* Coliforms *Streptococcus* *Anaerobic cocci*	Clind & Am Cefox ± Am
	I.V. Catheter	*Staphylococcus aureus* Coliforms Yeast	Ceph ± Am Amphotericin B (fungi)

± alone or with
Am = aminoglycoside
Amp = ampicillin
Carb = carbenicillin
Cefox = cefoxitin
Ceph = cephalosporin
Clind = clindamycin
Naf = nafcillin
Pen = penicillin G
Chlor = chloramphenicol
Mt = metronidazole

agent when the microbiology of bacteremia cannot be predicted on clinical grounds, (2) it covers polymicrobic bacteremia which is not infrequently seen in ill surgical patients,[183,184] (3) certain combinations are synergistic in killing some pathogens (e.g., carbenicillin and an aminoglycoside for *Pseudomonas*). There is a trend towards improved outcome in patients with gram-negative bacteremia treated with two effective antimicrobial agents,[185] but this is not without risk, as some combinations are more toxic.[186,187] Hence, the gravity of the patient's illness must justify these increased potential risks.

Staphylococcal bacteremia continues to be a serious problem in the surgical patient. It may represent a simple catheter associated sepsis or a deep-seated staphylococcal infection. The duration of therapy will depend upon a number of factors: the probable source of infection, whether the bacteremia was continuous, and the clinical status of the patient. In general, when there is a removable focus of infection such as an intravenous catheter or an abscess, a short course of antibiotic therapy can be employed, while patients with deep-seated infections such as osteomyelitis, mediastinitis, or endocarditis require 4 to 6 weeks of intravenous therapy. These generalizations can be made because the risk of endocarditis in persons *without* underlying valvular heart disease is relatively low in patients with bacteremia and a definable focus of infection.[188] If there is no definable focus of infection and the patient has continuous bacteremia, the likelihood that there is an intravascular focus of infection, that is, endocarditis, is high. There has been recent interest in employing measurements of anti-teichoic acid antibodies to aid in discriminating between uncomplicated bacteremia and bacteremia representing deep-seated infection. High titers of such antibodies usually indicate endocarditis or deep infection (i.e., requiring 4 to 6 weeks of therapy), while low levels are thought to indicate uncomplicated bacteremia.[189] However, the predictive value of such a measurement in an individual patient is at present unknown and broad application of this technique must await further methodological progress and evaluation in a greater number of patients.

Septic Shock

The therapy of gram-negative septic shock can be divided into four components: antimicrobial therapy, volume replacement, steroids, and surgical drainage. Antimicrobial therapy is summarized above under presumptive therapy of bacteremia. The important principle is high doses of an appropriate drug administered intravenously.

Aggressive volume replacement is an important aspect of early therapy, because there is loss of effective circulating blood volume due to splanchnic pooling and vasodilatation. Capillary leakage potentiates these effects. Preexisting volume deficits and poor myocardial function may cause mild hypotension to progress to severe septic shock. Large volumes of fluid replacement are required in order to prevent stagnant anoxia and lactic acidosis. Oliguria is not a contraindication to vigorous fluid administration when hypotension is present; such conditions require monitoring of central venous or pulmonary artery pressures. Fluid therapy in the form of either crystalloid (electrolyte solution) or colloid (plasma, albumin) should be given in sufficient quantities to maintain a central venous pressure of 12 to 14 cm of water or a pulmonary artery pressure of 12 to 16 torr. It is controversial whether crystalloid or colloid is the preferred form of volume replacement. A satisfactory approach is to use large amounts of crystalloid combined with small, judicious amounts of colloid.

When the blood pressure remains low despite fluid replacement, vasoactive drugs are needed. The preferred agent is the endogenous catecholamine, dopamine. This drug increases myocardial contractility and causes nonadrenergic vasodilatation of the renal and mesenteric vasculature. The expected result is a slight increase in the blood pressure, decreased or unchanged heart rate, increased cardiac output, and increased renal and mesenteric blood flow. The drug is most effective when the circulating blood volume has been restored. The dosage is 2 to 40 μg/kg of body weight per minute. When infused at rates greater than 20 μg/kg/min, the drug acts principally as an alpha-adrenergic vasoconstrictor. Vasoconstrictive agents such as levarterenol (Levophed) and metaraminol (Aramine) are not used routinely because septic patients are already under intense alpha-adrenergic stimulation. In extreme situations, isoproterenol can be used in dosages of 2 to 8 μg/min. This drug increases the cardiac output by its chronotropic and inotropic cardiac effects. It also causes vasodilatation of the arteriolar and venous systems, thereby improving the microcirculation.

The use of steroids in the treatment of septic shock remains controversial. Experimental studies in animals have been criticized for not being relevant to human physiology. The human studies are faulty because they are retrospective or lack appropriate controls. However, Shumer recently published a randomized prospective study of the use of steroids in the treatment of septic shock.[190] In his 86 saline treated control subjects, the mortality rate was 38.4 percent (33/86); in the steroid treated patients, it was 10.4 percent (9/86). Methylprednisolone (30 mg/kg) or dexamethasone (3 mg/kg) were equally effective. The steroids were administered as a bolus over 5 to 10 minutes through a large intravenous catheter. Administration of a single bolus was repeated, if necessary, four hours later. Although this study is said to be flawed, particularly with respect to the definition of septic shock, the results are impressive. Based on this study and in view of the low toxicity of short-term steroids, pharmacologic dosages of corticosteroids are recommended for patients in septic shock.

Drainage of the septic focus, when present, remains a cardinal surgical dictum. The effect of drainage and debridement is removal of large numbers of microorganisms from a protected environment. The usual situation is a deep-seated abscess or phlegmon in which microorganisms produce an environment which is hostile to the host's defenses and inviolate to penetration by antimicrobial agents.

Infections with Intravenous Catheters

The introduction of polyethylene intravenous catheters in the early 1960s ushered in a new era in the treatment of seriously ill patients. However, it also provided a new portal of entry for infection. The development of hyperalimentation and prolonged intravenous catheterization further complicated an already serious breach of normal defenses.

The major causes of catheter infections are: (1) faulty technique in decontaminating the skin and preparing the dressing when originally inserting the catheter, and (2) breakdown in sterility of the intravenous system when changing the bottles or intravenous lines.

The infection may originate in the catheter itself or, in the case of hyperalimentation, in the liquid formula or the filtering apparatus. The most common organisms are *Staphylococcus* and gram-negative bacilli such as *Klebsiella, Pseudomonas,* and *Serratia.* Fungi such as *Candida* also have been recognized as offending pathogens.

There are three types of infections seen with indwelling intravenous catheters. The first is transient bacteremia which clears spontaneously following removal of the source of infection, that is, the catheter. In this type of infection, the organisms recovered in the blood culture can also be cultured from the portion of the catheter at the puncture site. The second type is septic thrombophlebitis at the site of the catheter. This situation usually requires systemic antimicrobial therapy. If the bacteremia persists despite antibiotic therapy, surgical excision of the vein may be necessary. Such cases of suppurative thrombophlebitis may be occult in that there may be no overlying erythema or warmth. However, there is usually a palpable mass from which pus can be expressed from the puncture site by "milking" the vein or can be aspirated by a small needle inserted into the cord. The third and most catastrophic infection associated with intravenous catheters is metastatic seeding from the catheter site. The heart valves are particularly at risk and iatrogenic endocarditis can follow a catheter induced bacteremia, particularly in patients with a pre-existing valvular heart disease.

The decision to institute antimicrobial therapy for catheter-related infections is dictated by the clinical condition of the patient. If the fever and toxicity promptly respond to removal of the catheter, no further therapy is required. However, patients with persistent clinical symptoms of bacteremia following removal of the catheter should receive systemic antimicrobial therapy. An empiric regime to cover staphylococci and hospital-acquired gram-negative bacteria includes a semisynthetic penicillin or cephalosporin plus an aminoglycoside (see Table 9).

KAISER, DRUG THERAPY: ANTIMICROBIAL PROPHYLAXIS IN SURGERY, 315: 1129, OCT 1986

Fungemia associated with an intravenous catheter should be treated by removal of the device. If symptoms of sepsis persist or fungi are isolated from normally sterile locations, then systemic therapy with amphotericin B should be instituted.

Patients who become bacteremic often require the placement of *new* intravenous lines, either central or peripheral, because of hemodynamic instability. If urgently required, their placement should not be delayed even in the face of sepsis. A central intravenous line for total parenteral nutrition is rarely, if ever, required on an emergency basis and their placement is best delayed until antibiotics have been given for 24 to 48 hours or blood cultures are sterile.

PROPHYLACTIC ANTIBIOTICS

Opinions concerning the use of prophylactic antibiotics in surgery vary from affirmations of enlightened patient management to accusations of reckless polypharmacy. To understand these dissenting viewpoints, precise definitions are required.

Operative procedures are classified as *clean, potentially contaminated,* or *contaminated.* Antibiotics are considered *prophylactic* when they are used either in clean or potentially contaminated operations with the expectation of preventing infections in the postoperative period. The term is not appropriate for cases with established bacterial contamination since these situations more precisely involve *therapy* for infection. For example, the term *antibiotic prophylaxis* can be applied to elective colon surgery, but *antibiotic treatment* is used for a perforated appendix.

Guidelines for Use of Prophylactic Antibiotics

The decision to employ prophylactic antibiotics should be based upon knowledge of the possible advantages weighed against the potential dangers. Guidelines for use of prophylactic antibiotics in surgery are as follows:

1. *The operation should entail significant risk for contamination and postoperative infection.* Clean procedures that have a low incidence of infection such as thyroidectomy, mastectomy, and hernia repair should not be considered for prophylactic antibiotics. On the other hand, procedures involving grafts and prosthetic devices have a high risk of inadvertant contamination in the perioperative period. Additionally, antimicrobial prophylaxis may be beneficial in operative procedures that penetrate an area which harbors a luxuriant microflora. Hysterectomies, colonic resections, and head and neck procedures which enter the oropharyngeal cavity, are situations which may be appropriate. (In the case of colon operations, a suitable bowel preparation may be preferred to systemic antibiotics.)

2. *Ideally, the infecting bacteria should be well-defined.* The prophylactic antibiotic should have a narrow spectrum, being most active against the anticipated strains. These criteria are best satisfied in cardiac and vascular surgery where there is a high risk of infections due to gram-positive cocci such as staphylococci, pneumococci, and streptococci. Antibiotics with a limited spectrum such as penicillins and cephalosporins can be used in these situations.

3. *The antibiotic should be present in critical tissues in effective concentrations at the time of incision.* Experimental studies by Burke have shown that antibiotic therapy should be initiated

several hours prior to surgery in order to achieve adequate levels at the site of incision.[191] If the drugs are started during the procedure there may be a delay in delivery of the drug to the relevant site.

4. *Prophylaxis should be short-term and primarily perioperative.* It should be emphasized that the rationale for prophylactic antibiotics is protection during the operation and in the immediate postoperative period. Prolonged use of such drugs merely increases the risk of superinfection but does not reduce the subsequent incidence of septic complications.

5. *Broad spectrum antibiotics used for treating resistant microorganisms should not be used prophylactically.* The widespread use of such agents will encourage resistance within the hospital flora and thereby render these agents ineffective for the treatment of nosocomial infections.[192] Drugs with a narrow spectrum are preferred, the more potent agents should be reserved for life-threatening infections.

Risks in Use of Prophylactic Antibiotics

A balanced assessment of prophylactic antibiotics must consider the risk of widespread use of these agents. The potential dangers are harm to the individual patient receiving the drug and harm to the hospital environment where patients are exposed to nosocomial pathogens. The major risks are listed below:

1. *Untoward effects to the patient can be either allergic or toxic.* For example, patients treated with penicillin may develop a rash or fever as a manifestation of allergy. On the other hand, patients receiving tetracycline can experience direct toxicity to the liver, kidney, or gastrointestinal tract.

2. *The prophylactic antibiotic may induce resistant microorganisms in the host's microflora.*[193] Sites at greatest risk for changes in the flora are the oropharynx and the gastrointestinal tract. Overgrowth is most commonly seen with resistant gram-negative bacilli such as *Pseudomonas, Proteus,* and *Klebsiella* and *Serratia,* staphylococci, and fungi.[194]

3. *The impact of the use of the prophylactic antibiotic on the possible emergence of multiply resistant bacteria in the hospital flora must be considered.*[195] An entire hospital, or specific units within a hospital, may become colonized with resistant strains of bacteria due to antibiotic pressure.[196] Currently, many gram-negative bacilli have developed resistance to carbenicillin and to aminoglycosides such as kanamycin and, to a lesser extent, gentamicin.

4. *Extensive use of prophylactic antibiotics may produce delays in the diagnosis of occult infections.* Intra-abdominal abscesses, especially in the subdiaphragmatic space or the pelvis, may simmer for weeks to months following the use of prophylactic antibiotics. Indolent and often atypical presentations of these infections may occur. By the time the infection is obvious, the patient has been weakened and debilitated so that the prognosis is often grave. Additionally, the microorganisms causing these occult infections may be resistant to conventional antibiotics.

Controlled studies are available to define the indications for use of prophylactic antibiotics in several operative procedures. In other areas, however, such studies are not available. Common usage and custom, rather than scientific judgment, are often the major reasons for using these drugs. Having stated these caveats, it would appear that antibiotics have gained acceptance in certain surgical procedures for protection against the subsequent development of infection.

Cardiac Surgery

Valve replacement and procedures requiring cardiopulmonary bypass carry a risk of postoperative infection of approximately 5 to 15 percent in patients not receiving prophylactic antibiotics. The risk of endocarditis or endarteritis is 1 to 3 percent when a bypass is not used. Most infections are due to staphylococci, particularly *S. epidermidis;* pneumococci have also been encountered. Several studies have suggested that use of prophylactic antibiotics substantially reduces this risk of infection.[28,29,197] A rational approach would employ a single drug, for example, a semisynthetic penicillin or a cephalosporin. The antibiotic should be started one to two hours prior to surgery and continued for approximately 24 to 48 hours thereafter or until all chest tubes are out. With cefazolin, 1 gm preoperatively and 1 gm every eight hours postoperatively can be employed. The dose of cephalothin should be 2 gm every six hours because of the lower blood levels and shorter half-life. An alternative would be an antistaphylococcal penicillin such as oxacillin or nafcillin.

Vascular Surgery Involving Grafts

The risk of infection in vascular surgery due to gram-positive cocci, particularly staphylococci, has been amply documented.[32] A recent randomized, prospective, and double-blind study compared use of cefazolin with use of a placebo in 565 arterial reconstructive operations. A significant reduction in infections was demonstrated in the cefazolin group for procedures with the greatest risk for infection: abdominal aortic resection, aortofemoral bypass, and femoral-lower leg bypass. There was no benefit in brachiocephalic operations. The most common organisms were *S. aureus* and gram-negative bacilli, alone or mixed. A regime of prophylactic antibiotics, as described above for cardiac surgery, should be employed.[198] A more recent report has confirmed these findings. The investigators reported that a 4 dose regimen of perioperative cephradine significantly reduced the infection rate in vascular procedures with a groin wound.[215]

Gastrointestinal Surgery

The frequency of postoperative wound sepsis after elective colonic resection approaches 40 percent in carefully studied patients. This risk can be reduced to 6 to 10 percent by the administration of appropriate antimicrobial agents in the preoperative period.[199] The approach we prefer is an oral regimen of neomycin and erythromycin along with an effective mechanical preparation of the colon. Three doses of 1 gm of each drug should be given beginning 18 to 24 hours before surgery. Parenteral cephalosporins alone fail to reduce the rate of septic complications.[200] It is unknown if parenteral antibiotics combined with oral neomycin and erythromycin will further reduce the risk of infection. At present, many would argue against such antibiotic use. When colonic surgery is more urgent, due to obstruction or ischemic bowel disease, parenteral therapy with a cephalosporin should be given. In these situations there is no time for effective oral antibiotic regimens and there may be occult bowel perforation. If found, "treatment" is a more appropriate term and broad spectrum coverage is then warranted.

Operations on bowel segments where there is "fecalization" of the flora should be approached as are colon resections. This would include ileal surgery for Crohn's disease and correction of a blind loop.

Nichols has made a compelling arguement that certain patients who undergo gastroduodenal surgery benefit from parenteral administration of cephalosporins perioperatively. This benefit is restricted to those with compromised bacterial inhibiting factors (bleeding or obstructed duodenal ulcer or gastric ulcer or malignancy).[216]

Operative removal of gallstones, in the uncomplicated case, is not accompanied by an appreciable risk of infection. Hence, we would not recommend use of prophylactic antibiotics for such procedures. However, in the elderly patient or in those with obstruction there is a higher rate of bacterial contamination of the bile and subsequent wound infection, and parenteral antibiotic prophylaxis with a cephalosporin should be given.[201] Patients with acute cholecystitis or cholangitis have active infection and antibiotics should be given as therapy for established sepsis.

Obstetric and Gynecologic Surgery

Several studies have demonstrated that the incidence of vaginal cuff infections is reduced in patients undergoing vaginal hysterectomy by the use of perioperative antibiotics.[27] Some studies report that premenopausal women undergoing this procedure have the greatest incidence of postoperative sepsis. We recommend cefazolin since it gives prolonged blood levels, possesses a wide spectrum of antimicrobial activity, and has been used successfully in several institutions.[202] The drug should be administered in an intravenous dose of 1 gm every eight hours for three doses beginning two hours prior to surgery. The risk of infection is probably lower in abdominal hysterectomies, and demonstrating a beneficial effect of antibiotic administration has been more difficult. There are now data that establish the value of prophylactic perioperative cefazolin (3 doses) in reducing wound and pelvic infections and febrile morbidity after abdominal hysterectomy.[217]

Cesarean sections are more frequently performed in recent years and account for nearly 10 percent of all deliveries in the U.S. Between 5 to 30 percent of these procedures are complicated by a postoperative infectious complication (urinary tract infection, endometritis, wound infection). Perhaps in part due to the increased numbers of patients at risk, several investigations have evaluated the role of prophylactic antibiotics in reducing the incidence of postoperative endometritis and febrile morbidity. One group found no significant reduction (in cefazolin-treated versus placebo-treated patients) of febrile morbidity, although there was a favorable trend toward fewer infections in those given antibiotics.[204] Others have demonstrated a substantial decrease in the incidence of infection with antibiotic combinations (a penicillin and kanamycin) or with a cephalosporin or cefoxitin alone.[205–208] We favor the administration of cefazolin or cefoxitin. The prophylaxis can be started when the umbilical cord is clamped so as to avoid masking neonatal sepsis.

Total Joint (Hip, Knee, Elbow) Replacement

An antistaphylococcal drug, either a semisynthetic penicillin (oxacillin or nafcillin) or cephalosporin is recommended by most authorities for such procedures.[202,203] Antibiotics are used perioperatively as in vascular surgery. A multicenter, randomized, double-blind study of 2137 patients undergoing hip replacement has recently been published.[218] The investigators reported a reduction in hip infections from 3.3 percent (placebo treated) to 0.9 percent (antibiotic treated), thereby establishing the value of the regimen utilized (perioperative cefazolin, 1 gm every six hours for five days). No statistically significant benefit was seen in patients who underwent surgery in hypersterile operating rooms, as the infection rate was only 0.8 percent (placebo treated) in this subgroup. In other elective orthopedic procedures, prophylactic antibiotics are not indicated.

Genitourinary Tract Procedures

Although cystoscopy frequently induces transient bacteremia, the prevailing view is that prophylaxis is needed only in patients with rheumatic or congenital heart disease. Patients with urinary tract infection defined by bacilluria greater than 10^5/ml can be treated with appropriate antimicrobial agents prior to the urological procedure which is then performed during the course of therapy.

Prophylactic antibiotics have no place in the prevention of urinary tract infections associated with indwelling catheters.[112,209] Use of an antimicrobial agent in this situation just serves to select more resistant organisms which colonize the urine. Urinary tract colonization associated with indwelling catheters is delayed with a closed drainage system.

Neurosurgical Procedures

There is a unanimity of opinion that prophylactic antibiotics should be given to patients undergoing placement of an intraventricular shunt. This is not based upon properly performed clinical studies but seems reasonable due to the devastating consequences of infection and by analogy with other procedures involving implantation of a foreign body (i.e., valve prostheses or total hip replacements). Clean neurosurgical procedures without the placement of foreign material require no parenteral prophylaxis. One study has shown that prolonged (>6 hours) microneurosurgical procedures are accompanied by an appreciable risk of infection and a group given prophylactic clindamycin had fewer infections than a group of patients receiving placebos.[210]

Prophylaxis for Bacterial Endocarditis

Patients with valvular heart disease, either acquired or congenital, or with prosthetic valves are at increased risk of developing endocarditis following bacterial invasion of the bloodstream. Since certain dental and surgical procedures produce transient bacteremia, prophylactic antimicrobial agents have been recommended. It should be noted, however, that there are no controlled studies in man to prove the effectiveness of such prophylaxis. The recommendations of the American Heart Association[211] and the Medical Letter[202] are given in Table 10.

An entirely oral regimen for patients who are not allergic to penicillin substitutes 2 gm of penicillin V orally for the parenteral penicillin. Patients with prosthetic heart

TABLE 10. Prophylaxis for Bacterial Endocarditis Recommended by the American Heart Association[211] and the Medical Letter[202]*

Patient without Known Allergy	*Patient with Penicillin Allergy*
Dental and Upper Respiratory Tract Procedures	
Aqueous penicillin G (1 million units, IV or IM) and procaine penicillin G (600,000 units, IM) ½ to 1 hr before procedure. Then penicillin V, 500 mg po q 6h for 8 doses.	Erythromycin (1 gm orally) 1½ to 2 hrs before procedure. Then 500 mg po q 6h for 8 doses.
Gastrointestinal and Genitourinary Procedures	
Ampicillin (1 gm IM or IV) and gentamicin (1.5 mg/kg IM or IV) ½ to 1 hr before procedure. Then repeat 8 and 16 hrs later.	Vancomycin (1 gm IV) and streptomycin (1 gm IM) ½ to 1 hr before procedure. Repeat at 12 hours.

*Consult references for full recommendations.

valves are at a special risk of endocarditis and many experts recommend including an aminoglycoside even for dental or respiratory tract procedures. Some would also recommend addition of an aminoglycoside for those patients taking continuous oral penicillin for rheumatic fever prophylaxis, as their oral flora becomes more penicillin resistant.

Prophylaxis with Other Implanted Prostheses

There is an ever-growing population of patients with implanted artificial joints or vascular prostheses. Late infections of these devices occur but the pathogenesis is unknown. One might wonder if such patients should be subject to prophylaxis for dental or genitourinary tract procedures as are patients with valvular heart disease, in an effort to prevent infection. There are no data which demonstrate a salutary effect of prophylactic antibiotics in this situation so the physician must use clinical judgment in the individual patient. If the consequences of infection would be devastating, it is reasonable to administer a prophylactic cephalosporin (e.g., cefazolin, 1 gm IV q 8h for 3 doses) with the knowledge that its efficacy is presently unproven.

ANTIMICROBIAL AGENTS

Although agents with antimicrobial activity have been empirically used for centuries, the "modern" era of chemotherapy began with the development and introduction of sulfonamides and penicillin. Over the ensuing decades, there have been enormous gains in our understanding of the mechanisms of antimicrobial action and the epidemiology and the mechanisms of resistance to antibiotics. With these advances has come the recognition of untoward effects due to use of these drugs, both for the patient and the community, and the recognition of "new" diseases directly due to antimicrobial agents (e.g., chloramphenicol-related aplastic anemia, antibiotic-associated pseudomembranous colitis).

The development of new antimicrobial agents continues in part because the microbes and the diseases they cause are not static. The very presence of antimicrobial agents creates selective pressures for resistant organisms to become prevalent. In addition, greater understanding of the diversity of organisms that singly or in combination cause infections has spawned the need for new antimicrobial agents. We have seen in recent years the introduction of a "new" drug for an "old" infection (cefoxitin in intraabdominal abscess) and the rediscovery of an "old" drug for a "new" infection (erythromycin therapy of legionnaire's disease). No doubt the practitioner sometimes feels bewildered by the numerous antimicrobial agents available and seeks ways of choosing among them. The basic principles remain: (1) determining the identity of the infecting organism(s), (2) recognizing the antimicrobial spectrum of the antibiotic(s) to be given, and (3) understanding the pharmacology and toxicities of the agent so to avoid untoward reactions. The above sections have dealt extensively with the bacteriology to be expected at various sites, this section will summarize the activities, dosages, and toxicities of selected antimicrobial agents.

Penicillins

The penicillins interfere with bacterial cell wall synthesis and effect killing of susceptible pathogens (Table 11). The precise mechanisms of their action is only beginning to be understood. The penicillins share a basic nucleus on which are substituted various moieties which endow the individual penicillins with different degrees of gastrointestinal absorption, resistance to hydrolysis, and antimicrobial activity. Other than nafcillin, which is excreted to a notable degree in the bile, the penicillins are eliminated by renal mechanisms. When glomerular filtration is severely decreased, major reductions in the dosages administered are required. The major side effects are allergic, varying from simple rashes to anaphylaxis.

The penicillins and cephalosporins can be collectively referred to as beta-lactam antibiotics. The most common type of resistance clinically encountered is due to beta-lactamases, which hydrolyze the beta-lactam ring, producing an inactive byproduct. These can be chromosomally or plasmid-mediated. The beta-lactamases have variable avidity for different substrates, resulting in unique susceptibilities to each of the beta-lactam agents. Occasional bacteria are resistant because they lack a penicillin-binding protein, while in gram-negative bacteria the outer membrane complex can present a diffusion barrier for beta-lactams, so they cannot reach the site to which they bind.

Cephalosporins

The cephalosporins, like the penicillins, have a basic nucleus on which various substitutions can be placed. The resultant antibiotics vary in their absorption, serum protein binding, extent of distribution, and antibiotic spectrum. They are bactericidal. They enjoy wide use because of their efficacy, safety, and broad spectrum against most gram-positive and many gram-negative bacilli. They are excreted by the kidneys, necessitating adjustment in dose with advanced degrees of renal insufficiency. The major side effects are allergic; rashes, drug fever, and eosinophilia occur in up to 5 percent of treatment courses. There is an approximate 10 to 15 percent incidence of cross-allerginicity in patients who are allergic to penicillin, and the cephalosporins should not be administered

TABLE 11. Penicillins

Agent	*Route*	*Usual Dose*	*Selected Susceptible Pathogens*
Natural Penicillins			
Penicillin G	PO, IM, IV	IM, IV, 1.2–24 megaunits/day	Streptococci (incl. *S.pneumoniae* except enterococci)
Penicillin V	PO	1–2 gm/day	*Neisseria gonorrhoeae* (most)[1]
			Neisseria meningitidis
			Clostridia
			Other anaerobes (except *Bacteroides fragilis*)
			Pasteurella multocida
Aminopenicillins			
Ampicillin	PO, IM, IV	PO, 1–4 gm/day	Enterococci (U.T.I.)
		IM, IV, 2–12 gm/day	*Hemophilus influenzae* (most)[2]
Amoxicillin	PO	1–4 gm/day	*Escherichia coli* (many)
			Proteus mirabilis
			Salmonella
			Shigella
			Listeria
Penicillinase-Resistant Penicillins			
Nafcillin	IV, IM	IM, IV, 2–12 gm/day	*Staphylococcus aureus*
Methicillin	IV, IM		
Oxacillin	PO, IM, IV	PO, 1–4 gm/day	
Cloxacillin	PO		
Dicloxacillin	PO		
Antipseudomonal Penicillins			
Carbenicillin	IM, IV	IM, IV, 4–30 gm/day	*Pseudomonas aeruginosa*[3]
Ticarcillin	IM, IV	IM, IV, 2–24 gm/day	
Indanyl—Carbenicillin[4]	PO	PO, 1.2–2.4 gm/day	

[1]Penicillinase-producing gonococci are resistant to treatment; alternative agents are spectinomycin, tetracycline, or cefoxitin.

[2]Beta-lactamase producing *Hemophilus influenzae* account for 5 to 15% of isolates; alternative drugs are cefamandole, chloramphenicol, or trimethoprim-sulfamethoxazole.

[3]An antipseudomonal penicillin should not be used alone in serious pseudomonal infections.

[4]Useful only in urinary tract infections due to susceptible pathogens.

to patients who have experienced anaphylaxis or giant urticarial reactions from penicillins.

Cephalosporins are useful agents in several situations. They can be given to patients who are allergic to penicillins, when a penicillin would be the antimicrobial agent of choice (e.g., pneumococcal pneumonia). In circumstances where the infection could be due to one of a number of pathogens and a penicillin might not cover all the possibilities, the broader spectrum of cephalosporins is an advantage (e.g. biliary sepsis). They are the agents of choice in certain situations when penicillin resistance is found (e.g., cefamandole therapy in pneumonia due to beta-lactamase producing *H. influenzae*). In general, they should not be used for central nervous system infections (poor penetration) or infections due to enterococcus or pseudomonas organisms (poor activity). The older cephalosporins, cephalothin, cefazolin, cephaloridine, cepharadine, and cephapirin, are generally more active against susceptible gram-positive cocci than cefamandole, cefoxitin or cefotaxime. These newer agents have special attributes which make them useful in selected circumstances (Table 12).

There are several oral cephalosporins available. Indications for their use in hospitalized patients are limited (see Table 13).

Aminoglycosides

The aminoglycosides share certain properties: negligible oral absorption, poor CSF penetration, renal excretion, and some degree of nephrotoxicity and ototoxicity. They have become invaluable agents for the treatment of severe gram-negative bacillary infections (Table 14). As opposed to penicillins and cephalosporins, their therapeutic margin is narrow. Thus toxicity is a major problem with their use. It appears that measuring serum concentrations and altering the dose to achieve therapeutic and avoid toxic levels can minimize but not eliminate ototoxic and nephrotoxic reactions.

TABLE 12. Parenterally-Administered Cephalosporins

Agent	*Usual Dose (gm/day)*	*Route*	*Remarks*
Cephaloridine (Loridine)	2–4	IV or IM	Nephrotoxic, avoid
Cephalothin (Keflin)	2–12	IV	Best antistaphylococcal activity
Cefazolin (Ancef, Kefzol)	1.5–6	IV or IM	Can be given q 8h due to longer half-life
Cephradine (Velosef, Anspor)	2–8	IV or IM	Only agent with oral and parenteral form
Cephapirin (Cefadyl)	2–12	IV	Similar to cephalothin
Cefamandole (Mandol)	2–12	IV or IM	Best against *Hemophilus influenzae,* active against many *Enterobacter*
Cefoxitin (Mefoxin)	2–8	IV or IM	A cephamycin; only agent with good activity against *Bacteroides fragilis*
Cefotaxime (Claforan)	2–12	IV or IM	Active against some strains of *P. aeruginosa;* expensive

TABLE 13. Orally-Administered Cephalosporins*

Agent	*Usual Dose*	*Remarks*
Cephalexin (Keflex)	0.25–1 gm q 6h	Active against gram-positive cocci (except enterococci) and selected gram-negative bacilli
Cephradine (Velosef, Anspor)	0.25–1 gm q 6h	Oral and parenteral form
Cephaloglycin (Kafocin)	0.25–1 gm q 6h	Poorly absorbed
Cefadroxil (Duricef)	0.25–1 gm q 12h	Long half-life allows twice daily dosing
Cefaclor (Ceclor)	0.25–1 gm q 8h	Increased activity against *Hemophilus influenzae*

*Most gram-positive bacterial infections can be treated with a penicillin (unless the patient is allergic) or erythromycin. Orally administered drugs should not be employed for hospitalized patients with severe gram-positive or gram-negative infections. They are useful in urinary tract infection and to complete therapy when parenteral antimicrobial agents are no longer necessary.

The aminoglycosides have little or no activity against anaerobic bacteria and very poor activity against many facultative streptococci. Although active against *S. aureus* in vitro, they are inferior to the antistaphylococcal penicillins, vancomycin, or the cephalosporins in the treatment of staphylococcal infections. The aminoglycosides kill bacteria by binding to the ribosomes and interfering with essential protein synthesis. The major mechanism of resistance is via the production of enzymes that modify the aminoglycosides.

Tetracyclines

The tetracyclines (Table 15) are exceptionally broad-spectrum agents, with activity against gram-positive and gram-negative bacteria, *Mycoplasma, Rickettsia,* chlamydia, and some protozoa. However, they have become less useful than in prior years due to widespread bacterial resistance, which is often plasmid-mediated. The tetracyclines are primarily bacteriostatic agents. They work by binding to the ribosome and preventing protein synthesis. Resistance to the tetracyclines involves a block in their penetration into the cell.

The tetracyclines rarely produce serious untoward reactions. Minor gastrointestinal disturbances are not infrequent. They should not be used in patients with renal insufficiency for they will increase azotemia. An exception is doxycycline which is excreted by extra-renal mechanisms (gastrointestinal tract). Use of tetracyclines should be

TABLE 14. Aminoglycosides*

Agent	*Daily Dose*	*Usual Dosage Interval*	*Desired Serum Levels (μg/ml)*		*Remarks*
			Peak	*Trough*	
Streptomycin	1–2 gm	q 12h	25–30	5	Useful in infections due to enterococci, *Mycobacterium tuberculosis, Yersinia pestis, Francisella tularensis*
Gentamicin	3–5 mg/kg	q 8h	5–8	2	
Tobramycin	3–5 mg/kg	q 8h	5–8	2	Perhaps less nephrotoxic than gentamicin
Kanamycin	15 mg/kg	q 8h	15–25	5	Widespread resistance in nosocomial gram-negative bacilli
Amikacin	15 mg/kg	q 8h	15–25	5	Infrequent resistance at present
Neomycin oral	2–4 gm	q 6h	0	0	Used in portal-systemic encephalopathy

*Of the aminoglycosides, streptomycin is the most vestibulotoxic, while neomycin is the most nephrotoxic. The other agents all have some degree of ototoxic and nephrotoxic potential, although human and animal studies indicate tobramycin appears less nephrotoxic than the other agents.

TABLE 15. Tetracyclines

Agent	*Usual Daily Dose*	*Dose Interval*	*Half-life (hours)*	*Remarks*
Tetracycline	1–2 gm	q 6–8h	10	Least expensive
Chlortetracycline	1–2 gm	q 6–8h	7	Little difference from tetracycline
Oxytetracycline	1–2 gm	q 6–8h	9	Little difference from tetracycline
Demeclocycline	300–600 mg	q 12–24h	15	Used in syndrome of inappropriate antidiuretic hormone secretion
Minocycline	100–200 mg	q 12–24h	17	High frequency of vestibular side effects
Doxycycline	100–200 mg	q 12–24h	15	Can be used in usual dose with renal insufficiency

avoided in pregnant women or in young children for they can cause irreversible discoloration of the teeth. Perhaps because they are inexpensive, they are widely prescribed. However, they are the drug of choice in only a few infections (cholera, brucellosis, chlamydial infections, rickettsiosis, melioidosis, relapsing fever). They are acceptable alternatives to penicillins (in the allergic patient) for infections due to *N. gonorrhoeae*, spirochetes, *H. influenzae*, and *S. pneumoniae*.

Chloramphenicol

Chloramphenicol (Table 16) is a bacteriostatic antibiotic that works by binding to the 50S unit of the bacterial ribosome, preventing peptide chain elongation. The drug can be bactericidal against *S. pneumoniae* and *H. influenzae*. Its spectrum is broad, but the indications for its use are limited, since irreversible aplastic anemia can occur after its use, albeit rarely. It penetrates the central nervous system well and hence it is quite useful in the treatment of brain abscess and in the treatment of pneumococcal, meningococcal, or hemophilus meningitis in the penicillin-allergic patient. Chloramphenicol is active against most anaerobic bacteria, but the alternative agents clindamycin, cefoxitin, or metronidazole are usually preferred. Chloramphenicol is metabolized by the liver and the inactive glucuronic acid conjugates are excreted by the kidneys. Little or no modification is required in renal insufficiency, while in patients with advanced degrees of hepatic dysfunction, the drug should be avoided or the conventional dose reduced by 50 percent. There has been renewed interest in the use of the drug to treat ampicillin-resistant *Hemophilus influenzae* infections. It is the treatment of choice for meningitis due to such pathogens. Its other major use is in the treatment of typhoid fever. Many consider it the treatment of choice, although ampicillin (if sensitive) and trimethoprim-sulfamethoxazole are suitable alternatives.

Resistance to chloramphenicol is mediated through the production of an enzyme (chloramphenicol acetylase) which inactivates the compound. This is frequently a plasmid-mediated function and, hence, chloramphenicol resistance is widely disseminated in aerobic gram-negative bacilli. Dose-related anemia frequently occurs during therapy but is reversible upon discontinuation of the drug. Idiosyncratic aplastic anemia complicates the course of treatment in 1 case in 25,000 to 40,000.

TABLE 16. Chloramphenicol

Agent	*Route*	*Usual Dose (mg q 6h)*	*Remarks*
Chloramphenicol	PO IV	250–500 500–1000	Bitter taste
Chloramphenicol palmitate	PO	250–500	Tasteless oral suspension
Chloramphenicol sodium succinate	IV	500–1000	Rapidly hydrolyzed to free chloramphenicol

Sulfonamides and Trimethoprim

The sulfonamides (Table 17) were the first chemical agents introduced for the treatment of systemic infections. There have been thousands of sulfonamides synthesized, but only a few have proved useful in clinical practice. They inhibit bacterial metabolism by competing with para-aminobenzoic acid (PABA), a factor required for folic acid synthesis. Resistance has been associated with an altered enzyme with a lower affinity for sulfonamides or overproduction of PABA. The drugs are metabolized to some degree in the liver and free and conjugated forms are excreted by renal mechanisms. The doses used should be reduced in renal insufficiency. Side effects include gastrointestinal disturbances, hemolytic anemia, and severe allergic hypersensitivity reactions. Crystalluria is infrequent with the more soluble sulfonamides.

Trimethoprim is an aminopyridine that inhibits bacterial dihydrofolate reductase. It has considerable antimicrobial activity alone and has recently been approved for use in the treatment of urinary tract infections due to susceptible pathogens. It has enjoyed the widest use in combination with sulfamethoxazole. The sequential inhibition of two

TABLE 17. Selected Sulfonamides and Trimethoprim

Agent	*Route*	*Usual Dose*	*Half-life (hours)*	*Remarks*
Sulfisoxazole (Gantrisin, generic)	PO, IV	2–8 gm/day	6	Usual agent of choice
Sulfadiazine (generic)	PO, IV	1–4 gm/day	17	Useful in meningococcal prophylaxis, if susceptible
Sulfamethoxazole (Gantanol)	PO	1–4 gm/day	11	Can be given q 12h
Trimethoprim–sulfamethoxazole (Bactrim, Septra)	PO			For *Pneumocystis carinii* infection the dose is: 20 mg/kg/day of trimethoprim and 100 mg/kg/day of sulfamethoxazole
Single strength, 400 mg sulfamethoxazole and 80 mg trimethoprim		2 tabs q 12h		
Double strength, 800 mg sulfamethoxazole and 160 mg trimethoprim		1 tab q 12h		
Suspension, 400 mg of sulfamethoxazole and 80 mg trimethoprim per 10 cc		10–20 cc q 12h		
Trimethoprim (Trimpex) (Proloprim)	PO	100 mg q 12h	10	Newly released. Will be useful in the sulfa and penicillin allergic patient

*A parenteral form of trimethoprim–sulfamethoxazole is now available. Its use should be strongly considered in proven *P. carinii* infections (available from manufacturer).

steps in folic acid synthesis produces antimicrobial synergy. The drug is excreted by the kidneys and dose reductions are required with advanced degrees of renal insufficiency. The drug can interfere with human folate metabolism producing megaloblastic changes or various cytopenias. These can be overcome by administering folinic acid.

The primary indications for use of sulfonamides are lower urinary tract infections and nocardiosis. The fixed combination of trimethoprim-sulfamethoxazole is useful in prostatitis, urinary tract infections, purulent bronchitis, infections due to ampicillin resistant *H. influenzae,* salmonellal infections, and in pneumonia due to *Pneumocystis carinii.* Sulfisoxazole is usually the sulfonamide of choice for the treatment of systemic or urinary tract infections.

Erythromycin and Clindamycin

Erythromycin is a macrolide antibiotic that inhibits bacterial protein synthesis by binding to the 50S portion of the ribosome. Resistance to its antibacterial activity is due to poor intracellular penetration *(Enterobacteriaceae)* or ribosomal alterations that prevent binding (gram-positive cocci). It is the treatment of choice for infection due to *Mycoplasma pneumoniae* and *Legionella pneumophila.* It is effective against most streptococci, clostridia, *Neisseria,* and many *H. influenzae* and community-acquired staphylococci. Treponemes are sensitive. Activity against anaerobes is erratic. It is useful in the treatment of gram-positive coccal infections in the penicillin-allergic patients and in mycoplasma infections and legionellosis. Neither renal nor hepatic excretion account for the disappearance of the active drug. Dose reduction in renal insufficiency is not required. In combination with neomycin, erythromycin has been shown to reduce the rate of septic complications when administered prophylactically to patients undergoing colorectal surgery.

The various congeners differ in the degree of gastrointestinal absorption and in the degree to which food interferes with absorption. Gastrointestinal side effects are common during therapy but serious toxicity is rare. Cholestatic hepatitis occurs only with the estolate derivative. The drug cannot be given intramuscularly due to severe pain. Phlebitis is common during intravenous therapy of severe infections (Table 18).

Clindamycin (Table 19) is a chlorinated derivative of lincomycin. It is chemically unrelated to erythromycin but has a similar spectrum of action against streptococci and staphylococci. It has poor activity against *Neisseria, H. influenzae,* and enterococci but has excellent activity against most anaerobes. This activity against anaerobic bacteria underlies its chief use, serious anaerobic infections. Some nonperfringens clostridia and peptococci are resistant.

It inhibits bacterial protein synthesis at the level of the 50S ribosomal unit. Resistance is presumed to involve altered ribosomal binding. Plasmid-mediated resistance has been described in gram-positive cocci and *B. fragilis.* It is well absorbed orally and is well tolerated when given intravenously. It received considerable notoriety as a cause of pseudomembranous colitis, now known to be caused by *C. difficile,* but most cases of this complication are related to use of other antimicrobial agents. Nonetheless, diarrhea and colitis can complicate use of clindamycin and this is the major untoward reaction. The half-life of two to three hours is unaffected by renal failure but is prolonged in hepatic insufficiency.

TABLE 18. Erythromycins

Agent	*Route*	*Usual Dose (gm/day)*	*Expected* Peak Serum Levels (μg/ml)*	*Remarks*
Erythromycin base (E-Mycin)	PO	1–2	1–2	Generic least expensive; enteric coated to resist acid
Erythromycin estolate (Ilosone)	PO	1–2	1–2	Avoid, can cause cholestatic hepatitis
Erythromycin ethylsuccinate (Pediamycin)	PO	1–2	1–2	
Erythromycin stearate (Pfizer-E)	PO	1–2	1–2	
Erythromycin lactobionate	IV	1–2	8–10	Phlebogenic
Erythromycin gluceptate	IV	1–2	8–10	Phlebogenic

*After a 500 mg dose orally (fasting-state) or IV.

TABLE 19. Clindamycin

Agent	*Route*	*Dose (mg q 6h)*	*Expected Peak Serum Levels* (μg/ml)*	*Remarks*
Clindamycin hydrochloride	PO	150–300	3–5	Little effect of food on absorption
Clindamycin phosphate	IV, IM	300–600	IM, 3–5 IV, 10–12	Hydrolyzed to free hydrochloride in blood

*Levels are after a 300 mg (PO or IM) or 600 mg (IV) dose.

The major indications for clindamycin therapy are serious infections involving anaerobic bacteria, usually arising in the abdominal cavity or female pelvis. Although effective in the therapy of many staphylococcal or streptococcal infections, erythromycin and vancomycin are the preferred alternatives in the penicillin allergic patient.

Vancomycin

Vancomycin is a narrow spectrum antimicrobial agent with activity limited to gram-positive organisms. Its main advantage is activity against penicillin-resistant and cephalosporin-resistant gram-positive cocci and bacilli including *S. aureus, S. epidermidis,* streptococci, enterococci, anaerobic cocci, and clostridia. Vancomycin inhibits biosynthesis of peptidoglycan. Resistance in gram-positive bacteria is unusual. Vancomycin is not absorbed from the gastrointestinal tract and doses of 500 mg every six hours give levels up to 25,000 μg/gm of stool. The compound is only available for intravenous infusion because intramuscular injection is extremely painful. After 1 gm dosages, it is widely distributed to all body fluids except the bile and CSF and it is primarily excreted by the kidneys. The recommended dose for adults is 1 gm intravenously every 12 hours.

The indications for the use of systemic vancomycin include: (1) staphylococcal shunt infections in renal dialysis patients, (2) staphylococcal endocarditis or deep-seated staphylococcal infection, and (3) streptococcal endocarditis including enterococcal endocarditis in patients with a penicillin allergy. Oral vancomycin therapy has been used in the past for staphylococcal enterocolitis and has been recently shown to be efficacious in the treatment of antibiotic-associated pseudomembranous colitis due to *C. difficile.* The dosage for oral therapy is 1 to 2 gm/day. Major adverse reactions include auditory nerve damage, chills and fever, and hypotension on rapid intravenous infusion. The compound has a rather noxious taste which can be masked by various syrups when oral therapy is required. Nephrotoxicity is unusual.

Amphotericin B

Amphotericin B is an antifungal, antimicrobial agent which possesses no activity against bacteria. It is the single most effective agent for the treatment of deep-seated fungal infections including blastomycosis, histoplasmosis, cryptococcosis, candidiasis, sporotrichosis, aspergillosis, mucormycosis, and coccidioidomycosis. It is combined with flucytosine for the treatment of cryptococcal meningitis and disseminated *Torulopsis glabrata* infections. Amphotericin B is insoluble in aqueous solutions and is kept in suspension by the addition of bile salts to the intravenous preparation. The pharmacology of the agent is poorly understood. It is given only by slow intravenous infusion, and limited data indicate that it is widely distributed in all tissues except that its concentration is low in both the central nervous system and the eye. The route of excretion is not well understood, but no adjustment in dosages are needed in established renal failure.

Amphotericin B is used in the surgical patient to treat disseminated fungal infections, usually *Candida* or *Torulopsis,* which are seen most often in patients who have received long-term broad-spectrum antimicrobial agents or in those receiving total parenteral nutrition. The use of this agent in combination with flucytosine should be attempted only with the help of an infectious disease specialist because monitoring of serum levels of flucytosine is necessary to prevent lethal bone marrow suppression. Guidelines for the administration of amphotericin have been derived empirically for the most part and differ from one center to another. An initial dose of 1 mg should be given to test for potential adverse reactions. The dose is then increased in increments of 5, 10, 20, 40 and 60 mg until a total dose of 0.5 to 1.0 mg/kg/day is achieved. If severe adverse reactions occur (including chills, tachycardia, hypotension, tachypnea, or severe phlebitis), the addition of small amounts of heparin and hydrocortisone to the solution may decrease the incidence of these side effects. The daily and total dosage vary greatly. In general, low-dose therapy of 200 to 500 mg has been satisfactory for the treatment of

Candida and *Torulopsis* infections while higher total doses of 2 to 5 gm are necessary for treating deep-seated fungal infections such as cryptococcosis, histoplasmosis, and coccidioidomycosis.

The major adverse reactions include immediate toxicity with fever, tachycardia, hypotension, and tachypnea upon infusion or delayed toxicities of renal failure and bone marrow suppression. During therapy a dose-related decrement in glomerular filtration is to be expected, with most patients developing a serum creatinine of 2 to 3 mg/dl. This reverses upon discontinuation of the drug. Similarly, most patients develop anemia, with hematocrits at 28 to 32 percent, during prolonged therapy. This, too, is reversible. With intrathecal administration of this agent for fungal meningitis there may be a rather exuberant arachnoiditis. This is obviated by the placement of devices such as Omaya reservoirs for the direct delivery of the drug to the ventricles or cisterna. Amphotericin irrigations have been used in abscesses harboring fungi and in fungal infections of bone and joints, but the efficacy of this procedure has not been validated. The instillation of amphotericin B into the urinary bladder has been shown to be effective in eliminating candidal cystitis.

Metronidazole

Metronidazole has substantial in vitro activity against anerobic bacteria[219] and has recently been approved for use in the United States for the treatment of anerobic infections. It is active against most strains of *Bacteroides, Fusobacteria* and *Clostridia. P. acnes* and *Actinomyces* are resistant. Comparative prospective studies have demonstrated that when combined with an aminoglycoside it has produced results equivalent to Clindamycin and an aminoglyside in the treatment of serious intra-abdominal and pelvic infections. It is well absorbed orally with serum levels of 20–30 μg/ml with regimens of 500 mg q.i.d. The recommended intravenous dosage is 15 mg/kg (loading dose) followed by an infusion of 7.5 mg/kg every six hours. The half life is approximately 8 hours; as elimination of the drug is by metabolism no reduction in dose is required for those with decreased creatinine clearance. The most serious side effects of the drug are convulsions and peripheral neuropathy. Its use can also be complicated by a "Disulfiram-like" reaction if ethanol is ingested.

REFERENCES

1. Hospital Infections Branch, Bureau of Epidemiology, Center for Disease Control: *Trends in Surgical Wound Infection Rates—United States MMWR,* Jan 25, 1980, pp. 27–29.
2. Bartlett, JG, and Finegold, SM: *Anerobic infections of the lung and pleural space.* Am Rev Resp Dis 110:56, 1974.
3. Finland, M, and Barnes, MW: *Changing ecology of acute bacterial empyema: occurence and mortality at Boston City Hospital during 12 selected years from 1935–1972.* J Infect Dis 137:274, 1978.
4. Bartlett, JG, Gorbach, SL, Thadepalli, H, *et al.: The bacteriology of empyema.* Lancet 1:338, 1974.
5. Murray, PR, and Washington, JA: *Microscopic and bacteriologic analysis of expectorated sputum.* Mayo Clin Proc 50:339, 1975.
6. O'Keefe, JP, Bartlett, JG, Tally, FP, et al.: *An heuristic approach to hospital acquired pneumonia.* (Presented to the American Federation for Clinical Research Annual Meeting, Atlantic City, May 1975) Clin Res 24:350, 1976.

7. Johanson, WG, Pierce, AK, and Sanford, JP: *Changing pharyngeal bacterial flora of hospitalized patients: emergence of gram-negative bacilli.* N Eng J Med 281:1137, 1969.

8. Johanson, WG, Pierce, AK, Sanford, JP, et al.: *Nosocomial respiratory infection with gram-negative bacilli: the significance of colonization of the respiratory tract.* Ann Intern Med 77:701, 1972.

9. Keefer, CS: *Acute and chronic mediastinitis.* Arch Intern Med 62:109, 1938.

10. Neuhof, H: *Acute infections of the mediastinum with special reference to mediastinal suppuration.* J Thorac Surg 6:194, 1936.

11. Moncada, R, Warpeha, R, Pickleman, J, et al.: *Mediastinitis from odontogenic and deep cervical infection.* Chest 73:497, 1978.

12. Howell, HS, Prinz, RA, Pickleman, JR: *Anaerobic mediastinitis.* Surg Gynecol Obstet 143:353, 1976.

13. Bartlett, JG, and Gorbach, SL: *Anaerobic infections of the head and neck.* Otolaryngol Clin North Am 9:655, 1976.

14. Cryer, PE, and Kissane, J (eds.): *Abdominal pain, vomiting, fever and pleural effusion.* Am J Med 60:107, 1976.

15. Campbell, TC, Andrews, JL, and Neptune, WB: *Spontaneous rupture of the esophagus.* JAMA 235:526, 1976.

16. Loop, FD: *Trauma to the esophagus.* Cleve Clin Q 42:175, 1975.

17. Engelman, R, Williams, D, Gouge, TH, et al.: *Mediastinitis following open-heart surgery.* Arch Surg 107:772, 1973.

18. Wray, TM, Bryant, RE, and Killen, DA: *Sternal osteomyelitis and costochondritis after median sternotomy.* J Thorac Cardiovasc Surg 65:227, 1973.

19. Sanfelippo, PM, and Danielson, GK: *Complications associated with median sternotomy.* J Thorac Cardiovasc Surg 63:420, 1972.

20. Sutherland, RD, Martinez, HE, Guynes, WA, et al.: *Postoperative chest wound infections in patients requiring coronary bypass. A controlled study evaluating prophylactic antibiotics.* J Thorac Cardiovasc Surg 73:944, 1977.

21. Kluge, R, Calia, F, McLaughlin, J, et al.: *Sources of contamination in open-heart surgery.* JAMA 230:1415, 1974.

22. Rosendorf, LL, Daicoff, G, and Baer, H: *Sources of gram-negative infection after open-heart surgery.* J Thorac Cardiovasc Surg 67:195, 1974.

23. Smith, PW, Peterson, RJ, and Ferlic, RM: *Gallium scan in sternal osteomyelitis.* Am J Radiol 132:840, 1979.

24. Thurer, RJ, Bognolo, D, Vargas, A, et al.: *The management of mediastinal infection following cardiac surgery.* J Thorac Cardiovasc Surg 68:962, 1974.

25. Watanakunakorn, C: *Prosthetic valve endocarditis.* Prog Cardiovasc Dis 22:181, 1979.

26. Karchmer, AW, Dismukes, WD, Johnson, JR, et al.: *Staphylcoccus epidermidis prosthetic value endocarditis.* (Abstract) Presented at the 19th Interscience Conference on Antimicrobial Agents and Chemotherapy, Boston, October 1979.

27. Hirschmann, JV, and Inui, TS: *Antimicrobial prophylaxis: a critique of recent trials.* Rev Infect Dis 2:1, 1980.

28. Conte, JE, Cohen, SN, Roe, BB, et al.: *Antibiotic prophylaxis and cardiac surgery: a prospective, double-blind comparison of single-dose versus multiple-dose regimens.* Ann Intern Med 76:943, 1972.

29. Goldmann, DA, Hopkins, CC, Karchmer, AW, et al.: *Cephalothin prophylaxis in cardiac value surgery: a prospective, double-blind, comparison of two-day and six-day regimens.* J Thorac Cardiovasc Surg 73:470, 1979.

30. Kluge, RM, Calia, FM, McLaughlin, JS, et al.: *Serum antibiotic concentrations pre- and post-cardiopulmonary bypass.* Antimicrob Agents Chemother 4:270, 1973.

31. Szilagyi, DE, Smith, RF, Elliott, JP, et al.: *Infection in arterial reconstruction with synthetic grafts.* Ann Surg 176:321, 1972.

32. Willworth, BM, and Waldhausen, JA: *Infection of arterial prostheses.* Surg Gynecol Obstet 139:446, 1974.

33. Fry, WJ: *Vascular prosthesis infection.* Surg Clinic North Am 52:1419, 1972.

34. Moore, WS: *Experimental studies relating to sepsis in prosthetic vascular grafting,* in Duma, RJ (ed.): *Infections of Prosthetic Heart Valves and Vascular Grafts.* Baltimore: University Park Press, 1977.

35. Delgado, DG, and Cobbs, CG: *Infection of prosthetic valves and intravascular devices,* in Mandell, GL, Douglas, RG, and Bennett, JE (eds.): *Principles and Practice of Infectious Diseases.* New York: John Wiley and Sons, 1979.

36. Diethrick, EB, Noon, GP, Liddicoat, JE, et al.: *Treatment of infected aorto-femoral prostheses.* Surgery 68:1044, 1970.
37. Popovsky, J, and Singer, S: *Infected prosthetic grafts. Local therapy with graft preservation.* Arch Surg 115:203, 1980.
38. Nsouli, K, Lazarus, M, Schoenbaum, SC, et al.: *Bacteremic infections in hemodialysis.* Arch Intern Med 139:1255, 1979.
39. Onorato, IM, Axelrod, JL, Lorch, JA, et al.: *Fungal infections of dialysis fistulae.* Ann Intern Med 91:50, 1979.
40. Kirmani, N, Tuazon, C, Murray, H, et al.: *Staphylococcus aureus carriage rate of patients receiving long-term hemodialysis.* Arch Intern Med 138:1657, 1978.
41. Dobkin, JR, Miller, MG, and Steigbigel, NH: *Septicemia in patients on chronic hemodialysis.* Ann Intern Med 88:28, 1978.
42. Barcenas, CG, Fuller, TJ, Elms, J, et al.: *Staphylococcal sepsis in patients on chronic hemodialysis regimens.* Arch Intern Med 136:1131, 1976.
43. Eykyn, S, Phillips, I, and Evans, J: *Vancomycin for staphylococcal shunt infections in patients on regular hemodialysis.* Br Med J 2:80, 1970.
44. Gorbach, SL, and Bartlett, JG: *Anaerobic infections.* N Engl J Med 290:1177, 1974.
45. Tally, FP, and Gorbach, SL: *Clinical aspects of anaerobic infection.* J Infection (Suppl.) 1:25, 1979.
46. Gorbach, SL: *Treatment of intra-abdominal sepsis,* in Finegold, SM, Bartlett, JG, Chow, AW, et al.: *Management of Anaerobic Infections.* Ann Intern Med 83:375, 1975.
47. Finegold, SM: *Therapy for infections due to anaerobic bacteria: an overview.* J Infect Dis (Suppl.) 135:S25, 1977.
48. Weinstein, WM, Onderdonk, AB, Bartlett, JG, et al.: *Experimental intra-abdominal abscesses in rats: development of an experimental model.* Infect Immun 10:1250, 1974.
49. Onderdonk, AB, Weinstein, WM, Sullivan-Siegler, NM, et al.: *Experimental intra-abdominal abscesses in rats: quantitative bacteriology of infected animals.* Infect Immun 10:1256, 1974.
50. Louie, TJ, Onderdonk, AB, Gorbach, SL, et al.: *Therapy for experimental intra-abdominal sepsis: comparison of four cephalosporins, clindamycin and gentamicin.* J Infect Dis (Suppl.) 135:S18, 1977.
51. Thadepalli, H, Gorbach, SL, Broillo, PN, et al.: *Abdominal trauma, anaerobes, and antibiotics.* Surg Gynecol Obstet 137:270, 1973.
52. Bartlett, JG, Miao, P, and Gorbach, SL: *Empiric treatment with clindamycin and gentamicin of suspected sepsis due to anaerobic and aerobic bacteria.* J Infect Dis (Suppl.) 135:S80, 1977.
53. Swenson, RM, and Lorber, B: *Clindamycin and carbenicillin in treatment of patients with intraabdominal and female genital tract infections.* J Infect Dis (Suppl.) 135:S40-S45, 1977.
54. Chow, AW, and Guze, LB: *Bacteroidaceae bacteremia: clinical experience with 112 patients.* Medicine 53:93, 1974.
55. Harding, GK, Marrie, TJ, Buckwold, F, et al.: *A controlled comparison of ticarcillin, clindamycin, and chloramphenicol in the therapy of anaerobic infections.* J Inf Dis 142:384, 1980.
56. Thadepalli, H, Gorbach, SL, and Bartlett, JG: *Apparent failure of chloramphenicol in the treatment of anaerobic infections.* Curr Therap Res 22:421, 1977.
57. Louie, TJ, Bartlett, JG, Onderdonk, AB, et al.: *Failure of chloramphenicol therapy of experimental intraabdominal abscesses.* (Abstract) Presented at the 17th Interscience Conference on Antimicrobial Agents and Chemotherapy, New York, October 1977.
58. Eykyn, SJ, and Phillips, I: *Metronidazole and anaerobic sepsis.* Br Med J 2:1418, 1976.
59. Kirby, BD, Busch, DF, Citron, DM, et al.: *Cefoxitin for treatment of infection due to anaerobic bacteria.* Rev Infect Dis 1:113, 1979.
60. Ribner, BS, Billiard, BS, and Freimer, EH: *Treatment of significant bacterial infections in adults with cefoxitin.* Rev Infect Dis 1:152, 1979.
61. Tally, FP, McGowan, K, Kellum, JM, et al.: *A randomized comparison of cefoxitin with or without amikacin and clindamycin plus amikacin in surgical sepsis.* Ann Surg 193:318, 1981.
62. Drusano, G, Warren, JT, Saah, A, et al.: *Cefoxitin versus clindamycin and gentamicin for penicillin-resistant anaerobic infections.* (Abstract) Presented at the 19th Interscience conference on Antimicrobial Agents and Chemotherapy, Boston, October 1979.

63. EDLUNE, YA, MOLLSTEDT, BO, AND OUCHTERLONY, G: *Bacteriological investigation of the biliary system and liver in biliary tract disease correlated to clinical data and microstructure of the gallbladder and liver.* Acta Chir Scand 116:461, 1958.

64. LYKKEGAARD-NIELSEN, M, AND JUSTESEN, T: *Anaerobic and aerobic bacteriological studies in biliary tract disease.* Scand J Gastroenterol 11:437, 1976.

65. SHIMADA, K, INAMATSU, T, AND YAMASHIRO, M: *Anaerobic bacteria in biliary disease in elderly patients.* J Infect Dis 135:850, 1977.

66. ENGLAND, DM, AND ROSENBLATT, JE: *Anaerobes in human biliary tracts.* J Clin Microbiol 6:494, 1977.

67. BOURGAULT, AM, ENGLAND, DM, ROSENBLATT, JE, ET AL.: *Clinical characteristics of anaerobic bactibilia.* Arch Intern Med 139:1346, 1979.

68. LAPIS, JL, ORLANDO, RC, MITTELSTAEDT, CA, ET AL.: *Ultrasonography in the diagnosis of obstructive jaundice.* Ann Intern Med 89:61, 1978.

69. TAYLOR, KJ, ROSENFIELD, AT, AND SPIRO, HW: *Diagnostic accuracy of grey scale ultrasonography for the jaundiced patient.* Arch Intern Med 139:60, 1979.

70. HUANG, T, BASS, JA, AND WILLIAMS, RD: *The significance of biliary pressure in cholangitis.* Arch Surg 98:629, 1969.

71. DE LA MAZA, L, NAEIM, F, AND BERMAN, L: *The changing etiology of liver abscess.* JAMA 227:161, 1974.

72. RUBIN, RH, SWARTZ, MN, AND MALT, R: *Hepatic abscess: change in clinical, bacteriologic and therapeutic aspects.* Am J Med 57:601, 1974.

73. SABBAJ, J, SUTTER, VL, AND FINEGOLD, SM: *Anaerobic pyogenic liver abscess.* Ann Intern Med 77:629, 1972.

74. ALTEMEIER, WA: *Liver abscess: the etiologic role of anaerobic bacteria,* in BALOWS, A, DE HAAN, R, DOWELL, V, ET AL. (eds.): *Anaerobic Bacteria: Role in Disease.* Springfield, Ill.: Charles C Thomas, 1974.

75. ADAMS, EB, AND MACLEOD, IN: *Invasive amebiasis. II. Amebic liver abscess and its complications.* Medicine 56:325, 1977.

76. KROGSTAD, DJ, SPENCER, HC, AND HEALY, GR: *Amebiasis.* N Engl J Med 298:262, 1978.

77. CONN, HD, AND FESSEL, JM: *Spontaneous bacterial peritonitis in cirrhosis: variations on a theme.* Medicine 50:161, 1971.

78. HARKEN, AH, AND SCHOCHAT, SJ: *Gram-positive peritonitis in children.* Am J Surg 125:769, 1973.

79. BARTLETT, JG, CHANG, TW, GURWITH, M, ET AL.: *Antibiotic-associated pseudomembranous colitis due to toxin-producing clostridia.* N Engl J Med 298:530, 1978.

80. BARTLETT, JG: *Antibiotic-associated pseudomembranous colitis.* Rev Infect Dis 1:530, 1979.

81. KEIGHLEY, MRB, BURDON, DW, ARABI, Y, ET AL.: *Randomized trial of vancomycin for pseudomembranous colitis and post-operative diarrhea.* Br Med J 2:1667, 1978.

82. HUMPHREY, CD, CONDON, CW, CANTEY, JR, ET AL.: *Partial purification of a toxin found in hampsters with antibiotic-associated colitis (AAC): reversible binding of the toxin by cholestyramine.* Gastroenterology 74:1046, 1978.

83. BARTLETT, JG, ONDERDONK, AB, DRUDE, E, ET AL.: *Quantitative bacteriology of the vaginal flora.* J Infect Dis 136:271, 1977.

84. THADEPALLI, H, GORBACH, SL, AND KEITH, L: *Anaerobic infections of the female genital tract: bacteriologic and therapeutic aspects.* Am J Obstet Gynecol 117:1034, 1973.

85. HALL, WL, SOBEL, AI, JONES, CP, ET AL.: *Anerobic post-operative pelvic infection.* Obstet Gynecol 80:1, 1967.

86. SWEET, RL, AND LEDGER, WJ: *Puerperal infectious morbidity—a two year review.* Am J Obstet Gynecol 117:1093, 1973.

87. GIBBS, RS, O'DELL, TN, MACGREGOR, RR, ET AL.: *Puerperal endometritis: a prospective microbiologic study.* Am J Obstet Gynecol 121:919, 1975.

88. ROTHERAM, EB, AND SCHICK, SF: *Non-clostridial anaerobic bacteria in septic abortion.* Am J Med 46:80, 1969.

89. DIZEREGA, G, YONEKURA, L, ROY, S, ET AL.: *A comparison of clindamycin-gentamicin and penicillin-gentamicin in the treatment of post-cesarean section endomyometritis.* Am J Obstet Gynecol 134:236, 1979.

90. LEDGER, WJ, AND PETERSON, WP: *The use of heparin in the management of pelvic thrombophlebitis.* Surg Gynecol Obstet 131:1115, 1970.

91. BRENNER, RW, AND GEHRING, SW: *Pelvic actinomycosis in the presence of an endocervical contraceptive device.* Obstet Gynecol 29: 71, 1967.

92. Schiffer, MA, Elquezabal, A, Sultana, M, et al.: *Actinomycosis infections associated with intrauterine devices.* Obstet Gynecol 45:67, 1975.

93. Luff, RD, Gupta, PK, Spence, MR, et al.: *Pelvic actinomycosis and the intrauterine contraceptive device.* Am J Clin Path 69:581, 1978.

94. Kaye, D: *Symposium on urinary tract infection: host defense mechanisms in the urinary tract.* Urol Clin North Am 2:407, 1975.

95. Sanford, JP: *Urinary tract symptoms and infections.* Ann Rev Med 26:485, 1975.

96. Fang, LST, Tolkoff-Rubin, NE, and Rubin, RH: *Localization and antibiotic management of urinary tract infection.* Ann Rev Med 30:225, 1979.

97. Musher, DM, Thorsteinsson, SB, and Airola, II, VM: *Quantitative urinalysis: diagnosing urinary tract infection in men.* JAMA 236:2069, 1976.

98. Glew, RH, and Moellering, RC, Jr.: *Effect of protein binding on the activity of penicillins in combination with gentamicin against enterococci.* Antimicrob Agents Chemother 15:87, 1979.

99. Ronald, AR, Boutros, P, and Mourtada, H: *Bacteriuria localization and response to single-dose therapy in women.* JAMA 235:1854, 1976.

100. Ludwig, P, Buckwold, F, Harding, G, et al.: *Single-dose therapy of acute cystitis in females: a prospective randomized comparison of four regimens.* (Abstract) Presented at the 19th Interscience Conference on Antimicrobial Agents and Chemotherapy. Boston, October 1979.

101. Charlton, CAC, Crowther, A, Davies, JG, et al.: *Three-day and ten-day chemotherapy for urinary tract infections in general practice.* Br Med J 1:124, 1976.

102. Fang, LS, Tolkoff-Rubin, NE, and Rubin, RH: *Efficacy of single-dose and conventional amoxicillin therapy in urinary-tract infection localized by the antibody-coated bacteria technic.* N Engl J Med 298:413, 1978.

103. Thomas, V, Shelokov, A, and Forland, M: *Antibody-coated bacteria in the urine and the site of urinary-tract infection.* New Engl J Med 290:588, 1974.

104. Jones, ST, Smith, JW, and Sanford, JP: *Localization of urinary-tract infections by detection of antibody-coated bacteria in urine sediment.* N Engl J Med 290:591, 1974.

105. Harding, GKM, Marrie, TJ, Ronald, AR, et al.: *Urinary tract infection localization in women.* JAMA 240:1147, 1978.

106. Hawthorne, NJ, Kurtz, SB, Anhalt, JP, et al.: *Accuracy of antibody-coated-bacteria test in recurrent urinary tract infections.* Mayo Clin Proc 53:651, 1978.

107. Stamm, WE: *Guidelines for prevention of catheter-associated urinary tract infections.* Ann Intern Med 82:386, 1975.

108. Garibaldi, RA, Burke, JP, Dickman, ML, et al.: *Factors predisposing to bacteriuria during indwelling urethral catheterization.* N Engl J Med 291:215, 1974.

109. Gonick, P, Falkner, B, Schwartz, A, et al.: *Bacteriuria in the catheterized patient: cystitis or pyelonephritis?* JAMA 233:253, 1975.

110. Gross, PA, Harkavy, LM, Barden, GE, et al.: *Positive Foley catheter tip cultures—fact or fancy?* JAMA 228:72, 1974.

111. Britt, MR, Garibaldi, RA, Miller, WA, et al.: *Antimicrobial prophylaxis for catheter-associated bacteriuria.* Antimicrob Agent Chemother 11:240, 1977.

112. Warren, JW, Platt, R, Thomas, RJ, et al.: *Antibiotic irrigation and catheter-associated urinary tract infections.* N Engl J Med 299:570, 1978.

113. Vainrub, B, and Musher, DM: *Lack of effect of methenamine in suppression of, or prophylaxis against, chronic urinary infection.* Antimicrob Agent Chemother 12:625, 1977.

114. Meares, EM, Jr.: *Prostatitis: a review.* Urol Clin North Am 2:3, 1975.

115. Stamey, TA: *Chronic bacterial prostatitis.* Hospital Practice 5:49, 1971.

116. Oosterlinck, W, Wallijn, E, and Wijndaele, JJ: *The concentration of doxycycline in human prostate gland and its role in the treatment of prostatitis.* Scand J Infect Dis (Suppl.) 9:85, 1976.

117. Dow, D: *Trimethoprim-sulfamethoxazole in the treatment of chronic prostatitis.* J Can Med Assoc 112:26S, 1975.

118. DRACH, GW: *Trimethoprim/sulfamethoxazole therapy of chronic bacterial prostatitis.* J Urol 111:637, 1974.

119. BERGER, RE, ALEXANDER, ER, MONDA, GD, ET AL.: *Chlamydia trachomatis as a cause of acute "idiopathic" epididymitis.* N Engl J Med 298:201, 1978.

120. HARNISCH, JP, BERGER, RE, ALEXANDER, ER, ET AL.: *Aetiology of acute epididymitis.* Lancet 1:819, 1977.

121. MURPHY, JF, FRED, HL, AND CARLSON, V: *Renal and perirenal gas in a diabetic man.* JAMA 237:801, 1977.

122. SPAGNOLA, AM: *Emphysematous pyelonephritis: a report of two cases.* Am J Med 64:840, 1978.

123. MOORE, CA, AND GANGAI, MP: *Renal cortical abscess.* J Urol 98:303, 1967.

124. THORLEY, JD, JONES, SR, AND SANFORD, JP: *Perinephric abscess.* Medicine 6:441, 1974.

125. SALVATIERRA, O, JR., BUCKLEW, WB, AND MORROW, JW: *Perinephric abscess: a report of 71 cases.* J Urol 98:296, 1967.

126. SCHIFF, M, JR., GLICKMAN, M, WEISS, RM, ET AL.: *Antibiotic treatment of renal carbuncle.* Ann Intern Med 87:305, 1977.

127. PEDERSON, JF, HANCKE, S, AND KRISTENSEN, JK: *Renal carbuncle: antibiotic therapy governed by ultrasonically guided aspiration.* J Urol 109:777, 1973.

128. MONCRIEF, JA: *Medical progress: burns.* N Engl J Med 288:444, 1973.

129. LAW, EJ, KIM, OJ, STIERITZ, DD, ET AL.: *Experience with systemic candidiasis in the burned patient.* J Trauma 12:543, 1972.

130. MONCRIEF, JA, LINDBERG, RB, SWITZER, WE, ET AL.: *Use of topical antibacterial therapy in the treatment of the burn wound.* Arch Surg 92:558, 1966.

131. DAVIS, WA, KANE, JG, AND GARAGUSI, VF: *Human aeromonas infections: a review of the literature.* Medicine 57:267, 1978.

132. WASHINGTON, JA: *Aeromonas hydrophila in clinical bacteriologic specimens.* Ann Intern Med 76:611, 1972.

133. JOHNSON, RH, AND RUMANS, LW: *Unusual infections caused by Pasteurella multocida.* JAMA 237:146, 1977.

134. SWARTZ, M: *Cellulitis and superficial infections,* in MANDELL, GL, DOUGLAS, RG, AND BENNET, JE (eds.): *Principles and Practice of Infectious Diseases.* New York: John Wiley and Sons, 1979, pp. 797–812.

135. FLICK, MR, AND CLUFF, LE: *Pseudomonas bacteremia: review of 108 cases.* Am J Med 60:501, 1976.

136. GORBACH, SL, AND THADEPALLI, H: *Isolation of clostridium in human infections: evaluation of 114 cases.* J Infect Dis (Suppl.) 131:S81, 1975.

137. GORBACH, SL: *Other clostridium species (including gas gangrene),* in MANDELL, GL, DOUGLAS, RG, AND BENNET, JE (eds.): *Principles and Practice of Infectious Diseases.* New York: John Wiley and Sons, 1979, pp. 1876–1885.

138. JONDRZEJEWSKI, JW, JONES, SR, NEWCOMBE, RL, ET AL.: *Nontraumatic clostridial myonecrosis.* Am J Med 65:542, 1978.

139. WEBB, D, AND THADEPALLI, H: *Skin and soft tissue polymicrobial infections from intravenous abuse of drugs.* West J Med 179:200, 1979.

140. REA, WJ, AND WYRICK, WJ: *Necrotizing fasciitis.* Ann Surg 172:957, 1970.

141. STONE, HH, AND MARTIN, JD: *Synergistic necrotizing cellulitis.* Ann Surg 175:702, 1972.

142. SWARTZ, MN: *Myositis,* in MANDELL, GL, DOUGLAS, RG, AND BENNET, JE (eds.): *Principles and Practice of Infectious Diseases.* New York: John Wiley and Sons, 1979, pp. 818–823.

143. MELENEY, FL: *Clinical Aspects and Treatment of Surgical Infections.* Philadelphia: WB Saunders, 1949.

144. GARTENBERG, G, BOLTONE, EJ, KEUSCH, GT, ET AL.: *Hospital-acquired mucormycosis (Rhizopus rhizopodiformis) of skin and subcutaneous tissue.* N Engl J Med 299:1115, 1978.

145. SHELDON, DL, AND JOHNSON, WC: *Cutaneous mucormycosis.* JAMA 241:1032, 1979.

146. *Atypical Mycobacteria Wound Infections.* Morbid Mortal Weekly Report. pp. 238-239, Aug 6, 1976

147. BARZA, M: *Gas gangrene and similar anaerobic soft tissue infections,* in CONN, HF (ed.): *Current Therapy.* Philadelphia: WB Saunders, 1977, pp. 27–31.

148. FLORA, DJ: *Management of anaerobic soft tissue infections,* in FINEGOLD, SM, BARTLETT, JG, CHOW, AW, ET AL.: *Management of Anaerobic Infections.* Ann Intern Med 63:381, 1975.

149. Carmel, PW, Fraser, RAR, and Stein, BM: *Aseptic meningitis following posterior fossa surgery in children.* J Neurosurg 41:44, 1974.

150. Troost, BT, Walker, JE, and Cherington, M: *Hypoglycorrhachia associated with subarachnoid hemorrhage.* Arch Neurol 19:438, 1968.

151. Ford, LT, and Key, JA: *An evaluation of myelography in the diagnosis of intervertebral-disc lesions in the low back.* J Bone Joint Surg 32A:257, 1950.

152. Fischer, GW, Brenz, RW, Alden, ER, et al.: *Lumbar punctures and meningitis.* Am J Dis Child 129:590, 1975.

153. Petersdorf, RG, Swarner, DR, and Garcia, M: *Studies on the pathogenesis of meningitis: II. Development of meningitis during pneumococcal bacteremia.* J Clin Invest 41:320, 1962.

154. Leech, PF, and Paterson, A: *Conservative and operative management for cerebrospinal-fluid leakage after closed head injury.* Lancet 1:1013, 1973.

155. Hand, WL, and Sanford, JP: *Posttraumatic bacterial meningitis.* Ann Intern Med 72:869, 1970.

156. Levin, S, Nelson, K, Spies, HW, et al.: *Pneumococcal meningitis: the problem of the unseen cerebrospinal fluid leak.* Am J Med Sci 264:319, 1972.

157. Yoshikawa, TT, Chow, AW, and Guze, LB: *Role of anaerobic bacteria in subdural empyema: report of four cases and review of 327 cases from the English literature.* Am J Med 58:99, 1975.

158. Buckwold, FJ, Hand, R, and Hansebout, RR: *Hospital-acquired bacterial meningitis in neurosurgical patients.* J Neurosurg 46:494, 1977.

159. Kaiser, AB, and McGee, ZA: *Aminoglycoside therapy of gram-negative bacillary meningitis.* N Engl J Med 293:1215, 1975.

160. Rahal, JJ, Jr., Hyams, PJ, Simberkoff, MS, et al.: *Combined intrathecal and intramuscular gentamicin for gram-negative meningitis: pharmacologic study of 21 patients.* N Engl J Med 290:1394, 1974.

161. McCkacken, GH, Mize, SG, and Threlkeld, N: *Intraventricular gentamicin therapy in gram-negative bacillary meningitis of infancy.* Lancet 1:787, 1980.

162. Schoenbaum, SC, Gardner, P, and Shillito, J: *Infections of cerebrospinal fluid shunts: epidemiology, clinical manifestations, and therapy.* J Infect Dis 131:543, 1975.

163. Shurtleff, DB, Foltz, EL, Weeks, RD et al.: *Therapy of Staphylococcus epidermidis: infections associated with cerebrospinal fluid shunts.* Pediatrics 53:55, 1974.

164. Myers, MG, and Schoenbaum, SC: *Shunt fluid aspiration: an adjunct in the diagnosis of cerebrospinal fluid shunt infection.* Am J Dis Child 129:220, 1975.

165. Skinner, PR, Taylor, AJ, and Coakham, H: *Propionibacteria as a cause of shunt and postneurosurgical infections.* J Clin Path 31:1085, 1978.

166. Beeler, BA, Crowder, JG, Smith, JW, et al.: *Propionibacterium acnes: pathogen in central nervous system shunt infection: report of three cases including immune complex glomerulonephritis.* Am J Med 61:935, 1976.

167. McLaurin, RL: *Infected cerebrospinal fluid shunts.* Surg Neurol 1:191, 1973.

168. Stickler, GB, Shin, MH, Burke, EC, et al.: *Diffuse glomerulonephritis associated with infected ventriculoatrial shunt.* N Engl J Med 279:1077, 1968.

169. Dobrin, RS, Kay, NK, Quie, PG, et al.: *The role of complement, immunoglobulin and bacterial antigen in coagulase-negative staphylococcal shunt nephritis.* Am J Med 59:660, 1975.

170. Brewer, NS, MacCarty, CS, and Wellman, WE: *Brain abscess: a review of recent experience.* Ann Intern Med 92:571, 1975.

171. Ingham, HR, Kalbag, RM, Tharagonnet, D, et al.: *Abscesses of the frontal lobe of the brain secondary to covert dental sepsis.* Lancet 2:479, 1978.

172. Warner, JF, Perkins, RL, and Cordero, L: *Metronidazole therapy of anaerobic bacteremia, meningitis and brain abscess.* Arch Intern Med 139:167, 1979.

173. Kaufman, DM, and Leeds, NE: *Computed tomography (CT) in the diagnosis of intracranial abscesses: brain abscess, subdural empyema, and epidural empyema.* Neurology 27:1069, 1977.

174. Heineman, HS, Braude, AI, and Osterholm, JL: *Intracranial suppurative disease: early presumptive diagnosis and successful treatment without surgery.* JAMA 218:1542, 1971.

175. Rotherham, EB, Jr., and Kessler, LA: *Use of computerized tomography in the nonsurgical management of brain abscess.* Arch Neurol 36:25, 1979.

176. Baker, AS, Ojemann, RG, Swartz, MN, et al.: *Spinal epidural abscess.* N Engl J Med 293:463, 1975.

177. Schlossberg, D, and Shulman, JA: *Spinal epidural abscess.* South Med J 70:669, 1977.

178. McGowan, JE, Barnes, MW, and Finland, M: *Bacteremia at Boston City Hospital: occurrence and mortality during 12 selected years (1935–1972), with special reference to hospital-aquired cases.* J Infect Dis 132:316, 1975.

179. Young, LS, Martin, WJ, Meyer, RD, et al.: *Gram-negative rod bacteremia: microbiologic, immunologic, and therapeutic consideration.* Ann Intern Med 86:456, 1977.

180. Gunnar, RM, Loeb, HS, Winslow, ES, et al.: *Hemodynamic measurements in bacteremic and septic shock in man.* J Infect Dis 128:287, 1973.

181. McCabe, WR: *Gram-negative bacteremia.* Adv Intern Med 19:135, 1974.

182. DuPont, HL, and Spink, WW: *Infections due to gram-negative organisms: an analysis of 860 patients with bacteremia at the Univ of Minnesota Medical Center 1958–1966.* Medicine 48:307, 1969.

183. Kiani, D, Quinn, EL, Burch, KH, et al.: *The increasing importance of polymicrobic bacteremia.* JAMA 242:1044, 1979.

184. Roselle, GA, and Watanakunakorn, C: *Polymicrobial bacteremia.* JAMA 242:2411, 1979.

185. Anderson, ET, Young, LS, and Hewitt, W: *Antimicrobial synergism in the therapy of gram-negative rod bacteremia.* Chemotherapy 24:45, 1978.

186. Wade, JC, Smith, CR, Petty, BG, et al.: *Cephalothin plus an aminoglycoside is more nephrotoxic than methicillin plus an aminoglycoside.* Lancet 2:604, 1978.

187. Marsh, FP: *Do cephalosporins potentiate or antagonize aminoglycoside nephrotoxicity.* J Antimicrob Chemother 4:103, 1978.

188. Iannini, PB, and Crossley, K: *Therapy of Staphylococcus aureus bacteremia associated with a removable focus of infection.* Ann Intern Med 84:588, 1976.

189. Tuazon, C, and Sheagren, JN: *Teichoic acid antibodies in the diagnosis of serious infections with Staphyloccus aureus.* Ann Intern Med 84:543, 1976.

190. Schumer, W: *Steroids in the treatment of clinical septic shock.* Ann Surg 184:333, 1976.

191. Burke, JR: *The effective period of preventive antibiotic action in experimental incisions and dermal lesions.* Surgery 50:161, 1961.

192. Finland, M: *Nosocomial epidemics seriatum.* Arch Intern Med 137:585, 1977.

193. Louria, DB, and Kaminski, T: *The effects of four antimicrobial drug regimens on sputum superinfection in hospitalized patients.* Am Rev Resp Dis 85:649, 1962.

194. Finland, M: *Hospital-aquired infections: the problems of methicillin-resistant Staphylococcus aureus and infections with Klebsiella pneumonia.* Am J Med Sci 264:207, 1972.

195. Simmons, HE, and Stolley, PD: *This is medical progress? Trends and consequences of antibiotic use in the United States.* JAMA 227:1023, 1974.

196. Thomas, FE, Jackson, RT, Melly, MA, et al.: *Sequential hospital-wide outbreaks of resistant Serratia and Klebsiella infections.* Arch Intern Med 137:581, 1977.

197. Goodman, JS, Schaffner, W, Collins, HA, et al.: *Infection after cardiovascular surgery: clinical study including examination of antimicrobial prophylaxis.* N Engl J Med 278:117, 1968.

198. Kaiser, AB, Clayson, KR, Mulhevin, JL, et al.: *Antibiotic prophylaxis in vascular surgery.* Ann Surg 188:283, 1978.

199. Clarke, J, Condon, M, Bartlett, JG, et al.: *Preoperative oral antibiotics reduce septic complications of colon operations: results of prospective, randomized double-blind clinical study.* Ann Surg 186:251, 1977.

200. Condon, RE, Bartlett, JG, Nichols, RL, et al.: *Preoperative prophylactic cephalothin fails to control septic complications of colorectal operations: results of controlled clinical trial.* Am J Surg 137:68, 1979.

201. Strachan, CJ, Black, J, Powis, SJ, et al.: *Prophylactic use of cephazolin against wound sepsis after cholecystectomy.* Br Med J 1:1254, 1977.

202. *Antimicrobial prophylaxis for surgery:* Medical Letter 21:73, 1979.

203. Chodak, GW, and Plaut, ME: *Use of systemic antibiotics for prophylaxis in surgery.* Arch Surg 112:326, 1977.

204. Kreutner, AK, Del Bene, VE, Delamar, D, et al.: *Perioperative antibiotic prophylaxis in cesarean section.* Obstet Gynecol 52:279, 1978.

205. Gibbs, RS, Hunt, JE, and Schwarz, RH: *A follow-up study on prophylactic antibiotics in cesarean section.* Am J Obstet Gynecol 117:419, 1973.

206. Weisberg, S, Edwards, L, and O'Leary, J: *Prophylactic antibiotics in cesarean section.* Obstet Gynecol 44:688, 1971.

207. Wong, R, Gee, CL, and Ledger, WJ: *Prophylactic use of cefazolin in monitored patients undergoing cesarean section.* Obstet Gynecol 51:407, 1978.

208. Larson, P, Nelson, KE, Ismail, M, et al.: *Double-blind study of cefoxitin prophylaxis of post-cesarean infection.* (Abstract) Presented at the 19th Interscience Conference on Antimicrobial Agents and Chemotherapy. Boston, October 1979.

209. Chodak, GW, and Plaut, ME: *Systemic antibiotics for prophylaxis in urologic surgery: a critical review.* J Urol 121:695, 1979.

210. Savitz, M, and Malis, L: *Prophylactic clindamycin for neurosurgical patients.* NY State J Med 76:64, 1976.

211. AHA Committee Report: *Prevention of bacterial endocarditis.* Circulation 56:139A, 1977.

212. Smith, JA, Skidmore, AG, Forward, AD, et al.: *Prospective, randomized, double-blind comparison of metronidazole and tobramycin with clindamycin and tobramycin in the treatment of intra-abdominal sepsis.* Ann Surg 192:213, 1980.

213. Gall, SA, Kohan, AP, Ayers, OM, et al.: *Intravenous metronidazole or clindamycin with tobramycin for therapy of pelvic infections.* Obstet Gynecol 57:51, 1981.

214. Hoverman, IV, Gentry, LO, Jones, DW, et al.: *Intrarenal abscess: report of 14 cases.* Arch Int Med 140:914, 1980.

215. Pitt, HA, Postier, RG, MacGowan, WA, et al.: *Prophylactic antibiotics in vascular surgery.* Ann Surg 192:356, 1980.

216. Nichols, RL: *Use of antibiotics in surgical practice.* Am J Med 70:686, 1981.

217. Polk, BF, Tager, IB, Shapiro, M, et al.: *Randomized clinical trial of perioperative cefazolin in preventing infection after hysterectomy.* Lancet 1:437, 1980.

218. Hill, C, Flamant, R, Mazas, F, et al.: *Prophylactic cefazolin versus placebo in total hip replacement.* Lancet 1:795, 1981.

219. Tally, FP, and Sullivan, CE: *Metronidazole: In vitro activity, pharmacology and efficacy in anerobic bacterial infections.* Pharmacotherapy, in press, 1981.

CHAPTER 9

NEUROLOGY

David Chad, M.D., F.R.C.P. (C), Henry Astarjian, M.D., and Theodore Munsat, M.D.

Occasionally, our surgical colleagues ask us to evaluate preoperative patients who have neurologic diseases. What special precautions, if any, need be taken with the slow moving, rigid man with Parkinson's disease; the spastic woman suffering from multiple sclerosis; or the child with muscular dystrophy?

Often we are asked to account for abnormalities in the postoperative period. Why is the elderly man still confused two weeks after his operation; how does one manage the intention myoclonus following cerebral anoxia; is a patient's leg weakness caused by a stroke or by compression neuropathy?

Attention to a patient's unstable cardiac and renal function in the perioperative period may distract the attending surgeon and consulting internist from disturbances of mental state, power, tone, and sensation. Even when appreciated, such disturbances superficially seem relatively unimportant when compared to abnormalities of blood pressure, pulse, and urine output. But when the function of other systems has stabilized, neurologic abnormalities may persist and become a cause of great concern for family and staff.

In this chapter, we hope to provide the surgeon and consulting internist with a better grasp of neurologic disorders in surgical patients. In the first section, the more common neurologic illnesses are briefly described, and some of the problems that these diseases may cause in the preoperative and postoperative periods are discussed. In the second section, we describe neurologic complications which are first detected in the postoperative period and how to anticipate, recognize, and manage them.

PRE-EXISTING NEUROLOGIC DISORDERS

Dementia

The descriptive term dementia refers to a loss of intellectual capacity due to any one of a number of causes. It is either chronic or subacute and frequently irreversible. It is usually encountered in the elderly and less commonly in the middle-aged. Alzheimer's disease accounts for about 60 percent of such patients. Because of memory impairment, the patient will have difficulty giving a clear and concise history. On careful questioning, it may become apparent that although the patient is oriented to time, place, and person, he cannot recall three objects at five minutes, satisfactorily subtract 7 from 100 serially, or describe how objects are similar or different. Early in the course of the disease, unable to answer simple questions, he may resent the mental status exam; while in the advanced stages, he may be unconcerned with what the examiner has to say and lie in bed, disoriented and disheveled.

It is important to recognize the demented patient in the preoperative period. A significant number of demented patients, perhaps 15 to 20 percent, have a correctable disorder, and another 20 to 25 percent have a treatable illness.[1] A careful physical examination, and laboratory investigation may reveal, for example, signs of chronic liver or renal disease, hypothyroidism, vasculitis, or pernicious anemia, that can present as dementia. If not done previously, computerized axial tomography (CT scan) should be employed to exclude intracranial space-taking masses and hydrocephalus. A lumbar puncture along with appropriate serologic studies should also be performed to rule out rare cases of chronic central nervous system infection caused by *Treponema pallidum* and various fungi.

Clinical approaches and laboratory studies will provide the physician with a preoperative baseline of the patients' cognitive function and, in some cases, may even elucidate the nature of the dementing process. As mentioned, the majority of patients with dementia suffer from Alzheimer's disease, a poorly understood degenerative brain disorder. Many may also have cerebrovascular atherosclerosis, but this is rarely the cause of dementia.[1] Preoperative definition and documentation of mental status is of major importance in understanding why a patient has become confused postoperatively. The demented patient is much more sensitive to metabolic derangements and drugs. He will very easily develop an altered mental state that may persist even after the metabolic disturbances have been corrected and drugs withdrawn. Familiar faces, reassurance, early mobilization, and at times small amounts of phenothiazines, will help return the patient to his preoperative status.

Cerebrovascular Disease

The patient with cerebrovascular disease often has widespread atherosclerosis affecting the heart and peripheral vessels. There is often coexisting hypertension, cardiac abnormalities, diabetes, and elevated blood lipids. In the patient about to undergo a major vascular procedure or in a diabetic, hypertensive patient admitted for major general surgery, there may be extensive carotid disease, despite the fact that the patient has never had a stroke. It behooves the physician to identify the person harboring such disease so that intraoperative and postoperative complications can be avoided.

THE SYMPTOMATIC PATIENT

There may be a history of transient monocular blindness or transient cerebral hemisphere attacks (transient ischemic attacks or TIAs). Such symptoms are associated with tight carotid artery stenosis in about 50 percent of patients with this history.[2] Bruits correlate with demonstrable carotid disease in about 60 percent of cases.[3] Evidence is accumulating that those symptomatic patients treated surgically will have a lower incidence of future stroke than patients managed conservatively. Today, it is generally agreed that of TIA patients without treatment, one-third will suffer a stroke, one-third will continue to have TIAs, and one-third will become asymptomatic. Cerebrovascular surgery can now be carried out quite safely with a very acceptable complication rate.[4]

Should a patient with TIAs undergo elective major general surgery with its risk of hypotension, the chance of having a stroke during and after surgery is probably increased (compared to an asymptomatic patient) if a hemodynamically significant carotid lesion is present. When there is time before a major procedure, a symptomatic patient should be studied with carotid angiography. If a tight stenotic lesion is demonstrated, many would advocate endarterectomy.

THE ASYMPTOMATIC BRUIT

What should be the approach to the patient with an asymptomatic bruit? This is a controversial question as the natural history of this condition is not known.[3] However, there are strong suggestions that an asymptomatic bruit is often a precursor to TIAs and stroke.[5] Although some have suggested that carotid artery evaluation is not necessary before major thoracic and abdominal procedures,[6] there is disagreement on this point. Some authors favor proceeding with angiography and, when appropriate, endarterectomy before or at the same time as another major vascular procedure.[7,8]

The most prudent approach is to first study the carotid artery with noninvasive tests, such as Doppler ultrasonography and ophthalmodynamometry.[9] If a hemodynamic change is detected, angiography should be performed. Negative tests are reassuring, but if bruits are bilateral and harsh or if the patient has extensive atherosclerosis elsewhere, angiography is indicated.[10]

ANTICOAGULANTS

Several factors must be considered in the patient receiving anticoagulants for the control of TIAs who is about to undergo surgery and is unable to continue taking medication by mouth. Although the usefulness of anticoagulants in the prevention of stroke in the TIA patient is uncertain,[11] there are patients in whom the incidence of TIAs decreases with the institution of anticoagulants and then increases again when they are withdrawn.[12] In these people, anticoagulants prove useful and effective for long-term therapy and should be continued until the patient has been free of attacks for 3 to 12 months.[13] In a stable (TIA free) patient, anticoagulation can be safely stopped during the perioperative period. In the last few years, patients have been receiving antiplatelet agents such as aspirin and Persantine for the prevention of TIAs and stroke. In stable patients, these drugs can be discontinued in the perioperative period.

Some TIAs are more serious harbingers of stroke than others.[14] Recent TIAs, long-lasting episodes, and the occurrence of face, arm, and leg paresis during an attack, strongly suggest that anticoagulants should not be discontinued, and that the patient should be switched to heparin during the preoperative and postoperative periods.

TRANSIENT NEUROLOGIC DISTURBANCES

Although the majority of TIAs are caused by factors related to carotid atherosclerosis, one must remember that other mechanisms may give rise to transient neurologic disturbances.[15] Heart disease, including arrhythmias and valvular abnormalities, produce classical "TIAs." So too do vasculitides, polycythemia, sickle cell disease, and central nervous system syphilis. Migraine, epilepsy, and intracranial masses can masquerade as TIAs. The preoperative patient who gives a history of episodic neurologic dysfunction needs a complete and thorough investigation so that a readily treatable disorder is not overlooked.

STABLE STROKE

The medically stable patient with mild to moderate neurologic deficit, known to have had a stroke in the past, can encounter difficulties postoperatively. If a metabolic disturbance arises, the previously mild deficit may be accentuated or a focal seizure might occur. Both are due to the unmasking of a structural lesion by a metabolic insult and will resolve as the insult is removed.

Seizure Disorders

The patient with a well-controlled seizure disorder who has only an occasional convulsion should not be difficult to manage in the perioperative period, and no special neurologic investigations need to be performed before surgery. One should be familiar with the potential toxic effects of the commonly used anticonvulsants.[16,17] The commonest ones result from inadvertent overdose and produce alterations in the mental status, ataxia, and gastrointestinal disturbances. Occasionally, other effects will develop such as liver dysfunction, anemia, neutropenia, coagulation abnormalities, and hypocalcemia. It is very important to recognize these in the patient about to undergo major surgery. One drug might have to be discontinued and another introduced so that seizure control is maintained (Table 1).

THE UNSTABLE PATIENT

If attacks of a seizure disorder have recently increased in frequency or changed in clinical form or if a new convulsive disorder has developed, then a search for the cause or causes

TABLE 1. Use of Antiepileptic Drugs

Drug	*Route of Administration*	*Usual Dose (mg/kg)*	*Therapeutic Range (μg/ml)*	*Toxic Level (μg/ml)*	*Indications (Seizure Types)*
Phenytoin	PO, IV	4–7*	10–20	> 20	1. Tonic-clonic‡ (grand mal) 2. Simple or complex partial‡ (focal)
Phenobarbital	PO, IV, IM	1–5*	20–40	> 40	1. Grand mal‡ 2. Focal‖
Carbamazepine	PO	7–15†	4–10	> 10	1. Grand mal§ 2. Focal‡
Primidone	PO	10–25†	7–15	> 40	1. Grand mal§ 2. Focal§
Ethosuximide	PO	20–30†	40–100	> 100	— Absence‡ (Petit mal)
Clonazepam	PO	0.1–0.2†	10–70	> 20	1. Myoclonus‡ 2. Petit mal§
Valproic acid	PO, PR	10–60†	50–150	> 100	1. Myoclonus‡ 2. Petit mal‡ 3. Grand mal§ 4. Focal§

*Single daily or divided doses
†Divided doses
‡Drug of choice
§Secondline drug
‖Thirdline drug
¶Principle metabolite, phenobarbital, is measured

of these problems must begin before surgery. The history is crucial. Eye witness accounts of the seizures will sometimes provide a clue to the manner in which change has occurred. For example, minor motor seizures (petit mal) may be joined in later life by major motor (grand mal) spells.

One must ensure that adequate amounts of appropriate anticonvulsant(s) have been used. Certain drugs are more effective in some types of epilepsy than others. For example, phenobarbital, an excellent drug for the control of major motor convulsions is not the drug of choice in petit mal epilepsy where ethosuximide is effective. The EEG can be of help in choosing the best combination of drugs.

Metabolic disturbances, drug intoxication, or medication withdrawal may be responsible for a change in seizure pattern or frequency. Serum electrolytes, blood glucose, hepatic and renal function, and urine and blood toxicology screens should be carried out. A common problem in a general hospital is alcohol-related seizures. In an alcoholic, convulsions will often raise the question whether the seizures are related to an underlying seizure disorder or whether they are part of the alcohol withdrawal syndrome alone. Are anticonvulsants needed in the preoperative and postoperative periods? The alcoholic with focal seizures, lateralizing neurologic abnormalities, or an abnormal EEG is likely to have an underlying convulsive disorder aggravated by alcohol and should be treated with an anticonvulsant such as phenytoin. On the other hand, the patient whose generalized seizures occur in a short burst of two to six over a period of several hours, between 7 and 48 hours after stopping or decreasing alcohol consumption, and whose EEG is relatively normal does not need to be treated.[19] At times, the distinction between these two clinical situations is difficult, and when there is little time to take an in-depth history and perform a detailed preoperative evaluation, it is wise to treat with phenytoin or phenobarbital and review the situation in more detail later when the atmosphere is more relaxed.

Lumbar puncture and CT scan should be performed if a satisfactory explanation for a change in seizure pattern or frequency cannot be found, if choice of anticonvulsant is appropriate and serum level therapeutic, or if no metabolic or drug related disturbances exist. These tests will identify central nervous system infections or new structural lesions.

POSTOPERATIVE MANAGEMENT WITH A KNOWN SEIZURE DISORDER

In the postoperative period, when the patient cannot take anything by mouth, phenytoin can be given intravenously.[17] The drug should be injected through a small catheter directly into a vein no faster than 50 mg/min. During infusion, heart rhythm and blood pressure should be monitored because of the low risk that bradyarrhythmias or hypotension will develop. The phenytoin may be given in divided doses or the total daily dose may be given once. It should not be given intramuscularly because absorption from muscle is erratic and incomplete. The patient who has been receiving phenobarbital may receive it either intravenously or intramuscularly in divided doses.

Because injectable forms are not available, patients who have been taking carbamazepine or primidone preoperatively for generalized and/or focal epilepsy, and are to have nothing by mouth, must be switched to either phenobarbital or phenytoin. Determination of serum drug levels will help maintain effective anticonvulsant concentrations and avoid toxicity as some drugs are discontinued and others introduced (see Table 1). A rectal form of valproic acid[20,21] exists so that this drug could be continued in the postoperative period. However, it is not yet commercially available in the U.S. Abrupt withdrawal of anticonvulsants postoperatively may lead to status epilepticus which is discussed below. Anticonvulsants should only be withdrawn after a careful review of the patient's seizure history and EEG records. If anticonvulsants are to be discontinued, the dose should be gradually reduced over a period of several months.

Parkinson's Disease

Parkinson's disease produces slowness of movement, rigidity, postural instability, and tremor. Dementia may be a part of the clinical picture, particularly in the advanced stages.

Symptoms respond to anticholinergics, antihistamines, and amantadine, as well as to L-dopa or L-dopa and carbidopa (Sinemet). Because of the high incidence of disabling side effects with prolonged use, L-dopa should be held in reserve and used only when symptoms interfere with daily living to a significant degree. After approximately two years of use, side effects include dyskinesias, "on-off" and "wearing-off" phenomena. L-dopa may also contribute to the dementia of parkinsonism.[22]

The preoperative patient who has had the disease for several years and is now on Sinemet in addition to anticholinergic drugs may have troubling dyskinesias and psychiatric or behavioral disturbances. Both symptoms lessen in intensity when the dose of Sinemet is reduced and the anticholinergic discontinued. Cardiac arrhythmias are exacerbated by L-dopa but probably not by Sinemet.[23]

In the postoperative period, early mobilization and physical therapy are important to avoid an increase in stiffness. Because of a tendency for orthostatic hypotension, care in moving patients from bed to chair is required. With a smooth postoperative course, medication should be resumed as soon as feasible. If well tolerated, it is probably wise to start at one-third the preoperative dose of each and work up to the full dose over a couple of days. Many patients have dysphagia caused by disordered esophageal motility and in these patients aspiration is a continual threat.

If the patient is unable to take anything by mouth, and rigidity combined with tremor creates difficulty in day to day care, small doses of anticholinergics (Cogentin, 0.75 mg) may be given intramuscularly. There is no parenteral preparation of L-dopa and it is ineffective when given by rectum.[24] (Interestingly, a drug holiday of five to seven days may benefit patients plagued by the side effects of L-dopa and Sinemet.)[25]

All of the drugs used to treat Parkinson's disease cause disturbances in mental state. Should a patient develop a confusional state in the postoperative period, medication may have to be discontinued or at least decreased in dose. Because they tend to produce a parkinsonian syndrome, phenothiazines and butyrophenones should not be used to treat disturbances of mood and behavior. Monoamine-oxidase inhibitors are contraindicated because they exaggerate central effects of L-dopa.[26] Tricyclic antidepressants may be given to ease depression.

Movement Disorders

Movement disorders may be very mild and occur in an otherwise healthy person or severe and associated with serious underlying systemic or central nervous system disease. Movement disorders include chorea, athetosis, dystonia, drug-induced syndromes, and tremor.[27]

The physician will have several concerns at the time of surgery. Does the movement disorder reflect a correctable underlying illness or drug effect that should be treated preoperatively? The tremor of thyrotoxicosis, the myoclonus seen in uremia, and the orofacialbuccal movements of phenothiazine-induced dyskinesias can be detected by careful clinical and laboratory evaluation. Is the patient receiving adequate doses of appropriate medication and how can control be best maintained in the postoperative period when the patient will be unable to take oral medication? General anesthesia will suppress all abnormal movements during surgery, but in the postoperative period, a tremor or myoclonic jerk might interfere with nursing care or threaten to separate sutures. If the oral, pharyngeal, or respiratory muscles are involved, the risk of aspiration is increased.

Patients with chorea will usually be receiving phenothiazines, those with dystonia, phenothiazines, and benzodiazepines, and patients with tardive dyskinesias, drugs which deplete catecholamines (reserpine) or those that increase acetylcholine (choline, lecithin, and deanol). Familial or essential tremor is treated with propranolol or diazepam, and the tremor of Parkinson's disease with amantadine, anticholinergics, or Sinemet. All can be given in full dose up until the day of surgery except perhaps for propranolol which should be slowly tapered off because of the possible adverse cardiovascular effects of abrupt withdrawal (see Chap. 3, Cardiology). All of these drugs should be resumed when the patient starts to eat, at half the original dose and then slowly increased to full dose as appropriate.

If movements are disabling during the postoperative period when the patient may have nothing by mouth, then small doses of phenothiazines and diazepam may be given parenterally for all of the disorders involving abnormal movements, except Parkinson's disease. Parenteral anticholinergics should *not* be given to the patient with tardive dyskinesias for they will exacerbate the movements.[28] Paradoxically, although the phenothiazines cause tardive dyskinesia, they may be effective as therapeutic agents.[28]

As mentioned above, movement disorders are occasionally indicators of underlying metabolic encephalopathy. Asterixis, although not truly an involuntary movement disorder, may be an early sign of uremic, hepatic, or pulmonary encephalopathy.[29] Tremulousness and myoclonus are also common accompaniments of confusional states and will subside as the underlying condition is corrected (see Etiology of Pathologic States, below).

Headache

PREOPERATIVE PERIOD

The patient with chronic recurrent headache, be it of the tension, migraine, or cluster variety, may be receiving any one or several of a large number of drugs, including simple analgesics, narcotics, ergot preparations, antidepressants, anticonvulsants, and propranolol. Most of these can be given until the time of surgery (with the exception of propranolol, as noted above) and then resumed in the postoperative period.

POSTOPERATIVE PERIOD

Occasionally, the stress of surgery will aggravate vascular headache. If oral ergot preparations cannot be given and the pain is severe, small amounts of ergotamine tartrate (Gynergen, 0.5 mg IM) or narcotic can be administered parenterally.

In the patient whose headache has changed significantly in character or who develops severe headache for the first time in the postoperative period, a careful search must be made for intracranial disorders[30] and systemic disease[31] such as hypertension. The patient should be observed for signs of central nervous system disturbance such as fever, confusion, seizures, and lateralizing abnormalities. At times, the physician will be faced with a patient with only headache and a vague disturbance in behavior and thinking. Such symptoms and signs require immediate evaluation, particularly in the person at risk for postoperative vascular and infectious central nervous system complications. A lumbar puncture should always be performed and a CT scan is usually needed (see Etiology of Pathologic States, below).

One special situation deserves mention. Postoperative headache will occasionally be seen following neck surgery for carotid endarterectomy.[32] Specific cerebral pathology must be excluded, but in many cases the headache, often of the cluster type, is a result of carotid artery manipulation. The headache may respond to propranolol.

Multiple Sclerosis

Multiple sclerosis is a chronic disease of white matter whose cause is unknown. Small areas of demyelination occur in the optic nerves, brain stem, and spinal cord. A patient may experience an attack of blindness or weakness and after a few days recover completely. Neurologic disturbances recur, but after several years, fixed deficits are the rule. After 25 years of illness, many patients are still able to walk, and almost one-third can still work.

Preoperative evaluation may be time consuming and difficult. Patients may have poor vision, slurred speech, weak clumsy hands, and a broad based ataxic gait. Disturbances of mood, ranging from depression to euphoria (particularly late in the illness) may be present.

Because of spasticity, the patient may be receiving diazepam, dantrolene, or baclofen. All have proved effective in relieving muscle spasm; however, the use of diazepam is limited by drowsiness and the use of dantrolene by muscle weakness and hepatitis.[33] Rarely, dantrolene may cause an allergic pneumonitis associated with fever and a pleural effusion. Baclofen is the most useful of the three.[34,35] Diazepam can be continued up to the time of surgery and then, if needed, given parenterally postoperatively if severe spasms occur and the patient cannot take anything by mouth. The other two drugs should not be abruptly discontinued, but rather, gradually tapered off before surgery. Some patients will be taking prednisone on admission, particularly if they have had a recent relapse. This drug should, of course, be continued through the operative period and beyond at increased dose in the form of injectable steroid (see Chap. 5, Endocrinology).

Prolonged inactivity following surgery should be avoided[36] as it can lead to decubiti and pneumonia resulting in a neurologic relapse. Recurring urinary tract infection, a consequence of bladder dysfunction, is another cause of neurologic deterioration and must be treated promptly. Less common complications of multiple sclerosis are gross cognitive disorders and seizures. Should these occur in the postoperative period, a careful search must be made for other etiologies.

Neuromuscular Disorders

MYASTHENIA GRAVIS

Myasthenia gravis is a disease causing weakness of eye movement, facial expression, swallowing, chewing, speaking, and breathing. The limb muscles may also be affected. The hallmark of the illness is fluctuation in strength occurring throughout the day and from day to day. Following exercise, weakness resolves after a short period of rest. Patients may feel quite strong in the morning, only to find themselves weak and exhausted in the evening.

The disease results from autoimmune damage to the acetylcholine receptor and the diminished number of receptors results in failure of neuromuscular transmission. The etiology is still unknown but much has been learned in recent years about the pathogenesis of the illness.[37]

Patients with myasthenia gravis will probably be receiving anticholinesterase medication and/or steroids. Many will have had a thymectomy. The anticholinesterase group of drugs (neostigmine, pyridostigmine) act by reducing the hydrolysis of acetylcholine, making more available for interaction with the acetylcholine receptor. They are given by mouth every three to five hours. Dose varies from patient to patient but optimal therapeutic effect with pyridostigmine is generally achieved between 60 to 150 mg. four times a day. Troublesome muscarinic side effects may be treated with small doses of atropine. Steroids are commonly used on a single morning dose alternate day regimen. Thymectomy is often beneficial. However, the benefits may not be seen for a number of years.

The pattern of involvement in myasthenia gravis may range from mild ocular deficit (ptosis and ophthalmoplegia) to severe generalized bulbar and limb weakness. In severely affected patients, the postoperative course may be marked by prolonged respiratory muscle weakness and ventilator dependence requiring tracheostomy.

If surgery is elective, efforts should be made to reach the optimum level of control preoperatively. Infection, hypokalemia, or disordered thyroid function should be treated appropriately. Obese patients should be urged to lose weight to avoid compounding respiratory problems in the postoperative period with atelectasis and pulmonary embolism. Certain drugs, such as procainamide, quinidine, quinine, and chlorpromazine exacerbate weakness in myasthenia gravis by further blocking neuromuscular transmission and they should not be used.[38] Anticholinesterase medication should not be given on the morning of surgery. Muscle relaxants and conventional gaseous anesthetic agents should be used with extreme care.[39] If possible, epidural anesthesia should be used to avoid the potential complications of inhalational anesthesia.

Postoperative care of the myasthenia gravis patient will require vigilance and skill. The requirement for anticholinesterase medication often drops dramatically immediately after surgery so that these drugs should not be given for the first few postoperative days. There is less of a tendency for excessive pulmonary secretions and diarrhea to develop when these drugs are withheld. When the drugs are reinstituted, it is wise to start with a third of the preoperative dose and gradually increase as tolerated to the full dose. If the patient has been on steroids, these can be given parenterally.

If an infection develops, great care must be exercised in choosing an antibiotic. The aminoglycosides, bacitracin, and colistin should not be used because they impair neuromuscular transmission by interfering with acetylcholine release.[38]

The patient should not be extubated until vital capacity is adequate and pulmonary infection has been treated. In the very unusual case of persistent postoperative ventilator dependence caused by respiratory muscle weakness, immunosuppressive agents and plasmaphoresis can be considered.[37,38]

OTHER NEUROMUSCULAR DISORDERS

Table 2 lists some postoperative complications of other neuromuscular disorders. Pneumonia is seen in many of these illnesses. Predisposing conditions include respiratory muscle weakness, dysphagia with aspiration, kyphoscoliosis, respiratory muscle myotonia, and impaired immunoglobulin production.[40] Should a patient with myotonic dystrophy develop pneumonia, aminoglycoside antibiotics should be used with great caution.[41]

Arrhythmias and congestive heart failure (CHF) also occur as postoperative complications.[42,43] Postpartum maternal complications and fetal distress are common in myotonic dystrophy.[44]

Myoglobinuria, a combination of pigmenturia, aching weak muscles, high serum enzymes (creatine phosphokinase or CPK), and often renal failure can be seen as a postoperative complication.[45] The disorder may be either sporadic or inherited. Alcoholics make up a substantial proportion of patients in the sporadic group.[39] A weak alcoholic person, particularly one who has been found in a state of stupor, exposed to the elements, must be observed carefully for the development of oliguria and CPK elevation during the perioperative period. (This acute alcoholic myopathy is distinguished from an insidiously developing painless and usually reversible proximal myopathy occasionally seen in people who drink to excess over a prolonged period.)[46] Similarly, patients

TABLE 2. Some Postoperative Complications of Selected Neuromuscular Disorders

Neuromuscular Disorder	*Complication*
I. *Sporadic Disorders*	
A. Amyotrophic lateral sclerosis	Pneumonia
B. Polymyositis, dermatomyositis	Pneumonia, arrhythmias
C. Acute alcoholic myopathy	Myoglobinuria
D. Diabetic neuropathy	Orthostatic hypotension
II. *Inherited Disorders*	
A. Spinal muscular atrophy	Pneumonia
B. Friedreich's ataxia	Pneumonia, congestive heart failure, arrhythmias
C. Duchenne type muscular dystrophy	Pneumonia, congestive heart failure, arrhythmias
D. Myotonic dystrophy	Pneumonia, arrhythmias, postpartum maternal complications and fetal distress
E. Glycogen and lipid metabolism defects	Myoglobinuria
F. Hypokalemic periodic paralysis	Quadriparesis
G. Family history of anesthesia-related myoglobinuria	Malignant hyperpyrexia

with inherited defects of glycogen (McArdle's disease) and fat (carnitine palmityl transferase deficiency) metabolism must be scrutinized for falling urine output, pigmenturia, and raised serum CPK after a major surgical procedure. Such patients must be kept well hydrated with glucose containing solutions. Treatment of myoglobinuria consists of maintaining adequate urine flow with the osmotic diuretic, mannitol.

Patients with hypokalemic periodic paralysis (who should be screened for hyperthyroidism) may develop hypokalemia and generalized weakness in response to stressful situations and carbohydrate loads. If infection is treated promptly in the postoperative period and electrolyte and glucose concentrations are kept as close to normal as possible, weakness may be prevented. Should an attack occur, treatment involves administration of potassium and, at times, acetazolamide.[47]

MALIGNANT HYPERTHERMIA

Malignant hyperthermia is a syndrome of generalized muscular rigidity, rapidly rising body temperature, hyperkalemia, severe metabolic acidosis, and myoglobinuria occurring upon exposure to certain volatile agents, ketamine and depolarizing relaxants.[48–50] It is a rare disorder (less than 1 in 15,000 general anesthesia cases) that has had a high mortality rate (70%). In about 40 percent of cases, it appears to be inherited as an autosomal dominant trait. Some patients at risk will have elevated muscle enzymes and on careful examination, mild abnormalities of muscle function will be found, suggesting a subclinical myopathy.[48] Unfortunately, at present, at least half of all susceptible patients cannot be identified by routine clinical and laboratory methods. However, more detailed screening for patients at risk has been proposed.[49] When identified, such patients can be anesthetized so that malignant hyperthermia is avoided.[49] As soon as the diagnosis is suspected, all anesthesia should be discontinued. Patients with the full blown syndrome require prompt treatment with hyperventilation with 100 percent oxygen, bicarbonate, cooling and diuretics.[49] Procaine, corticosteroids, glucose and Thorazine have been used successfully by some.[51] Dantrolene is the only known specific therapeutic agent. At the time of diagnosis it should be given intravenously 1 to 2 mg/kg, which may be repeated every 5 to 10 minutes, to a total dose of 10 mg/kg.[49] The drug should be continued orally for 24 hours following control of the disorder.[49]

DANTROLENE

NEUROLOGIC COMPLICATIONS DURING SURGERY AND IN THE POSTOPERATIVE PERIOD

Disorders of the Central Nervous System

DISORDERS OF THE BRAIN

The patient who does not completely awaken from general anesthesia or who experiences a postoperative lucid interval and then lapses into a confused state (associated perhaps with focal or multifocal signs) presents the physician with a great diagnostic challenge. Depression of consciousness indicates brain failure, and steps must be taken to identify and reverse pathophysiologic processes as quickly as possible before damage becomes irreversible.[52]

Before he can effectively treat his patient, the physician must be able to associate certain clinical presentations (pathologic states) with disordered function (lesions) at specific neuroanatomic sites and he must have a knowledge of the causes of such neurologic dysfunction.

Lesion Location and Pathologic States

Under normal conditions, man is attentive and responsive because the brain stem reticular activating system maintains the cerebral hemispheres in a state of arousal or wakefulness. He is cognizant of the world around him because his cerebral hemispheres are intact. Disturbances of the arousal mechanism (brain stem) or the content of consciousness (hemispheres) will produce a number of different clinical pictures.

Damage to the brain stem, diffuse loss of hemisphere tissue, or profound depression of hemisphere function, will result in *coma.* Depression of the cerebral hemispheres by any one of many metabolic disturbances (e.g., hyponatremia), while sparing underlying brain structure, will give rise to a state of *confusion* or *delirium* which is often readily reversible. Gradual generalized loss of cerebral tissue will lead to the insidious loss of intellectual function and progressively reduce the content of consciousness. This, the *demented state,* is usually associated with alertness until the end stage of the process is reached. If acute metabolic disturbances occur in the demented patient, a prolonged state of intense confusion may result. It will persist even when metabolic disturbances are later corrected and has been called a *"beclouded dementia."*[53]

When the hemispheres undergo focal damage, seizures and abnormalities in the motor and sensory systems frequently result. There may also be a loss of cognitive functions, such as language or constructional ability, and the content of consciousness may be reduced. In general, if only one hemisphere is affected, the level of wakefulness will remain unimpaired. However, if the pathologic process damages both hemispheres or if loss of tissue is associated with a metabolic disturbance as in ischemic anoxia, then *focal or multifocal abnormalities* and *confusion* will coexist.

Etiology of Pathologic States

CAUSES OF COMA. *Brain stem damage* is not often encountered in the postoperative period. The commonest causes are pontine hemorrhage[54] and basilar artery occlusion leading to brain stem infarction.[55] The chronically hypertensive patient is particularly at risk.

Hemorrhage in the pons may cause hyperthermia, small pupils, decerebrate posturing (extension of arms and legs), and absence of oculocephalic (doll's eyes) and corneal responses. These signs give way to hypotension, irregular respirations, and death. Care is supportive and symptomatic.

Infarction causes multiple cranial nerve abnormalities admixed with long tract findings. Because infarction tends to spare the more dorsal and rostral part of the brain stem, arousal pathways may remain intact, and the patient may be aware but unable to communicate because of paralysis.[56] Very careful clinical evaluation and an EEG will be needed to diagnose this condition. With expert nursing care, patients may show slow improvement.

Another rather unusual brain stem disease is central pontine myelinolysis.[57] The underlying lesion is a large area of demyelination in the central pons. Patients become stuporous and develop cranial nerve abnormalities and quadraplegia. The patient at risk is the malnourished alcoholic who is being vigorously rehydrated postoperatively and develops severe electrolyte disturbances. It has also been described in the renal transplant patient.[29]

Another group of complications result from *hemispheric damage.* When cerebral blood flow is compromised for a prolonged period (as in cardiac arrest), a severe form of ischemic-anoxic encephalopathy may result. Patients may be unresponsive for days, only to develop much later a state of wakefulness with eye opening, sleep-wake cycles, and roving eye movements but without awareness and higher mental activity. Such a clinical picture has been called the persistent vegetative state (PVS) and is compatible with long periods of survival.[52]

Early in the comatose state, it is important to distinguish patients who will develop PVS from those who will recover or be left with mild to moderate disability.[58] Certain signs predict poor outcome.[59] If at 12 and particularly 24 hours after occurrence of the cerebral damage there is an absence of pupillary responses, corneal reflexes, motor response, and deep tendon reflexes (DTRs), then death or PVS is likely. Decerebrate or decorticate responses at 24 or 48 hours have the same implication. Favorable outcome is suggested by roving eye movements at 12 to 24 hours and early purposeful motor responses. Steroids and dehydrating agents are probably of little value in improving the outcome of ischemic anoxia.

Many metabolic abnormalities will depress the function of the cerebral hemispheres. When *hemispheric dysfunction* is mild or moderate, confusion results and when profound, coma develops. The causes of these two conditions are often the same.

CAUSES OF CONFUSION (TABLE 3). Soon after surgery, often on the third postoperative day,[60] staff and family may note that the patient is not thinking clearly. He is inattentive, unable to follow more than one simple command, and cannot retain new information. He may be subdued and apathetic during the day and agitated at night. Generalized seizures may occur. Apart from higher function abnormalities the neurologic exam may be unremarkable. Confusion, when associated with excessive agitation, visual hallucinations, and complex delusions is called delirium.[52]

Much has been written about the differential diagnosis of this condition.[52] Confusional states result from widespread interference with brain metabolism. Many patients have correctable or at least treatable disorders (see Table 3).

The proper way to identify the cause of a confusional state, or metabolic encephalopathy, is to consider in turn each body system. Most frequently, two or more causes are operative. An adequate amount of blood, containing proper quantities of oxygen, glucose, and cofactors being effectively pumped to and perfused through the brain are prerequisites for normal brain function. Such conditions will only be met if the hemoglobin concentration is normal, the lungs are effectively exchanging gas, the patient is well nourished and euglycemic, there is no serious heart disease, and the small cerebral vessels are patent. Moreover, because cerebral metabolism is sensitive to a host of metabolic derangements, if brain function is to be preserved liver, kidney and endocrine

TABLE 3. Differential Diagnosis of Confusion in the Postoperative Period

Etiology	*Selected Factors Placing Patient at Risk*	*Diagnostic Tests*
	I. Without Focal Abnormalities	
A. Substrate Deficiency		
1. Hypoxia-ischemia	a. Carotid atherosclerosis especially when associated with intraoperative hypotension	Chest x-ray, EKG, blood gases (factors a through g)
	b. Poor cardiac and/or pulmonary reserve	
	c. Severe anemia	Complete blood count
	d. Open-heart surgery (multiple cerebral emboli)	CT scan
	e. Trauma (fat embolism)	Sputum and urine analysis for fat
	f. Cancer (DIC)	Prothrombin time, partial prothrombin time, platelets
	g. Underlying vasculitis	ESR
2. Hypoglycemia	a. Liver disease	Serum glucose, prothrombin time, (LFTs)
	b. Insulin treatment and inadequate nourishment	
3. Thiamine deficiency (Wernicke's encephalopathy)	a. Alcoholism	LFTs (factors a and b)
	b. Malnutrition	
B. Major Organ Failure		
1. Liver	a. Pre-existing liver disease	LFTs, serum ammonia, cerebrospinal fluid, glutamine (factors a through d)
	b. Intraoperative hypotension	
	c. Anesthetic hypersensitivity reaction	
	d. Abdominal surgery (cholangitis)	Blood cultures
2. Kidney	a. Pre-existing renal insufficiency (e.g., diabetes)	BUN, creatine, urinalysis (factors a through c)
	b. Intraoperative hypotension	
	c. Underlying muscle disease, alcoholism, (myoglobinuria)	Creatine phosphokinase, urinalysis for myoglobin
3. Endocrine*		
—Hypothyroidism (anemia, dementia weakness†)	(Infection, dehydration, cold exposure‡)	T_4, T_3RU Free T_4, TSH
—Hyperthyroidism (arrhythmia, weakness†)		T_4, T_3, T_3RU
—Hypoadrenalism (hypotension, hypoglycemia, weakness†)	Anticoagulation§ (hemorrhage into adrenals)	Serum and urinary corticosteroids
—Hyperadrenalism		Serum and urinary corticosteroids

*Dysfunction may not be suspected in preoperative period
†Unexplained abnormalities in the preoperative period
‡Factors which may bring endocrine disorder to light
§Increases risk of de novo hypoadrenalism

ARIEFF, HYPONATREMIA, CONVULSIONS, RESPIRATORY ARREST, AND PERMANENT BRAIN DAMAGE AFTER ELEC SURGERY IN HEALTHY WOMEN, N.E.J.M., 314: 1529, JUNE 12, 198

TABLE 3, *Continued*

Etiology	*Selected Factors Placing Patient at Risk*	*Diagnostic Tests*
C. Electrolyte, acid-base and osmotic disturbance		
1. Hyponatremia	a. Edemetous states	Serum and urine sodium and osmolality (factors a through e)
	b. Head trauma‖	
	c. Pulmonary infection‖	
	d. Certain drugs‖ (antidepressants, chlorpropamide, anesthetics)	
	e. Diuretics	
2. Hypernatremia	a. Diabetes (nonketotic hyperosmolar state)	Serum sodium, osmolality, and glucose (factors a and b)
	b. Tube feedings in the debilitated	
3. Hypokalemia	Diarrhea	Serum potassium, blood gases, and pH
4. Hypocalcemia	a. Following neck surgery	Serum calcium and phosphate (factors a through e)
	b. Short bowel syndrome	
	c. Chronic renal insufficiency	BUN, Creatine
	d. Acute pancreatitis	Amylase
	e. Multiple transfusions with citrated blood	
5. Hypercalcemia	a. Underlying tumor	Serum and phosphate (factors a through c)
	b. Hyperparathyroidism	
	c. Prolonged immobilization	
6. Hypomagnesemia	a. Alcoholism	Serum magnesium, calcium, phosphate, and potassium (factors a through e)
	b. Malnutrition	
	c. Short bowel syndrome	
	d. Parenteral alimentation	
	e. Intestinal bypass surgery	
7. Hypermagnesemia	Renal insufficiency	Serum magnesium, BUN, creatine
8. Hyperglycemia	a. Diabetes (non-ketotic hyperosmolar state)	Serum glucose and sodium (factors a and b)
	b. Parenteral alimentation	
9. Acidosis		
a. metabolic	a. Diabetes	Electrolytes, blood gases, pH
	b. Alcoholism	Serum glucose
	c. Drug ingestion	Toxicology screen
	d. Renal failure	BUN, Creatine
	e. Prolonged hypotension	Blood lactate
b. respiratory	Oxygen therapy in chronic bronchitis	Electrolytes, blood gases and pH, chest x-ray
10. Alkalosis		
a. metabolic	Gastric outlet obstruction	Electrolytes, blood gases and pH, urinary chloride

‖May induce SIADH

DIC = disseminated intravascular coagulation; ESR = erythrocyte sedimentation rate; LFTs = liver function tests; SIADH = syndrome of inappropriate antidiuretic hormone secretion; RU = resin uptake.

Sterns, Et Al, Osmotic Demyelination Syndrome Following Correction of Hyponatremia, N.E.J.M., 314:1535, June 12, 1986.

TABLE 3, *Continued*

Etiology	*Selected Factors Placing Patient at Risk*	*Diagnostic Tests*
b. respiratory	a. Sepsis	Electrolytes, blood gases and pH, urinary chloride, blood cultures
	b. Hepatic failure	Electrolytes, blood gases and pH, urinary chloride, LFTs
D. Drugs and toxins	a. Pre-existing liver disease	Serum and urine toxicology screen (factors a through c) LFTs
	b. Pre-existing kidney disease	BUN, Creatine
	c. Porphyria	Watson-Schwartz test
E. Infection	a. Lymphoma, leukemia	Blood cultures, lumbar puncture (factors a and b)
	b. Immunosuppressive drugs	
F. Psychiatric illness	a. Pre-existing psychiatric illness	See Chapter 11, Psychiatry
	b. Prolonged stay in intensive care	
	II. With Focal Abnormalities¶	
1. Stroke	a. Arrhythmias	EKG (factors a through e)
	b. Myocardial infarction	
	c. Open heart surgery	
	d. Carotid endarterectomy	
	e. Intraoperative hypotension	
2. Hemorrhage	a. Inadequate intraoperative blood pressure control	
	b. Unsuspected pheochromocytoma	Urinary catecholamine measurements
3. Subdural hematoma	a. Alcoholism	Prothrombin time, partial thromboplastin time, platelets (factors a and b)
	b Bleeding diathesis	
4. Abscess	a. Sepsis	Blood cultures (factors a through c)
	b. Immunosuppressive drugs	
	c. Intravenous drug abuse	
5. Tumor	Underlying malignancy	

¶All confused patients with focal abnormalities on neurologic exam or with focal seizures need a CT scan without contrast. If no abnormality is seen, the scan should be repeated with contrast. Some patients will require an angiogram.

function must be normal; there can be no excess of drugs or toxins; no serious systemic or central nervous system infection may exist; and finally, temperature, and ionic and acid-base environment of the brain must be normal.

Identifying the cause of a confusional state requires careful clinical examination not only of the nervous system but also all other organ systems. Laboratory study should be extensive as checks are made on all the categories of disease alluded to above. A lumbar puncture is essential. Infection of the central nervous system by bacteria, fungi, protozoa, or viruses may produce little more than a vague change in mental state. Careful pressure determination, cell count and differential, gram stain and routine culture, protein, sugar, and the test of the Venereal Disease Research Laboratories (VDRL) should be done on all patients. In some, India ink preparation, Ziehl-Nielsen stain, and culture for fungi and tuberculus bacillus will be necessary.

Certain patients are at increased risk of developing confusional states in the postoperative period.[61] These include alcoholics, trauma victims, patients with cancer, transplant patients, and those with hepatic porphyria. The *alcoholic* may develop delirium tremens (DTs) early in the postoperative period and extreme agitation will make management very difficult. His confusional state might be caused by Wernicke's encephalopathy, in which disordered mentation is coupled with ophthalmoplegia and nystagmus. (All alcoholics, confused or not, must be given thiamine before and after surgery.) Subdural hematoma, an everpresent threat to the alcoholic, might cause little more than confusion and not be seriously considered in the diagnosis because of the absence of focal signs. When a confusional state cannot be explained by metabolic aberrations, a CT scan and lumbar puncture must be performed.

The *trauma victim* is at risk for developing fat embolism.[62] Restlessness, confusion, dyspnea, and tachypnea may occur soon after trauma or be delayed some 72 hours, with a mean time of onset of 41 hours after injury. Patients may have fever, hypoxia, abnormal chest films, and a petechial rash on the shoulders, neck, and upper part of the thorax. The cerebrospinal fluid is normal, but fat can be detected in sputum and urine. Pathologic study provides evidence for fat emboli in the lung and in small cerebral vessels.

The patient with a *neoplasm,* particularly a lymphoma or leukemia, may develop nonmetastatic complications, producing a confusional state. Intravascular coagulation[63] leads to signs of generalized brain disease with confusion, disorientation, delirium, and convulsions. The coagulation abnormality may be mild. Pathologic study shows multifocal hemorrhagic and ischemic infarctions. Fibrin thrombi are found in small cerebral blood vessels. If the diagnosis is made early, administration of heparin may help. Another important complication is infection.[64] Meningitis caused by *Cryptococcus* and *Listeria* may produce little more than a confusional state and highlights the importance of an LP in all confused patients, especially those who are immunosuppressed.

The *transplant patient,* too, is a person with special vulnerabilities because of immunosuppression. If he develops a confusional state postoperatively, a vigorous search must be undertaken for infection[65] even if some metabolic abnormality might account for it. The mycoses *(Aspergillus, Phycomycetes, Candida,* and *Cryptococcus)*, protozoa *(Toxoplasma gondii)* viruses (cytomegalovirus and herpes virus), and bacteria *(Listeria monocytogenes)* are all important pathogens and are notoriously difficult to diagnose. Chest x-ray will often be abnormal, reflecting pulmonary involvement by the same organism. The Sabin-Feldman dye test for toxoplasmosis should be ordered. A lumbar puncture must be performed and the fluid carefully analyzed as described above. A finding of normal cerebrospinal fluid does not exclude intracranial infection. A CT scan will help to detect single or multiple abscesses.

Finally, a patient who develops the triad of confusion, abdominal pain, and neuropathy after receiving one or several of a large list of drugs,[66] including routinely used sedatives and anticonvulsants must be suspected of having *acute intermittent porphyria.*

In all patients with diffuse encephalopathy, the EEG correlates with the clinical state, becoming slower as the level of consciousness declines. It is a useful tool because it may help to point out a focal process superimposed upon a diffuse one.[67]

CAUSES OF FOCAL CEREBRAL DISORDERS (TABLE 3). As mentioned earlier, the focal cerebral disturbances may present with hemiparesis, seizures, or disorders of higher cortical function. If one hemisphere is damaged, wakefulness will not be disturbed, and confusional states will not occur. However, there are exceptions to this general principle: (1) A patient might have a focal lesion that distorts surrounding structures and creates bihemispheric dysfunction. Such a person might develop a state of quiet or agitated delirium. (2) Small focal lesions in the left posterior temporal area may not give rise to striking neurologic findings. However, the patient may produce spontaneous, fluent, aphasic language, with word and letter substitutions which might imitate a behavioral disorder or confusional state. (3) Acute confusional states may develop in patients with infarction in the territory of the right middle cerebral artery without the usual associated features of a stroke such as hemiparesis.[68] (4) Patients with focal deficits may become confused after a seizure because of depression of both hemispheres.

As in the diffuse disturbances of cerebral function, determination of the cause for a focal lesion will be easier if underlying predisposing conditions are recognized. In the patient with *cancer* a cerebral metastatic lesion or embolism from nonbacterial thrombotic endocarditis should be considered. The *immunocompromised person* or septic patient may develop a brain abscess. The *alcoholic* or *uremic patient* may harbor a subdural hematoma. The patient with *cardiac arrhythmias* (particularly atrial fibrillation) can suffer embolic cerebral infarction.

Specific surgical procedures may also increase the likelihood of intraoperative or postoperative stroke. The hypertensive patient with a mild recently acquired neurologic deficit who undergoes a *carotid endarterectomy* may develop a hemorrhagic infarction postoperatively in the area of the original lesion.[69] The patient who undergoes *open heart surgery* may develop cerebral emboli of calcium, fat, or air.[70] Another risk of open heart surgery and cardiopulmonary bypass is prolonged hypotension.[70,71] In the setting of advanced atherosclerosis and attendant carotid stenosis, ischemic infarction may occur in the terminal perfusion field of the anterior, middle, and posterior cerebral arteries. The damage, when restricted to the parieto-occipital areas, may cause disorders of cortical function without (or with minor) lateralized motor findings.[70] If the ischemic-anoxic damage is more extensive, gnostic disorders will be associated with amnesia, bibrachial paresis, and cortical blindness.[59]

Careful review of the clinical picture and laboratory data will often lead to a specific diagnosis. The EEG may show diffuse slowing with a superimposed slow and/or sharp focus and not add a great deal of information. Occasionally, a focal lesion caused by infarction will be associated with a confusional state because of periodic lateralized epileptiform discharges (PLEDs) from the affected hemisphere.[72] The EEG makes the diagnosis, and the disordered mental status will usually resolve in less than one week.

A CT scan can be most valuable in localizing and identifying space-taking masses.[73] It will distinguish infarct from hemorrhage and help in differentiating infarct from tumor and abscess.

Seizures in the Postoperative Period

As we have previously indicated, patients developing diffuse or focal cerebral disease in the postoperative period will commonly develop seizures. These may be focal and infrequent, giving the physician plenty of time to plan investigations and ponder the choice of appropriate anticonvulsants. Alternatively, they may be intense, generalized, and abundant, leading to status epilepticus. In status, convulsions are so frequent that consciousness is not regained. Status is more difficult to stop the longer it exists. When long-lasting, it may cause cerebral damage and jeopardize the patient's overall condition by raising temperature, stressing the cardiovascular system, and occasionally causing myoglobinuria. In such a situation, immediate therapy is necessary.[74]

THERAPY OF STATUS EPILEPTICUS (Table 4). As blood is being drawn for hematologic studies and chemistries, 50 cc of 50 percent glucose should be given in case the patient is hypoglycemic. Then, diazepam, 10 mg intravenously, should be given over five minutes, employing a cardiac monitor in older patients. If seizures persist after 10 minutes, another 10 mg of diazepam is given in a similar manner.

Phenytoin should be given next, whether or not the seizures have stopped. It is administered intravenously at a rate no faster than 50 mg/min to a total dose of between 1 and 1.5 gm (18 mg/kg).[75,76] Very rapid injection (greater than 50 mg/min) may be associated with bradycardia and depression of sinoatrial rhythm, thought to be secondary to the propylene glycol adjuvant. At a slower rate, phenytoin may actually protect the heart from the adverse effects of this chemical.[77]

Intravenous phenytoin enters the brain and achieves therapeutic levels very rapidly. After receiving a full loading dose, patients may develop a complete but reversible ophthalmoplegia.[78] If convulsions persist beyond 20 minutes following injection, phenobarbital should be given intravenously at a rate of 25 mg/min to a dose of 400 to 600 mg. Respiratory depressant effects may be delayed.[79] Equipment for intubation and ventilatory support must be available. If seizures have not stopped after 30 to 60 minutes, another 400 to 600 mg of phenobarbital can be given slowly if respiratory and circulatory function remain adequate.

Should seizures persist after administration of diazepam, phenytoin, and phenobarbital, one can use paraldehyde,[80] lidocaine,[81] amobarbital,[82] or valproate.[21] Last, general anesthesia may be necessary.

While treatment is in progress, an intensive search should be made for causative factors. All potential metabolic disturbances must be considered as described above and a lumbar puncture must be done to rule out infection. An acidosis (lactic) usually lasts for about one hour following the last convulsion.[83] If it persists for much longer, other causes than the convulsions must be sought. When tonic-clonic movements cease, an EEG may help to decide if status has in fact ended.

Once seizures have been controlled, serum drug levels will help guide the physician to the appropriate maintenance doses of phenytoin or other anticonvulsants (see Table 1).

Action Myoclonus

In the patient who has emerged from an hypoxic confusional state, action myoclonus may develop.[84] This is characterized by brief shock-like contractions of limbs as they engage in some activity and may greatly interfere with essential motor activities. Successful treatment has been reported with L-5-hydroxytryptophan,[85] clonazepam,[86] and valproate.[87]

TABLE 4. Drug Treatment of Status Epilepticus

Drug	*Dose/Route*	*Advantages/Disadvantages/Complications*
Diazepam (Valium)	10 mg IV over less than one minute	Fast-acting (lipid soluble), short half-life IV (½–4 hours). Respiratory depression occurs, especially if barbiturates must be added. Other complications are bradycardia and hypotension. Must add maintenance drug (phenytoin or phenobarbital) to prevent seizure recurrence
	THEN PROCEED TO PHENYTOIN	
Phenytoin (Dilantin)	1000–1500 mg (18 mg/kg) IV slowly, at rate not greater than 100 mg/min directly into vein (can't be given through dextrose solutions)	No respiratory depression or sedation. Drug levels in the brain are therapeutic within 30–60 min. Effective as maintenance drug. Hypotension and cardiac arrhythmias can occur
IF NOT EFFECTIVE WITHIN 10–15 MIN FOLLOWING TOTAL DOSE, PROCEED TO PHENOBARBITAL		
Phenobarbital	1000–1500 mg (18 mg/kg) IV slowly	Respiratory depression and hypotension common with increasing doses (have intubation and ventilatory support immediately available). Effective as maintenance drug
	IF ABOVE INEFFECTIVE, THE FOLLOWING THIRD-LINE DRUGS MAY BE EMPLOYED	
Paraldehyde	PR: 5–10 cc diluted in 2 volumes mineral oil *or* IM: 5–10 cc *or* IV: 5–10 cc dilute 50 cc normal saline (4% solution).	Decomposes with storage; can cause metabolic acidosis, pulmonary hemorrhage and cardiovascular depression
Lidocaine (Xylocaine)	50–100 mg IV. If effective, then 50–100 mg diluted in 250 cc 5% dextrose and infused at a rate of 1–2 mgm/min	Higher doses may cause convulsions. No cardiovascular system depression. Reduce dose for congestive failure or liver disease
	IF ABOVE INEFFECTIVE, MAY PROCEED IMMEDIATELY TO GENERAL ANESTHESIA	
Pentobarbital	100–500 mg IV slowly	Hypotension limiting factor; resp. depression routine
Thiopental	25–200 mg IV slowly, followed by 1 mg/min drip if needed	Brain half-life less than 30 min; hypotension the limiting factor; respiratory factor; respiratory depression routine
Amobarbital Sodium	200–1000 mg IV slowly	Hypotension limiting factor, resp. depression routine
Ether or halothane by inhalation		

DISORDERS OF THE SPINAL CORD

Damage to the spinal cord is an unusual postoperative complication. Ischemic myelopathy can follow profound hypotension in association with ischemic-hypoxic encephalopathy.[59] It can be seen with atherosclerotic aortic disease and after repair of aortic aneurysms above the origins of the renal arteries.[88] It is important to ensure that a cord disturbance is not produced by a correctable process like an epidural abscess or neoplasm. The clinical setting and x-rays will help make the correct diagnosis.

Disorders of the Motor Unit

Trauma often results in weakness or numbness in the territory of a root, plexus, or nerve. Much has been written on the diagnosis and management of traumatic neuropathies.[89] In the patient recovering from general surgery or obstetric or gynecologic procedures, limb weakness may be quite unexpected, causing alarm and confusion. It is often presumed that limb paresis and numbness are due to a stroke. The recognition of peripheral neuropathy may help to avoid costly and hazardous investigation. A rapid return to normal often follows conservative care.

UPPER LIMB NEUROPATHIES

Wrist drop indicates *radial nerve injury* at the level of the axilla or humerus and is common in alcoholics. Should there be an urgent need for surgery, this neuropathy may be easily overlooked. Weakness of the intrinsic hand muscles suggests damage to the *ulnar nerve,* which because of its location behind the medial epicondyle, may be compressed in patients whose arms are fixed in extension on the operating table.[90] A similar pattern of weakness is seen in the postoperative patient who is positioned in the steep Trendelenburg position with the arm hyperabducted, causing lower *brachial plexus* injury.[90,91]

LOWER LIMB NEUROPATHIES

Difficulty flexing the hip and extending the knee, along with aching in the groin and numbness of the anterior and medial thigh suggests *femoral neuropathy.* Such a combination of symptoms and signs might be the first clue to retroperitoneal hemorrhage (bleeding into the iliacus).[92,93] Bleeding may occur into the psoas muscle and give rise to more extensive weakness because of lumbar plexus compression.[92] Other causes of femoral neuropathy in the surgical patient are psoas abscess and compression by retroperitoneal neoplasm. In the postpartum patient, compression may occur from a prolonged period in the dorsal lithotomy position.[94]

Weakness of thigh adductors combined with pain and numbness along the inner aspect of the thigh indicates *obturator neuropathy,* seen after genitourinary operations. It is also seen in pregnant women positioned in the lithotomy position for a prolonged period of time. Weakness of foot extension combined with numbness of the dorsum of the foot indicates *common peroneal nerve injury.* The nerve is superficial as it wraps around the neck of the fibula and thus can be compressed in the postoperative patient bedridden for a long time.

Foot extensor paresis, plantar flexor weakness, hamstring weakness, and numbness on the sole of the foot and back of the leg suggests *sciatic neuropathy.* This occurs following intramuscular injections into the buttock near the sciatic nerve or in women who have been on the obstetric table for long periods. It also occurs in patients immobilized in the supine position for a long time. A similar pattern of weakness and sensory change may be seen when parts of the *lumbosacral plexus* are compressed by the fetal head,[94] tumor, or an iliac artery aneurysm.[95] In postoperative neuropathies, electromyographic and nerve conduction studies are helpful in localizing the lesion and determining the chances for recovery. A review of other encountered neuropathies is presented in Table 5.

DIFFUSE WEAKNESS

Metabolic Derangement

Diffuse weakness in the postoperative period is often the result of a metabolic derangement[103] such as hypokalemia (potassium < 2.5 mEq/L), hyperkalemia (potassium > 7 mEq/L), or hypophosphatemia (phosphate < 2 mg/dl). Although hypercalcemia (calcium > 12 mg/dl) and hypermagnesemia (magnesium > 7 mEq/L) are capable of producing weakness, the overwhelming clinical effect is usually an alteration in consciousness. Hypocalcemia (calcium < 7 mg/dl) or hypomagnesemia (magnesium < 1 mEq/L) produce tetany.

Drugs

Rarely, *drugs* are responsible for producing postoperative weakness.[104] Many different classes of drugs have been implicated (e.g., antibiotics, cardiovascular agents, and anticonvulsants). Affected patients generally have an underlying disturbance leading to defective neuromuscular transmission such as myasthenia gravis, electrolyte disturbance, or the "decreased safety factor" for neuromuscular transmission seen in the aged. Renal failure may increase the risk of drug-induced weakness. Treatment consists of

TABLE 5. Other Neuropathies Encountered in the Postoperative Patient

Nerve(s)	*Surgical Procedure*	*Clinical Presentation*
Facial	Carotid endarterectomy[96]	Lip weakness
Superior laryngeal	Carotid endarterectomy[96]	Vocal cord paralysis
Hypoglossal	Carotid Endarterectomy[96]	Tongue weakness
Greater auricular	Carotid endarterectomy[96]	Ear lobe numbness
Spinal accessory	Neck surgery other than the above[97]	Trapezius weakness (shoulder pain)
Long thoracic	Mastectomy[98]	Winged scapula
Thoracodorsal	Mastectomy[98]	Shoulder abductor weakness
Brachial plexus	Mastectomy and subclavian vein catheter insertion[99]	Upper limb weakness
Hypogastric and inferior hypogastric plexus	Pelvic surgery[100]	Impotence and bladder dysfunction
Genitofemoral	Adhesions following appendectomy[101]	Groin pain
Ilioinguinal	High flank incision[101]	Groin pain, direct hernia
Saphenous	Varicose vein stripping[102]	Medial foreleg numbness
Sural	Varicose vein stripping[102]	Lateral foot numbness

withdrawing the offending agent and supporting respiration. In severe cases, calcium infusion may be necessary to restore strength.

Myoglobinuria

Myoglobinuria,[45] an important cause of postoperative weakness, was discussed above. The physician must be aware of the many causes of this syndrome which include inherited diseases of muscle (metabolic myopathies and malignant hyperpyrexia) and acquired conditions such as status epilepticus, severe crush injury, agitation (requiring tight restraints), limb ischemia, metabolic depression (caused, for example, by drugs and hypothermia), and systemic infection. In the patient at risk, measurement of serum CPK and urine analysis for myoglobin should be performed.

Polyneuropathies

Polyneuropathies may occur in the postoperative period. Rarely, between one and four weeks following general surgery the Guillain-Barré syndrome develops.[105] Great care must be taken to ensure that ventilatory support is adequate. Most patients will recover spontaneously and are not helped by steroids. Another uncommon cause of generalized weakness is porphyric neuropathy,[66] developing sometimes as long as a month after surgery. This superficially resembles the Guillain-Barré syndrome; but with careful examination, biochemical studies, and electrical tests, one can be differentiated from the other. (The Guillain-Barré syndrome is associated with high cerebrospinal fluid protein and slow nerve conduction velocity; porphyric neuropathy is characterized by elevated levels of porphobilinogen in urine and blood with normal cerebrospinal fluid protein and nerve conduction velocity.) Treatment of porphyric neuropathy consists of administering large quantities of glucose and vitamin B_6. Careful attention to cardiac rhythm is mandatory because of involvement of the autonomic nervous system in this neuropathy (the autonomic nervous system is also affected in Guillain-Barré syndrome). Use of hematin for treatment of porphyria appears promising.[66]

Disorders of the Neuromuscular Junction

Finally, *disorders of the neuromuscular junction* may cause postoperative weakness. Care of the known myasthenic patient in the perioperative period is difficult and was reviewed above. At times an asymptomatic patient not known to have the disease undergoes surgery and appears profoundly weak in the postoperative period. As mentioned earlier, defective neuromuscular transmission is usually unmasked by drugs and electrolyte disturbances. When a pure motor neurologic syndrome occurs with greatest involvement of ocular, facial, and respiratory muscle, myasthenia gravis must be considered. Another condition affecting the neuromuscular junction and causing a similar syndrome is botulism. Rarely, it occurs in the postoperative period:[106] affected patients have suffered wounds contaminated with *Clostridium botulinum* and developed dysphagia and dyspnea within two weeks of injury. Treatment consists of supportive care, antitoxin administration, and wound debridement. A detailed discussion of acutely and subacutely developing weakness is available.[107]

REFERENCES

1. Wells, CE: *Role of stroke in dementia.* Stroke 9:1, 1978.
2. Pessin, MS, Duncan, GW, Mohr, JP, et al.: *Clinical and angiographic features of carotid transient ischemic attacks.* N Engl J Med 296:358, 1977.
3. Fields, WS: *The asymptomatic bruit—operate or not?* Stroke 9:269, 1978.
4. West, H, Burton, R, Roon, AJ, et al.: *Comparative risk of operation and expectant management for carotid artery disease.* Stroke 10:117, 1979.
5. Machleder, HI: *Strokes, transient ischemic attacks and asymptomatic bruits.* West J Med 130:205, 1979.
6. Treiman, RL, Foran, RF, Shore, EH, et al.: *Carotid bruit, significance in patients undergoing an abdominal aortic operation.* Arch Surg 106:803, 1973.
7. Bernhard, VM, Johnson, WD, and Peterson, JJ: *Carotid artery stenosis, association with surgery for coronary artery disease.* Arch Surg 105:837, 1972.
8. Mehigan, JT, Buch, WS, Pipkin, RD, et al.: *A planned approach to coexistent cerebrovascular disease in coronary artery by-pass candidates.* Arch Surg 112:1403, 1977.
9. Ackerman, RH: *A perspective on non-invasive diagnosis of carotid disease.* Neurology 29:615, 1979.
10. Thompson, JE, Patman, RD, and Talkington, CM: *Asymptomatic carotid bruit. Longterm outcome of patients having endarterectomy compared with unoperated controls.* Ann Surg 188:308, 1978.
11. Genton, E, Barnett, HJ, Fields, WS, et al.: Cerebral ischemia: the role of thrombosis and of antithrombotic therapy. Study group on antithrombotic therapy. Stroke 8(1):147–175, 1977.
12. Fisher, CM: *The use of anticoagulants in cerebral thrombosis.* Neurology 8:311, 1958.
13. Toole, JF, and Cole, M: *Ischemic cerebrovascular disease,* in Baker, AB, and Baker, LH (eds.): *Clinical Neurology.* New York: Harper and Row, 1977, p. 25.
14. Duncan, GW, Pessin, MS, Mohr, JP, et al.: *Transient cerebral ischemic attacks.* Adv Intern Med 21:1, 1976.
15. Mohr, JP, Fisher, CM, and Adams, RD: *Cerebrovascular diseases,* in Thorn, GW, et al. (eds): *Harrison's Principles of Internal Medicine,* ed. 8. New York: McGraw-Hill, 1977, pp. 1850–1852.
16. Solomon, GE, and Plum, F: *General treatment of epilepsy,* in *Clinical Management of Seizures: A Guide for the Physician.* Philadelphia: WB Saunders, 1976, pp. 96–123.
17. Bruni, J: *Recent advances in drug therapy for epilepsy.* Can Med Assoc J 120:817, 1979.
18. Adams, RD, and Victor, M: *Epilepsy and the convulsive states,* in *Principles of Neurology.* New York: McGraw-Hill, 1977, p. 227.
19. Victor, M, and Brausch, C: *The role of abstinence in the genesis of alcoholic epilepsy.* Epilepsia 8:1, 1967.
20. Mattson, RH, Cramer, JA, Williamson, PD, et al.: *Valproic acid in epilepsy: clinical and pharmocological effects.* Ann Neurol 3:20, 1978.
21. Vajda, FJE, Mihaly, GW, Miles, JL, et al.: *Rectal administration of sodium valproate in status epilepticus.* Neurology 28:897, 1978.
22. Fahn, S, and Calne, DB: *Considerations in the management of parkinsonism.* Neurology 28:5, 1978.
23. Franz, DN: *Centrally acting muscle relaxants, in* Goodman, LS, and Gilman, A (eds.): *The Pharmacological Basis of Therapeutics,* ed. 5. New York: MacMillan Pub. Co., 1975, p. 234.
24. Eisler, T, Eng, N, Plotkin, C, et al.: *Absorption of levodopa after rectal administration.* (Abstract) Neurology 29:552, 1979.
25. Weiner, WJ, Perlik, S, Keller, WC, et al.: *The role of a "drug holiday" in the management of Parkinson's disease.* Neurology 29:553, 1979.
26. Bianchine, JR: *Drug therapy of parkinsonism.* N Engl J Med 295:814, 1976.
27. Duvoisin, R: *Clinical diagnosis of the dyskinesias.* Med Clin North Am 56:1321, 1972.

28. Kobayashi, RM: *Drug therapy of tardive dyskinesias.* N Engl J Med 296:257, 1977.
29. Raskin, NH, and Fishman, RA: *Neurologic disorders in renal failure.* N Engl J Med 294:143, 1976.
30. Hatfield, WB: *Headache associated with metabolic and systemic disorders.* Med Clin North Am 62:451, 1978.
31. Raskin, N: *Headache associated with organic diseases of the nervous system.* Med Clin North Am 62:459, 1978.
32. Messert, B, and Black, JA: *Cluster headache, hemicrania and other head pains: morbidity of carotid endarterectomy.* Stroke 9:559, 1978.
33. Utili, R, Boitnott, JK, and Zimmerman, HJ: *Dantrolene-associated hepatic injury. Incidence and character.* Gastroenterology 72:610, 1977.
34. Sachais, BA, Logue, JN, and Carey, MS: *Baclofen, a new antispastic drug. A controlled multicenter trial in patients with multiple sclerosis.* Arch Neurology 34:422, 1977.
35. Levine, MC, and VanBrochlin, JD: *Lioresal (Baclofen) treatment of spasticity: a double-blind comparison study with Dantrolene and Diazepam.* (Abstract) Neurology 27:391, 1977.
36. Bauer, HJ: *Problems of symptomatic therapy in multiple sclerosis.* Neurology 28:8, 1978.
37. Drachman, DB: *Myasthenia gravis.* N Engl J Med 298:134, and 298:184, 1978.
38. Patten, BM: *Myasthenia gravis: review of diagnosis and management.* Muscle Nerve 1:190, 1978.
39. Rowland, LP, and Layzer, RB: *Muscular dystrophies, atrophies and related disease,* in Baker, AB, and Baker, LH (eds.): *Clinical Neurology.* New York: Harper and Row, 1977.
40. deBacker, M, Bergman, P, Perissono, A, et al.: *Respiratory failure and cardiac disturbances in myotonic dystrophy.* Eur J Intens Care Med 2:63, 1976.
41. Brown, BR, Walson, PD, and Taussig, LM: *Congenital metabolic diseases of pediatric patients: anesthetic implications.* Anesthesiology 43:197, 1975.
42. Wenger, NK: *Myocardial involvement in systemic disease,* in Hurst, JW, Logue, RB, Schlant, RC, et al. (eds.): *The Heart Arteries and Veins,* ed. 3 New York: McGraw Hill Co., 1974, pp. 1363–1366.
43. Adams, RD, and Salam, MZ: *Acute and subacute myopathic paralysis,* in Thorn, GW, et al. (eds): *Harrison's Principles of Internal Medicine,* ed. 8. New York: McGraw-Hill, 1977, p. 1987.
44. Webb, D, Muir, I, Faulkner, J., et al.: *Myotonia dystrophica: obstetric complications.* Am J Obstet Gynecol 132:265, 1978.
45. Rowland, LP, and Penn, AS: *Myoglobinuria.* Med Clin North Am 56:1233, 1972.
46. Ekbom, K, Hed, R, Kirsten, L, et al.: *Muscular affectations in chronic alcoholism.* Arch Neurol 10:449, 1964.
47. Vroom, RQ, Jarrell, MA, and Maren, TH: *Acetazolamide treatment of hypokalemic periodic paralysis. Probable mechanism of action.* Arch Neurol 32:385, 1975.
48. Brooke, MH: *Malignant hyperpyrexia,* in *A Clinician's View of Neuromuscular Diseases.* Baltimore: Williams & Wilkins Co., 1977, pp. 176–178.
49. Gronert, GA: *Malignant hyperthermia.* Anesthesiology 53:395, 1980.
50. Britt BA: *Etiology and pathophysiology of malignant hyperthermia.* Fed. Proc. 38:44, 1979.
51. Maisel, RH, Sessions, DG, and Miller, RN: *Malignant hyperpyrexia during general anesthesia. Successful management of a case.* Ann Otol Rhinol Laryngol 82:729, 1973.
52. Plum, F, and Posner, JB: *Diagnosis of Stupor and Coma,* ed. 2. Philadelphia: FA Davis Co., 1972.
53. Adams, RD, and Victor, M: *Delirium and other confusional states,* in *Principles of Neurology.* New York: McGraw-Hill Co., 1977, p. 267.
54. Cuneo, RA, and Caronna, JJ: *The neurologic complications of hypertension.* Med Clin North Am 61:565, 1977.
55. Archer, CR, and Horenstein, S: *Basilar artery occlusion; clinical and radiological correlation.* Stroke 8:383, 1977.
56. Nordgren, RE, Markesbery, WR, Fukuda, K, et al.: *Seven cases of cerebromedullospinal disconnection: the "locked-in" syndrome.* Neurology 21:1140, 1971.
57. Messert, B, Orrinson, WW, Hawkins, MJ et al.: *Central pontine myelinolysis. Considerations on etiology, diagnosis and treatment.* Neurology 29:147, 1979.
58. Allen, N: *Life or death of the brain after cardiac arrest.* Neurology 27:805, 1977.

59. Caronna, JJ, and Finklestein, S: *Neurological syndromes after cardiac arrest.* Stroke 9:517, 1978.
60. Morse, RM, and Litin, EM: *The anatomy of a delirium.* Am J Psychiat 128:143, 1971.
61. Mesulam, MM, and Geschwind, N: *Disordered mental states in the postoperative period.* Urol Clin North Am 3:199, 1976.
62. Dines, DE, Burgher, LW, and Okazaki, H: *The clinical and pathologic correlation of fat embolism syndrome.* Mayo Clin Proc 50:407, 1975.
63. Collins, RC, Al-Mondhiry, H, Chernik, NL, et al.: *Neurologic manifestations of intravascular coagulation in patients with cancer. A clinicopathologic analysis of 12 cases.* Neurology 25:795, 1975.
64. Chernik, NL, Armstrong, D, and Posner, JB: *Central nervous system infections in patients with cancer, changing patterns.* Cancer 40:268, 1977.
65. Hotson, JR, and Pedley, TA: *The neurological complications of cardiac transplantation.* Brain 99:673, 1976.
66. Sergay, SM: *Management of hepatic porphyria.* Med Clin North Am 63:453, 1979.
67. Obrecht, R, Okhomina, FOA, and Scott, DF: *Value of EEG in acute confusional states.* J Neurol Neurosurg Psychiatr 42:75, 1979.
68. Mesulan, MM, Waxman, SG, Geschwind, N, et al.: *Acute confusional states with right middle cerebral artery infarctions.* J Neurol Neurosurg Psychiatr 39:84, 1976.
69. Caplan, LR, Stillman, J, Ojemann, R, et al.: *Intracerebral hemorrhage following carotid endarterectomy: a hypertensive complication?* Stroke 9:457, 1978.
70. Gilman, S: *Cerebral disorders after open-heart operations.* N Engl J Med 272:489, 1965.
71. Tufo, HM, Ostfeld, AM, and Shekelle, R: *Central nervous system dysfunction following open-heart surgery.* JAMA 212:1333, 1970.
72. Markand, ON, and Daly, DD: *Pseudoperiodic lateralized paroxysmal discharges in electroencephalogram.* Neurology 21:975, 1971.
73. Weisberg, LA: *Computated tomography in the diagnosis of intracranial disease.* Ann Intern Med 91:87, 1979.
74. Simon, RP: *Emergency Medicine.* Los Altos: Ca.:, Lange Medical Pub., in press.
75. Wilder, BJ, Ramsay, RE, Willmore, LJ, et al.: *Efficacy of intravenous phenytoin in the treatment of status epilepticus: kinetics of central nervous system penetration.* Ann Neurol 1:511, 1977.
76. Cranford, RE, Leppik, IE, Patrick, B, et al.: *Intravenous phenytoin: clinical and pharmacokinetic aspects.* Neurology 28:874, 1978.
77. Louis, S, Kutt, H, and McDowell, F: *The cardiocirculatory changes caused by intravenous dilantin and its solvent.* Am Heart J 74:523, 1967.
78. Specter, RH, Davidoff, RA, and Schwartzman, RJ: *Phenytoin-induced ophthalmoplegia.* Neurology 26:1031, 1976.
79. Harvey, SC: *Hypnotics and sedatives,* in Goodman, LS, and Gilman A (eds.): *The Pharmacological Basis of Therapeutics,* ed. 5. New York: MacMillan Pub. Co., 1975, p. 112.
80. Harvey, SC: *Hypnotics and sedatives, miscellaneous agents,* in Goodman, LS, and Gilman, A (eds.): *The Pharmacological Basis of Therapeutics,* ed. 5. New York: MacMillan Pub. Co., 1975, p. 131.
81. Taverner, D, and Bain, WA: *Intravenous lignocaine as an anticonvulsant in status epilepticus and serial epilepsy.* Lancet 2:1145, 1958.
82. Bladin, PF: *Intracarotid treatment of status epilepticus.* Epilepsia 4:151, 1963.
83. Orringer, CE, Eustace, JC, Wunsch, CD et al.: *Natural history of lactic acidosis after grand mal seizures. A model for the study of an anion gap acidosis not associated with hyperkalemia.* N Engl J Med 297:795, 1977.
84. Lance, JW, and Adams, RD: *The syndrome of intention or action myoclonus as a sequel to hypoxic encephalopathy.* Brain 86:111, 1963.
85. Van Woert, MH, and Sethy, VH: *Therapy of intention myoclonus with L-5-hydroxytryptophan and a peripheral decarboxylase inhibitor, MK 486.* Neurology 25:135, 1975.
86. Goldberg, MA, and Dorman, JD: *Intention myoclonus: successful treatment with clonzaepam.* Neurology 26:24, 1976.
87. Fahn, S: *Post-anoxic action myoclonus: improvement with valproic acid.* N Engl J Med 299:313, 1978.

88. Siekert, RG, and Dale, AJD: *Vascular disease of the spinal cord,* in Goldensohn, E.S. and Appel, S (eds.): *Scientific Approaches to Clinical Neurology.* Philadelphia: Lea and Febiger, 1977, pp. 819–828.
89. Simeone, FA (ed.): *Symposium on operative nerve injuries and their repair.* Surg Clin North Am 52:00, 1972.
90. Artusio, JF: *Anesthesia and its immediate post-operative complications.* Surg Clin North Am 44:493, 1964.
91. Feringa, ER: *Plexus syndromes,* in Vinken, PJ, and Bruyn, GW (eds.): *Handbook of Clinical Neurology* (Vol. 2) *Localization in Clinical Neurology.* Amsterdam: North Holland Pub. Co., 1969, pp. 128–156.
92. Emery, S, and Ochoa, J: *Lumbar plexus neuropathy resulting from retroperitoneal hemorrhage.* Muscle and Nerve 1:330, 1978.
93. Cranberg, L: *Femoral neuropathy from iliac hematoma: report of a case.* Neurology 29:1071, 1979.
94. Aminoff, MJ: *Neurological disorders and pregnancy.* Am J Obstet Gynecol 132:325, 1978.
95. Kubacz, GL: *Femoral and sciatic compression neuropathy.* Br J Surg 58:580, 1971.
96. Verta, MJ, Applebaum, EL, McClusky, DA, et al.: *Cranial nerve injury during carotid endarterectomy.* Ann Surg 185:192, 1977.
97. Warpeka, RL: *Head and neck surgery.* Surg Clin North Am 57:1357, 1977.
98. Zintel, HA, and Nay, HR: *Post-operative complications of radical mastectomy.* Surg. Clin. North Am. 44(2):313–323, 1964.
99. Baker, RJ: *Monitoring in critically ill patients.* Surg Clin North Am 57:1139, 1977.
100. Lee, JF, Maurer, VM, and Black, GE: *Anatomic relations of pelvic autonomic nerves to pelvic operations.* Arch Surg 107:324, 1973.
101. Nakano, KK: *The entrapment neuropathies.* Muscle Nerve 1:264, 1978.
102. McNamara, MF, Takaki, HS, and Yao, JST: *Venous disease.* Surg Clin North Am 57:1201, 1977.
103. Young, RR, Reberg, J and Adams, RD: *Approach to clinical neurology,* in Thorn, GW, et al. (eds): *Harrison's Principles of Internal Medicine,* ed. 8. New York: McGraw-Hill, 1977, pp. 1974–1975.
104. Argov, Z, and Mastaglia, FL: *Disorders of neuromuscular transmission caused by drugs.* N Engl J Med 301:409, 1979.
105. Arnason, BG, and Asbury, AK: *Idiopathic polyneuritis after surgery.* Arch Neurol 18:500, 1968.
106. Merson, MH, and Dowell, VR: *Epidemiologic, clinical and laboratory aspects of wound botulism.* N Engl J Med 289:1005, 1973.
107. Layzer, RB: *Remediable neuromuscular disorders.* Primary Care 2:235, 1975.

Chapter 10

ONCOLOGY

Richard A. Rudders, M.D., and
Larry Nathanson, M.D.

This chapter focuses on the special needs of cancer patients undergoing surgery for diseases other than cancer. Patients with cancer may require surgical intervention in the course of their illness beyond the usual surgical aspects of cancer management. In view of the complex and often bewildering array of treatment programs in use today, it behooves the internist and surgeon alike to be aware of special considerations which cancer patients undergoing treatment require whenever surgery is contemplated. Patients with neoplastic disease demand more than customary and routine surgical management for a particular acute or elective problem. For example, during the intraoperative and postoperative period, the side effects of a particular anticancer drug may become manifest and pose a serious threat. Also, during a stressful period, the cancer patient has not only physical but special emotional needs. Cancer patients are often being actively counseled and supported by psychiatrists, social workers, and psychologists and it is extremely important that these relationships be maintained and increased during the perioperative period. Finally, total cancer care requires the advice of numerous disciplines and surgical decisions are no exception. The multidisciplinary approach to management is an absolute necessity in all phases of decision making in cancer patients.

DECISION MAKING IN CANCER PATIENTS

Whenever surgical intervention is considered in a cancer patient, the particular situation should be carefully analyzed. This may be a formal process as in "decision analysis" or, more frequently, informal. Several questions should be asked. First, what is the risk to the patient if there is no intervention versus the risk if a procedure is performed? Second, what is the anticipated benefit of the procedure and, finally, what are the alternatives? In classical medical teaching, this translates into "indications" or "contraindications" for a particular form of surgery. It should be pointed out that most rules of thumb applied to surgical questions assume a basically healthy patient with an indeterminate life expectancy. When such thinking is applied to cancer patients, the axioms often fail. In making what would otherwise be routine surgical decisions, one must always bear in mind the overall prognosis (the anticipated life expectancy), the current treatment program (chemotherapy, radiotherapy, or otherwise), and the desires of the patient. One or more of these factors may drastically alter the decision process so that in a given situation the decisions for non-cancer and cancer patients may be quite different. That a potential surgical event in the medical life of a given cancer patient must be viewed in the context of a life-threatening and often fatal illness is crucial and cannot be overemphasized.

There is virtue in considering surgical intervention under the two broad categories of acute and more chronic or elective indications. In acute life-threatening situations, the tendency is to proceed in the decision making process giving little weight to considerations such as overall prognosis. Although this is usually appropriate, in some circumstances it may not be. For instance, it may be more reasonable in certain patients to treat such things as acute cholecystitis, acute appendicitis, or bony fractures non-surgically. The decision to do so suggests either an unacceptable risk or cost relative to an alternative, even though the alternative may be considered inferior or not definitive treatment. An example might be an acute fracture of the hip in a bedridden patient with far-advanced breast cancer. If an extensive surgical procedure is contemplated, one must weigh the benefit (re-establishing function, i.e., weight-bearing) which may be relatively unimportant since in this case the patient is bedridden and the risk (which may be considerable) versus an alternative to surgery, which might be radiotherapy. Although joint stabilization will not occur with radiation treatment alone, pain palliation and/or local tumor control will likely be achieved. In any of these situations, what is required is a careful analysis of the problem and a plan based on the combined judgments of several disciplines.

Decisions regarding so-called "elective" surgery may be more difficult and less clear-cut. In general, as the overall prognosis worsens, one tends to defer elective surgery. One example might be asymptomatic gallstones in the elderly cancer patient. In such a case, elective cholecystectomy might be deferred. On the other hand, when the prognosis is intermediate (years) or excellent (indeterminate), decisions regarding elective surgery are more difficult. If anything, there is a tendency to delay such decisions in view of the generally pervasive negative feeling regarding the prognosis of cancer patients. In many situations, this may not be in the best interest of the patient. The individual with bothersome hernias which might incarcerate and who has a malignancy with a good prognosis may well benefit from surgical intervention.

The decision to perform surgery on a cancer patient requires a knowledge of the natural history and biologic behavior of tumors. Tumor metastases or syndromes related to tumor products when recognized may drastically alter the decision making process and if not recognized may cause great confusion with benign conditions. The following section details aspects of tumor behavior which are important in evaluating a cancer patient for surgery.

PREOPERATIVE EVALUATION

The preoperative evaluation of the patient with cancer may reveal findings in both the physical examination and laboratory testing which may influence the ability of the patient to tolerate surgery.

Evaluation of Metastatic Disease

Discovery of a previously unexpected site of metastasis alters the decision regarding surgery for noncancer related conditions. For example, a patient with an apparent "cure" after resection of a lung cancer was admitted for repair of a hernia. Careful history and physical examination raised the possibility of brain metastasis which was confirmed by CT scan. The limitation of life expectancy due to this metastasis precluded performing elective surgery on this patient and prevented further possible complications of the surgery and hospital stay. It is important, therefore, to know that certain neoplasms characteristically recur or metastasize to particular tissues. Table 1 lists important metastatic sites. Thus, soft tissue and bone metastases must be looked for by physical examination and bone scan in breast cancer patients. The melanoma patient with occult bleeding should have a careful evaluation of the gastrointestinal tract. Patients with cervical cancer and back pain must be evaluated for infiltrative disease involving the sacrum or nerve plexus. A careful examination of the liver in patients with gastrointestinal cancer is critical. In many cancers, a review of the peripheral blood smear may be a first clue to the presence of myelophthistic anemia signifying bone marrow involvement.

So-called tumor markers may also be helpful in looking for occult metastases.

TABLE 1. Frequent Sites of Metastases in Common Cancers

Cancer	*Metastatic Sites*
Breast	Chest wall, bone, liver, lung, brain
Lung	Liver, bone, brain (particularly oat cell)
Prostate	Bone, liver
Head and neck (squamous)	Lung, bone, liver
Gastrointestinal	Liver
Soft tissue, sarcomas	Locoregional, lungs, liver
Skin (excluding melanoma)	Rarely metastasize
Melanoma	Locoregional, lung, liver, brain, gastrointestinal tract
Cervix	Locoregional
Uterus	Locoregional
Ovary	Peritoneal seeding

Carcinoembryonic antigen (CEA) may be elevated in a variety of cancers, particularly gastrointestinal and breast.[1] Alpha fetoprotein is useful in the evaluation of the extent of disease in patients with hepatoma or testicular carcinoma.[2] The only evidence of occult metastases from tumors known to produce hormones may be the reappearance of elevated circulating hormone levels.[3,4]

Neurologic Effects of Cancer

Of all patients with malignant disease, 10 percent may have neurologic complications.[5] These may be classified into direct or indirect effects of tumor involvement in the central system.[5,6] It is important to distinguish between such direct and indirect effects preoperatively, because a tumor mass causing a direct effect (e.g., cord compression) may necessitate immediate therapy which may preclude surgery for an unrelated condition, whereas such surgery may be able to proceed if it were found that the neurologic syndrome (e.g., peripheral neuropathy) was an indirect effect of the cancer. Often it is necessary to perform procedures such as computerized axial tomography or myelography to exclude the presence of a tumor mass.

DIRECT NEUROLOGIC EFFECTS

Direct central nervous system effects may be due to primary brain tumors, solid tumors or lymphomas metastatic to the brain or spinal cord, or disorders of the sensory or motor systems including paraplegia resulting from epidural spinal cord compression. Pain, paraparesis, urinary or fecal incontinence, and mental and behavioral changes constitute the most disabling symptoms with which the cancer patient is afflicted.

Intracranial Effects

Approximately one-third of patients with intracranial metastases present with focal neurologic signs, one-third with behavioral or mental changes, and one-third with general symptoms which would include headache, seizures, or projectile vomiting.[5] Occasionally, metastatic tumors may spread from the skull or the subdural space. Carcinoma of the breast, neuroblastoma and Ewing's sarcoma in children, and other sarcomas in adults are examples of this type of spread. Sometimes, involvement of a venous sinus may be seen with papilledema and retinal hemorrhage. Skull films may show the presence of lesions extrinsic to the brain which involve it secondarily. Computerized tomography is the best technique for demonstrating intracranial lesions.

Spinal Cord Effects

In evaluating patients for back pain and suspected disc disease, spinal cord metastases must be considered. Spinal cord metastases are most commonly produced by extradural metastases compressing the spinal cord; intraparenchymal metastases are uncommon (the reverse of the case in the brain).[7] The most common primary tumors producing such lesions include cancer of the breast and lung, Hodgkin's disease, soft tissue sarcomas, and prostatic cancer. These tumors invade the vertebral column first and then grow into the epidural space producing spinal cord compression, although patients with lymphoma or neuroblastoma may exhibit invasion via the paravertebral lymph nodes near the nerve roots and through the intravertebral foramina. Metastases to the vertebral body with subsequent compression fracture can also lead to cord compression.

The most common symptom of cord compression is pain, usually localized to the area of tumor involvement. Occasionally, pain may radiate from the back to the front in a radicular distribution, or it may be unilateral. Weakness of the extremities and paresthesias of the feet are common signs and may include hyperactive reflex and extensor plantar responses in the lower extremities, and sensory loss to vibration and position sense. Progression may then occur and may include complete loss of motor power, sensation, and autonomic function below the level of the block. Cord compression is a neurologic emergency and necessitates an extremely rapid diagnostic evaluation followed by urgent treatment which includes surgical decompression, corticosteroids, and radiotherapy. Similar symptoms in cancer patients may be produced by transverse myelitis due to radiation therapy or as a remote effect of cancer. Epidural hemorrhage also must be considered.

Direct involvement of the peripheral nerves and roots, including the cauda equina, in the epidural space of the lumbosacral or brachial plexuses in paravertebral areas commonly occurs. Cauda equina involvement is common with carcinomas of the breast, prostate, and cervix and lumbosacral plexus dysfunction with carcinomas of the bladder, prostate, and cervix. Due to metastatic carcinoma or lymphoma, paravertebral lymph nodes may also compress the lumbosacral plexus and carcinoma of the breast and carcinoma of the lung are mainly responsible for brachial plexus involvement. Pain, which is usually constant and severe, is the first symptom of limited plexus compression and may then be accompanied by sensory and motor symptoms including weakness, atrophy, deep tendon reflex loss, and loss of sensation.

Meningeal metastases are most common in acute lymphatic leukemia[8] but also occur in carcinomas of the breast, lung, pancreas, stomach, and prostate. Meningeal seeding may produce localized symptoms due to primary involvement of either cerebral, cranial, or peripheral nerves. Cerebral symptoms arise from subarachnoid blockade and involve hydrocephalus with headache and papilledema and dementia. There may be seizures. Cranial nerve involvement results from blockade of the subarachnoid pathways transversed by cranial nerves. Diplopia and facial palsy are the most common symptoms. Peripheral nerve involvement results from meningeal infiltration of nerve roots supplying the trunk and extremities. It usually involves weakness, numbness, and if the cauda equina is infiltrated, bowel and bladder function loss. Later pain may result. The identification of tumor cells in the cerebral spinal fluid with elevation of cerebral spinal fluid protein and glucose depression usually makes the diagnosis. Occasionally, myelography may be helpful. The differential diagnosis includes peripheral neuropathy or carcinomatous neuropathies. Cryptococcal meningitis must also be ruled out.

Usually the presence of central nervous system (CNS) disease indicates a poor prognosis so that elective nontumor surgery is deferred. When emergency therapy must be performed and it is felt that benefits of surgery outweigh the risks, then high-dose dexamethasone may be useful to decrease cerebral edema allowing surgery to be performed. Radiotherapy is also useful. It is important to avoid intraoperative and postoperative hypotension and hypertension in such patients to prevent potentially fatal hemorrhage into these CNS sites of metastases. Anticoagulation is also to be avoided.

INDIRECT NEUROLOGIC EFFECTS OF CANCER

Metabolic or Toxic Encephalopathies

These may result from hyponatremia (inappropriate antidiuretic hormone [ADH] syndrome for example), hypertensive or uremic encephalopathy (carcinomas of the cervix or other pelvic carcinomas with ureteral obstruction), or sepsis related to immunosuppression and infectious diathesis.[6,9] Under these circumstances, patients are usually quiet, apathetic, withdrawn, and lethargic and occasionally may have seizures. Symptoms or signs are usually symmetric and generalized. Coma may supervene. Treatment is that of the underlying cause of the metabolic disease.

Central Nervous System Syndromes

These occur most commonly in tumors of the lung, female genital tract, and breast.[6,9,10] Initial symptoms include ataxia and incoordination. Nystagmus, dysarthria, and personality changes are common. Pyramidal tract signs may be present. Loss of Betz cells through the cerebellar cortex may occur, accounting for the cerebellar syndrome that is present. An amyotrophic lateral sclerosis-like syndrome is rarely seen with Hodgkin's disease.[11] Ophthalmoplegia, ocular palsy, involuntary movement, muscle weakness and wasting, and sensory impairment are present. Progressive multifocal leukoencephalopathy is a rare subacute disorder which occurs primarily with leukemia, lymphoma, and myeloma and which is characterized by disorders of behavior, thinking, and speech as well as motor and sensory abnormalities and follows a relentless course toward coma and death. Cerebrospinal fluid may be unremarkable and at postmortem characteristic histopathologic changes of multiple foci of demyelination and the presence of giant cells are noted. Dementia is a common accompaniment of malignancies and may occur in the absence of intracranial metastases. Diagnostic changes in the EEG may be present with pleocytosis in the cerebrospinal fluid. Its treatment is the treatment of the underlying tumor.

Peripheral Neuropathy

The peripheral neuropathies include motor, sensory, and mixed neuropathies. They may lead to paralysis or orthostatic hypotension and are diagnosed by the characteristic elevation of the cerebrospinal fluid protein with pleocytosis and lack of other possible causes.[6] Such a peripheral neuropathy needs to be distinguished from that caused by vincristine therapy (see below) and, of course, the other more common causes of peripheral neuropathies.

Myasthenic Syndromes

The myasthenic syndromes include the Eaton-Lambert syndrome and true myasthenia gravis, which may be seen with thymoma particularly of the lymphocytic type.[12] The Eaton-Lambert syndrome is characterized by signs of muscle weakness with severe involvement of the pelvic girdle, dysphagia, and dry mouth. It differs from classical myasthenia in that ocular involvement is rare, the cranial nerves are spared, the deep reflexes are affected, and sharp stimuli evoke no response. It occurs primarily with oat cell carcinoma and other intrathoracic tumors. Normal amplitude of response gradually increases with continuing stimulation, the reverse of what is seen in classic myasthenia. Patients with Eaton-Lambert syndrome are very sensitive to muscle relaxants used in anesthesia and to aminoglycoside antibiotics, and such agents should be used with great caution (see Chapt. 9, Neurology and 17, Anesthesiology). The perioperative management of patients with myasthenia gravis is discussed in Chapter 9.

Myositis

Polymyositis or dermatomyositis may accompany malignant disease.[13] Tumors associated with these diseases include those of the breast, cervix, gallbladder, lung, kidney, ovary, pancreas, and prostate. A characteristic differential point is the association of dermatomyositis with underlying malignancy in men over the age of 50, whereas classical dermatomyositis with no underlying malignancy predominates in adult women. The syndrome may either preceed or follow the diagnosis of malignancy, but all males over the age of 50 with dermatomyositis must be carefully evaluated to exclude underlying malignancy. Electromyograms may show pseudomyotonic responses and laboratory findings include elevations of creatinine, phosphokinase, sedimentation rate, lactic dehydrogenase (LDH), amylase, and serum glutamic-oxaloacetic transaminase (SGOT). Biopsy of the affected muscle may demonstrate fibronecrosis with some inflammation.

Skeletal Effects of Cancer

The most serious musculoskeletal complication of malignancy is bone fracture. A pathologic fracture relating to cancer must always be considered when the trauma inducing the fracture appears to be inconsequential. Metastatic breast cancer is the most common cause of pathologic fracture, but such fractures are also commonly seen with myeloma and malignancies of the lung, prostate, and kidney. Biopsy is the only definitive method of establishing the correct diagnosis. If the fracture is established as being related to cancer, surgical stabilization may be required which usually should be combined with radiotherapy to the fracture site. As discussed earlier, the decision to proceed with such surgery depends upon the prior ambulatory and overall status of the patient, since external stabilization procedures (braces and so forth) plus radiotherapy will often suffice for palliation of pain.

Cardiopulmonary Effects of Cancer

SUPERIOR VENA CAVA SYNDROME

The superior vena syndrome is a relatively uncommon medical emergency. It is characterized by shortness of breath, facial swelling, and swelling of the trunk or upper extremities. Chest pain, cough, and dyspnea are less frequently reported. Findings on physical examination include thoracic vein and neck vein distention, edema of the face and neck, tachypnea, plethora, and sometimes cyanosis. The syndrome can vary depending upon whether the site of obstruction is either at the superior vena cava itself or at the innominate or jugular veins draining into the superior vena cava. Vena cava syndrome is most often seen with malignancies (particularly lymphomas or lung cancer) but can be caused by benign conditions such as fibrosing mediastinitis, aortic aneurysms, or venocclusive disease. A biopsy may be hazardous in view of the markedly elevated venous pressure. A thin needle biopsy of associated neck nodes or masses can be done safely and may quickly establish the diagnosis. Many cases, however, defy all attempts at a definitive diagnosis. Immediate institution of therapy is necessary to reverse the venous and airway obstruction. Radiotherapy is the recognized treatment of choice for malignant conditions although in rare cases where radiotherapy may be contraindicated, the institution of chemotherapy with nitrogen mustard or cyclophosphamide may be appropriate. Obtaining a diagnosis prior to institution of treatment is crucial, but lifesaving therapy often takes precedence over obtaining a tissue diagnosis.

HYPERTROPHIC PULMONARY OSTEOARTHROPATHY

This syndrome has four components. In order of decreasing incidence, they are: (1) clubbing of the fingers, (2) pulmonary osteoarthropathy, (3) gynecomastia, and (4) pachydermoperiostosis.[13] Clubbing is characterized by alteration in the ungualphalangeal angle; the normal, slightly upward direction of the nail bed with respect to the distal phalanx gradually changes to a downward direction. Pressure on the nail plate produces a "floating nail" with increased springiness at the base of the nail with respect to the underlying bone. Osteoarthropathy is characterized by pain, tenderness, and enlargement of the extremities, the result of periarticular and periosteal proliferation. Polyarthritis may also be present, mimicking rheumatoid arthritis. The joints most commonly involved are knees, ankles, elbows, wrists, and metacarpophalangeal joints. This syndrome may herald the onset of the tumor and appear prior to its clinical diagnosis. Adenocarcinoma and epidermoid carcinoma of the lung are the neoplasms most commonly associated with pulmonary osteoarthropathy; however, any intrathoracic disease (including some benign disease) can produce this syndrome. Bilateral or unilateral gynecomastia has been reported in association with this syndrome or alone. Pachydermoperiostosis is an uncommon proliferation of connective tissues which is associated with leonine facies. The syndrome may also occur in hepatic disease.[14] The etiology of this syndrome is not clearcut, although it has been associated in some cases with increased production of human chorionic gonadotropin (HCG) by various tumors.

PLEURAL EFFUSIONS

Thoracocentesis is indicated when pleural effusions are present to improve respiratory status preoperatively. Sclerosing agents (quinacrine, tetracycline) or antitumor agents (thiotepa or bleomycin) intrapleurally may be helpful to prevent reaccumulation.[15]

INTERSTITIAL LUNG DISEASE

Interstitial lung disease in cancer patients may be due to lymphatic (or lymphangitic) spread of tumor. Prior exposure to chlorambucil, cyclophosphamide, Myleran, carmustine (BCNU) and bleomycin may give rise to severe pulmonary fibrosis (see below), and patients who have received these drugs should have a careful preoperative evaluation of respiratory function, including blood gases and pulmonary function testing.

CARDIAC PROBLEMS

Tumor originating in the thorax, especially lymphomas, and pulmonary and breast tumors, may occasionally involve the pericardium or even myocardium. Pericardial involvement including pericardial infusion may be a life-threatening problem. Such patients present with the characteristic findings of pericardial infusion or tamponade and must be treated with pericardiocentesis.[16] Treatment with chemotherapy and/or radiotherapy may help to prevent reaccumulation.

Prior therapy with adriamycin may cause a cardiomyopathy (see below) and fluids should be administered cautiously to such patients to avoid congestive heart failure.

Gastrointestinal Effects of Cancer

GASTROINTESTINAL OBSTRUCTION

Gastrointestinal obstruction, perforation, or bleeding may be difficult to diagnose in the cancer patient because of the necessity of distinguishing these problems from the side effects of radiotherapy or cytotoxic drugs therapy, the masking of symptoms by steroids and the neurologic involvement by tumors. Furthermore, the diagnosis may be made more difficult by the inability to subject a patient with underlying nutritional and other chronic illness to appropriate diagnostic maneuvers. The extent of diagnostic and therapeutic intervention must also be weighed against the prognosis in the individual in whom such treatment is being considered. Frequently, such patients must be treated with gastrointestinal suction, fluids, and other conservative supportive measures long past the point at which patients without malignant disease would have been operated upon.

BILIARY TRACT OBSTRUCTION

In patients with a history of malignancy, the development of jaundice should always alert the physician to the possibility of biliary tract obstruction. Obstructions of the biliary tract may be intrahepatic or extra hepatic. Most such obstructions are due to metastatic disease, although occasionally primary bile duct carcinoma or primary intrahepatic tumors may account for this obstruction. Those lesions within the hepatic parenchyma are inaccessible to surgery. Pancreatic carcinomas predominate in the group presenting with obstruction. Percutaneous transhepatic angiography and thin needle liver biopsy performed under radiologic direction may be useful diagnostic techniques.

MALNUTRITION

In cancer patients, nutritional deficiency resulting from defective digestion and absorption of nutrients and vitamins as well as minerals including iron often occurs.[17] Causative mechanisms include: (1) inadequate intake of nutrients; (2) insufficient hematopoietic intrinsic factor; (3) inadequate digestive enzymes in the bile; (4) improper mixing of foods, enzymes, and bile; (5) biochemical and enzymatic dysfunction of the mucosal cells; (6) intrinsic disease of the intestinal walls; (7) inadequate length of the normal intestinal surface; (8) altered intraluminal pressure or motility; (9) obstruction of the mesenteric blood vessels; and (10) alteration of the autonomic nervous system. For example, lymphoma may produce a malabsorption syndrome when the small bowel is extensively involved and may also produce intestinal obstruction or fistula formation. Fever, abdominal cramps, bleeding, hypochromic anemia, and abdominal mass are characteristic of the disease. Gastrointestinal carcinomas, including those of the stomach, pancreas, liver, and colon, may produce some degree of malabsorption. This is particularly true of the linitis plastica form of gastric carcinoma. In the case of pancreatic carcinoma with obstruction, there may be inadequate secretion of the exocrine enzymes of the pancreas, leading to an inadequate emulsification of fats and neutralization of acids. Obstruction of lymphatics may also be a factor in a variety of solid tumors.

PROTEIN-LOSING ENTEROPATHY

Protein-losing enteropathy results from secretion of protein into the gastrointestinal lumen. It may result from inflammation and ulceration of the gastrointestinal mucosa caused by carcinoma or lymphoma of the esophagus, stomach, or colon or, occasionally, by tumor metastatic to the bowel such as melanoma. In some cases, such as that of villous adenoma of the rectum, the mechanism by which protein and electrolytes are secreted into the bowel is clear. With other types of gastrointestinal cancer, lymphoma, lung cancer, or ovarian carcinoma, the mechanism by which such protein loss is produced may not be apparent.

THE ANOREXIA-CACHEXIA SYNDROME

The anorexia-cachexia syndrome is a virtually universal feature of the natural history of malignancies in humans.[18] Although its causal mechanisms are not fully understood, clinically it is characterized by: (1) anorexia,[19] which may be absolute or relative to increasing nutritional needs and may be accompanied by loss of taste sensation; (2) hypermetabolism with energy consumed exceeding available nutritional supply; and (3) wasting due to a negative balance of protein and fat in the body. The cachexia syndrome is probably responsible for a large proportion of cancer deaths in patients with solid tumors. Loss of muscle protein and muscle strength, impaired cellular respiration, and neuromyopathies when they occur may result in the failure of function of critical muscle masses. This failure may occur in areas of skeletal muscle, such as intercostal or abdominal muscles resulting in atelectasis in the lung and consequent pneumonias and death. Furthermore, such infections are compounded by the immunodeficient state seen in malnutrition.[20] They may also result in depletion of smooth muscle as in the urinary or intestinal tracts resulting in relative failure of the respective organs. Weight loss seen in the cachexia syndrome is poorly estimated by changes in total body weight as there is a relative increase in interstitial fluid retention which tends to neutralize the effect upon the body weight of depletion of muscle mass. Thus, muscle tone, strength, and appearance may be more important in estimating the degree of cachexia than total body weight.

Adaptive mechanisms (which tend to conserve muscle mass at the expense of adipose tissue) that are present in starving normal individuals tend to break down in cancer patients.[21] The rate of disappearance of infused labelled glucose in blood is slower in cancer patients than in the normal glucose loaded individual. Thus, in addition to an absolute decrease in intake, there is an inefficient utilization of those nutrients which are in fact absorbed. Such malnourished patients usually recover poorly after surgery (see Chap. 15, Nutrition).

Therapy of this cachectic state is difficult unless the underlying cancer may be successfully treated. The use of enteral and parenteral nutritional support[22] may be very helpful in the patient in whom malnutrition threatens the outcome of indicated surgery (see Chap. 15, Nutrition). However, in the absence of effective antitumor therapy, this means of treatment of cachexia has short-lived success. Other techniques that have been used to combat anorexia and cachexia include the use of glucose plus insulin infusions and androgenic steroids. Androgenic steroids tend to be relatively nontoxic in males and may be effective for a short time in increasing positive nitrogen balance and stimulating erythropoiesis temporarily in anemic patients. In the patient whose anorexia stems in part from depression, the use of antidepressant medications and psychiatric consultation may be helpful.

Renal Effects of Cancer

Renal failure in neoplastic disease may be due to tumor invasion and replacement of renal parenchyma or involvement of ureters and bladder causing obstruction. It is also possible to have renal failure from nephrotoxic substances synthesized by the tumor and secreted into the blood or from nephrotoxic breakdown products of rapid tumor lysis such as uric acid (see below).

The diseases most commonly associated with parenchymal destruction in the kidney are leukemia and lymphoma. However, serious reduction in renal function is rarely due to parenchymal invasion. Nephrotic syndrome has been associated with lymphoma and may result from production of immune complexes in that disease. Obstructive uropathy is a more common cause of severe impairment of renal function with tumors. This may be demonstrated at the time of intravenous or retrograde pyelography or with ultrasonography. Use of ureterostomy or ureteral stint may be useful, particularly in patients with relatively indolent tumors, as may be the case with cervical carcinoma or sarcoma.

Dehydration, production of immunoglobulins as in multiple myeloma, hypercalcemia, or hyperuricemia may all result in compromise of renal function generally due to glomerular and/or tubular damage. Here, reversal of the metabolic abnormality may be helpful, although irreversible damage can occur. Administration of x-ray contrast media to patients with multiple myeloma may precipitate renal failure, and such patients should always be well hydrated for such procedures in an attempt to avoid this catastrophe.

Ectopic Hormone Syndromes

The ectopic hormone syndromes discussed below are discussed in Chapter 5, Endocrinology in greater depth.

HYPERCALCEMIA

Hypercalcemia is the most common hormone abnormality associated with cancer.[23] Tumors most frequently associated with hypercalcemia are those of the breast and lung and myeloma in which osseous involvement is usually present. Hypercalcemia in some of these cases may result from the production of osteoclastic stimulating factors which in turn result in local bone resorption adjacent to deposits of tumor cells in bone.[24]

In addition, some tumors, particularly those of the lungs (squamous cell), head and neck, and kidney may produce hypercalcemia in the absence of any obvious metastatic tumor in bone. In these patients, there is evidence of ectopic production of parathyroid hormone (or parathyroid hormone-like substance) or some other factor such as prostaglandins.[25] The management of hypercalcemia with hydration, diuretics, and mithramycin is described in detail in Chapter 5.

CUSHING'S SYNDROME

Cushing's syndrome, due to ectopic secretion of adrenocorticotropic hormone (ACTH) by tumor cells is the second most common endocrinopathy in cancer.[26] The nonadrenal cancers most commonly associated with this syndrome are lung (oat cell carcinoma), pancreatic (islet cell carcinoma or adenocarcinoma), thymic and thyroid (medullary).[38] The onset of the syndrome is usually rapid and may be accompanied by clinical evidence of tumor. Because of this rapid onset, the typical signs and symptoms of Cushing's syndrome such as moon facies, buffalo hump, and striae, fail to appear. Pigmentation is usually present owing to concurrent secretion of lipotropin. Hypokalemia is almost always present and may cause marked weakness and hypokalemic nephropathy. (For further detail see Chap. 5).

SYNDROME OF INAPPROPRIATE ANTIDIURETIC HORMONE SECRETION

In this syndrome, the inappropriate release of ADH by tumor cells results in hyponatremia, increased urinary sodium excretion, and increased urine osmolality (in the face of serum hyposmolality) in the absence of signs of salt depletion.[27] The most common tumors associated with this problem are bronchogenic (predominantly oat cell carcinoma) and pancreatic.[28] Intracranial neoplasms may also cause this syndrome. Both vincristine and Cytoxan can be causes of this syndrome although it is usually seen in untreated tumor patients. Treatment with fluid restriction and tetracycline derivatives is described in Chapter 5, Endocrinology.

ISLET CELL HORMONE SYNDROMES

The islet cell hormone syndromes are all uncommon but are important in the differential diagnosis of a wide variety of symptoms often associated with other surgical diagnoses.[29,30] They include the production of insulin with accompanying hypoglycemia seen in beta cell tumors of the pancreas (insulinoma). Gastrin produced by neoplastic non-beta islet cells results in massive acid secretion in the stomach, multiple ulcerations of the duodenum and stomach, and severe diarrhea—the Zollinger-Ellison syndrome. Rarely, neoplastic islet cell production of vasoactive intestinal peptide (VIP) results in severe watery diarrhea usually associated with hypokalemia (pancreatic cholera syndrome). Carcinoid syndrome with its production of serotonin (5-hydroxytryptamine), kallikrein, and other vasoactive substances by argentaffin tumors of the small bowel, stomach, lung, or pancreatic islets also may result in episodic diarrhea along with flushing and sweating. These syndromes must be kept in mind when evaluating the surgical patient, especially when diarrhea is a predominant symptom or multiple upper gastrointestinal ulcerations are found.

Hematologic Effects of Cancer

ANEMIA

Anemia in the cancer patient may be due to hemorrhage, concurrent presence of infection or uremia (toxic depression), radiotherapy, chemotherapy, tumor invasion of the marrow (myelophthisis), inadequate nutrition, or hemolysis.[31] The work-up of the patient with anemia must include studies which will distinguish between these various types of anemias. Most anemic cancer patients, particularly those with mild anemia, however, will be found to have an anemia of "chronic disease," the pathogenesis of which is still unclear. In this situation, red cells are usually normocytic but may be normochromic or hypochromic. There is a characteristic slight elevation of reticulocyte count that is inappropriately low for the degree of anemia. Plasma iron is low and plasma iron binding capacity is mildly depressed or in the low-normal range. Thus, iron deficiency anemia is distinguished by its characteristic elevation of plasma iron binding capacity. (See Chapter 7, Hematology).

ERYTHROCYTOSIS

Erythrocytosis, a complication of neoplasia and defined as an elevation of red cell mass in the absence of thrombocytosis or leukocytosis, is commonly associated with hypernephroma, hepatoma, cerebellar hemangioblastoma, uterine fibromyoma, and carcinomas of the adrenal, ovary, lung, and thymus.[32] Erythrocytosis is also seen with such benign renal diseases as renal cysts, hydronephrosis, and adenomas.[33] Elevated levels of erythropoietin have been found in serum, urine, and cyst fluid and tumor extracts from such patients, supporting the view that this complication is a hormonally induced response. The erythropoietin production, however, could be secondary to renal hypoxia, particularly in patients with benign tumors of the kidney. Androgenic steroids, particularly in patients with adrenocortical carcinoma, may play a causative role in the development of this syndrome. Its treatment is first and foremost treatment of the underlying tumor. Phlebotomy is usually not necessary for control of the syndrome.

HYPERCOAGULABLE STATES

Migratory thrombophlebitis is observed in some patients with cancer, particularly those with lung, pancreas, or liver cancer.[34] Clinical features are those of a superficial migratory thrombophlebitis which has a modest inflammatory component and tends to be unresponsive to anticoagulants. The axilla, neck, and upper extremities may be involved rather than the lower extremities as is the classical pattern with nontumor associated thrombophlebitis.

Occasionally, cardiac valves may be involved in a similar process leading to a picture of nonbacterial thrombotic endocarditis.[35] Thrombus vegetations may break off, leading to arterial embolization and infarction of the viscera. The mechanism of this syndrome is unknown, although in some patients sporadic observation of increased thrombin or other clotting factors has been noted. The disseminated intravascular coagulopathy (DIC) syndrome is caused by release of thromboplastic substances into the blood stream in patients with tumors.[36] These substances trigger the formation of thrombin. (See Chapter 7, Hematology.)

HEMORRHAGE

Hemorrhage may be associated with metastatic cancer. Thrombocytopenia is frequently signaled by the presence of purpura including both petechiae and ecchymosis, gingival bleeding, hematuria, or gastrointestinal bleeding. The appearance in the peripheral blood of immature red cells and white cells (leukoerythroblastic pattern) with or without thrombocytopenia suggests the presence of bone marrow metastases. Platelet agglutination may also cause this picture. Such a phenomenon may be related to the autoimmune phenomenon triggered by the tumor. In leukemia and lymphoma, hemorrhage is a common cause of death and usually results from the reduction in bone marrow megakaryocytes with secondary thrombocytopenia and also from hypersplenism with platelet lysis and agglutination or inhibition of platelet function. In the former case, platelet transfusion is indicated. These should be initiated only with clinical evidence of bleeding (microscopic hematuria or petechiae) and may have to be repeated every other day until platelet counts above 25,000/mm^3 are observed. Disseminated intravascular coagulation (DIC) with hypofibrinogenemia or fibrinolysins may also be present as in prostatic carcinoma. (See also Chapter 7, Hematology.)

LEUKEMOID REACTION

A leukemoid reaction is defined as a nonleukemic peripheral leukocyte (usually neutrophil) response exceeding about 30,000 and usually accompanied by increased myeloblasts and promyelocytes.[37] Patients with breast, lung, and gastric cancer are most likely to develop the reaction especially if hepatic metastases are present. Marrow aspiration may show mild granulocytic hyperplasia with normal maturation of myeloid elements. Eosinophilia may also occur in a number of malignant diseases, particularly Hodgkin's disease, mycosis fungoides, and lung cancer. It is important to distinguish the eosinophilia of malignant disease from eosinophilic leukemia and/or various benign eosinophilic syndromes. A mild degree of monocytosis occasionally occurs in cancer (up to 15%) and must be differentiated from that in tuberculosis. Occasionally, carcinomas of the colon, stomach, breast, or lung produce a lymphocytic type of leukemoid reaction which can be distinguished from chronic lymphatic leukemia by the absence of splenomegaly, basophila, and Philadelphia chromosome and by the elevation of leukocyte alkaline phosphatase levels.

HYPERVISCOSITY SYNDROME

A hyperviscosity syndrome in neoplastic disease may accompany dysproteinemia.[38] Patients with hyperfibrinogenemia and Waldenström's macroglobulinemia also have a tendency toward thrombosis or hemorrhage. Hyperviscosity may also result from polycythemia or any process such as hypoxia, acidosis, or hypertonicity which tends to increase the rigidity of the red cell membrane. The renal tubular acidosis that may accompany such dysproteinemias[39] may contribute to this effect. Resultant effects include blood stasis and organ infarction. Plasmapheresis or phlebotomy may be beneficial to patients with these symptoms.

Amyloidosis

The development of amyloidosis may be associated with a variety of hematologic neoplasms, principally multiple myeloma or other plasma cell dyscrasias but also occasionally with macroglobulinemia and malignant lymphoma.[13] The common denominator is the synthesis of a monoclonal immunoglobulin or fragment (usually a light chain) by the tumor. This fragment is then incorporated into the amyloid fibril and deposited in a variety of tissues. The most common sites of deposition are liver, kidney, heart, and peripheral nerves although in extensive cases, amyloid is deposited in almost every organ site. Amyloidosis is an important and potentially lethal complication of plasma cell disorders. There is also a group of patients whose clinical presentation may be due to amyloidosis and the underlying plasma cell dyscrasia may be occult. Such patients have a relatively low body burden of tumor, but for unclear reasons, the output of amyloidogenic precursor protein is high and extensive amyloidosis results. It is important to recognize patients with amyloidosis since they are at greater risk during any operative procedure. The prime problems relate to renal and cardiac failure. These patients tend to develop cardiac arrhythmias and are exquisitely sensitive to digitalis which may paradoxically worsen the cardiac failure. In rare patients, circulating anticoagulants have also been described. It is reasonable to carefully evaluate cardiac and renal function and coagulation parameters in such patients.

Hyperuricemia

Elevated uric acid levels and even clinical attacks of gout are common with neoplastic disease.[13] This is related to the high cell turnover rate of tumors and the increased load of released nucleic acids which are metabolized to uric acid. Patients with myeloproliferative disorders are especially at risk but hyperuricemia may accompany lymphomas and chronic lymphocytic leukemia as well. Patients with nonhematopoietic tumors may exhibit hyperuricemia but the degree is usually moderate and gouty attacks are rare.

Hyperuricemia may also result from the treatment of neoplastic disease, particularly with chemotherapeutic agents. An effective cytolytic drug(s) may cause rapid lysis of a large number of tumor cells resulting in a rapidly rising uric acid level. Such a circumstance is usually observed in treatment of leukemias and lymphomas. Hyperuricemia must be recognized and dealt with because it may precipitate a gouty attack and/or cause renal failure if not controlled. For this reason, patients with leukemia-lymphoma receiving initial treatment, concomitantly receive the xanthine oxidase inhibitor, allopurinol, to block the conversion of xanthines to uric acid.

Patients with rapidly rising uric acid levels that are not controlled should not be operated upon until the uric acid has reached a safe level and urine output is maintained. Diuresis, urine alkalization, and uricosuric agents will promote the excretion of uric acid. Patients with established but modestly elevated uric acid levels should be carefully monitored and kept well hydrated during a surgical procedure.

CHEMOTHERAPY RELATED COMPLICATIONS

Patients who are receiving or have received chemotherapy treatment who undergo surgery require special consideration. Cytotoxic therapy, even when administered at a time distant to the surgical procedure, may profoundly influence the surgical risk. The effects of drugs may be those of direct toxicity or indirect via an intermediate mechanism. This section details drug related complications which are important to consider prior to a contemplated surgical procedure.

General Considerations

Virtually all forms of chemotherapy interfere with the ability of cells to proliferate either directly or indirectly. Drugs may interfere with cellular deoxyribonucleic acid (DNA), ribonucleic acid (RNA), or protein synthesis; destroy the mitotic apparatus; or bind to nuclear constituents causing disruption. Many of the newer agents, particularly those derived from bacterial or fungal sources, have extremely complex cellular actions which have not been completely characterized. However, it is obvious that the common denominator is disruption of cells, particularly proliferating cells.

Toxic reactions to virtually every class of drugs can be divided into two large categories. The first category contains the reactions related to effects of the drugs on normal tissues which are rapidly proliferating and hence are more likely to be affected by the particular drug. The bone marrow, skin, and gastrointestinal tract have high turnover rates and are extremely sensitive to the effects of chemotherapeutic agents. One result is the almost universal depression of blood cell counts which may be of quite rapid onset (hours) and persist for months after a dose of a given drug. Interference with normal gastrointestinal physiology results in nausea, vomiting, diarrhea, or even frank mucosal ulceration and hemorrhage. Both of these effects are common in varying degrees to virtually all chemotherapeutic agents in use today. In many circumstances, this form of toxicity is dose limiting and clinically most bothersome and/or potentially life-threatening to the patient. Fortunately, such reactions are usually reversible. The time to reverse this toxicity depends on the pharmacology of the particular drug, particularly its metabolic half-life and tissue distribution pattern. It should be noted, however, that bone marrow and gastrointestinal toxicity may be so severe that it is irreversible and ultimately fatal. A complete blood count, platelet count, and liver function tests should always be assessed preoperatively in all patients taking these drugs, and a knowledge of the anticipated duration of toxic effects is essential.

The second category of adverse reactions includes those which are peculiar to the drug itself. The individual spectrums of drug toxicity are at least partly due to individual patterns of tissue distribution and routes of metabolism and excretion. For instance, a drug which is excreted intact in the urine may exhibit renal or bladder toxicity prior to effects on other organs. Likewise, a drug which is concentrated in skin or lung and excreted slowly from these sites may show prominent skin and lung toxicity. Each drug shows a pattern of specific organ toxicity which is more or less unique. A knowledge of the important specific organ toxicities and their relationship to total drug dosage is vitally important if the additional stress of a surgical procedure is contemplated.

Specific Drug Toxicities

The following commonly used drugs were selected from the more comprehensive list in Table 2 because each has a specific type of toxicity in addition to the usual toxic effects on bone marrow and the gastrointestinal tract. In each instance, the toxicity described has proven to be clinically important and often dose limiting.

ALKYLATING AGENTS

The most commonly used and prototypical alkylating agent is cyclophosphamide (Cytoxan). Other members of this group which are commonly used include nitrogen mustard, melphalan, chlorambucil, and busulfan. These drugs are grouped together since they share a common mechanism of action. Alkylation involves cross linking of DNA

TABLE 2. Chemotherapeutic Agents by Class

			Toxicity			
Chemical Family	*Common Name*	*Route Of Administration*	*Gastrointestinal*	*Hematopoietic*	*Nadir of blood counts (days)*	*Special Toxicity*
Alkylating Agents						
Nitrogen mustards	Nitrogen mustard	Parenteral	4+	4+	(7–15)	
	Melphalan	Oral	1+	4+	(10–12)	
	Cyclophosphamide	Parenteral	3+	4+	(8–14)	Genitourinary lung (pulmonary Fibrosis)
		Oral	1+			
	Chlorambucil	Oral	1+	4+		
Alkyl sulfonates	Busulfan	Oral	1+	4+	(11–30)	Lung (pulmonary fibrosis), pseudoaddisonian syndrome
Triazines	DTIC	Parenteral	3+	4+		
Nitrosoureas	Carmustine (BCNU)	Parenteral	3+	4+	(26–30)	Lung (pulmonary fibrosis)
	Lomustine (CCNU)	Oral	2–3+	4+	(40–50)	
	Streptozotocin	Parenteral	3+	3+		Renal
Antimetabolites						
Anti-folic acid	Methotrexate	Oral Parenteral	4+	4+	(7–17)	Renal, lung (pulmonary fibrosis), liver
Antipyrimidine	5-Fluorouracil	Oral Parenteral	1+	3+	(7–14)	Central nervous system
	Cytosine arabinoside	Parenteral	1+	4+	(12–14)	
Antipurine	6-Mercaptopurine	Oral	1+	4+	(7)	
6-Thioguanine	Oral		1+	4+		
Natural Substances						
Plant alkaloids	Vincristine	Parenteral	1+	0		Neurologic
	Vinblastine	Parenteral	2+	4+	(5–9)	
Antibiotics	Actinomycin-D	Parenteral	4+	4+	(15)	
	Mithramycin	Parenteral	3+	4+		Hypocalcemia
	Daunomycin	Parenteral	3+	4+	(10–14)	Cardiac
	Adriamycin	Parenteral	3+	4+	(10–14)	Cardiac
	Bleomycin	Parenteral	1+	0–1+		Lung (pulmonary fibrosis)
	Mitomycin	Parenteral	3+	4+		

TABLE 2 *Continued*

Chemical Family	Common Name	Route Of Administration	Toxicity: Gastrointestinal	Toxicity: Hematopoietic	Toxicity: Nadir of blood counts (days)	Toxicity: Special Toxicity
Organometallic Compounds						
Platinum complexes	Cis-diaminedichloroplatinum	Parenteral	3+	3+	(3–7)	Renal, ototoxicity
Miscellaneous						
Substituted urea	Hydroxyurea	Oral	2+	4+	(5–7)	
Methylhydrazine derivative	Procarbazine	Oral	2+	3+	(25–36)	
	O, P-DDD	Oral	4+	1+		

1+ = mild
2–3+ = moderate
4+ = severe

base pairs at the guanine residue resulting in disruption of the DNA content of the cell and cell death. Although all cells are susceptible to alkylating agents, proliferating cells are more so.

Cyclophosphamide may be given orally or parenterally. It is metabolized by microsomal enzyme systems in the liver and active metabolites are excreted in the urine. It is not surprising, therefore, that in addition to marrow and gastrointestinal toxicity, genitourinary toxicity is a common problem. The genitourinary lesion is relatively unique consisting of acute hemorrhagic cystitis.[40] This can be a disabling and potentially life-threatening event. Bacterial superinfection and profound blood loss are not uncommon. Patients may require hospitalization and treatment with appropriate antibiotics and blood transfusion. Mild degrees of cystitis are common and not as difficult to manage. It has been shown, however, particularly in children, that the chronic long term use of cyclophosphamide may lead to bladder fibrosis and loss of function. It is thus wise to maintain urine flow at a high level during cyclophosphamide administration and check the urine periodically for evidence of occult cystitis. Fortunately, the toxic effects of cyclophosphamide are among the most predictable and clearly dose related of any drug. Following the last dose, the toxic effects of the drug usually have waned by 10 to 14 days with the nadir in blood count occurring at the end of the first week. Prolonged toxic effects are rare unless there is significant impairment of renal function. Dehydration is to be scrupulously avoided, and a brisk urine output is needed to avoid cystitis.

The toxic effects of the other alkylating agents are listed in Table 2. It should be pointed out that the hematopoietic toxicity of certain other alkylating agents such as melphalan and busulfan may be prolonged, lasting for weeks after the drugs have been discontinued, and they are, therefore, less predictable. Finally, the pulmonary fibrosis seen with cyclophosphamide and busulfan may cause severe impairment and in these patients close attention must be paid to pulmonary toilet and oxygenation.

NITROSOUREAS

The nitrosoureas are a group of naturally occuring and semisynthetic drugs. They have been grouped with the alkylating agents since at least part of their activity is based on the release of moieties which have alkylating activity. The physicochemical property of importance common to these compounds is high lipid solubility. Because of this unique property, these drugs penetrate the blood-brain barrier which is an effective barrier to most chemotherapeutic agents (at conventional dosages). For this reason, these drugs are used to treat brain tumors and meningeal involvement by leukemia or lymphoma.[41] These drugs are given parenterally or orally, depending on the preparation, and are rapidly metabolized, the metabolites being excreted in the urine for many days. It is believed that the binding of these active metabolites and their prolonged clearance are responsible for the major and dose limiting toxicity and delayed bone marrow depression.[40,42] Thrombocytopenia or leukopenia may been seen as late as four to five weeks after the administration of these drugs and may be quite severe. For this reason, these agents are given only once every four to six weeks and blood counts are monitored very carefully. This side effect is particularly hazardous since it is totally unpredictable and not necessarily dose related. The orally active agents, lomustine (CCNU) and Semustine (methyl-CCNU) have widely replaced carmustine (BCNU), which can only be given parenterally and is quite sclerosing to veins. The naturally occurring nitrosourea, Streptozotocin, is used principally to treat malignant pancreatic islet cell tumors since it has unique cytotoxicity for pancreatic islet cells.[43]

ANTHRACYCLINE ANTIBIOTICS (ADRIAMYCIN, DAUNOMYCIN)

Both Daunomycin and Adriamycin (doxorubicinital) are glycosidic anthracycline antibiotics derived from a species of *Streptomyces.* Both drugs have similar physiocochemical properties and toxicity patterns but surprisingly the spectrum of antitumor activity of each is quite different. Whereas, Adriamycin has significant activity in a variety of hematopoietic and nonhematopoietic malignancies, Daunomycin's major antitumor activity is limited to the leukemia-lymphoma group. For this reason, Daunomycin has essentially been dropped in favor of Adriamycin. A great variety of tumors are responsive to Adriamycin and it is widely used as an antineoplastic agent.

Adriamycin is usually given parenterally and is rapidly cleared from plasma. The drug is bound for prolonged periods of time to various tumors and metabolized slowly by the liver. Metabolites are excreted in the bile and a small percentage in the urine. It is apparent, therefore, that pre-existing hepatic impairment requires significant dose reduction. The toxic manifestations of these drugs are of particular interest. Gastrointestinal and hematopoietic toxicity are prominent features which peak at 10 to 14 days. However, these agents are unique in causing significant cardiac toxicity[44,45] which is manifested in two major clinical forms. For two to three days following drug administration, EKG abnormalities may occur which are usually transient and completely reversible. The most common abnormalities observed are supraventricular tachyarrhythmias, ventricular ectopy, and ST-T wave changes. It has been established that up to one-third of all patients receiving these drugs may show this form of acute cardiac toxicity. The more important form of cardiac toxicity is cardiomyopathy. This may be severe or fatal and is totally dose limiting. This syndrome is manifest as varying degrees of "pump" failure which can be refractory to measures usually employed to treat heart failure. Once clinically overt failure occurs, it may be rapidly progressive and fatal. The pathophysiology and clinical manifestations of Adriamycin cardiomyopathy are indistinguishable from other forms of cardiomyopathy. Direct toxicity of drug to cardiac muscle DNA has been postulated as a possible pathogenetic mechanism. However, at least one study has presented evidence that peroxidation of cardiac lipid is necessary to produce cardiomyopathy and this action is totally separate from the drugs antitumor action which interferes with cellular DNA by intercalation.[46] In any case, cardiomyopathy has proven to be a total dose limiting form of toxicity. Since the incidence of serious cardiac toxicity is 1 to 2 percent when the total dose is less than 500 mg/m^2 of body surface area, this is the currently recommended maximum total dose. Above a level of 550 mg/m^2, the incidence of cardiomyopathy may be as high as 30 percent. No reliable predictive test is available. Routine measurement of systolic ejection times may be of some value in detecting early cardiomyopathy prior to demonstrable clinical symptoms. The patient undergoing surgery who has previously received Adriamycin should be watched carefully for the development of heart failure. Central venous pressure or Swan-Ganz catheter monitoring and "cardiac anesthesia" should be employed in these high-risk patients.

ANTIMETABOLITES

These drugs interfere with specific loci in the metabolic sequence leading to DNA synthesis in proliferating cells. The prototype of this class, methotrexate, is a specific inhibitor of the enzyme dihydrofolate reductase thus depleting the pool of reduced folates available for incorporation into the thymidylate molecule. Pyrimidines, along with purine, are the major nucleotide building blocks of the DNA molecule.

Gastrointestinal and marrow toxicity are prominent, relatively short-lived (7 to 14 days) and predictable. Methotrexate has toxicity related to its in vivo metabolism and excretion pathway. Also, when methotrexate is given orally or parenterally, it has a significant enterohepatic circulation, and 90 percent is excreted as the intact molecule in the urine. Hepatotoxicity, common with chronic usage, appears clinically and histologically as a toxic hepatitis which may progress to cirrhosis. Renal toxicity is important and potentially life-threatening. Although renal toxicity is rarely seen at conventional dose levels, the widespread use of the technique of supralethal doses of methotrexate followed by the so-called leukovorin rescue had created significant problems related to renal function.[43] Potential renal injury, presumably due to direct toxicity, is very common at high dose levels and occurs very rapidly. Furthermore, if renal excretion is further impaired by renal injury, marrow and gastrointestinal toxicities may be severe and fatal in spite of attempts at "rescue." No matter what the dose level of methotrexate administered, the urine output must be maintained. In the special circumstance described where extremely high, potentially lethal doses are administered, a brisk, induced diuresis is maintained and carefully monitored until the serum concentration has fallen to a safe level. Since the drug is excreted rather rapidly in the urine, toxic side effects are usually not prolonged (less than two weeks). To avoid side effects, patients taking methotrexate should have a diuresis maintained intraoperatively and postoperatively.

VINCA ALKALOIDS

Vincristine and vinblastine are the two natural plant alkaloids derived from a species of periwinkle. These drugs disrupt the microtubular proteins of the mitotic spindle apparatus resulting in damage to the cell during the mitotic phase of the proliferative cell cycle. Although the two members of this class of drugs are closely related, their toxicities differ widely. Vinblastine has rather conventional marrow and gastrointestinal toxicity while vincristine does not. Vincristine, however, is a very potent neurotoxin. The neurotoxicity of vincristine is the single most prominent toxicity and is dose limiting. Neurotoxicity is manifested principally as a peripheral neuropathy although cranial nerves and autonomic nerves (particularly gastrointestinal) may be prominently involved. The first signs of neuropathy are paresthesias and numbness of the distal extremities. This may progress to loss of reflexes, motor weakness, and neuritic pain. Early lesions are reversible if use of the drug is discontinued. Permanent loss of reflexes and motor weakness is common with prolonged use. Vincristine is also very sclerosing and can only be given intravenously. Its serum half-life is extremely short and the principal route of excretion is the biliary tract. Patients who have received vincristine usually have no specific problems if they require surgery. Those receiving Velban should have preoperative blood counts.

BLEOMYCIN

Bleomycin is the generic name for a mixture of glycopeptides isolated from the fermentation products of a strain of *Streptomyces.* Bleomycin A is the major component of the commercially available preparation. Bleomycin is an extremely interesting agent since it has significant antitumor activity yet lacks the traditional hematopoietic toxicity which has proven dose limiting with most chemotherapeutic agents.[47,48] Similar to many other antibiotic-like compounds, the mechanism of action of bleomycin is complex. It is most likely that bleomycin's toxicity activity is related to disruption of DNA by chain scission and fragmentation. This drug is given parenterally and the metabolic fate is poorly understood. Bleomycin accumulates in certain normal tissues such as skin and lung and also in certain tumors. Other tissues with low concentrations of drug have been shown to possess high concentrations of a peptidase enzyme which rapidly inactivates the drug.[49] Small amounts of the drug are detectable in the urine for as long as one week after administration. Given this metabolic fate, it is not surprising that the major toxic reactions to bleomycin are seen in the skin and lung. Pulmonary toxicity is particularly noteworthy since it may be severe, irreversible, and fatal. The pulmonary toxicity has proven to be dose limiting. The current recommendation is not to exceed a total dose of 400 units of bleomycin. Below this level the risk of serious pulmonary fibrosis is quite low, while above it the risk may be as high as 20 to 30 percent. It is likely, however, that even at lower total doses of drug, some degree of subclinical toxicity and pulmonary fibrosis results. It is wise, therefore, to be cautious about the use of this drug in elderly patients or patients with chronic lung disease. The acute lung toxicity is dramatic and presents as an interstitial pneumonitis which is indistinguishable from other interstitial pneumonitides such as certain bacterial, fungal, or pneumonocystis pneumonias or tumor involvement of the lung.[50] For this reason, the diagnosis of bleomycin lung may be extremely difficult and a lung biopsy may be required to establish a definitive diagnosis. Although corticosteroids have been used to treat blemomycin lung, it is not clear whether they are efficacious. Unfortunately, no diagnostic test is clearly predictive of lung toxicity although pulmonary function tests may detect early interstitial fibrosis. Patients who have received this drug, therefore, may develop considerable respiratory problems in the operative setting and the preoperative pulmonary evaluation and care require special consideration.

CIS-DIAMINEDICHLOROPLATINUM

Cis-diaminedichloroplatinum (cis-DDP) is a member of a group of platinum coordination complexes which have potent antitumor activity in animal and human tumor systems. This new drug has recently enjoyed widespread use in the treatment of testicular, gynecologic, and head and neck cancers.[51]

Cis-DDP is administered as a parenteral infusion and courses are repeated at three to four week intervals. Following an intravenous dose, there is an initial rapid clearance of the drug from the plasma, but there is persistence of significant levels which decline slowly over a four to six day period. The drug is excreted chiefly in the urine and the urinary excretory pattern is also bimodal. Approximately 25 percent of the drug is excreted in the first 24 hours, and about half is recovered in the urine over the first five days. During this period, most of the drug is found to be concentrated in certain organs such as liver, spleen, lungs, and kidneys. The highest levels are seen in kidney.

Cis-DDP has a significant bone marrow, gastrointestinal, and ototoxicity but the major concern is renal impairment. Cis-DDP is extremely nephrotoxic and causes acute tubular necrosis and varying degrees of renal failure in both animals and man, which is dose related. This drug should not, therefore, be administered to individuals with renal impairment. In recent years, it has become clear that renal toxicity may be modified or prevented entirely at therapeutic doses of cis-DDP if some form of diuresis is employed concurrently with drug administration. Various programs currently employ combinations of intravenous hydration and forced diuresis with diuretics, mannitol, or a saline load before and during platinum administration. With such regimens, the incidence of serious nephrotoxicity has been dramatically reduced to acceptable levels. If nephrotoxicity occurs, it may persist for as long as three to four weeks if recovery occurs at all. Renal function, therefore, should be monitored in all patients who have received this drug.[52]

CORTICOSTEROIDS

Prednisone is often included in treatment regimens. Its side effects are discussed in Chapter 5, Endocrinology. It should be remembered that when patients take supraphysiologic doses of this drug for longer than a week, their hypothalamic-pituitary-adrenal axis may be suppressed. If such patients need surgery, they should be "covered" for the stress of surgery like any patient with Addison's disease (see Chap. 5, Endocrinology).

OTHER CHEMOTHERAPEUTIC AGENTS

Many other drugs are commonly used to treat cancer. Their toxicity patterns are not particularly unique and, therefore, are not discussed here in detail but they are listed in Table 2.

Other Drug Effects

In addition to the specific effects outlined above, chemotherapeutic agents have global effects on a great variety of normal physiologic processes. Some of these effects are presented in other chapters and will not be presented in detail here. It should be noted, however, that the areas of concern in surgical patients outlined in Table 3 may be profoundly affected by cancer treatment. These include electrolyte and water balance (particularly urate metabolism), immunodeficiency and infection, and hemorrhage and wound healing. Cytolytic drugs produce these effects indirectly as the result of tumor cell lysis or directly as the result of interference with normal homeostatic mechanisms. It is critical to be aware of potential problems and avoid their development if possible. For instance, if an elective operation is planned in a patient receiving cyclic chemotherapy, the procedure should be performed just *before* the next cycle at a time when the adverse drug effects are at a minimum. In this manner, the likelihood of the drug effecting the surgical course will be minimized. It is wise to remember, however, that some effects such as immunosuppression persist for a long time after use of the drug is discontinued. In such circumstances, there may be an increased risk to the patient undergoing a procedure which has to be considered.

Finally, a question which arises quite often is when to reinstitute drug treatment in a patient who has undergone surgery and use of the drug has been discontinued

TABLE 3. Other Effects of Chemotherapeutic Drugs

Category	*Examples*	*Mechanism*	*Treatment*
Electrolyte and water balance	Dehydration, hypokalemia, hyponatremia, urate nephropathy	Nausea/vomiting, diarrhea, cytolysis	Replacement therapy, allopurinol
Immunodeficiency	Infections	Suppression of T- and B-lymphocyte function	Discontinue drug, specific antibiotics
Hemorrhage	Depressed clotting factors, thrombocytopenia	Interference with synthesis, depressed platelet production	Discontinue drug, specific factor replacement
Wound healing	Dehiscence of wounds	Interference with inflammatory process and collagen formation	Discontinue drug

temporarily. In order to answer such a question, one has to consider both the potential toxic side effects of the drug(s) and the type of surgery involved. In general, since the potential for gastrointestinal toxicity is common, it may be unwise to give drugs in the immediate postoperative period. The result may be wound dehiscence or serious water and electrolyte disturbances. Unless there is urgency concerning reinstitution of treatment, chemotherapy should be delayed for a minimum of 7 to 10 days. When given earlier, the risk increases. With a knowledge of the potential risks and side effects of chemotherapeutic agents and a common sense approach, the vast majority of cancer patients may undergo surgical procedures which are routine in every respect.

REFERENCES

1. Wanebo, HJ, Bhaskar, R, Pinsky, CM, et al.: *Preoperative carcinoembryonic antigen level as a prognostic indicator in colorectal cancer.* N Engl J Med 299:448, 1978.
2. Schultz, H, Sell, A, Nordgaard-Pedersen, B, et al.: *Serum alpha-fetoprotein and human chorionic gonadotropin as markers for the effect of postoperative radiation therapy and/or chemotherapy in testicular cancer.* Cancer 42:2182, 1978.
3. Weintraub, B, and Rosen, S: *Ectopic production of the isolated beta subunit of human chorionic gonadotropin.* J Clin Invest 52:3135, 1973.
4. Baylin, SB, Weisburger, WR, Eggleston, JC, et al.: *Variable content of histaminase, L-dopa decarboxylase and calcitonin in small-cell carcinoma of the lung.* N Engl J Med 299:105, 1978.
5. Posner, J: *Neurologic complication of systemic cancer.* Med Clin North Am 55:625, 1971.
6. Horenstein, S: *Distant effect of neoplasms on the nervous system.* Postgrad Med 50:85, 1971.
7. White, WA, Patterson, RH, Jr, and Bergland, RM: *Role of surgery in the treatment of spinal cord compression by metastatic neoplasm.* Cancer 27:558, 1971.
8. Pochedly, C: *Neurologic manifestations in acute leukemia.* N.Y.S. Med. J. I:575, II:715, III:878, 1975.
9. Brain, RL, and Norris, FH, Jr (eds.): *The Remote Effects of Cancer in the Nervous System.* New York: Grune & Stratton, 1965.
10. Curries, S, Henson, RA, Morgan, HG, et al.: *The incidence of nonmetastatic neurologic syndromes of obscure origin in the reticuloses.* Brain 93:629, 1970.
11. Ultmann, JE, and Moran, E: *Clinical course and complications in Hodgkin's disease.* Arch Intern Med 131:332, 1973.
12. Fukuhara, N, Takamori, M, Gutman, L, et al.: *Eaton-Lambert syndrome: ultrastructural study of the motor end-plates.* Arch Neurol 27:67, 1972.
13. Mills, JA: *A spectrum of organ systems that respond to cancer: the joints and connective tissue.* Ann NY Acad Sci 230:443, 1974.
14. Epstein, O, Ajdukiewicz, AB, Dick, R, et al.: *Hypertrophic osteoarthropathy: clinical, roentgenologic, biochemical, hormonal and cardiorespiratory studies and review of the literature.* Amer J Med 67:88, 1979.
15. Anderson, B, Philpott, GW, and Ferguson, TB: *The treatment of malignant pleural effusions.* Cancer 33:916, 1974.
16. Fredrickson, RT, Cohen, LS, and Mullins, CB: *Pericardial windows or pericardiocentesis for pericardial effusions.* Amer Heart J 82:158, 1971.
17. Walter, L, Jr: *Effects of cancer on nutrition.* Cancer 43:2020, 1979.
18. Theologides, A: *Cancer cachexia.* Cancer 43:2004, 1979.
19. DeWys, WD: *Anorexia as a general effect of cancer.* Cancer 43:2013, 1979.
20. Harvey, KB, Bothe, A, Jr, and Blackburn, GI: *Nutritional assessment and patient outcome during oncological therapy.* Cancer 43:2065, 1979.
21. Waterhouse, C: *Nutritional changes in patients with cancer.* Int J Radiat Oncol Biol Phys 1:521, 1976.
22. Copeland, EM, III, Daly, JM, Ota, DM, et al.: *Nutrition, cancer, and intravenous hyperalimentation.* Cancer 43:2108, 1979.

23. TASHJIAN, AH: *Tumor humors and the hypercalcemia of cancer.* New Engl J Med 290:905, 1974.
24. MUNDY, GR, RICK, ME, TURCOTTE, R, ET AL.: *Pathogenesis of hypercalcemia in lymphosarcoma cell leukemia: role of an osteoclast activating factor-like substance and a mechanism of action for glucocorticoid therapy.* Am J Med 65:600, 1978.
25. BESARAB, A, AND CARO, JF: *Mechanism of hypercalcemia in malignancy.* Cancer 41:2276, 1978.
26. WOLFSEN, A, AND ODELL, WD: *ProACTH: use for early detection of lung cancer.* Am J Med 66:765, 1979.
27. BARTTER, FC, AND SCHWARTZ, WB: *Syndrome of inappropriate secretion of antidiuretic hormone.* Am J Med 42:790, 1967.
28. BAUMAUN, GL, EZEQUIEL, LA, AND DINGMAN, JF: *Plasma arginine vasopression in the syndrome of inappropriate ADH secretion.* Am J Med 52:19, 1972.
29. WALSH, JH, TOMPKINS, RK, TAYLOR, IL, ET AL.: *Gastrointestinal hormones in clinical disease: recent developments.* Ann Intern Med 90:817, 1979.
30. NATHANSON, L: *Remote Effects of Cancer on the Host,* in HORTON J, AND HILL, GJ (ed.): *Clinical Oncology* Philadelphia: W.B. Saunders, 1977, pp. 49–85.
31. CROWTHERS, D, AND BATEMAN, CJT: *Hematological aspects of systemic disease-malignant disease.* Clin Hematol 1:447, 1972.
32. THORLING, EB: *Paraneoplastic erythrocytosis and inappropriate erythropoietin production.* Scand J Hematol (Suppl.) 17:1, 1972.
33. MURPHY, GP, BRENDLER, H, AND MIRAND, EA: *Erythropoietin release from renal cell carcinomas grown in tissue culture.* Res Commun Chem Pathol Pharmacol 1:617, 1970.
34. DEYKIN, D: *Thrombogenesis.* New Engl J Med 283:636–644, 1970.
35. ROSEN, P, AND ARMSTRONG, D: *Nonbacterial thrombotic endocarditis in patients with malignant neoplastic disease.* Am J Med 54:23, 1973.
36. COLMAN, RW: *Disseminated intravascular coagulopathy.* Am J Med 52:679, 1972.
37. WEICK, JK, HAGEDORN, AB, LINMAN, JW: *Leukoerythroblastosis.* Mayo Clin Proc 49:110, 1974.
38. PERKINS, HA, MACKENZIE, MR, AND FRIDENBERG, HH: *Hemostatic defects in dysproteinemias.* Blood 35:695, 1970.
39. MORRIS, RC, AND FUDENBERG, HH: *Impaired renal acidification in patients with hypergammaglobulinemia.* Medicine 46:67, 1967.
40. YOUNG, CW, AND BURIHENAL, JH: *Cancer Chemotherapy.* Ann Rev Pharmacol 11:369, 1971.
41. WALKER, MD: *Nitrosoureas in central nervous system tumors.* Cancer Chemother Rep 4:21, 1973.
42. YOUNG, RC, DEVITA, VT, JR., SERPICK, AA, ET AL.: *Treatment of advanced Hodgkin's disease with* [*l, e bis (2-chloroethyl)-1 nitrosourea*] *BCNU.* N Engl J Med 285:475, 1971.
43. BRODER, LE, AND CARTER, SK: *Pancreatic islet cell carcinoma. II. Results of therapy with streptozotocin in 52 patients.* Ann Intern Med 79:108, 1973.
44. LIVINGSTON, RB, AND CARTER, SK: *Single Agents in Cancer Chemotherapy.* New York: Plenum Press, 1970.
45. BLUM, RH, AND CARTER, SK: *Adriamycin. A new anticancer drug with significant clinical activity.* Ann Intern Med 80:249, 1974.
46. MEYERS, CE, MCGUIRE, WP, LESS, RH, ET AL.: *Adriamycin: the role of lipid peroxidation in cardiac toxicity and tumor response.* Science 197:165, 1977.
47. YAGODA, A, MUKHERJI, B, YOUNG, C, ET AL.: *Bleomycin, an antitumor antibiotic. Clinical experience in 247 patients.* Ann Intern Med 77:861, 1972.
48. RUDDERS, RA: *The treatment of advanced malignant lymphomas with bleomycin.* Blood 40:317, 1972.
49. UMEZAWA, H: *Natural and artificial bleomycins, chemistry and antitumor activity.* Presented at the Symposium on Antibiotics IVPAC Medicinal Chemistry Section, Ste-Marguerite, Quebec, Canada, March 1–3, 1971.
50. RUDDERS, RA, AND HENSLEY, GT: *Bleomycin: pulmonary toxicity.* Chest 63:626, 1973.
51. *Proceedings of the Third International Symposium on Platinum Corrdination Complexes in Cancer Chemotherapy.* J Clin Hematol Oncol 7: no 1 and 2, 1977.
52. MADIAS, N, AND HARRINGTON, JT: *Platinum nephrotoxicity.* Am J Med 65:307, 1978.

Chapter 11

PSYCHIATRY

Richard S. Blacher, M.D., and
Mark E. Molitch, M.D.

The psychologic fears of the person undergoing surgery may not be fully appreciated by his medical attendants. The risks of anesthesia, exploration, mutilation, and even death, as imagined by the patient often far exceed the realistic dangers involved, yet the patient usually does not share his concerns with his physicians. Indeed, some patients who seem quite calm and contained clinically may reveal a level of anxiety close to psychosis upon psychologic testing.[1] Even routine procedures such as herniorrhaphy may mean something far different to the patient than to the physician, and the latter's assumption that certain medical information is common knowledge may hinder communication between physician and patient. Thus, one sees patients who may avoid herniorrhaphy for fear of losing their testes—not so strange a fear, since scrotal examination is used in the diagnosis—yet not reveal their reason to the physician. After such an operation, numerous patients have asked us, "What did they find?" indicating a concern over cancer, a diagnosis obviously not entertained by the surgeon. Most patients are concerned over the exploratory aspect of any procedure, especially surgery, a concern often not shared by the physicians, since they know that various serious and malignant conditions are not even remotely considered in the many situations. Yet their very confidence may contribute to a lack of understanding of the patient's real worries.

Anesthesia is an obvious hazard in the patient's view, and the assurance that he will be "put to sleep" may not be calming. Anticipation of the loss of self-control may be especially trying to some subjects.

From the patient's perspective there is no such thing as "minor" surgery. While most physicians appreciate the general fears of mutilation, exploration, and death, it must be remembered that each patient brings his own personal, past experiences to the situation, which may color the entire picture.

> A 27-year-old woman with intestinal obstruction secondary to a long-standing duodenal ulcer refused surgery. This had been unanticipated because of her willingness in undergoing several previous, successful operations—a cholecystectomy and caesarean delivery. Investigation of her history revealed that although she had told her physician that her father had had leukemia, he had in fact died during surgery for stomach cancer. She connected her own situation to his. Once time was spent clarifying the situation and reassuring the patient, she was able to accept the operation.

It is interesting that this patient had not revealed the true story to her surgeon, since she felt that by telling it she would be criticizing surgeons in general and she did not want to offend her own surgeon whom she liked. Patients often seem to find it easier to express their apprehensions about surgery to an internist, and this is not surprising for several reasons. First, the internist may be the primary physician with whom the patient has a long-standing relationship. Second, the fact that the internist does not wield the scalpel may make talking about the anxieties relating to surgery easier for the patient, as the patient often worries that such anxieties may offend the surgeon—as if the latter's skills were being doubted.

The three periods of surgery—preoperative, intraoperative, and postoperative—present different problems in psychological management as well as medical management. This chapter will discuss psychological management in each of these periods.

THE PREOPERATIVE PERIOD

The length of the preoperative period varies from virtually none in emergency situations with no time for psychologic preparation to lengthy periods with long drawn-out work-ups with their own attendant hazards. It is the impression of many experienced surgeons that patients who have undergone emergency surgery have more postoperative complications and difficulties than those who have had reasonable preparation and not only because optimal physiologic balance had been reached. The sudden necessity for accepting a major change in the image of one's body—either internal or external—may be difficult for some patients.

On the other hand, a protracted wait for major, somewhat elective surgery brings its own hazards. The optimal time is usually quite individual, depending on the patient's ability to live in a state of suspended animation. Thus a noted cardiac surgeon reported that when his own catheterization revealed to him the necessity for coronary bypass, he called in his team immediately and had his surgery performed the same day.[2] Although few patients would have the opportunity to exercise such a choice, not many would opt for such a rapid decision. Most patients require some time—often days or weeks—to accept such a procedure, and the time involved may be determined not only by the patients' personality and tolerance for waiting (balanced by the fear of surgery) but by the length and extent of symptoms and disability as well.

Paradoxically, if a disability has been long accepted, some intrapsychic rearrangement may be required before the patient can accept an operation that may return him to normal functioning. Having adjusted to the disability, the patient must now readjust. In some cases, the patient may have eagerly embraced the limitations imposed by his condition—almost as if receiving an honorable discharge from previous obligations. In such cases, repair of the defect may be experienced partly as an imposition, and the patient may have so much ambivalence as to render rehabilitation almost impossible despite the most enthusiastic efforts by his doctor. These cases are, of course, extremely frustrating.

Patients with the history of a serious psychiatric breakdown in the past invariably arouse the anxieties of their medical attendants. However, it has long been observed that patients with chronic, severe, psychologic difficulties may surprisingly function better than usual during serious illness. We have also seen this seemingly paradoxical reaction in patients admitted for surgery. These patients almost always weather a surgical experience without any untoward psychologic difficulties and require no special attention besides reference to the effects of the medication they may be taking.

Management of the Patient Taking Chronic Psychiatric Medications

The medications being taken by psychiatric patients present a problem that is best dealt with by joint consultation among the anesthesiologist, surgeon, internist, and psychiatrist. Since minor tranquilizers, phenothiazines, and lithium have profound physiologic effects, their use in the perioperative period must be evaluated carefully. Obviously, the primary emphasis must be on getting the patient safely through the anaesthesia and surgery.

MINOR TRANQUILIZERS AND SLEEPING PILLS

The benzodiazepines—diazepam (Valium), chlordiazepoxide (Librium), chlorazepate (Tranxene), clorazepate monopotassium (Azene), lorazepam (Ativan), oxazepam (Serax), and prazepam (Verstran, Centrax)—are the most widely prescribed medications in the United States and up to 15 percent of patients admitted to general medical and surgical services may be taking such medications.[3] These drugs are relatively free of side effects, the principal one being sedation, especially in the elderly, although ataxia may occur. There may also be a central nervous system (CNS) depressant effect, especially when other medications which are CNS depressants are given.[4, 5] Narcotics should therefore be given cautiously to such patients preoperatively. Unless the dosage of the chronic medication is very high or the length of use greater than four months, the abrupt discontinuation of these drugs will usually result in only a mild increase in anxiety. Therefore, they can be discontinued at the time of surgery and may be reinstituted if needed when the patient is again able to take medications orally. Withdrawal when doses are high or the period of use is longer than four months should be done under the guidance of a psychiatrist.

Meprobamate is less often used than the benzodiazepines for the treatment of anxiety states, but it is still prescribed fairly frequently. Although sedation is the most common side effect, marked cardiorespiratory depression has been reported with the

MEPROBAMATE WITHDRAWAL

drug,[4] especially when additional CNS depressants are given. Meprobamate may also induce hepatic microsomal drug metabolizing enzymes[6] and, therefore, larger doses of anticoagulants and analgesics may be needed in such patients. If meprobamate is stopped abruptly in the hospital, a mild abstinence syndrome may develop similar to that for barbiturates (see below). However, if the daily dose is greater than 2 g severe withdrawal symptoms such as hallucinations, anxiety, tremors, and grand mal seizures may occur within 36 to 48 hours of withdrawal.[7] To avoid precipitating a withdrawal syndrome in such patients in the perioperative period, they should be placed on a barbiturate such as pentobarbital which can be given in doses of 150 to 400 mg. every 6 hours.[8] The dosage should be increased if there is tremulousness, weakness, insomnia, and orthostatic hypotension or decreased if there are signs of intoxication (slurred speech, nystagmus, ataxia, sedation).[8] Once the patient is stabilized on this dosage and stable postoperatively the dose of pentobarbital can be reduced by 100 mg/day.[8] If symptoms of withdrawal take place, further reduction in dosage should be halted for 24 to 48 hours.[8] The substitution of pentobarbital can also be used for patients taking large doses of other sedatives and hypnotics such as methaqualone (Quaalude), glutethimide (Doriden), and ethchlorvynol (Placidyl). The actual withdrawal is best carried out under the supervision of someone experienced in the handling of such patients.

The barbiturates are even less commonly used as anxiolytic agents, but are still commonly employed as hypnotics. The barbiturates are direct central respiratory depressants and in high doses can also suppress hypercapneic and hypoxic respiratory drives.[7] Great caution should be used when these drugs are employed in patients with preexisting respiratory impairment or when other CNS depressants are added. As with meprobamate, barbiturates induce production of hepatic microsomal enzymes, resulting in accelerated metabolism of analgesics, anticoagulants, some antibiotics, and many other drugs, so that with concomitant administration, increased dosages may be needed and, with discontinuation of the barbiturate, decreased dosages may be needed. Patients using barbiturates chronically often develop physical dependence on these drugs. The abrupt withdrawal of barbiturates upon admission to the hospital or with surgery may precipitate a withdrawal syndrome which may vary from tremulousness, weakness, anxiety, and insomnia to grand mal seizures and delirium, depending upon the degree of dependence. These symptoms normally develop within 24 hours and may last up to four to eight days. Delirium, agitation, and fever may appear between days four to seven, thus mimicking an occult postoperative infection. Untreated, the barbiturate withdrawal syndrome can be fatal. Because of this withdrawal syndrome, patients who receive the equivalent of 0.6 gm of pentobarbital or greater daily should have their barbiturates continued into the postoperative period. They then can be withdrawn from barbiturates if desired by the method outlined above for meprobamate and other sedatives. Lower daily doses of barbiturates do not usually result in significant withdrawal symptoms and barbiturates need not be continued postoperatively.

NEUROLEPTIC AGENTS (ANTIPSYCHOTIC DRUGS)

There are several different drugs in this category and their effects on the patient going to surgery vary (Table 1). Patients receiving such drugs chronically will often carry

TABLE 1. Common Side Effects of Neuroleptic Agents*

Chemical Name (Trade Name)	Usual Oral Dosage (mg/day)	Relative frequency of major side effects: Sedative Activity	Orthostatic Hypotension	Anticholinergic Activity	Extrapyramidal Effects
PHENOTHIAZINES					
Aliphatic Compounds					
Chlorpromazine (Thorazine)	100–1,600	High	High	High	Intermediate
Piperidine Compounds					
Mesoridazine (Serentil)	100–400	High	High	High	Intermediate
Thioridazine (Mellaril)	100–800	High	High	High	Low
Piperazine Compounds					
Fluphenazine (Permitil, Prolixin)	2.5–20	Low	Low	Low to intermediate	High
Perphenazine (Trilafon)	8–64	Low	Low	Low to intermediate	High
Trifluoperazine (Stelazine)	5–60	Low	Low	Low to intermediate	High
THIOXANTHENES					
Aliphatic Compounds					
Chlorprothixene (Taractan)	100–600	High	High	High	Intermediate
Piperazine Compounds					
Thiothixene (Navane)	5–60	Low	Low	Low	High
BUTYROPHENONES					
Haloperidol (Haldol)	2–100	Low to intermediate	Low	Low	High
DIHYDROINDOLONES					
Molindone (Lidone, Moban)	50–225	Low	Low	Low	Intermediate
DIBENZOXAZEPINES					
Loxapine (Loxitane)	50–250	Intermediate	Intermediate	Intermediate	High

*Modified from Bernstein, J. G.[10]

diagnoses of schizophrenia, mania, psychotic depression, senile dementia, and organic brain syndrome. Although some of these drugs cause sedation with chronic usage, this is not a major problem.

Of greatest concern preoperatively is the effects of these drugs on the cardiovascular system. Orthostatic hypotension is common as a result of direct alpha-adrenergic blockade in the vessel walls and an inhibition of centrally mediated autonomic pressor reflexes.[9] Supine blood pressure may also be lowered.[10] Chlorpromazine, thioridazine, and chlorprothixene are the worst offenders in this regard.[10] The phenothiazines also have a direct depressant action on the myocardium and papillary muscle and have antiarrhythmic properties that are similar to those of quinidine.[9]

Characteristic changes in the electrocardiogram consist of P-R and Q-T prolongation, decreased T wave amplitude, ST segment depression, prominent U waves, and QRS prolongation in high dosages.[9] Additionally, several patients have been reported with ventricular and supraventricular tachycardia, ventricular fibrillation, premature ventricular contractions, AV conduction disturbances, and heart failure due to these drugs.[9, 11] Through their anticholinergic and hence vagolytic effects these drugs may also give rise to a resting tachycardia. Thus the patient going to surgery who is receiving these agents appears to be, at least theoretically, at increased risk for hypotension, congestive heart failure, or arrhythmias and should be monitored closely intraoperatively and postoperatively. It should be noted, however, that major adverse cardiac effects are very uncommon. Should hypotension develop, the best therapy would be intravenous fluids, preferably guided by pulmonary wedge pressure measurements; norepinephrine or methoxamine should be used if fluid administration fails to raise the blood pressure.[9] Ventricular arrhythmias should be treated in the same fashion as quinidine induced arrhythmias with lidocaine.[9] A temporary pacemaker may be needed for phenothiazine induced conduction difficulties.[9] Heart failure should respond to digitalis and diuretics.[9] Hemodynamic and cardiac depressant effects are far fewer with haloperidol, although hypotension may still be a problem.[10] An additional uncommon problem is that chlorpromazine and perhaps some of the other phenothiazines may reverse the antihypertensive properties of guanethidine.[6] The phenothiazines generally have a synergistic effect with narcotic analgesics both on analgesia and on respiratory depression.[7]

The phenothiazines have other noncardiovascular properties that may cause problems for patients going to surgery. All of these drugs can produce anticholinergic effects, that is, blurred vision, dry mouth, tachycardia, constipation, and urinary retention. Fecal impaction and even paralytic ileus may been seen,[5] perhaps causing confusion in patients with abdominal pain or after intra-abdominal surgery. Rarely, phenothiazine treatment causes an abnormality of temperature regulation resulting in an inability to maintain normal body temperature in the face of heat or cold.[12] In hot environments or with strenuous exercise (e.g., with a grand mal seizure), phenothiazine induced adrenergic and cholinergic blockade may cause impairment of cutaneous heat elimination resulting in severe hyperpyrexia.[12] On the other hand, chlorpromazine may facilitate cooling in patients with severe hyperpyrexias due to infection, general anesthesia, or CNS disorders, probably by direct effects on hypothalamic temperature control areas.[12]

All of these drugs also produce extrapyramidal side effects. Acute dystonic reactions will almost always occur within the first four days of therapy and are not usually a problem in chronic use; such reactions will usually respond to diphenhydramine (Benadryl) or diazepam (Valium). A chronic parkinsonian-like state consisting of motor retardation, masked facies, tremor, and rigidity may occur and most such patients will be treated concomitantly with an antiparkinsonian drug such as benztropine, procyclidine, trihexyphenidyl, orphenadrine, or chlorphenoxamine.[5] Tardive dyskinesia may occur as a late complication of long-term therapy. Phenothiazines may produce a lowering of the seizure threshold but long-term schizophrenics with seizure disorders do not have an increased frequency of seizures when treated with both phenothiazines and anticonvulsants.[5] Therefore, if a new predisposition to seizures develops (e.g., following brain surgery) in a patient on chronic phenothiazine therapy, anticonvulsants should first be added routinely and phenothiazines need not be discontinued. Obviously, if seizures become refractory to usual anticonvulsants then the need for phenothiazines will need to be reassessed. Temperature regulation may also be disrupted in patients taking phenothiazines, but this is rarely of clinical importance.

In general, it is appropriate to continue these drugs into the postoperative period to control psychotic behavior and to avoid any withdrawal symptoms such as insomnia, headaches, nausea, vomiting, abdominal pain, and restlessness. Preparations for intramuscular injection are available for chlorpromazine, promazine, triflupromazine, fluphenazine, perphenazine, trifluoperazine, thiothixene, chlorprothixene, and haloperidol when patients are to have nothing by mouth. Patients who develop congestive heart failure, hypotension, or arrhythmias infraoperatively or postoperatively should have their needs for neuroleptic agents reassessed and these agents should probably be discontinued. Psychiatric consultation would be helpful in this regard.

ANTIDEPRESSANTS

Tricyclic Antidepressants

These agents are commonly used for the treatment of depression and enuresis. The side effects of the six types of tricyclic antidepressants are similar with regard to their effects on the patient going to surgery. Postural hypotension may occur in some patients especially when there is pre-existing cardiovascular disease.[12] The cardiac effects are similar to those of phenothiazines and resemble those caused by quinidine (especially quinidine toxicity). ECG changes occur in about 20 percent of patients[9] and consist of P-R, Q-T, and QRS prolongation, T wave flattening, and ST segment depression, although such changes are more likely to occur in patients with pre-existing cardiac disease.[13–16] Atrioventricular conduction defects may also be seen[14,15] and patients with pre-existing bundle-branch block may experience a worsening degree of heart block.[15] A decrease in myocardial contractility may occur with these drugs[15] and congestive heart failure may be precipitated in susceptible individuals.[9,13] In one study of 39 patients with pre-existing cardiovascular disease receiving antidepressant medications, the ratio PEP/LVET (pre-ejection period/left ventricular ejection time) was significantly prolonged.[16] Supraventricular and ventricular arrhythmias may occur[9,11] but are not common at therapeutic dosages. There have also been reports of myocardial infarction and sudden death occurring in patients receiving tricyclic antidepressants but it is difficult to ascribe these events to the drug in most cases.[13,15] However, these studies do serve to emphasize the need for caution in the use of these drugs in older patients with cardiovascular disease. In addition to these effects, the anticholinergic effects of these drugs often give rise to a modest resting tachycardia. Although there is no specific data on the risk of patients receiving antidepressants going to surgery, it may be assumed that they will be at a mildly increased risk for hypotension, congestive heart failure, and arrhythmias which should be managed as discussed for the phenothiazines.

The tricyclic antidepressants all have anticholinergic properties that may give rise to decreased peristalsis, constipation, and even an ileus.[12] Urinary retention and blurring of vision may also occur.[12] Tricyclics may also lower the seizure threshold in susceptible individuals and can cause a fine tremor and tardive dyskinesia.[14]

The tricyclic antidepressants block the action of antihypertensive agents such as methyldopa and clonidine, which act centrally at the level of the alpha receptor, and guanethidine, which acts peripherally. Conversely, the antihypertensive agents propranolol and metoprolol may interfere with the action of the antidepressants.[14] Tricyclics in combination with lithium can cause postural hypotension, tremor, and seizures. When tricyclics are given to patients taking oral anticoagulants, an increased anticoagulant effect may occur, necessitating lowered doses of the anticoagulant.[14] If pressor amines are used intraoperatively or postoperatively an exaggerated blood pressure response may occur.[7] Additive cardiotoxicity may occur if tricyclics are used along with quinidine, procainamide, or disopyramide.

The patient receiving tricyclic antidepressants should either have the drug continued into the postoperative period or tapered off with psychiatric consultation over the few weeks prior to elective surgery. The abrupt discontinuation of tricyclic drugs may precipitate a withdrawal syndrome, consisting of malaise, chills, coryza, and muscle aching.[7] In the older individual who may have some pre-existing heart disease, it would seem prudent to taper off and discontinue the drugs prior to anesthesia and surgery to avoid cardiovascular complications.

Monoamine Oxidase Inhibitors

Monoamine oxidase (MAO) inhibitors are still used to treat some patients with depression. Pharmacologically they act to block the oxidative deamination of catecholamines and serotonin, resulting in increased intracellular amine levels, and many of the side effects have to do with the build up of catecholamines. The most severe side effect is orthostatic hypotension and these drugs have been used as antihypertensive agents. Usually the postural hypotension is not associated with a tachycardia, and there is a decrease in cardiac output with occasional fluid retention.[17] These effects on blood pressure and cardiac output may last for several days after discontinuation of the medication.[7,14,17] These drugs also have anticholinergic side effects such as dry mouth, blurred vision, urinary retention, and constipation similar to those discussed above for the phenothiazines and tricyclic antidepressants.[14] Convulsions have also been reported.[7]

Because of their interference with the amine oxidases, these drugs have important interactions with many drugs that may be given in the perioperative period. Use of all sympathomimetic agents must be avoided in patients receiving MAO inhibitors to avoid hypertensive crisis, fever, and cardiac arrhythmias. Such drugs include the sympathomimetic agents found in cold remedies and decongestants, tricyclic antidepressants, amphetamines, antihistamines, methylphenidate (Ritalin), L-dopa, bronchodilators used in intermittent, positive pressure breathing (IPPB) machines, the respiratory stimulant doxapram, and any catecholamine or catecholamine releaser used for blood pressure support such as norepinephrine, epinephrine, dopamine, isoproterenol, and ephedrine.[13,18] Special mention must be made of meperidine (Demerol) which can cause hypertensive crisis, seizures, and coma when given to patients receiving these drugs. Dextromethorphan, a meperidine analog commonly used as an antitussive in cold remedies, may also cause severe fever, seizures, and cerebral hypoxia.[18] The amine tyramine is capable of liberating stored catecholamines and is contained in some cheeses, beer, wine, pickled herring, coffee, yeast, chicken liver, bean pods, and canned figs. Such foods must be eliminated from the patient's diet. Hypertensive crises that occur with such drug combinations should be treated with the alpha-adrenergic blocking agent phentolamine intravenously as if treating a patient with a pheochromocytoma (see Chapter 5, Endocrinology). Cardiac arrhythmias should be treated with propranolol. Chlorpromazine may be useful for severe hypertension. MAO inhibitors may block the antihypertensive effect of guanethidine and alpha methyldopa.[18]

In addition to the effects described above which are due to the interference with catecholamine metabolism, MAO inhibitors also inhibit hepatic microsomal enzymes, resulting in delayed metabolism and therefore increased activity of oral hypoglycemic agents, barbiturates, sedatives, narcotics, anticoagulants, and succinylcholine.[18] A patient receiving MAO inhibitors should have them discontinued three to four weeks prior to any elective surgery, because of the drug interactions described above. The potential hazards of anesthesia induction and the necessity for the anesthesiologist to be able to administer symphathomimetic agents when needed far outweigh the benefits of continuing MAO inhibitor therapy until the time of surgery. If emergency surgery is necessary in a patient taking MAO inhibitors, that patient should be treated as if he had a known pheochromocytoma (see Chap. 5, Endocrinology). Such a patient should have constant ECG and intra-arterial blood pressure monitoring. Phentolamine or nitroprusside must be available for immediate administration via a stopcock and intravenous propranolol and lidocaine should also be available for immediate use for arrhythmias (see Chap. 5).

LITHIUM CARBONATE

Lithium, used in treatment of manic-depressive illness, has a number of potential side effects that may affect the patient going to surgery. Serum levels of lithium determined 12 hours after the last dose should be less than 1.5 mEq/L, the therapeutic range being 0.6 to 1.2 mEq/L.[19] Sodium depletion as a result of salt restriction, fever with excessive perspiration, diarrhea, or use of diuretics can result in renal lithium retention with the accumulation of toxic levels. Toxic levels may result in nausea, diarrhea, vomiting, head tremor, ataxia, rigidity, muscle twitching, and slurred speech. Severe toxicity may lead to aphasia, seizures, coma, cardiovascular collapse, and death, serum lithium levels usually being over 2 mEq/L.

Therapeutic levels of lithium may cause T wave depression on ECG.[20] Arrhythmias resulting from lithium are extraordinarily rare but premature ventricular contractions (PVCs) have been reported in one patient and reversible sinus node abnormalities in two.[20,21] Toxic levels of lithium rarely affect the cardiovascular system, transient T wave abnormalities occurring on ECG and borderline hypotension also being a problem.[20] Cardiovascular collapse may occur in cases of fatal toxicity where the symptoms are predominantly neurologic.[20] Therefore, as long as lithium levels are normal and there is no sign of neurologic toxicity, lithium appears to have little cardiovascular toxicity in individuals with or without heart disease. However, the development of congestive heart failure with decreased renal perfusion on the implementation of dietary salt restriction or diuretic therapy may cause lithium retention and toxicity.

Lithium may cause a nephrogenic diabetes insipidus (DI) at lithium levels within the therapeutic range.[22] Such patients are unable to concentrate their urine and, if unable to adjust their intake appropriately (e.g., intraoperatively or postoperatively), they may develop severe dehydration and hypernatremia. Such patients will need to have their intravenous administration of free water adjusted to match this augmented output (see Chap. 5). Although this nephrogenic DI is normally reversible, it may not be in every case.[23] In addition to the well-described nephrogenic DI, lithium may have other toxic effects on the renal tubules, glomeruli, and interstitium resulting in decreased glomerular filtration, but studies of these effects are not conclusive.[23]

Lithium therapy interferes with thyroid adenyl cyclase activity resulting in hypothyroidism in 5 to 10 percent of patients.[24] Because of this, thyroid function should be checked in all patients on chronic lithium therapy and if hypothyroidism is found, it should be managed similarly to other varieties of hypothyroidism (see Chap. 5). Lithium has also been shown to cause elevations in calcium, magnesium, and parathyroid hormone in some individuals.[19]

Of importance in the surgical patient is the neutrophilic leukocytosis that occurs[19] since this may cause confusion with respect to infection or perforation of a viscus and so forth. Lithium also may potentiate the action of anesthetics and muscle relaxants so that lower doses of these agents should be employed.[25] Haloperidol and phenothiazines may cause extrapyramidal symptoms and even delirium when given in high dosage to patients taking lithium.[19]

Therefore, because chronic lithium therapy has little cardiovascular toxicity, it need not be discontinued prior to surgery, although it should not be given the day of surgery. As noted, anesthetic and neuromuscular blocking agents should be used cautiously. Thyroid and renal function (overnight dehydration test) should be checked preoperatively and careful attention needs to be paid to fluid and electrolyte balance intraoperatively and postoperatively in patients with evidence of partial or complete nephrogenic diabetes insipidus. Should lithium toxicity occur, mild cases can be treated with intravenous hydration with saline and nasogastric suction, since lithium is secreted into the stomach, and osmotic diuretics such as mannitol and acetazolamide. Severe toxicity is treated with hemodialysis or peritoneal dialysis if the former is not available.[19]

Management of the Patient Abusing Drugs

Occasionally, patients who abuse a variety of licit or illicit drugs will need surgery. Such patients may be extremely demanding psychologically and formal psychiatric consultation is often useful in dealing with such patients. In addition, the drug abuse itself may pose problems for the patient and physicians taking care of such patients should remember that they may be taking more than one drug.

BARBITURATE ABUSE

Patients receiving the equivalent of 0.6 gm of pentobarbital daily or more are at risk for severe barbiturate withdrawal syndrome. With short acting barbiturates, symptoms of withdrawal begin in about 12 to 36 hours with seizures occurring within 48 hours. With longer acting barbiturates, seizures might not occur for six to eight days. As discussed earlier, the barbiturate should be continued into the postoperative period and the dose decreased by no more than 20 percent per day, usually 100 mg/day.[8,26] The problems of respiratory depression and hepatic microsomal enzyme induction were discussed earlier. When other sedatives or hypnotics are abused, the patient should be managed as if they had barbiturate abuse (see discussion of meprobamate above).

OPIATE ABUSE

Opiates all produce some degree of respiratory and cough depression which may be additive to the effects of other central nervous system depressants.[27] Severe orthostatic hypotension may occur due to peripheral vasodilatation. Acute opiate overdose should be treated with the opiate antagonist naloxone given intravenously in a 0.4 mg dose,[26] repeating as necessary.

An acute opiate abstinence syndrome may occur within 3 to 4 hours in patients withdrawn from meperidine but only after 8 to 12 hours in patients withdrawn from morphine or heroin. Symptoms begin with anxiety, apprehension, and restlessness and progress to rhinorrhea, lacrimation, vomiting, diarrhea, salivation, perspiration, aching, and piloerection; mydriasis, hyperpnea, fever, and hypertension may occur.[27] The opiate abstinence syndrome should be avoided in the patient requiring surgery or who has other acute medical problems. This may be accomplished by substituting methadone for the narcotic usually used. The dose of methadone depends upon the extent of the prior drug habit. It should be realized that many addicts will exaggerate the extent of their usage to obtain more methadone, and the extent to which "street" heroin is cut with other substances varies from city to city and supplier to supplier. The usual starting dose is 20 mg of methadone two to three times daily, the dose being increased if signs of withdrawal ensue.[28,29] Although the usual route of administration is oral, methadone can also be injected parenterally. If the actual dose of narcotic is known, 1 mg of methadone can be substituted for each 3 to 4 mg of morphine, 1 to 2 mg of heroin, 0.5 mg of hydromorphine, or 20 mg of meperidine.[28] Methadone should be continued into the postoperative period, and the patient then should be referred to a methadone clinic for rehabilitation and management. Unexplained coma in a patient receiving methadone should be assumed to be due to the surreptitious use of heroin until proven otherwise, and treatment with naloxone should be prompt to avoid respiratory depression.

AMPHETAMINE AND COCAINE ABUSE

Excessive doses of either amphetamines or cocaine may give rise to a toxic syndrome characterized by visual, auditory, or tactile hallucinations, picking and excoriation of the skin, and paranoid ideation. Surprisingly, sympathomimetic effects are usually not present.[29] Symptoms of amphetamine withdrawal include fatigue, depression, lethargy, weakness, and hyperphagia. No specific therapy is needed for amphetamine withdrawal, but it should be remembered that these individuals often abuse barbiturates, opiates, and other drugs, and the withdrawal syndromes for these other drugs may need management.

PSYCHEDELIC DRUGS

Patients who have recently received psychedelic drugs may display sympathomimetic features such as hypertension, tachycardia, tremor, piloerection, nausea, weakness, fever; pupillary dilation and hyperreflexia.[8] These findings may prove difficult to distinguish from what may be seen in the patient requiring emergency surgery. Mental status is usually altered. In the face of a threatening situation such as an accident or a forced visit to a hospital emergency room, individuals under the influence of these drugs may develop severe anxiety and tension and may panic.[8] Usually the effects begin to clear in about 12 hours.[8] Mounting anxiety in a patient may best be treated with reassurance and phenothiazines or barbiturate if necessary. No major physiologic disturbances result from the withdrawal of lysergic acid diethylamide (LSD) or other psychedelics.[8] Phencyclidine (PCP, angel dust) is occasionally mixed with marijuana and can produce sympathomimetic symptoms and mental changes similar to those seen with LSD. Excessive muscle activity and agitation resulting in muscle injury and myoglobinuria has been reported with phencyclidine use.[30]

The Immediate Preoperative Period

As the time for surgery approaches, the patient's level of concern often mounts, but then on the eve of the operation, his fears apparently abate. The major preoperative concerns of the patient can usually be alleviated if the staff promotes the feeling that he is in friendly hands. A preoperative visit by the anesthesiologist who will be present at the induction is more calming than sedation[31] and results in a smoother anesthesia with less agent required.

When an event other than his own medical status necessitates rescheduling the operation, the patient's reaction may be quite strong. He has girded himself for the ordeal but now must begin his preparation anew. The staff must realize that his disappointment is often intense, and the greatest tact is required in giving him the news. While most patients can understand the need for performing *emergency* operations in place of their partly elective ones, they cannot be expected to consider any case as more important than their own. We have seen a depression-prone man go into a profound depression when told, "We have to cancel your operation because a more serious case was just admitted."

THE INTRAOPERATIVE PERIOD

Once the patient is anesthetized, there is a tendency to deal with him as oblivious to stimuli, and operating room personnel may talk as if he could not possibly hear anything. Yet this may be far from the case. The anesthetized patient may well register significant statements uttered in the operating suite.[32] By the use of hypnosis, we have been able to recover the exact words of a threatening stimulus given to the patient under deep anesthesia.[33] How these stimuli may affect the patient clinically at a later time is not known and care must be taken to avoid any statements which would be disturbing to the patient if he were fully conscious.

The patients who wake during surgery while paralyzed by curare-like drugs often subsequently develop a syndrome of traumatic neurosis.[34,35] This is marked by (1) repetitive nightmares of a poorly disguised operative situation (e.g., "I'm on a table and people are sticking me with wires"), (2) a preoccupation with death and being buried alive, and (3) a fear of insanity. The patients may be brought to the physician's attention by the nurse who finds such patients wandering around at night seemingly confused. Clarifying to such patients that they were indeed awake during surgery has, in our experience, always resulted in the rapid disappearance of the symptoms.

THE IMMEDIATE POSTOPERATIVE PERIOD

Our cautionary remarks regarding the patient's capacity to understand and remember events occurring during surgery despite the appearance of sedation also apply to the immediate postoperative period in the recovery room. Close observation reveals that a seemingly obtunded patient is easily aroused and is interested in his condition.[36] When approached by strangers, he may exhibit a clear sensorium but a remarkably casual attitude—a manifestation of denial. When his own physician visits, he is usually interested in knowing the outcome of the surgery and is eager for reassurance. Even if the condition is malignant, the patient may want to know and have the chance to begin immediately coming to grips with his new situation.

THE INTERMEDIATE POSTOPERATIVE PERIOD

Organic Mental Difficulties

Every psychic reaction has multiple determinants. Even in clearly "organic" conditions, such as delirium, the patient's behavior may depend upon a variety of psychic factors, the understanding of which may help in management. For example, a 50-year-old woman with a portocaval shunt developed a delirium after surgery and attempted to remove tubes and drains. She was restrained by wrist straps and thereupon became markedly agitated. Her physician learned that as a young child she had been tied into bed while her mother went out, and the restraints had rekindled her early, distressing situation. While she could not be trusted with free access to the equipment, calm and repeated explanations for the restraint resulted in a striking abatement of the agitation. The confusion of such a patient may make it difficult for the patient to evaluate reality and this increases anxiety to a frightening degree by the misjudging of events in the hospital. This anxiety in turn makes the patient's ability to judge even worse, and so a vicious circle is created.

The treatment of organic confusion, aside from correcting the underlying cause, is in good measure psychologic. That is, the patient's environment is made as stable as possible—no or few changes in rooms, the presence of the same nurses and members of the family if possible, and the use of a night light so that there are visual clues rather than the confusion of darkness and strange shadows. Careful explanation of all procedures is very helpful.

That the psychic elements may determine the delirious patient's responses should not surprise us since we know that the response to a cerebral toxin such as alcohol is usually determined more by social demands and expectations than by the blood level of the drug. Thus in an emergency, the inebriated person may act fairly normal, while a few minutes before he had seemed very drunk. In addition, the acute, organically impaired patient is responding emotionally to the loss of his brain function—a most frightening state for most patients. Such patients can be reassured that with medical care they will recover their minds. This comforting observation will often have a dramatically soothing and quieting effect.

The underlying organic cause of the delirium must always be sought as discussed in Chapter 9, Neurology. It is important to underline the fact that an acute delirium may be the first sign of worsening of the patient's medical condition (the development of hypoxia, hyperglycemia, fever, and so forth).[37]

The Intensive Care Unit

The Intensive Care Unit (ICU) may be said to represent the most ambivalent situation in all of medicine for the patient. The patient knows he is there because his life is in danger, and this being the case he knows there is no safer place to be. So he longs for transfer out, as a sign that he is safe, yet fears to leave, lest the close attention be lost. Unscheduled transfer from a cardiac unit may be accompanied by anxiety, increase in catecholamine levels, increased arrythmias, and death.[38] Transfer from surgical units may be accompanied by anxiety also, but since such patients usually are not suffering from damaged myocardia, the outcomes are rarely fatal.

The surgical patient in the ICU is subjected to a rather strange environment. Surrounded by an array of space-age devices which emit sounds and blink lights, he lies immobilized, with tubes and wires inserted in every natural orifice and a number of manmade orifices as well. Often he is unable to speak and thus is unable to let his needs be known to the nurses. It is no wonder that this is a terrifying experience and one dealt with at times by a massive psychic withdrawal from reality into a psychosis. But *overt* psychotic reactions are not the rule, and the so-called "ICU psychosis" seems to depend more on the extent of illness and treatment than on the environment itself.[39,40] In an ICU treating various surgical conditions, it may be only the patients who have undergone open-heart surgery who become openly disturbed—and then only after the danger has passed and the patients are able to contemplate what they have gone through. Of course, such disturbances may be life-endangering, especially since they usually show both organic and psychologic elements and the psychosis may cause the patient to be unable to cooperate in his treatment. Interestingly, whereas delirious patients who have undergone general surgical procedures may remove catheters and intravenous lines, it is almost unheard of for postcardiotomy patients to handle their apparatus—indicating a level of awareness in patients seemingly out of contact with reality.

Treatment of disturbed ICU patients becomes an emergency matter. The most effective and safe therapy is the rapid administration of small, repeated doses of haloperidol until the disturbed behavior subsides. One can safely give 1 to 2 mg doses intravenously (the intravenous route for haloperidol administration has not yet been approved by the FDA) or intramuscularly every 30 to 60 minutes until the agitated patient is calm. This can be done even with elderly people. Higher doses may have to be given to larger and younger patients.

Psychologic Difficulties

The differentiation between organic and purely psychologic difficulties may be arbitrary, depending on the predominance of one or the other aspect, since both factors may be present in the postoperative period. The incidence of gross psychic sequelae to surgery in the form of psychosis varys in different studies from less than 1 percent[41] (when the statistics were gleaned from charts and the patients required psychiatric hospitalization) up to 22 percent[37] (when the patient population was interviewed by psychiatrists). This same contrast in incidence has been noted in a study of cardiac surgery where hidden psychoses were revealed only after careful interviewing.[39] The psychoses follow the usual classification of such disorders and range from organic psychosis to schizophrenia, with the surgery and hospitalization acting as a stressor in a person already vulnerable. From the physician's point of view, such major and obvious upheavals represent a small percentage of the psychic difficulties actually encountered, since such major psychotic reactions may not be overtly present in the patient's behavior in the hospital. However, less clearly defined problems may often present as problems in *medical* management rather than as purely psychologic conditions. Such a situation is seen for example, when depressions are manifested by the patient's inability to eat, to be mobilized, or to follow simple medical regimens. Needless to say, the continuation of such a syndrome may impair the patient's convalescence and lead to various undesirable medical sequelae such as poor wound healing, decubitus ulcers, or thrombophlebitis.

Depressions and Pseudodepressions

Many so-called depressions seen in hospitalized patients are in reality not depressions at all but grief reactions. These occur quite commonly following mutilating procedures and even after the loss of internal organs. The patient may react with a sense of loss to the removal of a body part (e.g., an extremity, breast), a function (e.g., blindness, paralysis), or even to the loss of a sense of bodily integrity (e.g., loss of an internal organ). These bodily losses are the equivalent to the loss of a close person, and a warm, sympathetic, and supportive attitude should be adopted by the staff. These grief reactions are usually self-limited and last a week or two. If they do not spontaneously remit in several weeks, then further exploration may be in order.

The cause of depressions may not be as obvious as that of grief reactions but nevertheless can usually be ascertained. A depression can be distinguished from grief by the latter's appropriateness in response to a loss and by the depression's self-critical quality—at times, to the point of suicidal ideation—and presence of guilt feelings. Grief is usually expressed directly; depression may present via vague physical symptoms or withdrawal accompanied by anorexia, constipation, and insomnia.

TYPES OF DEPRESSION

The Guilty Survivor

A 63-year-old machinist came to the surgeon because of increasing pains in the right arm and shoulder of four weeks duration. He chose to see the surgeon because the latter had performed a pioneer vascular procedure 15 years before and had saved the patient's life. The present pain also required heroic intervention according to the patient. Five years before, his wife had died of a slowly progressive malignancy, and he had suffered along with her.

As the oldest son in an old-fashioned Italian family, he assumed the role of head of the family when his parents died in their forties, and he took this responsibility seriously. One month before, he had buried his youngest brother after a seige of cancer involving the right arm and shoulder. He cried bitterly as he recounted this, saying, "It should have been me instead of him."

This man represents a type of depression that may occur after major surgery. It was clear that his symptoms involved the exact body region and started at the time of his brother's death. He had survived an extremely difficult procedure, but others in the family were not so lucky. This type of depression is not uncommonly seen after heart surgery, especially coronary artery bypass procedures[42] where the patient may be the sole survivor of a family riddled by coronary disease. The patient does not expect to survive, but instead of experiencing joy at coming through safely, he becomes paradoxically depressed. Here, guilt is aroused by the "quantitative view" of death—as if nature demands a certain tribute in the form of lives, and someone else's death can take the place of one's own. That he had survived at the expense of loved ones was felt by the man described above.

Such patients can often be readily treated, when such a history is elicited, by pointing out that the depression is paradoxical, and by expressing a realization that it's difficult to celebrate a victory over illness when people one loved have died of similar illnesses. If applicable, it may help to point out that these procedures were not available in the past when the other person died. Usually, the depression lifts in a short while if treated.

The Fearful Resenter

Another large group of depressed patients suffer from a fear of their own anger. Patients who develop surgical complications such as wound infections and those in whom a procedure is unsuccessful—such as cancer patients with recurrence—may find themselves in an untenable emotional situation. Angry that the doctors have let them down, they are not able to be consciously aware of their resentment since (1) they may genuinely like the surgeon and (2) they may fear that their anger may stimulate a like response from their doctor and a refusal by him to continue treatment. Therefore, their anger turns upon themselves and is seen clinically as a depression. Such patients can often be readily treated by the physician's suggesting that he would understand that they might be resentful at their plight. Such permission to be angry when given early may often abort the depression. Since medical treatments cannot be universally and unqualifiedly perfect, one can expect such depressions in a wide variety of situations.

Other Types of Psychologic Upheavals

Given the terrible stress the surgical patient faces, it is remarkable that we do not see greater numbers of overt psychologic disturbances. Occasionally, we see gross paranoid episodes. A somewhat paranoid patient may respond with paranoia because of stress, but more commonly we see such episodes in nonparanoid patients in the immediate postoperative periods, especially in the Intensive Care Unit.

More far-reaching in their consequences are a number of common but usually hidden psychologic consequences of serious surgical illness. These include a covert type of psychosis that the patient hides from the staff.[39] Quite often this takes the form of the psychotic paranoia mentioned above, that causes the patient to worry about his sanity. This paranoia stems from the fact that while the patient is completely dependent on the nurses for his life, he experiences their ministrations as painful, as indeed they are. Having to breath against a new incision, being moved, receiving injections, and especially having tracheal suction are terribly uncomfortable and the patient would prefer to be left alone. He finds himself becoming angry at the staff, especially the nurses, yet fears this anger and the anticipated retaliation. Instead of experiencing the anger, he may project it and begin to feel that the nurses are trying to kill him. His theme becomes, "I'm not angry at them; they're angry at me." But he tells no one since something in him realizes that his thoughts don't quite make sense. We have found it useful for those preparing the patient for surgery to point out that necessarily uncomfortable procedures will be carried out and that he will not like them. When pain must be inflicted, it is helpful to tell the patient in advance. In this way, he is given permission to be angry without fear of retribution, since he understands that the staff expects some reaction. The dynamics here are similar to those of the patient at a later stage who becomes depressed.

Another source of extreme anxiety is the varying degree of organic mental impairment that the patient may experience following major surgery, especially after heart surgery or the use of consciousness-clouding drugs. For fear of being considered insane, the patient will seek to hide the impairment, or by employing the mechanism of denial, the patient will not allow himself to become aware of the dysfunction. Some patients may become depressed or anxious because of the difficulty but do not voluntarily bring this to the physician's attention. It is worthwhile pointing out the problem and then reassuring the patient that this is a transient phenomenon. Demonstration of the difficulty is carried out by simple mental testing: asking the patient to name the presidents of the country in reverse order, to subtract 7 from 100 and continue subtracting 7s. While the patient may be amazed at this inability, when it occurs, he will be relieved to know that the physician anticipates the difficulty.

REHABILITATION PERIOD

Often the physician is confronted by patients who continue to suffer with disabilities long after what appears to be a successful surgery. Quite often such patients are those who had adjusted (at times eagerly) to a chronic disabling illness. These patients were mentioned above. Perhaps the most vexing problems are those chronically depressed patients who seem never to get better despite the most appropriate treatment. The removal of one cause for complaint is rapidly followed by the appearance of another symptom. Repeated visits to the doctor may eventually evoke irritability in the physician brought on by frustration of his desire to cure. Such patients, often referred to as "crocks"[43] or similar pejorative terms, can only be treated when the physician is willing to lower his therapeutic goals to conform with the patient's need. The doctor wants to heal, but the patient seeks to be treated. Such patients can be relatively successfully treated by the doctor who is willing to let the patient see him when he calls and treats him without enthusiasm. "I don't know if this will help, but we can try it," might be said on giving a prescription. The physician feels he walks a tightrope with such patients, on the one hand not wanting to perform unnecessary tests and procedures and on the other not wanting to miss a treatable organic lesion.

SUMMARY

While surgery may be an everyday occurrence to the medical staff, it is a unique and dramatic experience for the patient. The patient is faced with unfamiliar dangers: anesthesia, the surgery itself, the threat of mutilation or bodily change, the possible discovery of unknown disease, and even death. That most people are able to tolerate the experience with relative equanimity is remarkable; that some experience some degree of psychic decompensation is not strange. The physician's awareness of the patient's plight may well spell the difference between a successful outcome and the unhappy sequelae of slowed recovery, poor rehabilitation, or long-lasting emotional scars.

REFERENCES

1. Meyer, BC, Brown, F, and Levine A: *Observations of the House-Tree-Person Drawing Test before and after surgery.* Psychosom Med 17:428, 1955.
2. *A heart surgeon tells of his own coronary bypass.* Medical World News October 18, 1976, p. 52.
3. Uhlenhuth, EH, Balter, MB, and Lipman, RS: *Minor tranquilizers, clinical correlates of use in an urban population.* Arch Gen Psychiatry 35:650, 1978.
4. Zisook, S, and DeVaul, R: *Prescribing anxiolytics.* Drug Therapy 9:41, 1979.
5. Davis, JM, and Casper, RC: *Side effects of psychotropic drugs and their management,* in Clark, WG, and del Giudice, J (eds.): *Principles of Psychopharmacology.* New York: Academic Press, 1978, p. 479.
6. Haraszti, JS, and Davis, JM: *Psychotropic drug interactions,* in Clark, WG, and del Giudice, J (eds.): *Principles of Psychopharmacology.* New York: Academic Press, 1978, p. 495.
7. Byck, R: *Drugs and the treatment of psychiatric disorders,* in Goodman, LS, and Gilman, A (eds.): *The Pharmacological Basis of Therapeutics,* ed. 5. New York: MacMillan Publishing Co., 1975, p. 152.
8. Jaffe, JH: *Drug addiction and drug abuse,* in Goodman, LS, and Gilman A (eds.): *The Pharmacologic Basis of Therapeutics,* ed. 5. New York: MacMillan Publishing Co., 1975, p. 284.

9. Fowler, NO, McCall, D, Chou, T-C, et al.: *Electrocardiographic changes and cardiac arrhythmias in patients receiving psychotropic drugs.* Am J Cardiol 37:223, 1976.
10. Bernstein, JG: *Prescribing antipsychotics.* Drug Therapy 9:71, 1979.
11. Alexander, CS, and Nino, A: *Cardiovascular complications in young patients taking psychotropic drugs.* Am Heart J 78:757, 1969.
12. VanderKolk, BA, Shader, RI, and Greenblatt, DJ: *Autonomic effects of psychotropic drugs,* in Lipton, MA, DiMascio, A, and Killam, KF (eds.): *Psychopharmacology: A Generation of Progress.* New York: Raven Press, 1978, p. 1009.
13. Jefferson, JW: *A review of the cardiovascular effects and toxicity of tricyclic antidepressants.* Psychosom Med 37:160, 1975.
14. Rosenbaum, AN, Maruta, T, and Richelson, E: *Drugs that alter mood. Tricyclic agents and monoamine oxidase inhibitors.* Mayo Clin Proc 54:335, 1979.
15. Bigger, JT, Jr, Kantor, SJ, Glassman, AH, et al.: *Cardiovascular effects of tricyclic antidepressant drugs,* in Lipton, MA, DiMascio, A, and Killam, KF (eds.): *Psychopharmacology: A Generation of Progress.* New York: Raven Press, 1978, p. 1033.
16. Burckhardt, D, Raeder, E, Muller, V, et al.: *Cardiovascular effects of tricyclic and tetracyclic antidepressants.* JAMA 239:213, 1978.
17. Nickerson, M, and Ruedy, J: *Antihypertensive agents and the drug therapy of hypertension,* in Goodman, LS and Gilman, A (eds.): *The Pharmacologic Basis of Therapeutics,* ed. 5. New York: MacMillan Publishing Co., 1975, p. 705.
18. Marco, LA, Randels, PM, and Sexauer, JD: *A guide to drug interactions with psychotropic agents.* Drug Therapy 9:45, 1979.
19. Rosenbaum, AH, Maruta, T, and Richelson, E: *Drugs that alter mood, II Lithium.* Mayo Clin Proc 54:401, 1979.
20. Tilkian, AG, Schroeder, JS, Kao, JJ, et al.: *The cardiovascular effects of lithium in man.* Am J Med. 61:665, 1976.
21. Wilson, JR, Kraus, ES, Bailas, MM, et al.: *Reversible sinus-node abnormalities due to lithium carbonate therapy.* N Engl J Med 294:1223, 1976.
22. Cox, M, and Singer, I: *Lithium and water metabolism.* Am J Med 59:153, 1975.
23. Anon: *Lithium nephropathy.* Lancet 2:619, 1979.
24. Emerson, CH, Dyson, WL, and Utiger, RD: *Serum thyrotropin and thyroxine concentrations in patients receiving lithium carbonate.* J Clin Endocrinol Metab 36:338, 1973.
25. Havdala, HS, Borison, RL, and Diamond, BI:*Potential hazards and applications of lithium in anesthesiology.* Anesthesiology 50:534, 1979.
26. Evans, LEJ, Roscoe, P, Swainson, CP, et al.: *Treatment of drug overdosage with naloxone, a specific narcotic antagonist.* Lancet 1:452, 1973.
27. Mansky, PA: *Opiates: human psychopharmacology,* in Iversen, LL, Iversen, SD, and Snyder, SH (eds.): *Drugs of Abuse,* Vol. 12 in *Handbook of Psychopharmacology.* New York: Plennum Press, 1978, p. 95.
28. Jaffe, JH: *Treatment of drug abusers,* in Clark, WG, and del Giudice, J (eds.): *Principle of Psychopharmacology.* New York: Academic Press, 1970, p. 547.
29. Winkler, A: *Treatment of opioid addiction,* in Jarvik, ME (ed.): *Psychopharmacology in the Practice of Medicine.* New York: Appleton-Century-Crofts, 1977, p. 435.
30. Cogen, FC, Rigg, G, Simmons, JL, et al.: *Phencyclidine-associated acute rhabdomyolysis.* Ann Intern Med. 88:210, 1978.
31. Egbert, LD, Battit, GE, Turndorf, H, et al.: *The value of the preoperative visit by an anesthetist. A study of doctor-patient rapport.* JAMA 185:553, 1963.
32. Levinson, BW: *States of awareness during general anaesthesia.* Br J Anaesth 37:544, 1965.
33. Blacher, RS, and Winkelstein, C: Unpublished data.
34. Meyer, BC, and Blacher, RS: *A traumatic neurotic reaction induced by succinycholine chloride.* NY State J Med 61:1255, 1961.

35. Blacher, RS: *On awakening paralyzed during surgery.* JAMA 234:67, 1965.
36. Winkelstein, C, Blacher, RS, and Meyer, BC: *Psychiatric observation on surgical patients in recovery room.* NY State J Med 65:865, 1965.
37. Titchener, JL, Zwerling, I, Gottschalk, L, et al.: *Psychosis in surgical patients.* Surg Gynecol Obstet 102:59, 1959.
38. Klein, RF, Kliner, VA, Zipes, DP, et al.: *Transfer from a coronary care unit. Some adverse responses.* Arch Intern Med 122:104, 1968.
39. Blacher, RS: *The hidden psychosis of open-heart surgery—with a note on the sense of awe.* JAMA 222:305, 1972.
40. Sgroi, S, Holland, J, and Marwit, SJ: *Psychological Reactions to Catastrophic Illness.* Read before the Annual Meeting of The American Psychosomatic Society, Boston, March 30, 1968.
41. Knox, SJ: *Severe psychiatric disturbances in the post-operative period—A five year survey of Belfast hospitals.* J Mental Sci 107:1078, 1961.
42. Blacher, RS: *Paradoxical depression after heart surgery: a form of survivor syndrome.* Psychoanal Q 47:267, 1978.
43. Lipsitt, DR: *Medical and psychological characteristics of "crocks."* Psychiatry in Medicine 1:15, 1970.

Chapter 12

PULMONARY DISEASES

John Urbanetti, M.D., and Barry Fanburg, M.D.

Impairment of pulmonary function occurring postoperatively is one of the most frequent complications of surgical procedures. Several circumstances occurring during and after surgery account for this finding. For example, the common use of sedation or changes in serum electrolytes or pH may impair ventilatory drive. Similarly, ventilation may be limited because of surgically induced alterations in chest wall mechanics such as those occurring from pain or abdominal bindings. Restricted movement and a poor cough may account for retention of secretions, infection, and atelectasis. Fluid imbalance and diminished cardiac output may result in pulmonary interstitial and alveolar water accumulation. Fluid depletion and decreased venous tone may lead to poor and maldistributed pulmonary perfusion. Thus, the patient who is sedated, artificially ventilated, immobilized for a long period of time, dependent upon intravenous feeding, and disallowed the benefit of an adequate cough is prone to a wide variety of complications which may lead to poor gas exchange.

Several of the potential abnormalities referred to above may be guarded against by careful preoperative assessment and management. Others need rapid attention at the time of their occurrence. From a pulmonary standpoint, a markedly obese patient or a patient with asthma is quite a different subject for an operative procedure than a patient who has no medical abnormalities. There are varied approaches to the pulmonary management of the patient in the preoperative and postoperative periods and in some areas of management data are insufficient to permit unequivocal conclusions. In these cases, one must use intuitive guidelines based on indirectly obtained pathophysiologic information. The purpose of this chapter is to draw attention to the manner of assessing pulmonary aspects of surgical patients, to point out factors of risk for these patients, and to review approaches to their pulmonary management during the perioperative period.

HISTORY AND PHYSICAL ASSESSMENT; ROUTINE LABORATORY TESTS

A careful pulmonary history is invaluable in the preoperative assessment of the surgical patient. Particular attention should be paid to any history of dyspnea, either at rest or with exertion, cough, sputum production, hemoptysis, wheezing, chest pain, medications, or previous pulmonary disease. A smoking history should be obtained. The patient who has shortness of breath regularly with mild exertion such as that associated with dressing or walking up a few stairs is likely to have destructive lung disease and is certainly a considerably higher surgical risk than the patient who only has episodic shortness of breath that is due to bronchospasm since the latter condition is often reversible. The surgical risk of a patient with a recent episode of bronchospasm might be improved considerably by postponing the operation, if possible, until the bronchospasm has been adequately treated. Cigarette smoking and obesity considerably increase the risk of developing pulmonary complications secondary to surgery[1,2] and should be eliminated or reduced as much as possible prior to surgery.

Careful attention should be given to the patient's breathing pattern during the physical examination. The use of thoracic accessory and abdominal muscles in inhaling and exhaling respectively may immediately indicate an increased risk of pulmonary failure following surgery since the patient is already calling upon a reserve mechanism for maintaining ventilation and further reserve may be limited. Clubbing of the nailbeds and cyanosis should be noted. The patient should be evaluated for diminution in breath sounds, wheezes, rales, and hyper-resonance or dullness to percussion. Cardiac size should be assessed; attention should be paid to the loudness of pulmonary valve closure; and murmurs should be listened for. Assessment should be made for possible cor pulmonale, which would indicate advanced disease. General nutritional status should be evaluated and the patient should be weighed to obtain a baseline for comparison with weights after surgery.

Although there is current uncertainty about the relative risks from radiation and benefits of routine preoperative chest x-rays for children who do not have pulmonary symptoms, chest x-rays should be done for most preoperative patients. The x-ray may point to pulmonary infiltrates, pleural effusion, or congestive heart failure which will need to be evaluated further or corrected prior to surgery. It will also serve as a baseline for comparison with chest x-rays done later, at a time of suspected atelectasis or pneumonia. Although, at times of later evaluation for pulmonary embolus, it may seem that it would have been desirable to have done a lung scan prior to surgery, there appears to be insufficient justification to do this expensive and potentially hazardous procedure routinely. Cor pulmonale may be further assessed with an electrocardiogram and echocardiogram.

PREOPERATIVE EVALUATION OF PULMONARY FUNCTION

Pulmonary Function Tests—Lung Volumes and Flow Rates

We currently have at our disposal a large armamentarium of pulmonary function tests which can be used to assess the status of lung function prior to surgery. The final result of lung function, the arterial blood gas, is now routinely checked at the time of surgery, at least partly because these gases need to be monitored during surgery. However, it should be remembered that the preoperative blood gas determination may also be useful for assessing the significance of later postsurgical decreases in Pa_{O_2} (arterial oxygen pressure) or in Pa_{CO_2} (arterial carbon dioxide pressure). The need to evaluate other parameters of pulmonary function preoperatively and the specific tests to choose are less clear. It does seem reasonable to obtain at least some measurement of lung volumes and flow rates prior to surgery in all patients suspected of having pulmonary impairment because of the predictive power of these tests in assessing risks, operability, and therapeutic options.

The measurement of vital capacity (Fig. 1) is available and is easily obtained in most hospitals. Indirect measurements of residual volume and total lung capacity determinations are done by helium dilution, nitrogen washout, or plethysmography and require more instrumentation than the simple measurement of vital capacity. Although not necessary in most cases, measurements of residual volume and total lung capacity may be useful in some instances for a better definition of the type and extent of lung disease.

There are several methods for determining the velocity of air flow and for assessing airway obstruction. The expiratory flow rate may be determined at each instant of the inspiratory or expiratory ventilatory cycle with a pneumotachygraph and the vital capacity can be recorded during this maneuver. The recording, the so-called "flow-volume loop," is shown diagrammatically in Figure 2. Other measurements of expiratory flow are the FEV_1 (absolute volume of gas exhaled from total lung capacity in one second), the FEV_1/FVC ratio (percentage of forced vital capacity (FVC) exhaled in one second), the maximum mid-expiratory flow rate, and flow rates obtained during other portions of the exhaled forced vital capacity. Flow measurements may be made with varying densities of gases to differentiate large and small airway dysfunction. This procedure helps to localize airway disease by making use of the relatively more turbulent flow in larger airways which is reduced by low density gases. Although determination of diffusing capacity may be a useful diagnostic procedure, it usually does not add much to the

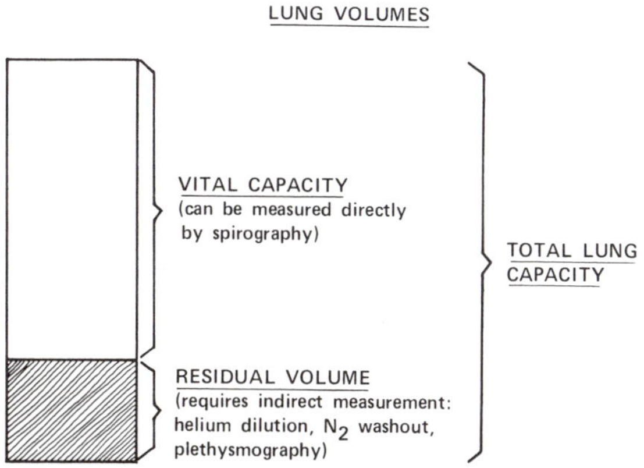

FIGURE 1. Lung Volumes: Total lung capacity is composed of the vital capacity plus the residual volume. Vital capacity is easily measured but can be influenced by the patient's effort. It may be decreased in restrictive or obstructive lung disease. Residual volume is more difficult to measure. It is usually increased in obstructive airway disease and decreased in restrictive disease.

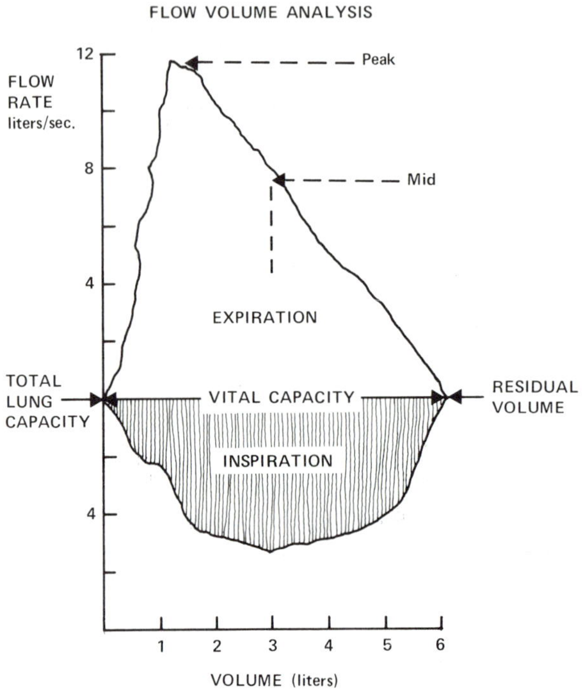

FIGURE 2. Flow-Volume Analysis: A flow-volume analysis provides a visual representation of flow rates at each instant of lung volume changes during inspiration and expiration. With calibration, one can determine the vital capacity, although it is not possible to obtain an absolute measurement of total lung capacity or residual volume from this analysis. Vital capacity is decreased with restrictive lung disease. Flow rates are decreased with obstructive disease.

management of the surgical patient. The measurement of maximum voluntary ventilation is done by having the patient exhale as much air as possible in a specified period of time. This requires achievement of the most efficient ventilatory rate and tidal volume. Diaphragmatic or chest wall muscle weakness and obstruction of expiratory flow rates are the major limitations to this maneuver.

Measurements of vital capacity and expiratory flow rates can be obtained simply and inexpensively without risk to the patient and should be done routinely in most preoperative evaluations where pulmonary impairment is suspected. For thoracic surgery and some other more complicated operations, one should have more complete measurements of the parameters of pulmonary function. The usefulness of these tests in patient evaluation and management will be discussed later.

Function Studies of Separate Lungs

In many cases involving thoracic surgery, it would be useful to know if pulmonary malfunction is unilateral and localized. This information might allow a speculation regarding the end result following resective surgery. Operations requiring resection of nonfunctioning lung would be expected to have little consequence, while operations with resection requiring removal of adjacent normal lung would be expected to have a deleterious effect on overall pulmonary function. Resection of an area of lung with a low ventilation-perfusion ratio may actually improve Pa_{O_2} levels since the resection would remove a location of "partial" shunting of poorly oxygenated blood. Often it is difficult to make this assessment with conventional pulmonary function tests.

Earlier methods to separate function of the individual lungs utilized intubation under general anesthesia with a Carlens double lumen tube which allowed measurement of gas exchange from each lung separately. The need for intubation has made this procedure unpopular and it is used very little today. Split function studies of ventilation-perfusion matching utilizing radionuclide scans are simpler to administer and are more generally used. For this procedure, a radionuclide is simply inhaled and administered intravenously in two separate maneuvers. Radioactivity is counted externally and the distribution of counts is evaluated. This method of testing will detect areas that are poorly ventilated or poorly perfused and an assessment of mismatching can be obtained. It can be assumed that areas that are both poorly ventilated and poorly perfused are probably not functional. However, these measurements do not allow quantitative assessment of gas exchange, and unless a clear-cut abnormality is found, interpretation in relation to surgical resection may be difficult.

Exercise Studies

Exercise studies allow assessment of the performance of the integrated cardiovascular and pulmonary systems under conditions of increased work load and give an indication of the patient's limitation under these circumstances. These studies may be useful in assessing a patient whose history of exercise intolerance is unclear and may help to determine what performance to anticipate from the patient following surgical resection of lung. With the exercise studies, minute ventilation, heart rate, and oxygen uptake can be determined by noninvasive procedures. Also, a measurement of oxygen saturation can be obtained with ear oximetry. A simple display of some parameters of exercise testing is shown in Figure 3. These values provide a more quantitative way of predicting the patient's postoperative limitation than can be obtained by simply observing the patient undergoing exercise. More complete measurements of the physiologic performance of the lungs and of gas exchange can be obtained by exercise studies with an indwelling catheter, but studies of this degree of sophistication are usually not necessary in the evaluation of the preoperative patient.

Blood Gases and Acid-Base Considerations

Arterial blood gases and pH measurements provide both an assessment of lung function and a baseline with which postoperative values can be compared. Although the composition of blood obtained with a pinprick following warming of an extremity may approximate that of capillary blood, more accurate measurements can be obtained from arterial puncture. Special care should be taken to assure adequate insulation of the sample from room air, rapid measurements, and cooling of the sample to limit glycolysis if measurements are to be delayed.

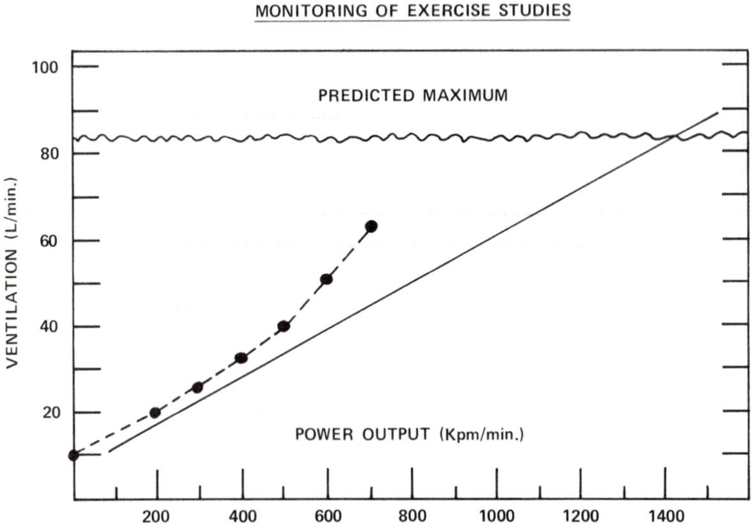

FIGURE 3. Monitoring of Exercise Studies: Studies are done either on a bicycle or a treadmill. Ventilation can be monitored with a mouthpiece and spirometer (from which gas exchanges can be determined). Ventilation is usually linear with increased work loads as demonstrated by the solid line and parallels oxygen consumption. Upward deviation of ventilation from linearity with low work loads is found with lung disease or with poor conditioning. The point of deviation from linearity may represent an anaerobic threshold where lactic acid accumulates in the blood. Monitoring should include an EKG and change in heart rate can be related to changes in ventilation. Arterial blood gases may be determined with the use of an arterial catheter for more complete measurements of gas exchange.

Pao_2 AND HYPOXEMIA

The Pao_2 is normally about 90 to 95 mm Hg in young individuals and decreases with increasing age in association with increases in ventilation-perfusion mismatching. Thus, the patient who is 70 years old may have a Pao_2 in the range of 70 to 75 mm Hg at atmospheric pressure under normal circumstances. Arterial hypoxemia may be caused by (1) alveolar hypoventilation, (2) diffusion defect, (3) ventilation-perfusion mismatching, and (4) arteriovenous shunting. When arterial hypoxemia is found in the preoperative patient, an attempt should be made to identify the cause for it.

Alveolar Hypoventilation

Alveolar hypoventilation is associated with an elevated $Paco_2$, as a reflection of inadequate elimination of CO_2 which is being constantly produced in the body. An elevated $Paco_2$ is, in turn, coupled with an elevated alveolar pressure of CO_2 ($P_{A}co_2$). According to the alveolar gas equation, $P_{A}co_2$ and alveolar oxygen pressure ($P_{A}o_2$) have a reciprocal relationship and an elevation in carbon dioxide pressure is associated with a lowering of oxygen pressure in both the alveolar space and in arterial blood. It is useful to think in terms of the alveolar–arterial oxygen pressure difference ($P[A\text{-}a]o_2$) as an indicator of the extent to which arterial hypoxemia results from alveolar hypoventilation alone as opposed to other factors such as ventilation-perfusion mismatching and a diffusion defect. There is normally a 5 to 10 mm Hg $P(A\text{-}a)O_2$ gradient secondary to physiologic "shunting" such as that from the thebesian veins. The $P(A\text{-}a)O_2$ gradient is calculated as indicated in Figure 4. Since the percentage of O_2 in dry room air at sea level is 20.9 percent, the partial pressure of O_2 in the upper airway is approximately 150 mm Hg. Reduction in P_AO_2 occurs concomitantly with accumulation of CO_2 in the alveoli, and an average alveolus maintains a P_AO_2 of approximately 100 mm Hg and a P_ACO_2 of approximately 40 mm Hg. An elevation in the $P(A\text{-}a)O_2$ gradient by more than 5 to 10 mm Hg at room air indicates that hypoxemia is not caused by hypoventilation alone but has an associated ventilation-perfusion mismatch and/or an associated diffusion defect. With hypoxemia secondary to hypoventilation alone, which occurs with normal lungs, the $P(A\text{-}a)O_2$ gradient remains normal. Hypoxemia secondary to alveolar hypoventilation and CO_2 retention alone is an uncommon finding in the preoperative setting except in some emergency situations, such as those where ventilation has been acutely depressed by sedation or other factors.

$$P_A O_2 = P_IO_2\dagger\ (\text{dry}) - \frac{Paco_2}{R^*}$$

$$P(A-a)O_2 \text{ gradient} = P_AO_2 - PaO_2$$

1. Determine P_IO_2 from known F_IO_2‡

For example, at 40% F_IO_2:

760	mm Hg = atmospheric pressure
−40	" " = water vapor (varies with temperature)
720	" " = dry atmospheric pressure
×.4	(F_IO_2 example)
288.0	mm Hg = partial pressure of inspired O_2

2. Measure $PaCO_2$ as estimate of P_ACO_2; estimate R

For example, with measured $PaCO_2 = 28$

$$\frac{PaCO_2}{R} = \frac{28}{.8} = 35$$

3. Hence, calculated $P_AO_2 = 288 - 35 = 253$ mm Hg

4. $P(A-a)O_2$ gradient = 253 mm Hg − measured PaO_2

*R = respiratory quotient assume to be 0.8 $\quad \frac{CO_2 \text{ Production}}{O_2 \text{ Uptake}}$

†P_IO_2 = partial pressure of inspired O_2

‡Fraction of inspired gas that is oxygen.

FIGURE 4. Calculation of Alveolar-Arterial Oxygen Pressure Gradient ($P[A-a]O_2$) This calculation is useful for the determination of the extent of the ventilation-perfusion mismatch. Hypoventilation alone does not produce an elevated $P(A-a)O_2$ gradient. Hence, a patient with normal lungs who has received a drug overdose which depresses ventilation does not have an elevated $P(A-a)O_2$ gradient, while intrinsic lung disease does usually result in an increased $P(A-a)O_2$ gradient.

Diffusion Defect

Defective diffusion of oxygen from the alveolus to the red blood cell is caused by interstitial processes or vascular diseases both of which increase the diffusion distance across the interstitium or by loss of alveolar-capillary surface area for gas exchange as occurs with emphysema. It is unusual for hypoxemia at rest to occur exclusively from a diffusion defect and when hypoxemia is present in a setting of interstitial disease it is most often due to a combined ventilation-perfusion mismatch and diffusion defect. Arterial hypoxemia as a result of a diffusion defect may become more pronounced with exercise since the combined diffusion defect and rapid capillary blood flow do not allow adequate time for equilibration of oxygen with hemoglobin. A diffusion defect as a possible cause for hypoxemia can be evaluated by measurement of single breath or steady state diffusing capacity with the gas, carbon monoxide. It should be kept in mind that lowered diffusing capacity can be caused by pulmonary vascular disease (such as pulmonary embolus) and lymphatic abnormalities (such as those occurring after lymphangiography) in addition to interstitial disease. The measurement of diffusing capacity may provide early detection of these abnormalities. Although the measurement of diffusing capacity does not play a major role in preoperative evaluation, it does occasionally detect a patient who has a greater than expected extent of lung disease.

Ventilation-Perfusion Mismatch

The most common cause for arterial hypoxemia is a ventilation-perfusion mismatch. This is a result of the high incidence of airway disease in the general population. The physiologic problem is that alveoli, on the average, are underventilated in relation to perfusion (Fig. 5) Hence, areas of the lung have increased venous admixture, (i.e., blood with hemoglobin that is less than 100% saturated). Because of the relatively flat portion of the oxygen-hemoglobin dissociation curve at hemoglobin saturations of greater than 90 percent, normally functioning alveoli cannot compensate for desaturated blood coming from areas of the lung which are hypoventilated, and underventilated areas of the lung are not helped by hyperventilation since there is a preferential distribution of ventilation to normally functioning lung. Recognition of ventilation-perfusion mismatch as a cause for hypoxemia requires the combination of an appropriate setting and the exclusion of other causes for hypoxemia. Therapy for patients with ventilation-perfusion mismatch must be directed toward the establishment of optimal patency of compromised airways (this will be discussed further under the section on Preoperative Treatment for Maximizing Lung Function).

Arteriovenous Shunting

Hypoxemia from diffusion defects and ventilation-perfusion mismatch can be corrected by the administration of 100 percent oxygen and with adequate time Pa_{O_2} can be raised, in both cases, to levels expected for normal persons breathing 100 percent oxygen. A true arteriovenous shunt cannot be corrected with 100 percent oxygen, because areas persist where oxygen does not reach the circulation. Hence, Pa_{O_2} will not be elevated to values

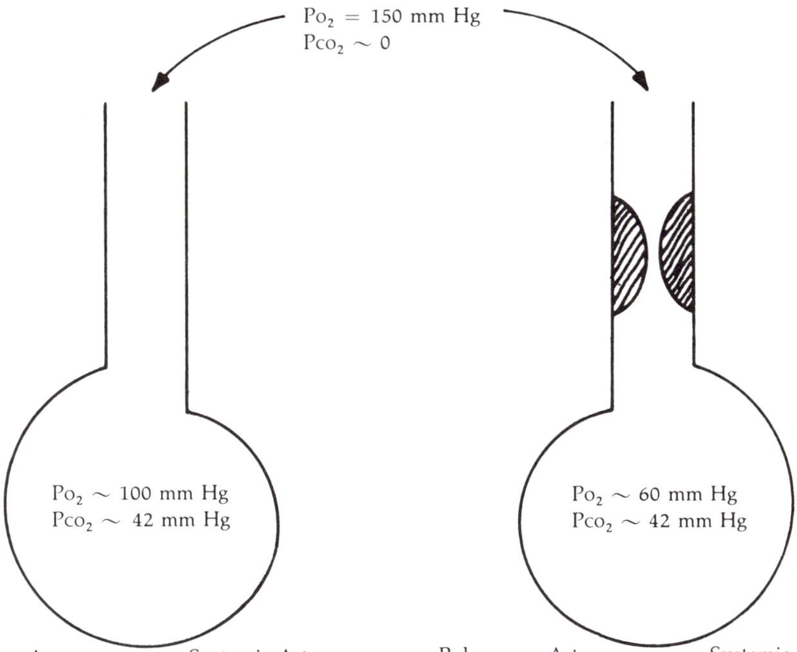

Pulmonary Artery		Systemic Artery
$Po_2 \sim 40$ mm Hg	→	$Po_2 \sim 90$ mm Hg
$Pco_2 \sim 44$ mm Hg	→	$Pco_2 \sim 42$ mm Hg

NORMAL

Pulmonary Artery		Systemic Artery
$Po_2 \sim 40$ mm Hg	→	$Po_2 \sim 50$ mm Hg
$Pco_2 \sim 44$ mm Hg	→	$Pco_2 \sim 42$ mm Hg

DECREASED VENTILATION-PERFUSION RATIO

FIGURE 5. Ventilation-Perfusion Mismatch Causing Arterial Hypoxemia: The only ventilation-perfusion mismatch that results in arterial hypoxemia is one in which ventilation is decreased relative to perfusion. Bronchoconstriction or airway plugging results in this type of mismatching. $Paco_2$ may not be influenced since CO_2 is highly soluble and eliminated by normally functioning alveoli. However, normally functioning alveoli cannot compensate for the mismatch in relation to Pao_2 since the oxygen-hemoglobin dissociation curve is already fully saturated for the perfusion of the normally functioning alveoli.

found in normal individuals breathing 100 percent oxygen. Shunting may occur at the cardiac or the pulmonary level. If shunting is suspected, the patient should be tested with 100 percent oxygen, breathing under conditions where exhaled nitrogen can be monitored to assure adequate intra-alveolar mixing of the 100 percent oxygen. Intrapulmonary arteriovenous shunting occurs most frequently with pneumonias, atelectasis, or alveolar collapse associated with respiratory distress syndrome, all of which may occur as postoperative complications. This subject will be covered more completely in the section on postoperative management.

$Paco_2$ and pH

$Paco_2$ and pH should be assessed preoperatively from the standpoints of both general evaluation of acid-base status and evaluation of lung function. The patients most likely to have CO_2 retention secondary to pulmonary malfunction are usually obvious from the history and physical examination. Nevertheless, it is not obvious from these parameters which of the patients with pulmonary disease do, indeed, have elevated levels of $Paco_2$. Measurement of $Paco_2$ must be coupled with bicarbonate and serum electrolyte determinations and information obtained in the history to make the most meaningful assessment of the findings. A full evaluation of acid-base status is discussed in Chapter 15, Fluid, Electrolyte, and Acid-Base Disorders. Elevated $Paco_2$ developed on the basis of pulmonary insufficiency should be considered to be a cautionary sign for any except the most simple of surgical procedures which can be managed by local anesthesia. The presence of hypercapnia forbodes a fragile patient for surgery. However, emergency surgery may have to be performed despite the elevated $Paco_2$. Lowered $Paco_2$ with an elevated pH and normal bicarbonate may be due to acute hyperventilation from anxiety associated with arterial puncture. Lowered $Paco_2$ may also occur on a chronic basis and is usually associated with metabolic acidosis, chronic anxiety, or liver or brain disease.

Operative Risk as Reflected by Lung Function Studies

Unfortunately, it is not possible to classify patients as operable or inoperable based on pulmonary function tests alone. One can only assign a relative risk from these tests. The findings on pulmonary function testing that do indicate a high risk for resective thoracic surgery both in morbidity and mortality include: a maximum voluntary ventilation or maximum breathing capacity of less than 50 percent of the predicted value; an FEV_1 of less than 50 percent of the predicted value; a maximum midexpiratory flow rate of less than 0.5 to 0.6 L/sec; a maximum expiratory flow rate of less than 100 L/min; a vital capacity of less than 1 L; a failure to improve vital capacity, forced vital capacity, or maximum midexpiratory flow rate as indicated above with bronchodilators, and an estimated postoperative FEV_1 of less than 0.8 to 1.0 L.[3–11] A mean pulmonary artery pressure greater than 35 mm Hg when the pulmonary artery to the affected side is occluded at the time of surgery is also associated with a high risk in thoracic resective surgery.[12] Many of these parameters were developed for resective thoracic surgery but can also be applied to other surgical procedures with the awareness that the frequency and severity of complications with these procedures will be less than with resective thoracic surgery. Upper abdominal surgery carries a high risk of development of pulmonary complications, since the procedure may interfere with diaphragmatic excursion and ventilation of lung bases. Obviously, any one of the pulmonary function parameters noted above carries less risk if the patient is to undergo an appendectomy rather than a pneumonectomy. It should be emphasized that except for resective thoracic surgery, none of these parameters are absolute contraindications to surgery and the benefits of surgery must always be weighed against the risks. Thus, there may be no choice but to operate on the patient with bowel obstruction with a vital capacity of less than 1 L and an elevated $Paco_2$. On the other hand, resective thoracic surgery can often be temporized when there is marked impairment of ventilatory function and other therapies, such as radiotherapy for cancer, can be used despite an awareness that these procedures are not likely to be curative.

Other Risk Factors

Other well defined risk factors[13–21] that do not contraindicate surgery but which are associated with increased perioperative pulmonary complications include: (1) obesity of 30 percent above ideal weight, (2) age greater than 60 years, (3) a current smoking history (inhalation of tobacco or other materials), (4) acute respiratory tract infection (viral or bacterial, upper or lower respiratory tract), (5) sepsis, and (6) malnutrition.

The combination of two or more of these risk factors including those of pulmonary function testing, may lead to clinically obvious pulmonary complication rates of over 80 percent for these patients.[22] Generally, an individual with any of these risk factors who is about to undergo general or spinal anesthesia should have preoperative assessment of and necessary therapy for the respiratory system. Baseline pulmonary function and arterial blood gases should be assessed and one or more of the therapeutic interventions noted in Table 1 and Figure 6 should be applied over whatever period of time is available before surgery.

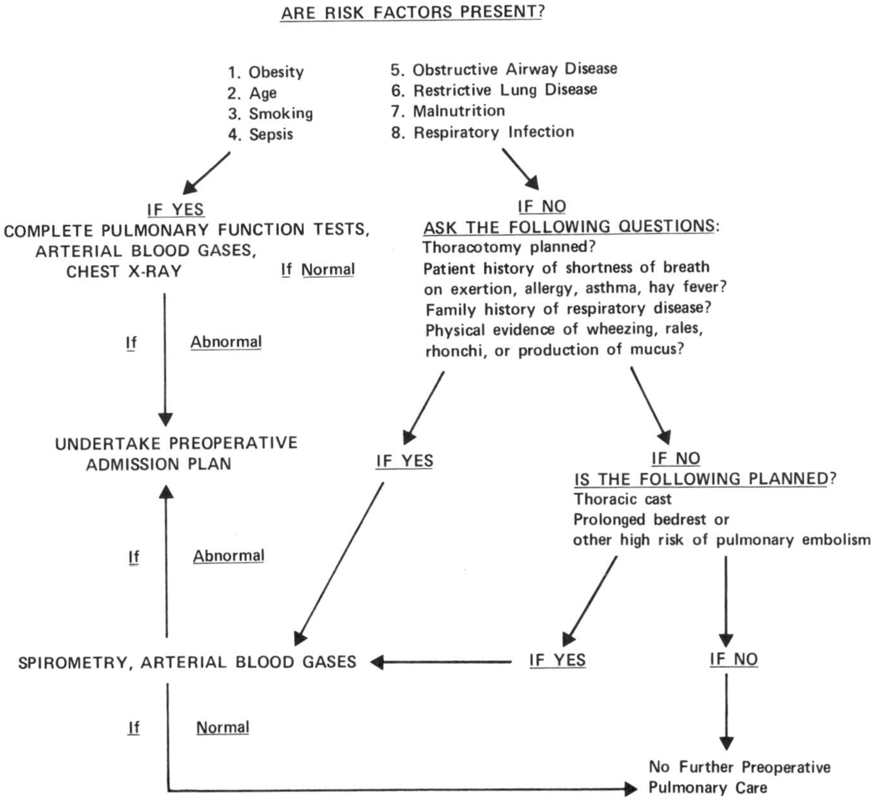

FIGURE 6. Flow Chart for Preoperative Care Plan.

TABLE 1. Presurgical Therapeutic Intervention

Ambulatory Therapy

A. Stop smoking (minimal effect but some utility in simply decreasing the number of cigarettes smoked)

B. Lose weight (no aggressive weight loss within one month of major surgery)

C. Treat bronchospasm (initiate therapy one month before surgery)

D. Treat excess mucus (initiate therapy one month before surgery)

E. Treat infection
   1. Culture sputum
   2. Treat with appropriate antibiotic (generally tetracycline or ampicillin at 250 mg. po q 6 hr, 2–4 weeks preoperatively)

F. Discontinue estrogen containing contraceptives

Therapy for Hospitalized Patient

Admit for 3 days of preoperative intensive pulmonary care.

Hospital Day 1:	A.	Repeat spirometry and arterial blood gas determination to assess efficacy of ambulatory therapy
	B.	Continue medications, maximize bronchodilators if indicated by spirometry
	C.	Assessment and instruction by chest physiotherapist
	D.	Chest physiotherapy treatment for excess mucus if present (2–4 times daily)
Hospital Day 2:	A.	Chest physiotherapy treatment (2–4 times daily)
Hospital Day 3: (Preoperative Day)	A.	Chest physiotherapy treatment (2–4 times daily)
	B.	No nocturnal sedatives or analgesics
	C.	Sputum culture as baseline
	D.	Continue normal intravenous hydration if necessary
	E.	Boost steroids if necessary (see Chap. 5, Endocrinology)
Operative Day:	A.	Shift to parenteral methylxanthines
	B.	Extubate routinely except for:
		1. Obesity: Continue intubation until patient fully awake
		2. Intraoperative or postoperative bronchospasm: Continue intubation until bronchospasm clearly under control
		3. Chronic obstructive pulmonary disease (moderately severe or worse): Continue intubation overnight postoperatively and until sedatives or narcotics can be minimized

PREOPERATIVE TREATMENT FOR MAXIMIZING LUNG FUNCTION

Oxygen Therapy

Problems related to oxygen therapy may occur perioperatively, intraoperatively, and postoperatively with the hypoxemic patient who is at substantially increased surgical risk due to the marginal nature of oxygen delivery to his most sensitive organs (brain, heart, and kidney). Of these sensitive organs, the cardiac response to longstanding hypoxemia has been best studied. Increases in pulmonary arterial pressure and pulmonary vascular resistance may occur, limiting cardiac reserve and predisposing the patient to congestive heart failure (Fig. 7). Pulmonary edema may also occur as a consequence of impaired left-ventricular function.

Since the ultimate concern of respiratory oxygen exchange is the adequacy of oxygen supply to the tissues, a number of interacting factors must be considered in order to assess the adequacy of tissue oxygen supply: 1) the Pa_{O_2}, (2) characteristics of the oxyhemoglobin dissociation curve, (3) hemoglobin concentration, (4) cardiac output, and (5) regional tissue perfusion. In the event that one of these factors is deficient, rendering the other steps "supernormal" is not likely to entirely make up for the deficiency. For instance, an individual limited by 40 percent carboxyhemoglobin may have a Pa_{O_2} of 150 mmHg and still show evidence of severe tissue hypoxemia. Since an abnormality of any one of these steps may render tissues hypoxic, assessment of the Pa_{O_2} alone may lead to an incorrect assumption of adequate oxygenation. Furthermore, since simple correction of a deficient Pa_{O_2} may not be sufficient to reverse evidence of tissue hypoxia, any evidence of tissue hypoxia should prompt assessment of each step in this chain in the event that "normalizing" the Pa_{O_2} does not correct the tissue hypoxia.

Assuming that the factors mentioned above as regulating delivery of oxygen to peripheral tissues are functioning normally, tissue hypoxia may be improved by the

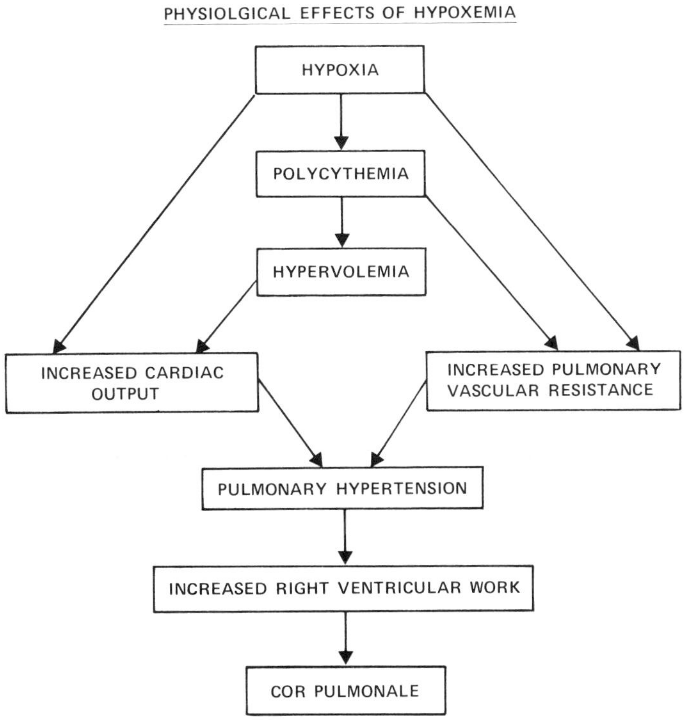

FIGURE 7. Physiologic Effects of Hypoxemia: Hypoxemia results in increased pulmonary vascular resistance (accentuated by acidosis), polycythemia, and increased cardiac output. Ultimately, pulmonary hypertension and right ventricular failure ensue. There may also be left ventricular failure probably secondary to decreased left ventricular contractility secondary to an undersupply of O_2 to heart muscles.

administration of oxygen by nasal prongs, face mask, or endotracheal tube. Delivery of known concentrations of oxygen is most effectively accomplished by Venturi-principle face mask or controlled endotracheal tube delivery systems.[23] Nasal prongs deliver an uncertain concentration of O_2 that is roughly gauged by the following values:

Flow rate, (liters/min)	Approximate Inspired O_2 Concentration (Percentage)
1	24
2	28
3–4	30
5–6	35

Flow rates above 5 to 6 L are generally found to be uncomfortable and a face mask may be required.

Face masks other than Venturi-type, due to their generally poor conformation to the face, rarely deliver stable concentrations of O_2. Only with the greatest attention to fit, high flow rates, and "reservoir bag" use can reliable inspired concentrations of 40 to 50 percent, be reached by this technique. The physician should not be misled to think that use of a "60, 70, or 100 percent" face mask (that is likely delivering lower concentrations) causes the patient's Pao_2 to correspond appropriately to the purported O_2 concentrations. The arterial PO_2 should always be measured.

Simple correction of oxygen deficiency by supplying supplemental oxygen may be associated with three potential complications (1) risk of ventilatory depression, (2) risk of pulmonary parenchymal atelectasis, and (3) risk of oxygen toxicity.

The ventilatory drive in normal individuals is only minimally oxygen-dependent. $Paco_2$ generally provides the major input to the respiratory center for ventilation control. However, certain individuals may demonstrate a lower than normal sensitivity to their own $Paco_2$ and if these individuals are exposed to an increased work of breathing (e.g., decreased compliance with congestive heart failure or increased airway resistance such as asthma) they may "allow" their $Paco_2$ to rise. Such individuals present clinically as "CO_2 retainers." The use of supplemental O_2 for these patients may cause them to hypoventilate once their oxygen needs are supplied, resulting in rapid and occasionally dangerous elevations in $Paco_2$. Therefore, in any individual whose initial $Paco_2$ is elevated, supplemental oxygen should be applied in gradually increasing steps (e.g., 24%, then 28%, then 30%) with $Paco_2$ measured shortly after each "step" increment in the fractional concentration of O_2 in inspired gas ($F\textsc{io}_2$). The $Paco_2$ may be safely allowed to increase to ranges of 60 to 70 mm Hg provided the pH is not less than 7.25.

Pulmonary parenchymal atelectasis occurs most commonly as the result of airway obstruction with subsequent reabsorption of trapped gas from the occluded distal air spaces. As higher oxygen concentrations are used, gas is absorbed from those occluded air spaces more quickly and subsequent collapse of those spaces may occur. Protection against such "high oxygen-induced atelectasis" is best obtained by insuring that individuals maintain large tidal volumes or are supported with small amounts of positive end-expiratory pressure (PEEP) during operative procedures and through the immediate postoperative period.

Oxygen is directly toxic to human tissue. In concentrations found in routine hospital settings, it is primarily toxic to the pulmonary parenchyma. An inspired concentration of 40 percent O_2 (FIO_2 = .4) is well tolerated for long periods. However, as the FIO_2 is increased above 60 percent, pulmonary mucosal and/or parenchymal damage becomes apparent in increasingly shorter periods of time. Fortunately, damaging concentrations of O_2 cannot usually be achieved by delivery of O_2 by various means to patients who are not intubated. Uninterrupted exposures to an FIO_2 of 100 percent may lead to evidence of pulmonary damage within 24 hours.[24] Although various experimental techniques are currently under investigation for prophylaxis of this complication (e.g., the use of antioxidants, steroids, and intermittent pre-exposure to high oxygen levels), restriction of supplemental oxygen to concentrations just sufficient to maintain a PaO_2 of 60 to 70 mm Hg seems to be advisable for patients with adequate hemoglobin and blood pressure.

The hemodynamic complications of chronic hypoxemia (increased pulmonary artery pressure, increased pulmonary vascular resistance, and polycythemia) generally do not respond to short term increases in FIO_2. There is increasing evidence that chronic long term "low-flow" oxygen therapy occasionally relieves these complications. Patients with such hemodynamic complications may benefit from a trial of several weeks of low-flow oxygen to maximize their pulmonary function prior to elective surgical procedures.[25]

In summary, oxygen therapy is utilized generally to maintain the PaO_2 at least at 50 to 60 mm Hg. Certain individuals in whom other causes of tissue hypoxia may be present may require assessment of the partial pressure of O_2 in mixed venous blood and/or cardiac output to better monitor tissue oxygen delivery.

Aerosol Therapy

Many of the abnormalities of the respiratory system can be viewed as occurring in a space that is accessible to topical therapy. Accordingly, a number of therapeutic substances have been manufactured or modified that theoretically take advantage of this topical route of administration. Aerosol deposition at various levels in the airway is largely dependent on particle size. Most commercially available devices for aerosolization produce particles of varied size that tend to distribute predominantly to the upper airways and trachea.[26] The instruments therefore fail to deliver substantial amounts of the aerosol to the more peripheral areas of primary concern. Ultrasonic nebulizers overcome this limitation to some extent, depositing a substantial portion of their aerosol more distally. However, since these devices may deposit exceptionally large quantities of fluid peripherally (3 to 6 ml water/min at maximum rate), excessive quantities of fluid may be retained.[27]

In addition to the mechanical difficulties of aerosol deposition, the patient's airways may themselves cause nonuniform deposition. Patients with airway diseases may have variable sites and degrees of obstruction that can direct gas flow (and hence the inhaled aerosols) away from certain areas of the lung. Other routes of drug administration in these situations may be more desirable. Certain aerosols, (e.g., water, acetylcysteine, disodium cromoglycate) may even induce a degree of bronchospasm, further exacerbating their maldistribution and the underlying disease. They should be used with caution in the face of underlying bronchospasm and rarely in the presence of progressive airway obstruction. Unless the patient is stable and has successfully used a given aerosol previously, aerosol therapy is recommended primarily for the administration of bronchodilators and in the restricted setting of chest physiotherapy.

Smoking Control

The risks of perioperative pulmonary complications directly correlate with an individual's current smoking history.[28] A history of current cigarette smoking increases the frequency of postoperative complications six to seven times that of nonsmoking controls.[22] Cigarette smoke may acutely lower the effectiveness of surfactant, decrease pulmonary compliance, increase airway resistance, inhibit ciliary function, and depress pulmonary macrophage metabolism and activity.[29–32] These abnormalities have been ascribed to cigarette smoking but are also seen with the inhalation of any tobacco product. The effects of smoking are to some extent reversible over a period of three to six weeks.[33] Cessation of smoking is accordingly recommended for at least that period of time preoperatively.

Carbon monoxide is one of the components of cigarette smoke. Heavy smokers may have 5 to 10 percent carboxyhemoglobin in the blood and in some cases up to 20 percent carboxyhemoglobin chronically present as a result of their smoking.[34] Exposure to heavy automobile traffic may raise the percentage of carboxyhemoglogin an additional 2 to 5 percent. Such combined exposures should be considered in the event of emergency surgery, recognizing that hemoglobin so combined is ineffective in oxygen transport. Cessation of exposure to carbon monoxide will reduce the risk from carboxyhemoglobin to negligible levels within 24 hours. Carbon monoxide elimination can be expedited, if necessary, with high inspired oxygen, and the risks of carboxyhemoglobin rendered negligible within six hours provided that the individual is asymptomatic initially. Firemen and those nonsmokers who occupy the same premises as smokers may also be at risk from carbon monoxide exposure.[35]

Obesity Control

Obesity is associated with a significantly increased incidence of postoperative pulmonary complications. Complication rates up to three times those of nonobese individuals are noted in some studies. Under ideal circumstances, preoperative weight loss resulting in a normal weight should be attempted. However, intensive dieting during the immediate preoperative period should be avoided, since studies have shown that the associated protein and phosphate depletion occurring with malnutrition may lead to poor tissue healing and respiratory failure.[36]

The obese patient should be assessed and treated preoperatively in a manner similar to all other high risk patients. Particular attention should be given to preoperative assessment of the possible presence of CO_2 retention (pickwickian syndrome). Patients with hypoventilation, secondary hypoxemia and CO_2 retention, polycythemia, and right heart failure are at particular risk of further respiratory failure.[37] Obese patients who do not retain CO_2 may demonstrate an increased work of breathing due to decreased lung and chest wall compliance,[38] increased ventilation due to increased metabolism, and less efficient respiratory musculature.[39] Most importantly, the abnormal thoracic mechanics may decrease the resting lung volume (the functional residual capacity or FRC). Ventilation to the lower lung zones may be severely compromised, particularly in the supine position (with the diaphragm elevated by intra-abdominal contents), and this may result in abnormal ventilation-perfusion relationships and hypoxemia.[40] These physiologic limitations may complicate intraoperative and postoperative oxygenation and weaning from artifical ventilation.

In the obese patient, epidural rather than general anesthesia may be particularly useful for minimizing postoperative complications.[41] Postoperative care should include upright positioning (to minimize basilar compression and atelectasis) and rapid and early ambulation (to minimize risk of venous thrombosis).

Physiotherapy

A wide variety of physical measures has been developed to enhance the expectoration and clearance of sputum and to retrain breathing patterns in individuals with respiratory disease. Application of these techniques to patients with underlying pulmonary disorders and other individuals at risk of surgical pulmonary complications has been found to significantly improve their postoperative morbidity and mortality.[42] The goals of the various techniques include:

1. Prevention or reversal of mechanical airways obstruction and/or atelectasis by:
   a. Assisting and preserving adequate depth and distribution of ventilation
   b. Assisting the removal of secretions from the tracheobronchial tree
   c. Maintaining full mobility of chest wall, shoulder girdle, spine, and abdominal musculature
2. Prevention of secondary complications of postoperative bed rest including:
   a. Postural defects
   b. Joint mobility limitations
   c. Reduced exercise tolerance
   d. Venous thrombosis

The techniques that have been developed for these purposes are generally applied in a coordinated program of preoperative assessment and instruction. Similar postoperative treatments are directed toward the same general goals and may be modified for specific problems or types of surgery as they are encountered.

Complete and efficient utilization of physiotherapy begins with the physician's evaluation of the patient's history, physical examination, and basic physiology. Evaluation of arterial blood gases, chest x-ray, and pulmonary function tests help the physiotherapists to direct their attention to specific areas of involvement and types of disorders. The physician's orders for physiotherapy should identify which of the specific goals is sought, the frequency and duration of treatments, and the specific contraindications (if any) to particular modalities of treatment.

Using the baseline data detailed above, the physiotherapist initially interviews the patient giving a detailed explanation of the proposed physiotherapy and its rationale.

Training of the patient in several techniques is undertaken—often including breathing exercises, bronchial drainage, chest percussion, and coughing exercises. Various maneuvers designed to treat the secondary complications of bed rest may be taught as well (i.e., leg exercises, arm and shoulder girdle movements, and body positioning to minimize pain and postural defects.

Certain of the techniques of physiotherapy may on occasion have undesirable physiologic consequences. Cough techniques can, by vagal reflex or rise in intrathoracic pressure, cause a decrease in cardiac output and should be used with caution for patients with unstable cardiovascular systems. For similar reasons, postural drainage may modify venous return, vagal tone, or central nervous system blood flow so as to cause dizziness, hypotension, or syncope in some patients and should be applied cautiously to the patient who has cardiovascular or neurologic instability. Similarly, the patient with a bleeding cerebral aneurysm may be at risk from increased intracranial pressure caused by cough. Cough techniques may also cause premature airway closure or collapse and should be applied with caution in patients with underlying obstructive airway disease, particularly if the technique is not productive of good results.

After initial assessment and training, patients with postoperative pulmonary risk factors should undergo regular physiotherapy treatments to assist in removal of secretions and/or to reinforce the initial training. Treatments should ideally begin as early as possible. The initial pulmonary function assessment is often performed at the same time as an outpatient preoperative surgical visit in order to permit hospitalization three to five days preoperatively for intensive physiotherapy (1 to 4 treatments/day if necessary). The physical therapist should enter an initial assessment and subsequent daily notes into the formal hospital record. Extensive discussion of the various techniques is beyond the scope of this chapter; however, the techniques are well documented in the *Brompton Hospital Guide to Chest Physiotherapy.*[43]

Intermittent Positive Pressure Ventilation

In addition to the use of the intermittent positive pressure breathing (IPPB) device as an aerosolizer, intermittent positive pressure breathing has been widely prescribed for the purposes of: (1). assisting respiration in order to decrease the work of breathing, (2) assisting respiration in order to provide hyperventilation, (3) decreasing right heart venous return (preload) and consequently treating pulmonary edema, and (4) stimulating cough and providing deep breathing sufficient to limit or to correct progressive atelectasis.

There is ample evidence that the "oxygen cost" of respiration is diminished by the use of IPPB.[44] For the normal individual, however, the respiratory work of breathing represents a very small percentage of total oxygen consumption and the benefit would be limited. For the individual with increased work of breathing (e.g., chronic obstructive pulmonary disease), intermittent relief of this work may only suffice to delay more specific or appropriate therapy of respiratory failure. A small savings in oxygen consumption may result from the use of IPPB, and the associated hyperventilation may also improve the Pa_{O_2} secondary to an improved P_{AO_2}. However, ventilation-perfusion changes during IPPB have been observed, which in some individuals may counteract this small improvement in Pa_{O_2}.[45] Whatever short term benefits accure, there is no evidence that gas exchange is improved for periods of greater than one hour, suggesting that the intermittency of this therapy is a primary limiting factor.[46,47] Hence, IPPB therapy is not recommended for reduction of work of breathing.

IPPB induced hyperventilation to improve CO_2 removal has been advocated. Although $Paco_2$ can be lowered temporarily, intermittent use of IPPB two to four times per day for periods of 10 to 20 minutes would be unlikely to provide significant long term improvement in an individual's elimination of CO_2.

Positive pressure ventilation of the lung by any technique in which intra-airway pressure is raised above right atrial pressure will tend to decrease venous return to the right heart in proportion to the duration and magnitude of the pressure applied. In extreme examples of positive pressure breathing (e.g., volume ventilation with added PEEP), the decrease in venous return to the right heart may superimpose on other physiologic effects of positive pressure ventilation to severely decrease the cardiac output. Careful application of the lower and intermittent pressures of IPPB may be useful in performing a mechanical "phlebotomy" of patients with pulmonary edema. Hence, this "side effect" of IPPB therapy may be occasionally useful in an emergency setting. IPPB in the awake patient, using current technology, has very little danger of producing an inadvertent major fall in cardiac output.

Pulmonary atelectasis has been shown to result from low tidal volume breathing such as breathing in a setting of thoracic pain or sedation. IPPB has been demonstrated to be effective in increasing the vital capacity of postoperative patients[48] thus preventing the collapse of small airways and alveoli. However, IPPB alone does not appear to be significantly better than a wide variety of other deep breathing methods in the treatment of postoperative atelectasis. Patients who are unable to independently cooperate with other techniques, however, may benefit from this device.

Other Mechanical Devices

Many additional mechanical devices have been utilized to improve preoperative and postoperative ventilatory function. These devices include various "incentive spirometers," flow measuring instruments, and "homemade" techniques such as the use of "blow bottles" and rubber glove inflation. Regular postoperative use of these devices has been shown to reduce the frequency of pulmonary complications by two-thirds.[49] Comparisons among the various devices are complicated by physiologic and technological factors, cost, patient compliance, and physician/nurse preference. The beneficial effects of all these devices are most likely related to the deep breathing maneuver necessary to activate them. Any method that ensures regular, deep breathing will minimize and likely reverse many of the postoperative pulmonary complications, provided that the patient is instructed in the use of these methods preoperatively and encouraged to continue them postoperatively.

Hydration

Water is almost universally present in therapeutic regimens designed to treat abnormalities of the respiratory tract. Dramatic changes in viscosity of mucus and ciliary action, in the absence of water, point out the importance of maintaining a normal state of hydration. In the normal individual, the state of hydration of the respiratory system is well protected by the nose and upper airway. Mild to moderate total body dehydration must occur before significant respiratory tract function abnormalities are noted. Most of the reported benefits from water vapor inhaled through intact upper airways are likely due to local hydration of this region. (Hence, humidification of oxygen during its delivery prevents local effects of drying). In an individual with a normal upper airway there is little evidence that inhaled water in any form alters the consistency of respiratory secretions.[50] Nebulized water vapor may be useful as an inducer of cough particularly if administered by ultrasonic nebulization. An occasional patient with hyper-reactive airways may demonstrate bronchospasm in response to nebulized water. Saline is considerably less irritating and is frequently used as the diluent for other nebulized substances. In a heated and concentrated form (20% hypertonic saline), inhalation of salt water is particularly useful for sputum induction.[51] Although nebulized water or saline is used for the induction of sputum, adequate hydration of the respiratory tract is most easily attained through oral or parenteral routes. All ambulatory patients with difficulties in clearance of secretions are encouraged to drink at least 1500 ml of fluids/day.

For individuals whose upper airway is bypassed (e.g. patients with tracheostomy or endotracheal tubes), supplemental humidifying devices are generally used. Inadequate humidification for 20 to 40 minutes generally results in severe decreases in ciliary motility and mucous clearance.[52] Humidifying devices should be checked regularly for proper function.

In summary, preoperative attention to hydration of the airway generally consists of insuring adequate systemic hydration of the patient. Nebulized or aerosolized water is used for cough induction or as a diluent for other aerosolized agents.

Mucokinetic Agents

The presence of sputum that is abnormally thick or tenacious most often reflects a state of inadequate patient hydration. If secretions are still thick and tenacious after adequate oral or parenteral hydration, various agents are available that may help thin the secretions sufficiently to expedite their removal. The direct instillation of saline through a nasopharyngeal catheter used for suctioning or as a part of endotracheal or tracheostomy tube care may be sufficient to promote cough and mobilize secretions effectively. Secretions that are persistently thick and purulent may be thinned with agents designed to break mucoprotein molecules into smaller, more soluble components. Of a wide variety of available drugs, the sulfhydryl bond reducing agents and the enzymatic agents seem most effective. Currently acetylcysteine is the most useful sulfhydryl bond reducing agent. This agent is most effective at an alkaline pH and, therefore, should not be mixed with a bronchodilator or acidic solution. Occasional complications of bronchospasm have been reported with its use. The likelihood of bronchospasm can be reduced by diluting the 20 percent solution to 5 to 10 percent with normal saline and by preceding its instillation with an aerosolized short acting bronchodilator (e.g., isoetharine). The short acting bronchodilator will, in addition, loosen secretions and open airways to this medication. Acetylcysteine inhibits the antibacterial action of a wide variety of penicillins and this should be considered with culture of the resultant sputum.[53]

Several enzymatic agents have also been shown to liquefy purulent secretions.

Among these are trypsin, chymotrypsin, streptokinase, streptodornase, and deoxyribonuclease. Of these enzymes, deoxyribonuclease is least irritating to tissues but still seems to be considerably more irritating than acetylcysteine. Deoxyribonuclease is most beneficial for lysis of thick purulent material (e.g., for patients with cystic fibrosis or lung abscess). The observation that naturally occurring proteases may contribute to the development of emphysema (α-1-antitrypsin deficiency) has prompted some individuals to regard deoxyribonuclease and other enzymatic agents as undesirable for routine mucolytic therapy.[54]

A variety of surface active agents has been studied for possible improvement of the kinetics of flow of mucus. Among these are sodium bicarbonate, dipalmitoyl lecithin, and ethanol. However, there is little evidence that use of any of these agents significantly improves clearance of mucus. Several oral agents have also been studied for purposes of clearance of mucus. Among these are ammonium salts, various volatile oils (e.g., elixir of terpin hydrate, eucalyptus oil, thymol), various creosote derivatives (e.g., guaiacol or guaifenesin). All of these substances are considered to be effective through vagal stimulation. Of this group, only the creosote derivatives have been shown to have a measurable effect. Even then, doses significantly higher than those routinely used may be necessary for a definite effect.[55] Several oral mucokinetic agents, including licorice, various plant oils, and organic and inorganic iodides, are considered to lower viscosity of secretions by a direct effect on the endobronchial mucosa. Of this group of agents the iodides seem most effective. Doses of 1 to 2 gm (10 to 20 drops) of a saturated solution of potassium iodide four times per day will measurably increase sputum volumes. Iodides should not be used in pregnant women or individuals with uncertain thyroid function. Adverse dermatologic and salivary gland effects are occasionally seen secondary to iodide sensitivity.

It is readily apparent that the choice of a mucokinetic agent lacks precision. Often the decision must be based on trial and error. A good basic approach is to first try to thin secretions with adequate hydration. If this is not successful, acetylcysteine may be tried. If this is still unsatisfactory, other agents may be tried.

Bronchodilators

The patient with bronchospastic or irritable airways should be assessed preoperatively by pulmonary function measurement of his flow rates with particular attention to bronchodilator responsiveness. Since the clinical assessment of bronchospasm is unreliable, any individual with a past history of repetitive pulmonary infection, regular smoking, childhood asthma, hayfever, or family history of allergic respiratory tract disease should be assessed with pulmonary function measurements. Most individuals who will benefit from use of bronchodilators can be identified by assessment of flow rates before and after administration of bronchodilators. Optimized dilatation of their airways will assist in clearance of mucus and minimize the likelihood of perioperative development of severe or complicating bronchospasm. These individuals may be treated initially with methylxanthines or beta-adrenergic agents. Systemic steroids may be added if intensive therapy with methylxanthines and sympathomimetics fails or if there is a contraindication to the use of the first two forms of therapy.

The most useful parameter of adequate therapy remains the pulmonary function test. The presence of bronchodilator-responsive obstructive airway disease can be demonstrated and quantitated. After the initiation of therapy, repeating the measurement of flow rate will permit demonstration of improvement. Retesting after Isuprel inhalation allows identification of any additional improvement that can be obtained with additional bronchodilators. Patients who have reversible bronchospasm are followed with repeated pulmonary function testing at two to four days after initiation of therapy and the dosage of the bronchodilator is modified as necessary.

The methylxanthines (theophylline and derivatives) are used for both initial and baseline therapy of bronchospasm. Serum theophylline levels of 10 to 20 μg/ml are effective and are associated with minimal side effects. Levels above this range are increasingly effective in relieving bronchospasm but are associated with increased risk of side effects. The occasional individual who benefits from higher serum levels must be monitored more closely.

The doses and preparations mentioned below should normally suffice to achieve effective serum levels. Patients with seemingly inadequate therapeutic response to theophylline should have a measurement of their serum theophylline level to confirm adequate dosage prior to changing to a supplemental bronchodilator.

The adjustment of methylxanthine dosage and type of preparation must take into account several variables. Firstly, various preparations have different effective or free theophylline equivalents. Hence, a change in preparation may have a substantial effect on theophylline serum levels, even though the amount of theophylline as listed by the manufacturers may be equivalent in the two preparations. Secondly, the pharmacokinetics of the drug are affected by a wide range of circumstances including:

1. Age: Both premature and elderly individuals seem less tolerant of "normal" dosage ranges; on the other hand, children up to the age of 16 to 17 years tolerate (and may require) higher than normal dosages.
2. Hepatic Enzymes: There may be a genetic determinant that is expressed as a rapid or slow metabolization of methylxanthines with dosage change required accordingly (serum level quantitation may help here). Smoking may induce hepatic enzymes to be more active. Underlying liver disease may impair the metabolic removal of methylxanthines and cause accumulation of the drug.
3. Different routes of administration may result in variable rate and extent of drug absorption. Oral absorption is most rapid on an empty stomach; fat or carbohydrate meals impair absorption to a greater extent than protein meals. Sustained release or enteric-coated preparations may have a very erratic absorption. Rectal preparations in solution are absorbed rapidly but suppository formulations may be absorbed very erratically.[56]

Loading doses of theophylline given to adults who have not received theophylline within the last 24 hours or more are 4 to 6 mg/kg of body weight, administered orally or intravenously over 15 to 20 minutes. Maintainence doses of theophylline of 0.5 to 1.0 mg/kg of body weight per hour generally provide adequate therapy if regularly assessed. Dosages of theophylline are noted in Table 2. Adjustments in these dosages can be made in light of the variables described above. Adequacy of dosage can be assessed and

TABLE 2. Theophylline Preparations

Preparation	Main Proprietary Product	Tablet Capsule (mg)	Sustained Release (mg)	Liquid (mg/15 ml)	Parenteral Preparation (mg)	Suppository/ Enema	Average Percentage of Theophylline	Approximate Dose to Yield 10 (mg) Free Theophylline	Notes
Theophylline (anhydrous)	Elixophyllin	100, 200	125, 250	80			100	10	Drugs of choice
	Slo-Phyllin	100, 200	60, 125, 250	80					
	Somophyllin	100, 200, 250				350/15 cc (as aminophylline)			
	Theo-Dur, Sustaire		100, 200, 300						
	Theolair	125, 250	250, 500						
	Theophyl	100, 225	125, 250	112.5					
Theophylline ethylenediamine (aminophylline)		100, 200			250, 500	100, 250, 350, 500	79–80	12	Main product for intravenous use
Theophylline monoethanolamines	Fleet	100, 200				250, 500, 250, 500	75	14	Particularly stable; liquid well-tolerated by rectum
Dihydroxypropyl theophylline (dyphylline)	Lufyllin	200, 400		100	250		70	14	Does not provide free theophylline but is equivalent to 70% theophylline
Theophylline cholinate (oxtriphylline)	Choledyl	100, 200, 400		300			64	16	Popular oral alternative
Theophyllin calcium salicylate	Quadrinal	130		195			48	21	Combination products with phenobarbital
	Verequad	130		195					

adjusted every hour if the medication is given intravenously or every 2 hours if it is administered orally.

Beta-adrenergic agents are currently employed in both acute and long-term therapy of bronchospasm in patients in whom methylxanthines alone fail to provide adequate control. Several routes of administration are available. The oral route is perhaps the safest, obviating a possible misuse of the spray and perhaps more effectively reaching obstructed airways not directly penetrated by a spray. Parenteral therapy is usually restricted to subcutaneous or intramuscular sites. Intravenous use of epinephrine or isoproterenol should be reserved for life-threatening bronchospasm. For parenteral use there is as yet no formulation that is demonstrably more effective than epinephrine. However, the alpha and $beta_1$ effects of epinephrine may be particularly undesirable in individuals with hypertension or diabetes. Epinephrine is not a particularly valuable drug for the routine treatment of adults with bronchospasm.

Inhalational agents are now available with relatively good $beta_2$ specificity. One such drug, isoetharine, is used primarily for purposes of bronchodilation prior to chest physiotherapy in a hospital setting in light of its brief one hour duration of action. For a longer (4 to 6 hour) duration of action, an inhaled formulation of metaproterenol is available. This drug is also available in oral formulation and can be most effectively used in a four to eight hourly dosage pattern. An occasionally associated muscular twitching and/or tremor can be best managed by decreasing the dosage and then gradually increasing the dosage to tolerated levels.

Bronchodilators may be stopped several hours prior to surgery or, if necessary in an unstable situation, they may be continued intravenously during surgery. Starting their administration when needed during surgery is always an option. One should be aware of possible arrhythmias associated with bronchodilators and alter the dose accordingly in the face of arrhythmias.

Corticosteroids are used in circumstances where methylxanthine and beta-active agents have failed or where they have produced significant side effects such as cardiac arrhythmias. They may also be useful where angina or cardiac arrhythmias make one hesitant to use other bronchodilators. An exceptionally wide variety of undesirable side effects prompts careful and circumspect use of long-term corticosteroids. Use of minimal levels required to achieve a particular degree of bronchodilation is necessary. Objective pulmonary function measurement of corticosteroid-induced improvement should be undertaken since subjective improvement is commonly seen as a nonspecific psychogenic steroidal effect. If patients are on long-term steroids, dosages should be temporarily increased to compensate for operative stress. Inhaled corticosteroids usually may be safely discontinued for short periods of time without ill effects since they have minimal systemic effects. In case of inability to inhale a nebulized steroid, oral or parenteral supplements may be given at the rough equivalent of 5 to 10 mg of prednisone per four puffs of spray (200 mcg. beclomethasone). This dose of prednisone likely exceeds that obtained systemically with beclomethasone and may cause some degree of adrenal suppression. In circumstances of acute bronchospasm, inhaled steroids should be discontinued and an oral or parenteral steroidal supplement should be utilized instead.

In summary, patients with bronchospasm, as demonstrated by physical assessment or the more sensitive pulmonary function techniques, benefit from preoperative use of bronchodilators in an effort to improve clearance of mucus and to minimize perioperative severe or complicating bronchospasm. It is important to minimize or eliminate various other factors which may trigger the bronchospasm (smoking, infection, and inhaled allergens) in addition to the use of bronchodilators. Methylxanthines are the drugs of choice for bronchodilatation and are occasionally supplemented with beta-adrenergic agents. Steroids, when routinely utilized by the patient, are normally continued and generally increased in the immediate preoperative hours when supplementation for a deficient hypophyseal-adrenal axis may be necessary (see Chap. 5, Endocrinology). Disodium cromoglycate can be safely discontinued prior to surgery.

Preoperative Management of Specific Chronic Lung Disease

Although many of the comments made above focus on the management of airway disease, they apply equally to a large number of other chronic lung diseases. Various types of restrictive lung disease should be treated optimally prior to surgery, if possible, so as to maximize lung function. For example, in patients with sarcoidosis, pulmonary function may be improved by treatment with steroids. Any patient with sarcoidosis who is being treated with steroids should have the therapy continued, and perhaps increased, in the perioperative period. Patients who have restrictive disease secondary to drug reactions (such as with bleomycin or busulfan) or radiation pneumonitis may benefit from maximal recovery from reversible components of the problem prior to surgery. A similar approach should apply to interstitial pneumonitis or fibrosis of unknown causes, although little reversibility may be achieved with therapy. In cases where there is no reversibility and surgery must be performed, the same general guidelines for preoperative management apply, but there may be no indication for airway therapy (i.e., bronchodilators, physical therapy, positive pressure breathing). On the other hand, with cases of bronchiectasis, treatment of the airways for optimal patency and management of infection may require prolonged and intensive care prior to surgery.

POSTOPERATIVE MANAGEMENT

General Procedures

Immediately following surgery, the patient who has undergone general anesthesia or any procedure associated with a prolonged period of limited ventilation is likely to have substantial microatelectasis (see Atelectasis below). All such patients should be assessed postoperatively with chest x-ray and arterial blood gas analysis. Obvious abnormalities of these parameters should be treated aggressively. Patients who are found preoperatively to have any of the pulmonary risk factors or abnormal results from chest x-ray, pulmonary function tests, or arterial blood gas analysis should be presumed to be at substantial risk of a postoperative pulmonary complication. Even if the patient's postoperative pulmonary parameters are stable, there may be benefit from treatment for presumed atelectasis.

Aggressive treatment includes particular attention to the effect of any of the postoperative risk factors (pain limiting deep breathing, narcotics, sedatives, body positioning which limits depth of inspiration, or increases in interstitial lung water), attention to the state of the airways, and attention to the degree of inflation of peripheral lung units.

The postoperative risk factors may compromise pulmonary function by limiting deep inspirations and further exacerbating atelectasis that may already be present. Pain from thoracic or abdominal procedures may limit a patient's efforts to breathe deeply, to cough, and to remove secretions.[57] While considerable attention has been paid to devising operative approaches that minimize postoperative pain, the ready availability of narcotics has drawn some emphasis from the observation that the pain contributes to postoperative pulmonary complications. The alternate observation that high-dose narcotics or sedatives increase the rate of pulmonary complications[58] suggests that chemical treatment of pain may be limited by its own side effects. Every attempt to reduce narcotic requirements through patient education and interpersonal rapport should be made. Further studies of the use of acupuncture for pain control may be useful.

The supine position for postoperative care may be desirable for purposes of cardiac output but may not be an ideal position for maximizing lung function. In the supine position, the diaphragm is elevated relative to lung volume, and tidal volumes are ordinarily smaller in this position. Additionally, the high diaphragm leads to a diminished functional residual capacity (FRC) which may result in the patient's breathing with some of his tidal volume in a region of "closing volume." This type of breathing results in ventilation-perfusion mismatching that may contribute to the patient's hypoxemia. Ideally, the patient should be positioned postoperatively in a semireclining or upright manner for maximal lung volume, particularly if the patient is obese.

Increases in interstitial lung water may produce complications by causing limitation of deep breathing which may result in hypoxemia. Every attempt to minimize congestive heart failure and other causes of increased interstitial lung water should be undertaken. It is important to note that the chest x-ray is not a sensitive measure of the presence or absence of interstitial lung water and/or fluid balance. This is particularly true in individuals who are undergoing positive pressure ventilation since the intrathoracic positive pressure may further delay radiologic evidence of increased interstitial lung water. A decrease in vital capacity or pulmonary compliance or an increase in $P(A\text{-}a)O_2$ gradient may be a more sensitive index of changes in interstitial lung water than the x-ray.

The state of the airways is best assessed postoperatively with a mechanical, objective measurement of flow rates. Auscultation alone is not sufficiently sensitive to determine whether variations in intensity of wheezing are due to a change in minute ventilation or to a change in airway diameter. Objective testing permits ready identification of bronchodilator responsiveness and accurate titration dosage of bronchodilator.

The inflation of the peripheral lung units will be more specifically discussed below under the heading of Atelectasis. Generally speaking, measures to promote an advantageous body position (more upright) and to improve the depth of respiration (tidal volume) are of significant value. Personnel or various devices which serve this end are all effective and probably should be used based on the assessment of total cost per therapeutic intervention. There is no evidence that IPPB devices or nebulization of saline are especially useful in decreasing the rate of postoperative complications.

The chest physiotherapist should be particularly alert to the development of complications in patients at increased risk of postoperative pulmonary complications. The daily parameters of pulmonary function are usually reviewed and noted in the patient's chart by the chest physiotherapist, thereby making the physiotherapist's visit valuable for both treatment and assessment.

Secretions

Respiratory secretions represent a complex admixture of the products of many different cells. Structures of the airways including goblet cells, mucous glands, seromucinous glands, and ciliated columnar cells all produce products which are carried by ciliary action to the oropharynx and in normal circumstances are swallowed. The products of alveolar cell secretions, most notably surfactant from the type II pneumonocyte, may be added to this mixture. This composite of secretions is cleared from lower airways at a rate of approximately one turnover every hour. Central airway clearance is somewhat faster than that occurring peripherally. Much foreign material, including infectious agents, is removed by scavenging macrophages.

Mucus aids the clearance of foreign material from the respiratory tract by trapping it and by assisting its mechanical removal by combined ciliary action and cough. Ciliated cells are found in all airways down to those of about 2 mm in diameter. These cells propel the mucus cephalad. The rate of movement is inhibited by several factors including cigarette smoke, oxygen concentrations above 25 percent, dry or cold air, viral infection, and increased viscosity of mucus such as that of mucoviscidosis.[59–61]

The concept of a double layer of mucus, a superficial viscid sheet (gel), and an underlying serous sheet (sol) in which the cilia beat to propel the superficial sheet, was proposed as early as 1934. Hydration of mucus is therefore an important factor in ciliary motion. Adequate hydration is ordinarily provided by a normal upper airway. Bypassing this airway with an endotracheal tube requires that careful attention be paid to the adequacy of humidity and temperature control. Both low temperature and humidity may trigger bronchospasm and are particularly likely to do so in patients with sensitive or "irritable" airways.[62] Mucus itself becomes an added factor in pulmonary disease when quantity or quality is changed. Trauma (e.g., smoking or repetitive tracheal suctioning), inflammation, and infection all promote hypersecretion of mucus. An individual may become aware of this hypersecretion and actively attempt its expectoration.

Flow rates of mucus seem to be increased by catecholamines and digitalis under experimental conditions.[63] The quantity of mucus also seems to be increased by several chemical agents including iodides (see section on mucokinetic agents above). The quality of mucus changes significantly in the presence of active infection or certain diseases (e.g., mucoviscidosis, familial dysautonomia) and may become thicker or more tenacious. Several chemical approaches may be taken in an attempt to "thin" these abnormal secretions as described above.

Mucus contains many proteins, analysis of which may provide an insight into immune or infectious mechanisms in the lung.[64] Various antibodies in mucus, particularly of the IgA type, may be present and may aid the body's initial response to infection.[65] Mucus also contains cells that may be useful diagnostically. Polymorphonuclear cells may be present during infection or inflammation. Noting the presence of intracellular bacteria may be particularly useful although gram stained preparations may contain bacteria simply overlying the stained cells. The presence of eosinophils is helpful in alerting the observer to the possible presence of allergic or immune responses. They may be particularly useful in alerting the physician to the presence of allergy in the patient suspected to have a usual chronic bronchitis or emphysema. Bronchoepithelial cells may appear in mucus as the result of a viral denudation of the tracheal mucosa. Histiocytes (macrophages) are normally seen in mucus and presumably function as bronchoalveolar scavengers, repositories of antibodies, and effectors of antimicrobial immunity. Macrophages should be seen in any sputum sample purportedly originating from the lower pulmonary tract.

Infectious agents can be identified in sputum samples. There are no firm criteria that can be applied to distinguish between colonization of the respiratory tract and "true" invasive infection. The predominance of a particular bacterial organism or evidence of fungal hyphal forms may be helpful in this assessment. As various techniques are developed to insure sampling of mucus with minimal upper airway contamination, the value of sputum culture will be increased. Since postoperative pneumonia occurs most commonly with bacterial organisms which were initially colonizing the respiratory tract and since most intubated patients become colonized within 72 hours of intubation,[66] it may be useful to periodically sample and culture the airway flora of all patients who are intubated for prolonged periods.

In summary, secretions play a role in lung defense and clearance mechanisms. When the secretions are abnormal in quantity or quality, they may promote airway obstruction and produce atelectasis. Attention to the quantity and quality of sputum may be valuable for early diagnosis and therapy of postoperative pulmonary infections.

MANAGEMENT OF SECRETIONS

In addition to forming a nidus for infection, secretions block air passages and interfere with optimal gas exchange. Any amount of interference with gas exchange may be detrimental to a patient whose pulmonary function is otherwise borderline. Therefore, regular suctioning of secretions is important with patients who are producing excessive amounts of them. Hydration and thinning of secretions helps with this process. At times intubation and/or bronchoscopy may be important for the adequate secretion removal. Additional details concerning secretions can be obtained from the text *Sputum Fundamentals and Clinical Pathology* edited by M. Dulfano.[67]

ATELECTASIS

The changes that occur in a segment of lung following bronchial occlusion have been well studied. Gas that is trapped distal to the obstruction is rapidly absorbed by the blood. O_2 tension falls to a greater extent than the concomitant rise in CO_2, and the resulting pressure in the gas space becomes less than atmospheric. In the case of body spaces with fixed walls such as the sinuses or middle ear, obstruction and pressure drop leads to a fluid transudation from surrounding capillaries. In the lung, the more mobile surrounding parenchyma may collapse into the space containing subatmospheric pressure in association with some transuded fluid, depending on the compliance of the surrounding lung. This collapse occurs over a period of hours if the occluded gas is room air. However, the collapse occurs within minutes if the occluded gas is pure oxygen in combination with some other rapidly absorbed gas such as the nitrous oxide utilized in anesthesia.

The oxygen saturation of the associated capillary blood will fall with acute occlusion of a lung segment. The resulting mixture of the hypoxic blood with normoxic blood from other lung units creates a venous admixture, or shunt, that if extensive, may result in cyanosis. Such an acute atelectasis usually produces only a transient shunt since the vascular supply to that area soon reflexively decreases as well and the blood is shifted to other, better ventilated lung units. Over a period of hours, the blood gases will often become normal at rest. Ordinarily, the patient will experience a concomitant increase in ventilation to the unaffected lung segments which may result (especially in the case of the massive atelectasis) in hypocapnia. A small improvement in Pa_{O_2} may result from this hyperventilation, but it usually is not sufficient to fully compensate for the decreased arterial oxygen tension. The normal lung has several protective mechanisms which interact to prevent complete collapse of a large segment. Collateral channels for ventilation exist at the alveolar level, thus permitting ventilation to occur, though diminished, even with localized obstruction. Surfactant, produced by type II cells in the alveoli, is a substance that reduces the surface forces of the liquid covering of peripheral airways and alveoli. In the absence of surfactant these surface forces would lead to alveolar and peripheral airway collapse. Deficiency of surfactant may be due to insufficient production (e.g., prematurity or pulmonary artery occlusion) or to its inactivation (e.g., pulmonary edema). The extent to which surfactant deficiency contributes to atelectasis has been difficult to quantify. Attempts to replace the deficient surfactant have not met with success.[68] Atelectasis, through a poorly understood reflex mechanism, promotes cough which, with its associated hyperinflation, helps relieve the atelectasis.

Therefore, atelectasis results from a combination of factors such as multiple occlusion of collaterals and/or loss of surfactant. Animal studies suggest surfactant production may decrease significantly after atelectasis perhaps leading to potentiation of the atelectasis. Occasional deep breaths ("sighs") appear to be important to maintain adequate surfactant activity.[69]

Atelectasis is the most frequently occurring postoperative pulmonary complication. Some evidence suggests that much of the atelectasis or at least its earlier stages may occur during surgery. The basal portions of the lung, particularly the posterior segments, are most susceptible to atelectasis. This may relate to the observation that a paralyzed or anesthetized patient with controlled ventilation shows a substantially decreased ventilation to his dependent lower lobes largely due to the hydrostatic forces applied to those lobes by the essentially liquid abdominal contents acting through a paralyzed, atonic diaphragm.[70] In this regard, the use of high volume ventilation during anesthesia may serve only to ventilate the nondependent portions of the lung and may fail to prevent atelectasis. Studies of the effects of intraoperative and immediately postoperative positioning to control the effects of paralyzed diaphragmatic compression of lung tissue have not been reported.

Several pulmonary physiologic changes occur following general anesthesia. Most may be viewed as the result of various degrees of atelectasis ranging from the "microatelectasis" reported by Bendixen[71] to gross radiologic or clinical evidence of lobar or whole lung collapse. A drop in vital capacity and functional residual capacity is commonly seen intraoperatively. The loss of volume may be as great as a 35 to 40 percent decrease from preoperative volumes. The functional residual capacity may be lowered below the closing volume (or that lung volume at which small peripheral airways begin to close). This leads to hypoventilation of large portions of lung tissue with subsequent hypoxemia. If the hypoventilation continues, small areas of alveolar closure persist. These areas may be too small to be identified radiologically but can be shown physiologically by noting decreasing lung compliance. The decreased compliance would then require increased ventilation pressure to achieve the same original volume of ventilation, and if such higher pressures were not utilized, further decreases in lung volume would follow with further atelectasis and hypoxemia.

Microatelectasis was clinically demonstrated by Bendixen[71] and is felt to be a major cause of intraoperative and postoperative hypoxemia. Reversal of the microatelectasis can ordinarily be accomplished with the careful hyperinflation that has become a common practice during operation. However, the superposition of other factors leading to atelectasis, such as those found in individuals with high risk of postoperative atelectasis, may make the routine techniques for reversal insufficient and larger degrees of postoperative atelectasis may appear.

Management of Atelectasis

PAIN

Drug therapy of pain must be balanced between adequate pain relief to allow full respiratory excursion and minimal drug dosage to avoid depression of respiratory drive. Current studies of psychologic aspects of pain may help with this dilemma.[72]

POSITION

Postoperative positioning that minimizes diaphragmatic compression of the bases of the lung is valuable, particularly in obese patients.[72,73] Frequent repositioning from side to side may be an effective alternative if the horizontal position seems necessary.

DEEP BREATHING

A variety of equipment (such as that for IPPB and incentive spirometry) and personnel (chest physiotherapists or respiratory therapists) has been brought to bear on the problem of producing sufficiently deep breaths. Minor degrees of atelectasis respond to any of a number of techniques that produce deep breaths. Despite many opinions, there are few objective data that document the uniform superiority of any particular technique in comparison to others, provided that the technique results in frequent and repetitive deep breaths.

RESISTANT ATELECTASIS

Suctioning both removes secretions directly and causes coughing and deep breathing. If not responsive to the above techniques, atelectasis may require more aggressive intervention. Direct bronchial suction and lavage (bronchoscopy) or application of positive end expiratory pressure with a face mask[74] or with intubation may be necessary. Newer techniques utilizing negative extrathoracic pressure are being developed and may provide a satisfactory alternative to the complications of positive pressure ventilation.[75]

Aspiration

Aspiration of foreign material into the lungs accounts for substantial perioperative morbidity and for nearly 15 percent of perioperative deaths.[76] Aspiration occurs commonly in an intensive care setting and is not entirely prevented by cuffed endotracheal tubes. In a perioperative setting, aspiration may occur as a result of chemically or mechanically induced incompetence of the normal glottic and pharyngeal protective mechanisms. Occasional gastroesophageal reflux may contribute to the likelihood of aspiration. Glottopharyngeal protective reflex mechanisms may be incompetent for considerable intervals of time after extubation.[77–79] Diabetics may be at particular risk if autonomic neuropathy of the vagus nerve causes delayed gastric emptying. Such patients may have full stomachs at the time of surgery even though they have not eaten since dinner the night before (see Chap. 5, Endocrinology).

The effects of aspiration are related to several characteristics of the aspirated material. Some fluids such as blood or saliva, produce little or no irritation of the airways or parenchyma. However, the acidity of gastric contents may cause bronchospasm and parenchymal damage. The degree of acidity is important, with a pH of 3.0 or higher causing little damage largely due to rapid tissue buffering of the acid. If a strongly acidic (pH $<$ 2.5) fluid is aspirated, a chemical pneumonitis appears with rapid onset of atelectasis, pulmonary parenchymal consolidation, and hemorrhagic exudation. The rapidity of damage is such that treatment with neutralizing or other lavage solutions is of little or no value unless performed within a few minutes of the observed aspiration.[80,81] The particulate matter in the aspirate contributes significantly to the degree of damage. Large pieces of food may cause immediate airway obstruction. Smaller particles and fibers distribute more peripherally, leading to segmental or peripheral atelectasis with consequent hypoxemia.

Controlling the effects of aspiration depends largely on its prevention which, in turn, largely depends on an awareness of its possibility. Use of cuffed endotracheal tubes may not entirely prevent aspiration since material collecting around the cuff may be aspirated when the tube is removed or the cuff deflated during routine nursing care. The most useful of a variety of prophylactic measures is lateral body positioning of patients and attention to the possibilities of gastric distention. The presence of a nasogastric tube does not assure gastric emptying and may in fact lead to recurrent reflux. Persistent aspiration should be investigated and consideration should be given to the possibilities of a patulous cardia and/or an intestinal obstruction.

MANAGEMENT OF ASPIRATION

Observed or suspected aspiration should be assessed with arterial blood gas sampling and a chest x-ray. A sample of fluid recovered from the airway may reveal a low pH (only if obtained within minutes of aspiration) and the presence of food or other gastric contents. Immediate bronchoscopy and lavage may be useful in management of aspiration. Lavage need not be undertaken with a neutralizing fluid but should be performed instead with small quantities of saline (5 to 10 cc) so as to prevent flooding of the remaining patent airways. Fiberoptic bronchoscopy may be performed easily if an endotracheal tube is in place.

The prophylactic use of antibiotics has not been shown to improve mortality or to reduce the risk of a secondary infection. A wide variety of organisms may be present in the aspirated material and use of specific prophylactic antibiotics will only serve to select out the more resistant organisms. Cultures should be obtained immediately and subsequent treatment directed toward clinical evidence of superinfection. It may be difficult to assess the presence of pneumonia in this setting, since fever, peripheral leukocytosis, and radiologic evidence of pneumonitis may each be present as a response to aspiration without bacterial superinfection.[82] The use of systemic steroids has been widely discussed; however, no adequate human trials are available. Animal model studies have shown no consistent benefit of steroids when given before or after aspiration.[83,84] We, therefore, use steroids only if they can be given immediately after aspiration and even then we do not have total confidence in their effectiveness. Aspiration, like other acute pulmonary toxic exposures may not produce obvious parenchymal or physiologic abnormalities for periods as long as 10 to 12 hours and may continue to produce progressive deterioration from the acute event alone for up to 24 hours. Accordingly, close monitoring with baseline arterial blood gases, chest x-ray and physical examination should be undertaken. Repetition of these studies at least 6 and 12 hours after aspiration is important. Long-term complications, including pneumonia, sepsis, empyema, and pulmonary abscess, are seen in up to one third of patients with observed aspiration.[85]

Pneumothorax

Pneumothorax may occur for a variety of reasons in the perioperative setting. The acute physiologic changes which occur depend on the degree and rapidity of collapse of the affected lung. Although the contralateral lung usually expands somewhat, the mediastinum more commonly shifts toward the unaffected lung which has a more negative pressure under ordinary circumstances. With progressive collapse of one lung, a significant fall in Pao_2 occurs due to ventilation perfusion imbalance. However, over the next several hours, the perfusion of that lung is gradually reduced and a normal Pao_2 is usually reached within 24 hours. Any residual hypoxemia is generally thought to be due to underlying disease in the unaffected lung. In circumstances of positive pressure ventilation or for individuals with vigorous cough, enough air may be forced into the pneumothorax to eventually reach positive pressure levels and cause progressive pulmonary collapse. Mediastinal shift and subsequent hypotension may occur which is thought to be due to limitation of mediastinal vascular flow.

An expiratory chest x-ray is the most sensitive tool for identifying a pneumothorax. By this technique cases of 5 to 10 percent pneumothorax may be detected. Cases of pneumothorax reaching the size of 15 to 25 percent of lung volume may present with clinical evidence of rapid shallow respirations. Cases of pneumothorax involving still larger lung volumes—25 to 50 percent—may show a hyperresonant note to percussion. If greater than 50 percent of lung volume is involved, physical examination may show evidence of hyperinflation of the chest with obvious delay of inspiration on that side.

In chest trauma, alveolar rupture may occur either secondary to rib fracture with penetration of the visceral pleura or secondary to parenchymal trauma. Air may either escape into the pleural space or dissect through the interstitium to the hilum and mediastinum. Subsequently, air may dissect from the mediastinum into the subcutaneous spaces, into unilateral or bilateral pneumothoraces, or into the peritoneum. The peritoneal gas may distribute over the mesentery and around the bowel wall (pneumatosis cystoides intestinalis) or simply collect subdiaphragmatically to simulate a perforated abdominal viscus. Pneumothoraces which occur in conjunction with thoracic trauma or ventilatory support (particularly in patients with airway disease) should be considered unstable and potentially life threatening. Establishment of an escape for accumulated air is important and may be accomplished through the placement of a chest tube.

There are special circumstances under which pneumothorax may occur. Occasionally, a tracheostomy tube will become displaced into the mediastinum with subsequent mediastinal emphysema and leakage of gas either into the subcutaneous tissues or pleural spaces. Endotracheal or tracheostomy tubes may perforate posteriorly through the trachea, directly into the mediastinum, and positive pressure ventilation may rapidly convert this perforation into a fatal tension pneumomediastinum. Pneumomediastinum may occur secondary to alveolar rupture in the presence of high positive pressure ventilation[86] or in association with necrotizing pneumonia. Pneumomediastinum may be most sensitively identified by a lateral chest x-ray. A crunching sound coincident with cardiac rhythm (Hamman's sign) may clinically indicate free gas in the pericardial tissues. A secondary bronchopleural fistula may result from the pneumothorax. In the event of chest trauma, additional rare causes of pneumothorax such as rupture of the esophagus and traumatic rupture of the larynx, trachea, or major bronchus should be considered. Traumatic esophageal rupture is commonly associated with a pleural effusion as well as a pneumothorax. Radiologic studies with contrast medium are helpful in establishing this diagnosis. Bronchial rupture is commonly associated with hemoptysis and may occur some minutes to hours after the acute trauma. Diagnosis and investigation of this problem is best undertaken with fiberoptic bronchoscopy.[87]

Bilateral pneumothoraces can often be tolerated, and if acquired slowly, the normal compensatory mechanisms will permit arterial blood gases to remain within normal limits. However, acute bilateral pneumothorax is a dangerous and frequently fatal condition requiring prompt therapy.

Chronic pneumothorax, even in the absence of pleural infection, may lead to substantial restriction of function of the underlying lung. Upon re-expansion, the lung will often continue to demonstrate restriction of vital capacity and flow rates. Decortication of the lung may return a substantial degree of function if the underlying parenchyma is otherwise normal as determined by pulmonary function testing.

Tension pneumothorax is defined as a pneumothorax in which the gas in the pleural space is under positive (greater than atmospheric) pressure throughout the entire respiratory cycle. When extreme, this positive pressure is transmitted to the mediastinal vessels and a decrease in cardiac output may result. It is distinctly uncommon to find tension pneumothorax in the absence of positive pressure ventilation or vigorous cough. Diagnosis of this particular condition can be made, if suspected, by the placement of a large needle in the second to third interspace anteriorly on the affected side. Outrushing air confirms the presence of pneumothorax. Outrushing air present only during exhalation indicates that a simple pneumothorax is present. Outrushing air throughout both the inspiratory and expiratory cycles indicates the presence of a tension pneumothorax. The needle for suctioning should be connected to an underwater seal and left in place until definitive therapy can be undertaken.

MANAGEMENT OF PNEUMOTHORAX

The severity of a pneumothorax depends on the underlying degree of illness of the patient. Patients who have had chest trauma, who are on ventilators, or who have a vigorous cough are considered to be at a greater risk of tension pneumothorax and are accordingly treated more vigorously. Small pneumothoraces (0 to 25%) are at little risk of tension pneumothorax and are generally treated conservatively with repeat assessment and chest x-ray. Larger pneumothoraces (25 to 50%) are often treated actively particularly when they are acute. If the patient is clinically asymptomatic, needle or catheter aspiration of the air may suffice. Larger thoracotomy tubes are often used, partly with the thought that they will induce a sufficient pleural reaction to cause adherence of visceral to parietal pleura and thus reduce the risk of future pneumothoraces. If the patient's blood pressure and arterial gases are stable, the chest tube is then connected to a direct underwater seal which acts as a one-way valve for escape of the trapped gases. Cessation of bubbling for a period of 8 to 12 hours is generally considered to indicate adequate seal of the leak and the chest tube is clamped for an additional 8 to 12 hours. The tube is removed if a subsequent expiratory chest x-ray shows no reaccumulation of the pneumothorax. On occasion, chest tubes placed for pneumothorax are connected to negative-pressure aspiration pumps for rapid gas removal from the pleural space. Rapid removal of trapped gas and re-expansion of underlying parenchyma may produce a unilateral pulmonary edema.[88] Re-expansion pulmonary edema most often occurs when the pneumothorax is large (greater than 50% of lung volume) and has been present for several days.[89] Re-expansion of pulmonary parenchyma shortly after the onset of pneumothorax will only rarely produce pulmonary edema.[90]

Pulmonary Infections

Postoperative pneumonia is a potentially serious complication with an associated significant mortality which may be as high as 70 percent in the case of some infections such as those with resistant *Pseudomonas* organisms.[91] The particular bacterial species responsible for the pneumonia almost uniformly originates from the bacterial population harbored by the patient. Aspiration of secretions and other material located in the oropharynx is a common occurrence during sleep or in the comatose patient.[66] Colonization of the lower respiratory tract may then occur, particularly in patients whose host defenses are compromised. Ventilated patients, with bypassed glottic defense mechanisms, are uniformly colonized within 72 hours of their intubation. The exact conditions underlying the development of an invasive infection are not clear, but the invading organism generally is the organism originally present in the airways as colonizer.[92]

MANAGEMENT OF PULMONARY INFECTIONS

Environmental sources should be controlled so as to reduce the likelihood of colonization with particularly resistant pathogens. The cleanliness of ventilating and environmental equipment and the isolation of infected patients or personnel should be routinely monitored by hospital infection control teams.

Aggressive attention to postoperative atelectasis and clearance of mucus reduces the likelihood of postoperative pneumonia. Prophylactic systemic antibiotics are of no value and in some studies are shown to increase the risk of nosocomial pneumonia.[93] Aerosolized antibiotics have been considered as a possible means of reducing the incidence of nosocomial infections.[94] Further studies on this subject are needed.

Clinical signs of increased cough, sputum production, fever, leukocytes, and pulmonary consolidation should prompt assessment of sputum by Gram stain and culture. Mucus should be assessed for evidence of pulmonary origin (presence of macrophages) and evidence of inflammatory response (leukocytosis, except in immune suppression). The presence of leukocytes in mucus is frequently seen as a response to the presence of an endotracheal tube. The predominant bacterial population will be a useful guide to the most likely infectious organism. Evidence of intraleukocytic bacteria is a stronger indication of pneumonia as opposed to colonization (be wary of bacteria overlying an occasional leukocyte on Gram stain). Appropriate antibiotics should be begun and routine treatment for atelectasis, clearance of secretions, and ventilatory support should be used. Further information regarding antibiotics will be covered in Chapter 8, Infectious Diseases.

The most useful parameters for assessing the progress of a pneumonia include fever, volume of mucus, and the P_A-ao_2 gradient. The chest x-ray may not be an accurate index of the degree of involvement or the rate of progression of the pneumonia and should not be used as a sole index of disease. Chest x-rays taken in intensive care units are frequently of less than optimal quality, are difficult to compare on a daily basis, and are commonly taken in a single view only. Every effort should be made to obtain x-rays with the patient in an upright position and full inspiration in appropriate views. Timing the x-ray with ventilator inspiration is useful.

Postoperative Bronchospasm

Postoperative bronchospasm, manifested clinically by wheezing, can be the result of a variety of insults and abnormalities. Patients with underlying airway irritability are at a greater risk of postoperative bronchospasm. Both asthmatic and bronchitic individuals may present bronchospastic responses to infection. Lack of humidification via endotracheal tube, aerosolized water vapor, and aerosolized irritant chemicals (e.g., acetylcysteine, deoxyribonuclease, disodium cromoglycate) may all trigger bronchospasm. Allergic individuals may demonstrate bronchospasm when exposed to an irritating chemical or to cigarette smoke. Occasionally shifting the administration of methylxanthines from an intravenous to an oral route will precipitate bronchospasm, partly due to fluctuating serum levels and partly due to the decreased free theophylline of several of the oral preparations noted previously. Aspirin or other salicylates may trigger an asthma attack in some patients. Coughing or laughing may also precipitate an asthmatic episode. Emotional stress is such a commonly observed triggering factor that asthma has been at times considered a purely psychosomatic disorder. A supportive and occasionally psychotherapeutic approach to individuals with a predominantly emotional component to their disease is most useful.

Bronchospasm is occasionally seen as a manifestation of sudden increases in interstitial lung water (early pulmonary edema). Clinically this finding is generally associated with other evidence of cardiac failure.

Pulmonary embolism may precipitate bronchospasm. This is likely due in part to the normal reflexive narrowing of airways that are underperfused and due in part to one or more of several active bronchoconstrictor agents released from the involved lung. The wheezing is rarely intense or lasts longer than a few hours.

Major decreases in lung volume with continued ventilation to that lung will cause turbulent gas flow in the resulting narrowed airways (wheezing). Pneumothorax, massive pleural effusion, or rapid growth of an air cyst in the involved lung may also be causative factors. Chest x-ray will be most useful in diagnosis. Aspiration, which may be unobserved, can precipitate bronchospasm through the toxic or obstructive effects of the aspirated material (see Aspiration above).

Obstruction of the upper airway caused by factors such as postextubation laryngospasm may result in dyspnea and wheezing. Prolonged endotracheal tube placement and tracheostomy both may lead to endobronchial granulomatous tissue overgrowths that cause wheezing or stridor. Tracheostomy performed with a "button" resection of cartilage often results in measurable narrowing of the airway by radiologic assessment. Soft tissue films of the neck, overpenetrated ("Bucky") views of the chest, midchest tomography, and computerized axial tomography scans will help visualize these lesions. Flow-volume loops will help assess their physiologic significance.

MANAGEMENT OF POSTOPERATIVE BRONCHOSPASM

Management of bronchospasm entails prediction and prophylaxis. Patients with any of the pulmonary risk factors or a history suggestive of airway disease should be investigated preoperatively for evidence of bronchospasm by obtaining flow-volume measurements. Although an occasional patient with hypersensitive airways will escape this screening (e.g., some patients with exercise induction of asthma), most individuals with irritable airways will be identified. Appropriate prophylaxis can be undertaken in the form of bronchodilation.

The appearance of bronchospasm postoperatively is investigated as suggested above. Most patients found to have peribronchial smooth muscle spasm will respond to methylxanthines, beta-active agents, or steroids as discussed earlier. Patients with severe preoperative bronchospasm or airway obstruction often benefit from a prolonged postoperative intubation of one or two additional days. Airway patency can be maximized then and extubation accomplished with a lower likelihood of complications.

Bronchoscopy and Fiberoptic Bronchoscopy

Bronchoscopy can be an exceptionally useful tool in the postoperative management of patients with difficult secretion clearance or aspiration of particulate matter. The more recently developed fiberoptic bronchoscope may be more widely used with less need for the heavy sedation or anesthesia that was required with the rigid bronchoscope. The fiberoptic bronchoscope can be successfully passed through the nasopharynx or via the endotracheal or tracheostomy tube and thus provides versatility with little patient discomfort. Physiologic changes may occur during bronchoscopy but are similar to those induced by routine suctioning except that bronchoscopy may continue for minutes as opposed to the 20 second or less interval for catheter suction. Arterial oxygen desaturation occurs almost routinely during bronchoscopy, the degree varying with the length of the procedure and amount of washing and suctioning performed. These effects may persist for four to six hours after the procedure. Oxygen supplementation is routinely provided during and after bronchoscopy for four to six hours. Arterial blood gases determinations should be obtained prior to bronchoscopy. A Pa_{O_2} of less than 50 mm Hg should be cause for an exceptional effort to maintain adequate oxygenation during bronchoscopy. Cardiac monitoring should be provided in these circumstances.

INDICATIONS FOR AND MANAGEMENT OF BRONCHOSCOPY

Respiratory secretions are at times sufficiently thick or obstructing to warrant bronchoscopic assessment and direct treatment (with the occasional use of acetylcysteine as a thinning agent). After insertion of the bronchoscope, airways should be observed for patency and gentle suction should be applied in airways that are occluded. Hemoptysis can be evaluated for site and cause by fiberoptic bronchoscopy and tampon or local application of a vasoconstricting agent can be used if hemoptysis is brisk.

Any deleterious effects on the airways of endotracheal tubes can be monitored with bronchoscopy and this information may be useful for making decisions about the removal of the endotracheal tube.[95] Another use for the fiberoptic bronchoscope is in the patient who is difficult to intubate. Here intubation can be more easily accomplished if an endotracheal tube is first placed over the bronchoscope and then inserted using the fiberoptic bronchoscope as a guide.

Sampling for cytology and tissue biopsy can also be performed through the bronchoscope. Bronchoscopy for sampling of infectious agents must take into account the possible upper airway contamination of the bronchoscope as it is passed into the peripheral airways. Unless special devices to prevent this contamination are used, bacterial culture results must be considered as possibly contaminated by upper airway organisms.

Respiratory Failure

Acute respiratory failure may be defined as the decompensation of respiratory homeostatic mechanisms resulting in inadequate gas exchange for the patient's metabolism. Adequacy of that gas exchange can be determined by assessing the patient's respiratory function with particular attention to criteria for respiratory support.

OXYGENATION

The measurement of Pa_{O_2} with knowledge of the inspired oxygen concentration and the Pa_{CO_2} allows calculation of the P_{A-aO_2} gradient, essentially a measure of the pulmonary function that summarizes the oxygen exchange capacity of the lung. This calculation should be performed as a very sensitive single index of the various pulmonary complications which may lead to acute respiratory failure. The method for doing the calculation was described previously in Figure 4. Factors other than Pa_{O_2} that influence O_2 delivery to peripheral tissue include O_2 carrying capacity of red blood cells, systemic blood pressure, and peripheral perfusion.

VENTILATION

The adequacy of ventilation is best assessed through measurement of the Pa_{CO_2}, as this is inversely proportional to the ventilation. Failure of adequate alveolar ventilation for CO_2 removal will be seen as an elevation in Pa_{CO_2}.

VENTILATORY RESERVE MECHANICS

Generally, individuals with a vital capacity of less than 15 cc/kg (normal 65 to 75 cc/kg) are incapable of adequate gas exchange. Inspiratory force measurements (normal 75 to 100 cm H_2O) reflect the muscular component of ventilation. Obtaining flow rate measurements (FEV_1/FVC or flow-volume loop) helps in assessing the airway limitations to ventilation, and compliance measurements reflect disease of the pulmonary parenchyma. It is not possible to obtain reliable flow rate measurements on the intubated patient with current technology.

MANAGEMENT OF RESPIRATORY FAILURE

Control of respiratory failure requires identification of the particular mechanism at fault. Respiratory failure can be identified as failure of either oxygenation, ventilation, or ventilatory reserve/mechanics.

Failure of adequate oxygenation can often be managed by the (relatively) simple expedient of oxygen supplementation. Intubation is occasionally necessary to provide inspired oxygen concentrations of 70 percent or more because of the technical limitations to delivery of such high concentrations by mask. Intubation may also be useful in permitting application of varying amounts of PEEP to relieve atelectasis and decrease shunting in some circumstances, as discussed above in the section on atelectasis. Decreased cardiac output resulting from PEEP may be a limiting factor.

Failure of ventilation can be managed with mechanical support. Positive pressure ventilation is commonly used. Complications of endotracheal tube placements and tracheostomies should be kept in mind. Occasionally, patients with uncomplicated muscular failure can be adequately ventilated with the assistance of several devices originally developed for patients with poliomyelitis (e.g., cuirass and tank ventilators, rocking bed, and pneumobelt).

Failure of ventilatory reserve/mechanics must be assessed and directly treated. Air flow limitations may be due to secretions, inflammation, or bronchospasm. Compliance (parenchymal "stiffness") limitations may be due to such reversible causes as pneumonic infiltrate, pulmonary edema, or abdominal distension. The specific etiology should be corrected if possible. Respiratory muscle discoordination has been receiving a good deal of attention. The inability to coordinate diaphragmatic motion with chest wall and abdominal muscular motion may be important in many individuals who present difficulties in weaning from the ventilator. Careful recording of gas flow, thoracic wall motion, and abdominal wall motion will permit identification of this disorder. The etiology and specific corrective actions are unknown. Spontaneous improvement will commonly be seen over several days. Weaning from the ventilator should be undertaken with the awareness that this discoordination may delay the weaning process.

Adult Respiratory Distress Syndrome

The adult respiratory distress syndrome (ARDS) is a clinically defined entity that combines a variety of pulmonary, cardiovascular, and other systemic insults into a picture of acute lung injury that may range from a mild pulmonary infiltrate to severe life-threatening respiratory failure. Signs of respiratory distress including dyspnea and cyanosis may appear in an individual with no severe pre-existing lung disease, often with a short period of latency. Physical examination may be remarkably normal despite severe parenchymal disease. Airway sounds may be only mildly impaired and there may be no crackles or wheezes characteristic of pulmonary edema. Radiologic and blood gas findings are compatible with a severe alveolar-interstitial process which morphologically consists of hyperemic dense parenchymal consolidation with hemorrhagic atelectasis and hyaline membranes. The associated physiology consists of abnormalities of compliance, ventilation-perfusion distribution, shunt, and diffusion and manifests itself as severe hypoxemia, frequently complicated by a decreased cardiac output, hypotension, and lactic acidosis.[96–98]

Diseases associated with ARDS, including other described causes of "noncardiac pulmonary edema," are listed in Table 3. Although the specific mechanism of lung injury has not been identified, several theories of pathogenesis have been advanced in consideration of varying patient populations presenting with the syndrome.

Sepsis is occasionally a precursor of ARDS. Experimental studies in animals have shown that injection of gram-negative endotoxin results in increased pulmonary lym-

TABLE 3. Causes of Adult Respiratory Distress Syndrome

Toxic Causes	Oxygen, ozone, phosgene, chlorine, sulfur dioxide, nitrogen dioxide, ammonia, endotoxin (sepsis), uremia
Aspiration	Aspiration of gastric contents or hydrocarbons (ethyl alcohol, kerosene), drowning (fresh/salt water)
Trauma	Fat embolism, trauma to central nervous system, lung contusion, radiation
Environmental Cause	High altitude
Circulatory Toxins	Transfusion reactions, blood product aggregates, pancreatitis, disseminated intravascular coagulation
Other	Hemorrhagic shock, rapid expansion of lung after thoracocentesis
Infections	Viral, rickettsial, *Mycoplasma,* parasitic

phatic flow—considered to be an index of capillary membrane injury.[99] Such capillary leaks are found in human endotoxin shock despite normal capillary wedge pressure and endotoxin is thought to be an important agent in the pathogenesis.[100]

Shock from any of several causes may be a contributing feature. Hemorrhagic, anaphylactic, or cardiogenic shock have all been shown at times to precede ARDS.[101] Data support an intravascular coagulopathy as the mechanism of injury in this group of disorders.[102, 103] Platelet and white blood cell (WBC) aggregates may occlude the pulmonary microcirculation, disintegrate and subsequently damage the endothelial wall due to release of local vasoactive substances and lysosomal substances.[104]

Multiple trauma, which is often associated with documented fat embolism, is commonly a precursor of ARDS.[105] Generally, the presentation of fat embolism is sufficiently distinctive to permit separate identification,[106] but ARDS may supervene without clear evidence of fat embolism.

Prolonged respirator care has been thought to be a contributing factor to ARDS.[107] The mechanical effects of ventilation may contribute through surfactant depletion by large respiratory excursions. High inspired O_2 tensions may be an additional contributing factor in this setting, since high O_2 concentrations have been clearly shown to be toxic to the lung parenchyma.[108] Such toxicity develops only over a period of time and generally at inspired oxygen concentrations $>$ 50 percent.[109] Most ARDS patients do not encounter these conditions until after the onset of disease. There is evidence, however, that high concentrations of inspired O_2 may further exacerbate the lung injury of ARDS.[110] Hence, efforts to maintain the lowest possible F_{IO_2} should be undertaken.

The possibility that various vasoactive agents or humoral factors could cause or contribute to ARDS has been studied. Vasconstrictors such as serotonin, adenosine triphosphate (ATP), and adenosine diphosphate (ADP) released from platelets may cause further local platelet aggregation as well as an increase in capillary pressure due to predominant pulmonary venous constriction, all leading to an increase in capillary permeability.[104] Pancreatitis may release lipolytic enzymes that damage surfactant[111] or are directly toxic to pulmonary endothelium, thereby increasing capillary permeability.[112] Surfactant itself may be decreased as a result of nonthoracic trauma,[113] but there is little evidence that this a major contributing factor in ARDS.

Perioperatively, ARDS is most commonly associated with complicating infections,[114] aspiration,[115] hypotension, cardiopulmonary bypass (see below), and central nervous system injury due to trauma.[116] Each of these seem to result in similar pathophysiologic changes which is perhaps best explained by the theory of increased capillary permeability and resulting transmembrane fluid "leak" into the interstitial space.[115,117]

Management of Adult Respiratory Distress Syndrome

Management of ARDS requires recognition and treatment of any identifiable underlying disorders leading to the ARDS. Appropriate support can then be provided to minimize the results of the respiratory failure.

At this time prevention of ARDS is possible in only isolated circumstances. Careful monitoring of Pa_{O_2} in patients at risk will permit use of the lowest possible F_{IO_2} to maintain adequate oxygenation. Measures attempting to preclude aspiration preoperatively and postoperatively are of value. However, even cuffed tracheostomy tubes do not completely prevent aspiration in the postoperative patient. Following extubation the laryngeal/glottal reflexes may not adequately protect the airway from aspiration and careful refeeding should be carried out.[77]

Treatment of the fully developed syndrome generally requires placement of an endotracheal tube to permit mechanical ventilation. Such tubes may be allowed to remain in place for 7 to 10 days if there are prospects for safe extubation within that period. Mechanical ventilation using tidal volumes of 12 to 15 cc/kg is most effective and should be applied with a volume ventilator that permits modification of flow rates and pressure wave forms. Inspired O_2 should be maintained at the lowest possible level consistent with adequate O_2 transport to the periphery. Sensitive manipulation of O_2 delivery often requires application of PEEP which reduces blood shunting past closed lung units and hence may dramatically improve oxygen transport to the arterial blood.[118] Generally 5 to 15 cm H_2O pressure is adequate to achieve this goal. Occasionally higher pressures are used,[119] but as pressures are increased the risk of severe decrease in cardiac output and possible pneumothorax increases appreciably. When PEEP is applied, the decrease in cardiac output which occurs may ultimately result in decreased O_2 delivery to the periphery despite an apparent increase in Pa_{O_2}.[120] Since systemic blood pressure may not be an adequate measure of cardiac output,[121] Swan-Ganz monitoring with thermal dilution measurements of cardiac output may be particularly useful in patients on PEEP. Determination of the most effective or "optimal" PEEP, keeping the above consideration in mind, is therefore achieved by careful assessment of systemic O_2 transport. It has been proposed that a useful approximation of the "optimal PEEP" may be found by ascertaining the compliance of the lung at various PEEP pressures and using the pressure at which the lung appears most compliant if cardiac output pressures are not available.[122] Generally, there is little or no airway disease associated with ARDS but attention should be paid to its possible presence since abnormal ventilation-perfusion ratios may contribute to the severe hypoxemia of ARDS. Bronchodilator therapy and modification of ventilator flow rates may both improve the ventilation-perfusion ratios. Also, it should be remembered that the content of hemoglobin contributes to O_2 delivery and any anemia may need to be corrected.

Nonventilatory treatment includes consideration of management of fluids, antibiotics, and steroids. Fluid management may be particularly difficult in ARDS as additional fluids may cause further sequestration of liquids in the lung via capillary permeability. Generally, fluid infusion is calculated to provide adequate cardiac filling pressures and adequate cardiac output (monitor cardiac output, urine output and blood pressure) while avoiding major increases in pulmonary wedge pressure.[123] Usually, wedge pressures greater than 20 to 25 mm Hg are associated with left ventricular failure. However, these pressures may be somewhat misleading and artificially elevated in patients with obstructive airway disease who are on ventilators with PEEP. Accurate assessment of the degree of transmission of alveolar pressure to the observed capillary wedge pressure cannot be made by simple removal of the patient from ventilatory support however briefly. There is no simple formula that permits reduction of clinical data into a single number indicating "failure." Fluid monitoring in the ventilated patient must still be assessed using all available data. Some degree of fluid restriction seems preferable, perhaps ideally to the extent of mild azotemia. There is no convincing evidence that colloid infusion is preferable to crystalloid infusion in these circumstances, presumably since the capillary "leak" is relatively large in molecular terms. There is some evidence that use of colloids increases sequestered lung water perhaps due to local increase in oncotic pressure.[124] Appropriate therapy of any congestive heart failure is critically important and a Swan-Ganz catheterization is necessary for proper assessment of heart failure.

Antibiotics used prophylactically are of no apparent benefit in ARDS and may simply serve to select a population of resistant organisms. While sepsis (endotoxin shock) may lead to ARDS, the frequency of sepsis as a primary cause of ARDS does not justify routine antibiotic therapy of all patients with ARDS. Secondary bacterial invasion of ARDS-damaged parenchyma should be approached as any other pneumonitis.

Routine use of steroids in a variety of doses has been strongly advocated. Data available to date are not convincing that the benefits of apparent reduction in lysosomal enzyme activity[125] or protection against oxygen toxicity[126] outweigh the potential risks of these agents. While awaiting further data, particularly in studies of methylprednisolone,[127] we do not routinely recommend use of these agents in ARDS.

As ARDS resolves, the patient can usually be weaned from the respirator in a manner similar to other long-term ventilator patients. Data concerning recovery rates and residual pulmonary function months and years after ARDS are now being collected.[128] Generally, there is persistent evidence of both mild restrictive and obstructive ventilatory defects which may compromise further lung function to a variable extent.

Pulmonary Embolic Disease

Pulmonary embolism has long been recognized as a complication of prolonged bedrest and surgical procedures. A relatively high mortality rate and serious risk of recurrence, particularly in untreated patients, have prompted studies of the origin and possible prophylaxis of pulmonary embolism. The diagnosis of pulmonary embolism may be particularly difficult. Pulmonary embolism may initially be suspected due to any of several observations. An approach to diagnostic evaluation and therapy of pulmonary embolus is outlined in Figure 8.

A number of conditions may be caused or exacerbated by the effects of pulmonary emboli. Dyspnea may result from an associated hypoxemia or from the hyperventilation necessary to accommodate the increased VD/VT (volume of dead space gas/tidal volume). Chest pain in this setting may result from pleural irritation due to parenchymal ischemia or from a secondary pulmonary hypertension. Hemoptysis secondary to pulmonary embolism results from hemorrhagic necrosis of ischemic pulmonary parenchyma. This is commonly associated with radiologic changes of a rapidly appearing alveolar infiltrate which characteristically clears by progressing to an interstitial pattern with subsequent resolution. Congestive heart failure without obvious cause may be a result of the hemodynamic effects of pulmonary embolism. Deterioration of patients with underlying chronic pulmonary disorders may occur as a result of further compromise of the pulmonary vascular bed by emboli. Generally when the development of any of the above signs or symptoms leads to concern of pulmonary emboli, anticoagulation therapy is commonly begun (except in patients with major contraindications, see Chap. 7, Hematology). Full and immediate anticoagulation is then followed by the collection of more definitive data.

Arterial blood gas analysis is generally performed. A room air Pa_{O_2} value greater

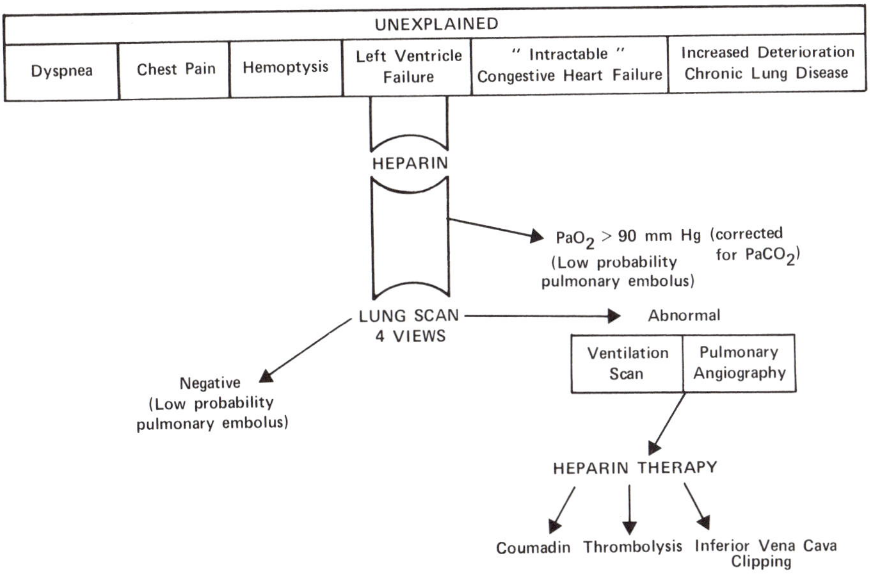

FIGURE 8. Scheme for Diagnostic Evaluation of Suspicion of Pulmonary Embolism: Many nonspecific and nondiagnostic symptoms may occur in association with pulmonary emboli. If pulmonary embolus is suspected and there is no contraindication, patients should be started on heparin immediately. A $Pa_{O_2} > 90$ mm Hg when corrected for Pa_{CO_2} is strong evidence against a pulmonary embolus. Also, a normal lung scan in four views makes pulmonary embolus highly unlikely. On the other hand, the lung scan may be difficult to evaluate in the presence of congestive heart failure, chronic obstructive lung disease, or asthma and pulmonary angiography may be necessary for an adequate diagnosis. (Modified from Sasahara, A.A.: *Current problems in pulmonary embolism: Introduction.* Prog in Cardiovasc Dis. 17:161, 1974).

than 90mm Hg (corrected for hyperventilation) is strong evidence against a clinically significant embolism. An electrocardiogram and a chest x-ray are taken for baseline data purposes only since these parameters are not particularly helpful in ruling out the possibility of embolism. Virtually all clinically significant emboli in individuals without obvious upper extremity disease or recent myocardial infarction originate from the deep leg or pelvic veins.[129] Assessment of these veins can be undertaken, and negative studies would be thought to reduce the statistical likelihood of pulmonary embolism. However, all venous assessment techniques are somewhat insensitive to abnormalities of the deep pelvic veins (see below).

Continued suspicion of pulmonary embolism then generally leads to use of the lung scan as a primary screening procedure. Lung scans, performed since the middle 1960s have not been shown to have a significant incidence of false negatives when performed in at least four views (anterior, posterior, and both laterals). Hence, a normal scan is particularly valuable in ruling out embolism. The lung scan occasionally shows a pattern of abnormality so typical of embolism that the diagnosis can be readily made. More often, however, the presence of underlying lung disease renders the test nonspecifically abnormal. Subsequent ventilation scanning or angiography may be necessary. Ventilation scanning techniques are still under development and are most useful for the assessment of large defects in the lung scan since such defects can result from localized ventilation abnormalities such as are seen in bullous disease. Smaller defects or remaining questions should be assessed by angiography, occasionally using selective dye injections and image magnification. Radiologic studies for the presence of emboli should be undertaken expeditiously since emboli may resolve within a few days, particularly if heparinization has been begun. Studies performed within the first three to five days of the acute episode are the most helpful.[130]

The diagnosis of embolism by radiography should lead to continued heparinization with the partial thromboplastin time (PTT) maintained at two to three times normal by continuous intravenous drip heparin therapy. The anticoagulation therapy is changed from heparin to Coumadin after 7 to 10 days and continued for three to six months unless an underlying cause can be identified and corrected.

Massive embolization has been treated at times by urokinase or streptokinase therapy[131] or suction embolectomy[132] for more rapid resolution of cardiovascular compromise. There is no evidence that these approaches are particularly useful in less severe degrees of embolism. The efficacy of emergency surgical embolectomy is still under discussion. Some authors regard the procedure as obsolete[133] while others feel that it continues to be valuable in patients who meet the criteria set forth by Sasahara for massive embolization requiring possible embolectomy.[134,135] The current infrequent use of this procedure will preclude early resolution of this question.

Occasionally venous interruption is used as an alternative to anticoagulation therapy. Generally thrombosis is first radiologically demonstrated peripheral to the proposed site of venous interruption. Immediate risk of death is reduced by venous interruption, but future recurrence of thrombosis of collateral channels is possible especially if underlying risk factors are not identified and treated.

Venous interruption, whether by clip, plication, or umbrella filtration is often undertaken for one of several reasons:[136]

1. Contraindication to anticoagulation
   a. Major surgery scheduled within one week, especially if in a closed space, for example, the spinal cord, central nervous system.
   b. Difficult anticoagulant management problems, for example, blood dyscrasias.
   c. Prior history of severe gastrointestinal bleeding or current intestinal bleeding.
2. Failure of anticoagulant trial: Recurrent documented embolism during anticoagulation therapy may be considered a failure if occurring several days after commencement of heparin therapy. Earlier recurrence may be due to release of old clots. Chest pain may recur simply due to bleeding into an older area of pulmonary infarct or extension of an embolus which has already occurred.
3. Continued predisposition to embolization, for example, patients with recurrent phlebitis.
4. Presence of other circumstances that have been proposed as relative indications for venous interruption, such as surviving a single episode of major embolism or suffering embolism early in pregnancy.

Venous interruption carries independent morbidity and mortality. A recent study reports a postoperative mortality of 8 percent and a frequency of postoperative recurrence of pulmonary emboli of 31 percent.[137] Umbrella insertion under local anesthesia appears to be a safer procedure but a mortality of about 1 percent is recognized due to central embolization of the device.[133]

The major difficulties in accurate diagnosis and therapy of pulmonary embolism listed above have called attention to deep venous thrombosis as a treatable and possibly preventable underlying disorder. The majority of clinically significant pulmonary emboli arise from venous thrombosis of the deep leg and pelvic veins. Unfortunately, clinical diagnosis of deep venous thrombosis (DVT) is difficult. While unilateral edema of the ankle can be a useful sign of DVT (50 to 80% positive correlation with phlebography [138,139]), significant pulmonary emboli are found at postmortem examination of patients with as little as a 5 to 10 percent incidence of clinical evidence of DVT.[140,141] More sensitive techniques for diagnosing DVT clearly show that half of pulmonary emboli may come from clinically silent extremities.[142,143]

A variety of techniques have been developed to identify DVT more accurately. Phlebography is considered the most specific technique. When carefully performed with a large quantity of dye and multiple view radiographic or cineradiographic technique, phlebography probably identifies up to 95 percent of peripheral thrombi. Filling of the upper thigh and deep pelvic veins may be incomplete, increasing the difficulty in interpretation at this site. The technique, nevertheless, remains the yardstick for other diagnostic interventions.[144] Occasional instances of dye-induced thrombophlebitis are recorded but are less likely with careful saline flushing of the veins and radiographic documentation of their subsequent clearing.

Plethysmography and ultrasound techniques both measure blood flow in the lower limbs. As a result they are primarily sensitive to larger vascular occlusions and may fail to detect small vessel disease, partial obstruction of larger vessels, or evidence of pelvic involvement. Both of these techniques show an 80 to 90 percent correlation with phlebography for large vein DVT and hence are particularly useful as noninvasive techniques for assessment of thromboses of these vessels.[144] However, their failure to detect small vessel disease precludes their use in the sensitive screening that may be of importance in prophylaxis (see below).

Thermography has been employed with good correlation with phlebography for large vein occlusions. The method is simple and easily repeated but unfortunately expensive at this time.[145] Radionuclide phlebography has been described[146] and would be especially useful since lung scanning would be possible with the same injection. However, the resolution of the scanning device (gamma camera) still does not approach that of phlebography. A wide variety of blood tests which utilize measurements of various clotting factors and/or their byproducts to assess ongoing thrombosis have been developed.[147–150] While these tests are still undergoing development, early clinical reports suggest a high degree of reliability in ruling out significant DVT.[151]

Radioactive (^{125}I) labeled fibrinogen tagging of venous thrombosis has been well studied. Since the Federal Drug Administration's release of labeled fibrinogen, this simple and very sensitive diagnostic test is increasingly available.[152,153] The disadvantages of this method include poor sensitivity in the upper thigh and pelvic region due to vascular background radiation and poor fibrinogen uptake (hence poor sensitivity) in older or retracting thrombosis.[154] Equipment cost, required technical expertise, and the delay necessary to pretreat with iodine for thyroid blocking all combine to make this test a poor choice for urgent clinical diagnostic problems. The test does serve as a sensitive screening device particularly for assessment of calf veins when plethysmography or ultrasound studies are normal.

It is important to note that the extreme sensitivity of labeled fibrinogen uptake allows identification of venous abnormalities of which the clinical significance is still unclear. Very few studies of the natural history of fibrinogen-detected DVT have been undertaken. Those that have been done[155,156] report up to 84 percent spontaneous lysis of DVT, propagation in less than 5 percent, and 1 percent embolization (two nonfatal cases). Nevertheless, it is this screening tool that has allowed identification of an exceptionally high rate of perioperative DVT (see below) and permitted study of the efficacy of prophylactic measures of treatment. Current enthusiasm for prophylaxis of thrombosis should be tempered by the recognition that only a few trials have demonstrated the effectiveness of this prophylaxis in diminishing the frequency of severe DVT, postphlebitic leg syndromes, or pulmonary embolism.

Treatment of established DVT is commonly undertaken by heparin anticoagulation therapy given by continuous intravenous infusion to maintain the partial thromboplastin time at 1½ to 2½ times normal control. Heparin is continued and once it is clear that the DVT is under clinical control, Coumadin is begun immediately with an overlap of 3 to 5 days.[157] There is some discussion in the literature regarding the presence of an increased risk of embolism from extensive iliofemoral thrombosis.[133,158] There appear to be no adequate studies to answer this question at the present time.

Prophylaxis of DVT is an area receiving intense study and debate. It is possible to establish a clinical listing of groups at statistically high risk for pulmonary emboli (see Table 4). Subsequent studies with radioactive labeled fibrinogen have demonstrated an exceptionally high frequency of DVT in these same groups.[159] Reduction of the incidence of DVT would be expected to reduce the incidence of pulmonary embolism and

TABLE 4. Factors Increasing Risk of Venous Thrombosis

1. Bedrest
2. Advanced age
3. Pelvic operations (gynecologic, urologic)*
4. Malignant disease
5. Obesity
6. Previous venous disease
7. Congestive heart failure
8. Pregnancy and estrogen containing contraceptives
9. Orthopedic procedures (hip surgery, lower limb fractures)* and other lower extremity trauma

*May require full dose (oral) anticoagulation (see text)

subsequent mortality in these groups at risk. While various protocols have been developed which clearly reduce the incidence of DVT, very few studies are available to demonstrate that the population under study subsequently benefits from a decreased incidence of pulmonary emboli. Best studied are patients with hip fractures who were first clearly shown to benefit from prophylactic anticoagulation in 1959.[160] The most common cause of postoperative death in patients following fracture and elective hip surgery is pulmonary embolism.[161] Full-dose anticoagulation clearly reduces the incidence of pulmonary embolism[162–164] while low-dose heparin does not.[165] Urologic surgery results in rates of DVT of 10 percent in transurethral prostatectomies and up to 50 percent in open prostatectomies.[166] Prophylactic anticoagulation clearly reduces the incidence of DVT and embolism[167] and full-dose anticoagulation can be used for open prostatectomies with adequate control of hemorrhage.[168] Low-dose anticoagulation should be employed with closed prostatectomies, particularly if other risk factors are present (see Table 4). An equivalent dose of parenteral anticoagulation (heparin) would be expected to achieve the same goal in these groups.

Lower dose parenteral anticoagulation ("minidose" heparin) has been shown to clearly reduce the incidence of DVT in several susceptible populations.[169] While firm evidence that the frequency of pulmonary emboli is equally reduced is still lacking, there is a strong clinical impression that such prophylaxis is warranted—particularly in light of ease of administration and freedom from complications. To be effective, this technique appears to be dependent on being begun prior to tissue injury.[170] It does not prevent DVT in certain groups (e.g., patients with hip fractures) which may require full oral anticoagulation (see Table 4). In other groups at risk, 5000 U of heparin is given subcutaneously two hours preoperatively and every eight hours subsequently until the patient is ambulatory. As there is no change in prothrombin time (PT) or PTT with these doses, assessment of these parameters is not routinely undertaken. Obesity should be corrected preoperatively if possible. Use of estrogen containing contraceptives should be discontinued one to two weeks preoperatively if possible.[171]

Intravenous administration of dextrans has been used as a method of preventing

DVT. Available data regarding the efficacy of this technique are conflicting.[172,173] As the incidence of hemorrhagic complications with this agent approach that of warfarin, it should only be used if heparin or warfarin are otherwise unacceptable.

Agents designed to suppress platelet activity are being intensively studied. Among these, aspirin and dipyridamole are of most interest. The available literature is not conclusive regarding the effectiveness of these agents in DVT. In instances where low-dose heparin might be used, aspirin seems to be somewhat effective. The effectiveness of aspirin and/or dipyridamole is not equal to that of warfarin for hip surgery prophylaxis.[174] Further studies of this area will likely continue to be confusing until the role of platelets in venous thrombosis is more clearly established.[175]

Pulmonary Rehabilitation

Patients who undergo thoracic or abdominal surgery commonly experience postoperative respiratory limitations which may be the direct result of surgery or of pulmonary postoperative complications. Rehabilitation of these patients to the level of the highest possible functional capacity should begin during the immediate postoperative period and should continue throughout subsequent hospitalization and convalescence.

The need for rehabilitation can often be predicted preoperatively by pulmonary function testing and assessment of existing limitations. An extrapolation to the postoperative state can then be made with the added knowledge of the extent of surgery. Patients undergoing thoracotomy and pulmonary resectional surgery are those most likely to require such planning. Patients with severe postoperative pulmonary complications often display prolonged or incomplete respiratory functional recovery and may also require rehabilitation. Rehabilitation is a natural extension of the chest physiotherapy that the patient experiences preoperatively. Commonly, it is the chest physiotherapist or nurse who initiates the planning necessary to develop and implement a program of pulmonary rehabilitation.

MANAGEMENT OF PULMONARY REHABILITATION

A program of pulmonary rehabilitation is generally instituted by a physician, physiotherapist, and a pulmonary nurse specialist as a team approach. Baseline pulmonary function is assessed and retraining of the disordered physiology is undertaken. Particular attention should be paid to abnormal or increased work of breathing. Obesity should be corrected and smoking should be discontinued. Obstructive airway disease and congestive heart failure should be treated. The patient's psychologic attitudes should be assessed and a "positive" outlook developed. Major degrees of depression are commonly seen in chronically limited respiratory patients, and such depression may be severe enough to require psychiatric intervention. The use of tranquilizers which may depress respiration should be avoided. It is extremely important that adequacy of the patient's daytime and nocturnal (sleep) arterial gases be assessed prior to assuming that emotional abnormalities are entirely psychiatric in origin. Individuals with chronic lung disease commonly hypoventilate at night and may consequently experience severe nocturnal hypoxemia. This hypoxemia may seriously disturb sleep and alter daytime emotional states.

Exercise reconditioning is an essential component of the rehabilitation process and has two goals:

1. To improve the muscular efficiency of peripheral musculature and, hence, reduce the amount of oxygen required for a given task.
2. To improve the individual's participation in his own care and rehabilitation.

Bicycling, use of a treadmill, and swimming are commonly used as therapeutic modalities. Clinical evidence for exercise intolerance at normal levels of activity includes: (1) diaphoresis, (2) cyanosis, diminished alertness, and uncoordination as evidence of hypoxemia, (3) severe dyspnea, (4) tachycardia disproportionate to the work level, and (5) "plateauing" or declining heart rate or blood pressure with increasing work load. Such "deconditioned" responses are commonly seen in patients whose physiologic capacity is less than 25 percent of predicted values. Their maximal exercise tolerance may be limited to 1 to 1.5 L of O_2 consumption per minute—roughly equivalent to that of light housework. Exercise training can often increase work tolerance by 50 percent or more. The daily activity of the more severely limited individual may need to be modified. Methods for minimizing work and maximizing the efficiency of such light activities as showering and shaving have been demonstrated.

Chronically administered low-flow oxygen may be of considerable use during rehabilitation. Oxygen supplementation often dramatically increases exercise tolerance. Several devices have been developed to permit oxygen delivery during ambulation. The patient's baseline arterial blood gases should be sampled at rest, during exercise, and during sleep if possible. Correction of the hypoxemia is undertaken with oxygen delivered by nasal cannula and the required flow rates are recorded. With a home ambulatory oxygen supply, the patient can administer the appropriate flow rate to maintain the state of improved oxygenation. Evidence to date suggests that 15 or more hours of low-flow oxygen per day are necessary for patients with significant hypoxemia to provide demonstrated long-term improvement in secondary polycythemia, exercise tolerance, and neuropsychiatric status.[176]

Postoperative Physiotherapy

Postoperative physiotherapy is routinely undertaken with patients recovering from thoracic surgery, general anesthesia, and any major procedure if the patient has particular risk of pulmonary complication (obesity, age, smoking history, obstructive airway disease, sepsis, malnutrition, acute respiratory infection). Additional mechanical and pharmacologic assistance may be sought to improve secretion removal and treat atelectasis, and, if necessary, is generally applied shortly before physiotherapy treatment to enhance results. Bronchodilators, in particular, are most efficiently applied just prior to scheduled physiotherapy.

Treatments should be most intensive immediately following operation. While nocturnal rest is important, even operations performed late in the day should be followed by aggressive chest physiotherapy. The specific modality used will depend on the assessment of pulmonary function. The therapist or nurse will ordinarily note the vital signs, results of chest tube drainage, blood gas results, chest x-ray data, quality and color of sputum, and the use of sedative or analgesic medications. A stethoscopic examination of the chest should be conducted before and after treatment to assess the changes that result from therapeutic maneuvers.

Occasionally nasotracheal (endotracheal if a tube is in place) suctioning will be found helpful in assisting with removal of secretions. Suctioning is facilitated by adequate patient hydration. The physician should be alert to the possible vagotonic and hypoxemic consequences of prolonged and vigorous suctioning. Postoperative coughing is generally encouraged but caution is urged in patients with unstable cardiovascular systems. Patients with pneumothorax may increase their air leak by forced coughing. In these patients, deep abdominal breathing and bronchial drainage techniques are preferable to energetic coughing exercises. Secretions are occasionally loosened in a sudden flood, particularly in lung abscess or bronchopleural fistula. Care must be taken that other portions of the lung are not infected or occluded by a "spill over." The occasional patient with a clotting disorder (excluding patients on low-dose heparin) should not be vigorously percussed as occasional pulmonary parenchymal or chest wall hematoma can result.

Patients with predominantly unilateral chest disease may become severely hypoxemic if the involved side is dependent while the patient is in the lateral position, and attention to the patient's tolerance of this position is necessary.

As the patient recovers and evidence of pulmonary complications diminishes or is lacking, the frequency of physiotherapy treatments is decreased. The patient, however, is encouraged to continue deep abdominal breathing exercises for periods of up to three to four weeks postoperatively. An occasional patient benefits from ambulatory visits to the Physiotherapy Department or home care visits by a trained visiting physiotherapist/nurse.

Special Cases

BURNS

Burn patients have several perioperative pulmonary risks that complicate their care. Upper airway burns occasionally occur secondary to the inhalation of heated gases. Usually these burns extend only a few centimeters into the airway because of the low heat content of the gases. However, with the inhalation of superheated steam or actual flame, the glottis may be damaged and intubation or tracheostomy may be necessary.[177] The various inhaled smokes and toxic gases may produce a severe tracheobronchitis with mucosal sloughing and distal hemorrhagic pulmonary edema. This may first become apparent clinically as late as 10 to 12 hours after the exposure and should be looked for by chest x-ray, assessment of arterial blood gases, and auscultation. Severe hypoxemia, hypercapnia, and combined respiratory and lactic acidosis may result.

Carbon monoxide exposure is commonly found in victims of fires. Inhalation results in high affinity binding to hemoglobin and a secondary shift of the oxyhemoglobin dissociation curve, both of which effectively render some percentage of the victim's hemoglobin (now carboxyhemoglobin) unable to transport oxygen. The arterial blood will nevertheless continue to demonstrate a "normal" Po_2, misleading the observer into thinking that an adequate oxygen content is present. Carbon monoxide dissociates steadily from its hemoglobin binding. This dissociation can be hastened by high levels of inspired oxygen, and the safety of the patient is enhanced within a few hours of exposure if 100 percent inspired O_2 is used.[178] Levels of 50 percent carboxyhemoglobin are commonly lethal. Levels of 5 to 15 percent carboxyhemoglobin are frequently found in heavy smokers and may present particular difficulties for the surgical patient with preexisting hypoxemia, anemia, or altered perfusion of critical organs.

Tracheostomies and chest tubes placed through burned skin have a very high incidence of complication by infection. Later complications of pneumonia and of pulmonary emboli occur frequently. Prophylaxis for pulmonary emboli is undertaken if hematologic parameters are normal. The hematogenous spread of organisms from burn sites is a common cause of pneumonia. Although typical burn therapy with mafenide creams has effectively suppressed hematogenous spread of these organisms, pneumonia occurs with equal frequency by the inhalational route.[179, 180]

CARDIAC SURGERY

Pulmonary complications are the most common cause of perioperative morbidity and mortality following cardiopulmonary bypass procedures.[181] Most of these complications seem to originate in the intraoperative and immediate postoperative period. Of greatest concern is the frequent appearance of a picture similar to ARDS that further stresses an already compromised patient. While a single unifying etiologic mechanism still escapes identification, several contributing factors have been identified.

Various clotting disorders have been associated with extracorporeal circulation which may lead to pulmonary parenchymal bleeding or capillary damage from disseminated intravascular coagulation.[182,183] Microembolization to the pulmonary vasculature has been demonstrated for a wide variety of both cellular and acellular components. Such material as degenerated platelets and polymorphonuclear cells, fibrin, and other protein aggregates might damage the capillary endothelium.[184–186] The use of Dacron blood filters seems to effectively diminish the frequency of these events.[187] Bypass circuit priming with crystalloid may exacerbate a tendency to interstitial edema. This can generally be controlled by the use of colloid or blood priming.[188] However, other studies suggest that homologous blood priming may lead to pulmonary capillary leukocyte migration and abnormalities of the Type II pneumonocytes—changes that correlate with pulmonary insufficiency in at least one study group. Such changes were not seen when autologous blood priming was undertaken.[189,190] Use of bubble oxygenation circuits may promote blood protein denaturation and cause release of free lipids. The former may lead to vascular sludging, the latter to fat microembolization, and both processes may damage the capillary microcirculation.[191]

The pulmonary artery is generally poorly, if at all, perfused during cardiopulmonary bypass. This may lead to a mild degree of pulmonary parenchymal hypoxemia sufficient to interfere with surfactant production.[192] However, subsequent studies of bypass perfusion of only one lung suggest that the perfusate rather than hypoxemia contributes to the pulmonary complications.[193]

The questions of oxygen toxicity, ventilator-pressure effects, and circulating toxins as a cause of the pulmonary complications are discussed in the literature referring to ARDS. A variety of abnormal responses of pulmonary vasculature during cardiopulmonary bypass have been described. Most notable are findings of increased pulmonary artery pressure in response to small air emboli[194] and in response to other measured and unmeasured components of the cardiopulmonary bypass perfusate.[195,196]

Less common pulmonary complications associated with cardiac surgery include compression of the left mainstem bronchus secondary to cardiomegaly. A decrease in local ventilation (Ewart's sign) and occasional collapse of the left lower lobe may result. Intraoperative positioning in the left lateral decubitus position may increase the likelihood of this complication. Use of beta-blocking agents intraoperatively and postoperatively may exacerbate bronchospasm in individuals with underlying bronchospastic disorders (asthma, bronchitis, and many individuals with seasonal rhinitis). While experience with the newer beta-blocking agents is limited, their respiratory side effects may be similar. Preoperative assessment of pulmonary function may be particularly useful here.

Management of Cardiac Surgery

The incidence of pulmonary complications in cardiopulmonary bypass surgery correlates with the length of bypass. There is some evidence that bypass exceeding a limit of 120 to 150 minutes in patients with normal lungs is followed by a rapid increase in complications.[197] The presence of abnormal lung function preoperatively leads to increased rates of complications; hence preoperative pulmonary function assessment is particularly useful.[197] Use of filtration devices (Dacron wool filters) reduces the incidence of pulmonary microemboli. No data on the resulting reduction of pulmonary complications is yet available. Studies of the pulmonary complications with various types of oxygenators provide ongoing data for modification of these devices. The use of membrane oxygenators seems to be advantageous compared to bubble oxygenators.[198,199] Careful attention to using priming solutions free of homologous blood has apparently reduced the incidence of pulmonary complications.[200]

Since cardiopulmonary bypass is, in a sense, uniformly stressful to pulmonary physiologic function with all patients sustaining some degree of pulmonary insult, careful preoperative assessment of pulmonary function with appropriate medical and physiotherapeutic intervention should be of great value.

MUSCLE DISORDERS

Myasthenia Gravis

Myasthenia gravis frequently presents perioperative complications that result from the underlying disease process. For unknown reasons, surgery seems to sensitize the patient with myasthenia to his normal anticholinesterase drugs. This may be partly related to the increase in endogenous steroids that occurs with any tissue trauma.[201] Since therapy with anticholinesterase compounds causes increased secretions and may in the immediate perioperative period precipitate a myasthenic crisis with "normal" doses, most authors recommend withholding these agents for 10 to 12 hours preoperatively and for up to three to four days postoperatively[202] with cautious reinstitution as the weaning and extubation process proceeds (see chap. 9, Neurology).

Patients with myasthenia gravis undergoing thymectomy have the superimposed risk of a high median sternotomy. Postoperative atelectasis and pneumonia may occur more frequently requiring assiduous attention to postoperative care. Intubation is commonly maintained for two to three days postoperatively, and particular care should be taken to avoid tracheostomy since patients may become dependent on long-term ventilatory support.

The myasthenic patient is particularly sensitive to a variety of drugs that may affect muscle action. Curare-like drugs may cause exceptionally prolonged paralysis.[203] Various antibiotics may have curare-like affects which can seriously inhibit the respiratory function of the myasthenic patient. Neomycin, kanamycin, colistin, streptomycin, and gentamicin are most commonly at fault in this respect. Neostigmine may reverse this effect.

Other Disorders Involving Respiratory Musculature

Muscular dystrophy, poliomyelitis, and tetanus may all present particular difficulties with postoperative weaning and pulmonary complications. Particular attention to the curariform effects of the various drugs noted above will assist in patient care. Respiratory paralysis may occur in patients with acute intermittent porphyria. In these patients, infections and a wide variety of drugs including ergot derivatives; antibiotics such as chloramphenicol, sulfonamides, and griseofulvin; barbiturates; phenytoin; glutethimide; and possibly chlordiazepoxide may precipitate paralysis. Weaning difficulties and atelectasis may result postoperatively (see chap. 7, Hematology).[204,205]

NARCOTIC ABUSE

Narcotic addicts have a substantially increased perioperative respiratory risk. Increased sensitivity to various infections has been well documented and unusual organisms are commonly seen in addicts, perhaps partly due to an associated leukopenia.[206] Although the pulmonary edema seen with heroin (and methadone) overdosage is a common cause of death,[207] it does not seem to predispose to later perioperative pulmonary edema. However, pulmonary function abnormalities may persist for several weeks after the acute edematous episode[208] increasing the risk of postoperative pulmonary complications. Similar pulmonary edema caused by pharmacologic overdose has been reported with chlordiazepoxide[209] and ethchlorvynol.[210] The pulmonary edema is treated by conventional measures.

Repetitive intravenous injection of various drugs which are often "cut" with talc may lead to a talc angiothrombosis with pulmonary artery hypertension.[211] Peripheral thrombophlebitis secondary to repetitive intravenous use of drugs may lead to septic thrombophlebitis and secondary pulmonary embolism.[212]

NEUROSURGERY

Acute pulmonary edema may occur following neurosurgical procedures and head trauma. The specific cause of the edema is not clearly understood but is likely related to a massive sympathetic hypothalamic discharge causing elevated pulmonary venous pressure and subsequent microvascular leakage.[213] The edema does not have a characteristic distribution and is often asymmetric. The time course of the edema may vary from one to several days. Its persistence, however, may indicate superimposed aspiration or infection. The pathophysiologic effects are similar to those of other causes of "noncardiac pulmonary edema" and should be treated similarly.

Neurosurgical procedures performed in the sitting position are also occasionally associated with venous air embolism. Right atrial monitoring by catheter sampling or fluoroscopic demonstration of air in the dural sinuses and internal jugular veins have documented occasional instances of substantial air embolism which, on at least one occasion, may have caused pulmonary edema.[214]

OBSTETRIC AND GYNECOLOGIC SURGERY

Amniotic fluid embolism causes respiratory failure as a presenting and frequently terminal event. The pulmonary vasculature is mechanically occluded by a combination of meconium and amniotic fluid. A reflex vasconstriction of the remaining pulmonary vasculature may also further compromise left atrial preload. Decreased left atrial preload, in association with a peripheral venous dilatation, may lead to a massive fall in cardiac output. Diagnosis may be made by right atrial or pulmonary artery sampling to document the presence of embolized material.[215,216]

Rarely, the diaphragm may rupture during delivery. The rupture is best diagnosed radiologically and expeditious repair will help preserve intestinal integrity.[217]

Pelvic sepsis may occur as a complication of pregnancy or various gynecologic procedures. If associated with a thrombophlebitis, the combined disease may present as multiple septic pulmonary emboli which commonly progress to cavitation.[212]

The risk of deep vein thrombosis and pulmonary embolism is significantly increased in postpartum or postsurgical gynecologic patients. Postpartum patients, especially if at risk for deep venous thrombosis (see Table 4 for other factors) benefit from low-dose heparin prophylaxis. Abdominal gynecologic surgery with pelvic dissection requires full-dose anticoagulation as prophylaxis.[218]

RADIATION THERAPY

Radiation therapy may be complicated by an early pneumonitis or late fibrosis further complicating surgical procedures. The dose of radiation previously administered, the lung volume affected, the time and type of radiation, and the duration of surgery contribute to the degree and number of complications. Chemotherapy presents a similar spectrum of complications with perhaps a greater incidence of infection secondary to associated hematopoietic cell damage and immune suppression. Combined radiation therapy and chemotherapy produce a higher complication rate.[219]

Ideally, surgical intervention after radiation therapy or chemotherapy should be delayed until tissue recovery is complete. Recovery of the immune defense system after chemotherapy or radiation may be adequate within two to four weeks and can be roughly assessed by the peripheral leukocyte count. The pulmonary effects of chemotherapy or radiation therapy directed to the chest may only first become manifest one to six months later. Since an increase in pulmonary postoperative complications may be expected, preoperative pulmonary function testing may be useful. Evidence of acute pneumonitis secondary to radiation may be best treated with corticosteroids, particularly if there is evidence of severe or progressive disease.[219]

REFERENCES

1. Morton, HJV: *Tobacco smoking and pulmonary complications after operation.* Lancet 1:368, 1944.
2. Choddoff, P. Margand, PMS, and Imbembo, AL: *Applied pulmonary physiology: morbid obesity and pulmonary function.* Crit Care Med 2:123, 1974.
3. Golebiowski, A, and Maidstone, K: *Pulmonary resection in patients over 70 years of age.* J Thorac Cardiovasc Surg 61:265, 1971.
4. Legge, JS, and Palmer, KNV: *Pulmonary function in bronchial carcinoma.* Thorax 28:588, 1973.
5. Karliner, JS, Coomaraswamy, R, and Williams, MH: *Relationship between pulmonary function studies and prognosis of patients undergoing pneumonectomy for carcinoma of the lung.* Dis Chest 54:112, 1968.
6. Mittman, C: *Assessment of operative risk in thoracic surgery.* Am Rev Resp Dis 84:197, 1961.
7. Higgins, GA, and Beebe, GW: *Bronchogenic carcinoma: factors in survival.* Arch Surg 94:539, 1967.
8. Uggla, LG: *Indications for and results of thoracic surgery with regard to respiratory and circulatory function tests.* Acta Chir Scand 111:197, 1956.
9. Kristersson, S, Lindell, SE, and Svanberg, L: *Prediction of pulmonary function loss due to pnemonectomy using ^{133}Xe-radiospirometry.* Chest 62:694, 1972.
10. Boushy, SF, Billig, DM, and North, LB: *Clinical course related to preoperative and postoperative pulmonary function in patients with bronchogenic carcinoma.* Chest 59:383, 1971.
11. Schwaber, JR: *Evaluation of respiratory status in surgical patients.* Surg Clin North Am 50:637, 1970.
12. Olsen, GN, and Block, AJ: *Pulmonary function testing in evaluation for pneumonectomy.* Hospital Practice 8:137, 1973.
13. Latimer, RG, Dickman, M, Day, WC, et al.: *Ventilatory patterns and pulmonary complications after upper abdominal surgery determined by preoperative and postoperative computerized spirometry and blood gas analysis.* Am J Surg 122:622, 1971.
14. Bendixen, HH, Sykes, MK, Todd, DP, and Surtees, MB: *Respiratory Care.* St. Louis: CV Mosby Co., 1965.
15. Dripps, RD, and Deming, MVN: *Postoperative atelectasis and pneumonia: diagnosis, etiology and management based upon 1,240 cases of upper abdominal surgery.* Ann Surg 124:94, 1946.
16. Gould, AB, Jr.: *Effect of obesity on respiratory complications following general anesthesia.* Anesth Analg 41:448, 1962.
17. Bunker, JP, Bendixen, HH, Sykes, MK, et al.: *A comparison of ether anesthesia with thiopental-nitrous oxide-succinylcholine for upper abdominal surgery.* Anesthesiology 20:745, 1959.
18. Chalon, T, Tayyab, MA, and Ramanathan, S: *Cytology of respiratory epithelium as a predictor of respiratory complications after operation.* Chest 67:32, 1975.
19. Rovenstine, EA, and Taylor, IB: *Postoperative respiratory complications: occurrence following 7,874 anesthesias.* Am J Med Sci 191:807, 1936.

20. Steward, DJ, and Sloan, IAJ: *Recent upper respiratory infection and pulmonary artery clamping in the etiology of postoperative respiratory complications.* Can Anaesth Soc J 16:57, 1969.
21. Meneely, GR, and Ferguson, JL: *Pulmonary evaluation and risk in patient preparation for anesthesia and surgery.* JAMA 175:1074, 1961.
22. Collins, CD, Darke, CS, and Knowelden, J: *Chest complications after upper abdominal surgery: their anticipation and prevention.* Br Med J 1:401, 1968.
23. Mithoefer, JC: *Indications for oxygen therapy in chronic obstructive pulmonary disease.* Am Rev Resp Dis 110:35, 1974.
24. Clark, J: *The toxicity of oxygen.* Am Rev Resp Dis 110:40, 1974.
25. American College of Chest Physicians: *Recommendations for continuous oxygen therapy in chronic obstructive lung disease. A statement by the Committee on Emphysema.* Chest 64:505, 1973.
26. Wolfsdorf, J, Swift, DL, and Avery, ME: *Mist therapy reconsidered: an evaluation of respiratory deposition on labelled water aerosols produced by jet and ultrasonic nebulizers.* Pediatrics 43:799, 1969.
27. Sladen, A, Laver, MB, and Pontoppidian, H: *Pulmonary complications and water retention in prolonged mechanical ventilation.* N Engl J Med 279:448, 1968.
28. Chalon, T, Tayyab, MA, and Ramanathan, S: *Cytology of respiratory epithelium as a predictor of respiratory complications after operation.* Chest 67:32, 1975.
29. Auerbach, O, Hammond, EC, Garfinkel, L, et al.: *Relation of smoking and age to emphysema: whole-lung section study.* N Engl J Med 286:853, 1972.
30. Miller, JM, and Sproule, BJ: *Acute effects of inhalation of cigarette smoke on mechanical properties of the lungs.* Am Rev Resp Dis 94:721, 1966.
31. Auerbach, O, Stout, AP, Hammond, EC, et al.: *Changes in bronchial epithelium in relation to cigarette smoking and in relation to lung cancer.* N Engl J Med 265:253, 1961.
32. Harris, JO, Swenson, EW, and Johnson, JE, III: *Human alveolar macrophages: comparison of phagocytic ability, glucose utilization and ultrastructure in smokers and nonsmokers.* J Clin Invest 49:2086, 1970.
33. Krumholz, RA, Chevalier, RB, and Ross, JC: *Changes in cardiopulmonary functions related to abstinence from smoking.* Ann Intern Med 62:197, 1965.
34. Conroy, JP: *Smoking and the anesthetic risk.* Anesth Analg 48:388, 1969.
35. Russell, MAH, Cole, PV, and Brown, E: *Absorption by nonsmokers of carbon monoxide from room air polluted by tobacco smoke.* Lancet 1:576, 1973.
36. Newman, JH, Neff, TA, Ziporin, P: *Acute respiratory failure associated with hypophosphatemia.* N Engl J Med 296:1101, 1977.
37. Burwell, CS, Robin, ED, Whaley, RD, et al.: *Extreme obesity associated with alveolar hypoventilation—a pickwickian syndrome.* Am J Med 21:311, 1956.
38. Sharp, JT, Henry, JP, Sweany, SK, et al.: *The total work of breathing in normal and obese men.* J Clin Invest 43:728, 1964.
39. Cherniak, RM, and Guenter, CA: *The efficiency of the respiratory muscles in obesity.* Can J Biochem Physiol 39:1215, 1961.
40. Said, SI: *Abnormalities of pulmonary gas exchange in obesity.* Ann Intern Med 53:1121, 1960.
41. Pflug, AE, Murphy, TM, Butler, SH, et al.: *The effects of postoperative peridural analgesia on pulmonary therapy and pulmonary complications.* Anesthesiology 41:8, 1974.
42. Bartlett, RH, Gazzariga, AB, and Geraghty, TR: *Respiratory maneuvers to prevent postoperative pulmonary complications: a critical review.* JAMA 224:1017, 1973.
43. Gaskell, DV, and Webber, BA: *The Brompton Hospital Guide to Chest Physiotherapy.* London: Blackwell Scientific Publications, 1977.
44. Sheldon, GP: *Pressure breathing in chronic obstructive lung disease.* Medicine 43:197, 1963.
45. Loke, J, and Anthonisen, NR: *Effect of intermittent positive pressure breathing on steady state chronic obstructive pulmonary disease.* Am Rev Resp Dis 110:178, 1974.

46. MILLER, RD, HEPPER, NGG: *The dangers and limitations of IPPB in managing diseases affecting ventilation.* in Ingelfinger, FJ, Ebert RV, Finland, M el al. (eds.): *Controversy in Internal Medicine-II.* Philadelphia; W. B. Saunders, 1974, p. 263.

47. BIRNBAUM, ML, CREE, EM, RASMUSSEN, H, ET AL.: *Effects of intermittent positive pressure breathing on emphysematous patients.* Am J Med 41:552, 1966.

48. CHENEY, FW, JR., NELSON, EJ, AND HORTON, WG: *The function of intermittent positive pressure breathing related to breathing patterns.* Am Rev Resp Dis 110:183, 1974.

49. BARTLETT, RH, BRENNAN, MC, GAZZANIGA, AB, ET AL.: *Studies on the pathogenesis and prevention of postoperative pulmonary complications.* Surg Gynecol Obstet 137:925, 1973.

50. DULFANO, MH, ADLER, K, AND WOOTEN, O: *Physical properties of sputum. IV. Effects of 100 percent humidity and water mist.* Am Rev Resp Dis 107:130, 1972.

51. MOULDING, T: *Precautions to prevent cross infection during use of heated aerosol inhalation equipment for sputum induction.* (Correspondence). Am Rev Resp Dis 90:968, 1964.

52. BURTON, JKD: *Effects of dry anaesthetic gases on the respiratory mucous membrane.* Lancet 1:235, 1962.

53. LAWSON, D, AND SAGGERS, BA: *N.A.C. and antibiotics in cystic fibrosis.* Br Med J 1:317, 1965.

54. BARTON, AD: *Aerosolized detergents and mucolytic agents in the treatment of stable chronic obstructive pulmonary disease.* Am Rev Resp Dis 110:104, 1974.

55. CHODOSH, S: *Objective sputum changes associated with glyceryl guaiacolate in chronic bronchial diseases.* Bull Physiopathol Respir 9:452, 1973.

56. ZIMENT, I: *Phosphodiesterase inhibitors. In Respiratory Pharmacology and Therapeutics,* ZIMENT, I (ed.): Philadelphia: WB Saunders Co., 1968, p. 190.

57. EGBERT, LD, LAVER, MB, AND BENDIXEN, HH: *The effect of site of operation and type of anesthesia upon the ability to cough in the postoperative period.* Surg Gynecol Obstet 115:295, 1962.

58. EGBERT, LD, AND BENDIXEN, HH: *Effect of morphine on breathing pattern: a possible factor in atelectasis.* JAMA 188:485, 1964.

59. HERS, JFP: *Disturbances of the ciliated epithelium due to influenza virus.* Am Rev Resp Dis (Suppl) 93:162, 1966.

60. LAURENZI, GA, YIN, S, AND GUARNERI, JJ: *Adverse effect of oxygen on tracheal mucus flow.* N Engl J Med 279:333, 1968.

61. BALLENGER, JJ: *Experimental effect of cigarette smoke in human respiratory cilia.* N Engl J Med 263:832, 1960.

62. ZEBALLOS, RJ, SHTURMAN-ELLSTEIN, R, MCNALLY, JF, JR., ET AL.: *The role of hyperventilation in exercise-induced bronchoconstriction.* Am Rev Resp Dis 118:877, 1978.

63. LAURENZI, GA: *Oxygen impairment of tracheal mucus flow: effect of catecholamines and digitalis.* Int Z Klin Pharmakol Ther Toxikol 4:433, 1971.

64. CRYSTAL, RG, FULMER, JD, ROBERTS, WC, ET AL.: *Idiopathic pulmonary fibrosis—clinical, histologic, radiographic, physiologic, scintigraphic, cytologic and biochemical aspects.* Ann Intern Med 85:769, 1976.

65. SMITH, CB, PURCELL, RH, BELLANTI, JA, ET AL.: *Protective effect of antibody to parainfluenza Type 1 virus.* N Engl J Med 275:1145, 1966.

66. JOHANSON, WG, PIERCE, AK, AND SANFORD, JP: *Changing pharyngeal bacterial flora of hospitalized patients: emergence of gram-negative bacilli.* N Engl J Med 281:1137, 1969.

67. DULFANO, MJ (ed.): *Sputum.* Springfield: Illinois, Charles C Thomas, 1973.

68. AVERY, ME: *Pharmacological approaches to the acceleration of fetal lung maturation.* Br Med Bull 31:13, 1975.

69. MEAD, J, AND COLLIER, C: *Relation of volume history of lungs to respiratory mechanics in anesthetized dogs.* J Appl Physiol 14:669, 1959.

70. BRYAN, AC: *Comments of a devil's advocate.* Am Rev Resp Dis 110:143, 1974.

71. BENDIXEN, HH, AND LAVER, MB: *Hypoxia in anesthesia, a Review.* Clin Pharmacol Ther 6:510, 1965.

72. PARBROOK, GD, STEEL, DF, AND DALRYMPLE, DG: *Factors predisposing to postoperative pain and pulmonary complications.* Br J Anaesth 45:21, 1973.

73. Bowen, TE, Fishback, ME, and Green, DC: *Treatment of refractory atelectasis.* Ann Thorac Surg 18:584, 1974.

74. Fowler, AA, III, Scoggins, WG, and ODonahue, WJ, Jr.: *Positive and expiratory pressure in management of lobar atelectasis.* Chest 74:497, 1978.

75. Krumpe, PE, Zidulka, A, Urbanetti, JS, et al.: *Comparison of the effects of continuous negative external chest pressure and positive end expiratory pressure on cardiac index in dogs.* Am Rev Resp Dis 115:39, 1977.

76. Edwards, G, Morton, HJV, Pask, EA, et al.: *Deaths associated with anaesthesia; report on 1,000 cases.* Anaesthesia 11:194, 1956.

77. Davis, FG, and Cullen, DJ: *Post-extubation aspiration following prolonged intubation.* Abstracts of scientific papers. Annual meeting of the American Society of Anesthesiologists, Washington, D. C., October 12–16, 1974, p. 181.

78. Claeys, DW, Lockhart, CH, and Hinckle, JE: *The effects of translaryngeal block and innovar on glottic competence.* Anesthesiology 38:485, 1973.

79. Cameron, JL, Reynolds, J, and Zuidema, GD: *Aspiration in patients with tracheostomies.* Surg Gynecol Obstet 136:68, 1973.

80. Cameron, JL, Anderson, RP, and Zuidema, GD: *Aspiration pneumonia—a clinical and experimental review.* J Surg Res 7:44, 1967.

81. Alexander, IG: *The ultrastructure of the pulmonary alveolar vessels in Mendelson's (acid pulmonary aspiration) syndrome.* Br J Anaesth 40:408, 1968.

82. Cameron, JL, Mitchell, WH, and Zuidema, GD: *Aspiration Pneumonia: clinical outcome following documented aspiration.* Arch Surg 106:49, 1973.

83. Downs, JB, Chapman, RL, Modell, JH, et al.: *An evaluation of steroid therapy in aspiration pneumonitis.* Anesthesiology 40:129, 1974.

84. Wilson, JW: *Treatment of prevention of pulmonary cellular damage with pharmacologic doses of corticosteroid.* Surg Gynecol Obstet 134:675, 1972.

85. Sladen, A, Zanca, P, and Hadnott, WH: *Aspiration pneumonitis—the sequelae.* Chest 59:448, 1971.

86. Kumar, A, Falke, KJ, Geffin, B, et al.: *Continuous positive pressure ventilation in acute respiratory failure: effects on hemodynamics and lung function.* N Engl J Med 283:1430, 1970.

87. Reynolds, J, and Christensen, EE: *Early radiologic signs of bronchial rupture.* Tex Med 64:50, 1968.

88. Ratliff, JL, Chavez, DM, Jamchuk, A, et al.: *Reexpansion pulmonary edema.* Chest 64:654, 1973.

89. Waqaruddin, M, and Bernstein, A: *Re-expansion pulmonary oedema.* Thorax 30:54, 1975.

90. Humphreys, RL, and Berne, AS: *Rapid re-expansion of pneumothorax: a cause of unilateral pulmonary edema.* Radiology 96:509, 1970.

91. Stevens, RM, Teres, D, Skillman, JJ, et al.: *Pneumonia in an intensive care unit. A 30-month experience.* Arch Intern Med 134:106, 1974.

92. Greenfield, S, Teres, D, Bushnell, LS, et al.: *Prevention of gram-negative bacillary pneumonia using aerosol polymixin as prophylaxis. I. Effect on the colonization pattern of the upper respiratory tract of seriously ill patients.* J Clin Invest 52:2935, 1973.

93. Tillotson, JR, and Finland, M: *Bacterial colonization and clinical superinfection of the respiratory tract complicating antibiotic treatment of pneumonia.* J Infect Dis 119:597, 1969.

94. Klick, JM, du Moulin, GC, Hedley-Whyte, J, et al.: *Prevention of gram-negative bacillary pneumonia using polymixin aerosol as prophylaxis. II. Effect on the incidence of pneumonia in seriously ill patients.* J Clin Invest 55:514, 1975.

95. Amikam, B, Landa, J, West, J, et al.: *Bronchofiberscopic observations of the tracheobronchial tree during intubation.* Am Rev Resp Dis 105:747, 1972.

96. Ashbaugh, DG, Bigelow, DB, Petty, TL, et al.: *Acute respiratory failure after surgery or trauma,* Petty, TL (ed.): in *Intensive and Rehabilitative Respiratory Care.* Philadelphia: Lea & Febiger, 1974, p. 190.

97. Martin, AM, Jr., Soloway, HB, and Simmons, RL: *Pathologic anatomy of the lungs following shock and trauma.* J Trauma 8:687, 1968.

98. Petty, TL, and Ashbaugh, DG: *The adult respiratory distress syndrome: clinical features, factors influencing prognosis and principles of management.* Chest 60:233, 1971.

99. Brigham, KL, Woolverton, WC, and Staub, NC: *Increased pulmonary vascular permeability after pseudomonas aeruginosa bacteremia in unanesthetized sheep.* Fed Proc 32:440, 1973.
100. MacLean, LD, Duff, JH, Scott, SM, et al.: *Treatment of shock in man based on hemodynamic diagnoses.* Surg Gynecol Obstet 120:1, 1965.
101. Edde, RE, and Burtis, BB: *Lung injury in anaphylactoid shock.* Chest 63:636, 1973.
102. Blaisdell, PW, and Scholobohm, RM: *The respiratory distress syndrome, a review.* Surgery 74:251, 1973.
103. Kwan, HC: *Disseminated intravascular coagulation.* Med Clin North Am 56:177, 1972.
104. Webb, WR: *Pulmonary complications of nonthoracic trauma: summary of the National Research Council Conference.* J Trauma 9:700, 1969.
105. Ashbaugh, DC, and Petty, TL: *The use of corticosteroids in the treatment of respiratory failure associated with massive fat embolism.* Surg Gynecol Obstet 123:493, 1966.
106. Vance, BM: *Significance of fat embolism.* Arch Surg 23:426, 1931.
107. Addington, WW, Cogell, DW, Baxley, ES, et al.: *The pulmonary edema of heroin toxicity—an example of the stiff lung syndrome.* Chest 62:199, 1972.
108. Hall, RM, and Margolin, FR: *Oxygen alveolopathy in adults.* Clin Radiol 23:11, 1972.
109. Nash, G, Blennerhassett, JB, and Pontoppidan, H: *Pulmonary lesions associated with oxygen therapy and artificial ventilation.* N Engl J Med 276:368, 1967.
110. Soloway, HB, Castillo, Y, and Martin, AM: *Adult hyaline membrane disease: relationships to oxygen therapy.* Ann Surg 168:937, 1968.
111. Zieve, L, and Vogel, WC: *Measurement of lecithinase A in serum and other body fluids.* J Lab Clin Med 57:586, 1961.
112. Rovner, AJ, and Westcott, JL: *Pulmonary edema and respiratory insufficiency in acute pancreatitis.* Radiology 118:513, 1976.
113. Greenfield, LF, Barkett, VM, and Coalson, JJ: *The role of surfactant in the pulmonary response to trauma.* J Trauma 8:735, 1968.
114. Ferstenfeld, JE, Schulster, DP, Ryte, MW, et al.: *Recognition and treatment of adult respiratory distress syndrome secondary to viral interstitial pneumonia.* Am J Med 58:709, 1975.
115. Robin, ED, Cross, CE, and Zellis, R: *Pulmonary edema.* N Engl J Med 288:239, 1973.
116. Moss, G, and Stein, AA: *The centrineurogenic etiology of the respiratory distress syndrome: protection by unilateral chronic pulmonary denervation in hemorrhagic shock.* J Trauma 16:361, 1976.
117. Pontoppidan, H, Geffin, B, and Lowenstein, E: *Acute respiratory failure in the adult.* N Engl J Med 287:690, 1978.
118. McIntyre, RW, Laws, AK, and Ramachandran, PR: *Positive expiratory pressure plateau: improved gas exchange during mechanical ventilation.* Can Anesthesia Soc J 16:477, 1969.
119. Kirby, RR, Downs, JB, Civetta, JM, et al.: *High level positive end expiratory pressure (PEEP) in acute respiratory insufficiency.* Chest 67:156, 1975.
120. Lutch, JS, and Murray, JF: *Continuous positive pressure ventilation on systemic oxygen transport and tissue oxygenation.* Ann Intern Med 76:193, 1972.
121. Harrison, L, Jr., Coalson, JJ, and Greenfield, LJ: *Effects of gram negative bacteremia on pulmonary capillaries and surfactant.* Fed Proc 28:400, 1969.
122. Suter, PM, Fairley, HB, and Isenberg, MP: *Optimum end expiratory pressure in patients with acute pulmonary failure.* N Engl J Med 292:284, 1975.
123. Swan, HJC, Ganz, W, and Forrester, J: *Catheterization of the heart in man with use of a flow directed balloon-tipped catheter.* N Engl J Med 283:447, 1970.
124. Holcroft, JW, and Trunkey, DD: *Extravascular lung water following hemorrhagic shock in the baboon: comparison between resuscitation with Ringer's lactate and plasmanate.* Ann Surg 180:408, 1974.
125. Wilson, JW: *Treatment or prevention of pulmonary cellular damage with pharmacologic doses of corticosteroid.* Surg Gynecol Obstet 134:675, 1972.

126. Sahebiami, H, Gacad, G, and Massaro, D: *Influence of corticosteroids on recovery from oxygen toxicity.* Am Rev Resp Dis 110:566, 1974.

127. Jones, RL, and King, EG: *The effects of methylprednisolone on oxygenation in experimental hypoxemic respiratory failure.* J Trauma 15:297, 1975.

128. Kolobow, T, Stool, E, Sacks, K, et al.: *Acute respiratory failure. Survival following ten days' support with a membrane lung.* J Thorac Cardiovasc Surg 69:947, 1975.

129. Kakkar, VV, Howe, CT, Flanc, C, et al.: *Natural history of postoperative deep-vein thrombosis.* Lancet 2:230, 1969.

130. Tow, DE, and Wagner, HN, Jr.: *Recovery of pulmonary arterial blood flow in patients with pulmonary embolism.* N Engl J Med 276:1053, 1967.

131. Marder, VJ: *The use of thrombolytic agents: choice of patient, drug administration, laboratory monitoring.* Ann Intern Med 90:802, 1979.

132. Scoggins, WG, and Greenfield, LJ: *Transvenous pulmonary embolectomy for acute massive pulmonary embolism.* Chest 71:213, 1977.

133. Sautter, RD: *Therapy for venous thrombosis and pulmonary embolism: Surgical approach to established disease,* in Fratantoni, J, and Wessler, S (ed.): *Prophylactic Therapy of Deep Vein Thrombosis and Pulmonary Embolism.* Bethesda: National Institutes of Health, 1975, p. 137.

134. Sasahara, AA, and Barsamian, EM: *Another look at pulmonary embolectomy.* Ann Thorac Surg 16:317, 1973.

135. Tibbutt, DA, Davies, JA, Anderson, JA, et al.: *Comparison by controlled clinical trial of streptokinase and heparin in treatment of life-threatening pulmonary embolism.* Br Med J 1:343, 1974.

136. Crane, C: *Venous interruption for pulmonary embolism: present status.* Prog Cardiovasc Dis 17:329, 1975.

137. Coupland, GAE, and Reeve, TS: *The sequelae of inferior vena caval interruption.* Aust NZ J Surg 45:245, 1975.

138. Cranley, JJ, Canos, AJ, and Sull, WJ: *The diagnosis of deep venous thrombosis: fallibility of clinical signs and symptoms.* Arch Surg 111:34, 1976.

139. McLachlin, JA, Richards, T, and Paterson, JC: *An evaluation of clinical signs in the diagnosis of venous thrombosis.* Arch Surg 85:738, 1962.

140. Welch, CE, and Faxon, HH: *Thrombophlebitis and pulmonary embolism.* JAMA 117:1502, 1941.

141. Coon, WW, and Coller, FA: *Clinical pathological correlation in thromboembolism.* Surg Gynecol Obstet 109:259, 1959.

142. Walker, MA: *The natural history of venous thromboembolism.* Br J Surg 59:753, 1972.

143. Kakkar, VV, Howe, CT, et al.: *Deep vein thrombosis of the leg: is there a high risk group?* Am J Surg 120:527, 1970.

144. Browse, N: *Diagnosis of deep-vein thrombosis.* Br Med Bull 34:163, 1978.

145. Bergqvist, D, Dahlgren, S, Efsing, O, et al.: *Thermographic diagnosis of deep vein thrombosis.* Br Med J 4:684, 1975.

146. Grollman, JH, Jr., Weber, MM, and Gomes, AS: *Phlebography and radionuclide clot localization in the lower extremities.* Radiol Clin North Am 14:2, 1976.

147. Gurewich, V, and Hutchinson, E: *Detection of intravascular coagulation by a serial dilution protamine sulfate test.* Ann Intern Med 75:895, 1971.

148. Ludlam, CA, Bolten, A, Moore, S, et al.: *New rapid method for diagnosis of deep vein thrombosis.* Lancet 2:259, 1975.

149. O'Brien, JR: *Heparin thrombin clotting time of platelet plasma in the diagnosis of deep venous thrombosis* (letter). Lancet 2:4579, 1975.

150. Hume, M, Sevitt, S, and Thomas, DP: *Venous Thrombosis and Pulmonary Embolism.* Cambridge: Harvard University Press, 1970.

151. Gurewich, V, Hume, A, and Patrick, M: *The laboratory diagnosis of venous thromboembolic disease by measurement of fibrinogen/fibrin degredation products and fibrin monomers.* Chest 64:585, 1973.

152. Flanc, C, Kakkar, VV, and Clarke, MD: *The detection of venous thrombosis of the legs using I^{125} fibrinogen.* Br J Surg 55:742, 1968.

153. Kakkar, VV: *The diagnosis of deep vein thrombosis using the I^{125} fibrinogen test.* Arch Surg 104:152, 1972.

154. Browse, NL, Clapham, WF, Croft, DN, et al.: *Diagnosis of established DVT with the I^{125} fibrinogen uptake test.* Br Med J 4:325, 1971.
155. Doouss, TW: *The clinical significance of venous thrombosis of the calf.* Br J Surg 63:377, 1976.
156. Hume, M, and Kuriakose, X: *I^{125} fibrinogen and the prevention of venous thrombosis.* Arch Surg 107:803, 1973.
157. Deykin, D: *Warfarin therapy.* N Engl J Med 283:691, 1970.
158. Browse, NL: *What should I do about deep vein thrombosis and pulmonary embolism?* Ann R Coll Surg Engl 59:138, 1977.
159. Morris, GK, and Mitchell, JRA: *Clinical management of venous thromboembolism.* Br Med Bull 34:169, 1978.
160. Sevitt, S, and Gallagher, NG: *Prevention of venous thrombosis and pulmonary embolism in injured patients.* Lancet 2:981, 1959.
161. Sevitt, S, and Gallagher, N: *Venous thrombosis and pulmonary embolism: a clinicopathological study in injured and burned patients.* Br J Surg 48:475, 1961.
162. Sevitt, S, and Gallagher, NG: *Prevention of venous thrombosis and pulmonary embolism in injured patients.* Lancet 2:981, 1959.
163. Neu, LT, Jr., Waterfield, JR, and Ash, CJ: *Prophylactic anticoagulant therapy in the orthopedic patient.* Ann Intern Med 62:463, 1965.
164. Eskeland, G, Solheim, K, Skjorten, F, et al.: *Anticoagulant prophylaxis, thromboembolism and mortality in elderly patients with hip fractures. A controlled clinical trial.* Acta Chir Scand 131:16, 1966.
165. Evarts, CM, and Alfidi, RJ: *Thromboembolism after total hip reconstruction: failure of low doses of heparin in prevention.* JAMA 225:515, 1973.
166. Nicolaides, AN, Field, ES, Kakkar, VV, et al.: *Prostatectomy and deep vein thrombosis.* Br J Surg 59:487, 1972.
167. Storm, O: *Suprapubic prostatectomy with peroperative (sic) dicumarol and epsilonaminocaproic acid prophylaxis.* Scand J Urol Nephrol 1:1, 1967.
168. Andersen, R, and Jensen, PB: *Prophylactic anticoagulation therapy in prostatic surgery.* Acta Chir Scand 132:444, 1966.
169. *International Multicentre Trial: prevention of fatal postoperative pulmonary embolism by low doses of heparin.* Lancet 2:45, 1975.
170. Morris, GK, and Mitchell, JRA: *The aetiology of acute pulmonary embolism and the identification of high risk groups.* Br Hosp Med 18:6, 1977.
171. Vessey, MP, and Mann, JI: *Female sex hormones and thrombosis—epidemiological aspects.* Br Med Bull 34:157, 1978.
172. Kline, A, Hughes, LE, Campbell, H, et al.: *Dextran 70 in prophylaxis of thromboembolic disease after surgery: a clinically oriented randomized double-blind trial.* Br Med J 2:109, 1975.
173. Brisman, R, Parks, LC, and Haller, JA, Jr.: *Dextran prophylaxis in surgery.* Ann Surg 174:137, 1971.
174. Turpie, AGG, and Hirsh, J: *Platelet suppressive therapy.* Br Med J 34:183, 1978.
175. Steele, PP, Weily, HS, and Genton, E: *Platelet survival and adhesiveness in recurrent venous thrombosis.* N Engl J Med 288:1148, 1973.
176. Block, AJ: *Low flow oxygen therapy—treatment of the ambulant outpatient.* Am Rev Resp Dis 110:71, 1974.
177. Pruitt, BA, Flemma, RJ, DiVincenti, FC, et al.: *Pulmonary complications in burn patients.* J Thorac Cardiovasc Surg 59:7, 1970.
178. Achauer, BM, Allyn, PA, Furnas, DW, et al.: *Pulmonary complications of burns: the major threat to the burn patient.* Ann Surg 177:311, 1973.
179. Pruitt, BA, Jr., DiVincenti, FC, Mason, AD, Jr., et al.: *The occurrence and significance of pneumonia and other pulmonary complications in burned patients: comparison of conventional and topical treatments.* J Trauma 10:519, 1970.
180. Mallory, TB, and Brickley, WJ: *Pathology: with special reference to the pulmonary lesions.* Ann Surg 117:865, 1943.
181. Dodrill, FD: *The effects of total body perfusion upon the lungs,* in Allen, JG (ed.): *Extracorporeal Circulation.* Springfield, Illinois: Charles C Thomas Co., 1958, p. 327.
182. Gomes, MMR, and McGoon, DC: *Bleeding patterns after open-heart surgery.* J Thorac Cardiovasc Surg 60:87, 1970.

183. Wilson, JW: *The pulmonary cellular and subcellular alterations of extracorporeal circulation.* Surg Clin North Am 54:1203, 1974.

184. Allardyce, DB, Yoshida, SN, and Ashmore, PG: *The importance of microembolism in the pathogenesis of organ dysfunction caused by prolonged use of the pump oxygenator.* J Thorac Cardiovasc Surg 52:706, 1966.

185. Ashmore, PG, Swank, RI, Gallery, R, et al.: *Effect of Dacron wool filtration on the microemboli phenomenon in extracorporeal circulation.* J Thorac Cardiovasc Surg 63:240, 1972.

186. Swank, RL, and Porter, GA: *Disappearance of microemboli transfused into patients during cardiopulmonary bypass.* Transfusion 3:192, 1963.

187. Connell, RS, Page, SU, Bartley, TD, et al.: *The effect on pulmonary ultrastructure of Dacron wool filtration during cariopulmonary bypass.* Ann Thorac Surg 15:217, 1973.

188. Long, DM, Sanchez, L, Varco, RL, et al.: *The use of low molecular weight dextran and serum albumin as plasma expanders in extracorporeal circulation.* Surgery 50:12, 1961.

189. Gadboys, HL, Slonim, R, and Litwak, RS: *Homologous blood syndrome—I, preliminary observations on its relationship to clinical cardiopulmonary bypass.* Ann Surg 156:793, 1962.

190. Rabelo, RC, Oleveira, SH, Tanaka, H, et al.: *The influence of the nature of the prime on postperfusion pulmonary changes.* J Thorac Cardiovasc Surg 66:782, 1973.

191. Lee, WH, Krumhaar, D, Fonkalsrud, EW, et al.: *Denaturation of plasma proteins as a cause of morbidity and death after intracardiac operations.* Surgery 50:29, 1961.

192. Balis, JU, Cox, WD, Pifarre, R, et al.: *The role of pulmonary hypoxia in the post perfusion lung syndrome.* Surg Forum 20:205, 1969.

193. Hahas, RA, Melrose, DG, Sykes, MK, et al.: *Postperfusion lung syndrome, role of circulatory exclusion.* Lancet 2:251, 1965.

194. Mandelbaum, I, and King, H: *Pulmonary air embolism.* Surg Forum 14:236, 1963.

195. Demos, MA, Strauss, RJ, Schnipper, LE, et al.: *Plasma serotonin levels during total cardiopulmonary bypass.* J Thorac Cardiovasc Surg 60:257, 1970.

196. Swan, H, and Meagher, DM: *Total body bypass in miniature pigs.* J Thorac Cardiovasc Surg 61:956, 1971.

197. Ratliff, NB, Young, WG, Jr., Hackel, DB, et al.: *Pulmonary injury secondary to extracorporeal circulation, an ultrastructural study.* J Thorac Cardiovas Surg 65:425, 1973.

198. Chopra, PS, Dufek, JH, Kroncke, GM, et al.: *Clinical comparison of the General Electric-Pierce membrane lung and bubble oxygenator for prolonged cardiopulmonary bypass.* Surgery 74:874, 1973.

199. Wright, JS, Fisk, GC, Torda, TA, et al.: *Some advantages of the membrane oxygenator for open heart surgery.* J Thorac Cardiovasc Surg 69:884, 1975.

200. Beall, AC, and Cooley, DA: *Physiologic studies during cardiopulmonary bypass eliminating heparinized blood.* Dis chest 47:7, 1965.

201. Vandam, LD, and Moore, FD: *Adrenocortical mechanisms related to anesthesia.* Anesthesiology 21:531, 1960.

202. Cohn, HE, Solit, RW, Schatz, NJ, et al.: *Surgical treatment in myasthenia gravis: a 27-year experience.* J Thorac Cardiovasc Surg 68:876, 1974.

203. Churchill-Davidson, HC, and Richardson, AT: *Myasthenic crisis: therapeutic use of d-tubocurarine.* Lancet 1:1221, 1957.

204. Tschudy, DP: *Porphyrin metabolism and the porphyrias,* in Bondy, PK, and Rosenberg, LE (eds.): *Duncan's Diseases of Metabolism. Vol. 1 in Genetics and Metabolism,* ed. 7. Philadelphia: WB Saunders, 1974, p. 775.

205. Berman, A, and Franklin, RL: *Precipitation of acute intermittent porphyria by griseofulvin therapy.* JAMA 192:1005, 1965.

206. Steinberg, AD, and Karliner, JS: *The clinical spectrum of heroin pulmonary edema.* Arch Intern Med 122:122, 1968.

207. Helpern, M, and Rho, YM: *Deaths from narcotism in New York City. Incidence, circumstances and post mortem findings.* NY State J Med 66:2391, 1966.

208. Light, RW, and Dunham, TR: *Severe slowly resolving heroin-induced pulmonary edema.* Chest 67:61, 1975.

209. Richman, S, and Harris, RD: *Acute pulmonary edema associated with Librium abuse: a case report.* Radiology 103:57, 1972.

210. Glauser, FL, Smith, WR, Caldwell, A, et al.: *Ethchlorvynol (Placidyl)-induced pulmonary edema.* Ann Intern Med 84:46, 1976.

211. Lamb, D, and Roberts, G: *Starch and talc emboli in drug addicts' lungs.* J Clin Path 25:876, 1972.

212. Fred, HL, Harle, TS: *Septic pulmonary embolism.* Dis Chest 55:483, 1969.

213. Sarnoff, SJ, and Sarnoff, LC: *Neurohemodynamics of pulmonary edema. II. The role of sympathetic pathways in the elevation of pulmonary and systemic vascular pressures following the intracisternal injection of fibrin.* Circulation 6:51, 1952.

214. Chandler, WF, Dimcheff, DG, and Taren, JA: *Acute pulmonary edema following venous air embolism during a neurosurgical procedure.* J Neurosurgery 40:400, 1974.

215. Resnick, R, Swartz, WH, Plumer, MH, et al.: *Amniotic fluid embolism with survival.* Obstet Gyn 47:295, 1976.

216. Masson, R: *Amniotic fluid embolism.* Am Rev Respir Dis. 120:187, 1979.

217. Creech, O, Jr., and Pearce, CW: *Stab and gunshot wounds of the chest.* Am J Surg 105:469, 1963.

218. Kakkar, VV, and Corrigan, TP: *Detection of deep vein thrombosis: survey and current status.* Prog Cardiovasc Dis 17:207, 1975.

219. Gross, NJ: *Pulmonary effects of radiation therapy.* Ann Intern Med 86:81, 1977.

Chapter 13

RENAL DISEASE AND HYPERTENSION

Jay B. Wish, M.D., and Jordan J. Cohen, M.D.

EVALUATION OF RENAL FUNCTION (TABLE 1)

Renal function can be divided into two major components: glomerular and tubular.

Glomerular Filtration

Glomerular filtration rate (GFR) can be estimated by assessing the renal clearance of a marker substance that is freely filtered but neither reabsorbed nor secreted by the tubules. Creatinine, a molecule produced by normal muscle metabolism, fulfills these criteria for estimating GFR: it is freely filtered and for practical purposes neither reabsorbed nor secreted by the tubules. Thus, the GFR can be approximated by the creatinine clearance (Ccr)

$$\text{Ccr} = \frac{\text{UcrV}}{\text{Pcr}}$$

where, Ucr = urinary creatinine concentration, V = urine flow rate, and Pcr = plasma creatinine concentration. In adult males with normal renal function, creatinine clearance is approximately 120 ml/minute or 180 L/day.

Creatinine has an important added advantage as a marker substance for glomerular filtration rate: it is produced by the body and eliminated in the urine at a fairly constant rate (15 to 20 mg/kg of body weight per day). Moreover, this rate is largely unaffected by hydration, diet, or catabolic state. Thus, under steady-state conditions, UcrV is nearly constant, and Ccr (i.e., GFR) is inversely proportional to Pcr. Therefore, serum creatinine concentration by itself is a fairly reliable indicator of GFR, and can be used as such. The

TABLE 1. Laboratory Evaluation of Renal Function

A. *BLOOD TESTS*
   a. *Urea Nitrogen:* readily available test (included on most 6-test chemistry profiles). Not as accurate an indicator of glomerular filtration rate (GFR) as serum creatinine.
   b. *Creatinine:* best single screening blood test for renal function. Can be used to approximate GFR (see text).

B. *CREATININE CLEARANCE*
   a. *24 Hour Urine Collection Method:* When used with simultaneous serum creatinine, accurately estimates GFR. Dependability limited by incomplete collections. Generally not necessary for routine evaluation of renal function.
   b. *Weight/Age Conversion Formula Methods* (See Text): Adequate in most cases to compute reductions in creatinine clearance so that appropriate drug dose modifications can be made.

C. *URINE TESTS*
   a. *Specific Gravity:* A reasonably good screening test for renal tubular function. First morning urine should have a value of 1.025 or greater.
   b. *pH:* little value as a screening test
   c. *Urinary Protein:*
      1. Dipstick Method: Reading of 1+ or greater on two occasions is indication for 24 hour urine protein determination
      2. 24 Hour Collection
         50 mg protein = upper limit of normal
         > 500 mg protein = signifies intrinsic renal disease
         > 2000 mg protein = suggests glomerular disease
         > 3500 mg protein = nephrotic range
   d. *Urinary Sediment*
      1. Cells
         > 4 RBC/hpf = abnormal
         > 4 WBC/hpf = abnormal
         > 1 renal tubular cell/hpf = abnormal
      2. Casts
         > 10 hyaline/coverslip = abnormal
         > 50 finely granular/coverslip = abnormal
         > 5 renal tubular cell casts/coverslip = abnormal
         Any red blood cell, white blood cell, hemoglobin, fatty or waxy casts = abnormal.
      3. Crystals = generally of little clinical significance, except in setting of acute deterioration in renal function.

Key:
RBC = White blood cells
hpf = High power field
WBC = White blood cells

normal serum creatinine concentration of approximately 1.0 mg/dl indicates a normal GFR of about 120 ml/minute. It is evident from the inverse relationship between serum creatinine concentration and GFR, however, that very small increases in serum creatinine concentration at the lower range of serum creatinine values signify large reductions in GFR.

Because muscle mass is the source of endogenous creatinine, and because muscle mass normally decreases with age, the serum creatinine concentration would be expected to fall with age if creatinine clearance remained unchanged. But renal function and creatinine clearance typically decline as part of the aging process; one study found that the mean creatinine clearance in a group of 35 healthy people aged 60 to 93 years was only 53 ± 10 ml/minute.[1]

In addition to age, sex and body weight are factors related to muscle mass. Although women have a 10 to 15 percent lower creatinine clearance on average than men of similar age and weight, serum creatinine concentrations are similar because women normally have less muscle mass.

Quick bedside estimation of creatinine clearance without collecting urine is often useful particularly when determining dose modifications of certain drugs in patients with impaired renal function. Cockroft and Gault[2] proposed the following formula for healthy adult males:

$$Ccr = \frac{(140\text{-age})\ (\text{weight [kg]})}{72 \times Pcr\ (\text{mg/dl})}$$

For adult females, the value obtained is multiplied by 0.85. This formula appears to have an acceptable margin of error for the rough estimates required by most clinical circumstances but may overestimate filtration rate when renal function is significantly impaired.[3]

Serum urea levels ("BUN") enjoyed favor as an index of GFR before the widespread availability of creatinine measurements. Because serum urea levels are influenced by many factors other than GFR (e.g., state of hydration) it is a much less satisfactory index of filtration rate than serum creatinine. Circumstances in which blood urea nitrogen may be elevated out of proportion to a decrease in GFR are listed in Table 2.

Tubular Function

In most forms of renal disease, tubular function declines more or less in parallel with the decline in GFR, and formal testing of tubular function is rarely necessary. Tubular functions that can be tested include: (1) concentrating ability, (2) diluting ability, (3)

TABLE 2. Causes of Elevation in Blood Urea Nitrogen Out of Proportion to Serum Creatinine

- A. Increased production of urea
  - 1. Increased protein intake
  - 2. Increased catabolism of body proteins
    - a. Shock or severe illness
    - b. Trauma or burns
    - c. Internal bleeding
    - d. Drugs
      - (1) Corticosteroids
      - (2) Tetracyclines
- B. Increased tubular reabsorption of urea
  - 1. Decreased urine flow rate due to decreased effective renal perfusion (prerenal azotemia)
  - 2. Decreased urine flow rate due to obstruction to urine flow (postrenal azotemia)

urinary acidification, (4) sodium conservation, (5) glucose transport, (6) phosphate reabsorption, and (7) amino acid reabsorption. Of these, only tests of concentrating ability —which have the greatest relevance for certain surgical patients—will be described.

The normal kidney can generate a urine with a concentration as high as 1,200 mOsm/kg H_2O during periods of relative or absolute water deprivation because of the influence of antidiuretic hormone. Thus, a normal kidney can excrete the typical daily solute load (approximately 500 mOsm) in as little as 400 ml of urine. As concentrating power falls, the obligate volume of urine required to excrete this relatively fixed daily osmolar load increases. If concentrating power is lost entirely, so that urine and plasma osmolality are similar (290 mOsm/kg H_2O), some 2 L of urine would be required to excrete the daily solute load.

The most accurate way to assess renal concentrating ability is to perform a water deprivation test: plasma and urine osmolalities are measured at frequent intervals until the urine concentration reaches 800 to 900 mOsm/kg H_2O or until plasma osmolality has risen substantially above normal (greater than 5%) or body weight has fallen by 5 percent. Such a test is too cumbersome to be performed as a routine screening procedure. A suitable alternative in most instances is to obtain a specific gravity measurement on the first voided urine following an overnight fast. A first morning urine specific gravity in excess of 1.025 is considered normal. A value less than 1.025 would merit repeat testing, a more formal test of urinary concentrating ability such as described above, or further evaluation of renal function.

Urinary concentrating ability is one of the most sensitive tests of renal function; its impairment may be the first clue to the presence of underlying renal disease. Recall that urine specific gravity may exceed 1.025 if abnormal quantities of glucose, protein, or iodine-containing compounds (radiocontrast media) are present in the urine even when concentrating power is impaired.

Examination of Urine

Routine analysis of the urine includes tests for specific gravity, urinary pH, presence of urinary protein and glucose, and microscopic examination of the urinary sediment.

URINARY pH

In only a few circumstances does the measurement of urinary pH on a random urine specimen provide useful clinical information. If urinary infection can be excluded, a urine pH in excess of 6.0 in the presence of systemic acidemia indicates an inability of the renal tubules to acidify the urine appropriately and is presumptive evidence of renal tubular acidosis. A markedly alkaline urine (pH > 7) in the presence of urinary tract infection would signify infection with a urea-splitting organism, most commonly *Proteus mirabilis.*

URINARY PROTEIN

The quantity of protein excreted in normal urine is less than 50 mg per 24 hours. Since routine screening tests for urinary protein (e.g., "dipstick" method) assess protein concentration rather than total daily protein in the urine, the results of such tests will also depend upon the volume of urine in which the protein is dissolved. Thus, a reading of "trace" or even "1+" proteinuria may not be abnormal in a very concentrated urine (specific gravity greater than 1.025). Conversely, a negative dipstick reading for protein in a very dilute urine does not necessarily indicate that 24-hour urinary protein excretion is normal. In such a circumstance, dipstick testing should be repeated on a urine specimen with a specific gravity of greater than 1.010.

Any patient with 1+ or greater proteinuria by dipstick testing should have a 24-hour urine collected for protein quantitation. The method commonly used for this determination, the turbidimetric sulfosalicylic acid method, is quite sensitive and will detect globulin as well as albumin. The dipstick method detects albumin alone and is not useful for the assessment of Bence Jones proteinuria or other immunoglobulinopathies. Although any 24-hour urinary protein excretion in excess of 50 mg may be considered abnormal, mild elevations in the range of 100 to 200 mg daily are not necessarily indicative of intrinsic renal disease and may be seen as a nonspecific reaction to febrile illness. Twenty-four hour urinary protein excretion in excess of 500 mg almost always signifies intrinsic renal disease, and greater than 2 gm is usually indicative of glomerular disease.

MICROSCOPIC EXAMINATION OF URINARY SEDIMENT

The usefulness of the urinary sediment examination in the detection and differential diagnosis of renal parenchymal disease cannot be overestimated. The urine to be examined should be fresh, clean (midstream catch), concentrated (first morning specimen preferred), and unrefrigerated. Approximately 10 ml of urine is placed into a conical centrifuge tube, and the specimen is spun for about 5 minutes. The supernatant is then carefully decanted. Using a glass pipette, one or two drops from the centrifuged "pulp" are aspirated and placed on a clean glass slide under a coverslip. It is preferable not to resuspend the sediment with a finger flick.

Normal urine may contain small numbers of red blood cells (0 to 4/high power field [hpf]), white blood cells (0 to 4/hpf), renal tubular cells (0 to 1/hpf), hyaline casts (0 to 10/coverslip), finely granular casts (0 to 50/coverslip), and even renal tubular cell casts (0 to 5/coverslip). The presence of greater numbers of the above elements is abnormal, as is the presence of any red blood cell casts, white blood cell casts, hemoglobin, fatty or waxy casts. The presence of red blood cell casts is generally diagnostic of primary glomerular disease, with greater numbers of these casts signifying more acute and active disease. Exudative glomerulonephritis may also show white blood cells and white blood cell casts, but the latter are more commonly seen in acute pyelonephritis and chronic interstitial renal disease. Pigmented casts may be seen whenever red blood cell casts are observed, but are also seen in acute tubular necrosis, especially when associated with hemolysis (hemoglobin casts) or muscle injury (myoglobin casts). A more characteristic finding in acute tubular necrosis is a marked increase in coarse granular casts, often broad and brown, as well as increased numbers of renal tubular cells with some in casts. Waxy and fatty casts are seen in the nephrotic syndrome, as well as in other types of chronic glomerulonephritis.

Crystals, particularly calcium oxalate, calcium phosphate, and uric acid, may be seen in the urinary sediment. In the setting of acute deterioration in renal function, such crystals may be helpful in the differential diagnosis, suggesting obstruction due to a stone or intrarenal precipitation of the crystalline substance.

THE UREMIC SYNDROME (UREMIA)

Definitions

The uremic syndrome is a clinical term referring to the symptomatic decline in renal function associated with a characteristic constellation of metabolic and physiologic abnormalities. The term is to be distinguished from azotemia, which merely denotes an elevated blood urea nitrogen level. The degree of azotemia may be disproportionately great with respect to the level of GFR when nitrogen turnover is increased, effective renal perfusion is compromised (prerenal azotemia), or urine flow is impaired (postrenal azotemia).[4]

The term renal insufficiency generally refers to an acute or chronic decrease in GFR, measured clinically as a serum creatinine concentration greater than normal or, more accurately, a creatinine clearance less than normal. The term renal failure, acute or chronic, refers to a more advanced stage of renal insufficiency, again defined as a decrease in GFR, sufficient to induce some or all of the metabolic and physiologic abnormalities of the uremic syndrome. When such abnormalities can no longer be managed conservatively by dietary manipulation and appropriate medications, the patient with chronic renal failure is said to have reached end-stage renal disease (ESRD).

Metabolic Abnormalities (Table 3)

WATER BALANCE

One of the first functions of the kidney to be impaired in renal insufficiency is the ability to concentrate the urine and to conserve water. In chronic renal insufficiency, this defect is probably due to a combination of distorted tubular architecture and osmotic diuresis secondary to the solutes that are retained in the plasma in the face of decreased GFR.[5] Solute diuresis also is likely to play a role in the decreased urinary diluting capacity seen in patients with renal insufficiency.[6] As renal insufficiency becomes more advanced, the range of urinary osmolarities, from dilute to concentrated, which the kidney can achieve becomes progressively more limited and ultimately narrows to a small range approximating the osmolarity of plasma.[7] As a result, the failing kidney cannot cope with large variations in daily water intake. Water consumed or given intravenously in excess of the kidney's limited ability to dilute the urine and excrete "free water" will be retained and the patient will become hyponatremic. Conversely, in the face of water restriction, solute diuresis and water excretion will continue, and the patient may become volume-depleted and hypotensive. Thus, in general, for the patient with advanced renal insufficiency, daily water intake should be around 2,500 ml; two liters to allow for the excretion of approximately 500 mOsm daily osmolar load in isotonic (290 mOsm/kg H_2O) urine and 500 ml for insensible losses.

TABLE 3. Metabolic Consequences of Renal Failure

A. Disorders of Water Balance	
1. Impaired urinary concentrating ability	→ intravascular volume depletion
2. Impaired urinary diluting capacity	→ hyponatremia
B. Disorders of Sodium Balance	
1. Renal salt wasting	→ intravascular volume depletion
2. Sodium retention	→ congestive heart failure → hypertension → peripheral edema
C. Abnormal Potassium Balance	
Decreased potassium excretory ability	→ hyperkalemia
D. Disorders of Acid-Base Balance	
1. Renal bicarbonate wasting 2. Decreased renal ammonia production	→ metabolic acidosis
E. Disorders of Divalent Ion Metabolism	
1. Phosphate retention 2. Impaired vitamin D activation 3. Secondary hyperparathyroidism	→ renal osteodystrophy metastatic calcification pruritus
F. Abnormal Nitrogen Metabolism	
1. Reduced renal nitrogen excretion	→ azotemia
2. Tissue catabolism 3. Urinary protein losses	→ cachexia and wasting
G. Altered Drug Metabolism	
1. Decreased renal excretion 2. Altered protein binding 3. Increased sensitivity of target organs 4. Metabolic loads	→ drug toxicity

SODIUM BALANCE

Normal individuals, in the face of sodium restriction or volume depletion, have the capacity to eliminate sodium almost completely from the urine. Thus, unless there are continued nonrenal routes of sodium loss, intravascular volume can be fairly well maintained. Almost all patients with chronic renal insufficiency and particularly those patients with disease primarily affecting the tubular architecture, such as medullary cystic disease, polycystic kidney disease, chronic interstitial nephritis, and chronic obstructive uropathy, waste sodium under certain circumstances. These patients are unable to reduce urinary sodium concentration below a relatively high fixed value, probably because of solute diuresis through remaining nephrons. Therefore, daily sodium intake should be maintained above 25 to 35 mEq in these patients, unless clinical edema (a sign of total body sodium overload) is present. Conversely, patients with advanced renal insufficiency are vulnerable to sodium retention and congestive heart failure if sodium intake is not sufficiently limited. Indeed, most patients with uremia are chronically volume expanded. Further sodium loading may exacerbate hypertension or precipitate congestive heart failure, and therefore most patients with advanced renal insufficiency should be cautioned against excessive salt intake. Bricker and associates recommend maintaining the existing level of salt intake if the patient has no signs of fluid overload (i.e., edema, pulmonary congestion, moderate or severe hypertension) when first observed.[8] Accelerated hypertension or the appearance of edema or sudden weight gain are indications for prompt reduction in the patient's daily salt intake.

POTASSIUM BALANCE

Most patients with chronic renal insufficiency retain their ability to excrete normal potassium loads even in the face of markedly reduced GFR. Hyperkalemia is seldom a complication of chronic renal failure except in the terminal stages or if there is marked oliguria. On the other hand, hyperkalemia is commonly seen in acute renal failure, both because of the frequent oliguria which limits potassium excretion and because these patients with acute renal failure are often acutely ill with marked catabolism that shifts potassium from the intracellular to the extracellular compartment. The systemic acidosis which accompanies renal failure also leads to a shift of potassium from the intracellular to the extracellular compartment, tending to raise the serum potassium level. However, there is evidence that chronic metabolic acidosis is associated with enhanced potassium excretion, even by the diseased kidney.[9]

There is a subset of patients with mild to moderate renal insufficiency who develop severe hyperkalemia despite normal potassium intake.[10] These patients have low plasma levels of renin and aldosterone ("hyporeninemic hypoaldosteronism") and show subnormal responses to various stimuli of the renin-angiotensin system. There is a high incidence of diabetes and primary tubulointerstitial disorders as the etiology of the renal disease in these patients. In most, the hyperkalemia can be controlled with dietary potassium restriction or with potent diuretic agents (e.g., furosemide, ethacrynic acid, thiazides). Occasionally, supplemental mineralcorticoid (e.g., Florinef) therapy is required.

Despite the ability of patients with advanced renal disease (GFR as low as 5% of normal) to increase potassium secretion per nephron sufficiently to maintain potassium homeostasis, even patients with only mild to moderate renal insufficiency may have difficulty excreting large potassium loads. "Potassium-sparing" diuretics such as spironolactone and triamterene, which further impair renal potassium excretion, should be used with extreme caution if any degree of renal insufficiency is present and are contraindicated entirely in patients whose creatinine clearance is reduced by 50 percent or more. Under no circumstances should potassium-sparing diuretics be given in combination with oral potassium supplements to any patient with renal insufficiency.

In the absence of hyperkalemia, it is not generally necessary to limit dietary potassium in patients with renal disease. Precautions regarding foods rich in potassium and salt substitutes that contain potassium may be in order. In patients with end-stage renal failure and those undergoing maintenance hemodialysis, dietary potassium intake should not exceed 70 mEq (3 gm) daily.

ACID-BASE BALANCE

Since one of the major functions of the kidney is the excretion of the endogenously produced acid from dietary protein (approximately 1 to 1.5 mEq of hydrogen ions/kg of body weight/day)[11] and the maintenance of acid-base homeostasis, one of the more important metabolic consequences of renal insufficiency is the retention of acid and the generation of a metabolic acidosis.

Normally, the kidneys are able to maintain plasma bicarbonate concentration at the appropriate physiologic level by reabsorbing virtually all filtered bicarbonate and by excreting an amount of acid equal to the endogenously generated load. The metabolic acidosis associated with uremia results from a progressive defect in the kidneys' ability both to reabsorb bicarbonate and to generate ammonia, the major urinary buffer for secreted hydrogen ion. Significant acidemia is uncommon until the GFR falls below 15 to 20 ml/minute, but intercurrent complications or any other abrupt demand for increased renal acid excretion may precipitate overt acidosis, reflecting the near maximal amounts of acid already being excreted per nephron.

In the dialysis patient with negligible GFR, plasma bicarbonate falls during the interdialytic period in accordance with the endogenous level of acid production. About one-half of the retained acid will be buffered in the extracellular fluid, reflected as a lowering of plasma bicarbonate, and the other half buffered intracellularly and by bone.

Respiratory responses lead to secondary hyperventilation, and blood pH may be restored to nearly normal values in patients with mild uremic acidosis. Such patients, with plasma bicarbonate in the range of 16 to 20 mEq/L usually do not require additional treatment for the acidosis per se. With more severe degrees of acidosis, lethargy, weakness, somnolence, cardiac irritability, and hyperkalemia may result. The retained hydrogen ions in uremia are partially absorbed by bone buffers which may contribute to uremic bone disease.

Blood gases from patients with uremic acidosis reveal a low pH and Pco_2, and serum electrolytes usually show an increase in the anion gap ($Na^+ - [HCO^- + Cl^-]$). Some patients with renal disease may have a metabolic acidosis with a normal or only slightly increased anion gap.[12] Such a pattern of hyperchloremic acidosis, classically found in the nonazotemic patient with renal tubular acidosis, is being seen more commonly in patients with advanced uremia. It has been proposed that the earlier use of phosphate binding gels and low protein (sulfur) diets may account for this changing anion pattern in uremic patients over recent years.[13]

Since the major source of retained acid in uremia is dietary protein, protein restriction (40 to 80 gm protein daily, depending upon severity) may prove to be sufficient therapy for the correction of moderate uremic acidosis. For more severe degrees of uremic acidosis, daily administration of alkali to titrate retained acid is indicated. If feasible, step by step increments of sodium bicarbonate, beginning with about 2.0 gm daily, is the preferred mode of therapy. Although it has been shown that sodium bicarbonate ingestion leads to significantly less sodium retention than equimolar amounts of sodium chloride ingestion,[14] if sodium bicarbonate therapy does lead to undesirable sodium retention, then sodium chloride intake should be appropriately reduced and/or diuretics administered to enhance sodium excretion. (See also Chap. 15, Fluid, Electrolyte and Acid-Base Disorders.)

CALCIUM AND PHOSPHORUS METABOLISM

As a general rule, derangements of divalent ion metabolism are much more characteristic of chronic rather than acute renal insufficiency. Fortunately, despite the very low serum calcium concentrations sometimes seen in renal failure, tetany and seizures are quite rare. Retention of phosphate due to decreased glomerular filtration leads to reciprocal lowering of serum calcium, which in turn stimulates parathyroid hormone (PTH) production. PTH promotes calcium reabsorption from bone and decreases renal calcium excretion, effects which tend to restore serum calcium concentration toward normal. In addition, a decreased ability of the diseased kidney to convert vitamin D to its active form impairs calcium absorption from the gut, aggravating the tendency toward hypocalcemia and the stimulation of PTH. The net result of this constellation of changes is "azotemic renal osteodystrophy." Pathologic features of this syndrome include osteomalacia due to decreased effective vitamin D, osteitis fibrosa due to secondary hyperparathyroidism, and osteosclerosis. These bone changes may result in fractures, skeletal deformities, growth retardation in children, and bone pain.

On occasion, plasma phosphate concentration may become so elevated that the calcium-phosphate solubility product is exceeded; this can occur even in the presence of hypocalcemia. The result may be metastatic soft tissue calcification. Although such extraskeletal calcification is most readily recognized in the skin, it frequently involves peripheral blood vessels, cornea, conjuctiva, periarticular tissue, viscera, and, most alarmingly, the conduction system of the heart. The latter may be fatal.[15]

Many studies indicate that phosphate retention is the single most important factor in the pathogenesis of renal osteodystrophy and secondary hyperparathyroidism.[16] Since phosphate is virtually ubiquitous among naturally occurring foods, it is extremely difficult to reduce phosphate absorption sufficiently by dietary restriction alone. Aluminum containing antacids, such as Amphojel, Basaljel, Aluminex, Dialume, and Alu-Caps, when taken in sufficient quantity at mealtime, provide a means for binding phosphate in the gut and preventing its absorption. Antacids containing magnesium are contraindicated since severe hypermagnesemia may result. Ideally, plasma phosphate should be maintained in the range of 3 to 4 mg/dl in nondialyzed patients with renal insufficiency and 4 to 5 mg/dl in dialyzed patients. Hypophosphatemia should be avoided, because it may lead to hemolytic anemia, myopathy, somatic cell dysfunction, and osteomalacia[17] (see Chap. 5, Endocrinology).

Equally important in the therapy of uremic osteodystrophy is an effort to establish a positive calcium balance by administering vitamin D. Measures designed to raise serum calcium should not be instituted until serum phosphorus is returned to normal because of the danger of metastatic calcification if the calcium-phosphorus product is allowed to rise unduly. The physiologic active form of vitamin D ($1,25[OH]_2D_3$) is now available commercially as Rocaltrol. This preparation appears to be the best available form of vitamin D supplementation for patients with renal failure.[18]

Daily intake of dietary calcium should approximate 1.0 to 1.5 gm. If dietary supplementation is required, calcium gluconate (9% calcium), calcium carbonate (40% calcium), or calcium lactate (13% calcium) may be used. For patients receiving chronic dialysis treatments, dialysate calcium concentration can be increased in an effort to improve calcium balance but dialysate concentrations greater than 6.5 to 7 mg/dl may result in metastatic calcification while producing negligible further improvement in uremic osteodystrophy.[19]

Even when all of the above measures are instituted, some patients with renal failure continue to suffer from symptomatic hyperparathyroidism. In such patients, subtotal parathyroidectomy may be considered.

NITROGEN METABOLISM

Although the blood urea nitrogen (BUN) is commonly used as a clinical index of GFR, the BUN is also influenced by urea loads (ingestion and/or catabolism of protein) and urine flow rate. Thus, for a given level of GFR, a reduction in dietary protein intake will result in a fall in BUN. In addition, the greater the reduction in GFR, the greater is the sensitivity of BUN to changes in protein intake. Restriction of dietary protein intake remains one of the most useful measures in the conservative management of renal failure because of the marked improvement in symptoms that often accompanies a reduced nitrogen load. Three important principles must be borne in mind, however, whenever such dietary manipulation is contemplated. First, an adequate total caloric intake must be insured to obviate increased catabolic turnover of endogenous protein. Second, dietary proteins vary considerably in the degree to which they can be used for anabolic purposes. Thus, it is possible to reduce total protein intake safely if "high biologic value" foods such as eggs and milk products are used. Third, an efficient diet must contain the minimum daily requirements of each essential amino acid, as well as a minimum quantity of "nonspecific" nitrogen.[20]

Using these specific principles, Giordano and Giovanetti developed a high biologic value, low protein (0.3 mg/kg body weight) diet for use in patients with renal failure. However, several problems have emerged with its use. First, nitrogen requirements vary considerably in patients with renal failure. Second, patients who come into nitrogen balance while ingesting the Giordano-Giovanetti diet may have accumulated nitrogen deficits too profound to repair fully. Third, such extremely low protein diets may be so unpalatable that compliance is impossible.

Kopple has introduced a diet containing 0.6 gm of protein/kg of body weight using a mixture of high biologic value protein and low quality protein to add variety. This improved patient acceptance, produced only a small increase in BUN, and resulted in positive nitrogen balance as reflected by a rise in serum albumin level and a gain in body weight.[21,22]

Although such proposed dietary formulae may serve as useful guidelines, no single nitrogen requirement can be applied to all uremic patients. The optimal diet for a given individual is one which will be eaten, minimizes protein intake, yet assures positive nitrogen balance. Successful dietary therapy may result in reduced gastrointestinal complaints (see below), reduced fatigue, apathy, cold intolerance, and improved physical activity. Because the negative nitrogen balance that results from over-restriction of dietary protein may have severe consequences (i.e., cachexia, impaired resistance to infection), dietary protein restriction should not be instituted until uremic symptoms appear or until moderately severe uremic acidosis develops. Even though urea itself produces few, if any, uremic symptoms and findings, the severity of the uremic state does correlate roughly with the BUN level; thus, this blood test has retained its usefulness as a chemical marker for uremia.

Gastrointestinal Manifestations (Table 4)

Anorexia is often among the earliest manifestations of uremia. Nausea and vomiting, especially upon arising in the morning, are also frequent complaints. Protracted vomiting may cause sodium, potassium, and volume depletion, to which the diseased kidneys have a limited ability to respond. Metabolic alkalosis, due to vomiting, may "mask" the uremic acidosis. Perhaps most importantly, volume depletion from gastrointestinal

TABLE 4. Clinical Manifestations of Renal Failure

A. *Gastrointestinal Manifestations*
   1. Non-specific → anorexia, nausea, vomiting
   2. Decreased oral intake, antacids → constipation
   3. Uremic mucositis → stomatitis, bloody diarrhea

B. *Cardiovascular Manifestations*
   1. Sodium retention → hypertension
   2. Sodium retention, hypertension, anemia → congestive heart failure
   3. Pericarditis

C. *Hematologic Abnormalities*
   1. Decreased erythropoietin levels } → anemia
   2. Bleeding diathesis } → anemia
   3. Shortened red blood cell survival } → anemia
   4. Platelet dysfunction → bleeding
   5. Abnormal white cell function → infections

D. *Nervous System Abnormalities*
   1. Peripheral neuropathy → weakness, sensory changes
   2. Encephalopathy → personality changes, dementia, movement disorders, coma
   3. Dialysis dysequilibrium syndrome → headache, vomiting, seizures
   4. Dialysis dementia syndrome → movement disorders, dementia, death

E. *Endocrine Abnormalities*
   1. Insulin resistance → glucose intolerance ("azotemic pseudodiabetes")
   2. Hyperlipidemia → ? accelerated atherogenesis
   3. Decreased triiodothyronine levels → "sick" euthyroid syndrome
   4. Decreased sexual function

losses may aggravate renal dysfunction and result in more severe uremia. Anorexia, nausea, and vomiting usually respond promptly to protein restriction or dialysis or both, suggesting that they are caused by toxic products of protein metabolism which are dialysable.

Uremia is commonly associated with constipation, probably due to a combination of decreased oral intake and the effects of the aluminum-containing antacids which are frequently prescribed to control hyperphosphatemia. On the other hand, some uremic patients develop diarrhea; when present, this symptom usually signifies uremic colitis, an ulcerating inflammatory process of unknown pathogenesis. Uremic colitis is also a cause of gastrointestinal bleeding and abdominal pain. Similar lesions may affect virtually any part of the gastrointestinal tract. In the mouth (uremic stomatitis) the lesions may range in severity from discrete superficial ulcerations to generalized erythema, exudation, and bleeding.[23]

Peptic ulcer disease appears to be more common in patients with chronic renal failure than in individuals with normal renal function. Basal as well as stimulated gastrin levels are known to be elevated in a majority of patients with renal failure, probably because of impaired clearance of the hormone; the kidney is a major site of deactivation of gastrin and other polypeptide hormones.[24] No significant correlation, however, has been found between basal or stimulated acid secretion and plasma gastrin levels. Indeed, it is not clear why elevated gastrin levels in this circumstance fail to activate feedback controls.

Pancreatitis is also more common in patients with chronic renal failure;[25] its diagnosis is often hampered, however, because serum amylase, the diagnostic hallmark of this disease, is elevated nonspecifically by decreased renal clearance.

Cardiovascular Manifestations (Table 4)

HYPERTENSION

Hypertension is undoubtedly the most common and perhaps the most important cardiovascular complication of chronic renal failure.[26] Hypertension may be the first clinical manifestation of renal parenchymal disease. As many as 5 percent of patients with newly diagnosed hypertension are found to have underlying renal parenchymal disease. Of patients with chronic renal failure, 80 percent or more have hypertension by the time they reach an advanced stage of their disease. In some patients, uncontrolled elevations of blood pressure may cause deterioration of renal function to accelerate. In patients with malignant hypertension, control of blood pressure may abort the development of renal insufficiency and even produce an improvement in renal function.

Positive sodium balance almost certainly plays a central role in the pathogenesis of the hypertension associated with chronic renal disease. The expansion of extracellular fluid volume that results from sodium retention is postulated to increase cardiac output, and thereby increase peripheral resistance through autoregulation.

Because sodium retention may be instrumental in producing hypertension in patients with renal disease, dietary sodium restriction and potent diuretics (e.g., furosemide) are thought by many to play an especially important role in the therapy of this form of hypertension. Less potent diuretics (e.g., thiazides) may not be effective in patients whose GFR is less than 40 ml/minute. Nondiuretic antihypertensive agents that have proven efficacious include propranolol, hydralazine, prazosin, methyldopa, and minoxidil.

CONGESTIVE HEART FAILURE

Sodium retention, hypertension, and anemia are among the several factors that often conspire to produce congestive heart failure in patients with chronic renal failure. Sodium retention results in extracellular volume overload and is frequently the major factor leading to cardiac decompensation. When this is so, controlled fluid removal by hemodialysis or other means may obviate the need for cardiac glycosides. Uncontrolled hypertension may eventuate in hypertensive cardiomyopathy, ischemic cardiomyopathy, or both. Cardiac function can often be improved by "unloading" the left ventricle with blood pressure reduction. The anemia of chronic renal disease places an additional strain on the heart which already may be compromised by volume overload, hypertension, and coronary vascular disease.

Whether uremia per se inhibits myocardial function producing so-called "uremic cardiomyopathy" is not settled.[27] Laboratory experiments using myocardial cell preparations have shown that severe uremia directly impairs some membrane functions (e.g., Na^+–K^+ATPase).[28]

The clinical presentation of congestive heart failure in the patient with renal disease is similar to that seen in other settings. Pulmonary edema may be the first manifestation; excessive intravascular volume is often the critical factor. Some contend that pulmonary edema can occur in renal failure without increased pulmonary vascular pressure (the "uremic lung syndrome") because of a primary increase in pulmonary capillary permeability.[29]

Management of congestive heart failure in patients with renal disease is focused primarily on removal of excessive extracellular fluid. In those with mild to moderate renal insufficiency, this may be accomplished by the use of potent diuretic agents in conjunction with dietary sodium restriction. In patients with more advanced renal failure, fluid removal via peritoneal dialysis or hemodialysis may be the only effective therapy. Digitalis preparations are usually not required if the congestive heart failure occurs in the absence of underlying heart disease. If needed, agents such as digoxin should be used cautiously and in reduced dosage because excretion occurs primarily by the kidneys.

PERICARDITIS

Uremic pericarditis is most commonly asymptomatic and is often discovered on physical examination as a cardiac rub, with or without hemodynamic changes. When pain occurs, it is typically pleuritic in nature and worse while lying down. The occurrence of uremic pericarditis is a clear indication for beginning hemodialysis. Indeed, as indications for chronic dialysis have become more liberal, its earlier use has reduced the frequency of uremic pericarditis in the nondialyzed patient.

When pericarditis develops in a patient already undergoing chronic hemodialysis, it is often a sign of inadequate dialysis. The incidence of pericarditis among dialysis patients may be as high as 10 to 20 percent,[30,31] with a mortality approaching 8 percent. Pericardial effusions under these circumstances are often hemorrhagic and may result in cardiac tamponade, constrictive pericarditis, congestive heart failure, or arrhythmias. Recurrent effusions unresponsive to increased dialysis and anti-inflammatory drugs (indomethacin, 25 mg every 6 hours and, in some cases, prednisone 30 to 40 mg, daily) constitute an indication for surgical intervention (i.e., pericardial window, subtotal or total pericardiectomy).

Hematologic Abnormalities (Table 4)

ANEMIA

Anemia occurs in the vast majority of patients with chronic renal insufficiency. Although it may be quite profound (hemoglobin as low as 5 to 7 gm/dl), it is often well-tolerated because of its gradual onset. The pathogenesis is multifactorial and includes decreased red blood cell (RBC) survival, ineffective erythropoiesis, and increased blood loss due to the bleeding diathesis that usually accompanies uremia.

Patients requiring chronic hemodialysis are subject to the additional problem of significant blood loss into the dialyzer. Depending upon dialysis volume and rinsing techniques, up to 33 ml of red blood cells may be lost per week on the dialysis membrane, ultimately leading to iron deficiency.[32] Additional blood loss occurs through sampling for laboratory tests.

Treatment of the anemia associated with chronic renal failure is not predictably successful, but certain measures should be attempted. Many patients with advanced renal disease and almost all chronic hemodialysis patients have some degree of iron deficiency. The status of iron stores is more accurately documented by serum ferritin levels than by serum iron and total iron binding capacity.[33] If oral iron therapy fails to reverse iron deficiency, parenteral iron therapy, generally given as 250 mg intramuscularly or intravenously, biweekly or monthly, is indicated. Because folic acid is dialyzable, it is generally given prophylactically to chronic dialysis patients. If anemia remains symptomatic despite iron and folate therapy, anabolic (androgen) steroid therapy may be tried.

Transfusion of packed red blood cells is the most direct means of increasing the hematocrit of patients with symptomatic anemia but carries the risk of hemochromatosis when employed frequently. Earlier fears that blood transfusion might sensitize patients to a variety of transplant antigens, thus jeopardizing the success of a future renal transplant, appear to be unfounded.[34]

COAGULOPATHY

The major hemostatic defect in uremic patients is due to a reversible platelet abnormality which can be corrected by hemodialysis or peritoneal dialysis. Both aggregation and release of platelet factor 3 are recognized to be abnormal. Neither abnormalities in plasma coagulation factors nor increased vascular fragility is felt to play a significant role in the uremic bleeding diathesis.[35]

Nervous System Changes (Table 4)

PERIPHERAL NEUROPATHY

The typical neuropathy that develops in patients with chronic renal failure is a distal, symmetrical mixed sensory motor polyneuropathy, affecting primarily the lower extremities. The pathogenesis is poorly understood. It is clinically and morphologically indistinguishable from the neuropathies seen in association with alcoholism, vitamin deficiencies, and diabetes. Muscle weakness usually does not develop until the sensory changes are well established. Following institution of dialysis, most patients show a rapid clinical improvement, most easily detected by a decrease in vibratory perception threshold.[36] Far advanced changes with paraplegia or quadraplegia may be resistant to dialysis.

CENTRAL NERVOUS SYSTEM DYSFUNCTION

Uremic encephalopathy shares many of the nonspecific clinical features characteristic of the metabolic encephalopathies accompanying liver failure, hypoxemia, severe acidosis, and drug toxicity. These include personality changes (particularly depression), poor judgment, lack of motivation, irritability, and memory loss. The earliest sign of uremic encephalopathy is often a clouding of the sensorium, characterized by impaired alertness, decreased attention span, memory lapses, and perceptual errors. This is commonly accompanied by disturbances of sleep patterns, with drowsiness during the day and insomnia at night. In more advanced stages, the encephalopathy may progress to a combination of amnesia, true delirium, dementia, overt psychosis, or coma. The mental abnormalities of uremia usually develop more rapidly in acute renal failure than in chronic renal failure, suggesting that it is more the rate of accumulation of uremic toxins than their blood level that is important in the pathogenesis of the encephalopathy.[37]

Movement disorders characteristic of other forms of metabolic encephalopathy are also seen with some frequency in uremia. These include asterixis, multifocal myoclonus, and, in severe acute uremia, focal or generalized seizures. Dialysis is the best treatment for all the clinical manifestations of uremic encephalopathy; both peritoneal dialysis and hemodialysis can produce improvement within several hours. If seizures occur, conventional anticonvulsant therapy should be given as well (see Table 5 for dosage modification). Other metabolic disturbances which might aggravate the encephalopathy (e.g., acidosis, hyponatremia, hypoxemia) should be looked for and corrected.[38]

Despite the efficacy of dialysis in improving the various manifestations of uremic encephalopathy, such therapy (especially hemodialysis) carries some risk of causing neurologic dysfunction. The so-called "dialysis dysequilibrium syndrome" can occur during or immediately after hemodialysis; it is characterized by headache, nausea, vomiting and, in severe cases, seizures. Its pathogenesis centers around the rapid removal of solutes from the plasma during an efficient dialysis which leads to an osmotic gradient between the blood and central nervous system. Hence, water moves into brain cells, resulting in cerebral edema.[39] The institution of hemodialysis earlier in the course of uremia, along with the use of less efficient dialyzers and shorter dialysis time for the first few treatments, has decreased the incidence of the dysequilibrium syndrome.

A slowly progressive, irreversible, and ultimately fatal encephalopathy has been reported to occur among some patients who have been treated with hemodialysis for several years. The syndrome, called dialysis dementia, is relatively rare but appears to occur in clusters. It is characterized by difficulty in speech and muscle coordination, followed by profound dementia and seizures. Electroencephalogram shows a characteristic slow, sharp triphasic and spike-wave pattern. The pathogenesis of the disorder is unclear; aluminum toxicity has been implicated[40] and refuted.[41] There is no known therapy.

Subdural hematomas, both acute and chronic, occur with increased frequency in hemodialysis patients, probably because of the systemic anticoagulation associated with the procedure.[42] As a rule, there is no history of trauma. Thus, the development of persistent headache, drowsiness, or delirium in a chronic hemodialysis patient should raise the possibility of subdural hematoma. Computerized tomography (CT scanning) has been very helpful in confirming this diagnosis.

Alterations in Endocrine Function (Table 4)

CARBOHYDRATE METABOLISM

Abnormalities of carbohydrate metabolism are characteristic of uremia and usually manifest themselves as glucose intolerance. Like adult onset diabetes mellitus, azotemic pseudodiabetes is associated with a hyperglycemic response to glucose loading. In contrast to true diabetes, however, fasting hyperglycemia is rarely noted in uremia. In fact, fasting hypoglycemia may occur in patients with advanced renal disease because of decreased renal gluconeogenesis.[43]

Under normal circumstances, 30 to 40 percent of circulating insulin is degraded by the kidney. As renal function deteriorates, the half-life of insulin is prolonged as the metabolic clearance rate is decreased. Thus, insulin-dependent diabetics frequently experience a decrease in their insulin requirements as renal failure supervenes. With time, the requirement for exogenous insulin may cease altogether in these patients.[44] Nondiabetic patients with hyperglycemia secondary to renal insufficiency generally do not require oral hypoglycemic or insulin therapy. Glucose loads are ultimately assimilated, albeit slowly, and under these circumstances, hyperglycemia per se does not appear to have adverse physiologic consequences.

LIPID METABOLISM

The incidence of type IV hyperlipidemia (hypertriglyceridemia) in chronic renal failure is quite high, affecting as many as 43 percent of non-nephrotic patients with renal disease.[45] The hypertriglyceridemia of renal disease results from a combination of increased hepatic production of triglyceride-rich very low-density lipoproteins (VLDL) and decreased peripheral removal of triglyceride.

Patients with advanced renal failure have an exceptionally high incidence of atherosclerotic cardiovascular disease.[46] Atherosclerotic cardiovascular disease is responsible for the majority of deaths among patients undergoing chronic hemodialysis. The precise contribution of hypertriglyceridemia to the evident acceleration of atherogenesis is not clear, but there is some evidence that uremia and dialysis increase the triglyceride content of high density lipoproteins (HDL).[47]

Plasma triglyceride levels can often be lowered effectively by dietary manipulation alone.[48] Should this fail due to poor patient compliance, clofibrate therapy may be considered. Clofibrate can reduce plasma triglyceride levels in uremia but its long-term risks and benefits remain to be evaluated.

THYROID FUNCTION

Abnormalities of thyroid function occur in almost all patients with chronic renal failure. The major defect of thyroid hormone metabolism in uremia appears to be impaired peripheral conversion of thyroxine (T_4) to triiodothyronine (T_3). Most patients with advanced renal insufficiency, whether undergoing maintenance hemodialysis or not, have normal or only slightly decreased serum levels of total T_4 and free T_4,[49] but more marked lowering of T_3 is typically found.[50] Thyroid-stimulating hormone (TSH) levels are usually normal in patients with renal disease. However, the responsiveness of TSH to stimulation by thyrotropin-releasing hormone (TRH) is impaired.[51] Despite these changes, most patients appear to be euythyroid clinically and, therefore, probably represent a variant of the euthyroid sick syndrome (see Chap. 5, Endocrinology).

Impairment of Host Defenses

Infection is directly responsible for the majority of deaths in patients who die as a result of acute renal failure, and infection is second only to cardiovascular complications as a cause of death among patients with chronic renal failure undergoing maintenance hemodialysis. The enhanced susceptibility to infection in uremia is attributable to numerous factors, the most significant of which is probably the inhibition of normal neutrophil function by uremic serum.[52] In addition, in vivo lymphocyte-monocyte function is decreased in uremia, as reflected by reduced delayed hypersensitivity skin test responses.[53] Furthermore, recognition of infections in patients with renal failure may be delayed because uremia reduces body temperature and suppresses the production of endogenous pyrogen by leukocytes. Cachexia and protein malnutrition in uremia may lead to reduced production of immunoglobulin and complement, further impairing host defenses.[54] Finally, the disruptive effects of uremia on mucosal barriers, the presence of external arteriovenous shunts, and the use of urinary and intravenous catheters in the acutely ill patient all predispose to infectious complications in uremia.

Altered Drug Metabolism in Renal Failure (Table 5)

Renal failure may modify the action of a wide variety of pharmacologic agents by several different mechanisms.[55] The most obvious of these is reduced renal clearance of the parent drug. Many drugs are metabolized to pharmacologically active compounds which are normally excreted in the urine. The accumulation of these active metabolites in renal failure can lead to toxicity if standard doses are administered. Mechanisms other than decreased renal clearance can also increase the levels of active drug in uremia. Thus, reduced levels of plasma binding proteins (especially in nephrotic syndrome) may cause an increase in unbound active drug at relatively low total plasma concentrations. Retention of compounds which compete with the drug for binding sites on plasma protein would also increase the concentration of active drug. A reduction in the apparent volume of distribution of the drug may occur because of the loss of normal binding sites in uremic body tissues.

Increased sensitivity to drugs, even at therapeutic plasma levels, can lead to toxic reactions in the uremic patient. Abnormalities of the blood-brain barrier in uremia can allow increased penetration of certain drugs into the central nervous system and result in potentially toxic reactions. Alterations of various target organs in uremia may lead to increased sensitivity of such organs to drugs. Gastrointestinal side effects of certain drugs may be more pronounced in renal failure because of the adverse effects of uremia itself on the gastrointestinal mucosa. Acetylsalicylic acid and similar agents may aggravate the platelet abnormality and enhance the hemorrhagic diathesis in renal failure. The direct effect of uremia on the central nervous system may predispose the patient with renal failure to increased cerebral toxicity from certain drugs.

Finally, the intake of certain electrolytes contained in pharmacologic preparations (e.g., sodium in carbenicillin, magnesium in antacids and in laxatives) may exceed the excretory capacity of the diseased kidney. Table 5 contains recommended dose modifications for agents frequently used in surgical patients. More comprehensive listings can be found elsewhere.[56–61]

SURGERY IN THE PATIENT WITH RENAL DISEASE

Surgery of a general nature in patients with chronic renal failure as well as surgery specifically related to the management of the uremic state or its complications is now commonplace. Procedures of the latter variety include insertion of arteriovenous shunts or creation of arteriovenous fistulas for dialysis, parathyroidectomy for symptomatic secondary hyperparathyroidism, pretransplant nephrectomy for infection or polycystic kidneys, pericardiectomy, splenectomy, laparotomy for gastrointestinal bleeding or intra-abdominal infection, and renal transplantation itself.

Many characteristics of the uremic state, even when treated by chronic dialysis, increase the risk of major surgery. This risk can be substantially reduced, however, by strict attention to the patient's preoperative, intraoperative, and postoperative status. Hata and associates[62] reported no perioperative or postoperative deaths among 17 dialysis patients requiring 26 operative procedures. Hampers and coworkers[63] reviewed 44 major operations on 33 patients requiring preoperative and postoperative dialysis; only 1 death occurred in the series. Lissos and associates[64] described 3 deaths among 76 patients on maintenance hemodialysis who underwent 98 surgical procedures. There were 2 deaths among 31 hemodialysis patients undergoing 40 elective and 9 emergency operations reported by Brenowitz and coworkers.[65] Haimov and associates[66] performed 58 general surgical and 9 major cardiovascular procedures on 66 chronic hemodialysis

TABLE 5. Guidelines for Drug Therapy in Patients with Impaired Renal Function

Agent	*Metabolism and Excretion (Minor Modes in Parenthesis)*	*Maintenance Schedule* Based on Creatinine Clearence (ml/min)* > *80 (normal)*	*–50†*	*50–10†*	*< 10†*	*Drug Removed by Dialysis (H, hemodialysis; P, peritoneal dialysis)*
Antimicrobial Agents						
Antimycotic drugs						
Amphotericin B	Nonrenal	q 24h	q 24h	q 24hr	0.5 mg/kg q 24h or 1.0 mg/kg q 48h	No (H,P)
5-fluorocytosine	Renal	25–50 mg/kg q 6hr	Unch‡	25–50 mg/kg q 12–24h	25 mg/kg q 24h	Yes (H,P)
Miconazole	Hepatic	q 8h	Unch	Unch	Unch	No (H)
Antituberculous drugs						
Ethambutol	Renal	15–25 mg/kg/day	Unch	7.5–15 mg/kg/day	5 mg/kg/day	Yes (H,P)
Isoniazid (INH)	Hepatic, renal	300–400 mg/day	Unch	Unch	200–300 mg/day	Yes (H,P)
Para-amino salicylate (PAS)	Renal, (hepatic)	q 8h	q 8h	q 12h	Not recommended	Yes (H)
Rifampin	Hepatic	q 24h	Unch	Unch	Unch	No
Aminoglycosides§						
Amikacin	Renal	5 mg/kg q 8hr	5 mg/kg q 12h	3–5 mg/kg q 12h	1–3 mg/kg q 12h	Yes (H,P)
Gentamicin	Renal	1–1.5 mg/kg q 8h	0.5–0.8 mg/kg q 8h	0.3–0.5 mg/kg q 8h	0.2 mg/kg q 8h	Yes (H,P)
Kanamycin	Renal	7.5 mg/kg q 12h	7.5 mg/kg q 18h	0.25 gm q 24–48h	7mg/kg q 5–7 days	Yes (H,P)
Neomycin	Renal	Not recommended for systemic use				Yes (H)
Tobramycin	Renal	1 mg/kg q 8h	0.5–0.75 mg/kg q 8h	0.25–0.5 mg/kg q 8h	0.1–0.2 mg/kg q 8h	Yes (H,P)
Streptomycin	Renal	0.5–1.0 gm q 12h	0.5–1.0 mg q 24h	0.5–1.0 gm q 2–3 days	0.5 gm q 3–4 days	Yes (H)
Cephalosporins						
Cefadroxil	Renal	0.5–1.0 gm q 12h	Unch	500 mg q 12–24h	500 mg q 36h	Yes (H)
Cefamandole	Renal	1–2 gm q 4–6h	0.75–1.5 gm q 6h	0.5–1.0 gm q 8h	0.25–0.75 gm q 12h	Yes (H), No (P)
Cefazolin	Renal	0.5–1.0 gm q 8–12h	Unch	250 mg q 6–12h	250 mg q 24–48h	Yes (H), No (P)
Cefoxitin	Renal	1–2 gm q 6–8h	1–2 gm q 8–12h	1–2 gm q 12–24h	0.5–1.0 gm q 24–48h	Yes (H), No (P)
Cephalexin	Renal	500 mg q 4–6h	Unch	500 mg q 8–12h	250 mg q 12–24h	Yes (H,P)
Cephalothin	Renal, (hepatic)	1–2 gm q 4–6h	Unch	1–2 gm q 6–8h	1–2 gm q 8–12h	Yes (H,P)

Cephapirin	Renal, hepatic	0.5–1.0 gm q 4–6h	Unch	0.5–1.0 gm q 8h	7.5–10 mg/kg q 8–12h	Yes (H)
Cephradine	Renal	0.5–1.0 gm q 6h	Unch	0.25–0.5 gm q 6h	0.25–0.5 gm q 12–24h	Yes (H,P)
Chloramphenicol	Hepatic, (renal)	q 6h	Unch	Unch	Unch	Yes (H), No (P)
Clindamycin	Hepatic, (renal)	q 6–8h	Unch	Unch	Unch	No (H,P)
Erythromycin	Hepatic	q 6h	Unch	Unch	Unch	No (H,P)
Lincomycin	Hepatic	q 6h	Unch	q 12h	0.5 gm q 24–36h	No (H,P)
Metronidazole	Hepatic, renal	q 8h	Unch	q 12h	q 24h	Yes (H)
Penicillins						
Amoxicillin	Renal	q 8h	Unch	q 12h Unch for UTI	q 16h Unch for UTI	Yes (H), No (P)
Ampicillin	Renal, (hepatic)	q 6h	q 6h	q 9h Unch for UTI	5–10 mg/kg q 24h Unch for UTI	Yes (H) No (P)
Carbenicillin	Renal, hepatic	4–6 gm q 4h	4–5 gm q 4h	2–4 gm q 6–12h	2 gm q 12h	Yes (H), No (P)
Isoxazolyl penicillins (oxacillin, cloxacillin, dicloxacillin, nafcillin)	Hepatic, renal	q 6h	Unch	Unch	Unch	No (H,P)
Methicillin	Renal, (hepatic)	q 4h	Unch	Unch	1–2 gm q 8–12h	No (H,P)
Penicillin G	Renal, (hepatic)	q 8h	Unch	Unch	q 10–12h <10–15 million units/day	Yes (H), No (P)
Ticarcillin		3 gm q 3–6h	2 gm q 4h	2 gm q 8h	2 gm q 12h	Yes (H,P)
Sulfamethoxazole with trimethoprim	Renal	q 12h	Unch	q 18h	q 24h	Yes (H,P)
Sulfisoxazole	Renal	q 6h	Unch	q 8–12h Unch for UTI	q 12–24h Unch for UTI	Yes (H,P)
Tetracyclines						
Doxycycline	Hepatic, renal	q 12h	Unch	Unch	Unch	No (H,P)
All others	Renal, hepatic	Varies with agent	Avoid in presence of decreased renal function			No (H,P)
Urinary antiseptics						
Methenamine mandelate	Hepatic, renal	q 6h	Unch	Not recommended		Unknown
Nalidixic acid	Hepatic, renal	q 8h	Unch	Not recommended		Unknown
Nitrofurantoin	Renal	q 8h	Unch	Not recommended		Yes (H)
Vancomycin	Renal	1 gm q 12h	1 gm 2–3 days	1 gm q 3–10 days	1 gm q 10–20 days	No (H,P)
Cardiovascular Agents						
Antiarrhythmic drugs						
Disopyramide	Renal	100–200 mg q 6h	Unch	100 mg q 10–20h	100 mg q 20–30h	Yes (H)
Lidocaine	Hepatic	1–4 mg/min IV infusion	Unch	Unch	Unch	No (H,P)

TABLE 5 *Continued*

Agent	*Metabolism and Excretion (Minor Modes in Parenthesis)*	*Maintenance Schedule* Based on Creatinine Clearence (ml/min)* > 80 (normal)	−50†	50–10†	< 10†	*Drug Removed by Dialysis (H, hemodialysis; P, peritoneal dialysis)*
Phenytoin	Hepatic	q 8h	Unch	Unch	Unch	No (H,P)
Procainamide	Renal, hepatic	q 3–4h	Unch	q 6–8h	q 8–12h	Yes (H)
Propranolol	Hepatic	q 6–12h	Unch	Unch	Unch	No (H)
Quinidine	Hepatic, (renal)	q 6h	Unch	Unch	Unch	Yes (H,P)
Antihypertensive drugs						
Clonidine	Nonrenal	q 12h	Unch	Unch	Unch	Unknown
Diazoxide	Hepatic	150–300 mg IV bolus	Unch	Unch	Unch	Yes (H,P)
Guanethidine	Hepatic, renal	q 24h	Unch	Unch	Unch	Unknown
Hydralazine	Hepatic	q 12h	Unch	Unch	Unch	No (H,P)
Methyldopa	Hepatic, renal	q 8–12h	Unch	Unch	q 12–18h	Yes (H,P)
Metoprolol	Hepatic	q 12h	Unch	Unch	Use with caution	Unknown
Minoxidil	Hepatic, (renal)	q 8h	Unch	Unch	Unch	Unknown
Nitroprusside	Nonrenal	0.5–8 μg/kg/min IV infusion	Use with caution, monitor thiocyanate levels			Yes (H,P)
Prazosin	Hepatic (renal)	q 8–12 h	Unch	Unch	Unch	Unknown
Reserpine	Extrarenal	q 24h	Unch	Unch	Reduce dose	No (H,P)
Cardiac glycosides						
Digitoxin	Hepatic, (renal)	q 24h	Unch	Unch	5 days/week	No (H,P)
Digoxin§	Renal	0.25 mg q 24h	Unch	0.125 mg q 24h	0.125 mg 5 days/week	No (H,P)
Diuretics						
Chlorthalidone	Renal, (non-renal)	q 24h	q 24h	Decreased effectiveness		Unknown
Ethacrynic acid	Hepatic	q 6h	Higher doses may be required		Not recommended	Unknown
Furosemide	Renal	q 6–12h	Higher doses may be required			No (H)
Mannitol	Renal	As indicated	Unch	Not recommended		Yes (H,P)
Mercurials	Renal	q 24h	Unch	Not recommended		Unknown
Metolazone	Renal	q 24h	Unch	Decreased effectiveness		No (H)
Spironolactone	Hepatic	q 6–12h	Use with caution	Not recommended		Unknown
Thiazides	Renal	q 12h	Unch	Decreased effectiveness		Unknown
Triamterene	Hepatic, (renal)	q 12h	Use with caution	Not recommended		Unknown

Sedative, Tranquilizer, and Analgesic Agents						
Acetaminophen	Hepatic	q 4h	Unch	Unch	Unch	Yes (H), No (P)
Aspirin	Renal, hepatic	q 4h	Unch	q 4–6h	Not recommended	Yes (H,P)
Barbiturates						
short-acting (pentobarbital, secobarbital)	Hepatic	qhs	Unch	Unch	Unch	No (H,P)
long-acting (phenobarbital, amobarbital)	Renal	q 8h	q 8h	q 12h	q 16h	Yes (H,P)
Benzodiazepines						
Chlordiazepoxide	Hepatic	q 6–8h	Unch	q 8–12h	q 12–24h	No (H)
Diazepam	Hepatic	q 8h	Unch	Unch	Unch for short term therapy	No (H)
Flurazepam	Hepatic	qhs	Unch	Unch	Unch	No (H)
Chloral hydrate	Hepatic	qhs	Unch	Unch	Unch	Unknown
Diphenhydramine	Hepatic	As indicated	Unch	Unch	Unch	Unknown
Haloperidol	Hepatic, (renal)	q 8h	Unch	Unch	Unch	Unknown
Meprobamate	Hepatic, (renal)	q 6h	q 6h	q 8–12h	q 12–18h	Yes (H,P)
Narcotic analgesics						
Codeine	Hepatic	q 4h	Unch	Unch	Unch	Unknown
Meperidine	Hepatic	q 4h	Unch	Unch	Not recommended for repeated use	Unknown
Methadone	Hepatic	As indicated	Unch	Unch	Unch	No (H,P)
Morphine	Hepatic	q 4h	Unch	Unch	Unch	Unknown
Naloxone	Hepatic	IV bolus	Unch	Unch	Unch	Unknown
Pentazocine	Hepatic, (renal)	q 4h	Unch	Unch	Unch	Unknown
Propoxyphene	Hepatic, (renal)	q 4h	Unch	Unch	Unch	No (H,P)
Phenothiazines	Hepatic, (renal)	q 6h	q 6h	q 8–12h	q12–18hr	No (H,P)
Tricyclic anti-depressants	Hepatic, (renal)	q 8h	Unch	Unch	Unch	No (H,P)
Miscellaneous Agents						
Anticoagulants						No, (H,P)
Heparin	Hepatic	q 4h bolus or IV infusion	Unch			No, (H,P)
Warfarin	Hepatic	q 24h	Unch	Use with caution because of Hemorrhagic tendency in uremia	Use with caution because of Hemorrhagic tendency in uremia	Unknown

TABLE 5 *Continued*

Agent	Metabolism and Excretion (Minor Modes in Parenthesis)	Maintenance Schedule* Based on Creatinine Clearence (ml/min) > 80 (normal)	–50†	50–10†	< 10†	Drug Removed by Dialysis (H, hemodialysis; P, peritoneal dialysis)
Anti-inflammatory drugs						
Colchicine	Renal, (hepatic)	q 12h	Unch	Unch	Avoid prolonged use	No (H,P)
Corticosteroids	Hepatic	As indicated	Unch	Unch	Unch	Unknown
Ibuprofen	Renal	q 6h	Unch	q 8h	q12hr	Unknown
Indomethacin	Hepatic	q 8h	Unch	Unch	Unch	Unknown
Phenylbutazone	Hepatic	q 8h	Unch	Unch	Use with caution	No (H,P)
Cimetidine	Renal	300 mg q 6h	Unch	300 mg q 6–8h	300 mg q 8–12hr	Yes (H)
Hypoglycemic drugs						
Acetohexamide	Renal, (hepatic)	q 12h	q 12–24h	Not recommended	Not recommended	Unknown
Chlorpropamide	Hepatic, (renal)	q 24h	q 24–36h	Not recommended	Not recommended	No (P)
Insulin (regular)	Hepatic, renal	As indicated	Unch	Insulin requirements decrease in uremia		No (H,P)
Tolbutamide	Hepatic, (renal)	q 8h	Unch	q 8–12h	q 12–24h	No (H)
Hypouricemic agents						
Allopurinol	Renal	q 24h	Unch	Unch	Unch	Probably yes (H,P)
Probenecid	Hepatic, (renal)	q 12h	Unch	Ineffective, not recommended		Unknown
Immunosuppressive drugs						
Azathioprine	Hepatic	q 24h	Unch	Unch	q 24–36h	Probably some (H,P)
Cyclophosphamide	Hepatic, (renal)	q 24h	Unch	Unch	Avoid or use with caution	Yes (H)
Methotrexate	Renal	Once weekly	Unch	75% of normal dose	50% of normal dose	Unknown
Theophylline	Hepatic	Constant IV infusion	Unch	Unch	Unch	Probably yes (H,P)

*When no dosage of drug is listed, use the dose conventionally prescribed for the specific indication.
†When a range of dosages and/or intervals is listed for a level of renal functional impairment, use the lower dose and/or a longer maintenance interval if the patient's creatinine clearance falls at the lower end of the clearance range for that column.
‡Unch = dose level and maintenance interval unchanged from normal
§Require usual loading doses at all degrees of renal failure; blood levels are best guide to therapy.
UTI = urinary tract infection

patients with a similar mortality rate. Lansing, and coworkers[67] reported upon five major cardiovascular operations on patients with end-stage renal disease with no deaths. Several reports document the fact that well-managed patients with chronic renal failure can tolerate major and minor surgery well and that mortality rates are well within reason.[62–67] Thus, renal failure should not be regarded as a contraindication to elective or emergency surgery.

The Patient Undergoing Chronic Dialysis (Table 6)

PREOPERATIVE CONSIDERATIONS

Most authors[62,63,65,66,68] agree that the final preoperative hemodialysis should be performed within 24 hrs of elective surgery. This strategy is thought to ameliorate the uremic bleeding diathesis by improving platelet function. An increased bleeding tendency due to rebound from the heparin used during dialysis does not seem to occur if dialysis is completed 6 to 12 hours prior to surgery.[69] Perhaps even more importantly, dialysis immediately prior to surgery removes potassium and lessens the risk of hyperkalemia, a common postoperative complication in such patients.[65] The presence of hyperkalemia preoperatively clearly increases intraoperative and postoperative risk, and

TABLE 6. Considerations in the Chronic Dialysis Patient Undergoing Surgery

Preoperative Considerations
1. Conduct final preoperative dialysis within 24 hours of elective surgery.
2. Control hyperkalemia if dialysis not possible.
3. Avoid excessive routine preoperative fluid restriction.
4. Restrict dietary protein and potassium for several days prior to surgery, if possible.
5. Correct anemia only if patient is elderly, has cardiac disease, or is undergoing open-heart surgery.
6. Recognize that use of prophylactic antibiotics controversial.
7. Modify dosages of drugs appropriately for renal failure.

Intraoperative Considerations
1. Use neuromuscular blocking agents with caution.
2. Maintain lightest plane of general anesthesia possible.
3. Insure adequate ventilation to compensate for metabolic acidosis.
4. Restrict intraoperative fluid administration to 0.5 ml/kg/hour plus measured losses.
5. Do not use potassium-containing intravenous solutions.
6. Pay meticulous attention to control of bleeding.
7. Position extremities to avoid thrombosis of dialysis access site.

Postoperative Considerations
1. Treat hyperkalemia, if necessary, with early postoperative dialysis.
2. Infuse low dose heparin during dialysis to minimize bleeding complications.
3. Monitor fluid status closely.
   A. Additional fluids may be necessary if large extravascular fluid shifts occur.
   B. Fluid overload should be treated with dialysis.
4. Keep skin sutures in place 8 to 14 days.
5. Monitor for signs of infection with vigilance; treat promptly with the most specific antimicrobial agent.
6. Modify dosages of drugs appropriately for renal failure.
7. Assure adequate nutrition, using hyperalimentation if prolonged gastrointestinal dysfunction occurs.

a preoperative serum potassium level higher than 5.5 mEq/l may be a contraindication to general anesthesia.[63] If circumstances require an immediate operation without benefit of dialysis, preoperative hyperkalemia should be treated emergently by the infusion of calcium, sodium bicarbonate, and glucose-insulin (see Chap. 15, Fluid, Electrolyte, and Acid Base Disorders). If possible, polystyrene sulfonate (Kayexalate) should be given by enema.

Hemodialysis in the 24 hours prior to surgery also tends to correct other physiologic disturbances in the patient with chronic renal failure. Adequate ultrafiltration can reduce the fluid overload responsible for congestive heart failure and hypertension, both of which increase the risk of anesthesia.[70] Correction of metabolic acid-base abnormalities by preoperative dialysis will allow more flexibility for artificial ventilation intraoperatively.

Preoperative volume depletion is common and especially hazardous in the patient with chronic renal failure. Even routine fluid restriction may be dangerous because of the urinary concentrating defect. Volume depletion from any cause can aggravate the renal vasoconstriction often induced by anesthesia,[69] leading to a further reduction in GFR; the result may be increased azotemia, acidosis, hyperkalemia, and hyperphosphatemia in the face of the unavoidable catabolic stress of surgery.

Tissue breakdown and increased catabolism during the postoperative period can lead to large nitrogen, potassium, and phosphate loads. The effects of these notable changes can be minimized by instituting dietary protein and potassium restriction several days before elective surgery. Potassium should be eliminated from intravenous solutions.

The chronic anemia which is present in nearly all patients with chronic renal failure is usually well-tolerated and, as a routine matter, need not be corrected. In one series[65], 12 percent of the patients had preoperative hematocrits of less than 20, and all tolerated surgery well. Patients with coronary artery disease, however, as well as those of advanced age, with decreased cardiac reserve and with the prospect of open-heart surgery should have their preoperative hematocrit increased to the range of 30% by transfusion if necessary. Special risks of transfusion in the patient with chronic renal disease should be borne in mind and include precipitation of congestive heart failure, hyperkalemia from the potassium load, and hepatitis. All of these risks can be reduced somewhat by the use of frozen, washed red blood cells. Ongoing blood losses should be replaced by transfusion prior to surgery. Because infections appear to be a more frequent postoperative problem in patients with chronic renal failure, routine preoperative administration of prophylactic antibiotics has been advocated.[65,68] Indeed, because patients with chronic renal failure are more susceptible to infections and because they often have additional sites for bacterial entry (e.g., dialysis access, disrupted mucosal barriers), the use of prophylactic antibiotics does have some a priori appeal. On the other hand, the prolonged circulation of broad spectrum antibiotics due to delayed excretion leads to a high incidence of secondary infection with organisms such as *Monilia,* resistant staphylococci, and *Pseudomonas.*[71] Because of this, the use of routine prophylactic antibiotics is discouraged by some.[66] Any infection, if present, should be treated with the most specific antibiotic possible, in doses adjusted according to the mode of drug excretion. Recall also that chronic hemodialysis patients have a high carrier rate for hepatitis-B virus, and hospital personnel should take appropriate precautions with regard to contact with and disposal of instruments.

The use of routine preoperative medications can pose problems in the patient with renal failure undergoing surgery. Medium-acting and long-acting barbiturates have a prolonged duration of action because of impaired clearance by the kidney; their use should be avoided or suitable dosage adjustments must be made. Short-acting barbiturates and most tranquilizers are metabolized primarily by the liver, and dosage modification of these agents is not required. Opiates and antihistamines are also metabolized largely by the liver but opiates potentiate water retention as a result of decreased renal blood flow and release of antidiuretic hormone. The resulting volume expansion may be poorly tolerated by the patient with renal failure. Urinary retention is common following the use of antihistaminic and anticholinergic agents, and the need to use an indwelling catheter may be prolonged with attendant increased risk of infection.

Many recommend the discontinuation of digitalis glycoside 24 hours prior to major surgery[65,66,68] because toxicity may be precipitated by perioperative fluctuations in potassium and calcium levels. Lidocaine may be used in ordinary doses, if necessary. In general, antihypertensive medications should be continued up to the time of surgery in their usual doses (see p. 499).[65] Some advocate that therapy with propranolol be discontinued gradually prior to surgery. Effective dialysis often adequately controls the hypertension accompanying chronic renal failure without medication.

INTRAOPERATIVE CONSIDERATIONS

The major risk of anesthesia in patients with chronic renal failure is depressed cardiac output. Adequate blood supply to tissues is crucial for normal oxidative metabolism in the face of the severe anemia typically present in these patients. Most inhalational anesthetics depress cardiac output. Susceptibility to agents that increase myocardial irritability (e.g., cyclopropane, ether) is enhanced by the effects of uremia on the myocardium. Methoxyflurane is known to produce acute renal failure and intrarenal precipitation of oxalate and should be avoided if renal failure is incomplete or potentially reversible. Regardless of the agent employed, most authors agree that the lightest possible plane of anesthesia should be maintained to minimize intraoperative risk.

Neuromuscular blocking agents have altered metabolism in uremia and their effects may be prolonged. Such agents should be used with extreme care. Succinylcholine may induce hyperkalemia intraoperatively, evidently related to a reduction in the transmembrane potential of the motor endplate with release of intracellular potassium.[72] In addition, the hydrolysis of succinylcholine is dependent upon plasma cholinesterase, the activity of which is known to be decreased in uremia.[73] Aminoglycoside antibiotics, particularly kanamycin, whose excretion is limited in renal failure, may further potentiate neuromuscular blockade.

Intubation prior to surgery may be complicated by bleeding because of the friable mucosa present in many uremic patients. If metabolic acidosis is present, as it commonly is, secondary hyperventilation should be maintained under anesthesia.

Dangerous volume expansion from injudicious fluid administration during surgery is common. Intraoperative fluid administration should be strictly limited to maintenance levels (e.g., 0.5 ml/kg of body weight per hour[68] or 20 to 30 ml/hour).[66] Losses should be measured and replaced with appropriate electrolyte solutions or blood. A central venous pressure monitor is generally recommended. Use of potassium-containing solutions during the intraoperative period is best avoided unless potassium depletion is known to be present. Intraoperative hypotension is generally tolerated very poorly, probably because of limited oxygen delivery secondary to anemia. Hypotension increases the risk of thrombosis of the dialysis access site, if present.

Intraoperative hemostasis is not usually a major problem in patients with chronic renal disease if preoperative dialysis has been adequate.[62,65,66] Meticulous attention to control of bleeding during the surgical procedure is, of course, required. The use of monofilament nonabsorbable suture material is recommended[68] and skin sutures should be allowed to remain in place for as long as twice normal time.

Thrombosis of the dialysis access site is a significant problem during and following major surgical procedures especially those done as emergencies.[65] Some believe the hypercoagulable state which follows surgery may play a role.[74] The incidence of thrombosis may be reduced by careful attention to the positioning of the appropriate extremity during the operation, avoiding excess pressure to the area, avoiding intravenous fluid administration and blood pressure measurements in the arm harboring the access site, and avoiding hypotension or dehydration.[66] In patients with Silastic cannula shunts, the use of a "heparin lock" may help keep the shunt open during surgery.[66] Despite these maneuvers, thrombosis of arteriovenous shunts and fistulas may still occur.

POSTOPERATIVE CONSIDERATIONS

Hyperkalemia is by far the most common complication among chronic dialysis patients undergoing major surgery. It occured in as many as 30 percent of patients in one series,[65] the majority becoming sufficiently hyperkalemic to require dialysis within 24 hours of surgery. Replacement fluid for patients with renal failure should not contain potassium unless appreciable deficits are evident, as ongoing catabolism alone may cause serum potassium to rise from normal or below to dangerously high levels. Volume overload is the second most common indication for dialysis within the first 24 to 48 hours following surgery. This complication can often be avoided by strict attention to fluid intake during the perioperative period. Volume overload may manifest itself as hypertension, congestive heart failure, or both. Postoperative fluid therapy should be limited to a maintenance rate of 10 ml/kg of body weight in 24 hours in addition to replacement of ongoing losses. Central venous or even pulmonary wedge (Swan-Ganz) pressure monitoring are extremely useful in assessing fluid requirements, especially when significant fluid shifts may be expected to occur. Hypertension that develops during or immediately after operation is usually caused by the infusion of excessive amounts of fluid.[66]

If possible, hemodialysis is best delayed in the immediate postoperative period because the use of heparin (required for the extracorporeal circuit) increases the risk of bleeding at the operative site. Even with the use of regional heparinization, hemorrhagic complications may occur due to "heparin rebound," a phenomenon that results from protamine sulfate being metabolized more rapidly than heparin.[75] Kjellstrand found that the continuous infusion of small amounts of heparin into the arterial line of the hemodialyzer provided sufficient anticoagulation in 98 percent of instances of dialysis and eliminated the need for protamine.[76]

Hata and coworkers[69] avoided hemodialysis in the early postoperative period by employing peritoneal dialysis through a Silastic peritoneal catheter placed at the time of the operation. The few septic complications of peritoneal dialysis in this series responded to removal of the catheter and to appropriate antibiotic therapy. The advantages of having a peritoneal catheter in place postoperatively are several: dialysis can be initiated immediately, the need for special access, personnel, or equipment is eliminated and anticoagulation is not required. Peritoneal dialysis may be effective even in the presence of abdominal drains or aortic grafts.[77]

Postoperative hypotension is not infrequent in patients with chronic renal failure. Brenowitz[65] noted an 8 percent incidence of postoperative hypotension that was unexplained by excessive fluid loss. The use of antihypertensive medications preoperatively may predispose to this complication,[78] but only half of Brenowitz's patients with postoperative unexplained hypotension had received such agents. Autonomic dysfunction may be present in patients with renal failure[79] and can interfere with normal reflex responses to hypotension. Indeed, patients who develop unexplained hypotension postoperatively may respond well to vasopressors but only poorly to volume expansion.[65]

Massive upper gastrointestinal bleeding can be a frustrating problem in chronic hemodialysis patients following major surgical procedures.[69] As many as 20 percent may develop this complication. If surgical intervention is required to control the upper gastrointestinal bleeding, the prognosis is grave.[69]

Wound healing may be adversely affected by uremia with its associated anemia and poor nutritional status in patients with renal failure.[71] Nonetheless, recent series of chronic hemodialysis patients undergoing major surgery have demonstrated that adequate dialysis results in satisfactory wound healing in most cases.[62,63,66] The role of anemia as an impediment to wound healing remains open to question.[80] Similarly, the precise contribution to defective wound healing of the poor nutritional status present in many uremic patients remains uncertain. Postoperative infections, particularly pneumonia and wound infections, occur with increased frequency in chronic dialysis patients, even those receiving optimal preparation for surgery.[63,65,66] The mechanisms by which uremia may impair host defenses have been discussed earlier in this chapter. Further disruption of skin and mucosal barriers through operative trauma, the presence of prosthetic devices and catheters, and various diagnostic and therapeutic manipulations all provide additional portals of entry for pathogenic organisms in the surgical patient.[63,65,66]

Early diagnosis is the key to the successful treatment of postoperative infections in the patient with renal failure. Infection may be particularly difficult to recognize in the uremic patient because fever and leukocytosis may be absent. Lethargy, disorientation, tachycardia, hypotension, and an unexplained aggravation of the uremic metabolic derangements (e.g., persistent hyperkalemia, azotemia, and/or acidosis despite dialysis) may be the only clues to the presence of infection. Once infection has been established, impaired host defenses may hasten the spread. Broad spectrum antibiotic coverage may be indicated until the offending organism is identified and its sensitivities known. The infection, once identified, should be treated with the most specific antimicrobial agent in doses modified, if necessary, for the renal failure. Enteric gram-negative organisms and *Staphyloccoccus aureus* are the most common pathogens associated with postoperative infections.

In summary, major surgical procedures can be successfully accomplished with modest increase in morbidity and mortality in well-managed chronic hemodialysis patients provided that certain principles of preoperative, intraoperative, and postoperative management are observed conscientiously.

The Patient with Renal Insufficiency (Table 7)

As summarized above, considerable experience with surgical procedures in the chronic dialysis patient has been reported in the literature. Less has been written, however, about surgical procedures in patients whose renal function is significantly reduced, but in whom chronic hemodialysis has not been required. Indeed, the nondialyzed patient with renal insufficiency may be more challenging to manage in the preoperative and postoperative period than the dialysis patient in view of the greater dependence on pharmacologic means to optimize plasma volume, blood pressure, and acid-base and electrolyte status in the former.

If the serum creatinine is less than 2.0 mg/dl (creatinine clearance may be greater than 50% of normal), the risk for surgery is not likely to be increased and no

TABLE 7. Considerations in the Patient with Renal Insufficiency Undergoing Surgery

Preoperative Considerations

1. Monitor closely for signs of volume depletion and treat as necessary with supplemental fluids.
2. Routine preoperative volume expansion with crystalloid recommended by many authors.
3. Routine preoperative use of diuretics (furosemide and/or mannitol) may be of value, but URINARY FLUID LOSSES MUST BE REPLACED.
4. Treat fluid overload and hyperkalemia if present; dialysis if necessary.
5. Correct anemia if patient is elderly, has cardiac disease, or is undergoing open-heart surgery.
6. Modify dosages of drugs appropriately for the degree of renal failure.

Intraoperative Considerations

1. Monitor hemodynamic parameters and fluid administration carefully.
2. Use muscle relaxants and long-acting barbiturates with caution.
3. Do not use methoxyflurane anesthesia.

Postoperative Considerations

1. Pay strict attention to state of hydration, fluid intake and output.
2. Routine use of diuretics (furosemide and/or mannitol) may be of value, but URINARY FLUID LOSSES MUST BE REPLACED.
3. If oliguria supervenes, trial of diuretics often appropriate, but BE SURE INTRAVASCULAR VOLUME STATUS IS ADEQUATE.
4. Monitor closely for signs of infection; treat promptly.
5. Do not allow fluid restrictions imposed by reduced urine output to interfere with patient nutrition. Use hyperalimentation if prolonged gastrointestinal dysfunction limits oral intake; remove excessive retained fluid with dialysis.
6. Modify dosages of drugs appropriately for the degree of renal failure.

special precautions need be taken. The level of renal functional impairment at which the risk of surgery is notably increased is difficult to quantify. It is axiomatic that azotemia has an adverse effect on surgical morbidity and mortality, but it is also true that surgery poses a threat to the remaining level of renal function. Thus, it is recommended that patients with a serum creatinine value greater than 2 mg/dl have a creatinine clearance determination made just prior to surgery to assess the precise degree of renal insufficiency and to serve as a baseline should renal function deteriorate.[81]

PREOPERATIVE CONSIDERATIONS

As noted above, the earliest functions of the kidney to be compromised in most renal diseases are the abilities to concentrate the urine appropriately and to conserve sodium properly. Thus, unlike the chronic dialysis patient who is at risk for fluid overload, the patient with mild to moderate renal insufficiency is at greater risk for volume depletion if appropriate precautions are not taken. For example, routine "NPO" orders for the preoperative patient with abnormal renal function may result in significant volume deficits and a further deterioration of renal function. Diuretic administration and gastrointestinal losses are the most common causes of chronic volume depletion in patients with renal insufficiency as in those with normal renal function. Frequent causes of acute volume depletion include bleeding, peritonitis, pancreatitis, burns, bowel obstruction, and systemic sepsis. Several days of successive tests, many of which entail fluid restriction, fasting, and enemas, can also cause significant fluid deficits to develop. Moreover, the tests themselves often result in fluid loss; examples include the osmotic diuresis produced by hyperosmotic intravascular contrast media and the gastrointestinal losses produced by hydrophilic barium enemas. A weight loss of 4 to 12 kg after some 5 days of testing is not uncommon.[82] Finally, nasogastric suction in the perioperative period can add significantly to the fluid deficit.

Preoperative volume depletion carries considerable risk for all patients, with or without renal insufficiency. If volume deficits are not repleted prior to surgery, the likelihood of developing postoperative acute renal failure is increased.[83] Thus, it is imperative that all patients be carefully assessed regarding preoperative volume status and that volume repletion be instituted where necessary. With increasing renal functional impairment, the ability of the patient to tolerate overhydration also decreases and so the use of central pressure monitoring devices such as central venous pressure (CVP) lines or Swan-Ganz catheters should be considered seriously to minimize the margin of error for fluid therapy.

Crystalloid administration, either alone[84] or in combination with potent diuretics (e.g., furosemide, mannitol)[82,85,86] has been advocated to insure an adequate state of hydration and urine flow prior to elective surgery in patients with moderate renal insufficiency. No single method is clearly superior. If diuretics are employed in the absence of volume surfeits however, it is imperative that urinary losses be replaced completely. Failure to do so will result in a contracted intravascular compartment. Use of a Swan-Ganz catheter is helpful in patients suspected of having cardiac decompensation to gauge pulmonary wedge pressure (see Chap. 3, Cardiology). If Swan-Ganz monitoring is not available, a CVP value in the range of 5 to 10 cm H_2O may be considered to reflect an optimal state of hydration.

The following recommendations for perioperative diuretic and fluid management have been proferred for patients with various degrees of renal insufficiency:[81]

FOR PATIENTS WITH SERUM CREATININE 2 TO 4 mg/dl. Preoperative: Furosemide, 40 mg intravenously on call to operating room. Intraoperative: Furosemide, 250 mg in 500 ml of 20 percent mannitol; administer at 20 ml/hour as needed to keep urine output between 100 and 200 ml/hour. Postoperative: Continue furosemide-mannitol drip for 24 hours. Replace *all* urinary losses with saline.

FOR PATIENTS WITH SERUM CREATININE GREATER THAN 4 mg/dl. Preoperative: Furosemide 80 to 500 mg intravenously on call to operating room. Intraoperative: Furosemide 500 mg to 1,000 mg in 500 ml of 20 percent mannitol; administer at 20 ml/hour to keep urine output between 100 and 200 ml/hour. Postoperative: Continue furosemide-mannitol drip for 24 hours. Replace *all* urinary fluid losses with saline.

Recall that a diuresis can be produced by contrast media used for arteriography or intravenous pyelography and by drugs which interfere with urinary concentrating ability; thus, the sine qua non of an adequate extracellular fluid volume is not an adequate urine output per se but a normal central venous (or pulmonary wedge) pressure.

If extracellular fluid *overload* requires treatment prior to surgery in the patient with renal insufficiency, higher than normal doses of potent diuretics, such as furosemide, are usually required. Furosemide administration usually results in some degree of natriuresis even in severe renal failure,[87] and is a relatively safe drug in high doses. Patients with serum creatinine greater than 4 mg/dl generally require a dose of at least 80 mg of this agent to produce an effect. If a given dose does not induce diuresis, it is generally pointless to repeat it; rather the dosage should be increased, by 50 or 100 percent, for the next trial until an effective dosage is found.

Although patients with mild to moderate renal insufficiency usually have sufficient tubular function to excrete a normal potassium load, preoperative hyperkalemia may be a problem especially in the face of trauma, hemolysis, or accelerated tissue catabolism. Standard therapy for hyperkalemia in the nondialysis patient is usually adequate to restore safe levels; in extreme circumstances, dialysis may be required for this reason alone. Serum potassium levels greater than 5.5 mEq/l are a relative contraindication to general anesthesia.

Chronic anemia is usually well-tolerated in nondialyzed patients with chronic renal insufficiency and need not be corrected preoperatively unless the patient is elderly, has coronary artery disease or decreased cardiac reserve, or is undergoing open heart surgery. In such circumstances, preoperative transfusions should be designed to restore hemoglobin levels up to 10 gm/dl or hematocrit to 30 percent.

INTRAOPERATIVE CONSIDERATIONS

Fluid administration should be monitored very carefully during surgery. A fine line is often tread between inadequate fluid replacement that may lead to intravascular volume depletion, oliguria, and possibly complete shutdown of the already compromised kidney and excessive fluid administration that can precipitate congestive heart failure, pulmonary edema, and hypoxemia. Hypotension resulting from blood loss is particularly hazardous because of the further reduction in renal function which may result. Patients with pre-existing renal disease, especially older patients, have decreased ability to recover from the oliguric renal failure induced by hypovolemia.[81]

As in the dialysis patient, muscle relaxants and long-acting barbiturates must be used with caution. Regimens of other drugs may have to be modified by reducing the dose or increasing the interval between doses as required by the degree of renal insufficiency. Even though most inhalational anesthetics carry some increased risk in the patient with renal disease, they can be used successfully in such patients. However, the risk of methoxyflurane nephrotoxicity appears to be increased substantially in patients with chronic renal insufficiency, and use of this agent should be avoided if possible.[88]

POSTOPERATIVE CONSIDERATIONS

Strict attention to the state of hydration should continue well into the postoperative period. Howard and Najarian[81] recommend maintaining a urine output above 100 ml/hour for the first 24 hours postoperative to provide a margin for sudden changes that may cause urine flow to fall. The patient should be weighed daily, and any significant weight change should be treated appropriately. Vital signs and central pressure monitor readings (CVP or Swan-Ganz) are also important parameters to follow. If urine output falls, the CVP should be maintained in the range of 5 to 10 cm H_2O to eliminate the possibility of volume depletion. If oliguria persists despite an optimal CVP, the urinary catheter should be checked by irrigation with a urethral syringe and changed if there is any question of patency. Assuming the CVP and other parameters verify that extracellular fluid volume is not depleted, a trial of diuretics may be attempted if oliguria persists. Howard and Najarian[81] recommend the slow administration of 20 to 40 mg furosemide intravenously, doubling the dose every two hours until a total dose of 500 mg is reached or until diuresis begins.

If urine output remains low and serum creatinine and BUN continue to rise, the presence of acute renal failure is established and dialysis must be contemplated. The postoperative patient is often quite catabolic, and blood urea nitrogen and serum potassium levels frequently rise rapidly in the presence of oliguria. Intravenous fluid administration should be reduced to match insensible and urinary losses. It may be possible to control hyperkalemia with conservative measures (e.g., glucose and insulin infusions, Kayexalate). Dialysis may be necessary to minimize the hazards of advancing uremia in the postoperative period and the decision to institute dialysis should be made relatively early. Peritoneal dialysis has been advocated as the dialytic procedure of choice during the early postoperative period because it avoids the risk of anticoagulation which is required for hemodialysis.[62] If trained personnel are available, however, hemodialysis can be performed safely with low-dose heparin infusion into the arterial line of the dialyzer[76] or with regional heparinization using protamine sulfate to produce sufficient anticoagulation for dialysis without increasing the risk of hemorrhage. Recall that more rapid metabolism of protamine may occur during periods of increased catabolism, resulting in the dissociation of heparin from the protamine-heparin complex and increased bleeding tendency.[75] The management of the patient with acute postoperative deterioration in renal function is discussed more extensively below.

Other postoperative problems such as infection, impaired would healing, and gastrointestinal bleeding, discussed in the preceding section on the chronic dialysis patient undergoing surgery, must be considered in the patient with mild to moderate renal insufficiency, especially if postoperative decompensation of renal function occurs. Care must be taken to identify and treat infection promptly and not to allow fluid restrictions imposed by reduced urine output to interfere with patient nutrition. Finally, it must be kept in mind that the dosages of many drugs given during the postoperative period for infection, gastrointestinal disturbance, cardiac problems, and the like will have to be appropriately reduced for the level of residual renal function.

The Renal Transplant Recipient

The primary consideration that sets the transplant patient apart from other patients with renal disease is the presence of chronic immunosuppression. Experience has shown that surgical procedures can be performed successfully with only a modest increase in risk in patients from this group if appropriate precautions are taken.

Within six months after transplantation, the doses of immunosuppressive drugs are, as a rule, relatively low. The usual drug regimen is (1) azathioprine (Imuran), 50 to 150 mg once daily by mouth and (2) prednisone 10 to 30 mg once daily by mouth. If the graft is functioning well, no dietary restriction is required except possibly modest salt restriction. Some transplant patients also require antihypertensive drugs (usually thiazides, propranolol, methyldopa, or hydralazine) for blood pressure elevation that may or may not be related to persistent renal dysfunction.

Hirsche and Woods[89] reported their experience with 24 elective surgical procedures performed on 21 renal transplant recipients. A majority of the operations were undertaken for conditions related to the renal transplant or complications of chronic corticosteroid therapy. The patients were prepared with intravenous methylprednisolone, 500 to 1,000 mg, given after induction of anesthesia during a two to four minute period. Smaller doses, rapidly tapered off, were employed during the postoperative period. Prophylactic antibiotics were used routinely, and furosemide with aggressive intravenous hydration were utilized intraoperatively to maintain a high urine output. All patients in this series survived surgery. There were no wound infections and there was no detrimental effect of the surgery on allograft function in any patient. The authors concluded that normal indications for elective surgery should be followed in renal transplant patients.

Kountz and coworkers[90] reported upon a series of 67 operations in 162 renal transplant patients. Most of the operations (71 percent) were necessary to correct complications directly related to the transplant procedure, and 21 percent were related to complications of immunosuppression or uremia. General anesthesia was used in all but five of the procedures. Additional doses of steroids beyond the maintenance levels were not given prior to, during, or after the operations in this series. Prophylactic antibiotics were given only if there was manipulation of the urinary tract or if the procedure was quite lengthy. Of the total number of procedures performed, 40 percent were classified as "emergency" (e.g., gastrointestinal bleeding, abscess, thrombosis, hematoma formation).

The mortality rate in this series was 30 percent but was confined for the most part (80%) to the group undergoing "emergency" procedures. Urologic problems, often complicated by sepsis, accounted for the majority of total complications. The time interval between transplantation and subsequent elective or emergency surgery did not appear to influence mortality. The donor source had no effect in predicting whether an allograft recipient would require posttransplant operative procedures, but recipients of kidneys from living relatives seemed to have lower overall morbidity and mortality rates, likely correlating with their lower dosage of immunosuppressive drugs. Neither living-related nor cadaveric allograft recipients had a higher than expected morbidity from wound infections or bleeding, considering the presence of chronic immunosuppressive therapy. Despite the high mortality experienced in this series, Kountz and colleagues conclude that immunosuppressed patients should not be denied surgery but in fact should be operated upon earlier than might otherwise be indicated to minimize the risks of the immunosuppressed state.

Stuart and coworkers[91] and Flamenbaum and Leslie[92] recommend the administration of additional hydrocortisone in the preoperative preparation and in the early postoperative period. To prevent adrenal insufficiency in those patients whose hypothalamic-pituitary-adrenal axis has been suppressed, 300 mg of hydrocortisone or its equivalent should be given daily. An intravenous form of azathioprine is available and may be substituted for the oral form on a milligram for milligram basis while the patient is receiving nothing by mouth. No apparent harm is done, however, if azathioprine is omitted for two to three days.

Since the transplanted kidney generally lies in the iliac fossa in an extraperitoneal plane, its presence usually does not interfere with intra-abdominal surgery, cesarean section, or even normal vaginal delivery. Stuart and coworkers[91] found no increased incidence of postoperative wound infection among renal transplant patients despite the presence of immunosuppressive drugs. Routine prophylactic antibiotics are not recommended in these patients for uncontaminated surgical fields. Systemic antibiotics are recommended when contamination is likely as well as for dental and oral surgery procedures.

ACUTE RENAL FAILURE IN THE SURGICAL PATIENT

The development of acute deterioration of renal function is a common event in the surgical patient. Acute renal failure (ARF) is defined as a sudden decrease in renal function and is generally reflected by a rise in BUN and serum creatinine. Notable changes in daily urine volume may or may not occur. ARF may occur in the patient with previously normal renal function or in the patient with underlying renal insufficiency (so-called "acute-on-chronic" renal failure). In the latter circumstance, the degree of reversibility of renal failure may be difficult to establish unless baseline renal function tests had been obtained.

Acute deterioration of renal function among hospitalized patients is probably more common than previously recognized. We recently studied prospectively the incidence of acute renal insufficiency in our institution and found that of all general medical and surgical admissions over a five-month period (2,419 patients), 106 patients (4%) developed a rise in serum creatinine by approximately 20 percent or more during the hospital stay.[93] Of these patients, 18 percent developed acute renal insufficiency postoperatively, without a history of other factors predisposing to renal failure such as hypotension, septicemia, or administration of nephrotoxic agents. Other series have also demonstrated that surgery is an important cause of acute renal insufficiency, accounting for 24 to 54 percent of cases of renal failure.[94–97] Among those surgical patients in whom a specific renal insult can be identified, sepsis has superseded shock as the most common cause of acute renal insufficiency.[98]

Terminology and Classification

The term "acute renal failure" refers to a sudden deterioration in renal function from any cause. The term "acute tubular necrosis" is usually reserved for that subset of patients in whom a self-limited form of acute renal failure occurs following shock, sepsis, trauma (including surgery), and the use of certain toxic agents. Acute tubular necrosis (ATN) is generally (but not always) characterized by a period of diminished urine output, increasing azotemia, and an inability to form a concentrated or dilute urine. The name tubular necrosis implies the presence of damage to the renal tubular epithelial cells, but on pathologic examination such damage is not universally present in patients with the clinical syndrome.[99] Despite intensive investigation, the precise pathogenesis of the decrease in glomerular filtration rate associated with acute tubular necrosis remains unclear.

Anuria is defined as a urine volume of less than 50 ml/day. Such marked reductions in urine flow rarely result from ATN and suggest the presence of some other conditions (e.g., bilateral cortical necrosis, rapidly progressive glomerulonephritis, obstructive uropathy, bilateral renal arterial occlusion).

Oliguria is defined as a daily urine output of less than 400 ml. This level of urine flow represents the minimal amount of urine in which the normal daily solute load (about 500 mOsm) can be excreted if the urine is maximally concentrated (1,200 mOsm/kg H_2O). Thus, progressive solute retention and azotemia necessarily develop if daily urine output is less than 400 ml, even if concentrating power is intact.

Renal failure associated with daily urine volumes of 400 to 1,000 ml is termed "nonoliguric." True polyuria, defined as a daily urine output of greater than 1 to 2 L, occurs only rarely in the setting of acute renal failure but may be seen when renal failure is due to nephrotoxic agents, particularly methoxyflurane or hypercalcemia.

Table 8 lists the most common causes of acute renal failure in the surgical patient in terms of the usual degree of reversibility. As with most arbitrary classifications, there is some overlap among categories. For example, acute glomerulonephritis may be reversible or irreversible, depending upon the severity of pathologic changes. Also ischemic renal damage may be readily reversible ("prerenal" azotemia), self-limited (classical acute tubular necrosis), or irreversible (cortical necrosis).

Approach to the Patient with Acute Renal Failure (Table 9)

The primary goal in the initial evaluation of the patient with acute renal failure is to exclude those disorders for which prompt, specific therapy may be curative. This would

TABLE 8. Causes of Acute Renal Failure (ARF)

I. *Reversible ARF*
   A. Decreased effective renal perfusion
   B. Extrarenal obstruction to urine flow

II. *Self-limited ARF*
   A. Acute tubular necrosis (ATN)
      1. Ischemic ATN: Shock, sepsis, "postoperative"
      2. Nephrotoxic ATN
         a. Drugs
         b. Radiocontrast media
         c. Pigment: Hemoglobin, myoglobin
   B. Acute interstitial inflammation: Allergic, infectious
   C. Intrarenal obstruction to urine flow: Drugs, uric acid
   D. Acute glomerulonephritis syndromes

III. *Irreversible ARF*
   A. Renal cortical necrosis
   B. Certain nephrotoxins: Methoxyflurane
   C. Large vessel occlusion
   D. Microvascular occlusion
      1. Malignant hypertension
      2. Some rapidly progressive glomerulonephritis-vasculitis syndromes
      3. Atheroembolic renal disease

include the physiologic oliguria and "prerenal" azotemia accompanying a decrease in effective renal perfusion, as well as the changes in urine volume and "postrenal" azotemia accompanying an extrarenal obstruction to urine flow. Obstruction of the urinary tract at the bladder outlet, particularly in men with prostatic hypertrophy, is probably the most common cause of a sudden, and often total, cessation in urine output. In the postoperative patient, sustained effects of anticholinergic agents or urethral swelling due to instrumentation may produce an impediment to bladder outflow as well. Therefore, as a general rule, the oliguric patient should be examined promptly for possible bladder distention. Even patients with indwelling catheters should be examined, as catheters may become obstructed. If there is any question about bladder distention, an echographic examination of the bladder or straight catheterization should be performed. Although upper urinary tract obstruction is a much less common cause of oliguria in the absence of a solitary kidney, this possibility should be evaluated by abdominal echography. If echography fails to exclude urinary tract obstruction as a cause of acute renal failure, other diagnostic procedures should be considered including radionuclide scanning,[100,101] intravenous pyelography,[102] and retrograde pyelography. The risks associated with the latter two procedures must be balanced against the likelihood of finding a correctable form of obstruction, as judged by the clinical setting and other available data.

In addition to assessing bladder distention, the physical examination should focus on the signs both of intravascular volume depletion and of volume overload. Useful signs include blood pressure and pulse (especially postural changes), jugular venous distention, skin turgor, moistness of skin and mucous membranes, pulmonary rales, gallop

TABLE 9. Clinical Approach to the Patient with Acute Renal Failure

I. *Rule-out Urinary Obstruction*
   - A. Physical examination: Bladder distention
   - B. Straight bladder catheterization or irrigation of indwelling catheter
   - C. Ultrasound of urinary system
   - D. If necessary
     1. Radionuclide scanning
     2. Intravenous urography
     3. Retrograde pyelography

II. *Assessment of Patient's Volume Status*
   - A. History: Intake and output, daily weight, drugs
   - B. Physical examination
     1. Blood pressure and pulse, postural changes
     2. Skin moistness, turgor, edema
     3. Cardiovascular exam: Jugular venous distention, gallop rhythm, pulmonary congestion
     4. Moistness of mucuous membranes
   - C. Central venous pressure determination, if necessary
   - D. "Fluid challenge" if overt signs of volume depletion present

III. *Laboratory Determinations*
   - A. Routine blood chemistries
     1. Rate of rise in blood urea nitrogen and serum creatinine
     2. Electrolyte abnormalities
   - B. Routine urinalysis
     1. Specific gravity
     2. Presence of protein or heme
     3. Examination of sediment
   - C. If previous renal function status unknown, abdominal x-ray to assess kidney size, presence of opacities
   - D. Special diagnostic indices (Table 10)

rhythm, and edema. If volume depletion is suspected, a fluid "challenge" of 500 to 1,000 ml of normal saline may be given intravenously over one to three hours. If urine output fails to increase, it may be useful to place a central venous catheter and continue saline infusion until the CVP exceeds 10 cm H_2O.

The presence of salt and water surfeits (as evidenced by peripheral edema, pulmonary congestion, gallop rhythm, ascites) does not exclude decreased effective renal perfusion as the cause of acute renal insufficiency. Indeed, patients with congestive heart failure or hypoalbuminemia, due to hepatic disease or nephrosis, commonly have diminished effective intraarterial blood volume and are therefore subject to the development of renal ischemia. Similarly, the absence of any overt physical signs of intravascular volume depletion, particularly in the postoperative or septic patient, does not exclude a decrease in effective renal perfusion.

A crucial step in the approach to the patient with acute renal failure is a careful examination of the urine. A routine urinalysis, which should be done by the physician, often provides many essential clues to the etiology of acute renal failure. A high urinary specific gravity, greater than 1.025 (in the absence of marked proteinuria, glycosuria, or radiocontrast media), is inconsistent with acute tubular necrosis or obstructive uropathy, and suggests "prerenal" azotemia. Heavy proteinuria is highly suggestive of glomerular disease. Moderate proteinuria may be seen with almost any type of parenchymal renal disease including acute tubular necrosis. Uncomplicated "prerenal" azotemia or extrarenal urinary obstruction is not characteristically accompanied by significant proteinuria. (A possible exception to this rule is severe congestive heart failure in which modest proteinuria may be seen.) Finding an abundance of crystals in the urinary sediment may point to intrarenal precipitation or extrarenal obstruction due to stone. If the diagnosis of allergic interstitial nephritis is suspected in a patient with fever, rash, and oliguric renal failure, the demonstration of eosinophils on a Wright's stained smear of the urinary sediment can help to confirm the diagnosis.

In general, urinary sediment in "prerenal" azotemia and obstructive uropathy is unremarkable. In acute tubular necrosis, sediment abnormalities are more typically found in patients with oliguria than those with nonoliguric renal failure. In oliguric renal failure due to ATN, at least some of the typical sediment abnormalities are found in about 80 percent of patients. These include renal tubular cells and casts, coarse granular pigmented casts, and a moderate number of red and white blood cells. Gross hematuria is unusual in acute tubular necrosis and, in the presence of severe oliguria, suggests renal arterial occlusion. The urinary sediment in acute pyelonephritis typically shows many white blood cells and white blood cell casts. The presence of clots, pyogenic debris, or necrotic tissue in the urine suggests urinary tract obstruction in the patient with acute renal failure.

A positive "dipstick" test for heme or a gross reddish or brownish pigmentation of the specimen in the absence of red blood cells in the sediment of a freshly voided urine is suggestive of renal failure due to hemoglobinuria or myoglobinuria.

Diagnostic Indices for Distinguishing Acute Tubular Necrosis from "Prerenal" Azotemia (Table 10)

The hallmark of acute tubular necrosis is a diminished ability to concentrate the urine and to conserve sodium. In contrast, a reduction in effective renal perfusion without tubular damage ("prerenal" azotemia) results in the elaboration of a concentrated urine

TABLE 10. Diagnostic Indices in Acute Renal Failure

	Prerenal Azotemia	*Oliguric Acute Tubular Necrosis*
Urine osmolarity	> 500 mOsm/kg H_2O or > 100 more than plasma	< 350 mOsm/kg H_2O or ≤ plasma
Urine to plasma creatinine ratio	> 40	< 20
Urine to plasma urea nitrogen ratio	> 8	< 3
Urine sodium concentration	< 20 mEq/L	> 40 mEq/L
Fractional excretion of sodium	< 1.0%	> 1.0%
Renal failure index	< 1.0	> 1.0

that is relatively free of sodium. These distinctions in the quality (not the quantity) of urine formed provide the basis for the diagnostic indices currently used in the evaluation of acute renal failure.

Urine osmolarity is the most specific measure of urinary concentrating ability. Although a urine to plasma osmolarity ratio (U/P osmolarity) greater than 2:1 is typical of prerenal azotemia and a ratio less than 1.1:1 is typical of established tubular necrosis,[103] the distinction is not absolute. Moreover, osmolarity determinations are frequently not available. The urine to plasma creatinine ratio (U/P creatinine) provides similar information; a U/P creatinine ratio of more than 40 is suggestive of prerenal azotemia, whereas a ratio of less than 20 is more consistent with established ATN.[104] The urine to plasma concentration ratio for urea is less specific as an index for concentrating ability but a U/P urea ratio of more than 8 is more likely to be associated with prerenal azotemia, and a ratio of less than 3 with established ATN.[104]

Patients with prerenal azotemia without underlying intrinsic renal disease typically excrete urine with a sodium concentration of less than 20 mEq/l, and often less than 10 mEq/l. In contrast, patients with tubular necrosis generally excrete urine with a sodium concentration greater than 40 mEq/l.

In an effort to improve diagnostic accuracy, measures of concentrating ability and of sodium conserving ability may be combined into a single parameter. One such parameter is the fractional excretion of sodium (FE_{Na}) which is the ratio of sodium excreted to sodium filtered, as follows:[105]

$$FE_{Na} = \frac{\text{Na excreted}}{\text{Na filtered}} = \frac{U_{Na} \times V}{P_{Na} \times GFR}$$

Substituting creatinine clearance for GFR yields:

$$FE_{Na} = \frac{U_{Na} \times V}{P_{Na} \times \dfrac{U_{cr} \times V}{P_{cr}}} = \frac{U_{Na} \times Pcr}{P_{Na} \times Ucr} = \text{U/P sodium} \div \text{U/P creatinine}$$

where U_{Na} = urinary sodium concentration, V = urine flow rate, P_{Na} = plasma sodium concentration, GFR = glomerular filtration rate, U_{cr} = urinary creatine concentration, P_{cr} = plasma creatinine concentration, U/P sodium = urine to plasma sodium ratio, U/P creatinine = urine to plasma creatinine ratio.

In prerenal azotemia, FE_{Na} is generally less than 1 percent and in acute tubular necrosis, it is generally greater than 1 percent.[104] Because measurement of urine volume is not necessary, FE_{Na} can be determined rapidly using a "spot" urine and a blood sample drawn simultaneously.

The "renal failure index" (RFI) is another derived parameter designed to aid in discriminating between ATN and prerenal azotemia. It is closely related to FE_{Na} and is the quotient of U_{Na} divided by U/P creatinine. In a prospective study, 83 percent of patients with prerenal azotemia had an RFI of ≤ 1.0, while no patient with oliguric ATN had an RFI of ≤ 1.0.[104]

Specific Clinical Entities

This section will discuss several clinical situations that are frequently associated with acute renal failure in the surgical patient. It is important to recognize, however, that acute tubular necrosis is often a multifactorial event in which a combination of such factors as volume depletion, nephrotoxins, sepsis, and heme pigments may play additive roles in the pathogenesis.

POSTOPERATIVE ACUTE RENAL FAILURE

Acute tubular necrosis can occur following major surgery, even in the absence of obvious predisposing factors (e.g., overt hypotension, sepsis, the use of nephrotoxic agents). Patients undergoing major surgery are often volume depleted preoperatively as a result of diagnostic testing, restriction of oral intake, and ongoing fluid losses. As noted earlier, restoration of normal intravascular volume preoperatively is the single most important therapeutic maneuver in the prevention of postoperative renal failure. At one time, almost two-thirds of patients undergoing major surgery experienced at least a transient deterioration in renal function.[106] This figure has been reduced substantially over the past 20 years by more rigorous attention to fluid replacement.[107]

General anesthesia virtually always poses a threat to the kidney. The induction of general anesthesia is known to cause profound changes in renal hemodynamics and in water and electrolyte excretion.[108] During general anesthesia, renal blood flow may be depressed as a consequence of systemic hypotension, renal vasoconstriction, or both. Anesthetic agents increase the levels of circulating catecholamines, antidiuretic hormone, and angiotensin, all of which are potent vasoconstricting agents.[109–111] The net result is that renal autoregulation, which would normally maintain renal blood flow in the face of systemic hypotension, is disturbed, and renal blood flow is further compromised, often in the absence of overt systemic hypotension. Patients with sepsis are at further risk for developing acute renal failure because of reduced renal blood flow secondary to shock, endotoxic vasoconstriction, and occasionally intravascular coagulation (see next section).

Although intraoperative reductions in renal blood flow can be prevented or minimized by the preoperative administration of intravenous crystalloid solutions, such solutions are much less effective in restoring renal blood flow intraoperatively.[103]

Most postoperative and traumatized patients gain weight because of sequestration of fluid in the area of tissue injury and because of water retention due to the elevation in antidiuretic hormone level induced by general anesthesia. However, such weight gain can be deceptive and may mask serious intravascular volume deficits. A disproportionate deficit in plasma volume often occurs in the course of major surgery, thought to be secondary to a functional extracellular fluid volume deficit and losses of albumin from the intravascular compartment. In one report,[112] significant intravascular deficits occurred in every postoperative patient studied, with some deficits being as great as 50 percent of the preoperative plasma volume. Another study found average postoperative blood volume deficits of 8 percent following extensive vascular operations, despite aggressive intraoperative fluid therapy.[113] It has been demonstrated in experimental animals that hypotension secondary to intravascular volume loss induces a much greater fall in renal blood flow than a similar degree of hypotension due to cardiac failure.[114] Thus, hypotension itself may not be the only factor determining the intensity of renal vasoconstriction in the face of volume depletion, and an "adequate" blood pressure may not ensure the maintenance of renal blood flow under these circumstances.

Fluid deficits during the early postoperative period may be aggravated further by the transient polyuria that sometimes occurs immediately following surgery. The mechanism for postoperative polyuria is unclear, but one possibility is the shunting of renal blood flow from the cortex to medulla during general anesthesia. This could lead to a "washout" of medullary hypertonicity and an impairment of urinary concentrating ability.

Several surgical circumstances have been identified that increase the risk of developing ATN;[109] these include cardiopulmonary bypass, abdominal aortic surgery, major biliary tree surgery, lengthy or extensive surgical procedures in older patients, surgery in patients with pre-existing renal disease, and major trauma. According to some, pre-existing renal insufficiency is the single most important predisposing factor in the development of postoperative deterioration in renal function.[107]

The incidence of postoperative deterioration in renal function in cardiac surgery patients is approximately 30 percent.[115–119] Fortunately, the majority of such patients have a mild, reversible decline in renal function which generally returns to normal after a few days.[116,117] The development of any renal dysfunction following open heart surgery, however, appears to be a bad prognostic sign. Mortality is less than 2 percent among cardiac surgical patients who maintain normal renal function, compared to about 30 percent in patients whose postoperative serum creatinine increases to 2 mg/dl or higher.[117] This excess mortality is probably not related solely to renal dysfunction per se. Oliguria and azotemia in these patients are often secondary to low cardiac output which itself worsens prognosis. If azotemia is due to congestive heart failure, therapy should be directed at improving cardiac performance.

Risk factors for the development of renal failure following cardiac surgery include increased patient age, underlying renal disease, operations involving the tricuspid valve, preoperative cardiac arrest or severe congestive heart failure, and duration of the operation.[118]

Aortic aneurysm is frequently associated with renal dysfunction, at least in part because of the effects of cross-clamping the aorta. Obviously, if the aorta is cross-clamped proximal to the renal arteries, as may be necessary in some operations, renal perfusion will be impaired immediately and the risk of acute tubular necrosis increases substantially. The safe period for cross-clamping the aorta above the renal arteries is about 30 minutes if the kidneys are without pre-existing disease, less if prior renal dysfunction is evident. If longer periods of clamping are required, renal circulation should be maintained by some form of bypass.[120]

Cross-clamping of the aorta below the level of the renal arteries also induces significant changes in renal hemodynamics but the exact mechanism is not completely understood. The renal tubular damage induced by infrarenal aortic clamping in experimental animals appears to be mediated by shunting of renal blood flow away from the cortex,[121] a response that is most likely mediated by neural mechanisms.

Attempts to minimize the decrease in renal cortical blood flow associated with abdominal aortic surgery have included aggressive preoperative hydration and the use of mannitol infusions. Even with these precautions, acute renal failure remains a relatively frequent complication of abdominal aortic surgery,[122,123] especially when performed on an emergency basis.[120,124]

Atheromatous emboli to the kidney are another cause of acute renal failure following surgical manipulation of the aorta. In patients with severe atherosclerotic disease, the intima may be eroded and covered extensively by a friable, amorphous material containing cholesterol crystals. Spontaneous embolization of this material occurs but, more often, embolization follows operative aortic trauma or renal arteriography. Atheroembolism of some degree probably occurs frequently in such situations, but serious disturbances in renal function are rare. If oliguric renal failure results, the potential for recovery of renal function is slight. In some cases, the onset of renal failure is gradual, with renal function deteriorating slowly over a matter of months. The detection of atheromatous material in the retinal vessels or evidence of peripheral embolization may support the diagnosis but renal biopsy is the only sure way to make the diagnosis.[125]

ACUTE RENAL FAILURE ASSOCIATED WITH SEPSIS

Sepsis is the most common cause of acute renal failure insufficiency among surgical patients.[98] Infection often leads to acute tubular necrosis in the absence of overt hypotension or "septic shock," and renal failure in such cases may be erroneously ascribed to the use of potentially lifesaving antimicrobial agents.

For many years, renal dysfunction in sepsis was ascribed to a decrease in renal blood flow. However, recent studies have revealed that most cases of sepsis are accompanied by a hyperdynamic circulatory state, with increased cardiac output, decreased total peripheral resistance, and expanded extracellular fluid volume. Disturbances in antidiuretic hormone (ADH) regulation[126] along with increases in total renal blood flow (in direct proportion to cardiac output),[127,128] typically result in an increased urine volume during early sepsis. Persistent renal fluid losses, coupled with "leakage" of plasma volume into the extravascular compartment, may lead to a fall in effective circulatory volume, in renal blood flow, and in GFR which can eventuate in ATN.[129] Thus, an "adequate" urine output during the early septic period does not necessarily ensure a normal circulatory volume and may represent "inappropriate polyuria." Careful monitoring of intake and output is necessary, but a positive fluid balance and weight gain do not ensure adequate plasma volume. Urinary sodium concentration should be monitored periodically; a fall to less than 10 mEq/L suggests circulatory insufficiency. Monitoring of intravascular volume status with a Swan-Ganz catheter may be helpful, particularly in the presence of respiratory insufficiency, a common occurrence in the acutely ill patient. Although fluid replacement may cause respiratory function to deteriorate initially, the maintenance of renal function should enable adequate diuresis to occur once the sepsis is controlled and the extracellular fluid is mobilized. Respiratory function would be expected to improve as the extracellular fluid leaves the pulmonary third-space.[129]

In addition to altered hemodynamics, systemic infection may result in renal functional impairment through immunologic mechanisms. Proliferative glomerulonephritis, ranging in severity from focal to crescentic, is the usual renal pathologic lesion seen under these circumstances. Urinalysis generally reveals abnormalities typical of acute glomerulonephritis: moderate to heavy proteinuria with red blood cells and red blood cell casts in the sediment. Since the glomerulonephritis is felt to be mediated by immune complex deposition in the kidney, serologic studies will often reveal depression of serum complement.

Immune-complex glomerulonephritis has been associated with bacterial endocarditis[130] and infections of prosthetic shunts.[131] Of particular interest here is the association between acute glomerulonephritis and visceral abscesses.[132] The severity of infection-associated glomerulonephritis generally parallels that of the infection, and complete recovery of renal function may occur when the infection is eradicated. A delay in therapy, however, may result in the development of chronic irreversible renal failure. In patients with visceral abscesses, bacteremia appears not to be a prerequisite for the glomerulonephritis.

DRUG-INDUCED ACUTE RENAL FAILURE (TABLE 11)

Drug nephrotoxicity is estimated to cause as many as 20 to 30 percent of the instances of acute renal failure in teaching hospitals.[133] In acute renal failure due to drug nephrotoxicity, oliguria and urinary sediment findings may be minimal or absent. Consequently, the diagnosis may not be made until the process is far advanced.[134] Fortunately, withdrawal of the offending agent usually leads to recovery although four weeks or more may elapse before clinical improvement occurs.

The pathogenesis of the ARF due to drugs varies with the offending agent. Three general mechanisms are recognized: (1) direct tubular toxicity (acute tubular necrosis), (2) immunologic reactions (acute interstitial nephritis, acute necrotizing angiitis, acute glomerulonephritis), and 3) obstructive nephropathy. A fourth pathogenetic mechanism, suppression of GFR due to inhibition of renal prostaglandin synthesis, has been suggested.[135]

The aminoglycoside antibiotics produce acute renal failure by direct tubular toxicity. As in ischemic acute tubular necrosis, other factors may contribute (e.g., alterations in renal perfusion, changes in glomerular filtration, preglomerular vasoconstriction).[136,137] Renal failure can occur with these agents even when peak and trough levels are both meticulously maintained below the "toxic" ranges.[138] Factors which appear to predispose to nephrotoxicity incude (1) pre-existing renal disease, (2) advanced patient age, (3) volume depletion, and (4) prolonged therapy.[139] Proper dosage schedules should take into account *lean* body weight, creatinine clearance,[140] and hematocrit[141] because each of these can affect the serum level achieved following a given dose. Proteinuria and cylindruria often precede the development of oliguria or azotemia.[142] Cephalosporins,

TABLE 11. Patterns of Drug-Induced Acute Renal Failure

A. *Acute Tubular Necrosis*
   1. Aminoglycosides
   2. Amphotericin B
   3. Polymyxins
   4. Cephaloridine, ? cephalothin

B. *Hypersensitivity-Mediated Nephritis*
   1. Vasculitis–Glomerulonephritis
      a. Penicillin
      b. Sulfonamides
   2. *Acute (Allergic) Interstitial Nephritis*
      a. Penicillins (especially semi-synthetic)
      b. Diuretics (furosemide, thiazides)
      c. Allopurinol
      d. Anticonvulsants
      e. Other antimicrobials (sulfonamides, rifampin)

C. *Obstructive Nephropathy*
   1. Intratubular precipitation of drug
      a. Sulfonamides
      b. Methotrexate
   2. Intratubular precipitation of organic acids
      a. Uric acid: Cancer chemotherapy
      b. Oxalic acid: Methoxyflurane

D. *Reversible Decreases in Glomerular Filtration Rate—Nonsteroidal Anti-inflammatory Agents (Inhibitors of Prostaglandin Synthesis)*
   1. Indomethacin
   2. Aspirin
   3. Others

E. *Alterations in Renal Function Tests without True Decline in Renal Function*
   1. Elevation in blood urea nitrogen (increased catabolism)
      a. Tetracyclines
      b. Corticosteroids
   2. Elevation in serum creatinine: Trimethoprim, cimetidine

particularly cephalothin, have been shown to potentiate aminoglycoside nephrotoxicity in man,[143] although some animal studies have demonstrated a protective effect.[144] Clindamycin may also potentiate aminoglycoside nephrotoxicity in man.[145] Neomycin and kanamycin are the most toxic aminoglycosides followed by gentamicin, tobramycin, amikacin, netilmicin, and streptomycin, in that order.[144]

Amphotericin B, even in therapeutic doses, can cause proximal as well as distal tubular damage. Thus azotemia, renal tubular acidosis, hypokalemia, and urinary concentrating defect may result. Although dehydrated and elderly patients are particularly subject to the nephrotic effects of amphotericin, virtually all patients receiving the drug demonstrate some nephrotoxicity which is dose-related.[146]

Other antimicrobials that can cause acute tubular necrosis include polymyxin B, polymyxin E (colistin),[147] and, more rarely, cephalothin.[148–150] Preliminary experience with the newer cephalosporins, cefamandole and cefoxitin, suggests that they are less nephrotoxic than cephalothin.[148]

Agents in the penicillin class of antibiotics are most frequently associated with hypersensitivity reactions affecting the kidney. Acute interstitial nephritis is the most common form of renal injury due to the penicillins and is most often associated with the semisynthetic derivative methicillin.[151] Ampicillin, nafcillin, oxacillin, and penicillin have also been documented to cause this lesion as have many drugs of other types (e.g., furosemide, thiazide, allopurinol). Fever, skin rash, and eosinophilia may occur separately or in any combination in patients with allergic interstitial nephritis. When present, these findings are helpful in suggesting the correct diagnosis; in many instances, however, none of these systemic manifestations of allergy are evident.

Allergic interstitial nephritis is generally reversible when the offending drug is withdrawn. Corticosteroid therapy may hasten the recovery of renal function by reducing the inflammatory response. Penicillins can also induce a hypersensitivity angiitis and acute glomerulonephritis whether or not there is a history of adverse reaction to the drug.[152] The syndrome is usually self-limited, but corticosteroids may be of benefit.

Obstructive nephropathy related to drugs may be due to intratubular crystallization of the drug itself (e.g., poorly soluble sulfonamides,[146] methotrexate[133]) or to crystalluria induced by the drug therapy. The latter mechanism is best exemplified by the intratubular precipitation of uric acid which may be associated with the chemotherapy of hematologic malignancies.

Intratubular precipitation of oxalate, resulting in obstructive nephropathy, is a major mechanism in the nephrotoxicity associated with methoxyflurane.[153,154] The risk of methoxyflurane toxicity is increased by higher doses, prolonged anesthesia, and pre-existing renal insufficiency.[155] There is some evidence that methoxyflurane may potentiate the nephrotoxic effects of the aminoglycosides and cephalosporins, perhaps secondary to the changes in renal blood flow induced by the anesthetic.[156]

A reversible decline in GFR has been reported to result from administration of nonsteroidal anti-inflammatory agents that inhibit prostaglandin synthesis (e.g., aspirin, indomethacin). These agents appear to exert no deleterious effects on renal function in normal man but do so in some patients with severe liver disease and ascites, lupus erythematosus, primary glomerular disease, or advanced congestive heart failure. Marked sodium retention may accompany the reduction in glomerular filtration.[135]

There are several drugs which produce biochemical abnormalities suggestive of an impairment in renal function, but glomerular filtration rate is actually unaffected. The tetracyclines and corticosteroids, because of their catabolic effect on metabolism, cause increased breakdown of tissue protein, release of nitrogenous wastes, and a rise in blood urea nitrogen level independent of any changes in renal function. This accumulation of nitrogenous wastes may be sufficient to precipitate signs and symptoms of uremia in a patient with only a modest degree of pre-existing renal insufficiency. Trimethoprim, the antimicrobial agent which is combined with sulfamethoxazole in co-trimoxazole (Bactrim or Septra), alters renal handling of creatinine and can produce an elevation in serum creatinine independent of any changes in GFR.[157,158] The rise in serum creatinine through this mechanism is not deleterious in itself, as long as the clinician recognizes the cause and does not institute therapy for acute renal failure inappropriately.

RADIOCONTRAST-INDUCED ACUTE RENAL FAILURE

The incidence of acute renal failure following intravascular administration of radiocontrast agents is uncertain; estimates vary between 0.15 and 13 percent.[159] Most authors agree that pre-existing renal insufficiency, myeloma, and volume depletion are definite predisposing factors for radiocontrast-induced ARF. Diabetes mellitus has also been cited as a risk factor, but it is not clear whether this risk is additive to that associated with the degree of renal insufficiency.

Among the various types of radiocontrast studies, angiography appears to be the most likely to produce acute renal failure,[159] even when newer, "less toxic" contrast agents are used.[160] Renal failure has also been reported following intravenous pyelography, computerized axial tomography (CAT) scan with contrast, intravenous cholangiography, and double-dose oral cholecystography.

The pathogenesis of radiocontrast-induced ARF is multifactorial[161] involving both a direct toxic effect on the renal tubules and adverse hemodynamic alteration.

The clinical course of radiocontrast-induced ARF is generally characterized by the onset of oliguria within 12 to 24 hours after the contrast procedure.[162] The duration of the oliguria is usually less than 5 days and, although supportive dialysis may be required, the prognosis for recovery is good. The serum creatinine usually peaks 3 to 10 days after contrast exposure and returns to baseline levels in about 80 percent of cases.[163] Therapy consists of normal supportive measures for acute renal failure. Recommended preventative measures include adequate hydration before, during, and after the contrast procedure, minimizing the dose of contrast medium, and using alternative diagnostic techniques (e.g., ultrasonography, CAT scan without contrast) whenever possible in the high-risk patient.

HEME-PIGMENT ASSOCIATED ACUTE RENAL FAILURE (TABLE 12)

Myoglobinuria associated with severe muscle trauma and crush injuries is frequently complicated by acute renal failure. Myoglobin is a heme pigment, similar in structure to hemoglobin but much smaller in molecular weight and readily filtered by the glomerulus. If muscle injury occurs, the myoglobin which is released into the plasma is rapidly excreted in the urine, and plasma concentrations of myoglobin remain low. The presence of significant amounts of myoglobin gives the urine a characteristic brownish coloration and causes the urine "dip stick" test for heme to be positive. Because severe trauma is frequently associated with shock and infection, it may be difficult to specify the role of myoglobinuria per se in the production of acute renal failure. Myoglobinuria and volume depletion appear to have a synergistic effect on the kidney. Maintaining optimum fluid balance seems to reduce the incidence of ARF in the presence of myoglobinuria.

Volume depletion and muscle injury also lead to acute renal failure in situations of strenuous exercise complicated by heat stroke.[164–168] Myoglobinuric renal failure has

TABLE 12. Causes of Pigment Nephropathy

A. Myoglobinuria	*B. Hemoglobinuria*
1. Traumatic rhabdomyolysis	1. Transfusion reaction
a. Crush injuries	2. Other immunologic-mediated hemolytic anemias
b. Burns	3. Glucose-6-phosphate deficiency and
c. Electric shock	a. Oxidizing drugs
d. Hemodynamic compromise to muscle	b. Certain infections
2. Non-traumatic rhabdomyolysis	4. Infectious hemolysis: Malaria, clostridial sepsis
a. Physical exertion/heat stroke	5. Miscellaneous
b. Electrolyte abnormalities	a. Toxins: Arsenic
(1) Hypokalemia	b. Physical agents: Hypotonic solutions, burns
(2) Hypophosphatemia	c. Mechanical etiologies: Extra-corporeal circulation, prosthetic cardiac valves
(3) Hypernatremia	
c. Inflammatory muscle disease	
(1) "Collagen-vascular" diseases	
(2) Infections, especially viral	
d. Metabolic muscle disease	
(1) Enzyme deficiency syndromes	
(2) ? Paroxysmal myoglobinuria	
e. Toxins: Alcohol, barbiturates, narcotics, amphetamines, carbon monoxide	

been reported following muscle damage due to status epilepticus, burns, electrical injury,[169] and ischemia. Sufficient muscle ischemia to produce myoglobinuric renal failure has occurred after vena cava ligation.[170] Nontraumatic rhabdomyolysis can also cause myoglobinuric acute renal failure.[171–176]

The diagnosis of rhabdomyolysis is supported by finding elevated levels of creatine phosphokinase (CPK), lactic dehydrogenase (LDH), glutamic oxaloacetic transaminase (SGOT), and aldolase. When extensive tissue damage occurs in the presence of acute renal failure, striking changes suggestive of hypercatabolism often occur, including a rise in BUN of over 30 mg/dl/day, a rise in serum creatinine of over 1.0 mg/dl/day, a rise in serum potassium over 1 mEq/L/day, a serum uric acid level exceeding 15 mg/dl, a serum phosphate level exceeding 8 to 10 mg/dl, and a fall in serum bicarbonate of over 2 mEq/L/day.[177]

Severe hypocalcemia may occur during the early stages of the renal failure, probably because the marked hyperphosphatemia fosters deposition of calcium in the injured muscle tissue. During the later recovery stages, hypercalcemia may develop, possibly due to persistent secondary hyperparathyroidism[178–180] or to dissolution of dystrophic calcifications in the traumatized muscle.[181]

Acute intravascular hemolysis is a well-known cause of oliguric renal failure. In the surgical patient, transfusion of incompatible blood is the most frequent explanation for brisk hemolysis. Transfusion reactions may occur several hours after the administration of red blood cells so that the etiology of the subsequent oliguria may not be apparent.[182]

Acute hemolysis and rhabdomyolysis are frequently accompanied by hypotension and shock, which may independently contribute to the production of renal failure.

Therapy is therefore directed at maintaining adequate arterial blood pressure and extracellular fluid volume with intravenous fluids until the patient is stable hemodynamically. The prophylactic administration of mannitol is recommended to aid in volume expansion and to dilate constricted renal arterioles before the oliguric renal failure is established. Once established, the renal disease associated with hemoglobinuria or myoglobinuria is managed similarly to the other forms of acute tubular necrosis.

Clinical Course in Acute Tubular Necrosis

Figure 1 illustrates the typical clinical course in oliguric ATN. The clinical picture at the onset is determined primarily by the nature and severity of the acute illness which has precipitated the renal failure. The patient may have multiple symptoms related to the causal disease such as shock, cardiac failure, respiratory distress, fever, gastrointestinal bleeding, or neurologic dysfunction which may distract the physician's attention from the oliguria and progressive azotemia. Once acute renal dysfunction is discovered, the presence of the "reversibles" (e.g., urinary obstruction, decreased effective renal perfusion) must be excluded and a search for the specific diagnostic features of ATN undertaken (see p. 475).

The fluctuations in BUN during the oliguric period illustrated in Figure 1 represent the effects of intermittent hemodialysis (HD) The signs and symptoms of uremia in acute

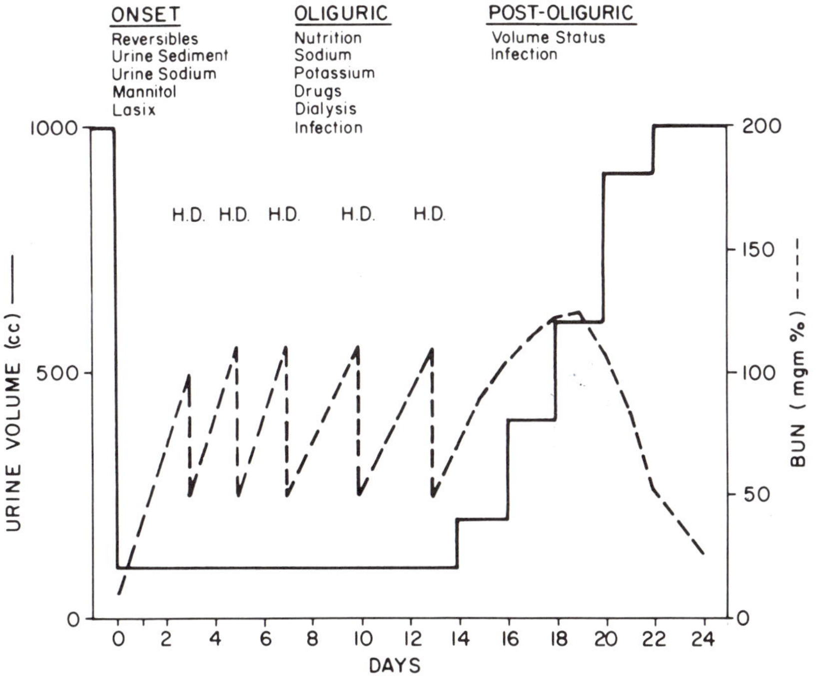

FIGURE 1. Typical clinical course in acute tubular necrosis. Note the effect on blood urea nitrogen (BUN) of intermittent hemodialysis (H.D.) treatments. The lists at the top of the figure refer to topics discussed in the text.

renal failure are identical to those in chronic renal failure but tend to occur at a lower BUN level in the former, presumably because the patient has not developed tolerance to the uremic toxins. Potentially serious manifestations of uremia include gastrointestinal bleeding, cardiac decompensation, and neuropsychiatric disturbances. The rapidity of development of uremic symptoms varies with the state of tissue catabolism; which tends to be increased in many of the illnesses which precipitate ATN. Daily dialysis is often required during the initial part of the oliguric phase in the hypercatabolic patient. As Figure 1 illustrates, however, the frequency of dialysis may often be reduced during the latter part of the oliguric phase, once intercurrent illnesses are controlled and the provision of adequate nutrition allows for a decrease in the rate of catabolism (see below).

Infection remains the highest cause of mortality in acute tubular necrosis, and it always must be of prime concern to the clinician managing an oliguric patient. The respiratory tract, urinary tract, and wounds are the most common sites of infection in acute renal failure, and septicemia occurs frequently. Indwelling bladder catheters should be removed once oliguric ATN is established as they merely provide a route of entry for pathogens which are not "washed out" by urine flow.

Respiratory failure is also a significant cause of mortality in oliguric renal failure. The injudicious administration of fluids may lead to pulmonary edema in the oliguric patient. A "shock lung" syndrome may develop in many of the same clinical situations that produce ATN (which may be likened to a "shock kidney"). In addition, the adult respiratory distress syndrome ("shock lung") is a common complication of trauma and septicemia; it is characterized by increased pulmonary capillary permeability leading to noncardiogenic pulmonary edema. The typically low central venous pressure in this syndrome may lead to an overly aggressive use of intravenous fluids in an attempt to treat the oliguria, further compounding the problems with respiratory function in this situation[183] (See Chapter 12, Pulmonary Diseases).

Dosage modifications are required for many therapeutic agents in the setting of acute renal failure to avoid toxicity. The effect of dialysis on excretion of the drug should also be considered. Recommendations regarding the use of specific drugs in renal failure are given in Table 5.

The typical duration of the oliguric period in acute tubular necrosis is 10 to 14 days. Oliguria may persist for as long as six to eight weeks with eventual recovery of renal function.[184] However, the persistence of oliguria for longer than 30 days or the development of anuria should suggest the presence of renal cortical necrosis. The risk of "permanent" ATN in the postoperative patient may be increased by advanced age (greater than 60 years), the use of nephrotoxic antibiotics, and the use of methoxyflurane anesthesia.[185] In at least 20 to 30 percent of cases of ATN, oliguria may never occur.[94] The diagnosis can be easily missed if biochemical monitoring of renal function is infrequent. Nonoliguric renal failure is generally seen following toxic rather than ischemic tubular injury and carries a significantly better prognosis.

The postoliguric phase of ATN begins when the daily urine output exceeds 400 ml. As illustrated in Figure 1, the BUN (and serum creatinine) may continue to rise for several days after the urine output begins to increase. Tubular dysfunction may also become apparent during this period, manifested by sodium wasting, urinary concentrating defect (polyuria), or a hyperchloremic metabolic acidosis. These tubular derangements may persist for several days following the return of normal glomerular function.[182]

During the postoliguric phase of ATN, volume status remains of concern because significant urinary water and electrolyte losses may occur. Approximately 20 percent of mortality in cases of ATN occurs during the postoliguric phase, with infection remaining the leading cause of death.

Treatment of Acute Tubular Necrosis

DIURETICS

The appeal of administering diuretics to the patient with acute oliguria is undeniable. Indeed, there are many reports that diuretics, when administered to selected patients at the appropriate time, may favorably influence the course of acute tubular necrosis. However, the indiscriminant use of diuretics in the setting of oliguria has its own risks, not the least of which is the precipitation of ATN in the patient with prerenal azotemia and marginally adequate effective renal perfusion. Nonetheless, many authors recommend the routine use of diuretics as a diagnostic and therapeutic maneuver in the patient with acute oliguria. This section will examine the evidence for and against such a recommendation.

Mannitol, an osmotic diuretic, is felt to have a beneficial effect upon the kidney in the setting of ATN because it can lead to increased GFR, a decrease in renin secretion, and a "washout" of tubular casts.[103] In addition, mannitol appears to produce a direct dilatation of renal arterioles and, if hypertonic mannitol is used, a shrinking of swollen glomerular capillary endothelial cells.[187] Mannitol may also induce diuresis in the absence of intravascular volume expansion and increases in renal blood flow.[188,189] In this respect, mannitol might be considered preferable to saline loading to increase urine output in the patient with marginal cardiac reserve.

Over the past 20 years, a number of reports have supported a role for mannitol in the prophylaxis (not treatment) of acute renal failure associated with trauma and high-risk surgery.[190–195] Mannitol infusion has been shown to minimize the deleterious changes in intrarenal hemodynamics which follow infrarenal aortic cross-clamping.[196] However, postsurgical oliguria can also be prevented by sustained preoperative and intraoperative hydration with saline.[197] Nevertheless, the impression that mannitol is useful in the prevention of oliguric renal failure has received wide acceptance, while the importance of adequate hydration per se has been less emphasized. Furthermore, as an extrapolation, the use of mannitol in the *treatment* of established oliguria has become popular in some quarters, despite scanty clinical evidence for its efficacy in this setting.

The use of mannitol is not without hazard. Its administration may result in an abrupt increase in plasma volume with precipitation of pulmonary edema. This is most likely to occur if there is a minimal or absent diuretic response, which is generally the case in established ATN. On the other hand, if mannitol does induce a brisk diuresis, volume depletion may occur if fluid losses are not monitored and replaced as necessary.

Furthermore, although urine volume may increase, this may not necessarily be associated with a therapeutic benefit.[198]

If mannitol is to be used as prophylaxis against renal failure in high-risk surgery (e.g., open heart, aortic, biliary), the dosage used should be the smallest which will maintain hourly urine volume between 50 and 100 ml[193] and no more than 100 gm (500 ml of a 20% solution) should be given in a 24-hour period. Urinary losses should be replaced with 0.45 percent saline containing 10 to 20 mEq of potassium per liter.

It has also been suggested that mannitol may be of benefit in the onset phase (no more than 50 hours after the insult) of oliguric renal failure if circulatory insufficiency has been ruled out or corrected, and especially if the urine to plasma osmolarity ratio is greater than 1.05.[199] Use of mannitol appears to be particularly promising in aborting or decreasing the severity of acute renal failure associated with muscle-crushing injuries, mismatched transfusion, rapid intravascular hemolysis, or acute hyperuricemia.[200] Maintaining urine flows of 2 to 4 L/day with mannitol for two or three days after such events is recommended.[200]

The "loop" diuretics, furosemide and ethacrynic acid, do not have the volume expanding effects of mannitol and hence do not carry the risk of precipitating pulmonary edema. On the other hand, if effective, the loop diuretics are likely to induce more volume depletion than does mannitol infusion. Therefore, if the use of furosemide or ethacrynic acid is to be considered in a patient with oliguria, it is important to correct any pre-existing intravascular volume deficit. Failure to do so might precipitate the development of ATN in a patient with otherwise reversible oliguria due to prerenal azotemia. Obviously, loop diuretics are preferable to mannitol in the treatment of oliguria associated with cardiac overload. Furosemide and ethacrynic acid, like mannitol, have a direct dilating effect on the renal arterioles, and successful diuresis may produce a "washout" of obstructing casts from the tubules. However, the loop diuretics do not decrease renin secretion nor have the theoretical advantage of improving capillary endothelial swelling.

Both furosemide and ethacrynic acid[201] are sufficiently potent to induce a diuresis in some cases of oliguria in which mannitol has been unsuccessful. But, as noted above, the induction of a diuresis in the oliguric patient does not necessarily indicate improved renal function[202] and may seriously reduce the circulatory volume, thereby aggravating renal failure.

If diuretics ever alter favorably the course of acute renal failure, it is only within the first day or two of oliguria that they do so.[199,203,204] This early period is thought by some to represent an interphase between prerenal azotemia and acute tubular necrosis, during which ATN has begun but is still reversible by pharmacologic means.[200] In fact, this phase is defined operationally by a diuretic response to mannitol or a loop diuretic in patients who have not responded to volume expansion alone.[205] Even if diuretic therapy during this period does not abort the establishment of ATN or directly improve renal function, it has been argued that a successful diuresis may "convert" oliguric renal failure to nonoliguric renal failure. In time, such a conversion might favorably alter the prognosis of ATN and might reduce the need for dialysis.

If a trial of diuretics is to be employed during the initial hours of oliguria, how aggressive to be with these agents is a matter of personal opinion. Most authors prefer to use mannitol first, in a single dose of 12.5 gm[92,198,206] or 25 gm[200] administered intravenously in a 25 percent solution over 5 to 10 minutes. An increase in urine output to over 30 ml/hour over the next 2 hours is a positive response and should be followed by the inclusion of mannitol in the maintenance intravenous fluids to maintain a comparable urine output.[92] A failure to respond to a single dose of mannitol might warrant consideration of a trial of furosemide. Most authors recommend starting with a furosemide dose of 200 to 250 mg[92,198,200,206] infused intravenously over 10 to 60 minutes. If no response occurs within two hours then a second dose twice as large as the first (400 to 500 mg) can be administered in a similar fashion. If no diuresis ensues, most authors would end the trial at that point. If a diuretic response to furosemide does occur, the dose can be repeated every 6 to 12 hrs to maintain a urine output greater than 30 ml/hour.

Although there are scattered reports of a beneficial effect of diuretics in patients with established acute renal failure,[207] most believe that diuretics are ineffective at this stage of the disease.[208–210] Moreover, ototoxicity may complicate the use of these agents in this setting.

In summary, diuretics appear to be useful in the prophylaxis of acute renal failure following trauma or certain high-risk operations. They may favorably alter the course of ATN if administered within the first few hours of the oliguria. In all cases, intravascular fluid deficits should be repaired before diuretic therapy is attempted, and attention to the maintenance of adequate intravascular volume following diuresis is essential. Diuretics are of no value in established acute renal failure.

MANAGEMENT OF FLUID AND ELECTROLYTE DISTURBANCES

The development of oliguric renal failure results in the disruption of the kidneys' ability to maintain a constant composition and volume of the body water and electrolytes and to excrete the nitrogenous end-products of protein catabolism. In many cases, conservative medical management can suffice to control the consequences of this disruption.

The most obvious result of oliguria is the inability to maintain normal water balance. Insensible losses continue and amount to about 12 ml/kg of body weight/day or about 850 ml/day in a 70 kg man. This rate of water loss is increased by fever, excessive sweating, and increased respiratory volumes. Insensible water loss is partially offset by the endogenous production of water during the oxidation of fat and protein. Normally, endogenous water production accounts for some 300 ml/day or about one-third the insensible loss. The rate is increased in states of rapid catabolism. The daily fluid requirement for the patient with renal failure, therefore, is equivalent to measured losses (from the gastrointestinal tract, drains, and urine) plus two-thirds of the estimated insensible water loss. The provision of water in excess of this amount would lead to volume expansion and hyponatremia. In patients with hypercatabolism, increased water of oxidation must be considered as intake. Accurate daily weights are an essential aid in designing proper fluid therapy.

In oliguric patients, the limited total caloric intake imposed by fluid restriction is usually insufficient to meet body demands, and most patients lose 0.3 to 0.4 kg of lean body mass per day due to catabolism of tissues.[211] Failure of the kidneys to excrete the end-products of tissue metabolism results in retention of nitrogenous compounds such as urea, creatinine, and uric acid; retention of nonvolatile acids such as sulfuric and phosphoric acid; and retention of the liberated intracellular ions potassium and magnesium. The rate at which these metabolites accumulate depends upon the rate of the body catabolism and the amount of residual renal function.

Azotemia usually progresses most rapidly during the first few days of oliguria. The appearance of the uremic syndrome, as discussed earlier in this chapter, is related both to the rate of nonprotein nitrogen accumulation as well as to the absolute level of the BUN. In the uremic syndrome associated with acute renal failure, the gastrointestinal and central nervous system manifestations tend to be predominant. The specific therapy for uremia is dialysis, and it is preferable not to wait until uremic symptoms appear in an otherwise debilitated and acutely ill patient. The rate of rise in the BUN may be somewhat offset by the provision of adequate calories to spare protein catabolism, but intercurrent infection, gastrointestinal bleeding, resorption of hematoma, or the persistence of devitalized tissue will tend to accelerate the progression to azotemia.

Metabolic acidosis almost always occurs in acute renal failure and is caused by failure of the kidneys to excrete hydrogen ions. The simultaneous retention of sulfate and phosphate leads to an increase in the "anion gap." The retained hydrogen to a large extent is buffered by bicarbonate, and the net result is a fall in plasma bicarbonate concentration. In a patient with normal catabolism (1 mEq/kg of body weight/day hydrogen ion production) and no renal excretion of acid, plasma bicarbonate should fall by about 2 mEq/L/day. This rate of decline is increased by hypercatabolism. Secondary hypocapnia normally minimizes the resultant acidemia and, as a general rule, specific therapy is not required. In the presence of hypercatabolism or limited respiratory reserve, however, severe acidemia (pH less than 7.20) may result. Because the administration of bicarbonate entails a sizable and potentially hazardous sodium load, dialysis is the frequently preferred method of therapy for severe metabolic acidosis associated with acute renal failure.

The sodium intake in acute renal failure should be limited to measured losses. This usually amounts to about 20 mEq/day in the patient with oliguria, more in the nonoliguric patient. The development of hyponatremia does not indicate inadequate provision of sodium but, rather, excessive retention of water. Moderate hyponatremia (serum sodium of 120 to 135 mEq/L) is usually asymptomatic and can be treated by more effective water restriction. Severe hyponatremia, however, may lead to serious central nervous system complications, and is an indication for dialysis in the patient with acute renal failure. Recall that hyponatremia may occur in the absence of true hypo-osmolarity if large amounts of administered mannitol have been retained. Cellular dehydration due to water shifts under these circumstances can be corrected by removal of the mannitol via dialysis.

Both hypertension and congestive heart failure often develop during acute renal failure because of excessive sodium and water administration. If congestive heart failure does not respond to fluid restriction, dialysis may be required. Hypertension can usually be controlled with conventional antihypertensive agents.

Hyperkalemia is the most feared metabolic complication of acute renal failure. It frequently occurs despite adherence to a potassium restricted intake, because potassium tends to shift from the intracellular to the extracellular fluid compartment as a result of tissue breakdown and metabolic acidosis. Transfusion of banked blood may be a major source of potassium. Hyponatremia, acidosis, and hypocalcemia enhance the cardiotoxic effects of hyperkalemia. Thus, a change in the electrocardiogram rather than the serum potassium level itself is the best indicator of potential toxicity. When EKG changes appear, specific therapy to reduce the serum potassium level and to protect the heart against the effects of potassium toxicity is mandatory. Although initial therapy with bicarbonate, calcium, glucose, insulin, and Kayexalate may be lifesaving, dialysis is generally required for the treatment of hyperkalemia associated with acute renal failure.

DIALYSIS

Specific indications for dialysis in acute renal failure include: hyperkalemia, fluid overload, hyponatremia, severe acidosis, and uremic complications such as bleeding, central nervous system manifestations, pericarditis, nausea, and vomiting. Of these, hyperkalemia is probably the most common indication in the acutely ill, hypercatabolic surgical patient with acute renal failure. However, rather than waiting for one or more of these potentially life-threatening complications to occur, most nephrologists now recommend that these abnormalities be prevented through the use of dialysis early in the course. Routine periodic dialysis simplifies management by liberalizing water and electrolyte restrictions and enhances the well-being of patients by minimizing the development of uremic symptoms. Perhaps even more importantly, by liberalizing fluid intake, aggressive dialysis allows for the provision of adequate calories and nutrition to minimize catabolism and promote wound healing.[96] If oral intake is possible, nutrition is improved because a more palatable diet can be provided and because gastrointestinal symptoms are minimized. The importance of nutrition in the treatment of acute renal failure is discussed in the next section.

The role of prophylactic dialysis in improving the morbidity and mortality of acute renal failure has been studied in several series. Unfortunately, most reports are based on historical controls, making it difficult to evaluate the role of other factors (e.g., better dialysis equipment, more potent antibiotics, increased experience). Nevertheless, the results of several retrospective studies suggest that the overall mortality associated with acute renal failure is reduced from about 55 percent to about 38 percent by prophylactic dialysis.[96,212,213] The frequency of uremic symptoms can also be decreased substantially with prophylactic dialysis.[96]

One controlled, prospective study of the effects of prophylactic hemodialysis among 18 severely traumatized combat patients showed a significant decrease in the incidence of major complications and mortality in the intensively dialyzed group.[214] In the intensively dialyzed group, BUN and serum creatinine were maintained below 70 and 5 mg/dl respectively, and 5 of 8 patients survived. In the routine dialysis group, dialysis was performed only when BUN and serum creatinine approached 150 and 10 mg/dl respectively, unless another clinical indication for dialysis arose. Only 2 of 10 patients in that group survived.

Dialysis therapy is indicated in approximately 50 percent of cases of acute renal failure.[215] Once the decision to employ dialysis therapy has been made, the choice between peritoneal dialysis or hemodialysis remains. Peritoneal dialysis offers several distinct advantages including widespread availability, technical simplicity, and ease in correcting states of overhydration. Specialized personnel, anticoagulation, and blood access are not required, and peritoneal dialysis can be performed with relative safety in patients with hemodynamic instability. Peritoneal dialysis is felt by some authors to be the treatment of choice in acute renal failure involving: (1) small children, (2) severe fluid overload, (3) gastrointestinal bleeding, (4) shock, (5) acute myocardial infarction, and (6) acute pancreatitis or peritonitis.[103] There are no absolute contraindications to peritoneal dialysis, but it may be technically difficult in a patient with multiple abdominal wounds or drains. Complications of peritoneal dialysis include peritonitis[216] and compromised pulmonary function due to elevation of the diaphragm by the dialysis fluid in patients with underlying lung disease. Peritoneal dialysis has certain disadvantages: it is inefficient, technical problems with drainage are common, patients must be immobilized, and significant protein losses occur which may aggravate malnutrition.

Hemodialysis is preferred if there is severe catabolism or the course of renal failure is prolonged. Prompt access to the blood stream can be obtained through the relatively simple surgical placement of an arteriovenous plastic cannula (Quinton-Scribner shunt) which can be used for repeated hemodialysis treatments. If shunt placement is not feasible or only few dialysis treatments are anticipated, catheters can be placed percutaneously into one or both femoral veins for blood access. This is a bedside procedure that can be performed by any experienced physician. Such catheters can be removed and replaced with each dialysis or may be left in place for two to three hemodialysis treatments, provided that adequate attention is given to bleeding and infection at the entry site.

NUTRITION

Optimal nutrition is of critical importance and is often overlooked in the treatment of acute renal failure. Proper dietary management, which is aimed at minimizing protein catabolism, not only limits the accumulation of nitrogenous wastes, nonvolatile acids, and potassium in the extracellular fluid compartment but also prevents malnutrition which can delay wound healing and decrease resistance to infection.

The first consideration in the dietary management of acute renal failure is to supply enough carbohydrate to obviate protein breakdown. Although a minimum of 100 gm of carbohydrate should be administered daily to avoid tissue protein being used as an energy source, an even larger carbohydrate intake is advantageous because the carbon fragments can be used in the production of nonessential amino acids. Since 1L of isotonic (5 %) glucose contains only 50 gm of carbohydrate, 2L would be required to satisfy even the minimum requirement. Therefore, in the oliguric patient taking nothing by mouth, glucose should be administered as a hypertonic (10 or 20 %) solution. If carbohydrates can be given by mouth, a preparation of equal parts Karo syrup and ginger ale, flavored with lemon juice and chilled provides a relatively palatable caloric source.[103]

The second consideration is to supply enough total calories (1800 to 2500 calories/day) and enough protein to restore positive nitrogen balance. The provision of calories as fat and 0.3 to 0.5 gm of high-quality protein per kilogram of body weight daily in the patient who is able to eat will often lead to a decrease in the BUN and symptomatic improvement even without dialysis. There is evidence that endogenous urea and other nitrogen-containing compounds can be "recycled" into the production of nonessential amino acids under the appropriate circumstances. Prerequisites for this include hydrolysis of urea into ammonia by gut bacteria, incorporation of ammonium ion into α-ketoglutarate to form glutamate, availability of α-keto precursors of nonessential amino acids, and transamination of the α-keto acid from glutamate.[217]

If the clinical circumstances preclude the possibility of oral intake, as is often the case in the surgical patient, these principles can be incorporated into the formulation of an appropriate regimen for parenteral nutrition. Indeed, by supplying the appropriate ratio of essential amino acids and calories in the form of hypertonic glucose, endogenous nitrogen can be used to create nonessential amino acids and develop a positive nitrogen balance; weight gain and wound healing can be promoted while BUN remains stable or decreases and the signs and symptoms of uremia improve.

The specific composition of total parenteral nutrition (TPN) in patients with acute renal failure must be tailored to the high energy requirements, the insulin resistance, and the negligible free water and urea clearance. This requires a hypertonic solution with a caloric/nitrogen ratio exceeding 450:1, and a high proportion of essential amino acids. Conventional protein hydrolysates should not be used for this purpose because they contain small polypeptides which cannot be efficiently utilized and may lead to a rapid rise in BUN. Conventional hyperalimentation solutions (e.g., Freamine) are better but less than ideal because they contain nonessential amino acids which may worsen azotemia in the presence of renal failure. "Renal failure fluid" (Freamine-E, Nephramine) which contains hypertonic glucose and the eight essential amino acids in appropriate concentrations[20] now appears to be the most effective preparation for minimizing azotemia and promoting positive nitrogen balance in patients with acute renal failure. The successful use of "renal failure fluid" in patients with acute renal failure has been reported.[218–221] In a randomized, double-blind, prospective study, the course of patients with acute renal failure treated with "renal failure fluid" was compared to those treated with hypertonic glucose alone.[222] A higher survival rate was noted among the group receiving renal failure fluid (75% vs. 44%), the survival difference being greatest among those patients with oliguria, requiring dialysis, or with infectious or hemorrhagic complications. Treatment with renal failure fluid was also noted to lower serum concentrations of magnesium, phosphate, and potassium, probably due to a shift of these ions intracellularly into regenerating tissue.[223] Others have also demonstrated lower morbidity and mortality among patients treated with parenteral nutrition.[224]

The positive effect of amino acid infusions has been confirmed at the cellular level.[225] Animals with ATN receiving amino acids showed enhanced regeneration of renal tubular cells and a more rapid improvement in renal function as compared to glucose-treated controls. In severely ill, catabolic patients with acute renal failure, the effect on mortality of "renal failure fluid" is less dramatic, probably due to complications from the underlying disease.[226,227]

The technique and the risks of parenteral hyperalimentation are discussed in Chapter 16, Nutrition. In the patient with a relative or absolute contraindication to central venous catheter placement, hypertonic glucose and amino acids can be administered through a peripheral vein. The complications of phlebitis and venous thrombosis can be minimized through the use of the "P-900" solution, so called because it is administered peripherally and has an osmolarity of 900, which is far in excess of that normally tolerated by peripheral veins. To each liter of solution, containing 65 gm of dextrose and 4 gm of nitrogen, is added 5 mg of cortisol and 500 units of heparin to reduce the incidence of phlebitis.[228] The efficacy of this solution in renal failure, though not as good as "renal failure fluid," is better than that of other peripherally administered, but isotonic, solutions. Intralipid, a fat emulsion supplying a large quantity of calories can also be administered through a peripheral vein (see Chap. 16). However, there is evidence that dextrose is a superior source of calories for patients with acute renal failure, possibly because it provides the carbon fragments necessary for the production of nonessential amino acids and recycling of urea nitrogen.[229]

Amino acids should be administered parenterally to all patients with acute renal failure of more than 2 to 3 days' duration who cannot take protein by mouth once the uremic state has been controlled by adequate dialysis and the BUN has been decreased to 70 to 80 mg/dl or less.[224] Amino acid infusions should not be continued during hemodialysis treatments, because the infused amino acids will be lost into the dialysate. If the patient is dialyzed vigorously, the BUN may fall to a level at which the pool of nitrogen is insufficient to provide substrate for the generation of nonessential amino acids. Therefore, in patients with BUN levels of less than 40 mg/dl, it may be necessary to give nonessential amino acids along with the essential amino acids.[224]

In summary, it appears that aggressive nutritional and dialysis therapy offers the greatest potential of improving the morbidity and mortality of acute renal failure, especially in the hypercatabolic surgical patient. The poor wound healing in uremia is particularly associated with nutritional deficiency,[230] and provision of adequate nutrition offers the best chance for postoperative and traumatized patients with renal failure to heal properly and promptly (see also Chap. 16, Nutrition).

Prognosis in Acute Tubular Necrosis

Despite major advances in therapy, mortality in patients with ATN remains substantial largely because the diseases that lead to renal failure are so often lethal. Properly treated, virtually no one should die of uremia or its associated metabolic disturbances.

Indeed, the failure to improve the survival figures in ATN despite increasing experience in management is probably due to a shift in the degree of severity of ATN in the patients encountered.[97,231] More older patients are undergoing surgery, and postoperative renal failure in the elderly patient carries a particularly grave prognosis. Patients with severe infections are being kept alive with potent new antibiotics and may develop renal failure due to sepsis or drug nephrotoxicity.

Sepsis continues to be the most frequent cause of death in ATN.[96,97,231,232] This may be due, at least in part, to the fact that patients with acute renal failure are now surviving long enough to become infected. Before dialysis was available, such patients more often succumbed earlier in the course of ATN to fluid and electrolyte abnormalities, shock, or hemorrhage.[233] The occurrence of sepsis is particularly ominous in the surgical patient following an abdominal operation. In a series of 114 consecutive patients with postoperative renal failure, only 12 percent of 51 patients whose clinical course was complicated by sepsis survived.[234] It is likely, therefore, that only better prevention and control of infection in acute renal failure will improve the survival rate significantly.

Other poor prognostic factors in ATN include the development of shock and respiratory failure requiring assisted ventilation,[235] gastrointestinal hemorrhage,[97] congestive heart failure,[232] ascites,[232] myocardial infarction,[236] and peritonitis.[236] The mortality from gastrointestinal hemorrhage can be significantly reduced by intensive prophylactic dialysis.[96]

As noted above, the mortality from nonoliguric ATN is considerably lower than that from oliguric ATN.[94] Early recognition of nonoliguric renal failure and its maintenance with adequate volume replacement have been reported to decrease mortality to as low as 7 percent.[237] The nonoliguric ATN associated with nephrotoxins (especially aminoglycoside antibiotics) seems to have a significantly better prognosis than the ATN associated with renal ischemic injury.[232]

It appears that even a relatively small deterioration in renal function may be an ominous prognostic sign in the acutely ill patient. In a prospective study of hospital-acquired renal insufficiency, those patients whose serum creatinine rose by as little as 3 mg/dl had a 64 percent mortality rate and an additional 12 percent required chronic dialysis.[93] In contrast, mortality was only 15 percent among those patients whose serum creatinine rose at least 20 percent but less than 3 mg/dl. These findings suggest the need for aggressive therapy to abort the progression of even a modest degree of renal failure.

Even though acute tubular necrosis is considered a self-limited disease, many patients who survive ATN do not recover completely. In one long-term study of ATN, 61 percent of survivors had renal function significantly below premorbid values.[95] Those who did experience "complete recovery" were, in general, younger (mean age 32) and had a shorter period of oliguria (mean 10 days) than those who had residual renal function impairment (mean age 52, mean length of oliguria 16 days). There were no significant differences in the maximal BUN or the mean number of dialyses in the two groups. In patients whose renal function did return to baseline during the four year follow-up period, "complete recovery" had occurred by three to six months. The presence of prior renal disease did not appear to affect the mortality rate or the subsequent return of renal function.

The frequency of persistent renal dysfunction has been confirmed following acute tubular necrosis. In a 2 to 15 year follow-up of 30 patients with ATN, abnormal endogenous creatinine clearance was found in 37 percent, and abnormal urinary concentrating ability was found in 47 percent. Those who had nephrotoxic ATN had a lower rate of persistent renal function abnormalities than those who had ischemic ATN. Nonetheless, most patients were clinically normal and had normal renal histology during the follow-up period. Two of these 30 patients had a progressive deterioration of renal function following recovery from ATN which was unexplained.[238]

In a large series of patients with postsurgical ATN, 9.5 percent of survivors experienced severe permanent renal failure.[185] These patients had pathologic evidence of renal fibrosis without cortical necrosis. Drug toxicity, in particular due to nephrotoxic antibiotics and methoxyflurane anesthesia, sometimes superimposed on ischemic ATN, may be responsible for the severity of these renal lesions.

The prognosis for recovery of renal function in ATN is thought by some to be predicted accurately by use of the ^{131}I-iodohippurate sodium renal scan. In one study, such scans were performed in 24 patients with ATN early in the acute illness.[239] Scans were read according to whether the renal image was prominent, faint, or absent within 30 minutes of radionuclide injection. All 10 patients with prominent images regained excellent renal function (average creatinine clearance 80 ml/minute). Of 7 patients with faint renal images, 6 recovered life-sustaining renal function (average creatinine clearance 25 ml/minute), whereas only 4 of 7 patients with absent renal images did so.

In conclusion, the mortality of acute renal failure in surgical patients remains high, and a significant number of those who survive will have residual renal impairment. Metabolic control of the seriously ill patient can be taxing, and early diagnosis and referral to a unit experienced in all aspects of acute renal failure offers the best prospect for recovery. Further improvement in morbidity and mortality rates is likely to stem more from preventative measures in high-risk patients than from improved treatment of established renal failure.

THE PATIENT WITH ARTERIAL HYPERTENSION (TABLE 13)

Hypertension is estimated to affect approximately 24,000,000 persons in the United States.[240] The untreated hypertensive male has a mortality rate seven times greater than that of the treated male with hypertension and ten times greater than that of the normotensive male. For females, the mortality rate of the untreated hypertensive is six times greater than that of the treated hypertensive and eight times greater than that of the normotensive woman.[241] Much of this excess mortality in the hypertensive patient is due to the complications of coronary artery disease and congestive heart failure, both of which are well-known and formidable surgical risk factors.[242,243]

The first part of this section will examine the three major mechanisms by which underlying arterial hypertension may increase surgical morbidity and mortality: the effect of hypertension upon the cardiovascular response to general anesthesia, the cardiovascular consequences of chronic hypertension and their contribution to surgical risk, and the interaction of various antihypertensive medications with anesthetic agents. The final parts of this section will deal with specific medical management of the patients with renovascular hypertension undergoing corrective surgery and the medical management of various hypertensive emergencies that may be encountered in the surgical patient.

Increased Surgical Risk in the Hypertensive Patient

EFFECT OF HYPERTENSION PER SE ON SURGICAL RISK

Despite indications of earlier studies to the contrary,[244] the hypertensive state per se has been clearly demonstrated to increase the risk of general anesthesia. The presence of high arterial pressures before anesthesia predisposes to the development of severe reductions in blood pressure intraoperatively, which are associated with electrocardiographic evidence of myocardial ischemia. In contrast, adequately treated hypertensive (and normotensive) patients develop no such problems while under anesthesia.[70] Cardiac output falls to the same degree (30%) in all groups, but baroreflex control of heart rate is

TABLE 13. Considerations in the Hypertensive Patient Undergoing Surgery

Preoperative Considerations
1. Careful history and physical examination. Supine and standing blood pressure measurements to assess blockade of postural responses due to therapy.
2. Routine determination of electrolytes, correction of abnormalities.
3. Assessment and correction of fluid deficits induced by diuretics.
4. Optimal control of hypertension preoperatively is desirable. If necessary, more aggressive antihypertensive therapy should be employed to achieve this.
5. In general, withdrawal of antihypertensive therapy prior to surgery is discouraged. See Table 14 for recommendations regarding specific agents.
6. Propranolol, given preoperatively, has been shown to suppress the adverse hemodynamic and metabolic responses to fear, laryngoscopy, and endotracheal intubation in selected patients.
Intraoperative Considerations
1. Continuous electrocardiographic monitoring before, during, and after anesethesia is essential. Dipolar monitoring with one lead on the manubrium sterni and the other lead at the V_5 precordial position permits observation of early ST segment deviations.
2. Premedication with atropine is recommended to avoid bradycardia in those patients taking adrenergic blockers (reserpine, guanethidine, propranolol).
3. Direct arterial pressure and central venous pressure or Swan-Ganz catheter monitoring are recommended in those patients with a history of coronary artery disease or left ventricular failure.
4. To minimize the hypertensive response to laryngoscopy and endotracheal intubation, wait until the patient is anesthetized before giving a muscle relaxant and intubating. Alternately, careful topical anesthesia may minimize the hypertensive response to endotracheal intubation.
5. For induction of anesthesia, the combination of a narcotic analgesic with a minimal dose of hypnotic, followed by maintenance anesthesia with nitrous oxide is recommended.
6. When artificial ventilation is necessary, minimize hypocapnia which can cause marked falls in blood pressure. Maintain Pco_2 in the range of the mid-30s by adjusting ventilation, adding CO_2 to the inspired gas mixture, or by using a closed circuit with partial rebreathing.
7. Treat hypotensive episodes during general anesthesia with fluid replacement, using pressor amines as a last resort.
8. Treat hypertensive episodes during anesthesia with nitroprusside administered by slow intravenous infusion.

significantly impaired in hypertensive patients both before and during anesthesia. Thus, the response to anesthesia depends more upon the pre-existing level of arterial blood pressure than whether or not the patient is being treated. For this reason, antihypertensive therapy should not be withdrawn prior to anesthesia without a compelling indication. Evidence indicates that the sustained hypocapnia associated with artificial ventilation during anesthesia (especially with halothane) contributes to the circulatory instability and that the use of partial rebreathing techniques may be warranted in selected patients.[245,246] Risks for hypertensive patients are increased during induction of anesthesia and subsequent intubation as they are during steady-state anesthesia.[247] During the induction and intubation phase, a significant number of hypertensive patients develop cardiac arrhythmias associated with sharp increases in blood pressure and heart rate and evidence of myocardial ischemia. This hypertensive response to intubation is no less frequent in patients receiving antihypertensive therapy with well-controlled preoperative blood pressures.

Foëx and Prys-Roberts[248] reviewed the subject of anesthesia in the hypertensive patient in 1974 and made the following recommendations: (1) Preoperative assessment and preparation should include a careful medical history, physical examination, full 12-lead electrocardiogram (preferably with exercise testing), and determination of serum electrolytes. The adequacy of antihypertensive therapy should be assessed with supine and standing blood pressure measurements in order to determine the extent of blockade of postural responses. Doses of antihypertensive medications should not be reduced preoperatively, even though blood pressure may fall while the patient is hospitalized. (2) Since there is no evidence that hypertensive patients require or benefit from more preoperative sedation than normotensive patients, increased dosages should not be given. Premedication with atropine is recommended routinely before induction of anesthesia to avoid bradycardia common in hypertensive patients, especially those taking reserpine, ganglionic blocking agents, or propranolol. (3) Continuous electrocardiographic monitoring before, during, and after anesthesia in hypertensive patients is essential and should be carried out. Direct arterial pressure and central venous pressure monitoring is also recommended, especially in those patients with a history of coronary disease or left ventricular failure. (4) For induction of anesthesia, no agent is entirely satisfactory in the hypertensive patient, but the combination of a narcotic analgesic with a minimal dose of hypnotic followed by maintenance anesthesia with nitrous oxide and oxygen is recommended. Ketamine has a tendency to cause hypertension even in normotensive patients, and its use is discouraged. (5) Since hypertensive patients react to laryngoscopy and endotracheal intubation with much greater elevations in blood pressure and heart rate than normotensive patients, these procedures should be performed with extra care. Careful topical anesthesia may minimize but does not suppress this response, although beta-adrenergic blockade may be effective in this regard. (6) When artificial ventilation is necessary, it is advisable to minimize hypocapnia by either adding CO_2 to the inspired gas mixture or by using a closed circuit with partial rebreathing. (7) Use of pressor amines is rarely indicated in the treatment of hypotension during anesthesia in hypertensive patients, since any further increase in resistance to ejection by the left ventricle will result in a reduction of blood flow, especially when the myocardium is depressed by anesthesia. Instead, fluid administration should be employed for blood pressure restoration. More recent clinical studies by Goldman and colleagues[243,249,250] have confirmed most of the observations and recommendations of Foëx and Prys-Roberts.

An increased tendency of the poorly controlled hypertensive patient to form hematomas has been described, particularly in the literature dealing with plastic and reconstructive surgery. Mara and Baker[251] reviewed 200 consecutive patients who had face lifts under local anesthesia and noted a 28 percent incidence of hematoma formation among those patients who had a diastolic blood pressure greater than 96 mm Hg at some time during their hospital stay. Hematoma formation did not occur in an additional 29 patients with elevated blood pressure in whom aggressive antihypertensive therapy with hydralazine was undertaken. Although the authors caution against the use of hydralazine in patients with a history of coronary or valvular heart disease, they found the drug to be generally safe, effective, and reliable for the acute and chronic lowering of blood pressure in the hypertensive patient undergoing plastic surgery. They recommend that hydralazine be used to control blood pressure for several weeks before undergoing elective operations in which hematomas are a serious risk.

EFFECT OF HYPERTENSIVE CARDIOVASCULAR DISEASE ON SURGICAL RISK

It is difficult to determine the relative contribution of hypertension per se and of its associated cardiovascular complications (e.g., coronary artery disease, congestive heart failure) to increased surgical risk. Pre-existing cardiac disease is well known to contribute substantially to surgical morbidity and mortality (see Chap. 3, Cardiology). It is interesting to note that, despite the observations of Prys-Roberts and Foëx regarding the adverse effect of underlying hypertension upon the cardiovascular response to general anesthesia, neither Manney and associates[242] nor Goldman and coworkers[243] implicated hypertension per se as an *independent* significant correlate of increased morbidity and mortality in the surgical patient.

Goldman and Caldera[249] explored this subject further in a 1979 follow-up to their series of 1001 consecutive patients undergoing noncardiac operations. Patients were grouped by preoperative blood pressure measurements and antihypertensive medications: group I, normotensive (diastolic pressure less than 90 mm Hg and systolic blood pressure less than 160 mm Hg); group II, normotensive but taking diuretics for reasons other than hypertension; group III, hypertension by history, now controlled with antihypertensive medications; group IV, hypertensive despite current use of antihypertensive medications; and group V, hypertensive, not taking antihypertensive medications. No patient had preoperative diastolic blood pressure greater than 120 mm Hg, or any evidence of accelerated or malignant hypertension. Despite markedly different mean preoperative systolic blood pressure values, the systolic pressures of patients in all five study groups fell to strikingly similar mean intraoperative nadir levels. Three other variables, however, did have independently significant correlations with lower intraoperative systolic pressures: lower preoperative systolic blood pressure values, the absence of renal or cerebrovascular complications of hypertension, and the use of halothane anesthesia. The need for intraoperative fluid challenge or adrenergic agents to maintain blood pressure did not correlate with preoperative blood pressure levels or medications but did correlate with the nature of the surgical procedure (e.g., extent of blood loss) and the use of halothane anesthesia.

On the other hand, normotensive patients (groups I and II) were significantly less likely to experience perioperative hypertension than were patients with histories of preoperative hypertension. However, hypertensive patients whose blood pressures had been normalized preoperatively with medications (group III) were just as likely to experience perioperative hypertensive episodes as patients who remained hypertensive preoperatively (groups IV and V). This is remarkably consistent with the observations of Prys-Roberts and coworkers[247] and confirms the impression that there is a hemodynamic instability in the hypertensive patient that persists despite what appears to be adequate pharmacologic blood pressure control. Indeed, Goldman and Caldera found that new hypertensive events were most common in those patients with histories of the severest hypertension, regardless of the success of preoperative in-hospital control. These findings would argue against the need for tight preoperative control and would imply that perioperative blood pressure lability may be as much a function of a patient's inherent vascular characteristics as of any modification of such characteristics by antihypertensive medication.

With regard to perioperative cardiac complications, there was no independent correlation with preoperative blood pressure status (groups I through V) in the Goldman and Caldera Study. All differences in the incidence of cardiac complications between the various groups could be explained entirely by two factors: (1) the calculated preoperative cardiac risk index score, taking into account the nine correlates enumerated in the 1977 report by Goldman and associates[243] (see Chap. 3, Cardiology) and (2) the development of a marked fall in blood pressure intraoperatively (defined as a decrease to less than 50% of preoperative level for any duration or a decrease of 33% for over 10 minutes). Unlike Prys-Roberts and colleagues,[70] who observed that preoperaive hypertension per se can predispose to such severe reductions in blood pressure under general anesthesia, Goldman and Caldera found no correlation between preoperative blood pressure status and the magnitude of intraoperative blood pressure reduction. These authors speculate that the hypertensive patients of Prys-Roberts and colleagues may have been at higher risk for general anesthesia than their own patients because the former had higher mean preoperative blood pressure values.

EFFECT OF ANTIHYPERTENSIVE THERAPY ON SURGICAL RISK (TABLE 14)

In the aggregate, the studies cited in the preceding sections suggest that aggressive preoperative blood pressure control in the hypertensive patient may decrease the incidence of severe reductions in intraoperative blood pressure, associated myocardial ischemia, and hematoma formation. It is apparent, however, that antihypertensive therapy does not decrease the likelihood that perioperative elevations in blood pressure will occur in patients with a history of hypertension. It is, therefore, reasonable to question whether the benefits of continuing antihypertensive therapy up to the time of surgery outweigh the risks, since these agents will often potentiate the vasodepressive effects of general anesthetic agents, inhibiting the ability of the cardiovascular system to respond to the stress of surgery.[252]

Indeed, the medical literature is replete with admonitions that various antihypertensive agents be withheld "two weeks prior to surgery to avoid the possibility of vascular collapse or cardiac arrhythmia during general anesthesia."[60] The emphasis on a "two-week period" originated in the 1950s with various reports that patients receiving reserpine, the most commonly used antihypertensive agent at the time, tolerated general anesthesia and surgery poorly. The two-week warning is appropriate pharmacokinetically for reserpine but does not apply to most other antihypertensive agents. Even for reserpine and other rauwolfia alkaloids, more recent studies have demonstrated that no special problems occur perioperatively when the agent is continued up to the time of surgery.[253,254] With the advent of many newer antihypertensive agents with fewer side effects, the once widespread use of reserpine has declined substantially over the past two decades. Each of the currently employed agents is discussed below.

Diuretics

Thiazide and related diuretics (chlorthalidone, metolazone) are the mainstays in the treatment of hypertension and generally the first agents to be tried in patients with

TABLE 14. Recommendations Regarding the Use of Specific Antihypertensive Agents in the Preoperative Patient

Agent	*Mechanism of Action*	*Usual Daily Dose*	*Recommendations*
Reserpine	Adrenergic blocking agent	0.1–0.5 mg once daily	May be continued up to the time of surgery.
Diuretics	Contraction of plasma volume Direct arteriolar dilatation	Hydrochlorthiazide 50 mg once or twice daily Metolazone 2.5–5.0 mg once daily Chlorthalidone 50–100 mg once daily Dosage of other agents in this group depends upon the specific drug used	Preoperative evaluation of volume status; correction of volume depletion with normal saline infusion. Preoperative determination of serum electrolytes, blood urea nitrogen and creatinine. Potassium replacement if serum K^+ level less than 3.0 mEq/l or less than 4.0 mEq/L in patient taking digitalis. May be continued up to time of surgery or may be discontinued up to 7 days prior to surgery if volume depletion is apparent. Thiazides often potentiate the response to skeletal muscle relaxants, so use the latter agents with care in patients taking thiazide.
Beta-blocking agents (propranolol, metoprolol)	Anti-adrenergic effect on the heart Central anti-adrenergic effect Anti-renin effect	Propranolol 80–240 mg in two divided doses Metoprolol 100–300 mg in two divided doses	Abrupt withdrawal in patients with coronary disease may precipitate acute coronary event. No adverse hemodynamic response to general anesthesia in patients taking beta blocking agents up to the time of surgery. Beta blockade may ameliorate the hypertensive response to laryngoscopy and endotracheal intubation. Therefore, beta blocking agents should be continued up to the time of surgery. Do not use methoxyflurane anesthesia in patients taking beta blocking agents.
Clonidine	Alpha-adrenergic agonist in vasomotor control center	0.2–0.8 mg in two divided doses	Abrupt withdrawal, particularly in patients with severe hypertension (daily clonidine dose > 1.0 mg) and renovascular hypertension, can precipitate hypertensive crisis. In general, it is not necessary to discontinue clonidine prior to surgery, but if patient is at risk for rebound hypertension (above) and a prolonged period during which clonidine cannot be given orally or by nasogastric tube is anticipated, then the drug should be

TABLE 14 *Continued*

Agent	*Mechanism of Action*	*Usual Daily Dose*	*Recommendations*
			slowly tapered off over the week prior to surgery, and another agent such as methydopa or hydralazine substituted.
Methyldopa	Alpha-adrenergic agonist in vasomotor control center	500–2000 mg in two or three divided doses	May be continued up to the time of surgery. Abrupt withdrawal may rarely produce rebound hypertension similar to that seen with clonidine withdrawal; but methyldopa, unlike clonidine, can be given parenterally in the patient taking nothing by mouth.
Prazosin	Peripheral postsynaptic alpha-adrenergic antagonist	3–20 mg in two or three divided doses	May be continued up to the time of surgery.
Hydralazine	Direct arterial smooth muscle relaxant	100–200 mg in two divided doses	May be continued up to the time of surgery. Can be given parenterally in the patient taking nothing by mouth.
Guanethidine	Blockade and depletion of catecholamines in the peripheral sympathetic neuron	25–50 mg once daily	In patients with moderate hypertension, discontinue guanethidine 2 weeks prior to surgery if problems with general anesthesia are anticipated; substitute another antihypertensive agent. In patients with severe hypertension, guanethidine should be continued up to the time of surgery. Anesthetic care should be intensified to compensate for impairment of normal circulatory reflex mechanisms.
Minoxidil	Direct arterial smooth muscle relaxant	2–40 mg in two divided doses	May be continued up to the time of surgery.

mild to moderate blood pressure elevation. In addition to the obvious contraction of extracellular fluid and plasma volumes, these agents appear to reduce blood pressure by other mechanisms. A fall in peripheral vascular resistance results from direct arteriolar dilitation and decreased receptor sensitivity to vasopressor substances such as angiotensin II.[255]

Most of the frequently encountered adverse effects of these diuretics are the consequences of the drug's effect, direct or indirect, on the kidney. Hypokalemia occurs in as many as 70 percent of patients taking thiazide and thiazide-like diuretics, with the highest incidence being seen in patients taking the longer acting agents (chlorthalidone, metolazone) or with high sodium intake. The majority of patients taking thiazides who have serum potassium levels greater than 3.0 mEq/L do not have significant whole-body potassium depletion and do not require routine potassium supplementation or potassium retaining drugs.[256] In patients receiving digitalis glycosides, however, it is prudent to restore serum potassium to about 4.0 mEq/L.

Thiazide diuretics may produce hyponatremia through a variety of mechanisms. Interference with the urinary diluting mechanism limits the ability to excrete free water. Although diuretic-induced hyponatremia is relatively uncommon in the absence of overt volume depletion or renal insufficiency, the clinician should be aware of this potentially dangerous complication of diuretic therapy.

Successful diuresis may lead to a reduction in plasma volume sufficient to decrease glomerular filtration rate and lead to prerenal azotemia. This is particularly true in patients being treated with diuretic agents for edematous conditions (congestive heart failure, cirrhosis with ascites, nephrotic syndrome), but it may also occur to a clinically significant degree in the hypertensive patient. Such a contraction of plasma volume may be of little or no consequence in the unanesthetized state but could present considerable problems in the maintenance of blood pressure during general anesthesia.

Any patient receiving diuretics should be evaluated carefully for intravascular volume status prior to surgery. Postural changes in blood pressure or pulse, dry skin and mucous membranes, poor skin turgor, and biochemical evidence of prerenal azotemia are all strongly suggestive of significant intravascular volume depletion. Such volume deficits should be overcome preoperatively with intravenous normal saline infusion. Diuretics should be discontinued if any evidence of volume depletion is present. Indeed in nonedematous patients, it is reasonable to withhold diuretics routinely for three to seven days prior to scheduled surgery.[257]

The thiazides are known to potentiate the response to skeletal muscle relaxants such as tubocurarine, gallamine, and succinylcholine.[258] Thiazide diuretics need not be discontinued for this reason prior to surgery but the dose of relaxant agents may require modification.

Propranolol

Beta-adrenergic blocking agents such as propranolol are effective in the treatment of angina pectoris, certain cardiac arrhythmias, hypertrophic subaortic stenosis, thyrotoxicosis, migraine, and hypertension. The antihypertensive effect of propranolol appears to have at least three components: an antirenin effect, an antiadrenergic effect on the heart, and a central antiadrenergic effect.

When considering the effect of propranolol upon the cardiovascular responses of the surgical patient, it is important to distinguish between those patients with intrinsic heart disease receiving propranolol for control of angina and those patients receiving propranolol for control of hypertension. The former group may have an increased risk for general anesthesia and major surgery because of previous myocardial infarction, arrhythmias, or congestive heart failure (i.e., unrelated to propranolol therapy per se). Moreover, there is very little evidence that patients being treated with propranolol for hypertension are at increased risk for surgery even when propranolol is continued up to the time of operation. The use of propranolol in the treatment of coronary artery disease and preoperative adjustments in propranolol dosage are discussed in Chapter 3, Cardiology.

Prys-Roberts[259] has also noted the beneficial effect of beta blockade upon the hypertension, tachycardia, and dysrhythmia associated with laryngoscopy and intubation in hypertensive patients. He observed no dysrhythmia or de novo electrocardiographic evidence of myocardial ischemia in 23 hypertensive patients undergoing surgery pretreated with a beta blocking agent. In contrast, dysrhythmia was noted in 41 percent and myocardial ischemia in 38 percent of hypertensive patients undergoing surgery who had not received beta blocking agents. Beta blocking agents such as propranolol are indeed effective antiarrhythmic agents in the awake as well as in the anesthetized patient, and they are the group of antihypertensive agents most effective in protecting the hypertensive patient against the effects of sympathetic overactivity due to laryngoscopy and endotracheal intubation. Foëx and Prys-Roberts suggest that the many benefits of beta blockade in the hypertensive patient undergoing general anesthesia may constitute a reason to employ such agents routinely in the perioperative period.[248]

Thus, currently available clinical and experimental data indicate that the use of beta blockers, such as propranolol, can be continued safely up to the time of surgery, whether the drug is being administered for hypertension or coronary artery disease. Propranolol therapy may actually improve the cardiovascular response to general anesthesia in the hypertensive patient. The anesthetist should know whether the patient is receiving propranolol at the time of surgery because the presence of beta blockade eliminates consideration of heart rate as a reliable indicator of hypovolemia during anesthesia. The hemodynamic responses (cardiac output, arterial pressure, heart rate) to acute hemorrhage and short periods of severe hypoxia are unaffected by beta blockade.[248]

The use of methoxyflurane anesthesia may be particularly hazardous in patients receiving beta blocking agents. Observations from experiments with dogs anesthetized with methoxyflurane indicate that a small dose of propranolol can cause extreme myocardial depression and death.[260]

Clonidine

Clonidine is a relatively new antihypertensive alpha-adrenergic agonist with a primary effect on the vasomotor center in the medullary portion of the brain. Clonidine is a good agent to use in patients with renal insufficiency because it has little effect on renal blood flow and GFR.

The antihypertensive response to clonidine can vary a great deal from patient to patient, and doses ranging from 0.2 to 2.4 mg daily may be required. The most common range is 0.2 to 0.8 mg daily, given in two doses. The most frequently encountered side effects with clonidine therapy are drowsiness (approximately 50%) and dry mouth (approximately 44%). Approximately 7 percent of patients discontinue use of the drug because of persistent undesirable side effects.[261] If toxicity due to overdose occurs, the adverse effects can be reversed with the alpha adrenergic blocking agent tolazoline, which passes the blood-brain barrier and can inhibit the central nervous system effects of clonidine.[257]

Abrupt withdrawal of clonidine may lead to markedly increased sympathetic outflow from the central nervous system, as manifested by severe hypertension (at or above pretreatment levels), anxiety, headache, nausea, vomiting, abdominal cramps, insomnia, tachycardia, premature ventricular contractions, and elevated urinary catecholamine excretion.[262] This reaction is relatively rare, considering that over 1.4 million people in the United States alone have been treated with clonidine and fewer than 3 dozen confirmed cases of adverse effects of withdrawal have been noted in the world literature.[261] Nonetheless, in the rare instances, the rebound hypertension may lead to a true hypertensive crisis (see Hypertensive Emergencies, page 582) and death. Effective treatment involves either reinstituting clonidine therapy, administration of an alpha adrenergic blocking agent (e.g., phentolamine) or administration of a direct smooth muscle relaxant (e.g., nitroprusside).

Whether or not to discontinue clonidine therapy prior to elective surgery depends upon many factors. There is no evidence that patients maintained on clonidine preoperatively and postoperatively do poorly with respect to their hemodynamic responses to general anesthesia. However, the drug should probably be tapered off slowly prior to elective surgery when a prolonged postoperative period of nasogastric suction is anticipated because clonidine is not available for parenteral use. Preoperative tapering is especially prudent in patients who require daily clonidine dosages of 1.0 mg or more or in whom renovascular hypertension is present. Such patients appear to be at the greatest risk for the development of rebound hypertension. The anesthetist should be aware that the surgical patient is taking clonidine, because the drug may potentiate the depressant effect of barbiturates, benzodiazepines, and other tranquilizers.

Methyldopa

Methyldopa is an extremely effective agent for the treatment of hypertension and is probably the most widely used antihypertensive drug after the diuretics. Because it lowers blood pressure without producing a fall in glomerular filtration rate or renal blood flow, it is considered by many the agent of choice for the treatment of hypertension associated with renal insufficiency. The mechanism of action of methyldopa is probably similar to that of clonidine: the major metabolite of methyldopa, alpha-methyl norepinephrine, is an alpha adrenergic agonist in the medullary region of the brain. As with clonidine, sympathetic output from the central nervous system is diminished and blood pressure falls as a result of decreased peripheral resistance, heart rate, and cardiac output. Methyldopa also lowers plasma renin levels in patients with essential hypertension as well as those with renal failure. Methyldopa, clonidine, prazosin, and hydralazine cause sodium and water retention by the kidney, which may offset the antihypertensive action. This effect can be minimized by concomitant administration of diuretics.

The usual dose of methyldopa is 500 to 2,000 mg daily, divided into two or three doses. The most common side effects are sedation, somnolence, and fatigue, which affect about 30 percent of patients taking the drug. Sedative effects often diminish after a week or two of therapy. Fatigue may persist but often is not recognized until the drug is withdrawn and a sense of well-being returns. More serious reactions to methyldopa include hepatic dysfunction (5%), drug fever (approximately 1%), and blood dyscrasias.

A positive Coomb's test occurs in 10 to 30 percent of patients taking methyldopa and may make crossmatching of blood difficult. Development of a positive direct Coomb's test is not an indication for discontinuing methyldopa therapy. If hemolytic anemia occurs (0.1 to 0.2%), then use of the drug must be discontinued immediately. Autoimmune thrombocytopenia and leukopenia resulting from methyldopa therapy have been reported but are exceedingly rare.

Abruptly discontinuing the use of methyldopa rarely results in a sympathetic discharge manifested by severe hypertension, tachycardia, headache, and nausea, similar to that seen in the "acute post-treatment" syndrome following withdrawal of clonidine.[263] Methyldopa does not appear to cause special problems intraoperatively or postoperatively[264] and should not be routinely withheld prior to elective surgery. Parenteral preparations are available.

Prazosin

Prazosin is a peripheral alpha-adrenergic antagonist which may have direct smooth muscle relaxant effect as well. Unlike other currently available alpha blocking agents (e.g., phenoxybenzamine and phentolamine), prazosin blocks only the postsynaptic alpha-adrenergic receptors. Because other alpha blocking agents interfere with norepinephrine action at both presynaptic and postsynaptic receptors, severe postural hypotension limits their usefulness in the long-term treatment of elevated blood pressure. Isolated blockade of postsynaptic receptors results in the much less dramatic hypotensive action of prazosin. A small percentage of patients have been reported to develop postural hypotension and even syncope, usually with the first dose of the drug.[265] However, postural dizziness is a continuing problem in only about 15 percent of patients taking the drug,[261] and this represents the most frequent adverse reaction to long-term prazosin therapy. Although prazosin has a vasodilator effect, it does not generally produce reflex tachycardia as other vasodilators (e.g., hydralazine) do.[266] Those who do develop tachycardia with prazosin use may benefit from the simultaneous administration of a beta-adrenergic blocking agent.[267]

The usual daily dosage for prazosin is 3 to 20 mg divided into two or three doses. It is recommended that therapy be started with 1 mg three times daily to minimize the postural dizziness and syncope that may accompany initial therapy. The dosage may then be increased slowly until satisfactory control of blood pressure is achieved. This drug has caused no special problems in patients undergoing general anesthesia and surgery, although it may block the response to vasopressors. No parenteral preparation is available.

Hydralazine

The predominant mechanism of action of hydralazine is a direct relaxing effect on arterial smooth muscle, leading to vasodilatation and a fall in peripheral resistance. Because hydralazine has little or no effect on venous smooth muscle, venous return to the heart is enhanced due to reflex venoconstriction. Reflex mechanisms also lead to an increase in heart rate, contractility, and cardiac output. Splanchnic, coronary, cerebral, and renal blood flow are increased. Vasodilatation also leads to an increase in plasma renin activity and to sodium and water retention by the kidneys. Propranolol has been shown to effectively block the reflex increase in cardiac output and elevated plasma renin activity associated with hydralazine therapy, potentiating its antihypertensive effect. Diuretics are often necessary to control the sodium retention which would otherwise blunt the effectiveness of hydralazine as an antihypertensive agent. Thus, hydralazine is seldom used alone, but when combined with a beta blocking agent and a diuretic in so-called "triple-therapy," it is extremely effective in moderate to severe hypertension. Hydralazine has the additional advantage of being available for parenteral use in severe hypertension (see below).

Many of the side effects of hydralazine are related to its direct or reflex mediated hemodynamic actions. The increase in heart rate, contractility, and preload (due to increased venous return) all augment myocardial oxygen requirements and may precipitate angina or other evidence of myocardial ischemia in the presence of coronary artery disease. Even though these effects are ameliorated by the concomitant administration of a beta blocking agent, coronary artery disease remains an important relative contraindication to the use of hydralazine.

A lupus-like syndrome has been associated with the use of hydralazine and has an incidence of 6 to 13 percent.[261] Various factors have been correlated with an increased incidence of lupus-type toxicity including duration of hydralazine therapy greater than six months, slow hepatic acetylation of the drug, and higher daily doses, generally 300 mg or greater. The syndrome can occur rarely with daily hydralazine doses of 200 mg or less. The development of a positive antinuclear antibody (ANA) blood test does not presage the development of a clinical lupus-like syndrome. Fortunately, even when the syndrome does develop, it rarely involves the kidneys and remits after discontinuing use of the drug. Interestingly, the use of hydralazine in patients with spontaneous systemic lupus erythematosus does not adversely affect the natural course of the disease.[60]

The usual daily dose of hydralazine is 100 to 200 mg, in two doses, generally in combination with a beta blocking agent and a diuretic. The continuation of hydralazine therapy up to the time of surgery appears to produce no special problems,[257] although it may reduce the pressor response to epinephrine. Because the drug can be administered parenterally, its use can be continued in the immediate postoperative period even when nothing can be taken by mouth.

Guanethidine

Guanethidine is a potent antihypertensive agent generally reserved for severe, accelerated, or malignant hypertension. It has a selective action at the peripheral sympathetic neuron to block the release and ultimately to deplete the nerve endings of catecholamines. This also interferes with normal circulatory reflexes, and the incidence of postural hypotension and dizziness with therapeutic doses of guanethidine is very high.[261] Because of these adverse reactions, guanethidine is most often employed as a "fourth-line" agent, after a patient with severe hypertension has failed to respond adequately to the combination of a diuretic, an adrenergic blocking agent, and a vasodilator. In such circumstances, therapy with the other agents is often best maintained, and a small dose of guanethidine (5 to 20 mg daily) added. Guanethidine often causes cardiac output to fall and hence may exacerbate cerebrovascular disease or pre-existing renal insufficiency.

The hypotensive effect of guanethidine is attenuated by the concomitant administration of tricyclic antidepressants, monoamine oxidase (MAO) inhibitors, and phenothiazines. Sympathomimetic drugs, such as those contained in over the counter cold remedies, also tend to nullify the hypotensive action of guanethidine. Since guanethidine sensitizes effector cells to catecholamines, administration of pressor agents such as dopamine or norepinephrine may result in an exaggerated hypertensive response.

Whether or not to continue guanethidine therapy up to the time of elective surgery is a matter of some controversy. Because guanethidine interferes with normal circulatory reflex mechanisms, patients taking the drug are clearly at increased risk for hypotension induced by general anesthesia or by fluid losses during surgery. Hence, Cheigh[60] recommends that guanethidine be routinely withheld for two weeks prior to elective surgery to minimize the possibility of vascular collapse or cardiac arrhythmia during anesthesia. However, if sufficient attention is paid to anesthetic response and fluid replacement during surgery, such risk can be minimized. Katz[257] favors continuing patients on guanethidine therapy up to the time of surgery for this reason, noting that the well-controlled hypertensive patient is a better surgical risk. McMahon[261] also emphasizes that the dangers of a hypertensive crisis, congestive heart failure, myocardial infarction, and stroke require continuation of antihypertensive drugs prior to surgery in the patient with severe hypertension. The problems arising from guanethidine-induced catecholamine depletion can be effectively offset during surgery by prompt replacement of fluid losses, use of atropine for bradyarrhythmias, and use of pressor agents in modified doses for hypotension.

Minoxidil

Minoxidil is a newly released drug effective for the treatment of severe hypertension. It is a potent direct vasodilator with a mechanism of action similar to that of hydralazine. Use of minoxidil has generally been reserved for patients whose blood pressure has not responded to a combination of other agents currently available, particularly those patients with severe hypertension associated with chronic renal insufficiency.[268,269] Although minoxidil is quite effective in reducing blood pressure, its use has been limited by a relatively high incidence of adverse reactions. It induces reflex tachycardia and salt retention as do other vasodilators. Hence, it should be administered with both a diuretic and an adrenergic blocking agent. Propranolol or metoprolol are the preferred adrenergic blocking agents for this purpose, but other agents such as methyldopa, clonidine, or guanethidine can be used if there is a contraindication to beta blockade such as severe congestive heart failure or obstructive lung disease.[270] Since many patients receiving minoxidil have advanced renal insufficiency, thiazide diuretics may not be potent enough to block the salt retaining effect; large doses of furosemide are often required under these circumstances. Minoxidil has been shown to improve renal function in some patients with pre-existing renal insufficiency.[271,272] This is related both to an increase in renal blood flow and improvement in the hypertension per se. On rare occasions, hypertensive dialysis patients treated with minoxidil have recovered sufficient renal function to allow discontinuation of dialysis.[273]

The risks of minoxidil therapy in the patient undergoing general anesthesia are uncertain because of limited experience with the drug. It is recommended that minoxidil therapy be continued up to the time of elective surgery and resumed postoperatively as soon as appropriate. No parenteral preparation is available.

The Patient with Renovascular Hypertension

Although renal artery stenosis is the most common surgically correctable form of hypertension, the incidence of renovascular disease is less than 5 percent of unselected hypertensive patients. Moreover, even a smaller fraction (1 to 2%) are surgical candidates. Stenosis is due to atherosclerosis in approximately two-thirds of cases (primarily in men, having a mean age of 50) and to fibromuscular dysplasia (primarily in women, having a mean age of 35) in the remaining one-third.

Preoperative preparation for corrective vascular surgery includes maintenance of pharmacologic control of blood pressure up to the time of surgery. Methyldopa has been recommended for this purpose because it is associated with minimal vasomotor instability, and if hypotension subsequently occurs, it can be quickly corrected by moderate volume expansion.[274] Use of clonidine should be avoided because the risk of accelerated hypertension due to the "acute post-treatment syndrome" is greater in patients with renovascular hypertension. Therefore, use of the drug should be tapered off slowly, and another agent (e.g., methyldopa) substituted during the week prior to surgery. Diuretic therapy in the immediate preoperative period should be minimized and accumulated sodium deficits should be repaired. If radiocontrast studies have been performed within the few days before surgery is scheduled, care must be taken to insure that renal function has not deteriorated. Surgery is best delayed until renal function is clearly optimal.

The actual surgical procedure employed depends upon the location and nature of the stenotic lesion. A nonoperative technique of arterial dilatation as an alternative to renovascular surgery has recently been reported. The technique, known as percutaneous transluminal angioplasty, involves the threading of a balloon-tipped catheter into the stenotic renal artery. Access is obtained percutaneously over a guiding wire entering the femoral artery, as with renal arteriography. Since dye can also be injected through the balloon-tipped catheter, contrast visualization of the artery is obtained as the catheter is advanced. With the balloon collapsed, the catheter tip is placed within the stenotic segment, then the balloon is inflated, dilating the stenotic portion of the renal artery with minimal trauma. Millan and colleagues have reported this technique to be effective in the dilatation of renal artery stenosis due to fibromuscular dysplasia.[275,276] In their experience, the procedure was followed by a prompt fall in the patients' blood pressure to normal and normalization of peripheral and renal venous renin levels. Grüntzig and associates[277] reported similar success in the use of this technique in the dilatation of a stenotic renal artery affected by atherosclerosis. Although experience with this technique is limited, it offers promise in selected patients with renovascular hypertension.

HIGH RATE OF RESTENOSIS – RICHARD DEAN 1982.

TABLE 15. Parenteral Agents Commonly Used in the Treatment of Hypertensive Emergencies

Agent	*Dosage*	*Advantages*	*Disadvantages*	*Indications*	*Contraindications*
Sodium nitroprusside	0.5–8.0 μ g/kg/min constant IV infusion	Predictably effective Generally safe Rapid onset of action Rapid dissipation of effect when therapy is stopped Decreases venous return so cardiac stimulation is minimal	Close monitoring of blood pressure and infusion rate are essential Potential of thiocyanate toxicity with prolonged use Solution is unstable and must be protected from light	Malignant hypertension Hypertensive encephalopathy Hypertension associated with intracranial hemorrhage or cardiac decompensation Aortic dissection	None
Diazoxide	300 mg or 5 mg/kg total dose IV bolus or infusion at 15 mg/min	Ease of administration Rapid onset of action Sustained effect if response occurs Monitoring in intensive care unit not required	Does not always produce a response Hypotensive effect cannot be precisely regulated Potential of overshoot in blood pressure response Reflex cardic stimulation may be hazardous in certain patients Significant salt and water retention Occasional nausea and vomiting	Uncomplicated malignant or premalignant hypertension Severe hypertension associated with renal insufficiency Hypertensive encephalopathy Toxemia of pregnancy Hypertension associated with acute nephritis	Intracranial hemorrhage Aortic dissection Coronary insufficiency Left ventricular failure

Trimethaphan camsylate	1–5 mg/min constant IV infusion	Rapid onset of action Rapid dissipation of effect when therapy is stopped Decreased venous return, cardiac output, and force of cardiac contractions	Close monitoring of blood pressure and infusion rate are essential Hypotensive effect may be variable and unpredictable Inhibition of pupillary reflexes makes neurologic assessment difficult Causes paralytic ileus and urinary retention with prolonged use Elevation of patient's head required for optimal anti-hypertensive effect	Aortic dissection Hypertension associated with acute left ventricular failure or intracranial hemorrhage Hypertensive encephalopathy	Relatively contraindicated in severe renaldisease
Hydralazine	10–20 mg IV or IM, repeated as necessary	Ease of administration Constant blood pressure monitoring not required Relative sparing of renal blood flow	Low rate of response in severest hypertension Delayed (20–30 min) onset of action Reflex cardiac stimulation may be hazardous in certain patients	Uncomplicated malignant or premalignant hypertension Severe uncomplicated postoperative hypertension Toxemia of pregnancy Hypertension associated with acute nephritis	Malignant hypertension with progressive renal insufficiency (not effective) Intracranial hemorrhage Aortic dissection Coronary insufficiency Left ventricular failure

Hypertensive Emergencies (Table 15)

Hypertension is a common occurrence in patients recovering from anesthesia and surgery, even in patients with no prior history of elevated blood pressure. In a study of 1844 recovery room admissions by Gal and Cooperman,[278] 3.3 percent had significant postoperative arterial hypertension. In over 40 percent of these episodes, the patient had no prior history of blood pressure elevation. Factors possibly contributing to postoperative hypertension include pain, emergence excitement, reaction to the endotracheal tube, hypercarbia, excess fluid administration, hypothermia and hypoxia. In 80 percent of the cases in this series,[278] the postoperative hypertension was mild and self-limited, lasting only two hours or so. But in the remaining 20 percent of cases, more severe and prolonged elevations in blood pressure occurred, leading in some to complications such as cardiac arrhythmias and congestive heart failure.

Patients recovering from cardiac surgery are at particular risk for the complications of postoperative hypertension. In such patients, hypertension may lead to impaired cardiac performance in the early postoperative period. Normalizing blood pressure in these patients has been shown to significantly reduce ventricular systolic wall tension, stroke work, and myocardial oxygen consumption, thereby improving cardiac performance.[279] For this reason, the routine use of after-load reducing agents such as nitroprusside and aggressive treatment of even mild elevations in blood pressure have been employed in postoperative cardiac and other high-risk surgical patients.[280]

In the routine postoperative patient, mild to moderate elevations in blood pressure can be treated effectively with the resumption of preoperative antihypertensive medication. If oral intake is precluded, parenteral methyldopa or hydralazine can be given for blood pressure control. In rare instances, hypertension will be much more severe postoperatively. The reason for this is unclear but may relate to a defect in central autoregulation in the hypertensive patient which is aggravated by the decrease in cerebral blood flow associated with general anesthesia. Additional factors include increased levels of circulating catecholamines due to pain, fear, the presence of an endotracheal tube, hypothermia, and hypoxemia. Surgical procedures which have been noted to have a higher incidence of postoperative hypertension include open heart[281] and carotid artery[282] surgery, correction of coarctation of the aorta,[283] and removal of pheochromocytoma.

Hypertensive emergencies requiring immediate lowering of blood pressure with the use of intravenous antihypertensive agents include malignant hypertension with progressive renal failure, hypertensive encephalopathy, hypertension associated with intracranial hemorrhage, hypertension associated with acute left ventricular failure and/or acute myocardial infarction, and aortic dissection.

GENERAL PRINCIPLES OF MANAGEMENT

Optimal medical management of any patient with a hypertensive emergency includes strict bed rest and confinement to an intensive care unit. Continuous monitoring of arterial blood pressure through the use of an indwelling arterial catheter is desirable. Fluid intake and output should be monitored carefully, and daily body weights obtained. Most patients with severe hypertension will benefit from the prompt intravenous administration of a potent diuretic agent (e.g., furosemide, 40 to 80 mg). Diuretics often improve intravascular volume overload (which is commonly present under these circumstances), offset the salt-retaining effect of vasodilator drugs, and may have a direct antihypertensive effect.[284] Serum electrolytes and renal function studies should be obtained frequently. Hypokalemia is frequently present as a result of markedly increased renin-angiotensin-aldosterone activity and may require potassium supplementation. Reduction of the blood pressure may produce transient renal functional impairment in the patient with renal disease because of decreased renal blood flow, but renal function should improve over the long term as normalization of blood pressure will allow for healing of the necrotizing renal arteriolitis.[285,286] Thus, aggressive antihypertensive therapy should be pursued regardless of the initial effect on renal function.

If oliguric renal failure supervenes in malignant hypertension, dialysis should be initiated to control the symptoms of uremia, to correct electrolyte disturbances, and to remove excess fluid which may be contributing to the hypertension. In rare instances, sufficient recovery of renal function may occur following the control of blood pressure to allow discontinuation of dialysis, although this may take up to a year.[273]

SPECIFIC ANTIHYPERTENSIVE AGENTS (TABLE 15)

Because the hypertensive emergency is a life-threatening situation, appropriate pharmacotherapeutic agents should be administered intravenously, have an immediate onset of action, and not adversely affect vital organs such as brain, heart, and kidneys. Each of the available agents has specific advantages and disadvantages that may recommend or contraindicate its use in a particular clinical situation.

Sodium Nitroprusside

Sodium nitroprusside (Nipride) is an extremely potent, rapidly acting, and predictably effective antihypertensive agent that has become the standard drug for treatment of hypertensive emergencies. Nitroprusside is a direct vasodilator, relaxing all vascular (arterial and venous) smooth muscle independent of autonomic innervation. When administered by intravenous infusion, the antihypertensive effect of nitroprusside is apparent within seconds and lasts only one to two minutes after the infusion is stopped. The extremely rapid clearance of the drug and dose-related antihypertensive effect mean that blood pressure can be titrated by adjusting the intravenous infusion rate. A constant rate infusion pump and an indwelling arterial catheter for constant monitoring of blood pressure are desirable but not essential if vigilant monitoring of blood pressure and infusion rate can be accomplished manually.

Sodium nitroprusside, by producing both arterial and venous dilatation, leads to decreased systemic resistance and decreased venous return, resulting in reduced stroke volume and cardiac output.[287] Activation of baroreceptor reflexes due to decreased arterial pressure will produce an increase in heart rate, but cardiac output generally remains below baseline levels. The decrease in cardiac output may lead to significant reductions in renal blood flow despite a decrease in renal vascular resistance, producing a reduction in creatinine clearance[288] and an increase in plasma renin activity.

Infusions of nitroprusside should be initiated at a rate of 0.5 μg/kg of body weight per minute then titrated upward until satisfactory control of blood pressure is achieved. An adequate hypotensive effect is generally obtained at infusion rates of less than 8 μg/kg/minute, but the response remains dose-related at higher levels as well. Almost all patients with severe hypertension respond to administration of nitroprusside if the agent is given in sufficient dosage. Although nitroprusside is relatively nontoxic, the major metabolite, thiocyanate, may produce adverse symptoms if allowed to accumulate. Thiocyanate toxicity is rare but can occur in patients in whom nitroprusside is administered for longer than three to four days, especially in the presence of renal insufficiency. Manifestations include weakness, nausea, tinnitus, psychosis, and hypothyroidism. Patients at risk should have thiocyanate levels monitored, and the nitroprusside infusion should be discontinued if levels exceed 10 μg/ml.[261]

Nitroprusside is supplied in 50 mg vials. The contents of one vial should be dissolved in 500 ml of 5 percent dextrose in water. The solution is sensitive to light, and the bottle and tubing should be covered with aluminum foil while hanging. If the solution turns dark brown or blue, it should be discarded.

As soon as nitroprusside therapy brings the blood pressure into the desired range, oral antihypertensive therapy should be initiated and efforts be made to wean the patient from the nitroprusside infusion.[289]

Diazoxide

Diazoxide (Hyperstat), a chemical relative of the thiazide diuretics, is also effective in hypertensive emergencies. In contrast to nitroprusside, it can be given as a single intravenous bolus injection without the need for an infusion pump or constant intra-arterial pressure monitoring. The hypotensive effect of diazoxide generally lasts from 4 to 10 hours,[290] often sufficient time to allow more conventional oral or intramuscular antihypertensive agents to exert their effects.

Diazoxide acts by directly dilating peripheral arterioles, with no significant effect on the venous circulation. This results in a lowering of peripheral vascular resistance and systolic and diastolic blood pressure, which is followed by stimulation of baroreceptors and an increase in sympathetic activity. The reflex sympathetic stimulation leads to increases in heart rate, stroke volume, inotropic influence, and cardiac output. These latter effects may be undesirable in a patient with limited cardiac reserve or coronary insufficiency since myocardial oxygen consumption will be increased. Because the force of cardiac ejection is also increased, diazoxide is contraindicated in the treatment of hypertension associated with aortic dissection.

Intense renal sodium retention is induced by treatment with diazoxide, due both to a transient fall in renal blood flow and GFR accompanying the reduction in blood pressure and to intrinsic sodium-retaining properties of the drug. Therefore, it is recommended that a diuretic, such as furosemide, 40 to 80 mg intravenously, be administered routinely just prior to diazoxide injection.

The antihypertensive effect of diazoxide is quite prompt, occuring within two to five minutes following the injection of an intravenous bolus. Blood pressure determinations should be done every 30 seconds following injection until the blood pressure stabilizes, then every five minutes for the next half hour. The patient should remain in the supine position throughout this initial period. Since the dose of diazoxide is fixed (300 mg or 5 mg/kg of body weight) and not titrated to the individual patient, episodes of hypotension may occur following therapy, although such occurrence is infrequent (< 5%).[261] Hypotensive episodes can be treated by elevation of the legs or, if severe, infusion of a pressor agent such as norepinephrine. On the other hand, if a satisfactory blood pressure response does not occur following a single injection of diazoxide, a second bolus should be given after 30 minutes. A total of 1200 mg may be given over a 24 hour period if necessary to maintain blood pressure control. Oral antihypertensive therapy should be initiated as soon as possible to minimize the necessity for repeated injections with diazoxide.

The intravenous injection of diazoxide is accompanied by nausea and vomiting in about 4 percent of patients.[261] Hyperglycemia occurs primarily in patients with a previous history of carbohydrate intolerance. It usually presents no problems and, if significant, can be treated effectively with insulin. More serious complications of diazoxide therapy, such as acute myocardial infarction or pulmonary edema, occur rarely (< 0.1%),[261] and primarily in patients with a prior history of coronary or valvular heart disease in whom use of the drug should be avoided.

Because of the reflex sympathetic stimulation and unpredictable hypotensive effect of diazoxide, it is not as versatile a drug as nitroprusside, which can be used in virtually any form of hypertensive emergency. Use of diazoxide is contraindicated in hypertensive emergencies associated with intracerebral hemorrhage, aortic dissection, myocardial infarction, or acute pulmonary edema. On the other hand, its potency and ease of administration make diazoxide particularly useful in the treatment of severe hypertension associated with impaired renal function, hypertensive encephalopathy, acute obstetrical hypertensive emergency, hypertensive crises associated with the "collagen-vascular" diseases, and uncomplicated but refractory cases of severe hypertension.[261] Diazoxide is not effective in the treatment of hypertension associated with pheochromocytoma.

Although most authors have emphasized the necessity of administering diazoxide by rapid intravenous injection for maximal antihypertensive effect,[291,292] a recent report has demonstrated the efficacy of diazoxide when given by intravenous infusion.[293] In this study, diazoxide was infused at a rate of 15 mg/minute up to a total amount of 5 mg/kg of body weight. This total is equivalent to the recommended dose for single bolus injection. Fifteen patients treated with diazoxide infusion had a fall in mean arterial pressure and sustained antihypertensive effect similar to that in 12 patients treated with a 300 mg bolus injection. The infusion was accompanied by a more gradual decline in blood pressure, which is felt to lower the risk of myocardial ischemia. The infusion technique allows for interruption of the procedure as soon as a satisfactory blood pressure level is achieved, minimizing the incidence of hypotension. Slow infusion can be repeated as necessary if inadequate response occurs or severe hypertension returns.

Trimethaphan Camsylate

Of the major pharmacologic agents currently used in the treatment of hypertensive emergencies, trimethaphan camsylate (Arfonad) is the oldest. It reduces blood pressure by competitively inhibiting the action of acetylcholine at postganglionic nerve terminals and preventing postsynaptic depolarization by "stabilization" of the membrane. A decrease in cardiac output may occur in hypertensive patients with decompensated heart failure or mitral valve disease. An insignificant increase in heart rate may be observed, most likely the result of incomplete autonomic blockade.[294] These characteristics make trimethaphan especially useful in the treatment of severe hypertension complicated by congestive heart failure or aortic dissection. Since renal blood flow may be significantly decreased and renal vascular resistance increased due to trimethaphan-induced hypotension and decreased cardiac output, use of the agent is not preferred in patients with renal insufficiency.

Trimethaphan is administered only by slow intravenous infusion. The standard preparation is 500 mg mixed in 500 to 1000 ml of 5 percent dextrose in water. The infusion is generally initiated at a rate of 0.25 to 0.50 mg/minute then titrated upward to achieve the desired hypotensive effect. The action of trimethaphan is immediate, and blood pressure should be monitored continuously via an intra-arterial catheter. Since the hypotensive effect is most pronounced when the patient is upright, the head of the bed should be elevated. As with nitroprusside, the duration of the drug's action is extremely short, and blood pressure will return to pretreatment levels within minutes of stopping the infusion. Therefore, if hypotension occurs in a patient being treated with trimethaphan, it can be reversed by discontinuing the drug and placing the patient in Trendelenburg's position.

Once satisfactory blood pressure control is achieved, oral antihypertensive therapy should be initiated and the infusion rate decreased or stopped as soon as possible. Prolonged therapy with trimethaphan may be accompanied by significant sodium retention and intravascular volume expansion, leading to an attenuation of the drug's effect. Concomitant diuretic therapy is therefore recommended.

Parasympathetic blockade by trimethaphan may lead to constipation, paralytic ileus, and urinary retention, particularly when administration of the drug is continued for more than 24 hours. In the postoperative patient, use of trimethaphan may prolong the duration of bowel and bladder paralysis. The use of trimethaphan is problematic in patients with hypertensive encephalopathy or intracerebral hemorrhage, since its ganglionic blocking effect will inhibit pupillary reflexes, making neurologic assessment difficult.[295]

Hydralazine

Intravenous administration of hydralazine (Apresoline) reduces blood pressure within 10 to 30 minutes and has been employed successfully in the treatment of hypertensive emergencies.[296] However, it should not be considered a first-line drug for the treatment of life-threatening complications of hypertension, because its antihypertensive effect is not immediate. Hydralazine is most useful in cases of accelerated hypertension associated with renal insufficiency (but not complicated malignant hypertension), acute glomerulonephritis, and toxemia of pregnancy, because it generally allows renal arterial blood flow to be maintained.

The usual parenteral dose of hydralazine is 10 to 20 mg, repeated as necessary. The duration of action ranges from 30 minutes to 9 hours. Diuretics and beta blocking agents should be given concomitantly to minimize the sodium retention and reflex sympathetic activity, respectively, that may attenuate the antihypertensive effect of hydralazine. As with diazoxide, the reflex increases in heart rate, stroke volume, and cardiac output contraindicate the use of hydralazine in the treatment of hypertension associated with intracranial hemorrhage, aortic dissection, acute myocardial infarction, and acute left ventricular failure.

Minoxidil

Minoxidil is an orally administered agent and, therefore, should not be considered a first-line drug in the treatment of hypertensive emergencies. However, it may be the only available oral antihypertensive drug sufficiently potent to allow weaning and discontinuation of parenteral agents in patients with extremely severe hypertension, especially when associated with advanced renal disease.[273,297] Minoxidil is the most potent oral antihypertensive agent currently available and its use will often produce satisfactory lowering of blood pressure in cases where combinations of other agents have failed.

REFERENCES

1. Friedman, SA, Raizner, AE, Rosen H, et al.: *Functional defects in the aging kidney.* Ann Intern Med 76:41, 1972.
2. Cockcroft, DW, and Gault, MH: *Prediction of creatinine clearance from serum creatinine.* Nephron 16:31, 1976.
3. Kim, KE, Onesti, G, Ramirez, O, et al.: *Creatinine clearance in renal disease. A reappraisal.* Br Med J 4:11, 1969.
4. Dossetor, JB: *Creatininemia versus uremia. The relative significance of blood urea nitrogen and serum creatinine concentrations in azotemia.* Ann Intern Med 65:1287, 1966.
5. Franklin, SS, Niall, JF, and Merrill, JP: *The influence of solute load on the isosthenuria of renal disease.* J Clin Invest 38:1005, 1959.
6. Kleeman, CR, Adams, DA, and Maxwell, MH: *An evaluation of maximal water diuresis in chronic renal disease: I. Normal solute intake.* J Lab Clin Med 58:169, 1961.
7. Bricker, NS, Dewey, RR, Lubowitz, H, et al.: *Observations on the concentrating and diluting mechanisms of the diseased kidney.* J Clin Invest 38:516, 1959.
8. Bricker, NS, Bourgoignie, JJ, and Weber, H: *The Renal Response to Progressive Nephron Loss,* in Brenner, BM, and Rector, FC, Jr. (eds.): *The Kidney.* Philadelphia: WB Saunders Company, 1976.
9. Gennari, FJ, and Cohen, JJ: *Role of the kidney in potassium homeostasis: lessons from acid-base disturbances.* Kidney Int 8:1, 1975.
10. Schambelan, M, Stockigt, JR, and Biglieri, EG: *Isolated hypoaldosteronism in adults: a renin deficiency syndrome.* N Engl J Med 287:573, 1972.
11. Relman, AS, Lennon, EJ, and Lemann, J, Jr.: *Endogenous production of fixed acid and the measurements of the net balance of acid in normal subjects.* J Clin Invest 40:1621, 1961.
12. Widmer, B, Gerhardt, RE, Harrington, JJ, et al.: *Serum electrolytes and acid-base composition with graded degrees of chronic renal failure.* Arch Intern Med 139:1099, 1979.
13. Gulyassy, PF, Yamauchi, H, and Depner, TA: *Conservative Management of Chronic Renal Failure,* in Earley, LE, and Gottschalk, CW (eds.): *Strauss and Welt's Diseases of the Kidney.* Boston: Little, Brown and Company, 1979.
14. Husted, FC, Nolph, KD, and Maher, JF: *$NaHCO_3$ and NaCl tolerance in chronic renal failure.* J Clin Invest 56:414, 1975.

15. KUZELA, DC, HUFFER, WE, CONGER, JD, ET AL.: *Soft tissue calcification in chronic dialysis patients.* Am J Pathol 86:403, 1977.

16. SLATOPOLSKY, E, RUTHERFORD, WE, HRUSKA, K, ET AL.: *How important is phosphate in the pathogenesis of renal osteodystrophy?* Arch Intern Med 138:848, 1978.

17. KNOCHEL, JP: *The pathophysiology and clinical characteristics of severe hypophosphatemia.* Arch Intern Med 137:203, 1977.

18. BRICKMAN, AS, COBURN, JW, FRIEDMAN, GR, ET AL.: *Comparison of effects of 1α-hydroxyvitamin D_3 and 1,25-dihydroxyvitamin D_3 in man. J Clin* Invest 57:1540, 1976.

19. DRÜEKE, T, BORIDER, PJ, MAN, NK, ET AL.: *Effects of high dialysate calcium concentration on bone remodeling, serum biochemistry, and parathyroid hormone in patients with renal osteodystrophy.* Kidney Int 11:267, 1977.

20. ROSE, WC, AND WIXON, RL: *The amino acid requirements of man: the role of nitrogen intake.* J Biol Chem 217:997, 1955.

21. KOPPLE, JD, AND COBURN, JW: *Metabolic studies of low protein diets in uremia. I. Nitrogen and potassium.* Medicine 52:583, 1973.

22. KOPPLE, JD: *Dietary Requirements,* in MASSRY, SG, AND SELLERS, AL (eds.): *Clinical Aspects of Uremia and Dialysis.* Springfield, Illinois: Charles C Thomas, 1976.

23. GRUSKIN, SE, TOLMAN, DE, AND WAGONER, RD: *Oral manifestations of uremia.* Minn Med 53:495, 1970.

24. KORMAN, MG, LAVER, MC, AND HANSKY, J: *Hypergastrinaemia in chronic renal failure.* Br Med J 1:209, 1972.

25. AVRAM, NM: *High prevalence of pancreatic disease in chronic renal failure.* Nephron 18:68, 1977.

26. DAVIDSON, RC, AND SCRIBNER, BH: *Cardiovascular manifestations of renal failure,* in EARLEY, LE, AND GOTTSCHALK, CW (eds.): *Strauss and Welt's Diseases of the Kidney.* Boston: Little, Brown and Company, 1979.

27. DRÜEKE, T, LAPAILLEUR, C, MEILHAC, B, ET AL.: *Congestive cardiomyopathy in uraemic patients on long-term dialysis.* Br Med J 1:350, 1977.

28. FEIHN, W, SEILER, D, AND HEIMBERG, K: *Transport ATPases of cardiac sarcolemma in experimental uremia.* Clin Chem Acta 73:93, 1976.

29. RACKOW, EC, FEIN, IA, SPRUNG, C, ET AL.: *Uremic pulmonary edema.* Am J Med 64:1084, 1978.

30. COMTY, CM, WATHEN, RL, AND SHAPIRO, FL: *Uremic percarditis.* Cardiovasc Clin 7(3):219, 1976.

31. MARINI, PV, AND HULL, AR: *Uremic pericarditis: a review of incidence and management.* Kidney Int 7(Suppl 2):S163, 1975.

32. FRIED, W: *Hematologic complications of chronic renal failure.* Med Clin North Am 62:1363, 1978.

33. HUSSEIN, S, PRIETO, J, O'SHEA, M, ET AL.: *Serum ferritin assay and iron status in chronic renal failure and haemodialysis.* Br Med J 1:545, 1975.

34. OPELZ, G, SENGAR, DPS, MICKEY, MR, ET AL.: *Effect of blood transfusions on subsequent renal transplants.* Transplant Proc 5:253, 1973.

35. RABINER, SF: *Bleeding Abnormalities,* in MASSRY, SG, AND SELLERS, AL (eds.): *Clinical Aspects of Uremia and Dialysis.* Springfield, Illinois: Charles C Thomas, 1976.

36. RASKIN, NH, AND FISHMAN, RA: *Neurologic disorders in renal failure.* N Engl J Med 294:204, 1976.

37. BOLTON, CF, JOHNSON, WJ, AND DYCK, PJ: *Neurologic manifestations of renal failure,* in EARLEY, LE, AND GOTTSCHALK, CW (eds.): *Strauss and Welt's Diseases of the Kidney.* Boston: Little, Brown and Company, 1979.

38. RASKIN, NH, AND FISHMAN, RA: *Neurologic disorders in renal failure.* N Engl J Med 294:143, 1976.

39. ARIEFF, AI, GUISADO, R, AND MASSRY, SG: *Uremic encephalopathy: studies on biochemical alterations in the brain.* Kidney Int 7(Suppl 2):S194, 1975.

40. ALFREY, AC, LEGENDRE, GR, AND KAEHNY, WD: *The dialysis encephalopathy syndrome: possible aluminum intoxication.* N Engl J Med 294:184, 1976.

41. ARIEFF, AI, COOPER, JD, ARMSTRONG, D, ET AL.: *Dementia, renal failure, and brain aluminum.* Ann Intern Med 90:741, 1979.

42. LEONARD, A, AND SHAPIRO, FL: *Subdural hematomas in regularly hemodialyzed patients.* Ann Intern Med 82:650, 1975.

43. Lim, VS, Kathpalia, SC, and Henriques, C: *Endocrine abnormalities associated with chronic renal failure.* Med Clin North Am 62:1341, 1978.

44. Westervelt, FB, Jr: *Metabolic and endocrine abnormalities. Part I: carbohydrate metabolism* in Massry, SG, and Sellers, AL (eds.): *Clinical Aspects of Uremia and Dialysis.* Springfield, Illinois: Charles C Thomas, 1976.

45. Wochos, DN, Anderson, CF, and Mitchell, JC, III: *Serum lipids in chronic renal failure.* Mayo Clin Proc 51:660, 1976.

46. Klein, KL, and Kurokawa, K: *Metabolic and endocrine alterations in end-stage renal failure.* Postgrad Med 64:99, 1978.

47. Brunzell, JD, Albers, JJ, Haas, LB, et al.: *Prevalence of serum lipid abnormalities in chronic hemodialysis.* Metabolism 26:903, 1977.

48. Sanfelippo, ML, Swenson, RS, and Reaven, GM: *Reduction of plasma triglycerides by diet in subjects with chronic renal failure.* Kidney Int 11:54, 1977.

49. Lim, VS, Fang, VS, Katz, AI, et al.: *Thyroid dysfunction in chronic renal failure: a study of the pituitary-thyroid axis and peripheral turnover kinetics of thyroxine and triiodothyronine.* J Clin Invest 60:522, 1977.

50. Spector, DA, Davis, PJ, Helderman, JH, et al.: *Thyroid function and metabolic state in chronic renal failure.* Ann Intern Med 85:724, 1976.

51. Czernichow, P, Danzet, MC, Broyer, M, et al.: *Abnormal TSH, PRL and GH responses to TSH releasing factor in chronic renal failure.* J Clin Endocrinol Metab 43:630, 1976.

52. Dobbelstein, H: *Immune system in uremia.* Nephron 17:409, 1976.

53. Byron, PR, Mallick, NP, and Taylor, G: *Immune potential in human uraemia. I. Relationship of glomerular filtration rate to depression of immune potential.* J Clin Pathol 29:765, 1976.

54. Casciani, CU, DeSimone, C, Bonini, S, et al.: *Immunological aspects of chronic uremia.* Kidney Int 13(Suppl 8):S49, 1978.

55. Rubin, AL, Stenzel, KH, and Reidenberg, MM (eds.): *Symposium on drug action and metabolism in renal failure.* Am J Med 62:459, 1977.

56. Bennett, WM, Singer, I, and Coggins, CH: *A practical guide to drug usage in adult patients with impaired renal function.* JAMA 214:1468, 1970.

57. Bennett, WM, Singer, I, and Coggins, CH: *Guide to drug usage in adult patients with impaired renal function: a supplement.* JAMA 223:991, 1973.

58. Bennett, WM, Singer, I, Golper, T, et al.: *Guidelines for drug therapy in renal failure.* Ann Intern Med 86:754, 1977.

59. Maffly, R, and Bennett, W: *Drug Therapy In Renal Disease,* in Rubenstein, E, and Federman, DD (eds.): *Scientific American Medicine.* New York: Scientific American, 1979.

60. Cheigh, JS: *Drug administration in renal failure.* Am J Med 62:555, 1977.

61. Anderson, RJ, Gambertoglio, JG, and Schrier, RW: *Fate of Drugs in Renal Failure,* in Brenner, BM, and Rector, FC (eds.): *The Kidney.* Philadelphia: WB Saunders Company, 1976.

62. Hata, M, Remmers, AR, Lindley, JD, et al.: *Surgical management of the dialysis patient.* Ann Surg 178:134, 1973.

63. Hampers, CL, Bailey, GL, Hager, EB, et al.: *Major surgery in patients on maintenance hemodialysis.* Am J Surg 115:747, 1968.

64. Lissos, I, VanBlerk, PJ, and Goldberg, B: *Surgical procedures in patients on maintenance hemodialysis.* S Afr Med J 46:850, 1972.

65. Brenowitz, JB, Williams, CD, and Edwards, WS: *Major surgery in patients with chronic renal failure.* Am J Surg 134:765, 1977.

66. Haimov, M, Glabman, S, Schupak, E, et al.: *General surgery in patients on maintenance hemodialysis.* Ann Surg 179:863, 1974.

67. Lansing, AM, Leb, DE, and Berman, LB: *Cardiovascular surgery in end-stage renal failure.* JAMA 204:682, 1968.

68. Silberman, H: *Renal failure and the surgeon.* Surg Gynecol Obstet 144:775, 1977.

69. Herrin, JT: *Preparation of the renal patient for surgery.* Int Anesthesiol Clin 13:183, 1975.

70. Prys-Roberts, C, Meloche, R, and Foëx, P: *Studies of anaesthesia in relation to hypertension. I. Cardiovascular responses of treated and untreated patients.* Br J Anaesth 43:122, 1971.

71. Schreiner, GE, and Maher, JF: *The patient with chronic renal failure and surgery.* Am J Cardiol 12:317, 1963.

72. Fahmy, NR, Gissen, AS, Savarese, JJ, et al.: *Decamethonium and serum potassium.* Anesthesiology 42:692, 1975.

73. Hesse, VE, Mostert, JW, Moore, RH, et al.: *Cholinesterase levels in man and renal allografted man.* J Surg Oncol 2:69, 1970.

74. Warren, R: *Medical progress: postoperative thrombophilia.* N Engl J Med 249:99, 1953.

75. Hampers, CL, Blaufox, MD, and Merrill, JP: *Anticoagulation rebound after hemodialysis.* N Engl J Med 275:776, 1966.

76. Kjellstrand, CM, and Buselmeier, TJ: *A simple method for anticoagulation during pre- and post-operative hemodialysis, avoiding rebound phenomenon.* Surgery 72:630, 1972.

77. Tzamaloukas, AH, Garella, S, and Chazan, JA: *Peritoneal dialysis for acute renal failure after major abdominal surgery.* Arch Surg 106:639, 1973.

78. Lissos, I, Goldberg, B, and VanBlerk, PJP: *Surgical procedures on patients in end-stage renal failure.* Br J Urol 45:359, 1973.

79. Kersh, ES, Kronfield, SJ, Propper, RW, et al.: *Autonomic insufficiency in uremia as a cause of hemodialysis-induced hypotension.* N Engl J Med 290:650, 1974.

80. Heughan, C, Grislis, G, and Hunt, TK: *The effect of anemia on wound healing.* Ann Surg 179:163, 1974.

81. Howard, RJ, and Najarian, JS: *Surgery in uremic patients: clinical guidelines.* Cardiovas Med 1:170, 1976.

82. Geis, WP, and Iwatsuki, G: *Acute and chronic renal failure.* Surg Clin North Am 57:1263, 1977.

83. Stone, AM, and Stahl, WM: *Effect of ethacryric acid and furosemide on renal function in hypovolemia.* Ann Surg 174:1, 1971.

84. Tasker, PRW, MacGregor, GA, and deWardener, HE: *Prophylactic use of intravenous saline in patients with chronic renal failure undergoing major surgery.* Lancet 2:911, 1974.

85. Bevan, DR, and Dudley, HAF: *Chronic renal failure and major surgery.* Lancet 2:1150, 1974.

86. Horsey, PJ: *Fluid balance after major surgery in chronic renal failure.* Lancet 2:1079, 1974.

87. Allison, MEM, and Kennedy, AC: *Diuretics in chronic renal disease: a study of high dosage furosemide.* Clin Sci 41:171, 1971.

88. Churchill, D, Knaak, J, Chirito, E, et al.: *Persisting renal insufficiency after methoxyflurane anesthesia: report of two cases and review of the literature.* Am J Med 56:575, 1974.

89. Hirsche, BL, and Woods, JE: *Experience with elective surgery in renal allograft recipients.* Am J Surg 127:730, 1974.

90. Leapman, SB, Vidne, BA, Butt, KM, et al.: *Elective and emergency surgery in renal transplant patients.* Ann Surg 183:266, 1976.

91. Stuart, FP, Simonian, SJ, and Hill, JL: *Special considerations in surgical management of patients on hemodialysis and after successful kidney transplantation.* Surg Clin North Am 56:15, 1976.

92. Flamenbaum, W, and Leslie, BR: *Diagnosis and management of renal failure in surgical patients.* Orth Clin North Am 9:845, 1978.

93. Bushinsky, DA, Wish, JB, Hou, SH, et al.: *Hospital-acquired renal insufficiency (1978–1979).* Kidney Int 16:875, 1979.

94. Anderson, RJ, Linas, SL, Berns, AS, et al.: *Nonoliguric acute renal failure.* N Engl J Med 296:1134, 1977.

95. Hall, JW, Johnson, WJ, Maher, FT, et al.: *Immediate and long-term prognosis in acute renal failure.* Ann Intern Med 73:515, 1970.

96. Kleinknecht, D, Jungers, P, Chanard, J, et al.: *Uremic and non-uremic complications in acute renal failure: evaluation of early and frequent dialysis on prognosis.* Kidney Int 1:190, 1972.

97. Kennedy, AC, Burton, JA, Luke, RG, et al.: *Factors affecting the prognosis in acute renal failure.* Q J Med 42:73, 1973.

98. Fischer, RP, and Polk, HJ: *Changing etiologic patterns of renal insufficiency in surgical patients.* Surg Gynecol Obstet 140:85, 1975.

99. OKEN, DE: *Nosologic considerations in the nomenclature of acute renal failure.* Nephron 8:505, 1971.

100. ORECKLIN, JR, AND BROSMAN, SA: *Current concepts in the diagnosis of acute renal failure.* J Urol 107:892, 1972.

101. BRITTON, KE, NIMMON, CC, WHITFIELD, HN, ET AL.: *Obstructive nephropathy: successful evaluation with radionuclides.* Lancet 1:905, 1979.

102. SHERWOOD, T, DOYLE, FH, BOULTON-JONES, M, ET AL.: *The intravenous urogram in acute renal failure.* Br J Radiol 47:368, 1974.

103. FRANKLIN, SS, AND MAXWELL, MH: *Acute renal failure,* in MAXWELL, MH, AND KLEEMAN, CR (eds.): *Clinical Disorders of Fluid and Electrolyte Metabolism,* ed 3. New York: McGraw-Hill Book Company, 1980.

104. MILLER, TR, ANDERSON, RJ, LINAS, SL, ET AL.: *Urinary diagnostic indices in acute renal failure. A prospective study.* Ann Intern Med 89:47, 1978.

105. ESPINEL, CH: *The FE_{Na} test. Use in the differential diagnosis of acute renal failure.* JAMA 236:579, 1976.

106. KRAGELUND, E: *Renal function after major surgery assessed on the basis of 24-hour creatinine clearance.* Acta Chir Scand 117:416, 1959.

107. FIGDOR, PP, HÖLTL, G, ZEKERT, F, ET AL.: *Changes in renal function associated with operations.* Int Nephrol 4:109, 1972.

108. DEUTSCH, S: *Effects of anesthetics on the kidney.* Surg Clin North Am 55:775, 1975.

109. COUSINS, MJ, AND MAZZE, RI: *Anaesthesia, surgery, and renal function. Immediate and delayed effects.* Anaesth Intensive Care 1:355, 1973.

110. PETTINGER, WA: *Anesthetics and the renin-angiotensin-aldosterone axis.* Anesthesiology 48:393, 1978.

111. MILLER, ED, LONGNECKER, DE, AND PEACH, MJ: *The regulatory function of the renin-angiotensin system during general anesthesia.* Anesthesiology 48:399, 1978.

112. HOYE, RC, BENNETT, SH, GEELHOED, GW, ET AL.: *Fluid volume and albumin kinetics occurring with major surgery.* JAMA 222:1255, 1972.

113. SØRENSEN, MB, AND ENGELL, HC: *Blood volume and hemodynamic changes in relation to extensive vascular operations.* Surg Gynecol Obstet 147:369, 1978.

114. GORFINKEL, HJ, SZIDON, JP, HIRSCH, LJ, ET AL.: *Renal performance in experimental cardiogenic shock.* Am J Physiol 222:1260, 1972.

115. ABEL, RM, WICK, J, BECK, CH, ET AL.: *Renal dysfunction following openheart operations.* Arch Surg 108:175, 1974.

116. BHAT, JG, GLUCK, MC, LOWENSTEIN, J, ET AL.: *Renal failure after open-heart surgery.* Ann Intern Med 87:677, 1976.

117. ABEL, RM, BUCKLEY, MJ, AUSTEN, WG, ET AL.: *Etiology, incidence, and prognosis of renal failure following cardiac operations.* J Thorac Cardiovasc Surg 71:323, 1976.

118. ABEL, RM, BUCKLEY, MJ, AUSTEN, WG, ET AL.: *Acute postoperative renal failure in cardiac surgical patients.* J Surg Res 20:341, 1976.

119. HEIMANN, H, BRAU, S, SAKURAI, H, ET AL.: *Acid-base changes in renal dysfunction following open-heart surgery.* Mt Sinai J Med 45:471, 1978.

120. SZILAGYI, DE, SMITH, RF, AND WHITCOMB, JG: *The kidneys in surgery of the abdominal aorta.* Arch Surg 79:252, 1959.

121. NANSON, EM, AND NOBLE, JG: *The effect on the kidneys of cross-clamping the abdominal aorta distal to the renal arteries.* Surgery 46:388, 1959.

122. GORE, I, AND HIRST, AE: *Atherosclerotic aneurysms of the abdominal aorta.* Prog Cardiovasc Dis 16:113, 1973.

123. LUFT, FC, HAMBURGER, RJ, DYER, JK, ET AL.: *Acute renal failure following operation for aortic aneurysm.* Surg Gynecol Obstet 141:374, 1975.

124. SPYRON, P, JONES, N, AND MATSUMOTO, T: *Pathophysiology and management of hypotension following declamping of abdominal aorta.* Ann Surg 176:805, 1972.

125. KASSIRER, JP: *Thombosis and embolism of the renal vessels,* in EARLEY, LE, AND GOTTSCHALK, CW (eds.): *Strauss and Welt's Diseases of The Kidney.* Boston: Little, Brown and Company, 1979.

126. HERMRECK, AS, BERG, RA, RUHLEN, JR, ET AL.: *Renal response in sepsis.* Arch Surg 107:169, 1973.

127. LUCAS, CE, RECTOR, FE, WERNER, M, ET AL.: *Altered renal homeostasis with acute sepsis.* Arch Surg 106:444, 1973.

128. Rector, F, Goyal, S, Rosenberg, IK, et al.: *Sepsis: a mechanism for vasodilatation in the kidney.* Ann Surg 178:222, 1973.

129. Lucas, CE: *The renal response to acute injury and sepsis.* Surg Clin North Am 56:953, 1976.

130. Gutman, RA, Striker, GE, Guilland, BC, et al.: *The immune complex glomerulonephritis of bacterial endocarditis.* Medicine 51:1, 1972.

131. Eknoyen, G, and Dillman, RO: *Renal complications of infectious diseases.* Med Clin North Am 52:979, 1978.

132. Beaufils, M, Morel-Maroger, L, Sraer, JD, et al.: *Acute renal failure of glomerular origin during visceral abscesses.* N Engl J Med 295:185, 1976.

133. Bennett, WM, Plamp, C, and Porter, GA: *Drug-related syndromes in clinical nephrology.* Ann Intern Med 87:582, 1977.

134. Gary, NE, Buzzeo, L, Salaki, J, et al.: *Gentamicin associated acute renal failure.* Arch Intern Med 136:1101, 1976.

135. Dunn, MJ, and Zambraski, EJ: *The effects on the kidney of drugs which inhibit prostaglandin synthesis.* Kidney Int 18:609, 1980.

136. Baylis, C, Rennke, HR, and Brenner, BM: *Mechanisms of the defect in glomerular filtration associated with gentamicin administration.* Kidney Int 12:344, 1977.

137. Hollenberg, NK, Adams, DF, Oken, DE, et al.: *Acute renal failure due to nephrotoxins.* N Engl J Med 282:1329, 1970.

138. Bennett, WM, Gilbert, DN, Houghton, D, et al.: *Gentamicin nephrotoxicity—morphologic and pharmacologic features.* West J Med 126:65, 1977.

139. Kahlmeter, G, Hallberg, T, and Kamme, C: *Gentamicin and tobramycin in patients with various infections—nephrotoxicity.* J Antimicrob Chemother 4(Suppl A):47, 1978.

140. Carlson, GC, Scheiner, E, Colaco, FM, et al.: *Nephrotoxic antibiotics in patients with renal failure.* Crit Care Med 7:1, 1979.

141. Riff, LJ, and Jackson, GG: *Pharmacology of gentamicin in man.* J Infect Dis 124(Suppl):S98, 1971.

142. Schentag, JJ, Jusko, WJ, and Plaut, ME: *Comparative tests for aminoglycoside nephrotoxicity.* Clin Pharmacol Ther 23:128, 1978.

143. Wade, JC, Smith, CR, Petty, BG, et al.: *Cephalothin plus an aminoglycoside is more nephrotoxic than methicillin plus an aminoglycoside.* Lancet 2:604, 1978.

144. Barza, M, Pinn, V, Tanguay, P, et al.: *Nephrotoxicity of newer cephalosporins and aminoglycosides alone and in combination in the rat model.* J Antimicrob Chemother 4(Suppl A):59, 1978.

145. Butkus, DE, deTorrente, A, and Terman, DS: *Renal failure following gentamicin in combination with clindamycin.* Nephron 17:307, 1976.

146. Appel, GB, and Neu, HC: *The nephrotoxicity of antimicrobial agents.* N Engl J Med 296:784, 1977.

147. Appel, GB, and Neu, HC: *The nephrotoxicity of antimicrobial agents.* N Engl J Med 296:722, 1977.

148. Barza, M: *The nephrotoxicity of cephalosporins: an overview.* J Infect Dis 137(Suppl):S60, 1978.

149. Barrientos, A, Bello, I, and Gutierrez-Millet, V: *Renal failure and cephalothin.* Ann Intern Med 84:612, 1976.

150. Simpson, IJ: *Nephrotoxicity and acute renal failure associated with cephalothin and cephaloridine.* NZ Med J 74:312, 1971.

151. Ditlove, J, Weidmann, P, Bernstein, M, et al.: *Methicillin nephritis.* Medicine 56:483, 1977.

152. Appel, GB, and Neu, HC: *The nephrotoxicity of antimicrobial agents.* N Engl J Med 296:663, 1977.

153. Frascino, JA, Vanamee, P, and Rosen, PP: *Renal oxalosis and azotemia after methoxyflurane anesthesia.* N Engl J Med 283:676, 1970.

154. Mazze, RI, Trudell, JR, and Cousins, MB: *Methoxyflurane metabolism and renal dysfunction: clinical correlation in man.* Anesthesiology 35:247, 1971.

155. Cousins, MB, and Mazze, RI: *Methoxyflurane nephrotoxicity: a study of dose response in man.* JAMA 225:1611, 1973.

156. Mazze, RI, and Cousins, MB: *Combined nephrotoxicity of gentamicin and methoxyflurane anesthesia: a case report.* Br J Anaesth 45:394, 1973.

157. Berglund, F, Killander, J, and Pompeius, R: *The effect of trimethoprimsulfamethoxazole on the renal excretion of creatinine in man.* J Urol 114:802, 1975.

158. SHOUVAL, D, LIGUMSKY, M, AND BEN-ISHAY, D: *Effect of co-trimoxazole on normal creatinine clearance.* Lancet 1:244, 1978.

159. BYRD, L, AND SHERMAN, RL: *Radiocontrast-induced acute renal failure: a clinical and pathophysiologic review.* Medicine 58:270, 1979.

160. PORT, FK, WAGONER, RD, AND FULTON, RE: *Acute renal failure after arteriography.* Am J Roentgenol 121:544, 1974.

161. HENEGHAN, M: *Contrast-induced acute renal failure.* Am J Roentgenol 113:1113, 1978.

162. ALEXANDER, RD, BERKES, SL, AND ABUELO, JG: *Contrast media-induced oliguric renal failure.* Arch Intern Med 138:381, 1978.

163. ANSARI, Z, AND BALDWIN, DS: *Acute renal failure due to radio-contrast agents.* Nephron 17:28, 1976.

164. KNOCHEL, JP: *Environmental heat illness. An eclectic review.* Arch Intern Med 133:841, 1974.

165. HAMILTON, RW, GARDNER, LB, PENN, AS, ET AL.: *Acute tubular necrosis caused by exercise induced myoglobinuria.* Arch Intern Med 77:77, 1972.

166. SCHRIER, RW, HENDERSON, HS, TISHER, CC, ET AL.: *Nephropathy associated with heat stress and exercise.* Ann Intern Med 67:356, 1967.

167. SCHRIER, RW, HANO, J, KELLER, HI, ET AL.: *Renal, metabolic, and circulatory responses to heat and exercise.* Ann Intern Med 73:213, 1970.

168. KNOCHEL, JP, DOTIN, LN, AND HAMBURGER, RJ: *Heat stress, exercise and muscle injury: effects on urate metabolism and renal function.* Ann Intern Med 81:321, 1974.

169. YOST, JW, AND HOLMES, FF: *Myoglobinuria following lightning stroke.* JAMA 228:1147, 1974.

170. OLIVERO, J, AND AYUS, JC: *Rhabdomyolysis and acute myoglobinuric renal failure. Complications of inferior vena cava ligation.* Arch Intern Med 138:1548, 1978.

171. KNOCHEL, JP: *Rhabdomyolysis and effects of potassium deficiency on muscle structure and function.* Cardiovas Med 3:247, 1978.

172. KNOCHEL, JP, BARCENAS, C, COTTON, JR, ET AL.: *Hypophosphatemia and rhabdomyolysis.* J Clin Invest 62:1240, 1978.

173. DOMINIC, JA, KOCH, M, GUTHRIE, GP, ET AL.: *Primary aldosteronism presenting as myoglobinuric acute renal failure.* Arch Intern Med 138:1433, 1978.

174. ULVILA, JM, AND NESSAN, VJ: *Hypernatremia with myoglobinuria.* Am J Med Sci 265:79, 1973.

175. SLOAN, MF, FRANKS, AJ, EXLEY, KA, ET AL.: *Acute renal failure due to polymyositis.* Br Med J 2:1457, 1978.

176. GRÜNFELD, JP, GANEVAL, D, CHANARD, J, ET AL.: *Acute renal failure in McArdle's disease.* N Engl J Med 286:1237, 1972.

177. SCHRIER, RW: *Acute renal failure.* Kidney Int 15:205, 1979.

178. SEGAL, AJ, MILLER, M, AND MOSES, AM: *Hypercalcemia during the diuretic phase of acute renal failure.* Ann Intern Med 68:1066, 1968.

179. LEONARD, CD, AND EICHNER, ER: *Acute renal failure and transient hypercalcemia in idiopathic rhabdomyolysis.* JAMA 211:1539, 1970.

180. DEMORGAN, NP, AND WATERHOUSE, C: *A case of tertiary hyperparathyroid crisis.* Am J Med Sci 256:322, 1968.

181. DETORRENTE, A, BERL, T, COHN, PD, ET AL.: *Hypercalcemia of acute renal failure. Clinical significance and pathogenesis.* Am J Med 61:119, 1976.

182. MELTZ, DJ, BERTLES, JF, DAVID, DS, ET AL.: *Delayed haemolytic transfusion reaction with renal failure.* Lancet 2:1348, 1971.

183. ZIMMERMAN, JE: *Respiratory failure complicating post-traumatic acute renal failure: etiology, clinical features, and management.* Ann Surg 174:12, 1971.

184. SIEGLER, RL, AND BLOOMER, HA: *Acute renal failure with prolonged oliguria.* JAMA 225:133, 1970.

185. MERINO, GE, BUSELMEIER, TJ, AND KJELLSTRAND, CM: *Postoperative chronic renal failure.* Ann Surg 182:37, 1975.

186. HOLLENBERG, NK, EPSTEIN, M, ROSEN, SM, ET AL.: *Acute oliguric renal failure in man: evidence for preferential renal cortical ischemia.* Medicine 47:455, 1968.

187. FLORES, J, DIBONA, DR, BECK, CH, ET AL.: *The role of cell swelling in ischemic renal damage and the protective effect of hypertonic solute.* J Clin Invest 51:118, 1972.

188. STAHL, WM: *Effect of mannitol on the kidney. Changes in intrarenal hemodynamics.* N Engl J Med 272:381, 1965.

189. WENDLING, MG, ECKSTEIN, JW, AND ABBOUD, FM: *Effects of mannitol on the renal circulation.* J Clin Lab Med 74:541, 1969.

190. BARRY, KG, COHEN, A, KNOCHEL, JP, ET AL.: *Mannitol infusion. II. The prevention of acute functional renal failure during resection of an aneurysm of the abdominal aorta.* N Engl J Med 264:967, 1961.

191. BARRY, KG, AND BERMAN, AR: *Mannitol infusion. III. The acute effect of the intravenous infusion of mannitol on blood and plasma volumes.* N Engl J Med 264:1085, 1961.

192. BARRY, KG, COHEN, A, AND LEBLANC, P: *Mannitolization. I. The prevention and therapy of oliguria associated with cross-clamping of the abdominal aorta.* Surgery 50:335, 1961.

193. BARRY, KG: *Post-traumatic renal shutdown in humans: its prevention and treatment by the intravenous infusion of mannitol.* Milit Med 128:224, 1963.

194. DOBERNECK, RC, MAZZE, RI, SCHWARTZ, FD, ET AL.: *Effect of hypertonic mannitol infusion on renal clearances in humans with normal or diseased kidneys.* J Urol 91:123, 1964.

195. SEITZMAN, DM, MAZZE, RI, SCHWARTZ, FD, ET AL.: *Mannitol diuresis: a method of renal protection during surgery.* J Urol 90:139, 1962.

196. ABBOTT, WM, AND AUSTEN, WG: *The reversal of renal cortical ischemia during aortic occlusion by mannitol.* J Surg Res 16:482, 1974.

197. BARRY, KG, MAZZE, RI, AND SCHWARTZ, FD: *Prevention of surgical oliguria and renal-hemodynamic suppression by sustained hydration.* N Engl J Med 270:1371, 1964.

198. FINN, WF: *Acute Renal Failure,* in EARLEY, LE, AND GOTTSCHALK, CW (eds.): *Strauss and Welt's Diseases of The Kidney.* Boston: Little, Brown and Company, 1979.

199. LUKE, RG, BRIGGS, JD, ALLISON, MEM, ET AL.: *Factors determining response to mannitol in acute renal failure.* Am J Med Sci 259:168, 1970.

200. LEVINSKY, NG, AND ALEXANDER, EA: *Acute Renal Failure,* in BRENNER, BM, AND RECTOR, FC (eds.): The Kidney. Philadelphia: WB Saunders Co., 1976.

201. AUGER, RG, DAYTON, DA, HARRISON, CE, ET AL.: *Use of ethacrynic acid in mannitol-resistant oliguric renal failure.* JAMA 206:891, 1968.

202. BRADLEY, VE, SHIER, MR, LUCAS, CF, ET AL.: *Renal hemodynamic response to furosemide in septic and injured patients.* Surgery 79:549, 1976.

203. KJELLSTRAND, CM: *Ethacrynic acid in acute tubular necrosis.* Nephron 9:337, 1972.

204. LUKE, RG, LINTON, AL, BRIGGS, JD, ET AL.: *Mannitol therapy in acute renal failure.* Lancet 1:980, 1965.

205. BAEK, SM, BROWN, RS, AND SHOEMAKER, WC: *Early prediction of acute renal failure and recovery: II. Renal function response to furosemide.* Ann Surg 178:605, 1973.

206. PATAK, RV, LIFSCHITZ, MD, AND STEIN, JH: *Acute renal failure: clinical aspects and pathophysiology.* Cardiovas Med 4:19, 1979.

207. CANTAROVICH, F, GALLI, C, BENEDETTI, L, ET AL.: *High dose furosemide in established acute renal failure.* Br Med J 3:449, 1973.

208. GANEVAL, D, KLEINKNECHT, D, GONZALES-DUQUE, LA: *High-dose furosemide in renal failure.* Br Med J 1:244, 1974.

209. KLEINKNECHT, D, GANEVAL, D, GONZALEZ-DUQUE, LA, ET AL.: *Furosemide in acute oliguric renal failure. A controlled trial.* Nephron 17:51, 1976.

210. EPSTEIN, M, SCHNEIDER, NS, AND BEFELER, B: *Effect of intrarenal furosemide on renal function and intrarenal hemodynamics in acute renal failure.* Am J Med 58:510, 1975.

211. GRIFFITH, GL, MAULL, KI, AND COLEMAN, C: *Acute reversible intrinsic renal failure.* Surg Gynecol Obstet 146:631, 1978.

212. TESCHAN, PE, BAXTER, CR, O'BRIEN, TF, ET AL.: *Prophylactic hemodialysis in the treatment of acute renal failure.* Ann Intern Med 53:992, 1960.

213. FISHER, RP, GRIFFEN, WV, AND CLARK, DS: *Early dialysis in the treatment of acute renal failure.* Surg Gynecol Obstet 123:1019, 1966.

214. CONGER, JD: *A controlled evaluation of prophylactic dialysis in acute renal failure.* J Trauma 15:1056, 1975.

215. GABOW, PA, ANDERSON, RJ, AND SCHRIER, RW: *Acute renal failure.* Cardiovas Med 2:1161, 1977.

216. TENCKHOFF, H: *Peritoneal dialysis today: a new look.* Nephron 12:420, 1974.

217. GALLINA, DL, AND DOMINIQUEZ, JM: *Human utilization of urea nitrogen in low caloric diets.* J Nutr 101:1029, 1971.

218. ABBOTT, WM, ABEL, RM, AND FISCHER, JE: *Treatment of acute renal insufficiency after aortoiliac surgery.* Arch Surg 103:590, 1971.

219. ABEL, RM, ABBOTT, WM, AND FISCHER, JE: *Acute renal failure. Treatment without dialysis by total parenteral nutrition.* Arch Surg 103:513, 1971.

220. ABEL, RM, ABBOTT, WM, BECK, CH, ET AL.: *Essential L-amino acids for hyperalimentation in patients with disordered nitrogen metabolism.* Am J Surg 128:317, 1974.

221. ABEL, RM, SHIH, VE, ABBOTT, WM, ET AL.: *Amino acid metabolism in acute renal failure: influence of intravenous essential L-amino acid hyperalimentation therapy.* Ann Surg 180:350, 1974.

222. ABEL, RM, BECK, CH, ABBOTT, WM, ET AL.: *Improved survival from acute renal failure after treatment with intravenous essential L-amino acids and glucose.* N Engl J Med 288:695, 1973.

223. ABEL, RM, ABBOTT, WM, AND FISCHER, JE: *Intravenous essential L-amino acids and hypertonic dextrose in patients with acute renal failure. Effects on serum potassium, phosphate, and magnesium.* Am J Surg 123:632, 1972.

224. BERGSTRÖM, J, FÜRST, P, HUTTMAN, E, ET AL.: *Parenteral nutrition in uremia.* Acta Anaesth Scand (Suppl 55):147, 1974.

225. TOBACK, FG: *Amino acid enhancement of renal regeneration after acute tubular necrosis.* Kidney Int 12:193, 1977.

226. LEONARD, CD, LUKE, RG, AND SIEGEL, RR: *Parenteral essential amino acids in acute renal failure.* Urology 6:154, 1975.

227. ASBACH, HW, STOECKEL, H, SCHÜLER, HW, ET AL.: *The treatment of hypercatabolic acute renal failure by adequate nutrition and haemodialysis.* Acta Anaesth Scand 18:255, 1974.

228. FREEMAN, JB: *Peripheral parenteral nutrition.* Can J Surg 21:489, 1978.

229. CORAN, AG, AND HERMAN, CM: *The use of parenteral alimentation in renal failure: the effect of an intravenous fat emulsion and essential amino acids on dogs undergoing bilateral nephrectomy.* J Ped Surg 7:21, 1972.

230. KURSH, ED, KLEIN, L, SCHMITT, J, ET AL.: *The effect of uremia on wound tensile strength and collagen formation.* J Surg Res 23:37, 1977.

231. SCOTT, RB, CAMERON, JS, OGG, CS, ET AL.: *Why the persistently high mortality in acute renal failure?* Lancet 2:75, 1972.

232. MINUTH, AN, TERRELL, JB, AND SUKI, WN: *Acute renal failure: a study of the course and prognosis of 104 patients and the role of furosemide.* Am J Med Sci 271:317, 1976.

233. MARSHALL, VC: *Acute renal failure in surgical patients.* Br J Surg 58:17, 1971.

234. BAEK, SM, MAKABALI, GG, AND SHOEMAKER, WC: *Clinical determinants of survival from postoperative renal failure.* Surg Gynecol Obstet 140:685, 1975.

235. CHAPMAN, A, AND LEGRAIN, M: *Acute tubular necrosis and interstitial nephritis,* in HAMBURGER, J, CROSNIER, J, AND GRÜNFELD, JP (eds.): *Nephrology.* New York: John Wiley and Sons, 1979.

236. MCMURRAY, SD, LUFT, FC, MAXWELL, DR, ET AL.: *Prevailing patterns and predictor variables in patients with acute tubular necrosis.* Arch Intern Med 138:950, 1978.

237. BROOKS, DH, AND SCHULHOFF, JW: *Acute nonoliguric renal failure in the postoperative patient.* Crit Care Med 4:193, 1976.

238. LEWERS, DT, MATHEW, TH, MAHER, JF, ET AL.: *Long-term follow-up of renal function and histology after acute tubular necrosis.* Ann Intern Med 73:523, 1970.

239. HARWOOD, TH, HIESTERMAN, DR, ROBINSON, RG, ET AL.: *Prognosis for recovery of function in acute renal failure.* Arch Intern Med 136:916, 1976.

240. *National Health Examination Survey. United States, 1960–1962.* National Center for Health Statistics, Series 11, Department of Health, Education and Welfare, Washington, D.C., 1964.

241. STORM-MATHISEN, H, LÖKEN, H, AND RIAN, U: *Complications in treated arterial hypertension.* Clin Sci Mol Med 45:205, 1973.

242. MANNEY, FM, EBERT, PA, AND SABISTON, DC: *Postoperative myocardial infarction: a study of predisposing factors, diagnosis and mortality in a high risk group of surgical patients.* Ann Surg 172:497, 1970.

243. Goldman, L, Caldera, DL, Nussbaum, SR, et al.: *Multifactional index of cardiac risk in non-cardiac surgical procedures.* N Engl J Med 297:845, 1977.

244. Moyer, JH, Brest, AN, and Nathanson, D: *Medical considerations in the hypertensive patient undergoing surgery.* Am J Cardiol 12:286, 1963.

245. Foëx, P, Meloche, R, and Prys-Roberts, C: *Studies of anaesthesia in relation to hypertension. III. Pulmonary gas exchange during spontaneous ventilation.* Br J Anaesth 43:644, 1971.

246. Prys-Roberts, C, Foëx, P, Greene, CT, and Waterhouse, TD: *Studies of anaesthesia in relation to hypertension. IV. The effects of artificial ventilation on the circulation and pulmonary gas exchanges.* Br J Anaesth 44:335, 1972.

247. Prys-Roberts, C, Greene, LT, Meloche, R, and Foëx, P: *Studies of anaesthesia in relation to hypertension. II. Hemodynamic consequences of induction and endotracheal intubation.* Br J Anaesth 43:531, 1971.

248. Foëx, P, and Prys-Roberts, C: *Anaesthesia and the hypertensive patient.* Br J Anaesth 46:575, 1974.

249. Goldman, L, and Caldera, DL: *Risks of general anesthesia and elective operation in the hypertensive patient.* Anesthesiology 50:285, 1979.

250. Goldman, L, Caldera, DL, Southwick, FS, et al.: *Cardiac factors and complications in non-cardiac surgery.* Medicine 57:357, 1978.

251. Mara, JF, and Baker, JL: *Hypertension and hematomas: prophylaxis with Apresoline.* Br J Plast Surg 30:169, 1977.

252. Rawlins, MD: *Drug interactions and anaesthesia.* Br J Anaesth 50:689, 1978.

253. Katz, RL, Weintraub, HD, and Papper, EM: *Anesthesia, surgery and rauwolfia.* Anesthesiology 25:142, 1964.

254. Alper, MH, Flacke, W, and Krayer, O: *Pharmacology of reserpine and its implications for anesthesia.* Anesthesiology 24:524, 1963.

255. Weinberger, MH, Ramsdell, JW, Rosner, DR, et al.: *Effect of chlorothiazide and sodium on vascular responsiveness to angiotensin II.* Am J Physiol 223:1049, 1972.

256. Kassirer, JP, and Harrington, JT: *Diuretics and potassium metabolism: a reassessment of the need, effectiveness and safety of potassium therapy.* Kidney Int 11:505, 1977.

257. Katz, RL: *Hazardous effects of drugs in hypertensive patients scheduled for elective surgery.* Cardiovas Med 3:1185, 1978.

258. Goddard, JF, and Phillips, OC: *The influence of non-anesthetic drugs on the course of anesthesia.* Pa Med J 68:48, 1965.

259. Prys-Roberts, C: *Medical problems of surgical pateints. Hypertension and ischaemic heart disease.* Ann R Col Surg Engl 58:465, 1976.

260. Viljoen, JF: *Guest discussion.* Anesth Analg (Cleve)54:577, 1975.

261. McMahon, FG: *Management of Essential Hypertension.* Mt. Kisco, New York: Futura Publishing Company, 1978.

262. Hansson, L, Hunyor, SN, Julius, S, et al.: *Blood pressure crisis following withdrawal of clonidine, with special reference to arterial and urinary catecholamine levels, and suggestions for acute management.* Am Heart J 85:605, 1973.

263. Frewin, DB, and Penhall, RK: *Rebound hypertension after sudden discontinuation of methyldopa therapy.* Med J Aust 1:659, 1977.

264. Nies, AS: *Adverse reactions and interactions limiting the use of antihypertensive drugs.* Am J Med 58:493, 1975.

265. Graham, RM, Thornell, IR, Gain, JM, et al.: *Prazosin: the first dose phenomenon.* Br Med J 2:1293, 1976.

266. Lowenstein, J, and Steele, JM: *Prazosin: mechanism of action and role in antihypertensive therapy.* Cardiovas Med 4:885, 1979.

267. Gault, CL: *Drug therapy of hypertension.* Med Clin North Am 62:1273, 1978.

268. Mitchell, HC, and Pettinger, WA: *Long-term treatment of refractory hypertensive patients with minoxidil.* JAMA 239:2131, 1978.

269. Keusch, GW, Weidmann, P, Campese, V, et al.: *Minoxidil therapy in refractory hypertension: analysis of 155 patients.* Nephron 21:1, 1978.

270. Nies, AS: *Clinical pharmacology of antihypertensive drugs.* Med Clin North Am 61:675, 1977.

271. Ryan, JR, Jain, AK, and McMahon, FG: *Minoxidil treatment of severe hypertension.* Curr Ther Res 17:68, 1975.

272. LOWENTHAL, DT, ONESTI, G, MUTTERPERL, R, ET AL.: *Long-term clinical effects, bioavailability and kinetics of minoxidil in relation to renal function.* J Clin Pharmacol 18:500, 1978.

273. LUFT, FC, BLOCH, R, SZWED, JJ, ET AL.: *Minoxidil treatment of malignant hypertension: recovery of renal function.* JAMA 240:1985, 1978.

274. DEAN, RH, AND FOSTER, JH: *Surgical management of renovascular hypertension in older patients.* Med Clin North Am 61:643, 1977.

275. MILLAN, VF, MAST, WE, AND MADIAS, NE: *Non-surgical treatment of severe hypertension due to renal artery intimal fibroplasia by percutaneous transluminal angioplasty.* N Engl J Med 300:1371, 1979.

276. MILLAN, VE, AND MADIAS, NE: *Percutaneous transluminal angioplasty for severe renovascular hypertension due to renal-artery medial fibroplasia.* Lancet 1:993, 1979.

277. GRÜNTZIG, A, KUHLMANN, U, VETTER, W, ET AL.: *Treatment of renovascular hypertension with percutaneous transluminal dilatation of a renal-artery stenosis.* Lancet 1:801, 1978.

278. GAL, TJ, AND COOPERMAN, LH: *Hypertension in the immediate postoperative period.* Br J Anaesth 47:70, 1975.

279. KOUCHOUKOS, NT, SHEPPARD, LC, AND KIRKLIN, JW: *Effect of alterations in arterial pressure on cardiac performance early after open intracardiac operations.* J Thorac Cardiovasc Surg 64:563, 1972.

280. SHEPPARD, LC, AND SAYERS, BM: *Dynamic analysis of the blood pressure response to hypotensive agents, studied in postoperative cardiac surgical patients.* Comput Biomed Res 10:237, 1977.

281. DAGGETT, WM, LAPPAS, DG, AND POWELL, WJ: *Pharmacology of the cardiovascular system in the surgical patient,* in SABISTON, DC (ed.): *Davis-Christopher Textbook of Surgery.* Philadelphia: WB Saunders Company, 1977.

282. GIFFORD, RW: *Management and treatment of malignant hypertension and hypertensive emergencies,* in GENEST, J, KOIW, E, AND KUCHEL, O (eds.): *Hypertension: Pathophysiology and Management.* New York: McGraw-Hill Book Company, 1977.

283. VERSKA, JJ, DEQUATTRO, V, AND WOOLLEY, MM: *Coarctation of the aorta: the abdominal pain syndrome and paradoxical hypertension.* J Thorac Cardiovasc Surg 58:746, 1969.

284. WERTHEIMER, L, FINNERTY, F, BERCU, BA, ET AL.: *Furosemide in essential hypertension.* Arch Intern Med 127:934, 1971.

285. WOODS, JW, BLYTHE, WB, AND HUFFINES, WD: *Management of malignant hypertension complicated by renal insufficiency.* N Engl J Med 291:10, 1974.

286. MAMDANI, BH, LIM, VS, MAHURKAR, SD: *Recovery from prolonged renal failure in patients with accelerated hypertension.* N Engl J Med 291:1343, 1974.

287. PALMER, RF, AND LASSETER, KC: *Sodium nitroprusside.* N Engl J Med 292:294, 1975.

288. BEHINA, R, SIQUEIRA, EB, AND BRUNNER, EA: *Sodium nitroprusside-induced hypotension: effect on renal function.* Anesth Analg 57:521, 1978.

289. AHEARN, DJ, AND GRIM, CE: *Treatment of malignant hypertension with sodium nitroprusside.* Arch Intern Med 113:187, 1974.

290. KOCH-WESER, J: *Diazoxide.* N Engl J Med 294:1271, 1976.

291. MROCZEK, WJ, LEIBEL, BA, DAVIDOV, M, ET AL.: *The importance of rapid administration of diazoxide in accelerated hypertension.* N Engl J Med 285:603, 1971.

292. MOSER, M: *Diazoxide—an effective vasodilator in accelerated hypertension.* Am Heart J 87:791, 1974.

293. THIEN, TA, HUYSMANS, FTM, GERLAG, PGG, ET AL.: *Diazoxide infusion in severe hypertension and hypertensive crisis.* Clin Pharmacol Ther 25:795, 1979.

294. BHATIA, SK, AND FROHLICH, ED: *Hemodynamic comparison of agents useful in hypertensive emergencies.* Am Heart J 85:367, 1973.

295. THOMSON, GE: *The recognition and treatment of hypertensive emergencies.* Drug Therapy:24, April, 1979.

296. ROMANKIEWICZ, JA: *Pharmacology and clinical use of drugs in hypertensive emergencies.* Am J Hosp Pharm 34:185, 1977.

297. WOOD, BC, SHARMA, JN, AND CROUCH, TT: *Oral minoxidil in the treatment of hypertensive crisis.* JAMA 241:163, 1979.

Chapter 14

RHEUMATOLOGY

Raymond E.H. Partridge, M.D.

The rheumatic diseases are among the most common conditions encountered causing pain and loss of physical function and, in some instances, widespread systemic disease. The incidental finding of a musculoskeletal syndrome, arthritis, or connective tissue disease is a relatively common occurrence in patients about to undergo surgery for unrelated conditions. Radiographic evidence of osteoarthritis is almost universal in the older age group and about one-third of these patients are symptomatic. The incidence of probable or definite rheumatoid arthritis, as defined by the American Rheumatology Association criteria, increases steadily with age and may exceed 10 percent of those over age 65. Gout and pseudogout are seen frequently and patients with either disease are prone to develop acute crystal-induced synovitis after surgery. Some of the less common conditions may have specific problems that effect surgery, for instance, the presence of circulating anticoagulants in systemic lupus erythematosus.[1]

The last decade has also seen a large increase in the number of joint reconstructive procedures performed in crippled patients with rheumatoid arthritis and osteoarthritis. A reasonable knowledge, therefore, is required of rheumatic diseases, their complications, and the problems that may arise as a result of antirheumatic drug therapy. The possible effects of corticosteroids, nonsteroidal antiinflammatory drugs, penicillamine, and immunosuppressive or cytotoxic drugs on wound healing, blood coagulation, and response to infectious agents may influence the decision to operate or may cause problems in the postoperative period. Fortunately, the great majority of patients with rheumatic diseases tolerate surgical procedures well with few serious complications and with only minor problems relating to pain and joint stiffness during the postoperative period of mobilization and ambulation.

RHEUMATOID ARTHRITIS (RA)

Rheumatoid arthritis is a peripheral, symmetrical inflammatory arthritis leading to progressive cartilage destruction, joint deformity, and loss of function, with vasculitis and systemic disease affecting other organ systems in a small proportion of patients. Joint inflammation is mediated by immune complexes that activate synovial fluid complement;[2] circulating rheumatoid factors are found in 75 to 80 percent of patients. Serum complement is usually normal or elevated but moderate serum complement depression occurs in severe systemic disease and vasculitis.[3] A moderate normocytic, normochromic anemia, and elevated erythrocyte sedimentation rate are present during active disease. Generalized osteoporosis, sometimes severe, is found in crippled and poorly mobile patients. The process of joint destruction and deformity takes place over a number of years, and in the early stages of the disease few complications will be encountered after surgery. In long-standing disease the length of hospitalization may be influenced by the presence of an active polyarthritis and deformities causing difficulties in postoperative rehabilitation or by extra-articular involvement.

Preoperative Evaluation

Functional capacity can deteriorate rapidly in severely crippled rheumatoid patients who are confined to bed without motion in the postoperative period. A detailed knowledge of preoperative joint function and deformity is necessary for well planned postoperative rehabilitation. Too often these factors are not evaluated adequately, and when patients are not making satisfactory postoperative progress in mobility and ability to administer self care, the absence of an accurate assessment of the preoperative physical state make the goals of rehabilitation more difficult to define.

In all patients undergoing elective surgery, preoperative evaluation of the extent of joint disease should be undertaken.[4] This will include noting the presence or absence of swelling, the presence of deformity and limitation of joint motion, and the degree of muscle wasting. A simple assessment of functional capacity should also be made, particularly the ability to walk with or without assistance, to move around in bed unaided, and to stand from a sitting position. If possible, appropriate assessments should be undertaken with the assistance of a physical therapist who will then be in a position to assist the nursing staff in devising a suitable program for postoperative maintenance of joint function. An evaluation of musculoskeletal problems by the nursing staff and physicians will also help in the correct positioning of deformed joints in an operating room when the patient is under anesthesia and avoid unnecessary stress and forceful manipulation.

A careful search should be made for manifestations of systemic disease which may complicate management.

SKIN LESIONS

The skin in a patient with long-standing rheumatoid arthritis is often thin and atrophic. Loss of dermal collagen is enhanced if corticosteroids have been used in treatment.[5]

Ischemic ulcers may be present above the ankle and over the malleoli, usually as a result of vasculitis, but may be enhanced by external pressure. Rheumatoid nodules over extensor surfaces, particularly on the elbows and buttocks, are sometimes complicated by local tissue breakdown, ulceration of the skin, and infection and may be a potential source of a postoperative systemic infection. Small rheumatoid fistuli may be seen on the upper surface of the metatarsal heads and around the toes.[6] These factors are particularly important in patients undergoing orthopedic joint reconstruction in which metal and plastic prostheses cemented in place with methyl methacrylate are at risk for infection unless measures are taken to eradicate infected lesions prior to surgery. The presence of vasculitic lesions on the skin should alert the examiner to the presence of extra-articular inflammation in other organs.

RHEUMATOID HEART DISEASE

Clinically significant rheumatoid heart disease is uncommon, although pathologically all layers of the heart may be involved with small granulomata and fibrosis. Rheumatoid nodules of the mitral and aortic valves may cause valvular incompetence in patients with long-standing seropositive rheumatoid arthritis.[7] Small pericardial effusions can be demonstrated in nearly half the patients by echocardiography and radiography,[8] but tamponade and pericardial constriction causing heart failure are rarely encountered. QRS voltage is not significantly reduced in these cases and ST-T wave changes are nonspecific. Heart block and arrhythmias may occur but one cannot be sure that they are due to rheumatoid arthritis. A formal cardiologic evaluation is indicated preoperatively if cardiac enlargement is present radiographically, if there is a heart murmur, or if arrhythmia or abnormalities are present on an electrocardiogram.

RHEUMATOID LUNG DISEASE

Rheumatoid lung disease of several different patterns is probably an integral part of the rheumatoid process and increases in frequency in rheumatoid disease of long duration. Interstitial fibrosis,[9] pleuritis with or without effusion,[10] rheumatoid nodules of lung[11] or pleura, and rheumatoid vasculitis are the most common manifestations of rheumatoid lung disease. Unrelated lung conditions including pneumonia, emphysema, bronchitis, and bronchiectasis are said to be more common in rheumatoid patients then in age-matched controls.[12] Impairment of pulmonary diffusing capacity was seen in 40 percent of patients in one study,[13] although most patients were asymptomatic and over one-half had normal chest radiographs. Lung function studies showed decreased lung capacity, decreased vital capacity, and arterial hypoxemia. Evidence of obstructive lung disease is also seen and is exaggerated by cigarette smoking.[14] Diffuse interstitial fibrosis appears radiographically as soft, fluffy patches of infiltrate of a fine reticular nodular pattern at the lung bases. Late disease appears as cysts and honeycombing of the lung. Most patients with early disease are asymptomatic, but coarse rales may be heard at the lung bases. Dyspnea, cyanosis, and clubbing are uncommon and characteristic of late disease. Asymptomatic patients with normal chest radiographs do not need routine pulmonary function tests unless cardiopulmonary surgery is being performed. Lung function studies should be done in patients with longstanding rheumatoid arthritis prior to surgery, particularly if there is exertional dyspnea or if chest radiographic abnormalities are present. These should include tests of ventilation, diffusing capacity, and arterial blood gases. Moderate or severe impairment of lung function, while not an absolute bar to surgery, may influence choice of anesthetic or the decision to perform certain types of elective reconstructive procedures.

ANEMIA

A moderate anemia with low serum iron and low total iron binding capacity is seen in the majority of patients with active rheumatoid disease. The hemoglobin value does not usually fall below 10 gm/dl.[15] If the degree of anemia is greater than this, a search for additional causes should be made. Iron deficiency anemia (in which case the total iron binding capacity will be elevated) due to occult blood loss from the gastrointestinal tract is the most usual cause. There appears to be no increased risk in operating on patients who have adapted to hemoglobin values as low as 10.5 gm/dl but those with lower values should be transfused a few days preoperatively.[16]

OSTEOPOROSIS

Osteoporosis is common in patients with rheumatoid arthritis and is worse in those with progressive deformities and poor mobility. Postmenopausal women are particularly affected and prolonged use of corticosteroids will make generalized osteoporosis worse. Extreme degrees of osteoporosis can be seen in patients with long-standing disease who have been confined to bed for lengthy periods and spontaneous fractures can occur. Careful handling of these patients by the nursing staff and aides is essential and is particularly important for the unconscious patient during and after surgery. Fractures of osteoporotic bone can sometimes occur by forcibly manipulating a limb if severe limitation of joint motion is present.

CERVICAL SPINE INVOLVEMENT

Rheumatoid involvement of the cervical spine is seen in 25 to 30 percent of patients with destructive seropositive disease of long duration.[17] Inflammation of the bursae between the transverse ligament of the atlas and the odontoid process of the axis causes erosion of the bone and ligament attenuation permitting excessive anterior subluxation of the atlas on the axis in cervical spine flexion. Descent of C_1 on C_2 is sometimes seen with a vertical rise of the odontoid into the foramen magnum and rarely, destruction of the odontoid process results in posterior subluxation of C_1 on C_2. Narrowing of the spinal canal may eventually result in cervical myelopathy in a proportion of affected individuals.[18] Fortunately, the anteroposterior diameter of the spinal canal in the upper cervical region is considerably greater than the diameter of the spinal cord, and anterior atlantoaxial subluxation of 10 mm or more is often seen without evidence of cord compression. Many patients are asymptomatic but some have neck pain or pain radiating into the occiput and lower mastoid region. Early signs of cord compression include proprioceptive loss in the hands, moderate hyperreflexia, and positive Babinski's signs.[17] Later, gross neurologic deficit and functional impairment may be present. Although cervical cord trauma leading to neurologic damage during induction of anesthesia or during a surgical procedure is very rare, the surgical team must be aware of the potential problems of an unstable cervical spine in an unconscious patient to avoid unnecessary manipulation of head and neck. Routine lateral cervical spine radiographs in flexion and extension should be taken in rheumatoid patients, particularly those with severe disease. The maximum distance between the posterior surface of the anterior arch of the atlas and the odontoid peg in full neck flexion is 2 to 3 mm as measured radiographically in normal subjects. The use of a soft cervical collar for rheumatoid patients being transported to the operating room serves as a reminder to the operating room staff and anesthesiologist of the presence of a rheumatoid cervical spine.[19] Postoperatively, soft cervical collar is useful in patients with neck or occipital pain and may subsequently be recommended as prophylaxis against cord involvement. Surgical stabilization of atlantoaxial subluxation is not required unless neurologic deficit is present.

OCULAR MANIFESTATIONS

Episcleritis, scleritis, and rheumatoid nodules of the sclera are uncommon[20] and cause no problem to the surgeon. Keratoconjunctivitis sicca (Sjögren's syndrome) occurs in more than 10 percent of rheumatoid patients and may be complicated by corneal abrasion and ulceration. In these patients, the use of artificial tears every two to three hours in the immediate postoperative period will avoid potential complications.

LARYNGEAL INVOLVEMENT

Involvement of cervical spine, larynx, and temporomandibular joints in rheumatoid patients comprise a triad of hazards for the anesthesiologist. Twenty-five percent of patients are said to have cricoarytenoid joint involvement,[21] but clinical problems may not be identified unless the patient is questioned closely. Pain, sometimes radiating to the ear, fullness in the throat on speaking, dyspnea, hoarseness, and occasionally inspiratory stridor may be present. The larynx may be tender to pressure. Cricoarytenoid arthritis produces progressive narrowing and fixation of the vocal cords in adduction causing narrowing of the airway. The diagnosis is confirmed by indirect laryngoscopy which may show immobilized cords in adduction with redness and swelling overlying the arytenoids. Difficulties in preoperative intubation may be encountered requiring a smaller endotracheal tube. Very rarely, preoperative tracheostomy for surgical anesthesia has been required. Postoperatively, extubation should be delayed until the patient is alert. Laryngeal edema as a result of intubation or postoperative respiratory infection poses a considerable risk. Humidified oxygen, antibiotics to control infection, and a short course of corticosteroids may be helpful. Emergency tracheostomy may rarely be required.[22]

Postoperative care

A severe exacerbation of arthritis is uncommon following surgery but increased pain and stiffness can occur following withdrawal of nonsteroidal anti-inflammatory drugs in the postoperative period. Patients receiving oral corticosteroids must receive an equivalent parenteral dose if oral administration is not possible. Other anti-inflammatory drugs that are part of the patients' individual treatment programs should be restarted as soon after surgery as possible. Physical therapy, including passive range of motion exercises for all joints and active bed exercises, must be instituted to prevent joint contractures which can develop *rapidly* in severely debilitated patients. Isometric quadriceps exercises will help to prevent knee contractures. Light ankle splints are preferable to a bed board in the control of foot position and prevention of equinus contracture. Nodules and bony prominences must be protected against ulceration (more common in patients with severe RA). Early postoperative mobilization is essential to minimize loss of function. Many patients with rheumatoid arthritis have a reduced functional capacity that may be temporarily reduced further following major general surgery or orthopedic procedures to upper and lower limbs. A social evaluation must be done before the patient is discharged from the hospital to ascertain that adequate home assistance is available or the patient is able to function independently.

Wound healing

A number of factors might predispose to impairment of wound healing in patients with rheumatoid arthritis including low serum albumin levels, vasculitis, wound hematomas secondary to nonsteroidal drug therapy, and the known effect of corticosteroids. A study by Garner and Mowatt[16] on 100 rheumatoid arthritis patients compared with 100 matched controls with osteoarthritis showed only minor differences in wound healing. Corticosteroid therapy was associated with some increase in wound infection and there was a significant delay in wound healing if corticosteroids had been given for more than three years. No difference between rheumatoid factor positive and negative patients was noted. D-penicillamine, which inhibits collagen cross-linking, is also associated with some delay in wound healing.[23]

Infections

Postoperative infections are probably not increased in rheumatoid arthritis patients who are not receiving corticosteroids although an increased incidence of chest[12] and joint[24] infection has been noted in rheumatoid arthritis patients, possibly related to reduced leukocyte chemotactic activity. Certainly the possibility of septic arthritis should be considered in the differential diagnosis of postoperative exacerbation of joint inflammation. Arthrocentesis and synovial fluid culture is essential in these cases.

Thromboembolism

Thromboembolism and deep venous thrombosis have been studied in patients undergoing lower limb joint replacement.[25] The incidence of deep venous thrombosis is lower in patients with rheumatoid arthritis than with osteoarthritis, although there was no clear correlation with drug therapy. Different authorities have favored warfarin, low-dose heparin,[26] or low molecular weight dextran. Preoperative and postoperative low-dose aspirin, 600 mg twice daily, has been shown to reduce the thromboembolic complications following total hip or knee replacement[27] and is considered the current treatment of choice for prophylaxis of emboli by many authorities.

SYSTEMIC LUPUS ERYTHEMATOSUS (SLE)

Systemic lupus erythematosus is a disease of generalized inflammation characterized by the presence in the serum of autoantibodies to nuclear constituents and circulating immune complexes. Complement-fixing antibodies to native DNA are present in many patients. Women between the ages of 15 to 45 years are principally affected. An erythematous malar rash, polyarthritis, glomerulonephritis, polyserositis, vasculitis, and central nervous system disease are the most frequent clinical manifestations of the disease. A moderate normochromic, normocytic anemia and mild leukopenia are present in many patients[28] and a Coombs-positive hemolytic anemia is found in some cases. Severe thrombocytopenia with purpura occurs in about 5 percent.[29]

Major surgery is occasionally necessary during the course of SLE and intra-abdominal catastrophes from vasculitis may occur requiring emergency intervention. Needle biopsy of the kidney is performed with some frequency. Later in the course of the disease, reconstructive surgery and joint replacement may be necessary for avascular necrosis of bone secondary to corticosteroid therapy. SLE is predominantly a disease of women during the childbearing years, and some may require surgical intervention during pregnancy. Complications following surgery in SLE are few but there is increased risk of postoperative infection and some patients react adversely to drugs. Many patients are treated with corticosteroids, sometimes in prolonged, high doses, which will delay wound healing, increase the risk of infection, and suppress the adrenopituitary axis.

Preoperative Evaluation

A hematologic and coagulation profile is essential in patients requiring surgery. If prothrombin time (PT) or partial thromboplastin time (PTT) are abnormal, specific factor assays are necessary to characterize the nature of the abnormality (see below). If time permits prior to surgery, an evaluation of inflammatory disease activity, immunologic status, and essential organ function should be done. The development of complications in the postoperative period might be due to activation of lupus disease activity, drugs, infection, or other conditions unrelated to SLE. A complete blood count, erythrocyte sedimentation rate, anti-DNA antibody titer, total hemolytic complement, C_3 and C_4 levels, and an immune complex assay are useful evaluations of disease activity. Unless the values are known prior to surgery, there may be difficulty in the interpretation of test values in the postoperative period.

LUPUS NEPHRITIS

Clinical evidence of renal disease is present in more than 50 percent of patients with SLE and usually develops within the first 12 months.[30] The severity of lupus nephritis is variable but a number of patients with diffuse proliferative or membranous glomerulonephritis will develop chronic renal insufficiency at a later stage of the disease. Acute renal failure during the course of SLE is rare. The presence of lupus nephritis in a patient requiring surgery may present special problems for the surgeon. Worsening of renal function indicated by a rise in serum creatinine or oliguria in the postoperative period is more likely to be caused by factors other than an acute exacerbation of lupus nephritis. Prerenal azotemia from depletion of extracellular fluid volume must be recognized early and treated. Acute tubular necrosis (ATN) may follow loss or sequestration of extracellular fluid, hypotension, incompatible blood transfusion, gram-negative sepsis, and the postoperative administration of drugs. Antibiotics including cephalothin, gentamicin, kanamycin, and vancomycin, have been incriminated as causal agents of ATN. Aspirin[31] and other nonsteroidal anti-inflammatory drugs[32] may reduce renal function, perhaps related to prostaglandin synthetase inhibition. An exacerbation of lupus nephritis as a cause of renal failure may be indicated by a fall in serum complement, a rise in anti-DNA antibody, and increased urinary sediment even if other renal complications are known to be present. An increased dose of corticosteroids will be required. High dose "pulses" of methylprednisolone (1 g daily IV for 3 days) have been used to treat severe exacerbation of lupus nephritis[33] but should only be considered when other therapy has failed. The management of renal failure is discussed in detail in Chapter 13, Renal Disease and Hypertension.

GASTROINTESTINAL DISEASE

Abdominal pain, often with nausea and vomiting are relatively common in acute SLE and frequent in childhood.[34] Cramping abdominal pain may indicate increased disease activity. Generalized nonspecific tenderness is present; guarding and rebound tenderness is absent. Mesenteric arteritis leading to bowel infarction and intestinal perforation occurring during active SLE is associated with localized and rebound tenderness and guarding.[35] Emergency surgical intervention is essential. Acute abdominal emergencies due to appendicitis, diverticulitis, peptic ulcer perforation, ruptured ovarian cysts, and other causes may occur during active or inactive SLE and must be differentiated from abdominal crises associated with the disease. The symptoms and signs of an acute abdomen caused by perforation of a hollow viscus may be modified by high-dose corticosteroid therapy. Pancreatitis associated with vasculitis occurs during active SLE and may respond to corticosteroid therapy.[36]

Lupus Anticoagulants

A circulating lupus anticoagulant identified by prolongation of the partial thromboplastin time and slight prolongation of the prothombin time is present in about 9 percent of patients with SLE.[37] The abnormalities of PT and PTT are not corrected by addition of equal volumes of normal plasma to the patients' plasma and in some cases the anticoagulant is present in high titer. Bleeding and clotting times are normal. The lupus anticoagulant may be an antibody against phospholipid required for the coagulation sequence and may account for the strong correlation with false-positive tests for syphilis in SLE.[1] The action of lupus anticoagulant is undoubtedly complex and the exact site of action is uncertain. An absolute decrease in prothrombin concentration has been described in a small number of SLE patients in association with the lupus anticoagulant.[38] Inhibitors against Factors VIII,[39] IX, XI,[40] and XII have been described in some patients with SLE.

Accelerated platelet destruction from antiplatelet antibodies causes thrombocytopenia in about one-third of patients with SLE although severe thrombocytopenia with purpura occurs in about 5 percent.[29] Bone marrow aspiration shows normal or increased megakaryocytes although a decrease in megakaryocytes has been reported in one patient.[41]

The lupus anticoagulant alone is not associated with a bleeding diathesis and major surgery may be performed without risk of hemorrhage.[37,42] The presence of inhibitors against specific clotting factors, an absolute decrease in prothrombin level, and thrombocytopenia are all associated with increased risk of bleeding and require corrective measures before surgery is undertaken.[1,39]

Evaluation and treatment

The presence of the lupus anticoagulant alone is benign and requires no treatment.[1] Inhibitors of specific clotting factors and thrombocytopenia may respond to prednisone, 60 mg daily over a 3 week period.[41] Prothrombin deficiency may not respond to corticosteroid therapy.[43] Platelet transfusion has been used as an emergency measure in thrombocytopenic SLE patients as an adjunct to corticosteroid therapy.[1] Platelets from 1 U of blood should raise the platelet count by 5,000 to 10,000 for two to four days.[44] Survival time of transfused platelets may be shortened by immune destruction in SLE and serial platelet counts over 24 hours are necessary to estimate survival. Cytotoxic drugs and splenectomy have been used for correction of thrombocytopenia in resistant cases.

Factors responsible for thrombocytopenia and clotting factor inhibition have been demonstrated in some cases to be circulating antibodies of the IgG class. Plasmapheresis has been used to reduce the levels of circulating antibodies and immune complexes in patients with SLE[45] and to remove inhibitors of Factor VIII in a patient with hemophilia.[46] Plasma exchange might be considered in emergency situations in the treatment of SLE complicated by thrombocytopenia and abnormal coagulation profiles. Fibrinogen levels after plasmapheresis return to normal within 48 hours, but the effect on antibody levels may be prolonged, allowing a time period when the risk of postsurgical bleeding is diminished. In the recent experience of this author, a rise in platelet count to normal was seen in 2 patients with SLE and thrombocytopenia after four 50 percent plasma exchanges, but the effect on circulating anticoagulants was less certain.

The observation that SLE may become more active after surgery has been suggested by Ropes.[47] This may be prevented by using increased doses of corticosteroids during surgery and in the immediate postoperative period for 2 weeks.[48] Increased disease activity may occur during pregnancy, following abortion, and postpartum requiring higher doses of corticosteroids to regain control of the disease.[49] Acute polyserositis after an extensive burn has been noted, probably reflecting an antigenic stimulus from tissue breakdown.[50]

All SLE patients should be observed carefully for infections in the postoperative period. Blood, urine, and wound cultures must be obtained if postoperative fever occurs. Prophylactic antibiotics should not be given routinely unless dental surgery is being performed.

Allergic reactions to drugs may be more common in patients with SLE including drug fever and rash from ampicillin[51] and acute anaplylaxis from ibuprofen.[52] Acute exacerbation of SLE has been observed after treatment of urinary tract infection with sulfisoxazole (Gantrisin).[29] None of these drugs should be used in the treatment of SLE if adequate substitutes are available. Prolonged administration of corticosteroids may delay normal healing and predispose patients to bacterial infections.

DERMATOMYOSITIS AND POLYMYOSITIS

Adults with dermatomyositis and polymyositis may require surgery for a number of reasons, including surgical removal of a neoplasm that is associated with the adult disease in about 10 percent of cases. Weakness is variable, but shoulder girdle and hip girdle weakness may make postoperative management and ambulation difficult. Involvement of pharyngeal muscles causes pooling of saliva in the valecular and pyriform sinuses, dysphagia, and dysphonia. The patient may be unable to swallow saliva and is at risk for the development of inhalation pneumonia or lung abscess. Respiratory muscle weakness may occur in severe cases but generally respiratory function is only mildly affected. Radiographically a mild pulmonary fibrosis may be present. Cardiac muscle involvement is reflected in an abnormal electrocardiogram in about 50 percent of patients, the most frequent abnormalities being nonspecific ST-T wave changes, bundle-branch block, and arrhythmias.[53] None of these abnormalities are likely to be significant in the postoperative period.

Pharyngeal muscle involvement is more likely to be present in patients with untreated or active disease and in patients refractory to corticosteroid therapy. Patients undergoing surgery requiring the use of general anesthesia should be evaluated for posterior pharyngeal muscle involvement by barium studies or esophagogram. Many patients with dermatomyositis will be undergoing treatment with corticosteroids and will require increased doses during the operative procedure and in the immediate postoperative period.

OTHER CONNECTIVE TISSUE DISEASES

Neither scleroderma or mixed connective tissue disease appear to be associated with significant postoperative complications. Impairment of lung diffusing capacity and pulmonary fibrosis is present in many cases and should be evaluated preoperatively but the impairment is rarely severe enough to cause significant problems during or after surgery. Corrective surgery for finger contractures has been described with only slight delay in wound healing,[54] although the risk of poor healing may increase with severe ischemia. Involvement of the gastrointestinal tract may sometimes require surgical intervention including nondilatable esophageal stricture[55] and adynamic ileus leading to obstruction. If possible, episodes of subacute obstruction should be managed conservatively with intubation and decompression but bowel resection is required in some cases.[56] Pneumatosis cystoides intestinalis[56] with submucous gaseous cysts may cause obstruction or pneumoperitoneum from cyst rupture. Abdominal wound healing does not appear to be significantly altered in scleroderma, but the risk of postoperative ileus is probably high if the gastrointestinal tract is involved.

SERONEGATIVE POLYARTHRITIS

Juvenile Rheumatoid Arthritis

Restriction of cervical spinal motion occurs in nearly 50 percent of children with polyarticular juvenile rheumatoid arthritis (JRA). Apophysial joint narrowing and fusion of the upper cervical vertebra progressing to impairment of cervical extension may cause serious difficulties in intubation in a few children. Flexion and extension radiographs of the cervical spine should be obtained prior to anesthesia in children with limited neck motion. Modification of the usual methods of anesthetic administration may be required.[57]

Ankylosing Spondylitis

Cervical spine involvement in patients with ankylosing spondylitis may progress to cervical fusion. Reduction in cervical spinal extension and sometimes severe flexion deformity may occur. Similar difficulties in intubation may be encountered as mentioned above. Limited chest expansion occurs in most patients with ankylosing spondylitis. Significant impairment of respiratory function is rare and postoperative chest complications do not appear to be greater than expected.

GOUT

Hyperuricemia (plasma urate levels above 7 mg/dl) is a common condition resulting from several different mechanisms including de novo overproduction of urate, renal disease, and drug administration (commonly diuretics). Individuals with hyperuricemia of long duration are at risk for development of acute gouty arthritis as a result of crystallization of monosodium urate crystals in and around joints. An acute gouty attack is usually monarthric, the first metatarsophalangeal joint being involved in 60 percent of first attacks followed in frequency by tarsal joints, ankles, heels, knees, wrists, fingers, and elbows. Joint swelling and redness may resemble a cellulitis. Systemic signs of inflammation occur in some patients including fever, leukocytosis, and elevation of the erythrocyte sedimentation rate. Pain and tenderness are usually severe, reaching a maximum within a few hours.[58] An attack may be precipitated in hyperuricemic or gouty individuals by several events including use of certain drugs, trauma, starvation, and surgery. The risk of postoperative gout in these patients is high. Linton and Talbott[59] described acute postoperative gout following surgery for removal of tophi in more than 80 percent of 22 gouty patients who were not receiving prophylactic colchicine, although the attack rate after other surgical procedures may be less. A gouty attack usually occurs between the third and fifth postoperative day and less commonly thereafter. The mechanism of postoperative gout is uncertain. A rapid rate of change of plasma urate level correlates with the development of acute gout, and it has been postulated that there is a disturbance in the dynamic equilibrium of urate in the postoperative period. No consistent change in plasma urate level after surgery has been observed, although a two to threefold increase in urinary uric acid excretion from the second or third postoperative day has been reported following abdominal surgery implying a transient alteration of urate metabolism.[60]

Plasma urate levels should be measured preoperatively. For individuals with a prior history of gouty attacks and those with plasma urate levels greater than 9 mg/dl, colchicine, 0.5 mg twice a day, orally, for three days prior to surgery may prevent postoperative gout.

The diagnosis of acute gout should be suspected in patients who develop a monoarticular arthritis or polyarthritis of the lower limb joints in the first few days after surgery. Confirmation of the diagnosis should be attempted in all cases, including those with apparently typical podagra, by synovial fluid aspiration and demonstration of negatively birefringent intracellular crystals in synovial fluid leukocytes by compensated polarized light microscopy. Only a drop of two of synovial fluid is required. In cases of polyarticular gout, arthrocentesis of more than one joint may be necessary to demonstrate crystals and confirm the diagnosis. Plasma urate levels alone may be misleading as acute gouty attacks can occur at times when the level is normal and hyperuricemia may be unrelated to arthritis.

A wide range of drugs are available for treatment of acute gout. Colchicine given orally, 0.5 mg every hour, is the traditional treatment for gout,[61] but there is a high incidence of gastrointestinal toxicity in elderly patients in whom electrolyte imbalance and dehydration may occur. Intravenous colchicine, 1.0 mg (2 ml) as a single dose followed by 0.5 mg every six hours to a maximum of 3 mg in 24 hours avoids gastrointestinal disturbance in most patients and has been recommended for postoperative patients unable to take oral medication. Severe local tissue irritation can occur from extravasation. This route must not be used in patients with renal impairment.

For patients able to take oral medication, nonsteroidal anti-inflammatory drugs are very effective. Naproxen 1.0 g,[62] fenoprofen (2.4 g),[63] ibuprofen (2.4 g), or indomethacin (300 mg) in divided doses in the first 24 hours followed by smaller maintenance doses over the next few days have low toxicity and are preferred to oral colchicine. A single joint with proven gouty inflammation by diagnostic arthrocentesis may be treated by injection of a single dose of intra-articular corticosteroid.

Antihyperuricemic agents, allopurinol and uricosuric drugs, have no place in the treatment of the acute attack. A decision to use these agents must be deferred until all signs of acute gout have subsided.

ARTICULAR CHONDROCALCINOSIS (PSEUDOGOUT)

The presence of microcrystalline deposits of calcium pyrophosphate dihydrate (CPPD) in articular cartilage is associated with self-limited attacks of inflammation in one, or occasionally two or three, joints. Most patients are 60 years of age or older. The knee joint is the site of more than 50 percent of acute attacks; wrists, elbows, ankles, shoulders, hips, and first metatarsophalangeal joints (pseudopodagra) may also be affected. The redness and swelling of the joint take longer to reach peak intensity than with gout; fever and leukocytosis may be present. Attacks are commonly precipitated by trauma, severe medical illness, and surgery, occurring after surgery in 9.4 percent of 106 patients with chondrocalcinosis in one series.[64]

Radiographic evidence of calcium deposition within the joint is often present. The diagnosis is confirmed by the identification of weakly positive birefringent crystals of calcium pyrophosphate within the leukocytes of an inflammatory synovial fluid. Hyperuricemia is present in 20 percent of patients with CPPD deposits and 5 percent of these also have articular urate deposits.[65] The distinction between gout and pseudogout can only be made by synovial fluid analysis and crystal indentification.

Removal of synovial fluid from the joint is often followed by amelioration of the attack. When CPPD crystals have been identified, local instillation of corticosteroid esters produces a rapid anti-inflammatory response. Oral administration of colchicine is not reliably effective, although success with intravenous colchicine is reported.[65] Nonsteroidal drugs, particularly indomethacin, are also effective and may be combined with intra-articular steroid injection.

PAGET'S DISEASE OF BONE

This disorder, which is more common in men over the age of 40, is usually a local, asymptomatic condition causing no disability either during or after surgery. Levels of plasma calcium and phosphorous are normal, as bone resorption and new bone formation are equal. If skeletal involvement is extensive, confinement to bed following surgery or during treatment of lower limb fractures reduces bone repair and may cause mobilization of calcium with hypercalcemia, hypercalciuria, and renal stones.[66] Frequent monitoring of plasma calcium values is necessary in the postoperative (or immobilization) period. Early ambulation should be the rule and usually leads to a fall in plasma calcium level. If early mobilization is impossible, hypercalcemia and hypercalciuria can usually be treated satisfactorily with a large fluid intake and neutral sodium phosphate, 5 to 6 gm daily with regular monitoring of plasma calcium, phosphorous, and blood urea nitrogen. Use of intravenous saline and furosemide is also effective in reducing hypercalcemia but the increase in urinary calcium excretion by this method could theoretically lead to renal stone formation (see Chapter 5, Endocrinology). High output cardiac failure from bone hypervascularity may be present in Paget's disease if more than 30 percent of the skeleton is affected. Postoperative fluid balance should be carefully monitored when cardiac failure is present.

ANTIRHEUMATIC DRUGS

Many patients suffering from a rheumatic disease take nonsteroidal anti-inflammatory and analgesic drugs on a chronic basis for relief of pain and stiffness; some may be on long-term corticosteroid therapy or may be receiving gold, penicillamine, cytotoxic agents or prophylactic drugs against gout. In most instances, the use of antirheumatic drugs presents no problem to the surgeon, but the potential side effects and toxicities of the major drug classes should be understood to limit the possibility of inappropriate administration or withdrawal in the preoperative and postoperative period. With the exception of corticosteroids, antirheumatic drugs can be stopped, if necessary, for several days before and after surgery without much harm to the patient apart from some increase in pain and stiffness. As a general rule, anti-inflammatory drugs should be resumed as soon as possible after surgery to facilitate rehabilitation. Table 1 shows a classification of antirheumatic drugs.

Effect of Antirheumatic Drugs on Platelets

The use of aspirin in small doses prolongs bleeding time up to two-fold[67] and has a minor effect on vitamin K dependent clotting factors.[68] Platelet aggregation is strongly inhibited by aspirin.[69] Acetylation of platelet cyclo-oxygenase by aspirin irreversibly inactivates the enzyme, thus inhibiting the prostaglandin production[70] that normally causes adenosine diphosphate (ADP) and serotonin release leading to platelet aggregation. Administration of 300 mg of aspirin will cause maximum inhibition which lasts for several days (the life span of the platelet).[71] In spite of this effect, there is little evidence of excessive bleeding at the time of surgery in patients taking aspirin, but as a precaution the drug should be discontinued for one week prior to elective surgery. Sodium salicylate and other salicylates lacking the acetyl radical do not affect platelet aggregation.[72] Other nonsteroidal anti-inflammatory drugs have a reversible effect on platelet aggregation for several hours,[73] the duration of effect being related to the plasma half-life of the drug.

Drug-Drug Interactions

Aspirin in excess of 3 g daily augments the hypoprothrombinemia associated with use of warfarin, and concomitant use of aspirin and with anticoagulants should be

TABLE 1. Antirheumatic Drug Classification

1. *Nonsteroidal Anti-inflammatory Drugs*	3. *Cytotoxic Agents*
Aspirin and salicylates	Cyclophosphamide
Propionic acids	Azathioprine
Ibuprofen	Methotrexate
Fenoprofen	
Naproxen	4. *Corticosteroids*
Indoles and related drugs	
Indomethacin	5. *Antihyperuricemic Drugs*
Tolmetin	Allopurinol
Sulindac	Probenecid
Pyrazolones	Sulfinpyrazone
Phenylbutazone	
Oxyphenbutazone	6. *Colchicine*
Fenamates	
Mefenamic acid	7. *Analgesics*
Meclofenamate sodium	Acetaminophen
	Propoxyphene
2. *Slow Acting Antirheumatic Drugs*	Pentazocine
Antimalarials	Zomepirac
Hydroxychloroquine	
Chloroquine	
Gold salts	
Gold sodium thiomalate	
Aurothioglucose	
Penicillamine	

avoided.[74] Phenylbutazone, choline salicylate, salsalate and other substituted salicylates have a similar effect. The propionic acid derivatives, indoles, and related drugs and the fenamates have little effect on warfarin binding but it is wise to check the prothrombin time daily for the first few days of combined administration. Phenylbutazone enhances the hypoglycemic action of sulfonylureas (chlorpropamide, tolbutamide) by displacement from albumin-binding sites.

Drugs such as barbiturates which increase liver microsomal enzyme metabolizing activity may reduce the efficacy of corticosteroids and *increase* the toxicity of cyclophosphamide. Allopurinol, by inhibiting xanthine oxidase, reduces the metabolism of 6-mercaptopurine formed from azathioprine and the dose of azathioprine must be reduced to 25 percent of the original value. The toxicity of methotrexate is enhanced by phenylbutazone and aspirin.

Other Drug Effects

The usual dosages and common side effects of antirheumatic drugs are listed in Tables 2 to 4. Administration of the patient's usual medication should be resumed postoperatively as soon as circumstances permit. Prolonged corticosteroid therapy and use of penicillamine may be associated with some delay in wound healing.[16,23] Corticosteroid administration suppresses the production of endogenous cortisol by the hypothalamic-pituitary-adrenal axis. Recovery of function after corticosteroid withdrawal takes place

TABLE 2. Nonsteroidal Anti-inflammatory Drugs

Drug	*Usual Effective Dose/Day*	*Drug Interactions*	*Effect on Platelets*	*Common Side Effects*
Aspirin	3–5 g	Warfarin, probenecid, corticosteroids	major	Gastritis, deafness, tinnitus, central nervous system (elderly), hepatotoxicity
Other salicylates	3–5 g	Warfarin	none	Tinnitus
Indomethacin	75–200 mg		moderate	Gastritis, prepyloric ulcer, central nervous system
Tolmetin	800–1600 mg		minor	Gastritis
Sulindac	300–400 mg		minor	Gastritis, diarrhea
Phenylbutazone	200–600 mg	Warfarin, sulfonylureas, phenytoin	minor	Gastritis, peptic ulcer, blood dyscrasia, fluid retention
Ibuprofen	800–3200 mg		minor	Gastritis, fluid retention, amblyopia
Naproxen	500–750 mg		minor	Gastrointestinal bleeding
Fenoprofen	1200–2400 mg		minor	Gastritis
Meclofenamate sodium	200–400 mg		minor	Diarrhea

slowly over several months, the actual time depending on the duration and dose of corticosteroids. The stress of surgery is not usually hazardous to those patients who have only received replacement doses of corticosteroids on a daily basis (prednisone, 5 mg or equivalent) provided this has been given as a morning dose.[75] As a precaution, however, additional corticosteroid therapy for three to four days over the operative and postoperative period is necessary for all patients on corticosteroid therapy and for those who have received oral corticosteroid within two years of the surgical procedure. Assessment of adrenal function is not usually performed postoperatively but an adrenocorticotropic hormone (ACTH) stimulation test may be performed if time permits prior to elective surgery. The abrupt withdrawal of corticosteroids is absolutely contraindicated in all patients either before or after surgery to avoid the risk of adrenal insufficiency and a relapse of the rheumatic disorder (see chapter 5, Endocrinology).

TABLE 3. Other Antirheumatic Drugs

Drug	*Usual Effective Dose*	*Drug Interactions*	*Common Side Effects*
Hydroxychloroquine	200–600 mg/day		Retinopathy, gastrointestinal effects, rash
Gold salts	50 mg/week		Pruritus, rash, stomatitis, proteinuria, marrow depression
Penicillamine	250–1500 mg/day	Azathioprine	Rash, fever, proteinuria, marrow depression, thrombocytopenia, "immunologic illness"
Cyclophosphamide	50–150 mg/day	Barbiturates, phenothiazines	Alopecia, gastrointestinal effects, hematuria, infections, marrow depression
Azathioprine	100–200 mg/day	Allopurinol	Marrow depression, gastrointestinal effects, infections
Methotrexate	10–25 mg/week	Aspirin, phenylbutazone	Gastrointestinal effects, hepatic toxicity
Corticosteroids	5–80 mg/day	Barbiturates	Cushing's syndrome, diabetes, osteoporosis, fracture, infections

TABLE 4. Antigout Drugs

Drug	*Usual Effective Dose*	*Drug Interactions*	*Common Side Effects*
Allopurinol	100–400 mg/day	Azathioprine, cyclophosphamide	Gastrointestinal effects
Probenecid	0.5–1.5 g/day	Aspirin	Gastrointestinal effects
Sulfinpyrazone	200–400 mg/day	Aspirin	Gastrointestinal effects
Colchicine	0.5–1.0 mg/day (prophylactically) 0.5 mg/hr (for acute gout)		Gastrointestinal effects, marrow suppression (rare)

REFERENCES

1. Rick, ME, and Hoyer, LW: *Hemostatic disorders in systemic lupus erythematosus.* Clin Rheum Dis 1:583, 1975.
2. Winchester, RJ, Agnello, V, and Kunkel, HG: *Gamma globulin complexes in synovial fluids of patients with rheumatoid arthritis.* Clin Exp Immunol 6:689, 1970.
3. Morgan, ES, Cass, RM, Lacox, RF, et al.: *A study of the relation of seronegative and seropositive rheumatoid arthritis to each other and to necrotizing vasculitis.* Am J Med 47:23, 1969.
4. McCann, V: *Pre-and post-operative management role of allied health professionals.* Orthop Clin North Am 6:881, 1975.
5. Grahame, R: *Elasticity of human skin in vitro: a study of the physical properties of the skin in rheumatoid arthritis and the effects of corticosteroids.* Ann Phys Med 10:130, 1969.
6. Shapiro, RF, Resnick, D, Castles, JJ, et al.: *Fistulization of rheumatoid joints, spectrum of identifiable syndromes.* Ann Rheum Dis 34:489, 1975.
7. Iveson, JMI, Thadani, V, Ionescu, M, et al.: *Aortic valve incompetence and replacement in rheumatoid arthritis.* Ann Rheum Dis 34:312, 1975.
8. Prakash, R, Atassi, A, Poske, R, et al.: *Prevalence of pericardial effusion and mitral-valve involvement in patients with rheumatoid arthritis without cardiac symptoms.* New Engl J Med 289:597, 1973.
9. Walker, WC, and Wright, V: *Diffuse intestital pulmonary fibrosis and rheumatoid arthritis.* Ann Rheum Dis 28:252, 1969.
10. Walker, WC, and Wright, V: *Rheumatoid pleuritis.* Ann Rheum Dis 26:467, 1967.
11. Walker, WC, and Wright, V, *Pulmonary lesions and rheumatoid arthritis.* Medicine 47:501, 1968.
12. Walker, WC, *Pulmonary infections and rheumatoid arthritis.* Q J Med 36:239, 1967.
13. Schernthaner, A, Scherako, O, Kolarz, G, et al.: *Seropositive rheumatoid arthritis associated with decreased diffusion capacity of the lung.* Ann Rheum Dis 35:258, 1976.
14. Collins, RL, Turner, RA, Johnson, AM, et al.: *Obstructive pulmonary disease in rheumatoid arthritis.* Arthritis Rheum 19:623, 1976.
15. Mowat, AG, *Rheumatoid arthritis and connective tissue diseases,* in Israels, MCG, and Delamore, IW (eds.): *Hematological Aspects of Systemic Disease.* Philadelphia: WB, Saunders, 1976, pp. 286–318.
16. Garner, RW, Mowat, AG, and Hazleman, BL: *Wound healing after operations on patients with rheumatoid arthritis.* J Bone Joint Surg 551B:134, 1973.
17. Hancock, DO: *The cervical spine in chronic rheumatoid arthritis.* Clin Rheum Dis 4:443, 1978.
18. Matthews, JA: *Atlanto-axial subluxation in rheumatoid arthritis. a 5-year follow-up study.* Ann Rheum Dis 33:526, 1974.
19. Mowat, AG: *Medical implications of orthopedic surgery in rheumatic diseases.* Clin Rheum Dis 4:249, 1978.
20. Jayson, MIV, and Jones, DEP: *Scleritis and rheumatoid arthritis.* Ann Rheum Dis 30:343, 1971.
21. Lofgren, RH, and Montgomery, WW: *Incidence of laryngeal involvement in rheumatoid arthritis.* N Engl J Med 263:193, 1962.
22. Polisar, IA, Burbank, B, Levitt, LM, et al.: *Bilateral midline fixation of cricoarytenoid joints as a serious medical emergency.* JAMA 172:901, 1960.
23. Schorn, D, and Mowat, AG: *Penicillamine in rheumatoid arthritis: wound healing, skin thickness and osteoporosis.* Rheum Rehab 16:223, 1977.
24. Baum, L: *Infection in rheumatoid arthritis.* Arthritis Rheum 14:135, 1971.
25. Kelsey, JL, Wood, PHN, and Charnley, J: *Prediction of thromboembolism following total hip replacement.* Clin Orthop 114:247, 1976.
26. Nicolaides, AN, Dupont, PA, Desai, S, et al.: *Small doses of subcutaneous heparin in preventing deep venous thrombosis after major surgery.* Lancet 11:890, 1972.
27. McKenna, R, Bachmann, F, and Kaushal, SP: *Thromboembolic disease in patients undergoing knee replacement.* J Bone Joint Surg 58A:928, 1976.

28. Budman, DR, and Steinberg, AD: *Hematologic aspects of systemic lupus erythematosus.* Ann Intern Med 86:220, 1977.

29. Rothfield, NM: *Systemic lupus erythematosis: clinical and laboratory aspects,* in McCarty, DJ (ed.): *Arthritis and Allied Conditions.* Philadelphia: Lea & Febiger, 1979.

30. Rothfield, NF: *The kidney in lupus erythematosus.* Contrib Nephrol 7:128, 1977.

31. Kimberly, RP, and Plotz, PH: *Aspirin-induced depression of renal function.* N Engl J Med 296:418, 1977.

32. Kimberly, RP, Bowden, RF, Kaiser, HR, et al.: *Reduction of renal function by newer nonsteroidal anti-inflammatory drugs.* Am J Med 64:804, 1978.

33. Cathcart, ES, Edelson, BA, Scheinberg, MA, et al.: *Beneficial effects of methylprednisolone "pulse" therapy in diffuse proliferative lupus nephritis.* Lancet 1:163, 1976.

34. Meislin, AG, and Rothfield, NF, *Systemic lupus erythematosus in childhood.* Pediatrics 42:37, 1968.

35. Zizic, T, Shulman, LE, and Stevens, MD: *Colonic perforations in systemic lupus erythematosus.* Medicine 54:411, 1975.

36. Seijert, GG, Heinz, N, and Ruffman, A: *Pancreatitis in visceral lupus erythematosus.* Gastroenterologia 107:317, 1967.

37. Feinstein, DL, and Rapaport, SI, *Aquired inhibitors of blood coagulation.* Prog Hemost Thromb 1:75, 1972.

38. Veltkamp, JJ, Kerkhoven, P, and Loeliger, EA: *Circulating anticoagulant in disseminated lupus erythematosus.* Hemostasis 2:253, 1974.

39. Robboy, JJ, Lewis, EJ, Schur, PH, et al.: *Circulating anticoagulants to factor VIII.* Am J Med 49:742, 1970.

40. Castro, O, Farber, LR, and Clyne, LP: *Circulating anticoagulants against factors IX and XI in systemic lupus erythematosus.* Ann Intern Med 77:543, 1972.

41. Griner, PF, and Hoyer, LW: *Amegakaryocytic thrombocytopenia in systemic lupus erythematosus.* Arch Intern Med 125:328, 1970.

42. Margolius, A, Jr., Jackson, DP, and Ratnoff, OD: *Circulating anticoagulants: a study of 40 cases and a review of the literature.* Medicine 40:145, 1961.

43. Gonea, PF, Herdman, R, and Bridges, RA: *The coagulation abnormalities in systemic lupus erythematosus.* thrombosis diathesis Haemarrhagica 20:456, 1968.

44. Mollison, PL: *Blood Transfusion in Clinical Medicine.* Oxford: Blackwell Scientific Publications, 1972, p. 79.

45. Moran, CJ, Parry, HF, Mowbray, J, et al.: *Plasmaphoresis in systemic lupus erythematosus.* Br Med J 1:1573, 1977.

46. Edson, JR, McArthur, JR, Branda, RF, et al.: *Successful management of a subjural hematoma in a hemophiliac with an anti-factor VIII antibody.* Blood 41:113, 1973.

47. Ropes, MW: *Systemic Lupus Erythematosus.* Cambridge, Massachusetts: Harvard University Press, 1976.

48. Rothfield, NF: *Clinical features of systemic lupus erythematosus,* in Kelley, WN, Harris, Ed, Ruddy, S, et al. (eds.): *Textbook of Rheumatology.* Philadelphia: WB Saunders Co., 1981.

49. Zurier, RB: *Systemic lupus erythematosus and pregnancy.* Clin Rheum Dis 1:613, 1975.

50. Partridge, REH: (in preparation).

51. Dubois, EL: *Lupus erythematosus,* ed. 2. Los Angeles: University of Southern California Press, 1974, p. 612.

52. Partridge, REH: *Anaphylactic reactions to ibuprofen in patients with systemic lupus erythematosus.* In preparation, 1980.

53. Bohan, A, Peters, JB, Bowman, RS, et al.: *A computer-assisted analysis of 153 patients with polymyositis and dermatomyositis.* Medicine 56:255, 1977.

54. Lipscomb, PR, Simons, GW, and Winkelmann, RK: *Surgery for sclerodactylia of the hand. Experience with six cases.* J Bone Joint Surg 51:1112, 1969.

55. Henderson, RD, and Pearson, FG: *Surgical management of esophageal scleroderma.* J Thorac Cardiovasc Surg 66:686, 1973.

56. Nelson, SW: *Extraluminal gas collections due to diseases of the gastrointestinal tract.* Am J Roentgen 115:225, 1972.

57. Pahle, JA, Kass, E, and Munthe, E: *Orthopedic surgery for childhood arthritis.* Clin Rheum Dis 4:425, 1978.

58. Wyngarden, JB, and Holmes, EW, *Clinical gout and the pathogenesis of hyperuricemia,* in McCarty, DJ (ed.): *Arthritis and Allied Conditions.* Philadelphia, Lea & Febiger, 1979.

59. Linton, RR, and Talbott, JH: *The surgical treatment of tophaceous gout.* Ann Surg 117:161, 1943.

60. Smith, ML, and Scott, JT: *Uric acid excretion and surgery.* Ann Rheum Dis 31:102, 1972.

61. Wallace, SL: *Treatment of the acute attack of gout.* Clin Rheum Dis 3:133, 1977.

62. Wilkens, RF, Case, JB, and Huis, FJ: *The treatment of acute gout with Naprosen.* J Clin Pharmacol 15:363, 1975.

63. Wallace, SL: *Colchicine and new anti-inflammatory drugs for the treatment of gout.* Arthritis Rheum 18:847, 1975.

64. O'Duffy, JD: *Clinical studies of acute pseudogout attacks.* Arthritis Rheum (Suppl) 19:349, 1976.

65. McCarty, DL: *Calcium pyrophosphate crystal deposition disease: pseudogout: articular chondrocalcinosis,* in McCarty, DJ (ed.): *Arthritis and Allied Conditions.* Philadelphia: Lea & Febiger, 1979.

66. Howell, DS: *Metabolic bone disease,* in McCarty, DJ (ed.): *Arthritis and Allied Conditions.* Philadelphia: Lea & Febiger, 1979.

67. Bick, RL, Adams, T, and Schmalhorst, WR: *Bleeding times, platelet adhesion and aspirin.* Am J Clin Pathol 65:69, 1976.

68. Gast, LF: *Influence of aspirin on hemostatic parameters.* Ann Rheum Dis 23:500, 1964.

69. Weiss, HJ, and Aledort, LM: *Impaired platelet/connective tissue reaction in man after aspirin ingestion.* Lancet 2:495, 1967.

70. Roth, AJ, Stanford, N, and Majerus, PW: *Acetylation of prostaglandin synthetase by aspirin.* Proc Natl Acad. Sci USA 72:3073, 1975.

71. Burch, JW, Stanford, N, and Majerus, PW: *Inhibition of platelet prostaglandin synthetase by oral aspirin.* J Clin Invest 61:314, 1978.

72. Weiss, HJ, Aledort, LM, and Kochwa, S: *The effect of salicylates on the hemostatic properties of platelets in man.* J Clin Invest 47:2169, 1968.

73. Fossgreen, J: *Ketoprofen. A new nonsteroidal anti-inflammatory agent.* Scand J Rheumatol (Suppl) 14:7, 1976.

74. O'Reilly, RA, Sahud, MA, and Aggeler, PM: *Impact of aspirin and chlorthalidone on the pharmacodynamics of oral anticoagulant drugs in man.* Ann NY Acad Sci 79:173, 1971.

75. Danowski, TS, Bonessi, JV, Sabeh, G, et al.: *Probability of pituitary-adrenal unresponsiveness after steroid therapy.* Ann Intern Med 61:11, 1964.

Chapter 15

FLUID, ELECTROLYTE, AND ACID-BASE DISORDERS

David A. Bushinsky, M.D., and
Jordan J. Cohen, M.D.

The surgical patient is at an increased risk for the development of a wide variety of fluid, electrolyte, and acid-base disorders. In normal man, a broad range of fluid intake can be tolerated because the kidney is able to concentrate and dilute the urine appropriately to maintain a nearly constant plasma osmolality. Likewise, a varied intake of sodium, potassium, or other electrolytes can be tolerated because of regulated renal electrolyte excretion. In the surgical patient, however, excessive demands are often placed upon the kidney by large fluid and electrolyte losses or by unavoidable or injudicious intake. Moreover, the metabolic load for excretion is often increased by a high rate of catabolism.[1] At the same time, renal perfusion may be diminished or renal parenchymal injury may be present. Thus, the kidney may be severely hampered in its ability to maintain homeostasis. The physician's task is to identify the specific fluid and electrolyte stresses that are being placed upon the kidney and the extent to which renal responses to these stresses may have been compromised. From these considerations, a rational plan for adjusting input and influencing output can be formulated.

BODY SPACES

Prior to discussing alterations in body fluid and electrolyte balance, a brief review of the normal body space compartments and fluid and electrolyte requirements is in order. In the adult male, water accounts for 50 to 60 percent of body weight.[2] Skeletal muscle and solid viscera contain approximately 70 percent water by weight whereas fat contains little water. Thus, on average, adult females having relatively more fatty tissue contain a somewhat smaller percentage of water, usually about 45 to 55 percent of body weight.

By the same token, obese individuals have a smaller percentage of total body water than lean, muscular individuals.

Approximately two-thirds of total body water resides within cells (about 40% of body weight), whereas approximately one-third makes up the extracellular space (about 20% of body weight). The extracellular space is further divided into plasma (about 4% of body weight) and interstitial fluid (about 16% of body weight). The compartmentalization of body fluids depends upon the hydrostatic and oncotic pressure gradients between blood and interstitial fluid and upon the transport mechanisms and permeability characteristics of cell membranes.

FLUID REQUIREMENTS

Under normal circumstances of temperature and humidity, approximately 200 to 400 ml of water are lost through the lungs, 300 to 600 ml through the skin, and 100 to 200 ml in the feces each day.[3] Such losses are termed "insensible." The normal osmotic load requiring excretion each day is approximately 600 mOsm.[4] Because healthy kidneys can concentrate the urine to about 1200 mOsm/kg H_2O, this solute load requires the excretion of a minimum of approximately 500 ml of urine each day. Thus, the normal person requires approximately 1400 ml of water each day to balance unavoidable losses. Approximately 200 to 400 ml of this water requirement is available from the oxidation of protein, carbohydrate, and fat. This leaves a requirement of slightly over 1 L of water that must be provided from exogenous sources daily.

An elevation of body temperature increases water losses through hyperventilation and perspiration. Febrile patients lose approximately 100 ml of additional fluid per degree Farenheit of temperature elevation per day.[4] Warm environments that result in profuse sweating increase skin losses by approximately 100 ml per day per degree elevation in ambient temperature above 85° Farenheit.[4] Urinary solute load increases during catabolism and may reach levels higher than 1200 mOsm each day.[5] This increased solute load increases the minimum rate of urine flow. Thus, a catabolic, febrile patient in a warm environment may have a baseline water requirement of 4 or 5 L per day. A portion of such increased water losses may be balanced by increased endogenous water formation.[6]

OSMOLALITY

The osmolality of the body fluids normally varies by no more than 2 percent around its mean value of about 285 mOsm/kg H_2O. This precise osmotic control is achieved by the thirst mechanism and by the regulated release of antidiuretic hormone (ADH).[7] An increase in body fluid osmolality causes the release of antidiuretic hormone which acts on the kidney to permit the absorption of solute-free water in the distal tubule. The resultant excretion of hypertonic urine leads to a dilution of body fluids and a decrease in serum osmolality. In addition, an increase in osmolality stimulates thirst which results in correction of hyperosmolality if water is available. A decrease in plasma osmolality inhibits antidiuretic hormone release resulting in the excretion of a dilute urine and an increase in plasma osmolality. The normal kidney has an extremely large reserve capacity for the excretion of a water load. Given normal urinary diluting capacity, up to 20 L of solute free water can be excreted each day if required by excessive intake.

A decrease in the maximum urinary concentrating or diluting capacity limits the range of fluid intake within which normal osmolality can be maintained. An impairment in urinary diluting ability can result in hyponatremia whereas an impairment in concentrating ability can result in hypernatremia. These abnormalities of fluid regulation are common among surgical patients.

Hyponatremia

FACTITIOUS OR PSEUDOHYPONATREMIA

As implied above, hyponatremia generally signifies the presence of hypo-osmolality, and the hypo-osmolality is the focal point for diagnosis and treatment. One should bear in mind, however, that on occasion hyponatremia occurs in conjunction with a normal osmolality or even with an increased osmolality. Hyponatremia with normal osmolality occurs in patients with severe hyperlipidemia or marked hyperproteinemia. In these conditions, the fraction of plasma which is aqueous (approximately 93% normally) is reduced by the presence of large molecular weight, nonaqueous material. Sodium (and all other solutes) is confined to the aqueous portion of the plasma, but its concentration is expressed per unit volume of whole plasma. Hence, sodium concentration will appear to be low under these circumstances when, in fact, its concentration per liter of plasma water is normal. The finding of a normal value for plasma osmolality (eg., freezing point depression) in the face of a low serum sodium concentration confirms the presence of pseudohyponatremia.

Hyponatremia with increased osmolality results from the presence of a large concentration of some osmotically active solute confined to the extracellular fluid. Such solutes as glucose and mannitol are sufficiently small (molecular weight 180 for each) to exert a sizable osmotic effect at abnormally high but achievable plasma concentrations. The exclusively extracellular distribution of these solutes causes water to be drawn from cells and, in consequence, sodium concentration falls. The hallmark of this condition is an elevated serum osmolality in the face of a low serum sodium concentration.

TRUE HYPONATREMIA

Because the normal kidney can excrete up to 20 L of solute free water each day, an enormous increase in water intake is required to produce hyponatremia in the presence of normal diluting capacity. Thus, some impairment in diluting capacity is the root cause of true hyponatremia in the vast majority of instances. Such impairment is commonly referred to as a water excreting defect. Water excreting defects may result from (1) generalized renal insufficiency, (2) decreased delivery of filtrate to the diluting segment of the nephron, (3) a defect in solute reabsorption in the ascending limb of Henle's loop, and (4) an elevated level of antidiuretic hormone.

Manifestations of hyponatremia vary with its magnitude and with the rapidity of its development.[8–12] Symptoms of mild and slowly developing hyponatremia include disordered taste sensation, easy fatigability, and dyspnea on exertion. More striking symptoms include nausea, vomiting, and abdominal cramps. Neurologic manifestations are the most worrisome and include weakness, lethargy, restlessness, confusion, seizures, and coma. These neurologic manifestations, often referred to as "water intoxication," rarely occur if serum sodium concentration remains above 125 mEq/L, even when hyponatremia develops acutely. Conversely, neurologic symptoms may be mild or absent when serum sodium is as low as 100 to 110 mEq/L if the disorder has developed very gradually.

It is helpful to categorize patients with hyponatremia with reference to their apparent extracellular fluid (ECF) volume. Thus, hyponatremia may occur in association with extracellular fluid volume depletion, modest extracellular volume excess (no edema), and marked extracellular fluid volume excess (edema).[13]

Hypovolemic Hyponatremia

Hyponatremia associated with extracellular fluid volume depletion signifies the presence of a large deficit of total body water with a disproportionately larger deficit of total body sodium. This is *not* to say that hyponatremia associated with volume depletion results directly from loss of hypertonic fluid as such from the body. In point of fact, this rarely if ever is the cause of frank hyponatremia. Rather, hyponatremia in conjunction with volume depletion arises because of an obstacle to water excretion created by the loss of isotonic fluid. Isotonic losses, whether from the kidney, from the gastrointestinal tract, or into internal "third" spaces, retards the formation of a dilute urine both by a direct and an indirect, ADH-mediated effect on the kidney. The depletion of ECF volume leads directly to a stimulus to proximal sodium reabsorption which reduces the delivery of filtrate to the distal nephron and thereby limits the "raw material" available for the creation of solute free water at the ascending limb of Henle's loop. Diminished distal delivery also increases the opportunity for passive back-diffusion of the free water that is generated because of prolonged contact time within the collecting duct during passage through the hypertonic medulla. Volume depletion is also a potent, "nonosmotic" stimulus to ADH release and may override the inhibiting effects of hypo-osmolality. The net result of these changes is that ingested or administered water tends to be retained as the body endeavors to "protect volume at the expense of osmolality."

Hypovolemia is, of course, a frequent occurrence in surgical patients and is the most common antecedent to the development of hyponatremia in this group because hypotonic fluids are often administered in large quantities before adequate salt repletion has been achieved. Volume depletion due to renal losses is most often the consequence of diuretic administration. Special note should be made concerning the use of diuretics to promote urine flow in the postoperative period. All too often, volume depletion and hyponatremia are the consequence because of the unrecognized negative sodium balance that results. Diuretic induced potassium depletion may also cause hyponatremia by mechanisms that are not clear.[14] In addition to overzealous use of diuretics, sodium depletion due to renal losses can occur in metabolic alkalosis (see p. 648), adrenal insufficiency, and certain intrinsic renal diseases, most notably those in which tubulointerstitial damage has occurred (e.g., analgesic abuse nephropathy, medullary cystic disease).[15] In addition, if sodium intake is severely restricted, patients with chronic renal insufficiency of almost any cause may become volume depleted due to inadequate renal sodium conservation.[16] Sodium deficits in surgical patients are even more commonly the result of gastrointestinal losses. Typical electrolyte composition of gastrointestinal secretion is shown in Table 1.[17] The sequestration of extracellular fluid at sites of injury or inflammation ("third space") is also frequent among surgical patients and is often overlooked.[17] A measurement of urinary sodium concentration is often helpful in differentiating between renal and extrarenal sodium losses. In the former, values generally exceed 20 mEq/L, whereas in extrarenal sodium losses, values typically fall below 10 mEq/L and are often as low as 2 to 4 mEq/L.

The treatment of hypovolemic hyponatremia should focus on restoration of extracellular fluid volume. In general, isotonic sodium chloride is the most appropriate fluid for initial volume replacement. The rate of administration and the total quantity required for full correction of deficits varies widely in accordance with the clinical circumstances. Careful monitoring of vital signs and bedside examination usually suffice to gauge the adequacy of therapy. If a recent body weight obtained under circumstances of normovolemia is available, it can be used as a target for replacement therapy. When more precise guidelines are required, a central venous catheter or a Swan-Ganz catheter may be utilized to monitor central pressures. Hypotonic fluids should not be used until adequate volume repletion has permitted normal diluting capacity to be restored.

Hypervolemic Hyponatremia

Hyponatremia is often accompanied by frank edema. In this setting, total body sodium is invariably increased but total body water is increased to an even greater extent. Patients with hyponatremia due to renal failure fall into this category. In such patients, surfeits of water disproportionately large with respect to those of sodium often develop. The retention of both sodium and water is simply the consequence of the inability of the damaged kidney to keep pace with normal excretory demands.

TABLE 1. Mean Electrolyte Content of Gastrointestinal Secretions (mEq/L)

Secretion or Source	*Sodium*	*Potassium*	*Chloride*	*Bicarbonate*
Saliva	10	26	10	30
Stomach	50	10	130	1
Duodenum	140	5	80	10
Ileum	140	5	104	30
Bile	145	5	100	35
Pancreatic	140	5	75	115

Modified from Shires and Canizaro.[17]

In the absence of renal failure, the mechanisms responsible for hyponatremia in edema-forming states are similar to those in hypovolemia. Edema-forming states are characterized by a reduction in the "effective" extracellular fluid volume, that is, in that portion of the extracellular volume linked physiologically with renal homeostatic mechanisms. Thus, a marked reduction in effective extracellular fluid volume due to congestive heart failure, nephrotic syndrome, and possibly hepatic cirrhosis causes an impairment in water excretion because it results in precisely the same effects on the kidney as does true volume depletion.[18] Proximal tubular sodium reabsorption is stimulated, thereby limiting the rate at which filtrate is delivered to the distal diluting segments of the nephron and increasing passive back-diffusion of water into the medullary interstitium. In addition, antidiuretic hormone release is enhanced by the nonosmolar stimulus of the apparent reduction in extracellular volume. Both of these changes limit the excretion of solute-free water and foster the development of hyponatremia when water intake is maintained.

The underlying tendency of edematous patients to develop hyponatremia may be aggravated by the added stresses placed on water homeostasis by a wide variety of surgical conditions. Sudden reductions in extracellular volume from modest losses of body fluids as well as sudden but modest increases in free water intake in the perioperative period may cause notable hyponatremia in such patients.

Ideally, treatment of hyponatremia associated with edema should focus on reversing the underlying disorder. Restricting water intake to less than 800 to 1500 ml/day is often necessary; provision of additional sodium is rarely required. It is obvious that additional sodium will have the unwanted effect of aggravating the degree of edema. In rare circumstances, however, the symptoms of hyponatremia are sufficiently severe to justify the administration of hypertonic saline to achieve a more rapid improvement in plasma osmolality.

Normovolemic Hyponatremia

The occurrence of hyponatremia in association with an apparently normal extracellular fluid volume (i.e., in the absence of frank hypovolemia or edema) is characteristic of those conditions in which excessive amounts of antidiuretic hormone are present or in which the kidney is excessively sensitive to the hormone's effect. In either event, hyponatremia results from a failure of the kidney to elaborate an appropriately dilute urine for the prevailing rate of water intake.

PHYSIOLOGIC AND PHARMACOLOGIC ANTIDIURESIS. Numerous physiologic stimuli to ADH release other than hyperosmolality or volume depletion are recognized. Pain[19] and emotional stress[20] are among the more important and both are, of course, commonly present in the postoperative period. Several pharmacologic agents are also known to stimulate ADH release or to heighten the sensitivity of the kidney to antidiuretic effects of the hormone (Table 2).[21,22] Many of these agents are commonly used in the perioperative period. Thus, antidiuresis during and immediately following surgery is extremely common[41] and, in the face of injudicious administration of solute-free water, can account for significant hyponatremia. Such physiologic and/or pharmacologic

TABLE 2. Drugs Causing Water Retention

Drug	*Reference*
Primarily by Stimulating ADH Release	
Isoproterenol	23
Halothane	24
Ether	24
Cyclopropane	24
Thiopental	24
Nitrous oxide	24
Morphine	25,26
Barbiturates	27
Nicotine	28,29
Acetylcholine	22
Carbamazepine	30
Clofibrate	31
Vincristine	32
Cyclophosphamide	33
Primarily by Facilitating Peripheral Action of ADH	
Chlorpropamide	34,35
Tolbutamide (large dose)	36
Diazoxide	37
Indomethacin	38
Oxytocin	39,40

Modified from Miller and Moses.[21]

antidiuresis is usually short-lived and can be treated effectively with modest water restriction and the discontinuation of un-needed drugs.

SYNDROME OF INAPPROPRIATE ANTIDIURETIC HORMONE SECRETION (SIADH). The more commonly encountered causes of SIADH are listed in Table 3. The hallmark of this syndrome is persistent antidiuresis due to the peripheral elaboration of ADH (or an ADH-like substance) or to a pathologic stimulus to the central release of ADH. Chronic water retention tends to increase the size of all body fluid compartments.

TABLE 3. Causes of Syndrome of Inappropriate ADH (SIADH)

Central nervous system disorders	*Malignant tumors*
Brain tumor or abscess	Carcinoma of the lung
Subdural or subarachnoid hemorrhage	Carcinoma of the duodenum
Guillain-Barré syndrome	Carcinoma of the pancreas
Skull fracture	
Cerebral atrophy	*Pulmonary disorders*
Seizure disorders	Tuberculosis
Herpes simplex encephalitis	Abscess
Tuberculous or purulent meningitis	Aspergillosis
Acute intermittent porphyria	Viral pneumonia
	Bacterial pneumonia

The resultant expansion of extracellular volume leads to an inhibition of renal sodium reabsorption and a consequent natriuresis. The diagnostic criteria for establishing the presence of SIADH include (1) persistent hyponatremia, (2) normal renal function, (3) normal adrenal and thyroid function, and (4) inappropriately concentrated urine (urine osmolality is usually greater than 150 mOsm/kg H_2O). Typically, appreciable quantities of sodium are present in the urine (>20 to 30 mEq/L), reflecting the excretion of the normal daily sodium intake. In the sodium-restricted patient, however, urinary sodium excretion may fall to negligible levels.[42,43]

Many of the conditions associated with SIADH are encountered among surgical patients (see Table 3). Mild forms of this syndrome may not be manifested by notable preoperative hyponatremia but may severely limit the amount of solute-free water that can be administered before significant hypo-osmolality supervenes. Even "routine" intravenous infusions of dextrose and water for purposes of preoperative or postoperative hydration may exceed the capacity of such patients to excrete free water.

Satisfactory treatment of hyponatremia due to SIADH can often be accomplished by modest water restriction alone. If symptoms of water intoxication are present, infusion of small amounts of hypertonic (3 to 5%) saline should be considered. The risks of congestive heart failure from volume overload can be minimized by the simultaneous administration of a potent diuretic (e.g., furosemide, ethacrynic acid).[44] The net result of such combined therapy is the loss of solute-free fluid from the body and the restitution of a normal complement of sodium. Generally speaking, treatment should be continued until serum sodium concentration rises above 130 mEq/L. Long term management of persistent SIADH may be facilitated by the chronic administration of demeclocycline[45] or lithium,[46] agents known to interfere with the action of ADH on the kidney. Demeclocycline is both more efficacious and better tolerated than lithium in most patients[47–49] but appears to carry substantial risk in patients with liver disease.[50]

Hypernatremia

Hypernatremia is invariably associated with hyperosmolality. Hypernatremia may result from (1) inadequate fluid intake, (2) increased water loss, or (3) administration of hypertonic saline (Table 4).

The clinical manifestations of hypernatremia are confined almost exclusively to the central nervous system and include lethargy and coma.[8] Muscle irritability and convulsions are unusual.[51] The degree of central nervous system depression is a function both of the magnitude of the hyperosmolality and of the rate at which it develops; the more rapid the development of hypernatremia, the more likely symptoms are to occur.

DECREASED WATER INTAKE

Most instances of hypernatremia among surgical patients fall in this category. As noted above, obligatory water requirements are often increased in the surgical patient due to increased insensible losses and to the increased urinary solute load secondary to heightened catabolism. Incomplete replacement of such solute poor water losses results in progressive concentration of body fluids, even if renal concentrating ability is completely normal. Any impairment in renal concentrating ability will, of course, aggravate the

TABLE 4. Hypernatremic Disorders

Inadequate fluid intake
Water deprivation in the postoperative or comatose patient

Increased water excretion
Renal
  Central diabetes insipidus
  Nephrogenic diabetes insipidus
  Osmotic diuresis
Nonrenal
  Pulmonary, gastrointestinal, or cutaneous water loss in excess of sodium chloride

Hypertonic saline administration
Hypertonic saline administration faster than renal sodium chloride excretion

tendency to hyperosmolality. If thirst mechanisms are intact, and if free access to water is not impeded, water ingestion will keep pace with the body's needs.[52] However, in the presence of coma or other circumstances limiting free access to water, water needs must be met by appropriate therapeutic administration.

INCREASED WATER LOSS

Polyuric States

Polyuria can result from a wide variety of conditions (see Table 5).[53] Polyuric disorders result in hypernatremia, of course, only when water intake is insufficient to balance the urinary losses.

Both *central* diabetes inspidus and nephrogenic diabetes insipidus result in the excretion of large quantities of dilute urine. Among surgical patients, important causes of central diabetes insipidus include head trauma and certain neurosurgical procedures. A detailed discussion of diabetes insipidus can be found in Chapter 5, Endocrinology.

Brisk osmotic diuresis occurs most commonly in uncontrolled diabetes (intense glycosuria) or following the administration of large quantities of mannitol. In addition, the abrupt relief of renal failure is often accompanied by an osmotic diuresis due to the rapid excretion of urea and other retained solutes. During brisk osmotic diuresis, the urinary loss of water may far exceed the loss of sodium and attendant anions.[54] The consequence is the net removal of water from the body at a rate in excess of the loss of body solute. As a consequence, hypernatremia typically supervenes. Thus, urinary losses engendered by osmotic diuresis must be replaced with appropriate hypotonic fluids.

Extrarenal Water Losses

Hypertonic nasogastric feedings that are incompletely absorbed may result in significant water losses through the gastrointestinal tract.[55] In addition, increased water loss from

TABLE 5. Polyuric Disorders

Condition	*Possible Cause*
	Central Diabetes Insipidus
Head trauma, skull fractures, orbital trauma	Histiocytosis X
Pituitary surgery	Sickle cell disease
Craniopharyngioma, cerebral tumors	Encephalitis
Metastatic tumors	Meningitis
Granulomas	Vascular, aneurysms
Sarcoid	Hypoxic "brain death"
Tuberculosis	Optic atrophy, nerve deafness, diabetes mellitus, and diabetes insipidus
Lues	Leukemia
	Nephrogenic Diabetes Insipidus
Congenital condition	Following successful renal transplant
Hypercalcemia	Diuretic phase of acute tubular necrosis
Hypokalemia	Hypergammaglobulinemic disorders
Lithium intoxication	Multiple myeloma
Phenacetin nephropathy	Sarcoid
Demethylchlortetracycline	Sjögren's syndrome
Propoxyphene intoxication	Amyloidosis
Methoxyfluorane	Sickle cell anemia
Uric acid nephropathy	Interstitial nephritis
Medullary cystic disease	Acute renal artery stenosis
Following relief of urinary tract obstruction	
	Osmotic Diuresis
Mannitol	Glucose
Urea	Diabetes mellitus out of control
Chronic renal failure	Nonketotic hyperglycemic hyperosmolar coma
Diuretic phase of acute tubular necrosis	Sodium
Relief of urinary tract obstruction	Diuretics
Successful renal transplant	Excessive administration of sodium-containing intravenous fluids
High protein tube feeding	Chloride and other anions
Intravenous hyperalimentation	Hypertonic enemas
	Cholestyramine

Modified from Fichman.[53]

the body may occur in patients with extensive cutaneous burns, especially in patients treated with hyperosmotic topical solutions (e.g., Betadine)[56], and in patients treated with certain oral agents such as lactulose[57] and cholestyramine,[58] both of which can obligate large volumes of water in the stool.

ADMINISTRATION OF HYPERTONIC SALINE

Hypernatremia may, of course, result from the inadvertent administration of excessive quantities of hypertonic saline in the treatment of hyponatremia. A more common cause of iatrogenic hypernatremia is the administration of hypertonic sodium bicarbonate solutions in the treatment of severe metabolic acidosis, as during cardiopulmonary arrest.[59,60] The absorption of hypertonic saline used to induce abortion has also been reported to cause hypernatremia.[61]

TREATMENT OF HYPERNATREMIA

The principal concern during the treatment of hypernatremia is to avoid overly rapid restoration of normal plasma osmolality. The risk of rapid correction stems from the tendency of the brain to swell as plasma osmolality is reduced.[62–64] The intracellular solute content of brain increases during the development of hypernatremia because of the creation of so-called idiogenic osmoles. This adaptive mechanism allows the brain to maintain a more nearly normal volume in the face of marked total body water deficits. As water deficits are repaired, however, a lag in the disappearance of such idiogenic osmoles renders the brain susceptible to sudden swelling. Thus, moderate to severe hypernatremia (e.g., serum sodium concentration > 160 mEq/L) should be corrected gradually over the course of 48 hours or more. During the treatment of hyponatremia, if neurologic status improves and then deteriorates, cerebral edema should be suspected even if the serum sodium and osmolality remain above normal.[52] Hypertonic mannitol or saline should then be immediately administered. If hypernatremia is associated with extracellular fluid volume deficits, such deficits can be restored rapidly with isotonic solutions.

POTASSIUM

Normal Potassium Balance

Potassium balance is normally maintained in the face of continuous variations in intake because appropriate adjustments in renal excretion occur. Under normal circumstances, all but a small amount of potassium entering the gastrointestinal tract is absorbed.[65] Skin losses are negligible unless the volume of sweat is very large.[66] The kidney can normally adjust the amount of potassium excreted over a very wide range (from about 5 to 1,000 mEq/day). Such variations in potassium excretion reflect changes in the secretion of the cation across the renal tubular epithelium. Renal excretion is largely independent of the glomerular filtration rate and the amount of potassium filtered. Virtually all filtered potassium is reabsorbed during passage through the nephron, regulation of excretion taking place within the distal tubule and collecting duct where potassium ions are secreted into the tubular lumen.

Table 6 depicts the distribution of body potassium. Only a small fraction of body potassium resides in the extracellular compartment. Thus, potassium entering the body must pass into the intracellular compartment prior to being excreted so that plasma potassium concentration can remain within the normal range of 3.5 to 5 mEq/L. Two hormones, insulin and aldosterone, strongly influence the cellular uptake of potassium.[67,68] Insulin levels rise promptly following large potassium loads; a parallel increase in glucagon secretion apparently offsets the otherwise hypoglycemic effect of the increased insulin levels. How cellular uptake of potassium is facilitated by insulin is not

TABLE 6. Body Potassium Distribution in the "Average" Young Adult Male

Distribution	*Body Weight (mEq/kg)*
Total body potassium	53.8
Intracellular	48.3
Extracellular	5.5
Plasma	0.2
Interstitial—lymph	0.5
Transcellular	0.5
Bone	4.1
Dense connective tissue	0.2

Modified from Edelman and Leibman.[2]

completely known, but the mechanism appears to be independent of glucose uptake. Aldosterone secretion is also stimulated by potassium loading, an effect that appears to be mediated directly by plasma potassium concentration on the adrenal glands.

Potassium Depletion and Hypokalemia

True potassium depletion is defined as a reduction in total body potassium not accompanied by an equivalent change in nitrogen balance. In most cases, the finding of hypokalemia (serum potassium < 3.5 mEq/L) establishes the presence of a potassium deficit.[69] The degree of the deficit, however, is often difficult to predict from the decrement in plasma potassium concentration because superimposed factors can affect transcellular potassium distribution. On the one hand, hypokalemia may result entirely from a shift of potassium into cells without any loss from the body. Such shifts may occur in association with acute alkalemia or in the crisis of hypokalemic familial periodic paralysis. On the other hand, appreciable potassium deficits may be present in the face of normal or even elevated serum potassium concentrations. A notable example is the patient with diabetic ketoacidosis in which the acid-base disturbance and the hyperosmolality may cause a substantial shift of potassium out of cells.

CAUSES

There are three mechanisms capable of producing potassium depletion: decreased intake, increased renal excretion, and extrarenal losses (see Table 7). Each is commonly encountered among surgical patients.

Dietary deprivation alone is a rare cause of symptomatic potassium depletion among nonhospitalized individuals because potassium is present in such a wide variety of foods.[71] Long periods of potassium deprivation occasionally occur in certain hospitalized

TABLE 7. Classification of Hypokalemic Disorders

I. Inadequate dietary intake
II. Increased renal excretion
  A. Diuretics
  B. Metabolic alkalosis
  C. Antibiotics: Carbenicillin, amphotericin B, gentamicin
  D. Magnesium deficiency
  E. Diabetic ketoacidosis
  F. Mineralocorticoid excess
    1. Primary aldosteronism
      a. Adenoma
      b. Bilateral hyperplasia
    2. Cushing's syndrome
      a. Primary adrenal disease
      b. Secondary to nonendocrine tumor
    3. Accelerated hypertension
    4. Renal vascular hypertension
    5. Renin producing tumor
    6. Adrenogenital syndrome
    7. Licorice excess
  G. Bartter's syndrome
  H. Renal tubular acidosis
  I. Acute hyperventilation
  J. Starvation
  K. Acute leukemia
III. Extrarenal losses
  A. Vomiting
  B. Gastric drainage
  C. Diarrhea of various causes
  D. Chronic laxative abuse
  E. Villous adenoma of the colon
  F. Ureterosigmoidostomy

Modified from Kunau and Stein.[70]

surgical patients receiving little or no oral intake and maintained on potassium-poor intravenous fluids. Under such circumstances, sizable potassium deficits may emerge.

Renal potassium losses may result from many causes, as indicated in Table 7. Of special relevance for the surgical patient are diuretics, acid-base disturbances, antibiotics, and magnesium deficiency. Most of the potent diuretics (e.g. furosemide, ethacrynic acid, thiazides) cause an immediate increase in renal potassium excretion while promoting excretion of sodium. Despite the brisk kaliuresis seen on initiation of diuretic therapy, a significant potassium deficit seldom accumulates even with continued treatment if electrolyte intake is adequate and other kaliuretic factors are absent.[72] Edematous patients who respond adequately to diuretic therapy are at much greater risk of developing significant potassium deficits because some potassium loss may continue as long as the diuresis persists.[14] Diuretic-induced potassium losses may be minimized by the simultaneous administration of potassium-sparing agents (e.g. spironolactone, triamterene).

Osmotic diuresis, resulting from an excess of non-reabsorbable solute within the tubular lumen (e.g., glucose, mannitol) invariably increases renal excretion of potassium. Urinary potassium losses of 10 to 20 mEq typically occur within two to three hours after initiating an osmotic diuresis with mannitol.[73] In diabetic patients, as much as 150 mEq of potassium may be lost within the first day after insulin therapy is discontinued, even in the absence of frank ketoacidosis.[74]

Metabolic alkalosis is a frequent occurrence in surgical patients (see p. 565) and is almost always associated with potassium depletion. Of special importance in this regard is the metabolic alkalosis following loss of gastric fluid via nasogastric suction or vomiting. When hydrochloric acid is lost from the stomach, bicarbonate replaces some of the chloride previously reabsorbed by the renal tubule along with sodium. As a result, the capacity of the proximal tubule to reabsorb bicarbonate is transiently exceeded by the bicarbonate load so that there is increased delivery of bicarbonate along with sodium to the distal nephron. Some of the accompanying sodium is lost in the urine with bicarbonate and some is reabsorbed in exchange for potassium. This stimulus to potassium secretion will continue as long as the metabolic alkalosis and associated chloride deficits are present. Potassium deficits in the range of 300 to 500 mEq are commonly encountered during gastric alkalosis.[75]

Certain antibiotics are capable of producing sizable renal potassium losses. Amphotericin B causes kaliuresis presumably by direct injury to renal transport processes and a reduction in renal potassium reabsorption. Serum potassium levels may fall below 2.5 mEq/L with cumulative doses of amphotericin B of less than 1 gm.[76] Carbenicillin leads to significant hypokalemia in approximately 10 percent of patients treated with this agent;[77] the kaliuretic effect of this antibiotic stems from its being a nonreabsorbable anion often given in large doses. Gentamicin may lead to potassium depletion in association with renal magnesium wasting.[78]

Patients with magnesium deficiency have excessive renal excretion of potassium which can be corrected only after replenishment of body magnesium.[79]

Extrarenal loss of potassium through the gastrointestinal tract is by far the most common cause of potassium depletion among surgical patients. Potassium concentration of gastric fluid is relatively low (approximately 10 mEq/L) and fluctuates within a narrow range. Thus, protracted vomiting and gastric drainage result in some direct loss of potassium but, as noted above, the major factor in producing hypokalemia under these circumstances is related to the augmented renal potassium losses secondary to metabolic alkalosis. By contrast, sizable intestinal potassium losses can result from loss of small intestinal fluid or from diarrhea. Special mention should be made of villous adenomas of the colon; these tumors may cause severe hypokalemia because they secrete a mucus-containing fluid that is very rich in potassium.[80,81] Patients with ureterosigmoidostomies also frequently become potassium depleted due to the relentless exchange of potassium for sodium by the colonic mucosa.[82]

The route of potassium loss is generally apparent from the clinical setting. In evaluating hypokalemia of uncertain origin, however, a measurement of urinary potassium concentration is frequently helpful. A low urinary potassium concentration (less than 10 to 15 mEq/L) signifies near maximal renal conservation, implying that the depletion has occurred by an extrarenal mechanism; furthermore, it has probably been present for several days. The exception to this generalization is the patient who has been treated with diuretics and recently discontinued their use. Therefore, a low urinary potassium concentration is strong evidence for extrarenal potassium depletion only in the absence of recent diuretic treatment. On the other hand, if urinary potassium concentration is high (greater than 30 to 40 mEq/L) signifying inadequate renal conservation, it is likely that the kidney itself is the source of the potassium loss.

MANIFESTATIONS

Many patients tolerate a moderate degree of potassium depletion (loss of 5 to 10% of body potassium) with no outward signs. Larger deficits are usually symptomatic and the symptoms are similar irrespective of the cause of the potassium losses. The important clinical manifestations relate to disturbed neuromuscular functions and reflect altered electrical properties of cell membranes.

Skeletal muscle weakness is an early manifestation.[83] Limb muscles tend to be affected initially, trunk and respiratory muscles later.[84] An extreme degree of potassium depletion may culminate in generalized areflexia, paralysis, and death from respiratory muscle failure. Smooth muscle dysfunction also occurs and probably explains the paralytic ileus and gastric dilatation occasionally seen in potassium deficient patients. Severe potassium depletion may cause significant structural damage to skeletal muscle and can produce frank rhabdomyolysis and myoglobinuria. Potassium depletion of lesser degree may potentiate the rhabdomyolysis associated with strenuous exercise or other precipitating factors.

Cardiac manifestations of hypokalemia include abnormalities in conduction and rhythmicity. Electrocardiographic abnormalities include depression of ST segments, lowered T wave voltage, and increased U wave voltage.[85] These EKG changes are nonspecific and are not invariably present in potassium depleted patients. A more important hazard of potassium depletion in cardiac patients is that it can provoke digitalis intoxication.

Potassium deficits can induce a variety of functional and structural changes in the kidney, the most significant of which is an interference with the effect of antidiuretic hormone. As a result, the kidney is unable to elaborate a maximally concentrated urine. Occasionally, polyuria and secondary polydypsia are the first clues to the presence of severe potassium depletion.[86]

MANAGEMENT

The repair of potassium deficits must be undertaken with great care. Since the magnitude of the potassium loss is not readily measurable clinically, the exact amount required for replacement cannot be predetermined. However, the serum potassium level provides a useful endpoint for replacement therapy. In practice, potassium supplements are generally recommended until normal serum potassium levels are re-established. Because administered potassium must first traverse the extracellular compartment before reaching the depleted cells, transient hyperkalemia may be induced even in the face of profound potassium deficits. Thus, the benefits of rapidly reversing serious functional disturbances of potassium depletion must be balanced against the risk of cardiotoxic serum potassium concentrations. As a general rule, it is better to err on the side of caution and repair deficits slowly. If rapid repair is necessary, it is important that serum potassium concentration be measured frequently and that the electrocardiogram be monitored to detect early signs of hyperkalemia.

Oral potassium supplementation is preferable whenever possible; gradual absorption following oral administration minimizes the risk of inducing transient hyperkalemia. Under most circumstances, potassium should be replaced as the chloride salt because the presence of coexisting chloride deficits limits the ability of the kidney to retain administered potassium. When potassium is infused intravenously, the rate of administration should not exceed 20 mEq/hour and no more than 100 to 150 mEq should be given per day unless the degree of potassium deficiency is life-threatening.

Potassium Surfeits and Hyperkalemia

Hyperkalemia is defined as a serum potassium concentration greater than 5.0 to 5.5 mEq/L. A factitious elevation of serum potassium can result from the lysis of cells in the blood sample. The most common cause of factitious hyperkalemia is hemolysis due to improper technique in blood collection, handling, or storage. Other causes are a very severe thrombocytosis[87] or leukocytosis.[88]

CAUSES

The causes of hyperkalemia can be classified into three groups (see Table 8): increased excretory burden, decreased excretory capacity, and altered transcellular distribution. In normal individuals, abrupt oral administration of as little as 50 mEq of potassium (less than 2% of normal body potassium) transiently increases plasma potassium concentration by 0.5 to 1.0 mEq/L.[89] In some instances, the oral administration of only 100 to 200 mEq can elevate plasma potassium concentration to dangerously high levels of 7 to 8 mEq/L.[89] Nevertheless, it is very uncommon for *sustained* hyperkalemia to occur solely as a result of dietary potassium excess. An iatrogenic increase in potassium intake, on the other hand, is a well-recognized cause of significant hyperkalemia. In a large group of patients receiving oral or intravenous potassium chloride supplements, fully 4 percent developed notable hyperkalemia.[72] Inadvertent potassium loading can occur as a result of high-dose potassium penicillin therapy (approximately 1.5 mEq potassium/1,000,000 U) or during treatment with potassium-containing salt substitutes.

Surgical patients are at special risk of hyperkalemia from a sudden breakdown of tissues. Because cellular potassium concentration averages 150 mEq/L of cell water, tissue breakdown can release enough potassium to overwhelm normal homeostatic mechanisms regulating extracellular potassium.[2] When new cell formation is thwarted (e.g., dietary protein deprivation), the net addition of potassium resulting from unopposed catabolism may contribute substantially to extracellular potassium. Much greater potassium loads are delivered to the body fluids when cell breakdown is accelerated by

TABLE 8. Classification of Hyperkalemia

- I. In vitro hemolysis
  - A. Improper collection of blood
  - B. Hematologic disorders with increased white blood cell or platelet count
- II. Increased excretory burden
  - A. Oral or intravenous potassium chloride
  - B. Potassium containing drugs
  - C. Tissue damage: Trauma, burns, rhabdomyolysis
  - D. Destruction of tumor tissue
  - E. Transfusion
- III. Decreased excretory capacity
  - A. Acute renal failure
  - B. Chronic renal failure
  - C. Potassium sparing diuretics
  - D. Mineralocorticoid deficiency
    1. Addison's disease
    2. Bilateral adrenalectomy
    3. Hypoaldosteronism
  - E. After renal transplantation
- IV. Altered transcellular distribution
  - A. Acidosis
  - B. Succinylcholine
  - C. Arginine infusion
  - D. Digitalis overdose
  - E. Hyperkalemic periodic paralysis
  - F. Hyperosmolality

Modified from Kunau and Stein.[70]

trauma due to crush injuries, burns, or major surgery. Intravascular hemolysis of native or transfused blood constitutes another common source of potassium requiring excretion. In the absence of brisk hemolysis, blood transfusions actually tend to result in a fall in serum potassium due to re-uptake of potassium by transfused cells and possibly to the alkalinizing effects of citrate when used as an anticoagulant.[90,91] As with exogenous potassium loads, cellular potassium loads seldom result in serious hyperkalemia when renal function is intact. However, renal function is frequently reduced in precisely those patients who experience accelerated rates of cell breakdown.

The most frequent causes of clinical hyperkalemia fall into the category of reduced excretory capacity. Acute oliguric renal failure is the prototypical example (see Chap 13, Renal Disease and Hypertension). Not only is renal potassium excretion virtually absent during acute renal failure, the excretory burden of potassium is often increased by exogenous potassium loads, frank tissue breakdown due to trauma, or the catabolic effects of surgery or sepsis. In this circumstance, life-threatening hyperkalemia rather than fluid overload or uremic toxicity becomes the major concern[92] (the management of acute renal failure is discussed in detail in Chap. 13, Renal Disease and Hypertension).

Most patients with stable chronic renal insufficiency keep up with daily demands for potassium excretion surprisingly well, unless the excretory burden is increased significantly or unless the excretory capacity is further reduced.[93] Therefore, when hyperkalemia is encountered in a patient with chronic renal insufficiency, a detailed dietary and drug history should be obtained. Special attention should be paid to the possible use of potassium-rich foods, to the ingestion of potassium-containing salt substitutes, and to the administration of potassium sparing diuretics (e.g., spironolactone, triamterene).[94]

Patients with less severe degrees of chronic renal insufficiency occasionally develop significant hyperkalemia. In many instances, this problem is related to the syndrome of hyporeninemic hypoaldosteronism. In most such cases, there is a component of chronic interstitial renal disease and about half of these patients prove to be diabetic. The hyperkalemia is frequently accompanied by moderate hyperchloremic metabolic acidosis. The mechanism of hyperkalemia in this syndrome is not completely understood.[15,95,96] Approximately one-third of patients receiving renal transplants also develop hyperkalemia presumably due to a decreased excretory ability of the graft.[97]

Hyperkalemia due to transcellular redistribution of potassium can result from several causes (See Table 8). Acute metabolic acidosis may result in hyperkalemia because of a shift of potassium from cells to the extracellular compartment.[98] Respiratory acidosis is much less likely to produce an important increase in serum potassium concentration. Several drugs can induce transient hyperkalemia by altering internal potassium distribution. Succinylcholine, by inhibiting cell membrane repolarization and cellular potassium uptake, typically causes plasma potassium concentration to rise slightly.[99] This effect may be greatly aggravated in the presence of trauma, burns, or neuromuscular disease, and life-threatening hyperkalemia may result.[100] Arginine monohydrochloride (and other cationic amino acids) cause a transient slight shift of potassium from cells. This agent is occasionally used as a source of hydrogen ions in the treatment of metabolic alkalosis and as a diagnostic stimulus for the release of growth hormone. Although of little clinical consequence when normal homeostatic mechanisms are intact, the hyperkalemia induced by use of arginine monohydrochloride may be of serious magnitude in the presence of modest renal insufficiency.[101] Digitalis poisoning due to massive overdose can also cause hyperkalemia.[102]

CLINICAL MANIFESTATIONS

All of the clinically important manifestations of hyperkalemia, like those of hypokalemia, relate to interference with the electrophysiologic events underlying nerve conduction and muscle contraction. In the presence of hyperkalemia, the ratio of intracellular to extracellular potassium is decreased, and as a result the resting membrane potential is reduced toward threshold level, delaying depolarization and hastening repolarization. These changes result in a reduced conduction velocity and contribute to the observed increase in myocardial excitability.

Cardiac tissue is exceptionally vulnerable to hyperkalemia. Both the specialized conduction tissue (Purkinje system) and the atrial and ventricular muscle fibers themselves are affected. The electrocardiogram is an invaluable adjunct to the measurement of serum potassium in recognizing and managing this electrolyte disturbance. Because the progression to fatal cardiac toxicity is unpredictable and often swift, the presence of any of the electrocardiographic changes associated with hyperkalemia is an indication for immediate treatment. The earliest and most specific electrocardiographic change is symmetrical peaking or "tenting" of the T wave. Thereafter, the characteristic widening of the QRS complex and lengthening of the P-R interval may appear.[103] Second-degree heart block may occasionally supervene. Atrial standstill may follow with a complete disappearance of the P wave. As ventricular conduction time continues to lengthen, the QRS complex widens further and may merge with the T wave, producing a premorbid "sine wave" pattern.[104]

As a general rule, there is a relationship between the magnitude of hyperkalemia and cardiotoxicity but the rate at which hyperkalemia develops is also a determining factor. When hyperkalemia appears abruptly (e.g., acute renal failure, acute metabolic acidosis, intravenous infusion of potassium), evidence of cardiotoxicity may develop with serum potassium concentrations no higher than 6 to 7 mEq/L. When hyperkalemia evolves more slowly, (e.g., chronic renal failure, adrenal insufficiency, use of potassium sparing diuretics), cardiac manifestations may be minimal or absent with serum potassium concentrations as high as 8 or 9 mEq/L.

TREATMENT OF HYPERKALEMIA

The abrupt onset of hyperkalemia constitutes a true medical emergency. Whenever possible, the underlying cause should be corrected. Because electrocardiographic changes provide the most reliable index of the severity of potassium intoxication, the electrocardiogram should be monitored throughout to gauge the effectiveness of therapy. If the electrocardiogram reveals only peaking of the T waves and if the serum potassium concentration is no higher than 6 mEq/L, restriction of dietary potassium and liberalization of dietary sodium may be sufficient unless oliguric renal failure is present. More vigorous therapeutic intervention is required if the serum potassium concentration is greater than 7 mEq/L or if more severe electrocardiographic changes are present. Fortunately, several measures are available for reversing life-threatening potassium toxicity and many can be undertaken simultaneously. As noted in Table 9, these measures fall into three general categories: immediate reversal of membrane effects, transfer of potassium into cells, and removal of potassium from the body.

The infusion of calcium ions can produce an immediate lessening of the cardiotoxicity of hyperkalemia. Calcium's beneficial effects depend upon its ability to restore a

TABLE 9. Treatment of Hyperkalemia

Immediate reversal of membrane effects
Calcium
Transfer of potassium into cells
Insulin and glucose
Sodium bicarbonate
Removal of potassium from the body
Diuretics (potassium wasting)
Cation exchange resins (Kayexalate®)
Hemodialysis
Peritoneal dialysis

more normal difference between threshold and resting membrane potentials rather than on altering the internal distribution of potassium. Calcium gluconate is the agent of choice for this purpose; 10 to 30 ml of 10 percent solution may be administered intravenously over a period of a few minutes. A similar amount of calcium gluconate may be added to 1 L of a glucose solution and administered more slowly as a continuous infusion. The beneficial effects of calcium infusions are transient and serve only to "buy time" for the institution of more lasting maneuvers.

Inducing a redistribution of potassium from extracellular to intracellular compartments can also reduce the immediate danger of cardiotoxicity. There are two principal approaches: stimulating insulin release and rapid alkalinization of the extracellular fluid. Release of insulin, which augments cellular uptake of potassium, can be stimulated by the administration of glucose. A solution of 50 ml of 50 percent glucose can be administered intravenously and followed by a continuous infusion of a 10 percent glucose solution. If renal failure is present, continuous infusion of more concentrated glucose solutions (25 to 50%) may be undertaken but requires placement of a central venous catheter to avoid local osmotic damage. The administration of 10 to 20 U of regular insulin per 100 gm of glucose is generally advised to ensure maximal potassium uptake, although this may not be necessary in the absence of diabetes. Administration of sodium bicarbonate to alkalinize body fluids also promotes transfer of potassium into cells. This maneuver is especially efficacious when metabolic acidosis is wholly or partially responsible for the hyperkalemia. Under these circumstances, at least one or two ampules of sodium bicarbonate (approximately 50 mEq/ampule) can be administered intravenously over a 5 to 10 minute period. The total amount of bicarbonate and the rapidity with which additional quantities should be administered depends upon the cause and severity of the acidosis. Even when serum bicarbonate is normal, however, the administration of one or two ampules of sodium bicarbonate is not hazardous and will lessen the severity of cardiotoxicity.[105]

The removal of some potassium from the body is generally required. Because impaired renal excretion of potassium is so frequently the cause of hyperkalemia, attention should be directed at improving overall renal function whenever possible. The use of proximal or loop diuretics (furosemide, ethacrynic acid) may help facilitate potassium excretion. Certainly, all drugs that impede potassium excretion should be discontinued and potassium ingestion should be curtailed. When renal excretion cannot be increased promptly, the most desirable alternative is to involve the gastrointestinal tract in potassium removal. Cation exchange resins are very effective for this purpose. Sodium polystyrene sulfonate (Kayexalate) can be given orally (20 to 30 gm in an aqueous suspension) or by retention enema (50 to 100 gm in 200 ml of water). An appropriate amount of 70 percent sorbitol should be administered concomitantly to increase the amount of fluid entering the bowel, thereby facilitating exchange and preventing constipation. Certain surgical conditions (e.g., recent colonic surgery) may preclude the use of cation exchange resins by either route. Moreover, the rate of potassium removal by cation exchange resins may be too slow if the potassium burden is great (e.g., crush injury, extensive burns). Under these circumstances, hemodialysis may be required. Hemodialysis can remove as much as 25 to 50 mEq of potassium per hour. Peritoneal dialysis is a less desirable alternative because the efficiency of potassium removal is much less. No more than 10 to 15 mEq of potassium can generally be removed per hour with this technique.

ACID-BASE DISORDERS

Clinical disturbances of acid-base balance are reflected by changes in the carbonic acid-bicarbonate buffer system. The following equations are used for describing the equilibrium state in this system in blood:[106,107]

$$pH = 6.1 + \log \frac{[HCO_3^-]}{0.03\ Paco_2}$$

$$[H^+] = 24 \times \frac{Paco_2}{[HCO_3^-]}$$

These are equivalent mathematical expressions, differing only in the units chosen to express blood acidity: millequivalents per liter of hydrogen ion in one and pH in the other (Table 10). In each case, carbonic acid concentration is expressed as the partial pressure of carbon dioxide ($Paco_2$) in millimeters of mercury and plasma bicarbonate concentration (HCO_3) directly in millequivalents per liter. In either expression, the level of acidity is determined by the ratio of these two physiologic variables. The factors governing each of these physiologic variables and, hence, impinging on plasma acidity are listed in Table 11.

Serum bicarbonate is not measured as such in the clinical laboratory but is estimated from the total carbon dioxide content or calculated from the pH and $Paco_2$. Acid-base data should be obtained from arterial blood samples whenever possible, but venous blood samples collected without stasis can provide sufficiently reliable information for many clinical purposes.

Before continuing the discussion, certain terms should be defined. *Acidemia* signifies an increase in plasma hydrogen ion concentration (decrease in pH), whereas *alkalemia* signifies a decrease in plasma hydrogen ion concentration (increase in pH). The terms *acidosis* and *alkalosis* are used to describe primary pathophysiologic processes that tend to alter acidity through one or more of the factors listed in Table 11. The term *metabolic*

TABLE 10. pH and Hydrogen Ion Concentration Equivalents

pH	*H⁺ (nEq/L)*	*pH*	*H⁺ (nEq/L)*
7.70	20	7.25	56
7.65	22	7.20	63
7.60	25	7.15	71
7.55	28	7.10	79
7.50	32	7.05	89
7.45	35	7.00	100
7.40	40	6.95	112
7.35	45	6.90	126
7.30	50		

TABLE 11. Physiologic Factors Impinging on Plasma Acidity

Through plasma bicarbonate concentration
Rate of hydrogen ion input
Rate of renal acid excretion
Rate of hydrogen ion or bicarbonate ion loss via the gastrointestinal tract
Availability of nonbicarbonate buffers
Space of distribution for bicarbonate
Through plasma carbon dioxide tension
Rate of carbon dioxide production
Rate of alveolar ventilation

Modified from Cohen.[108]

describes an acid-base disturbance initiated by a change in bicarbonate concentration; the term *respiratory* describes a disturbance initiated by a change in P_{CO_2}. Each initiating (primary) process, whether metabolic or respiratory, sets in motion secondary physiologic responses that alter the level of the opposing variable. The metabolic disturbances induce a ventilatory response that alters P_{CO_2} and minimizes the impact on acidity. Respiratory disturbances result in an immediate titration of tissue buffers that acutely alters the level of bicarbonate. If the respiratory disturbance is prolonged (a few days or more), a change in renal acid excretion and bicarbonate reabsorption occurs which results in further adjustments in acid-base equilibrium. Respiratory disturbances are therefore classified into acute and chronic subgroups.

The magnitude of each of these secondary physiologic responses (ventilatory, buffer, and renal) is roughly proportional to the magnitude of the initiating primary disorder. Thus, an appropriate range of physiologic responses can be defined for each class of acid-base disturbance, as detailed below.

A *simple acid-base disturbance* involves one primary process and its appropriate physiologic response. In a *mixed acid-base disturbance* two or more primary processes coexist. Because these processes may have either additive or nullifying effects on plasma acidity, mixed acid-base disturbances may produce dramatically extreme deviations in hydrogen ion concentration or disarmingly minor or undetectable deviations.

Metabolic Acidosis

Metabolic acidosis is the acid-base disturbance initiated by a reduction in bicarbonate concentration. The resulting increase in hydrogen ion concentration leads to an increase in alveolar ventilation and a reduction in carbon dioxide tension. The decrement of carbon dioxide tension observed in patients with simple metabolic acidosis is roughly proportional to the decrement in plasma bicarbonate concentration. On the average, each 1 mEq/L reduction in bicarbonate concentration in patients with stable metabolic acidosis is associated with a 1.0 to 1.3 mm Hg reduction in Pa_{CO_2}.[109]

The pathophysiologic processes that result in metabolic acidosis can be classified into two groups: those involving a loss of body bicarbonate as such and those involving the addition of a strong acid that consumes bicarbonate during the process of buffering. The degree to which plasma bicarbonate falls during metabolic acidosis is a function not only of the magnitude of the bicarbonate loss or of the acid load but of the time interval over which the offending process occurs and of the speed with which the kidney is able to replenish bicarbonate stores.

CAUSES OF METABOLIC ACIDOSIS

The major causes of this acid-base disturbance are listed in Table 12 and can be classified into two groups according to the presence or absence of an elevated concentration of undetermined anions. The undetermined anion concentration, often referred to as the anion gap, can be defined as the difference between serum sodium concentration and the sum of serum chloride and total carbon dioxide concentrations.[111] The normal undetermined anion concentration, defined in this way, ranges between 8 to 12 mEq/L. As noted in Table 12, the causes of metabolic acidosis associated with a normal undetermined anion concentration can be subclassified as follows: A loss of bicarbonate as such, an abnormality of renal tubular hydrogen ion secretion with well preserved glomerular function; and the addition of hydrochloric acid to body fluids.

The loss of bicarbonate as a cause of metabolic acidosis is of particular relevance to the surgical patient. Bicarbonate can be lost from the body either through the gastrointestinal tract or the kidney. The most common cause of gastrointestinal bicarbonate loss is diarrhea during which bicarbonate derived from pancreatic and intestinal secretions is incompletely absorbed. Bicarbonate concentration of diarrheic stools is almost always higher than that of plasma and may reach levels exceeding 70 to 80 mEq/L. Infants and young children are particularly prone to develop acidosis as a result of

TABLE 12. Causes of Metabolic Acidosis

Undetermined Anion Concentration	
Normal	*Elevated*
Loss of bicarbonate	Overproduction of organic acids
Diarrhea	Lactic acidosis
Small bowel losses	Diabetic ketoacidosis
Ureterosigmoidostomy	Alcoholic ketoacidosis
Ileal loop bladder	Prolonged starvation
Carbonic anhydrase inhibitors	Methyl alcohol ingestion
Dilutional acidosis	Ethylene glycol ingestion
Disproportionate failure of renal tubular function	Paraldehyde ingestion
Renal tubular acidosis	Salicylate intoxication
Tubulointerstitial renal disease	Renal insufficiency
Urinary tract obstruction	
Addition of hydrochloric acid	
Ammonium chloride	
Lysine hydrochloride	
Arginine hydrochloride	

Modified from Cohen and Kassirer.[110]

diarrhea because of the relatively large bicarbonate losses in proportion to bicarbonate stores that occur over a short time. Small bowel losses of bicarbonate may also occur via drainage through tubes or fistulae.

Significant metabolic acidosis caused in part by the loss of bicarbonate is a frequent complication of patients with ureterosigmoidostomy. The temporary retention of chloride-rich urine in the sigmoid colon results in the reabsorption of chloride in exchange for extracellular bicarbonate, which is subsequently evacuated with the stool. Reabsorption of urinary ammonium as well as renal damage from infection and other causes may also contribute importantly to the development of acidosis in these patients. Frequent enemas or the use of rectal tubes to reduce contact time between urine and colonic mucosa may reduce the tendency towards acidosis in this circumstance. Urinary diversion via an ileal conduit is associated with a much lower incidence of metabolic complications. Unless stomal obstruction develops, external drainage of the urine is usually sufficiently prompt to avoid significant bicarbonate loss.

The enzyme carbonic anhydrase is necessary for normal renal bicarbonate reabsorption. Inhibition of this enzyme can result in sufficient bicarbonatruria to cause metabolic acidosis. Acetazolamide (Diamox®), the most commonly employed carbonic anhydrase inhibitor, is used occasionally as a diuretic and more frequently to lower intraocular pressure in patients with glaucoma.

Mild metabolic acidosis can result from a marked and sudden increase in the space of bicarbonate distribution, which causes existing bicarbonate to be diluted or "lost" into a larger volume. Such dilutional acidosis is occasionally seen during rapid re-expansion of the severely volume contracted patient when such re-expansion is accomplished with saline or other fluids lacking in bicarbonate or equivalent base.[112]

Several varieties of congenital and acquired renal tubular diseases result in sufficient limitation of bicarbonate reabsorption or urinary acidification or both to cause frank metabolic acidosis. This group of disorders is referred to as renal tubular acidosis. Two main types of renal tubular acidosis are recognized: distal (classical, type I) and proximal (type II).[113,114]

In distal renal tubular acidosis, the terminal segments of the nephron are unable to sustain large transepithelial hydrogen ion concentration gradients. As a consequence, urinary hydrogen ion concentration remains relatively low (pH greater than 5.5) even after acid loading. Both the acidosis and the frequently associated hypokalemia generally are corrected by daily alkali therapy. Distal renal tubular acidosis may be primary (idiopathic) or secondary to hyperglobulinemia, hypercalcemia, amphotericin B toxicity, lithium, renal transplantation, or systemic lupus erythematosus (Table 13).

In proximal renal tubular acidosis, the major defect appears to be an inability to sustain a normal rate of bicarbonate reabsorption in the proximal tubule. When the filtered load of bicarbonate does not exceed this diminished capacity for bicarbonate reabsorption, urinary acidification is normal. Even large amounts of bicarbonate therapy may be ineffective in fully correcting the acidosis because the administered alkali is not reabsorbed by the kidney and rapidly escapes into the urine. Proximal renal tubular acidosis is frequently associated with other proximal tubular transport defects (Fanconi's syndrome) and may be seen with inborn errors of metabolism (cystinosis, Wilson's disease), heavy metal toxicity (lead), outdated tetracycline, multiple myeloma (with light chain proteinuria), or transplant rejection (see Table 13).

TABLE 13. Causes of Renal Tubular Acidosis

Type 1: Distal	*Type 2: Proximal*
Primary	Primary
Sporadic	Sporadic
Inherited	Inherited
Hyperglobulinemia	With Fanconi's syndrome
Hypercalcemia	Cystinosis
Amphotericin B toxicity	Wilson's disease
Lithium toxicity	Lead
Renal transplantation	Outdated tetracycline
	Multiple myeloma
	Amyloidosis
	Renal transplantation
	Vitamin D deficiency

Hyperchloremic metabolic acidosis occurring in association with hyperkalemia has been described in patients with hyporeninemic hypoaldosteronism. Most such patients have mild to moderate impairment of renal function due to some form of chronic interstitial disease; more than half are diabetic. Even in the absence of hyporeninemia, patients with a variety of tubular interstitial diseases (e.g., pyelonephritis, analgesic abuse nephropathy, chronic transplant rejection) or urinary tract obstruction may develop tubular dysfunction out of proportion to glomerular insufficiency and manifest persistent hyperchloremic acidosis.

Metabolic acidosis with a normal anion gap can also result from the addition of hydrochloric acid or a hydrochloric acid precursor to body fluids. Hydrochloric acid itself is occasionally administered intravenously in the treatment of severe metabolic alkalosis (see below). Excessive administration will, of course, result in metabolic acidosis. More commonly, this form of metabolic acidosis is the consequence of the administration of ammonium chloride or of the chloride salts of cationic amino acids (e.g., lysine, arginine). Such amino acids are contained in certain of the preparations used for hyperalimentation and total parenteral nutrition.[115] When metabolized, these amino acids yield hydrochloric acid.

The causes of metabolic acidosis associated with an elevated undetermined anion concentration can be subclassified into two groups, overproduction of organic acids and renal insufficiency (Table 12). A wide variety of organic acids may accumulate in the body fluids in association with certain disease states or in response to various toxins. Among surgical patients, lactic acidosis constitutes by far the most important cause of acidosis in this category.[116] Circulating lactic acid derives from the anerobic reduction of pyruvic acid by several tissues, (e.g., muscle, skin) and is metabolized to carbon dioxide and water largely by the liver and kidney. Normal plasma concentrations of lactate range between 1 and 2 mmol/L. Clinical lactic acidosis occurs most often as a result of tissue hypoxia which can increase the production of lactic acid dramatically. Hepatic dysfunction due to intrinsic liver disease or reduced hepatic circulation is frequently present in patients with lactic acidosis and may contribute importantly to the severity of the acid-base disturbance. The more common causes of lactic acidosis are listed in Table 14. Of particular relevance to the surgical patient are shock (e.g., blood loss, sepsis), seizures,[117] cardiac arrest, and cardiopulmonary bypass.[118,119]

TABLE 14. Causes of Lactic Acidosis

Overproduction of lactic acid
Excessive oxygen (energy) demands
Severe voluntary exercise
Prolonged general convulsions
Decreased oxygen delivery
Shock
Cardiac arrest
Cardiopulmonary bypass
Severe hypoxia ($Pa_{O_2} < 30–35$ mm Hg)
Very severe anemia
Interference with oxygen utilization
Phenformin
Isoniazid overdosage
Idiopathic ("spontaneous")
Diabetes mellitus
Leukemia
Other chronic diseases
Underutilization of lactic acid
Hepatic failure
Ethanol intoxication

Modified from Cohen and Kassirer.[110]

The occurrence of lactic acidosis often has grave prognostic significance, the eventual outcome depending largely on the reversibility of the underlying disease.[120] The onset of lactic acidosis is often abrupt, thus requiring the prompt institution of therapy. The rate of bicarbonate administration required to keep pace with the continuing rate of acid production in patients with lactic acidosis varies considerably and can be determined in individual instances only by monitoring acid-base parameters frequently. It is often necessary to administer such large quantities of bicarbonate (e.g., 100 to 300 mEq/hour) that the risk of marked hyperosmolality and serious vascular congestion is great. If concomitant diuretic therapy fails to produce adequate sodium and water losses, dialysis may be required to prevent or treat these complications. When dialysis therapy is necessary, additional alkali is provided by the diffusion of bicarbonate or bicarbonate precursor (e.g., acetate) from the dialysate into the circulation. Unfortunately, even prompt and vigorous therapy often fails to avert death unless treatment of the underlying cause is effective.

Ketoacidosis due to the over-production of acetoacetic acid and beta-hydroxybutyric acid occurs in diabetes mellitus, alcoholic ketoacidosis, and prolonged starvation. These metabolic derangements are discussed in Chapter 5, Endocrinology. The overproduction of organic acids occurs in association with various ingested toxins (see Table 12), is often life-threatening, and requires prompt alkali therapy as well as specific measures designed to increase the metabolism or clearance of the toxin in question.

The metabolic acidosis occurring in association with renal insufficiency results from the failure of renal tubular function to excrete the daily hydrogen ion load produced by endogenous acid production. Under normal dietary conditions, this endogenous acid production averages 1 mEq/kg of body weight per day in adults[121] and up to 3 mEq/kg of body weight per day in infants and young children.[122] During periods of increased catabolism, and after trauma or an operation, endogenous acid production can be markedly increased. The clinical consequences and management of acidosis associated with renal insufficiency are discussed in detail in Chapter 13, Renal Disease and Hypertension.

TREATMENT OF METABOLIC ACIDOSIS

Treatment of metabolic acidosis should center about removing the underlying cause, if possible, and providing adequate amounts of bicarbonate if necessary. If plasma bicarbonate concentration remains above 16 to 18 mEq/L and if the cause of the acidosis can be treated or is self-limited, bicarbonate replacement therapy may not be necessary because the normal kidney can replete body bicarbonate stores over a period of several days. If, however, the cause of the acidosis cannot be eliminated (e.g., chronic renal failure), long-term alkali therapy may be necessary. Bicarbonate, or an organic anion that can be converted to bicarbonate (e.g., citrate), may be administered orally for this purpose with the dose adjusted empirically to maintain the desired plasma bicarbonate concentration.

If bicarbonate concentration is markedly depressed ($<$ 10 mEq/L), rapid therapeutic intervention is advisable even if the underlying cause can be removed quickly (e.g., diabetic acidosis, certain forms of lactic adidosis). Among the compelling arguments favoring alkali therapy in patients with such severe degrees of metabolic acidosis is the substantial risk of abrupt worsening of the acidemia due either to further decrements in bicarbonate concentration or to even slight reduction in the magnitude of the respiratory response. For example, a patient with a plasma bicarbonate of 5 mEq/L and a $Paco_2$ of 10 mm Hg would have a hydrogen ion concentration of 48 mEq/L (pH 7.31). If ventilatory effort is not sustained (e.g., fatigue, sedative administration occur) and $Paco_2$ rises only slightly to 15 mm Hg, hydrogen ion concentration would rise to 72 mEq/L (pH 7.14), a life-threatening degree of acidemia.[123]

Rapid correction of metabolic acidosis is accomplished most reliably by the intravenous administration of sodium bicarbonate. As a general rule, therapy should be designed to replace no more than about one-half of the total bicarbonate deficit over the initial 12 hours of treatment in order to avoid the consequences of abrupt changes in extracellular acid-base equilibrium. In any event, plasma bicarbonate should not be raised above 14 to 16 mEq/L acutely. When this precaution is observed, tetany, altered mental status, and convulsions rarely occur. In estimating the amount of bicarbonate required to produce a desired increment in plasma bicarbonate concentration, the effect of nonbicarbonate buffers on the fate of administered bicarbonate must be considered. Because at least 50 percent of an administered bicarbonate load is dissipated immediately by hydrogen ions relinquished from nonbicarbonate buffers, a rough estimate of the dose of bicarbonate required can be obtained by multiplying the desired increment in plasma bicarbonate concentration by an apparent space of distribution at least twice as large as the normal extracellular fluid volume (i.e., approximately 40% of body weight).[124] The apparent space of bicarbonate distribution may be even larger in patients with severe metabolic acidosis (i.e., plasma bicarbonate less than 5 mEq/L).[125] Such estimates of bicarbonate requirements serve only as rough guidelines and must be adjusted to suit individual circumstances. This is particularly true when increased acid production (e.g., lactic acidosis) or bicarbonate losses (e.g., ongoing diarrhea) continue during the period of therapy.

Alkalinizing agents such as lactate (as in Ringer's lactate) offer no advantage over bicarbonate in the urgent treatment of the metabolic acidosis. Indeed, a potential disadvantage is their requirement for metabolic conversion, necessitating adequate cardiac and hepatic function. If cardiac or renal failure preclude administration of adequate amounts of bicarbonate (with sodium) it may be necessary, as noted above, to institute peritoneal dialysis or hemodialysis.

Metabolic Alkalosis

Metabolic alkalosis refers to those acid-base disturbances initiated by an elevation in plasma bicarbonate concentration. Metabolic alkalosis is frequently encountered among surgical patients because loss of gastric fluid and the administration of certain diuretic agents, the two major causes of this acid-base disturbance, are commonplace. Regardless of cause, metabolic alkalosis is typically associated with secondary hypoventilation and some elevation in $Paco_2$. This adaptive response of the respiratory system is analogous to the hyperventilation and secondary hypocapnia classically associated with metabolic acidosis. The magnitude of the secondary adjustments in carbon dioxide tension appear to be somewhat less than those generally associated with metabolic acidosis; on the average, each 1 mEq/L increment in plasma bicarbonate concentration in patients with simple metabolic alkalosis is associated with an approximately 0.5 to 0.7 mm Hg increment in $Paco_2$.[126] In patients with normal pulmonary function and only moderate degrees of metabolic alkalosis, the degree of secondary hypoventilation does not produce significant hypoxemia. In patients with underlying pulmonary insufficiency, however, as well as those with very severe metabolic alkalosis, the attendant hypoxemia may be of considerable clinical importance. This is especially true in patients requiring mechanical ventilation in whom an element of metabolic alkalosis may be a critical factor in perpetuating ventilator dependency.

Persistent elevation of plasma bicarbonate concentration implies the presence of some obstacle to the excretion of bicarbonate by the kidney. This axiom stems from the ease with which the normal kidney can eliminate surplus bicarbonate from the circulation when exogenous alkali is provided. Three principal mechanisms are recognized whereby surplus bicarbonate fails to be excreted by the kidney: (1) disproportionate deficit of body chloride coupled with increased renal sodium avidity (chloride responsive), (2) direct stimulation of renal bicarbonate reabsorption (chloride resistant), and (3) generalized reduction of renal function coupled with alkali administration. The common causes of metabolic alkalosis are classified according to these mechanisms in Table 15.

CAUSES OF METABOLIC ALKALOSIS

Disproportionate loss of body chloride coupled with increased renal sodium avidity is by far the most common mechanism accounting for sustained elevation of plasma bicarbonate concentration. The concurrence of chloride deficits coupled with a stimulus

TABLE 15. Causes of Metabolic Alkalosis

Disproportionate deficit of body chloride (chloride responsive)
Vomiting
Gastric suction
Diuretics
Villous adenoma of the colon
Abrupt relief of chronic hypercapnea
Direct stimulation of renal bicarbonate resorption (chloride resistant)
Hyperaldosteronism
Cushing's syndrome
Bartter's syndrome
Severe potassium depletion
Alkali administration with renal insufficiency
Milk alkali syndrome

Modified from Cohen and Kassirer[110]

to renal sodium conservation occurs as a consequence of gastric acid loss, renal losses induced by most potent diuretics (thiazides, furosemide, ethacrynic acid) and, less commonly, chloride losses in the stool (e.g., certain forms of villous adenoma of the colon). Sustained alkalosis occurs in these settings because renal bicarbonate reabsorption is accelerated as the kidney endeavors to conserve filtered sodium in the presence of an inadequate complement of filtered chloride (i.e., hypochloremia). The hallmark of this form of metabolic alkalosis is the excretion of a virtually chloride-free urine. As a corollary, the bicarbonate surplus is rapidly excreted into the urine following provision of adequate dietary or parenteral chloride salts. It is for this reason that these forms of metabolic alkalosis are commonly referred to as chloride responsive.

Gastric alkalosis deserves special mention because of its frequency among surgical patients. The magnitude of the alkalosis seen in these circumstances is, of course, dependent upon the quantity of hydrochloric acid lost from the body which, in turn, is a function of the quantity and degree of acidity of the gastric fluid. Gastric loss is responsible in virtually every instance of severe metabolic alkalosis (plasma bicarbonate level greater than 45 to 50 mEq/L). Patients with gastrin-secreting tumors are especially prone to the development of severe metabolic alkalosis owing to the large volume of intensely acid gastric juice that may be formed. The degree of alkalosis attendant upon nasogastric suction can be significantly reduced by the concurrent administration of cimetidine.[127]

Direct stimulation of renal bicarbonate reabsorption is a much less common cause of sustained metabolic alkalosis. This mechanism appears to play the major role in the metabolic alkalosis associated with various forms of mineralocorticosteroid excess and in rare patients with extremely severe potassium deficiency (see Table 14). As a general rule, patients with mineralocorticoid excess have only mild to moderate degrees of metabolic alkalosis. The acid-base disturbance is resistant to the usual dietary intake of chloride. As a result, abundant chloride is typically found in the urine in the face of sustained metabolic alkalosis. Appreciable potassium chloride supplements may, however, have a beneficial effect on the level of plasma bicarbonate. In rare instances, severe potassium depletion (serum potassium concentration less than 2 mEq/L) has been associated with chloride resistant metabolic alkalosis in the absence of hyperadrenocorticism.[132] Such patients regain the ability to conserve administered chloride normally after repair of the potassium deficit.

Generalized reduction of renal function due to acute or chronic renal failure can result in sustained metabolic alkalosis if exogenous alkali administration exceeds the excretory capacity of the kidney.[133] One example of this form of metabolic alkalosis occurs in patients with the milk-alkali syndrome in whom chronic ingestion of absorbable alkali has resulted in substantial renal functional impairment due to nephrocalcinosis.[134]

Treatment of gastric alkalosis and other forms of chloride responsive alkalosis, as implied above, requires the provision of adequate quantities of exogenous chloride.[128] Because potassium deficits virtually invariably accompany metabolic alkalosis, potassium chloride should generally be included in the replacement regimen. Indeed, in mild metabolic alkalosis such as that frequently induced by diuretic agents, chloride repletion may be accomplished entirely by administering the potassium salt. In the patient with frank volume deficits, however, an appreciable fraction of the chloride supplement should be provided as the sodium salt. In the rare patient with very severe metabolic alkalosis (plasma bicarbonate 45 to 50 mEq/L or pH greater than 7.65) more rapid dissipation of the bicarbonate surplus may be required and can be accomplished by the infusion of dilute hydrochloric acid or of the hydrochloric acid precursor, arginine monohydrochloride.[129,130] Hydrochloric acid can be infused via central venous catheter in a concentration of 100 mM/L (0.1 normal). Only approximately 50 percent of an infused acid load serves to titrate extracellular bicarbonate, the remainder being accommodated by nonbicarbonate buffers. Consequently, the quantity of acid required to affect a given reduction in plasma bicarbonate concentration can be estimated by assuming a space of distribution approximately twice as large as the true extracellular fluid volume. The following formula may be applied:

$$\text{acid (mEq) needed for correction of metabolic alkalosis} = \text{current } [HCO^-{}_3] - \text{desired } [HCO^-{}_3] \times \text{Body Weight(kg)} \times 0.40$$

If arginine monohydrochloride is employed as the source of hydrogen ion, careful monitoring of plasma potassium concentration is required. Arginine infusions cause a shift of potassium out of cells and, especially in the presence of renal insufficiency, can result in clinically significant hyperkalemia.[101,131] Arginine monohydrochloride may be given by peripheral vein; 300 ml of a 10 percent solution provides 143 mEq of hydrogen ion. In the presence of reasonably normal renal function, the adequacy of chloride repletion in patients with metabolic alkalosis is most easily confirmed by the appearance of abundant chloride in the urine.

Respiratory Acidosis

Respiratory acidosis refers to those acid-base disturbances initiated by an elevation in carbon dioxide tension (hypercapnia) and occurs whenever alveolar ventilation is reduced. The acidemia that results from hypercapnia causes a titration of tissue buffers and an immediate but very small increment in plasma bicarbonate concentration. An abrupt elevation of $Paco_2$ to levels of 80 to 90 mmHg (acute respiratory acidosis) is associated with an increment in plasma bicarbonate concentration no greater than 3 to 4 mEq/L.[135,136] Sustained elevations in $Paco_2$ (chronic respiratory acidosis) evoke an increase in renal acid excretion and bicarbonate reabsorption that leads to a much larger increment in plasma bicarbonate concentration. In simple, chronic respiratory acidosis (of at least 3 to 4 days duration), each millimeter of mercury increment in $Paco_2$ is associated with a mean increment in plasma bicarbonate concentration of approximately 0.3 to 0.4 mEq/L.[137,138]

Hypercapnia is always associated with some degree of hypoxemia (unless inspired oxygen concentration is increased). Thus, the manifestations of this acid-base disorder are to a considerable extent manifestations of reduced oxygen availability as well as of increased $Paco_2$. Symptoms depend not only on the magnitude of but also upon the rapidity with which the hypercapnia and hypoxia develop. As a general rule, chronic hypercapnia is better tolerated than acute hypercapnia of similar magnitude. Clinical manifestations include anxiety, marked breathlessness, and reduced mental capacity. Headaches and objective signs of cerebral edema may occur, possibly reflecting the vasodilating effects of carbon dioxide. Stupor and coma may supervene.[139]

CAUSES OF RESPIRATORY ACIDOSIS

The common clinical causes of respiratory acidosis are listed in Table 16 and are subdivided into those which are typically associated with abrupt, transient hypercapnia and those which tend to produce sustained elevations in carbon dioxide tension. Acute respiratory acidosis is frequently seen among surgical patients. Central suppression of ventilation (general anesthetics, narcotics), airway obstruction, acute intrapulmonary disease, and improperly adjusted ventilators are common occurrences. Treatment of acute respiratory acidosis, regardless of etiology, must be directed at prompt removal of the underlying cause. It is imperative to restore adequate ventilation swiftly in order to prevent severe hypoxemia and extreme acidemia. Intubation and mechanical ventilation are frequently required. Although the administration of bicarbonate may help blunt the

TABLE 16. Causes of Respiratory Acidosis

Acute	*Chronic*
General anesthesia	Obstructive pulmonary disease
Sedatives	Brain tumor
Cardiac arrest	Respiratory nerve damage
Pneumothorax	Primary myopathy involving respiratory muscles
Pulmonary edema	Restrictive disease of thorax
Severe pneumonia	Prolonged pneumonia
Bronchospasm	Primary alveolar hypoventilation
Laryngospasm	
Aspiration of foreign body	
Mechanical ventilators	

Modified from Cohen[108]

developing acidemia, such therapy is a temporizing maneuver at best and should not divert attention away from correcting the hypercapnia and attendant hypoxia.

Longstanding respiratory acidosis occurs in the great majority of instances as a result of underlying chronic obstructive pulmonary disease. Patients with chronic CO_2 retention from this and other causes are at increased risk from surgery and require very careful management during the perioperative period. A detailed discussion of the management of surgical patients with chronic lung disease can be found in Chapter 12, Pulmonary Diseases.

Respiratory Alkalosis

Respiratory alkalosis refers to those acid-base disturbances initiated by a reduction in carbon dioxide tension (hypocapnia) and occurs whenever alveolar ventilation is increased. The alkalemia that results from hypocapnia causes an immediate titration of tissue buffers and fall in plasma bicarbonate concentration. This decrement in plasma bicarbonate is somewhat greater in magnitude than the analogous increment in bicarbonate seen during acute respiratory acidosis of comparable severity. An abrupt reduction in $Paco_2$ to 20 to 25 mmHg is associated, on the average, with a 3 to 4 mEq/L fall in plasma bicarbonate concentration.[140] Prolonged reductions in $Paco_2$ (chronic respiratory alkalosis) evoke renal adaptive responses which cause a transient reduction in acid excretion and a sustained reduction in renal bicarbonate reabsorption. As a result, plasma bicarbonate concentration falls further in chronic respiratory alkalosis, each millimeter of mercury decrement in Pco_2 being associated with an approximately 0.4 to 0.5 mEq/L reduction in plasma bicarbonate concentration.[141]

Acute voluntary hyperventilation is associated with numbness and tingling of the hands, feet, and perioral area, carpal pedal spasm, and lightheadedness; Trousseau's sign may be positive. Most patients with respiratory alkalosis rarely complain of these symptoms. Tachycardia is often present but the blood pressure is usually unchanged.[142] The clinical picture is usually dominated by the findings associated with the underlying disorder.

CAUSES OF RESPIRATORY ALKALOSIS

Common causes of respiratory alkalosis are listed in Table 17. Unexplained acute respiratory alkalosis in the surgical patient should raise the suspicion of early gram-negative

TABLE 17. Causes of Respiratory Alkalosis

Anxiety, hysteria	Congestive heart failure
Fever	Pneumonia
Gram-negative septicemia	Mild pulmonary edema
Salicylate intoxication	Pulmonary emboli
Central nervous system diseases	Hypoxia
Cerebrovascular accident	Hepatic insufficiency
Trauma	Mechanical ventilators
Infection	
Tumor	

Modified from Cohen and Kassirer[110]

sepsis, mild pulmonary edema, pulmonary emboli, or anxiety. Acute respiratory alkalosis occurs frequently in critically ill patients and may signal an unfavorable outlook. Chronic respiratory alkalosis is seen less often among surgical patients. Persistent unexplained hyperventilation should prompt consideration of underlying hepatic insufficiency or primary central nervous system disease. The only effective treatment for respiratory alkalosis is removing the underlying cause.

Mixed Acid-Base Disturbances

Mixed acid-base disturbances occur when two or more simple acid-base disorders coexist. Such mixed disturbances are surprisingly common among hospitalized patients. The presence of a mixed acid-base disturbance is frequently suggested by a careful analysis of the acid-base values, themselves. Table 18 depicts the patterns of acid-base values typically encountered in simple acid-base disorders of variable magnitude. When the magnitude of the secondary change in $Paco_2$ or bicarbonate concentration (in the metabolic and respiratory disorders, respectively) is inappropriate with respect to the magnitude of the initiating process, the presence of a mixed disturbance should be considered. Even when a seemingly appropriate relation exists between an initiating disturbance and its anticipated secondary response, such a relationship may merely be the fortuitous consequence of a dual or even a triple acid-base abnormality. To avoid this diagnostic pitfall, clues to the presence of complicating acid-base disturbances should be sought from a close examination of other laboratory data (e.g., the unmeasured anion concentration) and particularly from the patient's history.

Certain mixed disturbances are characterized by a normal or near normal hydrogen ion concentration. Thus, the presence of both chronic respiratory acidosis and metabolic alkalosis or of both metabolic acidosis and respiratory alkalosis may be overlooked if one focuses only on the level of acidity and fails to appreciate the abnormalities in plasma bicarbonate concentration and $Paco_2$. It is also clear that other combinations of simple disturbances tend to cause extreme shifts in hydrogen ion concentration because bicarbonate concentration and $Paco_2$ are deviated in opposite directions. Thus, in patients with both metabolic acidosis and respiratory acidosis and in those with both metabolic alkalosis and respiratory alkalosis relatively small abnormalities in $Paco_2$ and bicarbonate concentration can produce alarmingly high or low hydrogen ion concentrations, respectively.

TABLE 18. Expected Compensation for Simple Acid-Base Disorders

Metabolic acidosis	$Paco_2$ should fall by 1.0 to 1.3 mm Hg for each 1 mEq/L fall in plasma HCO_3^- concentration
Metabolic alkalosis	$Paco_2$ should rise by 0.5 to 0.7 mm Hg for each 1 mEq/L rise in plasma HCO_3^- concentration
Acute respiratory acidosis	Plasma HCO_3^- concentration should not rise more than 3 to 4 mEq/L
Chronic respiratory acidosis	Plasma HCO_3^- concentration should rise by 0.3 to 0.4 mEq/L for each 1 mm Hg rise in $Paco_2$
Acute respiratory alkalosis	Plasma HCO_3^- concentration should not fall more than 3 to 4 mEq/L
Chronic respiratory alkalosis	Plasma HCO_3^- concentration should fall by 0.4 to 0.5 mEq/L for each 1 mm Hg fall in $Paco_2$

The following are frequently encountered examples of mixed acid-base disturbances:

RESPIRATORY ACIDOSIS AND METABOLIC ACIDOSIS

Elements of respiratory and metabolic acidosis frequently coexist in patients with cardiopulmonary arrest. Such patients often develop lactic acidosis because of poor tissue perfusion and hypercapnia because of inadequate ventilation. Patients with severe pulmonary edema may develop a similar picture. As noted above, this combination of disturbances may produce extreme degrees of acidemia, plasma hydrogen ion concentration occasionally reaching levels well in excess of 100 mEq/L (pH less than 7.0). Effective treatment usually requires intubation and mechanical ventilation and intravenous alkali therapy. The outlook is limited by the nature and severity of the underlying disease.

METABOLIC ALKALOSIS AND RESPIRATORY ACIDOSIS

This combination of disturbances is seen relatively frequently because patients with carbon dioxide retention secondary to severe pulmonary disease often develop metabolic alkalosis as a result of vomiting or diuretic administration. As noted earlier, an element of metabolic alkalosis in a patient with chronic CO_2 retention may critically reduce ventilatory drive. This factor may prevent weaning from mechanical ventilators or contribute importantly to underlying hypoxemia.

CHRONIC RESPIRATORY ACIDOSIS COMPLICATED BY A SUDDEN REDUCTION IN $Paco_2$

Patients with chronic hypercapnia have an elevated plasma bicarbonate concentration as a result of normal renal adaptation, as noted above. When such patients experience an abrupt reduction in $Paco_2$ (e.g., intubation, mechanical ventilation), alkalemia may ensue because plasma bicarbonate concentration will remain elevated until the kidney can excrete what is now an excessive amount of alkali. If the sudden reduction in $Paco_2$ results in a fall in hydrogen ion concentration to less than 25 to 30 mEq/L (pH greater than 7.60), coma, seizures, and even death can occur. Thus, in patients with moderate or severe respiratory acidosis who require intubation and mechanical ventilation, $Paco_2$ should be lowered gradually to prevent plasma hydrogen ion concentration from falling much below normal.[143] If such patients are treated with a chloride-free diet (e.g., low salt intake because of congestive heart failure), the kidneys will be unable to excrete the now surplus bicarbonate and a "post-hypercapnic" metabolic alkalosis will persist.

CHRONIC RESPIRATORY ACIDOSIS COMPLICATED BY A SUDDEN RISE IN $Paco_2$

Patients with chronic respiratory acidosis who develop abrupt further increments in $Paco_2$ (intercurrent pulmonary infection, congestive heart failure, excessive oxygen or sedative administration) require prompt attention because the degree of acidemia and hypoxemia may be severe. Treatment should be directed at the factors causing the acute respiratory failure; mechanical ventilation may be necessary. Administration of sodium bicarbonate should be avoided because the effect on acidity is only transient and because of the risk of volume overload.

METABOLIC ACIDOSIS AND RESPIRATORY ALKALOSIS

This mixed acid-base disturbance is common among patients with salicylate intoxication because of the independent effects of salicylates on both cellular metabolism and ventilation. Gram-negative sepsis can also produce this mixed acid-base disturbance because of the frequent occurrence of primary hyperventilation, on the one hand, and of lactic acidosis and/or renal failure, on the other.

MIXED METABOLIC ACIDOSIS AND ALKALOSIS

Patients with metabolic alkalosis occasionally evidence simultaneous metabolic acidosis. This mixed disturbance is seen most often in alcoholics in whom vomiting from gastritis is commonplace and in whom a predisposition to ketoacidosis and lactic acidosis is present. The diagnosis of mixed metabolic acidosis and alkalosis depends upon an accurate history and ancillary laboratory data. When the acidosis component of this mixed disturbance is associated with an increased anion gap, the diagnosis can be made by careful analysis of the plasma anionic composition. Under this circumstance, the unmeasured anion concentration will be elevated to a greater degree than anticipated from the observed change in plasma bicarbonate concentration. For example, a patient with gastric alkalosis who develops superimposed lactic acidosis may have the following laboratory findings: sodium 140 mEq/L, chloride 90 mEq/L, bicarbonate 10 mEq/L. The unmeasured anion concentration of 40 mEq/L is some 25 to 30 mEq higher than normal, yet the difference between the normal plasma bicarbonate (24 mEq/L) and the observed value (10 mEq/L) is only 14 mEq/L. Thus, the original plasma bicarbonate must have been significantly elevated (approximately 40 mEq/L) signifying that a metabolic alkalosis must have been present.

REFERENCES

1. Fitzgibbons, JP: *Fluid, electrolyte and acid-base management in the acutely traumatized patient.* Orth Clin North Am 9:627, 1978.
2. Edelman, IS, and Leibman, J: *Anatomy of body water and electrolytes.* Am J Med 27:256, 1959.
3. Maffly, RH: *The body fluids: volume, composition, and physical chemistry,* in Brenner, BM, and Rector FC, (eds.): *The Kidney.* Philadelphia, W.B. Saunders, Co., 1981, 76–115.
4. Randall, HT: *Fluid, electrolyte and acid-base balance.* Surg Clin North Am 56:1019, 1976.
5. Holden, WD, Krieger, H, Levey, S, et al: *The effect of nutrition on nitrogen metabolism in the surgical patient.* Ann Surg 146:563, 1957.
6. Moore, FD: *Common patterns of water and electrolyte change in injury, surgery and disease.* N Engl J Med 258:277, 325, 377, 427, 1958.
7. Harrington, JT, and Cohen, JJ: *Clinical disorders of urine concentration and dilution.* Arch Intern Med 131:810, 1973.

8. Arieff, AI, and Guisado, R: *Effects on the central nervous system of hypernatremic and hyponatremic states.* Kidney Int 10:104, 1976.
9. McCance, RA: *Experimental sodium chloride deficiency in man.* Proc R Soc Lond (Biol) 119:245, 1936.
10. Stormont, JM and Waterhouse, C: *The genesis of hyponatremia associated with marked overhydration and water intoxication.* Circulation 24:191, 1961.
11. Arieff, AI, Llach, F, and Massry, SG: *Neurological manifestations and morbidity of hyponatremia: correlation with brain water and electrolytes.* Medicine 55:121, 1976.
12. Lipsmeyer, E, and Ackerman, GL: *Irreversible brain damage after water intoxication.* JAMA 196:286, 1966.
13. Berl, T, Anderson, RJ, McDonald, KM, et al.: *Clinical disorders of water metabolism.* Kidney Int 10:117, 1976.
14. Fichman, MP, Vorherer, H, and Kleeman, CR: *Diuretic-induced hyponatremia.* Ann Intern Med 75:853, 1971.
15. Schrier, RW, and Regal, EM: *Influence of aldosterone on sodium, water and potassium metabolism in chronic renal disease.* Kidney Int 1:156, 1972.
16. Danovitch, GM, Bourgoignie, J, and Bricker, NS: *Reversibility of the "salt-losing" tendency of chronic renal failure.* N Engl J Med 296:14, 1977.
17. Shires, GT, and Canizaro, PC: *Fluid, electrolyte, and nutritional management of the surgical patient,* in Schwartz, SI (ed.): *Principles of Surgery.* New York: McGraw-Hill Book Co., 1979, pp. 65–97.
18. Berliner, RW, and Davidson, DG: *Production of hypertonic urine in the absence of antidiuretic hormone.* J Clin Invest 36:1416, 1957.
19. Moran, WH, Jr., Miltenberger, FW, Shuayb, WA, et al: *The relationship of antiduiretic hormone secretion to surgical stress.* Surgery 56:99, 1964.
20. Dubovsky, SL, Grabon, S, Berl, T, et al: *Syndrome of inappropriate secretion of antidiuretic hormone with exacerbated psychosis.* Ann Intern Med 79:551, 1973.
21. Miller, M, and Moses, A: *Drug-induced states of impaired water excretion.* Kidney Int 10:96, 1976.
22. Fichman, MP: *Role of cyclic nucleotides in the etiology and therapy of polyuric disorders,* in Volicer, L, (ed.): *Clinical Aspects of Cyclic Nucleotides.* New York: Spectrum Publications, 1977.
23. Berl, T, Cadnapaphornchai, P, and Harbottle, JA: *Mechanism of stimulation of vasopressin release during beta-adrenergic stimulation with isoproterenol.* J Clin Invest 53:857, 1974.
24. Fichman, MP: *Disorders of renal concentration and dilution,* in Gonick, HC, (ed.): *Current Nephrology.* Boston: Houghton Mifflin Co., 1977, pp. 57–98.
25. deBodo, RC: *The antidiuretic action of morphine and its mechanism.* J Pharmacol Exp Ther 82:74, 1944.
26. Schnieder, H, and Blackmore, EK: *The effect of nalorphine on the antidiuretic action of morphine in rat and man.* Br J Pharmacol 10:45, 1955.
27. deBodo, RC, and Prescott, KF: *The antidiuretic action of barbituarates (phenobarbital, amytal, pentobarbital) and the mechanism involved in this action.* J Pharmacol Exp Ther 85:222, 1945.
28. Burn, JH, Truelove, LH, and Burn, I: *The antidiuretic action of nicotine and smoking.* Br Med J 1:403, 1945.
29. Cadnapaphornchai, P, Boykin, JL, Berl, T, et al.: *Mechanism of effect of nicotine on renal water excretion.* Am J Physiol 227:1216, 1974.
30. Fliegel, KM, and Cole, CH: *Inappropriate antidiuresis during carbamazepine treatment.* Ann Intern Med 87:722, 1977.
31. Moses, AM, Howanitz, J, Van Gemert, M, et al.: *Clofibrate-induced antidiuresis.* J Clin Invest 52:535, 1973.
32. Fine, RN, Clarke, RR, and Shore, NA: *Hyponatremia and vincristine therapy: syndrome possibly resulting from inappropriate antidiuretic hormone secretion.* Am J Dis Child 112:256, 1966.
33. Steele, TH, Serpick, AA, and Block, JB: *Antidiuretic response to cyclosphosphamide in man.* J Pharmacol Exp Ther 185:245, 1973.
34. Weissman, PN, Shenkman, L, and Gregerman, RI: *Chlorpropamide hyponatremia: drug-induced inappropriate antidiuretic hormone activity.* N Engl J Med 284:65, 1971.
35. Nisbet, P: *Chlorpropamide-induced hyponatremia.* Br Med J 1:904, 1977.
36. Hagen, GA, and Frawley, TF: *Hyponatremia due to sulfonylurea compounds.* J Clin Endocrinol Metab 31:570, 1970.

37. Pohl, JEF, Thurston, H, and Swales, JD: *The antidiuretic action of diazoxide.* Clin Sci 42:145, 1972.

38. Anderson, RJ, Berl, T, McDonald, KM, et al: *In vivo evidence for an antagonism between vasopressin and prostaglandin in the mammalian kidney.* J Clin Invest 56:420, 1975.

39. Pittman, JG: *Water intoxication due to oxytocin: report of a case.* N Engl J Med 268:481, 1963.

40. Morgan, DB, Kirway, WA, Hancock, KW, et al: *Water intoxication and oxytocin infusion.* Br J Obstet Gynecol 84:6, 1977.

41. Hayes, MA: *Water and electrolyte therapy after operations.* N Engl J Med 278:1054, 1968.

42. Bartter, FC, and Schwartz, WB: *The syndrome of inappropriate secretion of anti-diuretic hormone.* Am J Med 42:790, 1967.

43. Nolph, KD, and Schrier, RW: *Sodium, potassium and water metabolism in the syndrome of inappropriate antidiuretic hormone secretion.* Am J Med 49:534, 1970.

44. Hantman, D, Rossier, B, Zohlman, R, et al: *Rapid correction of hyponatremia in syndrome of antiduiretic hormone secretion, an alternative therapy to hypertonic saline.* Ann Intern Med 78:870, 1973.

45. deTroyer, A, and Demanet, JC: *Correction of antidiuresis by demeclocycline.* N Engl J Med 293:915, 1975.

46. White, MG, and Fetner, CD: *Treatment of the syndrome of inappropriate secretion of antidiuretic hormone with lithium carbonate.* N Engl J Med 292:390, 1977.

47. Burrows, GD, Davis, B, and Kincaid-Smith, P: *Unique tubular lesion after lithium.* Lancet 1:1310, 1978.

48. Hestbech, J, Hansen, HE, Amdisen, A, et al: *Chronic renal lesions following longterm treatment with lithium.* Kidney Int 12:205, 1977.

49. Forrest, JN, Cox, M, Hong, C, et al.: *Superiority of demeclocycline over lithium in the treatment of chronic syndrome of inappropriate secretion of antidiuretic hormone.* N Engl J Med 298:173, 1978.

50. Carrilho, F, Bosch, J, Arroyo, V, et al.: *Renal failure associated with demeclocycline in cirrhosis.* Ann Intern Med 87:195, 1977.

51. Katzman, R, and Pappius, HM: *Hypernatremia and hyperosmolarity,* in *Brain Electrolytes and Fluid Metabolism.* Baltimore: Williams & Wilkins Co., 1973, pp. 278–290.

52. Feig, PU, and McCurdy, DK: *The hypertonic state.* N Engl J Med 297:1444, 1977.

53. Fichman, MP: *Disorders of renal concentration and dilution: hyponatremia and hypernatremia,* in Gonnick, HC (ed.): *Current Nephrology.* Boston: Houghton Mifflin, 1978, pp. 145–200.

54. Epstein, FM: *Disturbances in renal concentrating ability,* in Andreoli, TE, Grantham, JJ, and Rector, FC (eds.): *Disturbances in Body Fluid Osmolality.* Bethesda: American Physiological Society, 1977, pp. 251–266.

55. Engel, FL, and Jaeger, C: *Dehydration with hypernatremia, hyperchloremia and azotemia complicating nasogastric tube feeding.* Am J Med 17:196, 1954.

56. Scoggin, C, McClellan, JR, and Cary, JM: *Hypernatremia and acidosis in association with topical treatment of burns.* Lancet 1:959, 1977.

57. Kaupke, C, Sprague, T, and Gitnick, GL: *Hypernatremia after the administration of lactulose.* Ann Intern Med 86:745, 1977.

58. Primach, WA, Gartner, LM, McGurk, HE, et al: *Hypernatremia associated with cholestyramine therapy.* J Pediatr 90:1024, 1977.

59. Mattar, JA, Weil, MH, Shubin, H, et al.: *Cardiac arrest in the critically ill.* Am J Med 56:162, 1974.

60. Waters, WC, III, Hall, JD, and Schwartz, WB: *Spontaneous lactic acidosis.* Am J Med 35:781, 1963.

61. DeVillota, ED, Cavanilles, JM, Stein, L, et al.: *Hyperosmolal crises following infusion of hypertonic sodium chloride for purposes of therapeutic abortion.* Am J Med 55:116, 1973.

62. Finberg, L: *Hypernatremic (hypertonic) dehydration in infants.* N Engl J Med 289:196, 1973.

63. Hogan, GR, Dodge, PR, and Gill, SR: *Pathogenesis of seizures occurring during restoration of plasma tonicity to normal in animals previously chronically hypernatremic.* Pediatrics 43:54, 1969.

64. Arieff, AI, and Kleeman, CR: *Studies on mechanisms of cerebral edema in diabetic comas: effects of hyperglycemia and rapid lowering of plasma glucose in normal rabbits.* J Clin Invest 52:571, 1973.

65. Smith, FW, and Sleisinger, MH: *Physiology of the colon,* in Sleisinger, MH, and Fordstran, JS (eds.): *Gastrointestinal Disease.* Philadelphia: WB Saunders Co., 1978, pp. 1523–1548.

66. Ahlman, KL, Eränko, O, Karvenen, MJ, et al.: *Mineral composition of thermal sweat in healthy persons.* J Clin Endocrinol 13:773, 1953.

67. Hiatt, N, Yamakawa, T, and Davidson, MP: *Necessity for insulin in transfer of excess infused potassium to intracellular fluid.* Metabolism 23:43, 1974.

68. Alexander, EA, and Levinsky, NG: *An extrarenal mechanism of potassium adaptation.* J Clin Invest 47:740, 1968.

69. Schwartz, WB: *Potassium and the kidney.* N Engl J Med 253:601, 1955.

70. Kunau, RT, and Stein, JH: *Disorders of hypo and hyperkalemia.* Clin Nephrol 7:173, 1977.

71. Squires, RD, and Huth, EJ: *Experimental potassium depletion in normal human subjects: I. Relation of ionic intake to the renal conservation of potassium.* J Clin Invest 38:1134, 1959.

72. Kassirer, JP, and Harrington, JT: *Diuretics and potassium metabolism: a reassessment of the need, effectiveness and safety of potassium therapy.* Kidney Int 11:505, 1977.

73. Gennari, FJ, and Kassirer, JP: *Osmotic diuresis.* N Engl J Med 291:714, 1974.

74. Atchley, DW, Loeb, RF, Richards, DW, Jr, et al.: *On diabetic acidosis: a detailed study of electrolyte balance following the withdrawal and reestablishment of insulin therapy.* J Clin Invest 12:297, 1933.

75. Kassirer, JP, and Schwartz, WB: *The response of normal man to selective depletion of hydrochloric acid.* Am J Med 40:10, 1966.

76. Douglas, JB, and Healy, R: *Nephrotoxic effects of amphotericin B including renal tubular acidosis.* Am J Med 64:154, 1965.

77. Klastersky, J, Vanderkelen, B, Daneau, D, et al.: *Carbenicillin and hypokalemia.* Ann Intern Med 78:774, 1973.

78. Bar, RS, Wilson, HE, and Mazzaferri, EL: *Hypomagnesemic hypocalcemia secondary to renal magnesium wasting: a possible consequence of high dose gentamicin therapy.* Ann Intern Med 82:646, 1975.

79. Shils, ME: *Experimental human magnesium depletion.* Medicine 48:61, 1969.

80. Hodin, E, and Remington, JH: *Villous adenoma with severe electrolyte depletion.* Dis Colon Rectum 12:36, 1969.

81. Babior, BH: *Villous adenoma of the colon.* Am J Med 41:615, 1966.

82. Loughlin, JF: *Quadriplegia, hypopotassemia, and hyperchloremic acidosis after bilateral ureterosigmoidostomy.* N Engl J Med 254:329, 1956.

83. Duggin, GG, and Price, MA: *Hypokalemic muscular paresis in migratory Papua/New Guineans.* Lancet 1:649, 1974.

84. Holler, JW: *Potassium deficiency and diabetic acidosis.* JAMA 131:1186, 1946.

85. Surawicz, B: *Relation between the ECG and electrolytes.* Am Heart J 73:814, 1967.

86. Relman, AS, and Schwartz, WB: *The nephropathy of potassium depletion: clinical and pathological entity.* N Engl J Med 255:195, 1956.

87. Ingram, RH, Jr., and Seki, M: *Pseudohyperkalemia with thrombocytosis.* N Engl J Med 267:895, 1962.

88. Bronson, WR, DeVita, VT, Carbone, PP, et al.: *Pseudohyperkalemia due to release of potassium from white blood cells during clotting.* N Engl J Med 274:369, 1966.

89. Keith, NM, and Osterberg, AE: *Human tolerance for potassium.* Proc Staff Meet Mayo Clin 21:385, 1946.

90. Simon, GE, and Bove, JR: *The potassium load from blood transfusion.* Postgrad Med 49:61, 1971.

91. Collins, JA: *Massive blood transfusion,* in Cash, JD (ed.): *Clinics in Hematology, Blood Transfusion, and Blood Products.* Philadelphia: WB Saunders Co., 1976, p. 216.

92. Lordon, RE, and Burton, JR: *Post-traumatic renal failure in military personnel in Southeast Asia.* Am J Med 53:137, 1972.

93. Strauss, MB: *Acute renal insufficiency due to lower-nephron nephrosis.* N Engl J Med 293:693, 1948.

94. Cohen, AB: *Hyperkalemic effect of triamterene.* Ann Intern Med 65:521, 1966.

95. Schambelan, M, Stockigt, JR, and Biglieri, EG: *Isolated hypoaldosteronism in adults: a renin deficiency syndrome.* N Engl J Med 287:573, 1972.

96. Sebastian, A, Schambelan, M, Lindenfeld, S, et al.: *Amelioration of metabolic acidosis with fludrocortisone therapy in hyporeninemic hypoaldosteronism.* N Engl J Med 297:576, 1977.

97. DeFronzo, R, Goldberg, M, Cooke, CR, et al.: *Investigations into the mechanism of hyperkalemia following renal transplantation.* Kidney Int 11:365, 1977.

98. Burnell, JM, Villamil, MF, Uyeno, DT, et al.: *The effect in humans of extracellular pH change on the relationship between serum potassium concentration and intracellular potassium.* J Clin Invest 35:935, 1956.

99. Evers, WE, Racz, JB, and Dobkin, AB: *A study of plasma potassium and electrocardiographic changes after a single dose of succinylcholine.* Can Anaesth Soc J 16:273, 1969.

100. Cooperman, LH: *Succinylcholine induced hyperkalemia in neuromuscular disease.* JAMA 213:1867, 1970.

101. Bushinsky, DA, and Gennari, FJ: *Life-threatening hyperkalemia induced by arginine.* Ann Intern Med 89:632, 1978.

102. Reza, MJ, Kovick, RB, Shire, KI, et al.: *Massive intravenous digoxin overdosage.* N Engl J Med 291:777, 1974.

103. Finch, CA, Sawyer, CG, and Flynn, JM: *Clinical syndromes of potassium intoxication.* Am J Med 1:377, 1946.

104. Levine, HD: *Electrolyte imbalance and the ECG.* Mod Concepts Cardiovasc Dis 23:246, 1954.

105. Fraley, DS, and Adler, S: *Correction of hyperkalemia by bicarbonate despite constant blood pH.* Kidney Int 12:354, 1977.

106. Henderson, LJ: *The theory of neutrality regulation in the animal organism.* Am J Physiol 21:427, 1908.

107. Cohen, JJ: *A new acid-base nomogram featuring hydrogen ion concentration: Henderson revisited.* Ann Intern Med 66:159, 1967.

108. Cohen, JJ: *Disorders of hydrogen ion metabolism,* in Earley, LE, and Gottshalk, CW (eds.): *Strauss and Welt's Diseases of the Kidney.* Boston: Little Brown and Company, 1979, pp. 1543–1579.

109. Lennon, EG, and Lemann, J, Jr.: *Defense of hydrogen ion concentration in chronic metabolic acidosis.* Ann Intern Med 65:265, 1966.

110. Cohen, JJ, and Kassirer, JP: *Acid-base metabolism,* in Maxwell MH and Kleeman, CR (eds.): *Clinical Disorders of Fluid and Electrolyte Metabolism.* New York: McGraw-Hill Book Company, 1980, pp. 181–232.

111. Emmett, M, and Narins, RG: *Clinical use of the anion gap.* Medicine 56:38, 1977.

112. Garella, S, Chang, BS, and Kahn, SI: *Dilution acidosis and contraction alkalosis: review of a concept.* Kidney Int 8:279, 1975.

113. Narins, RG, and Goldberg, M: *Renal tubular acidosis: pathogenesis, diagnosis and treatment.* Disease-a-Month, March 1977.

114. Gennari, FJ, and Cohen, JJ: *Renal tubular acidosis.* Ann Rev Med 29:521, 1978.

115. Heird, WC, Dell, RB, and Driscoll, JM, Jr.: *Metabolic acidosis resulting from intravenous alimentation mixture containing synthetic amino acids.* N Engl J Med 287:943, 1972.

116. Oliva, PB: *Lactic acidosis.* Am J Med 48:209, 1970.

117. Orringer, CE, Eustance, JC, Wunsch, CD, et al.: *Natural history of lactic acidosis after grand mal seizure.* N Engl J Med 297:796, 1977.

118. Huckabee, WE: *Abnormal reacting blood lactate. I. The significance of hyperlactaemia in hospitalized patients.* Am J Med 30:833, 1961.

119. Huckabee, WE: *Abnormal reacting blood lactate. II. Lactic acidosis.* Am J Med 30:840, 1961.

120. Relman, AS: *Lactic acidosis,* in Brenner, BM, and Stein, JH (eds.): *Acid-Base and Potassium Homeostasis.* New York: Churchill Livingston, 1978, pp. 65–100.

121. Relman, AS: *Renal acidosis and renal excretion of acid in health and disease,* in Dock, W, and Snapper, I (eds.): *Advances in Internal Medicine.* Chicago: Year Book Medical Publishers, 1964, pp. 295–347.

122. Albert, MS, and Winters, RW: *Acid-base equilibrium of blood in normal infants.* Pediatrics 37:728, 1966.

123. Kassirer, JP: *Serious acid-base disorders.* N Engl J Med 291:773, 1974.

124. Schwartz, WB, Jensen, RL, and Relman, AS: *The deposition of acid administered to sodium-depleted subjects: the renal response and the role of whole body buffers.* J Clin Invest 33:587, 1954.

125. Garella, S, Dana, CL, and Chazan, JA: *Severity of metabolic acidosis as a determinant of bicarbonate requirements.* N Engl J Med 289:121, 1973.

126. von Ypersele de Strihou, C, and Farns, A: *The respiratory response to chronic metabolic alkalosis and acidosis in disease.* Clin Sci Mol Med 45:439, 1973.

127. Vaziri, ND, Barton, CH, Ness, R, et al.: *Special uses of cimetidine.* Ann Intern Med 88:266, 1978.

128. Kassirer, JP, and Schwartz, WB: *Correction of metabolic alkalosis in man without repair of potassium deficiency: a re-evaluation of the role of potassium.* Am J Med 40:19, 1966.

129. Abouna, GM, Veazey, PR, and Terry, DB, Jr.: *Intravenous infusion of hydrochloric acid for treatment of severe metabolic alkalosis.* Surgery 75:194, 1974.

130. Worthley, LIG: *The rational use of i.v. hydrochloric acid in the treatment of metabolic alkalosis.* Br J Anaesth 49:811, 1977.

131. Hertz, P, and Richardson, JA: *Arginine-induced hyperkalemia in renal failure patients.* Arch Intern Med 130:778, 1972.

132. Garella, S, Chazan, JA, and Cohen, JJ: *Saline resistant-metabolic alkalosis or "chloride-wasting nephropathy": report of four cases with severe potassium depletion.* Ann Intern Med 73:31, 1970.

133. Van Goidsenhoven, GMT, Gray, OV, and Prince, AV: *The effect of prolonged administration of large doses of sodium bicarbonate in man.* Clin Sci 13:383, 1954.

134. Punsar, S, and Somer, T: *The milk-alkali syndrome: a report of three illustrative cases and a review of the literature.* Acta Med Scand 173:435, 1963.

135. Giebisch, G, Berger, L, and Pitts, RF: *The extrarenal response to acute acid-base disturbances of respiratory origin.* J Clin Invest 34:231, 1955.

136. Brackett, NG, Jr., Cohen, JJ, and Schwartz, WB: *Carbon dioxide titration curve of normal man.* N Engl J Med 272:6, 1965.

137. Schwartz, WB, Brackett, NC, Jr., and Cohen, JJ: *The response of extracellular hydrogen ion concentration to graded degree of chronic hypercapnia.* J Clin Invest 44:291, 1965.

138. van Ypersele de Strihou, C, Brasseur, L, and de Coninck, J: *The "carbon dioxide response curve" for chronic hypercapnia in man.* N Engl J Med 275:117, 1966.

139. Dulfano, MJ, and Ishikawa, S: *Hypercapnia: mental changes and extrapulmonary complications. An expanded concept of the "CO_2 intoxication" syndrome.* Ann Intern Med 63:829, 1965.

140. Arbus, GS, Herbert, LA, Levesque, PR, et al: *Characterization and clinical applications of the "significance band" for acute respiratory alkalosis.* N Engl J Med 280:117, 1969.

141. Gennari, FJ, Goldstein, MB, and Schwartz, WB: *The nature of the renal adaptation to chronic hypocapnia.* J Clin Invest 51:1722, 1972.

142. Saltzman, H, Heyman, A, and Sieker, H: *Correlation of clinical and physiological manifestations of sustained hyperventilation.* N Engl J Med 268:1431, 1963.

143. Asmundsson, T, and Kilburn, KH: *Complications of acute respiratory failure.* Ann Intern Med 70:487, 1969.

Chapter 16

NUTRITION

Johanna Dwyer, D.Sc., and
Thomas O'Donnell, M. D.

Nutritional care of the surgical patient is a three-step process: (1) assessing the underlying nutritional state, (2) determining both the caloric and nitrogen *requirements* and *goals,* and (3) selecting the *route*—oral, enteral, or parenteral—and the *type* of nutritional repletion. The field of nutritional intervention is changing rapidly and some aspects may appear chaotic and contradictory. This chapter will acquaint the reader with a standardized approach to nutritional intervention in the surgical patient. The basic approach employed here relies on an understanding of the metabolic changes associated with surgical stress, but its simplified manner should not be interpreted as a failure to recognize the inherent complexity of the field. An exhaustive discussion of enteral and parenteral nutrition is beyond the scope of this chapter, and the reader is referred to the excellent texts by Ballinger,[1] Fischer,[2] and Schneider et al.[3]

SURGICAL STRESS AND THE METABOLIC RESPONSE

Energy Requirements

Why certain surgical patients require more calories or protein than others will be addressed in a general sense in subsequent sections. This section details the alterations in energy requirements and flux of substrate fuels (glucose, free fatty acids, ketone bodies, and amino acids) which occur with fasting and disease states. Once the unique metabolic demands of a particular disease state are appreciated, nutritional intervention can be appropriately tailored to that state. Table 1 contrasts the metabolic rates in several states: (1) patients convalescing from clean major surgical operations, (2) patients with major

TABLE 1. Circulatory and Metabolic Alteration in Various Surgical States* (Mean ± SEM)

	Post Operative Non-Infected State	Moderate to Severe Trauma: Hypovolemia and Shock	Moderate to Severe Trauma: Post shock	Sepsis: Low Output State	Sepsis: High Output State
Circulatory Alterations					
Mean arterial pressure (mm Hg)	81 ± 10	57 ± 10	78 ± 14	62 ± 9	89 ± 12
Cardiac index ($L/M^2/min$)	3.6 ± 0.3	1.7 ± 0.7	4.3 ± 1.0	1.9 ± 1.1	4.8 ± 1.6
Pulmonary arterial mean pressure (mm Hg)	18 ± 4	14 ± 4	21 ± 5	29 ± 5	28 ± 5
Pulmonary capillary wedge pressure (mm Hg)	8 ± 2	7 ± 5	12 ± 5	15 ± 5	13 ± 5
Metabolic Alterations					
Metabolic rate ($kcal/M^2/24$ hours)	980 ± 210		1131 ± 213	1040 ± 169	1240 ± 250
Body temperature (t°C)	38.2	36.4	38.7	37.3	39.4

*From Clowes, GHA, Jr., O'Donnell, TF, Blackburn, GL, et al.[183]

trauma, and (3) patients with sepsis. The basal metabolic rate or basal energy expenditure (BEE) is defined as the energy required at a specific time of day to maintain the vegetative bodily processes of the fasting and resting individual at thermal neutrality (20°C). The proverbial 70 kg man may burn 1 kilocalorie (kcal) of energy per minute at rest but with moderate activity this expenditure is increased up to 5 to 7½ kcal/minute. Table 1 shows that there is a significant difference in the energy requirements of the patient convalescing from clean major surgery in comparison to those of either traumatized or septic patients. In uneventful convalescence from major surgery, there are no abnormal respiratory demands and there is very little increase in energy expenditure. By contrast, with tissue injury and especially with sepsis the BEE may be increased 20 to 35 percent. We have found it important to categorize the responses to trauma or sepsis as: (1) the high output or hyperdynamic response or (2) the low output or hypodynamic response.[4] These are not static states and under the dynamics of disease one may phase into another. In the high output phase, cardiac index and peripheral blood flow may be elevated to at least 50 percent above basal values. In the high flow state, fever alone fails to account for the elevated caloric requirement. The energy expenditure is much greater than that predicted by the DuBoise formula (7% rise in metabolic rate for each one-half degree Centigrade of body temperature elevation). Increased work of respiration and possible uncoupling of phosphorylation may account for this difference. In thermal injury, there is the added factor of evaporative heat loss. In the low output state, the cardiovascular system is unable to meet the elevated circulatory demands so there is an inadequate perfusion of peripheral tissues, particularly muscle. Cardiac output may be only 30 to 90 percent of basal values. Metabolic heat production is not maintained to a sufficient degree to counteract ambient heat loss, so body temperature may drop to subnormal levels. Thus, the stress of trauma or sepsis greatly increases the caloric requirement in contrast to uncomplicated postoperative convalescence.

Endogenous Substrate Fuels (Table 2)

ENERGY SOURCES

There are three sources of endogenous fuel which may be utilized in times of fasting or stress: carbohydrate (glucose), fat (free fatty acids or ketone bodies), and protein (as amino acids). The carbohydrate source is the least abundant (1/100 of the caloric content of the fat stores), so liver and muscle glycogen usually is expended by 24 hours of fasting. The protein stores are contained centrally within the liver and peripherally within muscle. Some degradation of the protein stores (proteolysis) and subsequent oxidation of their constituent amino acids occurs during adaptation to fasting.[5] The carbon fragments of the amino acid products of peripheral protein oxidation (alanine and glutamine) are converted to glucose by the liver (gluconeogenesis). The resultant increase in urinary nitrogen excretion is an index of gluconeogenesis and therefore of proteolysis. A major aim of nutritional therapy is to reduce the use of endogenous protein stores, because protein is needed for synthesis of important acute phase proteins and enzymes as well as for muscle work (e.g., respiration).

TABLE 2. Arterial Insulin and Substrate Levels in Various Surgical Conditions* (Mean ± SEM)

	72 Hour Fast (n = 6)	*Post Operative Noninfected (n = 7)*	*High Flow Sepsis (n = 9)*	*Low Flow Sepsis (Septic Shock) (n = 9)*
Glucose (mM/L)	3.7 ± 0.3	5.0 ± 0.6	8.3 ± 0.6	7.2 ± 0.7
Lactate (mM/L)	0.6 ± .04	0.8 ± 0.1	1.9 ± .2	3.14 ± .74
Free fatty acids (mM/L)	1.2 ± .04	.84 ± .42	.65 ± .12	.96 ± .15
Ketone (mM/L)	2.0 ± 0.5	0.8 ± 0.02	.014 ± .004	.035 ± .007
Glycerol (mM/L)	0.17 ± 0.05	0.13 ± 0.05	0.14 ± .01	0.10 ± .02
Alanine (mM/L)	.18 ± .02	.28 ± .04	.27 ± .03	.43 ± .05
Insulin (mU/L)	10 ± 8	30 ± 9	46 ± 4	6 ± 1

*From Clowes, GHA, Jr., O'Donnell, TF, Blackburn, GL, et al.[183]
n = number of patients

FASTING

After 24 hours of fasting, glycogen is expended as a potential glucose source. Thereafter, fat and peripheral protein stores are the principal sources of energy fuels. Under the favorable influence of lowered serum levels of the antilipolytic hormone insulin, fat is released from fat stores in the form of free fatty acids and glycerol. Free fatty acids can be oxidized directly as fuel by muscle. After partial oxidation by the liver, ketone bodies also can be utilized as fuel by muscle and by certain sections of the brain. The branched-chain amino acids, leucine, isoleucine, and valine, are directly oxidized by muscle. The amino acid byproducts of this oxidative process, alanine and glutamine, are deaminated in the liver and the carbon skeletons are resynthesized to glucose. The endogenous use of branched-chain amino acids by muscle gradually decreases as adaptation to fasting occurs and fat stores become the principal fuel source.[5]

TRAUMA

Although arterial glucose levels are approximately 30 mg/dl higher in noninfected postoperative patients than in fasting subjects, glucose uptakes are similar.[6] On the other hand, lactate production by peripheral tissue is three times greater in the noninfected postoperative patient than in the fasting state. Thus, only one-half of the glucose uptake is completely oxidized in the postoperative patient. Concomitant with the enhanced anaerobic metabolism of glucose in the postoperative traumatic state, free fatty acids and ketone oxidation are reduced well below fasting values. Based on a calculation of the available fuel derived from glucose and fat, there would be an energy deficit. The endogenous oxidation of branched-chain amino acids fills this deficit.[7] The enhanced release of alanine and excretion of urinary nitrogen reflect the elevated protein oxidation.

SEPSIS

The substrate fuel pattern is different in high flow sepsis compared to the fasting or noninfected postoperative patient. Although the blood insulin level is increased four-fold over that in fasting, peripheral glucose uptake is comparable to that in fasting. This pattern is indicative of insulin resistance (more insulin required for a given glucose uptake). Incomplete oxidation of glucose is indicated by the four-fold increase in lactate production over fasting. In sepsis, approximately one-quarter of the glucose uptake is completely oxidized. In addition to the deficit in energy derived directly from glucose, lipolysis is decreased as denoted by the lowered glycerol release. Thus, utilization of free fatty acids is diminished and ketone body uptake is negligible. To avoid a peripheral energy fuel deficit, oxidation of peripheral protein is increased, as signified by a three-fold increase in alanine release and a greater negative nitrogen balance.[7]

Low Flow Sepsis

In low flow sepsis, glucose uptake is increased to the highest values observed for any of these states, but circulatory insufficiency and the resultant anaerobic conditions are associated with a five-fold increase in lactate production. Thus in low flow sepsis, less glucose is *completely oxidized* via the energy rich citric acid cycle than any other state. While the markedly elevated catecholamine levels are associated with increased free fatty acid levels, free fatty acid and ketone bodies are not utilized by tissue in amounts proportional to their availability. This suggests some selective blocking of free fatty acid utilization by peripheral tissues, perhaps induced by catecholamines. The potential energy fuel deficit is greater than that observed in high flow sepsis and is matched by further increases in the utilization of endogenous protein in the form of branched-chain amino acids.[7]

COMMON TYPES OF MALNUTRITION

Energy and Protein Depletion States

The finding that significant protein-calorie malnutrition was present in as many as 25 to 50 percent of medical and surgical patients who had undergone surgical or medical stresses while hospitalized for two weeks or longer came as a shock to many practicing surgeons in the mid-1970s.[9,23] A series of recent studies has confirmed this general finding and shown that increased vulnerability to infections and other complications are likely among such patients if nutritional support is not undertaken.[35] Nutritional support measures which are now available can prevent such sequelae in a large proportion of cases.

Three states have been identified in such patients. These bear some resemblance to the syndrome of protein-calorie malnutrition seen among malnourished children in developing countries:

1. VISCERAL ATTRITION. The term visceral attrition is used to describe the loss of labile protein stores of the viscera (e.g., liver, pancreas, and gut mucosa). Visceral attrition usually results from a combination of severe catabolic stress coupled with diets or intravenous feeding inadequate to maintain energy or nitrogen balance. It requires biochemical assessment for diagnosis. The labile protein stores in the visceral tissues are the first affected when semistarvation or stress increase protein catabolism. Skeletal muscle stores respond less rapidly, and connective tissue and brain protein undergo relatively little change in starvation.[20] The loss of visceral protein accounts for the increased rate of nitrogen excretion first seen following starvation or trauma. If the endocrine milieu is favorable, alterations in protein turnover occur, with the result that in a stressed state skeletal muscle reserves are then moved to the liver to support protein synthesis and visceral stores are spared. If the shift fails to occur, eventually the synthesis of liver proteins deteriorates. For this reason, serum proteins such as albumin or transferrin and cellular immune function are usually depressed in visceral attrition. If such indices are not assessed, this form of malnutrition is difficult to recognize since anthropometric measurements often remain in the normal range. However, if the stresses and hypercatabolism are long continued, they lead to cellular and fat losses in roughly equivalent amounts and are accompanied by losses of body water with eventual development of a weight deficit.[21] Fat stores alone afford little protection; obese patients

may also develop acute visceral attrition while their body fat remains above normal levels.

2. CACHEXIA OR EMACIATION. The terms cachexia and emaciation are used to describe the wasted patient. This condition is frequently present on admission to the hospital and is the result of mild catabolic stress coupled with inadequate intakes over a long period.

3. MIXED STATES. Mixed states most usually result from some major stress such as heart failure, trauma, or major surgery which increases protein catabolism in a patient who is already marasmic, particularly if semistarvation regimens are employed when the stress ensues.

MICRONUTRIENT DEPLETION

With the single exception of iron deficiency anemia which is common in premenopausal females and the aged of both sexes, vitamin and mineral deficiencies are usually present in association with energy and protein depletion states rather than by themselves. The vast majority of surgical patients who are malnourished are either obese or undernourished and starved. Other classical deficiencies are very rare indeed.

COMPLICATIONS RESULTING FROM MALNUTRITION

Several complications result from malnutrition (particularly protein and calorie depletion) in surgical patients. Progressive weight loss, weakness, and apathy are among the most obvious.[9–12,14,15,22–24] Depressed ventilatory responses to hypoxia[25] and increased incidence of decubiti at pressure points[26] have also been demonstrated. Depressed cell-mediated immunity which may be associated with increased rates of infection,[27–30] particularly of gram-negative sepsis, impaired wound healing, wound disruption,[30–33] and greater incidence of bowel fistulae[34] has been related to malnutrition as well. Also evident are a decreased response to chemotherapy for infection and certain forms of cancer[35,36] and decreased tolerance for radiation therapy.[24] Obesity[37] and nutritional deficiency diseases[38] increase operative risks and delay postoperative recovery. While some of these metabolic changes are inevitable, nutritional support of surgical patients, especially the stressed patient, can prevent unnecessary complications.

MODERN NUTRITIONAL ASSESSMENT AND SUPPORT TECHNIQUES

Evidence is already available that careful nutritional assessment and preoperative conditioning for surgery using the newer nutritional support techniques pays dividends in terms of successful surgical outcomes. For example, a recent study showed that use of total parenteral nutrition augmented gastric mucosal regeneration, allowing a more rapid return to normal physiologic secretory patterns and better maintenance of protective gastric mucosal mechanisms than the usual administration of postoperative fluids and glucose solution.[31] Appropriate surgery, nutritional support, and medical treatment can help to reverse cachexia in cancer patients.[39,40] Inasmuch as good nutritional status is necessary for the maintenance of an intact immune system, *some* failures of immune response can be prevented[41] by nutritional support.

Continual monitoring and more individualized nutritional support in the postoperative recovery period decreases the likelihood of infections and other complications and shortens lengths of stay in the hospital. In contrast, failure to pay attention to the patient's nutritional status may nullify the beneficial effects of sophisticated, brilliantly executed surgery and otherwise adequate postoperative care.

Presurgical Deterioration in Nutritional Status

Many patients referred to the surgeon are already in a nutritionally depleted state. Some of these conditions are unavoidable. Fortunately, a number of new developments make it possible for the surgeon to correct or ameliorate malnutrition secondary to disease. These advances include:

1. Techniques of nutritional assessment suitable for ill and hospitalized patients
2. Techniques of nutrient delivery suitable for hospitalized and ambulatory patients who do not respond to usual oral routes.
   a. Cannulation of central veins to permit infusion of hypertonic nutrient solutions.
   b. Better methods of peripheral hyperalimentation using lipid or "protein sparing" solutions.
   c. Improved techniques of tube feeding.
   d. Better techniques for administering defined bulk-free formula enteral diets.
3. Greater availability of suitable products for providing needed nutrients.
   a. Amino acids and protein hydrolysates.
   b. Safe lipid emulsions for intravenous administration.
   c. Bulk-free formula enteral diets.
   d. Other special enteral diets.
4. Greater fundamental knowledge of the nutrient needs of surgical patients.

If the diagnosis permits postponement of surgery, it is worthwhile to replete the patient at least partially using these measures to decrease morbidity.

Period of Semistarvation before or after Surgery

PREOPERATIVE PERIOD

Preoperative diagnostic studies and the actual surgical procedures may require that the patient abstain from food in the immediate preoperative and postoperative periods. However, in the past few decades the length of time that the patient is kept in a semistarved state may have inadvertently been increased by changes in the practice of medicine. Diagnostic procedures have become much more involved and prolonged.

Many of these involve fasting or result in missed meals, causing what one patient sourly called "diagnostic starvation."[42] The stress and anxiety experienced by the patient awaiting surgery as well as the disease process itself may also take their tolls on appetite and result in inadequate intakes. In addition, in the past few decades surgical procedures have become possible for many hitherto inoperable conditions. Patients suffering from these disorders often come to surgery malnourished and semistarved and have very long and complicated postoperative courses. If the surgical procedure requires several days of semistarvation postoperatively and complications lengthen this period, a state of chronic malnutrition may ensue, slowing recovery and compromising medical treatment. Patients in such a state contrast sharply with those who undergo surgery well-nourished and sustain the short period of starvation following surgery with no obvious ill effects.[43]

PROBLEMS IN THE IMMEDIATE POSTOPERATIVE PERIOD

The starving individual differs from the postoperative patient who has received no alimentation for several days, because the latter has sustained injury and trauma. Surgery produces significant metabolic alterations[4,21,44,45] including an increase in basal metabolism (hypermetabolism) and mobilization of metabolic fuels, particularly of visceral and skeletal muscle protein, during the acute phase of recovery immediately following the surgical procedure.[16,36,46–55]

After injury, the contribution to total energy expenditure from protein is approximately 16 percent[56] in contrast to perhaps half that amount in a nonstressed state.[57] Since increased catabolism of protein as well as energy also occurs in the postoperative period, unless deficits are expeditiously repleted, the risks of both energy and protein depletion are considerable.

Infections and Sepsis

The postoperative patient who develops complications involving a localized infection or sepsis runs great risks of nutritional depletion, even when effective antibiotic therapy is available.[58,59] The major consequences of infectious disease are a further increase in basal metabolic rate and peripheral resistance to the action of insulin.

The negative balances of energy, nitrogen, potassium, magnesium, zinc, and sulfur which are also sometimes observed result from several contributory factors. These include fever, diarrhea, vomiting, anorexia which decreases food intake, and alterations in endocrine responses. The gradual development of nitrogen sparing adaptive mechanisms which cut body nitrogen losses in the urine and feces as simple starvation proceeds are absent in febrile starving patients. As a result, nitrogen losses remain high, hypermetabolism persists, and depletion of energy and protein stores may occur rapidly. While fever is certainly not the cause of hypermetabolism in sepsis and more profound metabolic changes are responsible, the effects of the sequelae of fever on nutrient stores can lead to profound disturbances secondary to it. The more severe or longer the illness is, the greater the absolute loss of nutrients is likely to be. Functional inefficiencies in metabolism also lead to nutrient wastage. Increased utilization of vitamins may precipitate deficiency states if the infection is long continued.[60–62]

Surgery Which Compromises Digestion and Absorption

Operative procedures, their complications, and associated medical problems which directly affect the integrity or function of the gastrointestinal tract are particularly likely to jeopardize nutritional status. Energy and protein as well as vitamin and mineral depletion may result. Nutrition related difficulties are particularly common among patients who have undergone the operations discussed below.

1. EXTENSIVE RESECTIONS OF THE HEAD AND NECK. These procedures may be associated with difficulties in consuming sufficient food by usual oral routes to meet energy needs.

2. PARTIAL AND TOTAL GASTRECTOMY. These patients may often present for surgery in a malnourished state because of long-standing difficulties in gastrointestinal function and the extensive series of diagnostic workups they may have undergone. Risks of malnutrition are further heightened by the trauma and catabolic effects of the surgery itself and subsequent derangements of gastrointestinal function which persist after the immediate postoperative period. Dysphagia and substernal pain may be present in the first few weeks due to trauma to the lower esophagus during surgery. These difficulties and an early sensation of fullness contribute to loss of appetite and weight. Dumping syndrome may occur. Other late manifestations resulting from surgery include steatorrhea which is sometimes due to either discoordination in gastric and gallbladder emptying or bacterial overgrowth in the small intestine. Virtually all total gastrectomy patients and a third of partial gastrectomy patients malabsorb iron. Vitamin B_{12} deficiency occurs in 10 percent of patients and folic acid deficiency in 1 percent.

In view of these known difficulties, total parenteral nutritional support may be advisable in the two weeks after surgery with careful monitoring of progress as the patient is changed over to enteral routes. Much of the weight loss which persists even several months after surgery is due to inadequate postdischarge management. Oral and parenteral supplementation coupled with careful dietetic guidance following discharge can do much to help the patient overcome these problems.

3. EXTENSIVE RESECTIONS OF THE SMALL INTESTINE. Resections of the ileocecal valve, distal ileum, and more than half of the small intestine are commonly associated with malabsorption due to short bowel syndrome. The extent of the resection, its site, and the presence of diseased segments which are retained influence its severity. The malabsorption often involves all nutrients and, even after recovery, it may continue for protein, fat, carbohydrate, water and fat soluble vitamins, iron, calcium, and magnesium.

In the first week or more following surgery, rigorous parenteral nutritional support is mandatory, with particular attention paid to fluid and electrolyte levels since early postoperative fluid loss is great. Even after use of the enteral route has been resumed, a carefully tailored therapeutic diet involving frequent meals high in protein with carbohydrate and fat to tolerance, oral mineral and vitamin supplements, and parenteral injections of vitamin B_{12} are likely to be necessary.

4. BLIND LOOP SYNDROMES. Surgical procedures or other conditions which form blind loops of the small intestine may be associated with bacterial growth in the upper

small intestine. This situation may result in malabsorption of fat, fat soluble vitamins, minerals such as calcium and magnesium which are excreted as soaps when fat malabsorption occurs, and vitamin B_{12}. If surgical revisions or antibiotics do not prove efficacious in curing the condition, medium chain triglycerides may be used. This form of fat does not require conjugated bile salts for absorption. In blind loop syndrome, the conjugated bile salts may be deconjugated owing to the lush bacterial overgrowth and thus are unavailable so that fat is malabsorbed and steatorrhea ensues. Use of medium chain triglycerides circumvents this problem. Vitamin B_{12} status may be preserved by parenteral administration.

5. OSTOMIES OR FISTULAE. The exudative losses and potential problems with malabsorption and infection make it extremely important to watch patients with ostomies or fistulae closely.

Coexisting Medical Problems

The presence of a large number of pre-existing medical problems increases the probability of malnutrition in surgical patients. Some of the more commonly encountered conditions are summarized in Table 3. This is especially true if the conditions have not been adequately managed prior to surgery.

TABLE 3. Medical Problems in Surgical Patients Causing Increased Risk of Nutritional or Other Complications

1. *Ingestion, Digestion, and Absorption Compromised or Likely to Be Inadequate*
   Neurologic disorders decreasing ability to eat or impairing motility of stomach
   Small or large tumors of gastrointestinal tract producing partial or complete obstruction, malabsorption, and possibly hypermetabolism
   Gastrointestinal malfunction as in pancreatic insufficiency, celiac disease, Crohn's disease
   Chronic alcoholism

2. *Impaired Absorption*
   Diseases of the liver, gallbladder, or pancreas altering digestive enzyme secretions

3. *Inadequate Metabolism of Nutrients but no Malabsorption*
   Chronic renal failure
   Chronic liver failure
   Carcinoma outside of the gastrointestinal tract, such as endocrine tumors
   Major trauma
   Cutaneous burns
   Congenital anomalies in infants (risks are especially increased due to inadequate reserves)
   Poorly controlled diabetes mellitus

4. *Increased Need for Nutrients*
   Pregnancy, lactation
   Infancy, especially prematurity
   Adolescents at puberty

5. *Increased Loss of Nutrients*
   Hyperthyroidism
   Exudative losses of protein and energy as by enterocutaneous fistulas or abscesses, burns

NUTRITIONAL ASSESSMENT OF THE PATIENT

The nutritional review of the patient follows the stepwise scheme of screening, assessment, development of the nutritional support plan, selection of appropriate intervention measures, evaluation, and follow-up. The process is similar regardless of which point in the care cycle the physician encounters the patient although specifics may vary.

Screening

Screening permits the physician to review the large number of patients he sees each day for the presence of characteristics which indicate a high risk for poor nutritional status. Tables 4 and 5 present some easily observed characteristics which, if present, merit further assessment.

TABLE 4. Factors Which May Predispose to Malnutrition

1. *Body Weight*
   Recent unplanned gain or loss of more than 10% of usual weight
   Usual body weight more than 20% over or under ideal
   Patient has no knowledge of usual weight but clothes are ill fitting
   Weight patient reports as usual is much (10 or more pounds) lower than actual weight

2. *Brief Diet History*
   Failure to eat for more than 10 days
   Reported anorexia, nausea, vomiting, disordered taste
   Poorly fitting dentures or edentulous
   Evidence income or meals inadequate for needs
   Disrupted family or cooking situation
   Lives alone and prepares own meals
   Eats more than half of meals away from home
   Special diet (diabetic, "bland," ulcer, etc.)
   Diet monotonous, limited, faddist
   Excessive alcohol intake or problem drinking
   Food allergies, intolerances

3. *Medications*
   Use of catabolic, immunosuppressive, anti-infective agents, or other drugs known to induce anorexia

4. *History*
   Chronic disease or previous surgery of gastrointestinal tract
   Chronic alcoholism
   Other chronic diseases which often involve rigid diets or nutritional consequences: Diabetes mellitus; hypertension; hyperlipidemia; coronary artery disease; chronic lung, renal, or liver disease; circulatory problems; neurologic disorders or paralysis; mental retardation; carcinoma
   Conditions involving increased needs: Fever, infection, trauma, burns, growth, pregnancy, endocrine conditions
   Conditions involving external losses: Fistulas; open wounds; draining abscesses or effusion; chronic blood loss; renal dialysis; exudative enteropathy; burns; malabsorption due to disease of gut wall, pancreas, bacterial overgrowth of upper gut, or surgical excision of intestine

5. *Previous Laboratory Test Results Indicative of Nutritional Problems:* Low hemoglobin, hematocrit, etc.

TABLE 5. Common Forms of Malnutrition in Surgical Patients

Type of Disorder	*Serum Proteins (Albumin, Transferrin)*	*Signs of Cellular Immune Function*	*Edema*	*Weight for Height*	*Fatness*	*Arm Muscle Circumference*	*Comments*
Visceral attrition	Depressed	Depressed	Variable	Normal	Normal	Normal	Edema is only present if serum albumin levels are less than 3g/dl If long continued weight, fatness and arm-muscle circumference may decrease
Cachexia, emaciation, or adult marasmus	Normal	Normal	No	Depressed	Depressed	Depressed	Serum proteins may be depressed late in its course
Mixed visceral attrition and adult marasmus	Depressed	Depressed	Variable	Depressed	Depressed	Depressed	

Assessment

Those patients who are found to be at nutritional risk on one or more of the screening factors deserve more careful and lengthy assessment of their nutritional status. This will furnish the basis for the nutritional support plan and the schedule for further monitoring. The assessment battery varies depending upon the suspected problem, but in general it includes physical measurements (anthropometry), dietary review, and biochemical and clinical tests. The objectives of assessment are, first, to determine what the problem is, and second, to obtain the information necessary for correcting it if this is possible.

CHANGES IN BODY COMPOSITION

Weight for Height and Weight Change

The single most useful tool for the nutritional assessment and monitoring of surgical patients is measured weight for height and its change over time. It furnishes a simple and easily obtained indication of changes in body mass. Daily measurement of weight is recommended for hospitalized patients.[63,64] Due account needs to be taken of edema, which may mask weight loss in acute visceral attrition and mixed depletion states. Since edema only becomes clinically evident after fluid accumulation has reached 10 percent or more of body weight, indirect indices which suggest its presence must be employed. These include examination of fluid intake and output and serum albumin (edema being likely if it is below 3 g/dl).

Depletion of Lean Body Mass

There is no single index available for clinical use which permits direct assessment of changes in lean body mass.[65] However, taken together, several simple measurements can provide a fairly good picture of changes which are taking place in that group of tissues.

ARM MUSCLE CIRCUMFERENCE. This measurement is derived from the measurement of the circumference of the arm (at a point midway between the acromial process and the olecranon on the upper arm [see Fig. 1]) and measurement of the triceps skinfold (see below) taken at the same point according to the following formula:

$$Cm = Ca - \pi s$$

where Cm = arm muscle circumference (cm)
Ca = arm circumference (cm)
π = 3.1416
s = triceps skinfold (mm)

Arm muscle circumference may also be determined by use of a nomogram (see Fig. 2).

The value obtained for arm muscle circumference is compared to sex and age specific

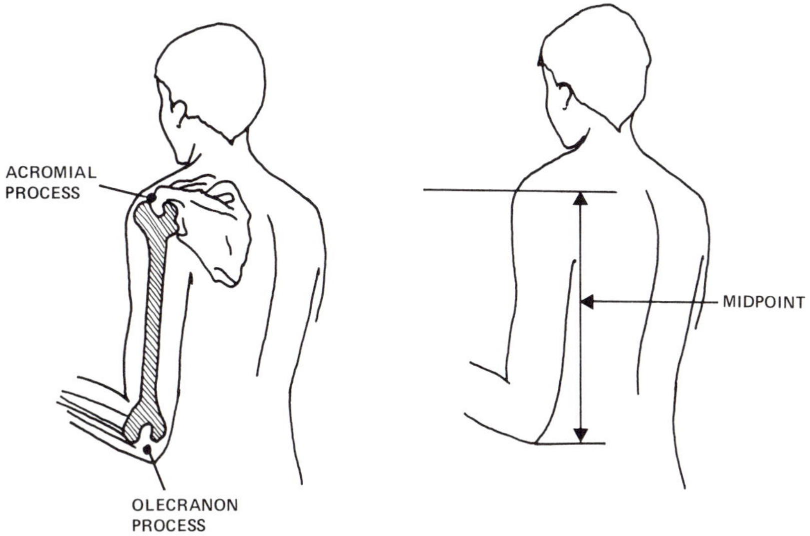

FIGURE 1. Arm Circumference is measured as follows: (1) Bare the patient's arm and have him bend it so his forearm is at a right angle with the hand across his stomach. (2) Locate the acromial process of the scapula and place your middle finger on its tip. Locate the olecranon on the ulna and place your other middle finger on it. (3) Estimate the midpoint of the upper arm over the triceps by extending your thumbs toward each other down the back of the arm directly in line with the elbow, keeping your middle fingers on the acromial process and the olecranon. (4) Mark the midpoint with a marking pen. It should be at the back of the arm directly in line with the elbow. (5) Measure circumference of arm at midpoint.

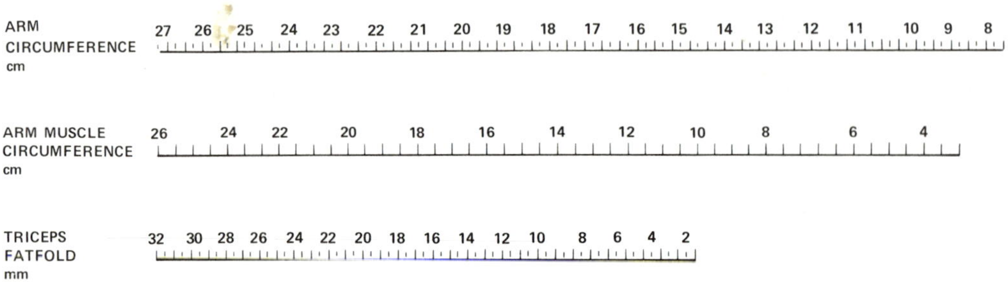

FIGURE 2. Nomogram for determination of arm muscle circumference. To obtain arm muscle circumference: (1) Position a ruler so it is touching the known values for arm circumference and fatfold. 2. Read off value on middle line for arm muscle circumference.

tables. Half or less than half of the normal value indicates decreased visceral and muscle protein.[12,15] Table 6 presents normative values.

Hematologic Indices

Hemoglobin, hematocit, and complete blood counts are useful in evaluating the presence of anemia.

Visceral Protein

Low serum albumin and, more specifically, serum transferrin levels also may indicate visceral protein deficits.[66] These secretory proteins have short half-lives and are therefore particularly sensitive to deficiencies of energy and amino acids. Synthesis slows during semistarvation. Low values may be due to many causes, such as increased losses in gastrointestinal or renal disease or decreased synthesis, as in liver failure, but if these other causes are ruled out, low values support a diagnosis of protein depletion. Transfer-

TABLE 6. Values for Midarm Circumference and Arm Muscle Circumference Indicative of Risk of Protein Energy Undernutrition*

		Percentage of Normal Standard			
	Normal Standard	*90% (mild protein deficiency)*	*80% (moderate protein deficiency)*	*70% (severe protein deficiency)*	*60% or less (critical protein deficiency)*
Midarm Circumference					
Males	29.3	26.3	23.4	20.5	17.6
Females	28.5	25.7	22.8	20.0	17.1
Arm Muscle Circumference					
Males	25.3	22.8	20.2	17.7	15.2
Females	23.2	20.9	18.6	16.2	13.9

*Adapted from Heymsfield, SF Bethel, RA, Ansley, JD, et al.[139] and Jelliffe, D. B.: *The Assessment of the Nutritional Status of the Community.* World Health Organization, Geneva, 1966.

rin, with a half-life of 8 days, is probably more sensitive than albumin, with a 14 day half-life.

Approximate Nitrogen Balance

Depletion of lean body mass can also be roughly assessed by calculation of intake and output of nitrogen sources.[26,67,68] The total of all enteral and parenteral alimentation is recorded and energy and nitrogen intakes are calculated to obtain a value for nitrogen intake.

Nitrogen output can be grossly assessed by collection of 24-hour urinary output and a laboratory determination of urinary urea nitrogen. To the value obtained an extra 3.5 gm is added to account for other bodily nitrogen losses which are harder to measure and thus assumed to be constant (2.0 g for stool losses, and 1.5 g for endogenous losses as by skin and hair). The method tends to overestimate nitrogen losses slightly but is close enough to be satisfactory for clinical purposes.[68]

If it is impossible to perform such measurements, the approximate values presented in Table 7 give a rough idea of deficits which can usually be expected in surgical patients.[69]

BLOOD UREA NITROGEN (BUN). If BUN is 8 mg/dl or less, inadequate protein intake is likely.

OTHER TESTS. Other indices, such as the creatinine-height index are not sufficiently accurate or specific as measures of malnutrition to merit consideration.[14,70–72]

DEPLETION OF ENERGY RESERVES

Energy reserves are assessed by observing changes in physical measurements such as body weight and fatness, by monitoring of energy intakes, and by calculations of resting metabolism, making allowance for losses which may be occurring owing to the disease process.

Triceps Skinfold Measurements

The assessment of fatfolds at either the triceps or subscapular sites is used by some workers to assess body fat content and to derive arm muscle circumferences. It permits more direct observation of the status of fat depots than body weight. If it is impossible to measure body weights on a regular basis in very ill patients, triceps and arm muscle diameters permit some assessment of body fat and muscle reserves. The triceps value obtained is compared to sex and age specific standardized values.[73] If triceps skinfold measurements are used, care should be taken to learn the proper procedures for taking measurements and the limitations which exist for very fat and extremely emaciated patients whose fatfolds are exceedingly difficult to assess.[74] Figure 3 illustrates the measurement of triceps skinfolds, and Table 8 presents triceps skinfold norms.

TABLE 7. Usual Increases in Nitrogen Excretion and Energy Outputs Seen in Surgical Patients*

Condition	*Urea Nitrogen Excretion (g/day)*	*Percentage of Energy Increase Over Resting Metabolism*
Major Burns (over 30% of body surface area)	12–18	145–220
Multiple trauma with patient on ventilator		150–175
Severe sepsis	11–14	140–170
Multiple trauma		130–155
Major injury or trauma	9.5–11.5	118–142
Long bone fracture		115–130
Infection,	9–11	110–130
Peritonitis		105–125
Elective surgery	7–9	90–110
Fever		110–130 (an increase of 1°C increases resting metabolism 10–13%)
Normal postoperative patient at rest		100–105
Normal patient at rest on usual diet	6–17 (depending on protein intake)	100–105
Starvation	203	85–100

*Adapted and expanded from Blackburn, GL, Bistrian, BR, Maini, BS, et al.: *Nutritional and metabolic assessment of the hospitalized patient.* J Parenteral Enteral Nutrition, 1:11, 1977.

TABLE 8. Values for Triceps Skinfolds Indicative of Risk of Protein-Energy Malnutrition*

Sex	*Normal Standard*	*Percentage of Normal Standard* 90%	80%	70%	60%
			Indicates mild to moderate energy depletion		
Male	12.5	11.3	10.0	8.8	7.5
Female	16.5	14.9	13.2	11.6	9.9

*Adapted from Heymsfield, SF, Bethel, RA, Ansley, JD, et al.[139] and Jelliffe, D. B.: *The Assessment of the Nutritional Status of the Community.* World Health Organization, Geneva, 1966.

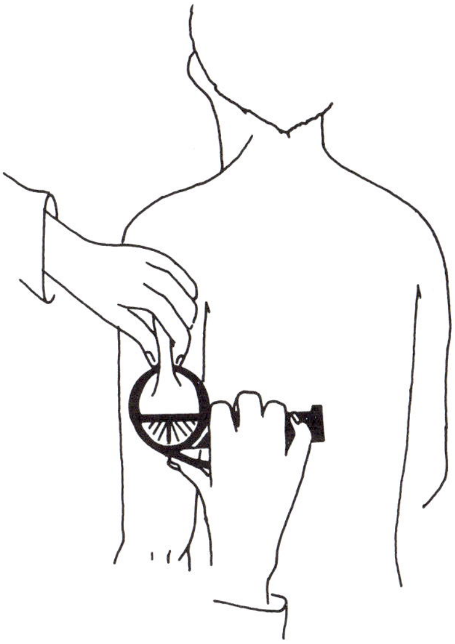

FIGURE 3. The triceps skinfold measurement is determined as follows: (1) Make sure patient's arm is hanging relaxed at his side. (2) Pick up the triceps skinfold: At the midpoint of the back of the upper arm, pick up the double fold of skin and fat with your thumb and forefinger about one centimeter above the mark you made when measuring arm circumference. (3) Take the measurement: Place the skinfold calipers over the fatfold and below your fingers directly at the mark where the fold is largest. Make sure that the pressure exerted on the fold is from the calipers, not your fingers. Release the calipers but continue to hold the fold. Take the reading 3 seconds after release of the calipers and record to 0.5 centimeters. Remove calipers, reapply, and obtain a duplicate reading. Use average. (Skinfold calipers can be ordered from Cambridge Scientific Industries, Inc., 101 Virginia Avenue, Cambridge, Maryland 21613.)

Energy Intakes

First an initial diet history should be taken to identify changes in appetite, weight, and food habits which suggest that nutrient intake has been reduced. Present energy intake is relatively easy to obtain for the hospitalized patient by recording all enteral and parenteral sources of alimentation actually consumed. A dietary history helps the physician to separate out weight loss due to diet from that due to the illness itself and may be particularly helpful in planning interventions for outpatients.

Energy Output

Direct measurement of resting metabolism is the most valid index of energy output. If this is not feasible, estimates of usual resting metabolism may be employed[75] making allowances for the extent of catabolism associated with the particular disease process or condition (see Table 7). Inspection of the patient may provide additional clues as to the degree of hypermetabolism. For example, the presence of tachycardia indicates that hypermetabolism may be present. Fever increases energy outputs by at least 10 percent per degree centigrade.

MICRONUTRIENT DEPLETION STATES

Most hospital clinical laboratories are not equipped to perform biochemical tests for all of the vitamin and mineral deficiency states which may conceivably develop in the surgical patient. The physician must rely upon dietary history, knowledge of present nutrient intakes, and the disease in question in assessing nutritional status in these respects. Fortunately, most vitamin and mineral deficiency diseases take weeks or months to develop so that, unless the patient is in a malnourished state prior to admission, this is unlikely to be an immediate problem. The reader is referred to several excellent recent references for specific information on the identification of classical deficiency diseases,[76] deficiencies which may arise due to drug-nutrient interactions,[68] and inadequate parenteral nutritional support after surgery.[1,2,78,79] If techniques such as total parenteral nutritional support are to be used, a detailed knowledge of the special requirements for vitamins and minerals administered by this route is necessary and the chemical laboratory must be capable of monitoring the complex nutritional problems which arise. Otherwise, the attending physician runs the risk of inadvertently producing micronutrient malnutrition by the application of incompletely understood therapeutic maneuvers.[78,79]

ALTERED IMMUNE FUNCTION

A depressed cell-mediated immune response has been observed in hospitalized adults with malnutrition. This state may be reversed upon nutritional repletion.[13,80] The most widely used tests are dinitrochlorobenzene (DNCB) sensitization by the Catalona technique and skin tests with recall antigens such as candida, streptokinase-streptodornase (Varidase, SK/SD), and mumps. The most common procedure is to use the recall antigens first and only then to proceed to DNCB, since the latter test gives a prominent delayed hypersensitivity response. Some workers have employed the differential and total serum lymphocyte counts to identify lymphopenia which may suggest impaired cell-mediated immunity. Other tests are still in the experimental state.[14,81] Delayed hypersensitivity skin testing appears to offer promise in ascertaining prognosis more precisely for those patients being considered for nutritional support.[35]

REFERRING PATIENTS TO OTHER FACILITIES

Whenever total parenteral nutrition or jejunostomy feeding are likely to be necessary, the physician must realistically examine the facilities at his or her disposal. In these situations, the only way to minimize complications is the presence of trained and experienced personnel and appropriate protocols which minimize the hazards of nutritional support. The greater the experience with the modified routes and diets for each specific phase in the disease process with each type of patient, the greater the likelihood of success.

The possibility of referring the patient requiring total parenteral nutrition to a hospital where a nutritional support service exists should be seriously considered if a nutritional support team is not available in the present hospital, if the risks associated with the use of total parenteral nutrition are greater than 5 percent, or if the procedure is performed so seldom that calculation of iatrogenic morbidity is not possible. Similar considerations apply for the management of tube feedings by jejunostomy.

DEVELOPING THE NUTRITIONAL SUPPORT PRESCRIPTION

The first step in the development of the nutritional support plan is to decide upon the objective. While the general goal of maintaining the best nutritional status possible is always constant, depending upon the phase of therapy and the patient's illness, immediate objectives vary from maintaining normal nutrient intakes to providing abundant supplies of nutrients to permit regeneration of tissue and rehabilitation of the patient who is in a depleted state. The second step in developing the care plan is to determine the levels of nutrients which must be provided. Third, the route of administration and nutrient sources which are to be utilized must be specified. Fourth, measurable targets and a plan for monitoring progress must be developed. The fifth and final step is implementation of the plan. This includes informing the patient of the rationale for the indicated therapy and answering his questions about it, writing necessary orders and explaining special procedures to other health care personnel involved in treatment, and adjusting the plan, if need be, as experience is gained from the patient's response to therapy.

Factors Relevant to Setting Appropriate Objectives

PRE-EXISTING NUTRITIONAL STATUS

If the patient's nutritional status is already depleted and it is possible to delay therapy such as surgery which involves induction of a semistarved state in the immediate preoperative and postoperative periods, treatment should be postponed until nutritional support measures to rehabilitate the patient have been instituted. If the patient is very obese, elective surgery should also be postponed until after weight reduction measures have brought body fatness down to levels associated with lesser risk of complications during anesthesia, surgery, and the postoperative period.[82]

TYPE OF SURGERY

The nutritional support measures necessary in the acute catabolic stage depend mostly upon the extent of tissue injury and the general health of the patient. Using Moore and Brennan's[83] classification of degrees of trauma, the following measures are suggested:

1. MINOR TISSUE INJURY WITHOUT VOLUME REDUCTION. Included in this category are such events as clean elective surgery, minor injuries such as sprains and fractures, minor vascular surgery, penetrating lacerations and wounds involving little muscle belly damage, and other operations not involving the major body cavities. One or two days of partial starvation are usually involved, but the starvation is transient and

the resulting changes in body composition are minimal. Special nutritional support other than provision of usual diets is not called for.

2. MODERATE TISSUE INJURY WITH TRANSIENT VOLUME REDUCTION. The operative procedures included here are clean, soft tissue operations without sepsis, major fractures, and penetrating wounds. Often the patient is subjected to partial starvation for from three days to a week, but complications may extend this period. Since glucose intolerance increases during stress, the usual doses of intravenous glucose may be inadequate for the stressed patient. Complete oxidation of glucose may be decreased in these states (see Table 2).

The need for nutritional support depends less on the tissue injury itself than upon the presence of other disease problems and complications. When the situation is complicated by the presence of such difficulties as congestive heart failure, other cardiac dysfunction, chronic liver or renal disease, or persistent fever, the catabolic response will be more prolonged and profound. Once fluid and electrolyte levels have been brought under control, nutritional support measures other than glucose alone need to be contemplated, since otherwise partial starvation may continue in the face of increased catabolism, severely depleting reserves.

When moderate tissue injury is uncomplicated, alterations in body composition as a result of the partial starvation are trivial, and usual procedures involving ordinary intravenous electrolytes and dextrose solution to provide 100 to 200 gm of glucose daily are adequate. However, this may not be the case for the stressed patient.

3. MASSIVE TISSUE INJURY WITH REDUCED VOLUME AND FLOW, PULMONARY INSUFFICIENCY, TISSUE ANOXIA, NECROSIS, AND SEPSIS. Included here are major burns, severe hemmorhage, extensive and severe trauma, and invasive infection. All involve prolonged partial starvation unless special measures are instituted. These states are characterized by profound protein catabolism (e.g., 14 to 30 gm/day), increased levels of fat mobilization to compensate for the greatly increased resting metabolic rate, and a powerful tendency to conserve water and salt, which may mask tissue wasting. Energy and protein depletion can rapidly ensue in view of the hypermetabolism if the patient is allowed to remain in a state of partial starvation. Thus, extensive nutrition support measures are called for.

PHASE OF RESPONSE TO SURGERY OR DISEASE

The objectives of nutritional support also vary depending upon which of these conditions obtain:

Acute Catabolic Response to Stress or Surgery

The presence of stress may be indicated by a heart rate above 100 beats/minute, a fever of 38°C, or a history of trauma, burns, or surgery. The postoperative patient's metabolism (like that of his febrile or burned peers) is characterized by a catabolic tendency which predominates at least for a brief period owing to endocrine alterations. The severity and length of the catabolic phase of response depends upon the type of operation or injury, its extent, the presence of infection, duration of immobilization, past and present nutritional status, concomitant chronic disease, age, and sex.[84] During this phase, even if energy and protein intakes are satisfactory, nitrogen excretion may exceed nitrogen intake, owing to increased tissue breakdown as a result of the trauma and perhaps also decreased protein synthesis.[85–87] The metabolic milieu is such that nitrogen loss is favored, especially after trauma and in the presence of fever or infection. Resting metabolism remains high and the adjustments usually seen in starvation which conserve body protein stores by the catabolism of an energy rich mixture of substrates from fat are less efficient. If the catabolic process continues to the point where a third of total body protein is lost, death occurs.[88]

Even in the face of adequate intakes, some endogenous protein sources will be utilized during the acute catabolic phase in an effort to repair the injury even if this is at the expense of other tissue. Even high energy, high protein nutritional support is unable to prevent nitrogen losses at the peak of the catabolic response period, but negative nitrogen balance and the risks of atrophy of skeletal muscle can be reduced.[84] If exogenous sources of energy and nitrogen are not available, losses will be greater, and a chronic state of posttraumatic starvation may ensue, leading to decreased muscle strength, poor respiratory capacity, and increased risks of bronchopneumonia.

In the first few days after surgery, the objective is to maintain a relative abundance of the circulating substrates needed to cope with the trauma and stress. Even if intakes are insufficient during this period, in the healthy, previously well nourished patient, endocrine alterations permitting mobilization of body energy and protein stores permit this.[16] Preoperative nutritional support of the patient so that he undergoes surgery in good nutritional status also helps to achieve adequate substrate supply. Postoperative support which permits rapid repletion of the stores which are being mobilized is also of assistance. Such postoperative nutritional support is mandatory for patients who are very ill, who have had extensive surgery, or who develop a major complication such as sepsis which may result in the persistence of the acute phase for days or even weeks longer than usual. Note that even for the well nourished patient, the objective of nutritional measures is to shorten the length of time during which a semistarved or fasted state exists as much as possible.

Adaptive Phase after Surgery

Once the acute catabolic phase is concluded, endocrine adjustments favor anabolism. The objective here is to continue to provide the circulating substrates necessary for healing and to achieve energy and nitrogen balances which are slightly positive to replete body stores.

Sepsis, Systemic Infections or Other Situations Involving Prolonged Stress

The objective here is to preserve nutritional status until the hypermetabolism which depletes energy and protein reserves (especially those of the viscera and skeletal muscle due to the stress of infection and fever) is brought under control. Since the patient is usually debilitated and the sheer bulk of nutrients which must be delivered to meet elevated needs is high, special routes of administration may be necessary. Once the infection has been brought under control, the objective becomes a fed state with sufficient supplies to permit rehabilitation of depleted reserves.

Sepsis, secondary to complex surgical procedures especially when nutritional status has already been depleted by severe disease, is a life threatening problem. Even vigorous antibiotic therapy is often ineffective. In skilled hands, a combination of appropriate antimicrobial therapy supplemented by vigorous nutritional support may be lifesaving.

Parenteral techniques employing central venous catheters carry considerable risk themselves because of the dangers of microbial contamination, thrombus formation, and other problems. Enteral routes also have difficulties such as induction of diarrhea, regurgitation, and hyperosmolar dehydration. Thus, it is absolutely mandatory that nutritional support be skillfully provided for such critically ill patients, even if this means transferring the patient to another facility.

The third line of defense is to rehabilitate or correct nutritional deficits, since those who are recovering from sepsis run much higher risks than normal of secondary infections during early convalescence.

Determining Amounts of Nutrients to Be Provided

The amounts of nutrients needed depend upon all of the following factors:

1. Present nutritional status, the extent of pre-existing nutritional depletion if it exists, and the specific nutrient deficits identified.
2. The phase of response to disease or injury.
3. Type of surgical procedure, which to a large extent determines the degree of trauma and stress.
4. The present rate of hypermetabolism which helps to predict the likelihood of future drains on nutrient reserves.
5. Presence of organ failure or secondary disease states such as cancer, pneumonia, or trauma which affect utilization of nutrients.
6. Age, sex, and size of the patient.
7. Presence of normal physiologic states which increase nutrient needs, such as pregnancy, lactation, or growth.

SPECIAL IMPORTANCE OF ENERGY AND PROTEIN

From the standpoint of planning nutritional support, the most difficult problem in managing the surgical patient is to assure that energy and protein needs are met. While micronutrient needs also may alter, and reserves may have become depleted since only small amounts of nutrients need to be delivered, their provision poses fewer problems. As a general rule, if prescriptions meet recommended allowances they are unlikely to become a problem unless parenteral routes are used for more than a week.

Energy Needs

LEVELS. The level of energy (caloric requirements) which must be provided will depend upon:

1. The extent of catabolism associated with the specific disease process.
2. The time which has elapsed since the onset of the disease process.
3. The nutritional state of the patient. When weight loss exceeds 10 percent of normal predicted body weight, it is likely that host responses may be impaired and rehabilitation measures are in order to remedy this.
4. Whether the goal is to maintain energy balance, to minimize weight loss in the patient following surgery or infection, or to achieve positive energy balance so as to restore body mass in a debilitated individual.

METHODS OF ASCERTAINMENT. There are a number of different methods for establishing energy needs, which are described at length elsewhere.[75] One method is outlined below:

1. *Determine basal energy needs under normal conditions.* If a direct determination of resting metabolism is not possible, the best procedure is to calculate what the energy need of the patient would be if he were in good health and to add assumptions to account for the stress due to the disease state. This is done as follows:
   a. Calculate *body surface* area from weight and height (since body weight in surgical patients often reflects fluid loss or gain, it alone is not an accurate reflection of body mass) (Fig. 4). If weight alone is available, assume the individual is of "normal" height and calculate approximate metabolic rate from Table 9.
   b. Read off the standard metabolic rate (e.g., basal metabolic expenditure) for a patient of that age and sex (Table 10).
   c. Multiply body surface area times metabolic rate to get *calories per day.*
2. *Allow for the hypermetabolism which may be induced by the disease state* (see Table 7).
3. *Add an extra 25 percent for a margin of safety.*
4. *To maintain energy balance,* multiply the resting rate obtained for the patient in health by the sum of the allowance for disease state and the margin of safety. Add the product to the resting rate in health for the resting rate in disease to maintain energy balance.
5. *To promote weight gain,* a reasonable goal is 1 to 2 pounds per week. Thus, an extra 500 to 1,000 kcal per day as well as a diet high in protective nutrients (protein, vitamins, and minerals) must be added to maintenance need determined in step 4.

Protein Needs

Body protein needs during illness are calculated by determining the minimal amount of nitrogen needed to achieve nitrogen equilibrium in health and the special allowance for the disease state is then added to it.

TABLE 9. Approximate Basal Metabolic Rates Determined from Body Weight

Weight (Kg)	*Kcal/day*	*Weight (Kg)*	*Kcal/day*
104	2280	62	1547
102	2247	60	1509
100	2214	58	1471
98	2180	56	1433
96	2147	54	1394
94	2113	52	1356
92	2079	50	1316
90	2045	48	1277
88	2011	46	1236
86	1977	44	1196
84	1942	42	1155
82	1907	40	1113
80	1872	38	1071
78	1837	36	1029
76	1802	34	986
74	1766	32	942
72	1730	30	897
70	1694	28	852
68	1658	26	806
66	1621	24	759
64	1584		

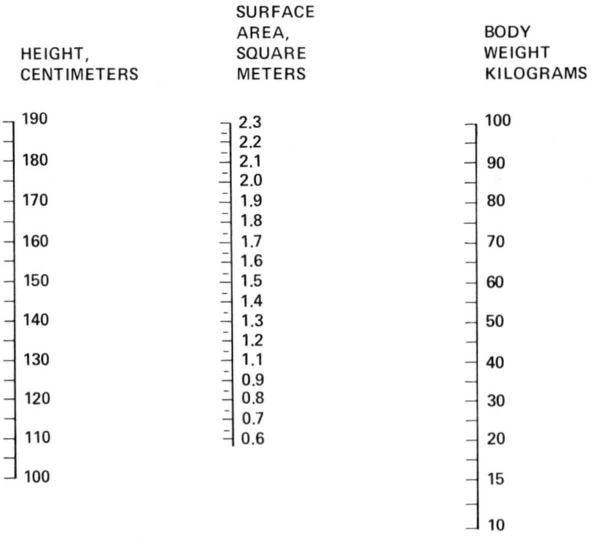

FIGURE 4. Nomogram for determining body surface area from height and weight. Adapted from Wilmore, DW.[95]

TABLE 10. Usual Metabolic Rates for Adult Patients of Different Ages*

Age (Years)	*Kcal/Body Surface Area(m^2)*	
	Males	*Females*
20	926	847
25	900	845
30	883	842
35	876	840
40	871	838
45	869	828
50	859	814
55	850	799
60	838	785
65	826	773
70	811	761
75 or over	797	751

*Adapted from Fleisch, A.: *Le metabolisme basal standard et su determination au moyen du Metabocalculator* Helv Med Acta 18:23, 1951.

NITROGEN TO CALORIE RATIOS. Since nutritional support in surgery often involves parenteral routes and utilizes amino acids or protein hydrolysates rather than naturally occuring sources of protein, statements of need in terms of grams of protein per kilogram are less useful than terms of reference dealing with amino acid nitrogen. Moreover, calculations of protein needs always assume that energy intakes are adequate, since if they are not the underlying assumptions are violated and the prescription is meaningless. For these reasons protein needs are expressed as nitrogen to calorie ratios and assume energy adequacy.

The ratio of a high quality source providing nitrogen is expressed as grams of nitrogen provided by the protein per day compared to total energy need per day. Since high quality protein is assumed to be 16 percent nitrogen, the grams of nitrogen provided are multiplied by 6.25 to obtain grams of protein. For example, the normal reference adult needs approximately 56 g of protein per day or 9.1 g of nitrogen (N) and 2,700 kcal. Therefore, the nitrogen to calorie ratio of the normal adult diet is:

$$\frac{9.1 \text{ g N/day}}{2{,}700 \text{ kcal}} = \frac{1}{301}$$

While ideal nitrogen to calorie ratios have not yet been validated or firmly established, these rules of thumb may nevertheless be helpful to the physician in clinical practice.

The nitrogen to calorie ratios for the diets of normal infants are 1:337 and for the diets of normal children 1:416.[89] The usual ratio in normal individuals is assumed to be approximately 1:300 to 1:350. In illness, since protein metabolism may be more inefficient, the nitrogen to calorie ratio varies from 1:100 to 1:200; 1:150 is thought to be optimal. For adults in the postoperative state 1:110 is used, and for those who are being stressed, 1:140.

During injury about 17 percent of total energy expenditure is from protein[56] in contrast to perhaps 8 percent (or a nitrogen to calorie ratio of 1:140 as opposed to 1:300) in a nonstressed state.[57] Based on these findings, it is assumed that protein intakes of 16 percent of total calories (assuming energy intakes of about 40 to 45 kcal/kg/day or 3,000 kcal total intake, of which 481 kcal or 120 g are derived from protein furnishing 20 g of nitrogen) yielding a nitrogen to calorie ratio of 1:150 should be appropriate for achieving positive nitrogen balance and restoring lean body mass in depleted, stressed adults (e.g., to achieve an *anabolic* state). In contrast, protein intakes as low as 8 percent of total calories (assuming energy intakes of about 30 to 35 kcal/kg/day or 2,700 kcal total intake of which 216 kcal or 54 g of protein furnish 8.8 g of nitrogen) yielding a nitrogen/calorie ratio of 1:300 are likely to be satisfactory for preserving body mass in nonstressed convalescent patients (e.g., to achieve a *maintenance* state).

However, these generalizations fall down in the face of disorders such as renal failure and liver failure in which nitrogen may accumulate.[90,91] In such states, desirable nitrogen/calorie ratios may range from 1:450 to 1:700.

Another special case is presented by the patient who is suffering from infectious disease or sepsis after surgery. The primary importance of providing for increased energy needs cannot be overemphasized for such patients since if these are not met, body protein will be catabolized to meet them and rapid depletion will ensue. Even in the best of circumstances when energy needs are provided for, the wastage and functional inefficiency characterizing the state will increase nitrogen losses. An allowance of 10 percent extra nitrogen per degree centigrade of fever may be used and is probably particularly appropriate if weight loss has already occurred.

While these general guidelines permit the physician to obtain a figure for protein needs which may be used for initial care planning, constant monitoring is essential so that intakes may be adjusted as appropriate. Nitrogen utilization is best estimated by measuring the daily urinary urea nitrogen loss as well as keeping track of the metabolic rate, nitrogen to calorie ratios, and nitrogen intakes. Since enteral and parenteral routes vary in the efficiency with which protein sources are utilized (enteral routes generally being more efficient), some care is needed in assuming that paper calculations and clinical realities will be one and the same. Finally, findings must be correlated to the degree of weight loss and changes in energy reserves.

Routes of Administration and Nutrient Sources to Be Utilized

The means of providing nutritional support today are much more sophisticated than they were even a few years ago. Nonetheless, the major routes remain the enteral (by mouth and/or gastrointestinal tract) and parenteral (venous) or mixtures of the two.

The most appropriate route and method of administration depends upon the following variables:

1. Degree and type of nutritional depletion already existing.
2. Phase of response to illness or injury and presence of hypercatabolism or sepsis.
3. Functional status of the gastrointestinal tract.
4. Presence of organ failure which alters abilities to handle fluids or nutrients.
5. Presence of secondary disease states.

6. Appetite of the patient.
7. Costs of the method chosen.
8. Risks.
9. Patient wishes, especially if choice is feasible among several modalities.
10. Experience and expertise of the hospital staff in using the method in question.

The characteristics of the major nutritional support modalities are reviewed in subsequent sections of this chapter in greater detail, but the complexity of the techniques and the variety of products on the market are now so great that it is impossible to cover all of the information necessary for optimum use. The reader is urged to review several of the excellent recent publications which do so.[16,17,21,43,55,56,57,75,92–114] In general, the aim of the nutritional support plan is to use the gastrointestinal tract whenever possible, since costs and risks are lower, and efficiency of nutrient utilization (especially visceral protein synthesis) is higher.[57] If the patient is able to eat, every advantage should be taken of this fact.

Forward Planning with Established Checkpoints

Regardless of the point at which the surgeon first sees the patient, it is important for him to map out the general nutritional support strategy to be employed and to establish the checkpoints at which signs of progress or lack of it in response to treatment are to be looked for. The hospital dietitian is an ally who should be called upon at the planning stage. The support measures chosen should be detailed on the chart or patient records.

For preoperative nutritional support or weight reduction measures which are undertaken prior to elective or semielective surgical procedures, a period of two or three weeks is usually required for objective responses such as alteration in transferrin levels, lymphocytes, or serum albumin or weight change to occur, and therefore, re-evaluation should not be done before this time unless the patient reports further deterioration in his status. If a satisfactory response has then been obtained, surgery can be scheduled. If not, treatment should be re-evaluated and additional time allowed for nutritional rehabilitation with weekly assessment thereafter.

Postoperatively, the high nutritional risk patient should be evaluated daily if not more frequently with special attention to his nutritional status. At the end of a week the patient should have entered the anabolic phase of recovery. If he has not, extensive nutritional support planning involving special enteral or parenteral routes must be considered. Depending upon the progress of the patient, monitoring thereafter varies, but in any event, a weekly review is called for as long as the patient is hospitalized.

Many patients are not fully rehabilitated from the nutritional standpoint at discharge. Those who need special therapeutic diets should be carefully instructed by the dietitian prior to discharge. A follow-up visit with the dietitian and the physician should be scheduled two weeks later for evaluation and further adjustment of diet to home conditions. Subsequent visits will depend upon patient progress, biweekly or monthly evaluations are called for thereafter.

The physician's forward planning of nutritional support for the patient will greatly benefit from discussion with the dietitian, nurse, and pharmacist as well as with other physician specialists involved in care of the patient.[115,116]

Follow-Up and Evaluation

Surgical practice is so busy that it is often easy to overlook the fact that routine audits of the outcomes of nutritional support can often improve the efficiency as well as the effectiveness of care and outcomes. At least once a year, such an audit should be carried out.

ENTERAL NUTRITIONAL SUPPORT

The goal of enteral nutritional support is to attain satisfactory nutritional status by provision of sufficient food to achieve maintenance or anabolism. Depending upon the functional status of the gastrointestinal tract, usual oral routes, tube, or tube and ostomy feedings may be required. Calorie and protein needs are calculated as listed previously.

Options Available

The options available today for providing a nutritionally complete diet to the patient enterally are many. The major categories available listed in order of their deviations from usual food intakes are these:

1. Oral
   a. Normal "house" diets
   b. Therapeutic "house" diets
   c. One of the above plus food modules or nutritional supplements
2. Either Oral or by Tube
   a. Meal replacements
   b. "Elemental" or defined formula diets
3. Tube
   Nasopharyngeal tube
4. Tube and Ostomy
   a. Esophagostomy
   b. Gastrostomy
   c. Jejunostomy

Table 11 presents a glossary of terms used to describe various formula feedings used, and Table 12 presents specific characteristics of representative products presently on the market.

Considerations Governing Selection

The nutritional support method of choice is the simplest means by which nutritional objectives can be achieved. When appetite is present and the gastrointestinal tract is functional, oral alimentation is always to be preferred. Even if it can only furnish a portion of total needs and back-up measures are necessary as well, the preference of the patient, the opportunity it provides for the patient to participate in his own therapy, its

TABLE 11. Glossary of Terms to Describe Formulas Used in Enteral Feeding

Term	*Description*
Complete formula	Provides at least the amount of energy, protein, essential fatty acids, vitamins, and minerals specified by the US Recommended Dietary Allowances for maintenance of nutritional status if fed in sufficient volume.
Incomplete or supplemental formulas	Lack one or more of the nutrients specified in the US Recommended Dietary Allowances. Used as supplementary feedings to augment nutrient intake.
Polymeric formulas	Contain mixtures of protein, fat, and carbohydrate in their high molecular weight, polymeric forms (e.g., whole proteins, triglycerides, starch, and disaccharides) and in proportions similar to those in normal diets. They are usually low in osmolality, provide 1 kcal/ml and require normal proteolytic, lipolytic and carbohydrate digestive capacity.
Modified polymeric formulas	Proportions or type of protein, fat, or carbohydrate are modified to allow for special needs (for example, low fat, high protein, lactose free) so that they differ in type or amount provided in comparison to normal diets. They usually provide 1 kcal/ml, are low in osmolality, and may be helpful if proteolytic, lipolytic, or carbohydrate digestive capacity is slightly compromised.
Monomeric formulas	Low molecular weight sources of protein and carbohydrate are provided (amino acids, oligosaccharides, or monosaccharides). They are nearly devoid of lipid and low in residue. Provide approximately 1 kcal/ml, are high in osmolality and do not require normal proteolytic or lipolytic digestive capacity.
Modular formulas	Concentrated sources (modules) of protein, fat, or carbohydrate which are high in calories and low in volume. Provide approximately 2 kcal/ml. Osmolality varies depending on whether polymeric or monomeric sources of nutrients are used. The modules are mixed to provide formulas with special properties needed when fluid restriction or organ failure is present.
Defined formula, elemental, chemically defined diets	Formula which is based only on purified products (such as egg albumin as a protein source, medium chain triglycerides as a lipid source). The chemical and physical composition of the mixture is easily defined because the elements or items used are few in number.
Undefined formula diet	Formulas based on homogenates of food items (such as milk, meat). The chemical and physical composition is somewhat more variable than that of defined formula diets.
Maintenance formula	Provides protein or amino acids in amounts usually required for maintenance of protein nutriture.
High nitrogen or "anabolic" formula	Provides protein or amino acids in amounts needed for repletion or rehabilitation.
Low residue formula	One which uses protein sources such as egg albumin, soy protein, or amino acids (which are low in residue) instead of a milk base (higher in residue).

TABLE 12. Common Formulas Available for Enteral Feeding (NOTE: Values are only approximate as formulas change constantly.)

Product Manufacturer	Form	Percentage of Calories at Standard Dilution: Carbohydrate	Protein	Fat	Kilocalories	Sodium (mEq)	Nitrogen to Calorie Ratio	mOsm	Purposes and Comments
Aminaid (McGaw)	Powder	67	4	29	2.0/ml	5.9/L	1:662	?	Supplementary feeding used for renal failure, low in electrolytes. Not a complete feeding (e.g., Recommended Dietary Allowances for vitamins, minerals, etc., are not met by it alone).
	Liquid	64	4	32	2.0/ml	5.8/L	1:864	1125/L	
Carnation Instant Breakfast (Pet Milk) when mixed with whole milk	Powder	50	22	25	1.1/ml	42.2/L	1:112	?	Complete liquid diet with undefined formula which is usually used as a supplementary feeding: completely meets Recommended Dietary Allowances if 1.4 L are consumed. Not appropriate for tube feeding.
Casec (Mead Johnson)	Powder	0	100		3.6/g	0.1/L	1:26	?	Modular supplementary feeding, can also be used in modular feedings as a protein source. Incomplete.
Citrotein (Doyle)	Liquid	74	24	3	6.3/ml	28.0/L	1:102	496/L	Polymeric supplementary feeding, also useful as a calorie source in modular feedings. Incomplete.
Compleat B (Doyle)	Liquid	48	16	36	1.0/ml	67.9/L	1:154	490/L	Complete defined formula diet for tube feedings. Completely meets Recommended Dietary Allowances if 1600 ml fed per day.
Controlyte (Doyle)		57		43	1.6/ml	21.0/L	0	?	Modular supplementary feeding, can also be used in modular feedings for a low protein, low electrolyte, calorie source. Incomplete.

TABLE 12 *Continued*

Product Manufacturer	Form	Percentage of Calories at Standard Dilution: Carbo-hydrate	Protein	Fat	Kilo-calories	Sodium (mEq)	Nitrogen to Calorie Ratio	mOsm	Purposes and Comments
Cutter 2 (Cutter) liquid	Liquid	49	15	36	1.0/ml	27.0/L	1:162	435–510 /L	Complete defined formula diet for tube feeding; complete if 2000 ml fed per day.
EMF (Control Drugs)	Liquid		100		2.0/ml	10.6/L	1:24	?	Modular feeding which is a protein source for modular feedings.
Ensure (Ross)	Liquid	55	14	31	1.0/ml	31.6/L	1:177	460/L	Polymeric complete defined formula diet also used as supplementary or tube feeding which is modified so as to be lactose free. Comes in several flavors. Complete if 1920 ml are fed per day.
Ensure Plus (Ross)	Liquid	53	15	32	1.5/ml	47.9/L	1:168	?	Polymeric complete defined formula diet high in calories per unit volume. Supplementary feeding or tube feeding complete if 1920 ml fed per day.
Flexical (Mead Johnson)	Powder	62	9	31	1.0/ml	26.1/L	1:268	723/L	Monomeric elemental diet low in residue and lactose free; complete if 2000 ml fed per day.
Gevral (Lederle)	Powder	27	68	5	3.5/g	65/kg	1:35	?	Modular polymeric supplementary feeding high in protein and calories. Used in solid form. Incomplete.
Hycal (Beecham)	Liquid	98	1	1	2.5/ml	3.8/L	0:100	?	Modular monomeric supplementary feeding used in modular feeds as a carbohydrate source low in electrolytes.
Isocal (Mead Johnson)	Liquid	50	13	38	1.1/ml	23.1/L	1:192	350/L	Polymeric defined formula used in tube feeding. Defined formula which is modified so as to be lactose free. Complete if 1920 ml is fed per day.

TABLE 12 *Continued*

Product Manufacturer	Form	Percentage of Calories at Standard Dilution: Carbohydrate	Protein	Fat	Kilocalories	Sodium (mEq)	Nitrogen to Calorie Ratio	mOsm	Purposes and Comments
Lipomul-Oral (Upjohn)	Liquid	1		99	6.0/ml	17.4/L	0:100	0	Modular fat source for modular supplementary feedings.
Lolactene (Doyle)	Powder	53	27	21	0.8/ml	38.3/L	1:93	F	Polymeric formula feeding which is low in lactose and residue. Complete if 1150 ml fed per day.
Lonalac (Mead Johnson)	Powder Liquid	30 29	21 21	50 50	0.7/ml 0.7/ml	1.2/L 1.1/L	1:115 1:116	?	Polymeric modular supplementary feeding high in protein and low in sodium, also used for modular feedings. Incomplete.
MCT Oil (Mead Johnson)	Liquid	0	0	100	7.7/ml	0	0:100	0	Modular feeding consisting of medium chain triglycerides furnishing easily absorbed fat and energy source for those suffering from malabsorption of fat. Incomplete.
Mertene (Doyle)	Liquid	46	24	30	1.0/ml	39.8/L	1:102	539	Polymeric defined formula diet.
Meritene (Doyle)	Powder milk	45	26	29	1.0/ml	39.7/L	1:95		Complete if 1200 ml fed per day.
Mull-Soy (Syntex)	Liquid	53	26	22	1.25/ml	38.0/L	1:128	670/kg	Polymeric modified formula diet low in lactose and residue and high in nitrogen. Complete if 1150 ml fed per day.
Neo-Mull-Soy (Syntex)	Liquid	32	11	48	1.5/ml	18.7/L	1:227	252/kg	Polymeric modified formula diet. Incomplete.
Nutramigen (Mead Johnson)	Liquid	62	13	35	0.7/ml	14.0/L	1:185	443/kg	Polymeric formula diet low in lactose and low in residue. Incomplete.
Polycose (Ross)	Powder	100	0	0	4/g	36/kg	0:100	570/L	Modular supplemental feeding high in carbohydrate (oligosaccharides) used in modular feedings.

TABLE 12 *Continued*

Product Manufacturer	Form	Percentage of Calories at Standard Dilution: Carbohydrate	Protein	Fat	Kilocalories	Sodium (mEq)	Nitrogen to Calorie Ratio	mOsm	Purposes and Comments
Portagen (Mead Johnson)	Powder	46	14	43	1.0/ml	20.4/L	1:175	?	Monomeric formula diet low in lactose with MCT Oil as fat source useful for malabsorption. Complete if 966 ml fed per day.
Precision LR (Doyle)	Powder	92	10	1	1.1/ml	30.5/L	1:256	610/L	Polymeric defined formula diet low in residue which is lactose, gluten, and cholesterol free. Complete if 1710 ml fed per day.
Precision HN (Doyle)	Powder	83	17	1	1.0/ml	40.6/L	1:146	580/L	Polymeric defined formula diet high in nitrogen, low in residue, lactose, gluten, and cholesterol. Complete if 2950 ml fed per day.
Precision Isotonic (Doyle)	Powder	60	12	28	1.0/ml	33.4/L	1:204	300/kg	Polymeric defined formula diet, low in residue, lactose, gluten, cholesterol, and purines. Complete if 1580 ml fed per day.
Precision Mod N (Doyle)	Powder	60	13	28	1.2/ml	44.8/L	1:192	?	Polymeric formula diet. Complete if 1650 ml fed per day.
Pregestimil (Mead Johnson)	Liquid	53	13	38	0.7/ml	13.0/L	1:187	539/L	Polymeric defined formula diet for infants.
Promis (Mead Johnson)	Powder	0	100	0	3.7/g	0.87/g	1:27	?	Modular supplemental feeding low in lactose used as a solid.
ProSobee (Mead Johnson)	Liquid	40	15	45	0.7/ml	18.0/L	1:162	258/kg	Polymeric modified formula diet.
Sustacal (Mead Johnson	Powder and milk	54	24	22	1.0/ml	40.5/L	1:102	?	Polymeric defined formula diet in vanilla and chocolate flavors. Complete if 1080 ml fed per day.
	Liquid	55	24	21	1.0/ml	40.2/L	1:103	625/L	
Sustagen (Mead Johnson)	Powder with water	68	24	8	1.7/ml	54/L	1:103	125/L	

TABLE 12 *Continued*

Product Manufacturer	*Form*	*Percentage of Calories at Standard Dilution* *Carbo-hydrate*	*Protein*	*Fat*	*Kilo-calories*	*Sodium (mEq)*	*Nitrogen to Calorie Ratio*	*mOsm*	*Purposes and Comments*
Vital (Ross)	Powder	74	17	9	1.0/ml	17/L	1:150	450/L	Protein delivery as free amino acids and peptides. Complete at 1500 ml.
Vivonex (Eaton)	Powder	90	8	1	1.0/ml	37.4/L	1:308	500/L (600–1200/L if flavored)	Monomeric elemental diet which is low in residue and free of lactose and gluten.
Vivonex HN (Eaton)	Powder	81	18	1	1.0/cc	33.5/L	1:133	844/L	Same as above but higher in protein. Complete if 3000 ml fed per day. Protein content is higher than in Vivonex regular formula.

safety in relation to alternatives, and its low cost give it a decided advantage over other forms of enteral therapy.

However, at times oral intakes are partially or totally contraindicated because of the disease process, surgery, inability or unwillingness of the patient to consume the diet, or a continued failure to achieve adequate intakes by this route which is severe enough to jeopardize the patient's nutritional status.[117,118] If this happens, a choice of special feeding method then must be made.

FOOD INTAKE BY ORAL ROUTE

Usual "House" Diets

The usual diets served in hospitals attempt to simulate the usual dietary patterns in this country: approximately 13 to 15 percent of total calories from protein (a nitrogen to calorie ratio of 1:207 to 1:165), 40 to 42 percent from fat, and 43 percent from carbohydrate. They are planned to meet or exceed all of the Recommended Dietary Allowances and usually provide several choices so that all patients can find something they will eat.

Therapeutic "House" Diets

Approximately 40 percent of patients in most large teaching hospitals are on one form of therapeutic diet or another. The most commonly ordered dietary modifications are routinely prepared by the hospital dietitians and incorporate a variety of modifications in texture (soft, clear liquids, etc.), macronutrients (calorie modifications, type or amount of fat, carbohydrate), electrolytes (low sodium), timing of meals (as in diabetes diets), low or high residue diets and other modifications ("bland" diets excluding coffee, spices, and alcohol). These diets also are planned to meet Recommended Dietary Allowances.

House Diets With Food Supplements

The diets already discussed are planned for maintenance. To adjust them to promote anabolism during periods of rehabilitation, several modifications can be made.

SNACKS. The addition of several snacks or special feedings makes it possible for most patients to increase their energy intakes substantially. Patients will often eat far more than anticipated if eating is made easy for them. Snacks inbetween meals are one way to augment energy intakes, especially if a variety of snacks which can be nibbled by the bedside are supplied. For the patient who has difficulties consuming large amounts of food in solid form, nutritionally complete liquid formula supplements flavored as the patient prefers may be useful if supplied in an ice bath at the bedside throughout the day where neither the patient nor the attendants forget it. Tube feeding should be instituted if after 48 hours the patient's oral intake continues to decline even after suitable snacks and nutritional supplements have been provided.

DIETARY SUPPLEMENT FORMULAS. The patient who lacks appetite and who requires protein or energy supplementation beyond levels of intake which he is able to meet through diet alone is a candidate for the so-called "nutritional supplements" which are now available. Table 12 presents a partial list of the products available. The simplest strategy to adopt for such patients is to provide the usual house diet adjusted to food preferences, taste, and special therapeutic requirements for meals. Liquid dietary supplements which are commercially produced and widely available and juices are provided at intervals between meals and for all fluids intake.

These liquid commercial products are designed to provide protein supplementation and thus have very low nitrogen to calorie ratios (e.g., 1:70 to 1:93). Special products are available which are low in sodium or lactose for those who require it. The high protein densities in a small volume of these products make them suitable for the debilitated patient since the bulk of food which must be eaten is small. Protein intakes can be further enhanced by adding calcium caseinate formula, whole fresh eggs, or powdered protein sources. Caloric density can be increased by the addition of medium chain triglyceride oil or other oils depending upon tolerance or glucose polymers such as dextrins (which provide carbohydrate without increasing sweetness or altering intraluminal tonicity). These products are available in a number of flavors which increases palatability and adds variety.

FOODS SUITABLE FOR EITHER ORAL OR TUBE FEEDING

Types of Feedings Available

Liquified foods possess the potential advantage of being suitable for either oral or tube feeding. The two major types of foods are usual meals which are mixed with fluid and put through a blender or pureed to a semiliquid consistency and commercially available liquid formulas.

LIQUIFIED DIETS. Liquified feedings produced in most hospitals usually consist of milk based formulas which are pureed with meat, vegetables, fruits, minerals, and vitamins. Commercially prepared purees of common foods are also available in a ready to feed form.

Their disadvantages for oral use are chiefly taste, color, texture, viscosity, and the tendency for larger particles to settle out if the mixtures are not drunk immediately. These difficulties are somewhat less important when such preparations are employed for tube feeding, but their consistency requires a large caliber tube for their administration to avoid clogging. Moreover, great care must be taken in preparation and storage of the hospital prepared diets since the products readily serve as a medium for bacterial growth. Other physical characteristics such as viscosity and osmolality which affect tolerance to tube feedings vary from recipe to recipe, as does nutrient adequacy. For these reasons in spite of their low cost, ready availability, and the fact that flexible recipes to meet each individual patient's special needs can be employed, they are not popular means of nutritional support in hospitals. However, for patients living at home who need liquid feedings high in nutrient density at low cost, liquified foods may still be useful.

DEFINED FORMULA DIETS. In the past decade, a whole range of liquid formula products have been developed which have acceptable taste, palatability, and other aesthetic qualities as well as the viscosity and texture to permit them to be used interchangeably for oral or tube feedings.[119–126] In contrast to liquified foods, the formulas are compounded from food constituents such as protein from soy or casein; carbohydrate from sucrose, lactose, or corn syrup solids; fat from various vegetable oils; and vitamins and minerals. Thus nutrient composition can be specified very precisely.

For oral use, their flavor, color and consistency make them more attractive to patients and for use in tube feedings their better flow, other physical characteristics, and ready to feed qualities offer distinct advantages over foods put through a blender or pureed.

The formulas vary widely in their taste, cost, energy content per unit volume (usually 1 kcal/ml), nitrogen to calorie ratios, sources of protein, energy and other constituents affecting tolerance, and the extent to which they provide nutritionally complete alimentation. Representative examples appear in Table 12.

A consultation with the dietitian prior to setting up the nutritional support plan will usually save the physician time and trouble in the end, as well as making for greater patient comfort. Therefore, only the major characteristics of these products will be reviewed here. Specific attributes and additional, more up-to-date information can be obtained by consultation with the dietitian.

Two general types of formulas are available: *Maintenance formulas* provide approximately 1 kcal/ml, a nitrogen to calorie ratio of 1:200 or 1:300, and, if fed as the sole source of food, 30 to 35 kcal/kg/day. Usually they furnish vitamins and minerals in sufficient amounts to meet Recommended Dietary Allowances. *High nitrogen formulas* are designed for patients who are in hypermetabolic states or who require sufficient nutrients to support anabolism. These formulas provide 1 kcal/ml with nitrogen to calorie ratios of 1:150, somewhat lower than usual diets or formulas. Ratios as low as 1:100 may be required for managing the severe stress of sepsis. If fed in sufficient quantity to provide 40 to 45 kcal/kg/day, anabolic needs may be met. Such elevated intakes are sometimes possible to achieve by oral routes if these products are used judiciously as meal replacements, snacks, and extra feedings but often partial or total tube feeding will be necessary.

FOOD INTAKE BY TUBE

Indications

Tube feeding is appropriate when the patient cannot or will not take food by mouth but his gastrointestinal tract is functional, or when appetite is insufficient to meet nutrient needs by oral routes alone. The simplest route for tube feeding is the nasogastric. New fine gauge Silastic tubes with mercury tips allow easy passage, flexibility, and greater patient comfort and are more suitable for long-term use than the earlier, less flexible, larger gauge, nonweighted rubber tubes. The gauge and type of tube must be calibrated to the viscosity of the formula passing through it. Some find the 42 inch, number 8 French pediatric nasojejunal tube useful for many adults, others prefer fine bore intravenous-type catheters. If there is concern about gastric emptying, a larger tube may be used and gastric residua monitored for a few days. Infusion pumps are helpful, especially when slow rates of feeding are desired. It is also wise to check for gastroesophageal reflux with a barium swallow to minimize chances of aspiration.

Choices and Forms of Feeds Available

In addition to the various types of maintenance and high nitrogen formulas which have already been described, three other choices are available if oral routes are bypassed: defined formula–low residue diets, special formulas for organ failure, and individually compounded formulas utilizing modular feedings. These latter products are not palatable enough for most patients to tolerate them by mouth, but if this is not an obstacle they may be used orally as well.

DEFINED FORMULA–LOW RESIDUE DIETS. These prepackaged formulas, also known as "elemental" or "chemically" defined diets, are low residue preparations designed for feedings by mouth or tube.[119] They usually contain L-amino acids or short chain peptides, dextrose or oligosaccharides as the main energy source, and a small amount of fat, either from medium chain triglycerides or some other source. Essential fatty acids, vitamins, and minerals are usually supplied in amounts sufficient to meet Recommended Allowances if sufficient formula is taken to provide for energy intakes. These formulas require little or no digestive processing before absorption, are virtually completely absorbed, and leave minimal residue. The early report that their use could reduce the concentration and types of microorganisms in the large bowel[120] has not been confirmed by more recent studies.[121–125] However, fecal volume is markedly reduced, and this may be helpful in cleansing the bowel prior to surgery. The hypothesis that a combination of oral antibiotics and these formulas may reduce enterically related infections in cancer patients or in those with bone marrow dysfunction has not been proven.[126] Another question is whether these preparations prevent intestinal epithelial damage to a greater extent than other types of oral feedings during chemotherapy.[127] Other uses of these formulas, summarized in Table 11, are better documented.[26,120,128]

SPECIAL FORMULAS FOR ORGAN FAILURE. A number of special formulas for patients with advanced renal failure are already available. Preparations are now being developed for use in patients with hepatic encephalopathy and certain other states. Another alternative if the patient's condition does not permit use of formula diets with a fixed composition is to deal with the problem by adjusting available formulas by dilutions and additions.

MODULAR FEEDINGS. These products are concentrated sources of carbohydrate or protein usually consisting of predigested protein and hydrolyzed starch or glucose polymers. They permit the physician or dietitian to compound liquid feedings with special characteristics if the need arises and an available formula is not suitable. By mixing these relatively pure sources of the macronutrients, a satisfactory balance with respect to type and amount of carbohydrate, protein, and fat as well as other constituents can be achieved. Clinically they are useful for the fluid restricted, hypermetabolic patient or the patient with renal failure for whom usual formulas are inappropriate in their protein, sodium, potassium, and fluid volume. Since they must be formulated individually, bacterial contamination must be guarded against, and the possibility of diarrhea or other evidence of intolerance secondary to untried combinations must also be considered. The assistance of the clinical pharmacist and the dietitian is valuable in compounding new formulas from these modular products, since they are aware of the particular attributes of the various components and how best to achieve a suitable final product.

Monitoring

To avoid aspiration, the patient should be fed in a sitting or semisitting position and the bed's head elevated to 30° above horizontal for at least one hour after each feed. A number of characteristics of formulas may affect the patient's tolerance to tube feeding. These include:

1. *Cleanliness* in formula preparation, storage, and equipment.
2. *Temperature* of the formula when it is administered. It is best tolerated if fed at room temperature.
3. *Volume and flow rate of feed.* Generally a dilute diet of 100 to 200 ml is administered initially as a bolus feeding through the barrel of a large syringe or funnel and the mixture allowed to flow into the stomach by gravity. After feedings the tube should be rinsed with water to prevent clogging. Over time, tolerance will build until 300 to 500 ml can be administered every two to four hours. The gastric contents should be aspirated to evaluate the residua before each feeding.

4. *Adequacy of fluid intake.* Additional water (the amount depending upon the formula used) must be given since most of the formulas are hypertonic and solute loads are sufficiently high to cause dehydration in the absence of free water.
5. *Osmolality of the feed.* Gastrointestinal adaption is usually satisfactory if the precautions mentioned above are taken. Altered gastrointestinal function due to lactose intolerance or malabsorption of fat may be responsible for diarrheas. When these problems occur, lactose free formulas, alternative forms of fat, or bulk-free chemically defined diets may be called for.

Enteral Hyperalimentation

Hyperalimentation simply means supplying nutrients in amounts in excess of the Recommended Dietary Allowances, whether by mouth, tube, intravenous feeding, or other means. The term "enteral hyperalimentation" is sometimes used to describe the technique of constant drip gavage using a high caloric density defined formula diet.[18] This technique has proven extremely useful when very large amounts of nutrients must be delivered, as is the case for many patients whose nutritional support must be designed to reverse depletion states. Special small, thin walled nasogastric tubes are employed with continuous pump infusions to furnish a constant drip gavage of high calorie, high nitrogen formulas. Intakes as high as 4,000 kcal and 16 gm of nitrogen per day are possible using these techniques. These techniques have been employed with patients suffering from a wide variety of disorders ranging from esophageal disease to inflammatory bowel disease.[129]

If chemically defined diets are supplied which are high in amino acids and readily absorbable carbohydrates, relatively large amounts of nutrients can be provided even to very debilitated patients with lesions in the lower intestine.

Cyclic enteral hyperalimentation is also employed. The cyclic technique, first used parenterally, involves providing hypertonic dextrose and amino acids for approximately 12 hours a day then providing saline or other dextrose free solutions the remainder of the time. Some workers now employ a similar technique for enteral hyperalimentation. It is useful in mobilizing the energy stored in the liver during the glucose phase, appears to reverse hepatic steatosis, and improves visceral function.[130]

Ostomies in Tube Feeding

When nasogastric intubation is impossible, surgical procedures may still make it possible to use the gastrointestinal tract if it is functional. The development of very fine bore intravenous type catheters, continuous infusion pumps, and the newer forms of formulas have increased the efficiency and effectiveness of feedings by these routes.[131–141]

ESOPHAGOSTOMY. Small esophagostomies for feeding are now possible due to the availability of fine gauge tubes. The incision required is cosmetically more acceptable to patients than the larger incisions required decades ago. Such a route offers an alternative to jejunostomy for gastrectomy patients.

GASTROSTOMY. This is the usual route employed if long term feeding will be necessary. If a patient is suspected of being at high risk prior to surgery, a feeding gastrostomy may be indicated. In nutritional support planning, the speed of gastric emptying must be taken into consideration in selecting the proper formula. Anticipatory guidance with respect to stoma care is also important.

JEJUNOSTOMY. Useful in cases of upper gastrointestinal obstruction, great care is necessary in planning nutritional support using this route. Needle catheter jejunostomies require formulas capable of flowing through very fine bore tubes. Tube placement is critical to assure adequate mixing of the ingesta with pancreatic juice and bile, otherwise maldigestion and malabsorption occur. The osmolarity of the formula must be low enough to prevent dumping syndrome due to hyperosmolar solutions entering the jejunum. The form of nutrients also must be adjusted: protein hydrolysates or amino acids which can be absorbed without pancreatic proteolytic enzymes and medium chain triglycerides which do not require high concentrations of bile salts and pancreatic lipase may be helpful in overcoming mixing problems.

Table 13 summarizes the indications, common problems, and therapies for various forms of tube feeding.[140,141]

COMBINED ENTERAL-PARENTERAL FEEDINGS

Indications

Often there is no reason to abandon the enteral route entirely if in and of itself it proves to be inadequate to sustain the critically ill patient's extremely high energy needs in the face of limited body fuel reserves. Many debilitated, malnourished, or emaciated postsurgical patients fall in this category, especially those who have not received feeding gastrostomies or jejunostomies in anticipation of possible postoperative problems. For such patients, constant drip tube feedings of suitable formulas, vitamins, and trace elements by slow infusion pump permit the gastrointestinal tract to be utilized to the limits of its capacity. Peripheral vein, or if needs be, central vein alimentation is used to deliver nutrients and fluids which cannot be provided in sufficient amounts by enteral routes.

Combined enteral and parenteral feedings may also be required for the patient being "weaned" from total parenteral nutritional support as he becomes rehabilitated.[135–137] The transition here varies depending upon the functional state of the gastrointestinal tract from tube or feeding ostomy to oral feedings. In any event, the transition from parenteral to enteral feedings should be gradual. The changeover time will depend upon patient tolerance but is usually at least three to seven days.

PARENTERAL NUTRITION

Perhaps no new development in nutrition has focused more attention on the relevance of nutrition to the surgical patient than the development of total parenteral nutrition. This method permits the delivery of adequate calories and protein to the patient totally

TABLE 13. Indications for Various Forms of Enteral Feeding and Ways to Correct Common Problems

Type of Feeding and Indications	*Contraindications*	*Complication*	*Therapy*
Usual Intake by Mouth			
Route of choice if gastrointestinal tract is functional, patient desires oral feeding, and appetite present	Obstruction, partial or total in lower gastrointestinal tract; impairment of swallowing mechanisms; ileus, fistulas, especially of upper gastrointestinal tract; coma, symptomatic exacerbation of disease with intake by mouth; severe diarrhea; severe vomiting; refusal or inability of patient to sustain satisfactory intakes by mouth; potential for aspiration, as during anesthesia, use of strong sedatives, during immediate postoperative period, with debilitated patients having depressed cough reflexes and/or preexisting pulmonary problems, or hiccoughs (which increase risk of aspiration); preparation of the gastrointestinal tract for surgery; malabsorption as when transit times are very rapid, pancreatic enzymes are low or absent, biliary secretion is decreased, mucosal function of bowel is altered due to disease, radiation injury, or surgery as in short bowel syndrome; protein-energy malnutrition with consequent anorexia.		

TABLE 13 *Continued*

Type of Feeding and Indications	*Contraindications*	*Complication*	*Therapy*
Chemically Defined (Elemental) Formula Diets Fed By Mouth			
Need for large loads of nutrients to be delivered when appetite is insufficient and gastrointestinal tract is functional, intestinal sounds are present, and stomach emptying is efficient.	Metabolic problems such as renal disease, corticosteroid therapy, etc., which make patients unable to tolerate amounts of nutrients or volume of formula required to meet nutritional needs.	Malabsorption; hyperosmolar, non-ketotic coma among diabetics; exacerbation of metabolic problems with renal and hepatic disorders; serious losses of water and electrolytes in patients with malabsorption secondary to bowel fistulas, damaged or resected small intestine.	Sometimes can be avoided by slow continuous feeding utilizing a pump; check protein levels; discontinue and use parenteral nutrition support.
Pancreatitis, pancreatic fistula or massive bowel resection with large intestinal fluid losses. Fistulas of the intestinal tract. Malabsorption not responding to other formulas. Lesions low in the gastrointestinal tract, such as inflammatory bowel disease, ulcerative colitis, Crohn's disease. Reduced length of small intestine with malabsorption.	Modifications by dilution and addition are sometimes, but not always, possible to avoid intestinal fluid loss.	Hyperosmotic hyperglycemic nonketotic dehydration.	Usually due to osmotic diuresis secondary to glucosuria; check to make sure overadministration has not occured to compensate for under administration at some other time. Check flow rate and slow it if it is overly rapid. Use insulin if necessary upon initiation and when caloric load is being increased; discontinue when feedings are discontinued. These complications are most usual when large loads of nutrients are fed to produce an anabolic state.
Enterocutaneous fistulas or inflammatory bowel disease making decreased stool bulk desirable.		Unpalatability	Feed by tube.

TABLE 13 *Continued*

Type of Feeding and Indications	*Contraindications*	*Complication*	*Therapy*
Need to decrease pancreatic, biliary, and gastrointestinal secretions.		Inadequate weight gain in a critically ill patient.	Most formulas are designed for normal needs, not hypermetabolic states, and are inadequate in nitrogen. Use high nitrogen formulas with continuous drip or pump infusion.
Transitional feeding when going from parenteral to enteral route.		Diarrhea	Infusion rate may be too rapid; start at low concentrations (e.g., 10–15%) and gradually build up concentration to 25% weight/volume (1Kcal/ml) using a slow continuous infusion rate.
Nasogastric Tube Feeding			
Patient is unable to tolerate oral feed owing to weakness or debilitation. Persistant lack of appetite.	Impaired gastric emptying; gastric retention; some degree of lower bowel obstruction; high risk of vomiting and potential aspiration; esophageal regurgitation; vomiting; high fistula in the gastrointestinal tract may not permit tube to reach below the level of the fistula; inadequate absorption; obstruction of small intestine or below; complete bowel obstruction.	Improper placement leading to increased reflux.	Tip of tube is best positioned in lower esophagus rather than stomach to avoid reflux when patient is supine.
		Sore throats and difficulties in swallowing.	Use of silicone elastomers (Silastic) of small gauge rather than rubber or polyethylene may give relief.
		Tube expelled on regurgitation or coughing.	Weight tube with mercury tip or bag.
		Difficulties in placement of tube.	Chill tube before insertion, insert with stylet, or insert with larger tube alongside it fitted into half of a gelatin capsule, then irrigate larger tube and withdraw it, leaving small tube properly positioned

TABLE 13 *Continued*

Type of Feeding and Indications	*Contraindications*	*Complication*	*Therapy*
Poor swallowing as with head/neck tumors causing pain or obstruction in deglutition or as in neurologic difficulties in swallowing.	Extreme debilitation, especially in patients having depressed cough reflexes, pre-existing pulmonary problems, because of risks of aspiration.	Plugging of tube.	Use formula which is more finely dispersed or a larger tube.
Severe persistent anorexia requiring some form of forced feeding.	Hiccoughs, increase risks of aspiration. Unsupervised use, as when patient removed from floor for tests and procedures.	Aspiration	Staff must always adhere to strict procedures, including a preliminary test of response with water, progressive increase with diluted formula at slow infusion rates while monitoring tolerance with patient in semiseated or upright position during feeding and shortly afterwards. Slow drop feeding from bag or bottle further decreases risk of aspiration.
Fistula of upper gastrointestinal tract requiring a tube to bypass it.	Comatose patient.		
Severe malabsorption requiring a formula fed slowly and continually to permit absorption.	Cosmetic, social, and psychologic problems among ambulatory or discharged patients from having a tube protruding from his nose (esophagostomy).		
Use of gastrointestinal tract to help maintain its structure and function, also to stimulate hyperplasia after resection of bowel.		Esophagitis	Use smaller tube.
		Cramps, diarrhea, vomiting or nausea.	Formula may be too cold, administer at room temperature. Delivery rate may be too fast. Slower feeding rates are generally best tolerated, and continuous drip is best of all.
Formula so unpalatable that patient cannot ingest adequate amounts by mouth.			
Patient resists oral feeding owing to psychologic problems.		Dumping syndrome with diarrhea	Excessive values of hyperosmolar solutions are reaching small intestine. Slow flow rate down.

TABLE 13 *Continued*

Type of Feeding and Indications	*Contraindications*	*Complication*	*Therapy*
		Hypo-osmolar malabsorption with diarrhea	Begin feeding with dilute solutions to tolerance of feeds high in glucose, then administer serum albumin parenterally if they are low to increase serum osmolarity. Finally, increase caloric concentration of the solution.
		Unidentifiable causes of diarrhea.	Add antidiarrhea agents such as opiates or diphenoxylate with atropine (Lomotil) to feeding solution, but monitor for intestinal sounds and fecal impaction and avoid overdosage which may give rise to paralytic ileus or massive pseudo-obstruction of the colon.
		Stricture	Use smaller tube.
		Inadequate weight gain	Causes are many, but patient may not be receiving all the formula which was ordered. Order monitoring of intake.
		Food borne illness	Bacterial contamination may have occured in preparation or from cans standing open at room temperature. Tube feeding equipment may be dirty. Check preparation, storage, and techniques.
Esophagostomy Tube			
Need for long term feeding.	Esophagitis, stricture		See stricture, above

TABLE 13 *Continued*

Type of Feeding and Indications	*Contraindications*	*Complication*	*Therapy*
Cosmetic considerations for discharged patient who objects to tube protruding from nose.			
Gastrointestinal tract functional.			
Partial gastrectomy or esophagogastrectomy with stomach up in chest requiring tube feeding.			
Enteral Hyperalimentation (Using Nasogastric Tube and Infusion Pump)			
Protein energy-malnutrition requiring nutritional rehabilitation rather than maintenance (e.g., 130–160% over normal levels) especially with severe or rapidly progressive moderate protein energy malnutrition.	Terminal (moribund) Severe gastrointestinal disturbance, such as intractable vomiting, hiccoughs, or bleeding in the upper gastrointestinal tract; lower bowel obstruction; pulmonary aspiration of stomach contents; esophageal erosion.	Clogging of tube lumen.	Flush tube with water, replace tube if problem persists.
		Vomiting, bloating and nausea.	Reduce flow rate. Add peripheral hyperalimentation if needed. Check for other complications.
		Diarrhea and cramping.	Reduce flow rate, dilute solution, check for other complications, consider need for revising formula, add antidiarrheal drug.
		Diarrhea with fat or protein malabsorption.	Consider constant infusion of formula which does not require proteolytic or lipolytic capacity to digest and which is low in dissachharides.
Gastric retention with usual nasogastric tube without pump.		Edema	Reduce sodium content of formula or slow flow rate.

TABLE 13 *Continued*

Type of Feeding and Indications	*Contraindications*	*Complication*	*Therapy*
		Condition requiring fluid restriction present (e.g., in some cardiac, hepatic, or renal disease).	Consider use of high caloric density formula of modular type tailored to patient's needs.
		Enterocutaneous fistula or inflammatory bowel disease requiring low residue feeds.	Use formula which is low in residue.
		Hyperglycemia and glucosuria.	Reduce flow, administer insulin
		Hypernatremia, hypercalcemia	Adjust electrolyte concentration of formula.
		Essential fatty acid deficiency.	Provide oral supplement of linoleic acid or Intralipid introvenously.
		Insufficient intake achieved owing to these or other complications to permit repletion.	Supplement enteral feeds with peripheral alimentation.
Gastrostomy Tube Need for long term tube feeding as a prophylactic measure during recovery from intestinal surgery which is likely to result in significant malabsorption.	Coma; obstruction of stomach as by tumor, etc.; inability to withstand surgery.		
Jejunostomy Tube: Obstruction at a level higher than the jejunum. Comatose patient.		Dumping syndrome. May be due to hyperosmolar solutions.	Avoid by initial infusion of formula at a reduced concentration and rate, increasing as tolerance is demonstrated. Also, use of formulas of low osmolarity with glucose oligosaccharides and some fat may help.

TABLE 13 *Continued*

Type of Feeding and Indications	*Contraindications*	*Complication*	*Therapy*
		Maldigestion and malabsorption	Often due to inadequate mixing of feeding with bile and pancreatic juice. Remedies include checking positioning of tube, use of pancreatic extract, use of medium chain triglycerides which are less dependent upon pancreatic lipase and bile salts for their digestion and oligosaccharides, protein hydrolysate, and free amino acids which can be absorbed without pancreatic extract or bile.

by an intravenous route. In general, this route is elected when the oral and enteral route cannot meet these needs.

Parenteral Caloric and Protein Needs

Preceding sections have detailed how energy expenditure and the patterns of substrate fuels varies with particular disease states. The following section will focus on the relationship of parenteral nutrition to caloric and protein needs. Although caloric need is discussed separately from protein requirements, it should be understood that they are intimately related. The technique of nitrogen balance which measures "nitrogen in" minus "nitrogen out" (urine, gut, other bodily fluids) permits assessment of protein dynamics. An individual can be kept in "positive nitrogen balance," which implies but does not confirm a net protein synthesis, by supplying either massive amounts of amino acids intravenously and very little carbohydrate or alternatively by giving massive amounts of carbohydrate and no protein. Since the standard American diet is composed of 50 percent carbohydrate, 35 percent fat, and 15 percent protein, teleologically the use of these extreme one substrate regimens would appear metabolically inefficient. Indeed, a balanced intravenous diet composed of fat, carbohydrate, and amino acids has been shown to be associated with incorporation of amino acids into both liver and peripheral tissue.

Parenteral caloric requirements can roughly be assessed by (1) determining the basal energy expenditure or basal metabolic rate (Table 14); (2) assessing the pre-existing nutritional deficit, and (3) recognising the caloric demands of the particular disease state. The basal energy expenditure or basal metabolic rate depends on age, sex, height, and

TABLE 14. Methods for Determining Caloric Requirements

A. RELATIONSHIP BETWEEN NITROGEN EXCRETION AND CALORIC REQUIREMENTS

Degree of Catabolism	*Urea-N/24 hr*	*Percentage of RME over Basal Metabolic Rate*	*Caloric Requirements (X BEE)**
1°, Normal	< 5	0	1.76 × BEE = parenteral 1.54 × BEE = enteral (1° and 2°)
2°, Mild	5–10	0–20	
3°, Moderate	10–15	20–50	2.2 × BEE = parenteral
4°, Severe	> 15	> 50	2.5 or > × BEE = parenteral

B. SIMPLIFIED AND IMMEDIATE ESTIMATION OF CALORIC AND PROTEIN REQUIREMENTS

Degree of Stress	*Calories (kcal/kg/24 hr)*	*Protein (g/kg/24 hr)*
None	30	1
Mild	35	1.5
Moderate	40	2
Severe	45–50	2.5

*BEE = basal energy expenditure (basal metabolic rate)

weight as shown in Tables 9 and 10. The additional calories which are required due to either a pre-existing nutritional deficit or the particular disease state are not as simply derived. Several methods for roughly calculating these latter requirements will be presented. Since measurements of metabolic expenditure by sophisticated calorimetry or by oxygen consumption are not used routinely for clinical assessment, one must rely on a very important relationship between nitrogen excretion and metabolic rate as shown in Table 14,A. It is well recognized that nitrogen excretion is not only related to metabolic rate but also depends on pre-existing nitrogen stores, nitrogen intake, and the ratio of nonprotein calories to nitrogen intake.[50] However, to calculate caloric requirements we ignore these theoretical considerations. Table 14,A outlines the relationship between nitrogen excretion, as measured by urinary urea nitrogen output in 24 hours, and metabolic rate.[16] The 24 hour urinary urea nitrogen output is obtained by multiplying the urea nitrogen concentration of an aliquot of urine by the 24 hour urinary volume (Table 15). Addition of 4 g, the constant nonurinary urea nitrogen loss, results in a rough estimate of *total nitrogen loss.* Based on this relationship, caloric requirements can be graded into four general categories dependent on the severity of the disease and the concomitant stress as discussed in the previous section. For mild degrees of catabolism, such as convalescence from clean surgery, urea nitrogen/24 hours is generally less than 10 g/24

TABLE 15. Calculation of Estimated Total Nitrogen Loss

	Example
Urine urea nitrogen = 6 g/L	
24-hr urine volume = 2 L	
∴ 24 hr urea nitrogen loss = 6 g/L × 2 L or 12 g	
if constant, nonurinary urea nitrogen loss = 4 g	
Approximate total nitrogen loss = 16 g/24 hr	

hours. The parenteral caloric requirements to maintain anabolism in this situation are nearly two times BEE, being 1.76. The value for the parenteral route is higher than the enteral requirement (1.5 × BEE). The lower caloric needs for the enteral regimen are probably related to a more efficient utilization of energy by the enterohepatic route.[50] As would be expected in high flow sepsis or major burns, the caloric requirements may rise to three times the BEE.

An alternative method for calculating caloric requirements is shown in Table 14,B. Energy requirements in a nonstressed individual will be maintained by supplying 30 kcal/kg of body weight/24 hours, while positive nitrogen balance and increased fat stores will be associated with a rate of 46 kcal/kg/24 hours.[147] In patients with mild to severe sepsis or with extensive burns, the requirements may be increased to as high as 60 kcal/kg/24 hours (Table 16).

Certainly there are shortcomings to these "cookbook" methods. The first was derived from a retrospective analysis of the relationship of the infusion rate of total parenteral nutrition to urinary nitrogen excretion.[16] The amount of calories required to keep the patient in positive nitrogen balance was ascertained. Subsequently that multiple times the individual's basal energy expenditure to maintain positive nitrogen balance was derived. Although these studies were controlled for the degree of stress, pre-existing nutritional deficits were not mentioned. However, recent studies using heavy carbon labelled glucose have validated the figure of 1.76 × BEE as a guide to caloric requirements in the nonstressed patient.[159] The second method was based on body weight and was derived from an analysis of exchangeable potassium data (K_e) in patients whose degree of stress and pre-existing malnutrition were not well documented. By regression analysis, a multiple times the body weight which assured a net positive K_e flux (protein synthesis) was derived.[147] Despite these drawbacks, both these methods attempt to tailor caloric requirements to the needs of the patient and the disease state.

Protein metabolism is in constant flux. While over 70 g of protein enters the gut per day as cells or enzymes, only 10 g is lost by stool per day. The rest of the protein is reabsorbed into the amino acid pool for subsequent protein synthesis. A 70 kg man generally consumes 90 g of protein a day. With provision of sufficient nonprotein energy, protein synthesis is comparable to or greater than protein breakdown. The amino acids tryptophan, lysine, threonine, methionine, and phenylalanine and the branched-chain amino acids leucine, isoleucine, and valine, are termed *essential*, because they cannot be formed endogenously by transamination as can the other amino acids. They are, there-

TABLE 16. Example of Planning Total Parenteral Nutritional Requirements

SUBJECT: 60 YEAR OLD 185 CM, 80 KG MAN WITH LATERAL DUODENAL FISTULA AND TEMPERATURE ELEVATION TO 38°C

STEP 1: CALCULATE DAILY VOLUME NEEDS

Nasogastric tube	1000 ml/24 hr	
Fistula	800 ml/24 hr	(via sump)
Insensible loss	1000 ml/24 hr	
Urine loss	1200 ml/24 hr	
Total	4000 ml/24 hr	

STEP 2. CALCULATE ELECTROLYTE NEEDS

(MEG)	Na^+	K^+	Cl^-
Nasogastric tube	60	10	120
Fistula	120	20	90
Insensible loss	20		20
Urine	40	10	40
Total	240	40	270

STEP 3. CALCULATE CALORIC NEEDS

METHOD 1 (Table 14) URINARY UREA LOSS = 10 g/24 hr

$2 \times$ BEE = 24 hr caloric needs

$2 \times$ 1680 kcal/24 hr = 3360

METHOD 2 (Table 14) MODERATE DEGREE OF CATABOLISM →

40 kcal/kg/24 hr

40×80 kg = 3200 kcal/24 hr

REQUIREMENTS: 4000 ml with 240 mEq Na, 40 K, 270 Cl and 3300 kcal

ORDERS: AFTER ACHIEVING GLUCOSE TOLERANCE DAY #3

	VOLUME (ml)	Na (mEq)	K (mEq)	Cl (mEq)	CALORIES
1000 ml TPN SOLUTION q 8 hrs →	3000	90	105	120	3060
500 ml D5/NS c̄ 15 mEq KCl q 12 hrs →	1000	154	30	154	170
24 HOUR TOTALS	4000	244	135	274	3230

fore, a dietary requirement, being important for maintaining nonspecific host resistance. The aromatic amino acids are building blocks for the central neurotransmitters.[68] The branched-chain amino acids, leucine, isoleucine and valine, are the only amino acids oxidized to a significant degree by muscle. Our earlier studies showed that these amino acids may be oxidized as a source of endogenous fuel during periods of stress such as trauma and sepsis.[6] Infusions of branched-chain amino acids have been associated with decreased peripheral proteolysis during the stress of fasting[148] or stress.[149] By competing with the aromatic amino acids at the blood-brain barrier, they may be helpful in the encephalopathy of hepatic failure.[150]

A simple method of calculating protein requirements is to supply 1 to 1.5 gm of protein/kg/24 hours for mild degrees of stress, and 2.5 gm of protein/kg/24 hours for moderate to severe stress (Table 14,B). A second but more detailed method requires calculation of the 24 hour urinary urea nitrogen output and addition of 4 grams to provide a rough estimate of total nitrogen loss (Table 15). Obviously the *nonurinary* urea nitrogen loss increases dramatically with intestinal fistulae or burns.

Nitrogen to Calorie Ratio

The intimate relationship between caloric and protein requirements determines "protein synthetic rates." The nitrogen to calorie ratio of standard total parenteral nutrition (TPN) solutions varies from 1:125 to 1:150. In severe stress, such as massive trauma, a ratio of 1:100 may be associated with greater rates of protein synthesis.[152] A recent important study emphasized how the nitrogen to calorie ratio should be tailored to the patient's changing disease state and degree of malnutrition.[152] In patients with moderate nutritional depletion, a nitrogen to calorie ratio of 1:150 (the standard TPN ratio in most institutions) maintains adequate nitrogen balance. In patients with severe nutritional depletion, a lower nitrogen to calorie ratio (1:100 or 125) appears more appropriate. The actual affects of this ratio on protein synthesis awaits labelled nitrogen flux studies employing varying nitrogen to calorie ratios.

Table 17 shows that the most common indications for total parenteral nutrition are related to compromised gut function.[155] A secondary consideration in the selection of a route is the amount of calories required for nutritional repletion and maintenance. In severe nutritional depletion and/or in severe stress states (extensive sepsis), it may be easier to supply the massive amounts of calories required by a parenteral rather than an enteral route.

Solutions Available for Parenteral Nutrition

Table 18 compares three forms of parenteral nutrition and support: (1) total parenteral nutrition (hyperalimentation), (2) intravenous (IV) fat regimen (fat, 5% glucose, and 3% amino acids), (3) "protein-sparing" solution (isotonic amino acids) with or without 5

TABLE 17. Indications for Total Parenteral Nutrition

Primary (Lifesaving) Indications	*Secondary (Life Supportive) Indications*
Enterocutaneous fistula	Malignancy
Gastrointestinal tract obstruction	Renal failure
Inflammatory bowel disease	Hepatic failure
"Short gut" syndrome	Severe malnutrition in the preoperative or postoperative patient
Malabsorption syndromes	Massive catabolism
Acute pancreatitis	

TABLE 18. Components of Parenteral Nutritional Support

Type	Protein			Nonprotein Calories			Osmolarity (mOsm/L)	Nonprotein Calorie:Nitrogen Ratio
	Source	G/L	Kcal/L	Source	G/L	Kcal/L		
Total parenteral nutrition	Amino acids	42.5	170	Dextrose (25%)	250	850	1850	125:1
Intravenous fat regimen	Amino acids	42.5	170	Intralipid (10%)	100	1100	280	106:1*
				Dextrose (5%)	50	170	830	
Protein-sparing solution	Amino acids	35	140	Endogenous fat	Variable		525	0:1
				±Dextrose (5%)	50	170	830	

*When given at the ratio of 2 L of 5% dextrose in water and 4.25% amino acids to 1 L Intralipid.

percent glucose solution. While protein in the form of amino acids is common to all three, the principal caloric source differs. In TPN, 20 to 30 percent glucose is the chief source of calories, while a combination of fat (10%) and glucose (5 to 10%) supplies calories in the intravenous fat regimen. The third form of parenteral support, "protein-sparing" solution, relies on the endogenous release of fat from lipid stores under the favorable influence of lowered serum insulin levels (i.e., mimicking the hormone-substrate relationships of adaptation to fasting).

Total Parenteral Nutrition

COMPOSITION (Table 19)

The solution for total parenteral nutrition is a mixture of 20 to 30 percent dextrose (glucose) and 4 to 5 percent crystalline amino acids. Added are 1 to 3 percent multiple vitamins, electrolytes, and trace elements. This solution provides 900 to 1000 kcal/1000 cc and 5.25 to 6 g of nitrogen (42.5 g of amino acids). Dextrose provides 850 Cal. In our institution, 35 mEq of sodium, 30 mEq of potassium, 5 mEq of calcium, 8 mEq of magnesium, 35 mEq of sodium, 30 mEq of phosphate, multivitamins, and trace elements are added to each 1000 cc. Table 20 compares the amino acid composition of domestically available crystalline amino acid solutions. Crystalline amino acid solutions are favored now over protein hydrolysate solutions for the following reasons: (1) the amino acid pattern is predictable and is not based on random cleavage of protein hydrolysate, (2) the ammonia content is lower, (3) the nitrogen is of a "higher biologic value," and (4) the potential for allergic reactions is lower.

TABLE 19. Individual Constituents of Various Parenteral Nutritional Solutions per 100 ml Solution

Constituent	*Total Paraenteral Nutrition*	*Intravenous Fat Regimen*	*Protein-Sparing Solution*
Amino acids (g)	42.5	42.5†	35
Dextrose (g)	250	50†	
Sodium (mEq)	30	30	25
Potassium (mEq)	40	40	15
Calcium (mEq)	5	5	
Magnesium (mEq)	8	8	5
Acetate (mEq)	40	40	54
Chloride (mEq)	35	35	25
Phosphate (mEq)	10	10	15
Multivitamin concentrate (ml)	1	1	*
Folic acid (μg)	300	300	*
Vitamin K_1 (μg)	300	300	
Vitamin B_{12} (μg)	3.3	3.3	*
Trace elements (ml)	1		

*Required weekly,
†Infused as nonlipid component of regimen.

TABLE 20. Individual Amino Acid Content of Crystalline Amino Acid Solutions

Amino Acids (g/100 ml)	Aminosyn (Abbott)			Freamine II (McGaw)	Travasol (Travenol)			Veinamine (Cutter)
	3.5%	5%	7%	8.5%	3.5%	5.5%	8.5%	8%
Essential								
L-Isoleucine	0.252	0.360	0.510	0.590	0.167	0.263	0.406	0.493
L-Leucine	0.329	0.470	0.660	0.770	0.216	0.340	0.526	0.347
L-Lysine	0.252*	0.360*	0.510*	0.870*	0.202†	0.318†	0.492†	0.667†
L-Methionine	0.140	0.200	0.280	0.450‡	0.202	0.318	0.492	0.427
L-Phenylalanine	0.154	0.220	0.310	0.480	0.216	0.340	0.526	0.400
L-Threonine	0.182	0.260	0.370	0.340	0.146	0.230	0.356	0.160
L-Tryptophan	0.056	0.080	0.120	0.130	0.063	0.099	0.152	0.080
L-Valine	0.280	0.400	0.560	0.560	0.160	0.252	0.390	0.253
Total Grams	*1.645*	*2.350*	*3.320*	*4.190*	*1.372*	*2.160*	*3.340*	*2.827*
Total Grams/Container	*15.270 /1000 ml*	*11.230 /500 ml*	*15.865 /500 ml*	*19.700 /500 ml*	*6.860 /500 ml*	*10.800 /500 ml*	*16.700 /500 ml*	*14.135 /500 ml*
Nonessential								
L-Histidine	0.105	0.105	0.210	0.240	0.153	0.241	0.372	0.237
L-Arginine	0.343	0.490	0.690	0.310	0.363	0.570	0.380	0.749
L-Glutamic acid	—	—	—	—	—	—	—	0.426
L-Aspartic acid	—	—	—	—	—	—	—	0.400
Glycine	0.448	0.640	0.900	1.700	0.725	1.140	0.760	3.387
L-Proline	0.300	0.430	0.610	0.950	0.146	0.230	0.356	0.107
L-Alanine	0.448	0.640	0.900	0.600	0.725	1.140	1.760	—
L-Serine	0.147	0.210	0.300	0.500	—	—	—	00
L-Cysteine	—	—	—	0.020	—	—	—	—
L-Tyrosine	0.031	0.044	0.066	—	0.014	0.022	0.034	—
Total Grams	*1.822*	*2.604*	*3.676*	*4.320*	*2.126*	*3.343*	*5.171*	*5.306*
Total Grams/Container	*18.220 /1000 ml*	*13.020 /500 ml*	*18.380 /500 ml*	*21.600 /500 ml*	*10.630 /500 ml*	*16.715 /500 ml*	*25.855 /500 ml*	*26.530 /500 ml*
% Essential amino acids	*47.4*	*47.4*	*47.4*	*49.2*	*39.2*	*39.2*	*39.2*	*47.7*

*As the acetate
†As the hydrochloride
‡As D1 methionine

There are three methods for preparing TPN solution: (1) bulk method, wherein anhydrous glucose is combined with a 5 percent amino acid solution; (2) stock solution, where 350 cc of 50 percent glucose is mixed with 750 cc of a 5 percent amino acid solution and 5 percent dextrose; and (3) a kit method employing 500 cc of 50 percent glucose and 500 cc of 8.5 percent amino acid solution. The first two methods mix the components under sterile conditions in a laminar flow hood, whereas the kit method permits sterile mixture of small lots of TPN under closed conditions and avoids the use of the laminar flow hood. Both the bulk and stock solution methods are useful in larger institutions where greater than 5 patients per day will be requiring TPN. By contrast, the kit method is readily utilizable in smaller community hospitals where only 2 to 3 isolated patients may be receiving TPN. Thus, 1 L of solution supplies 42.5 g of amino acids and 1020 Kcal/liter. The hypertonic mixture (1850 mOsm) has a nonprotein nitrogen to calorie ratio of 1:136. A dose of 2.5 L of TPN solution in a 24 hour period would supply a 70 kg man with approximately 2500 Kcal or approximately 36.5 kcal/kg of body weight/24 hours, the theoretical requirement for an unstressed individual.

INDICATIONS

Disease states in which TPN is indicated (see Table 16) can be divided into two general categories:[156] (1) those requiring primary therapy and (2) those requiring secondary therapy. The use of TPN as *primary therapy* implies TPN is lifesaving and without TPN the patient would not survive, while the use of TPN as *secondary therapy* suggests that TPN is supportive and not totally needed for patient survival. Abnormalities of gut function (e.g., intestinal fistula, short bowel syndrome) are the most frequent indications for primary therapy with TPN. Several other general indications, in addition to the type of disease, can be applied to the selection of TPN. Because of the high "start-up" cost and the 3 to 4 day delay to achieve maximum calorie intake, TPN usually should be undertaken when the patient will require greater than 7 to 10 days of parenteral nutrition. TPN is the therapy of choice in patients with both visceral and somatic protein depletion, as indicated by serum albumin levels of less than 3.5 g/dl, negative reactions to a battery of recall skin test antigens, and a decreased arm muscle circumference and/or creatinine height index. In patients with a recent preoperative weight loss greater than 10 lb. of body weight and moderate changes in these parameters, selection of TPN as the parenteral solution of choice should be individualized and depends upon: (1) age, older patients cannot withstand semistarvation as well as younger patients and (2) degree of operative or disease stress. In hypercatabolic states, caloric concentration becomes a major consideration. Since TPN has nearly twice the caloric density per unit volume of the 10 percent intravenous fat regimen, less volume of fluid is required for a given caloric load (see Table 18). TPN therefore is the *parenteral* solution of choice for significant nutritional depletion and marked catabolic states.

CATHETER INSERTION AND CARE

In our institution, we have favored the infraclavicular, subclavian route of catheter placement because the topography of the upper anterior chest permits easier maintenance of the catheter than the internal jugular location. Central catheter insertion should be approached like any surgical operation, as shown in Figure 5. Strict asepsis is imperative. The individual placing the catheter and his assistant should gown and wear both a mask and a cap. Since many of these patients have their catheters placed while in an intensive care unit environment, the patient should be walled off with curtains. Alternatively, central line insertion should be carried out in a special procedure room. This may further minimize septic complications. The patient is placed in a head down position with the feet elevated to fill the supracardiac major veins. A distended, external jugular vein is usually good clinical evidence that the subclavian vein also will be turgid. In addition, this position serves to prevent air embolus during catheter insertion. Several key anatomic landmarks are important in inserting the catheter: (1) the clavicle, (2) the sternal notch, and (3) the insertion of the anterior scalene muscle onto the first rib. The subclavian vein is drawn away from the clavicle if the patient hyperextends his back by pressing his shoulders to the bed. This can best be accomplished by placing a rolled towel between the two scapulae.

An area from the lower neck to the ipsilateral shoulder and infra-areolar region is

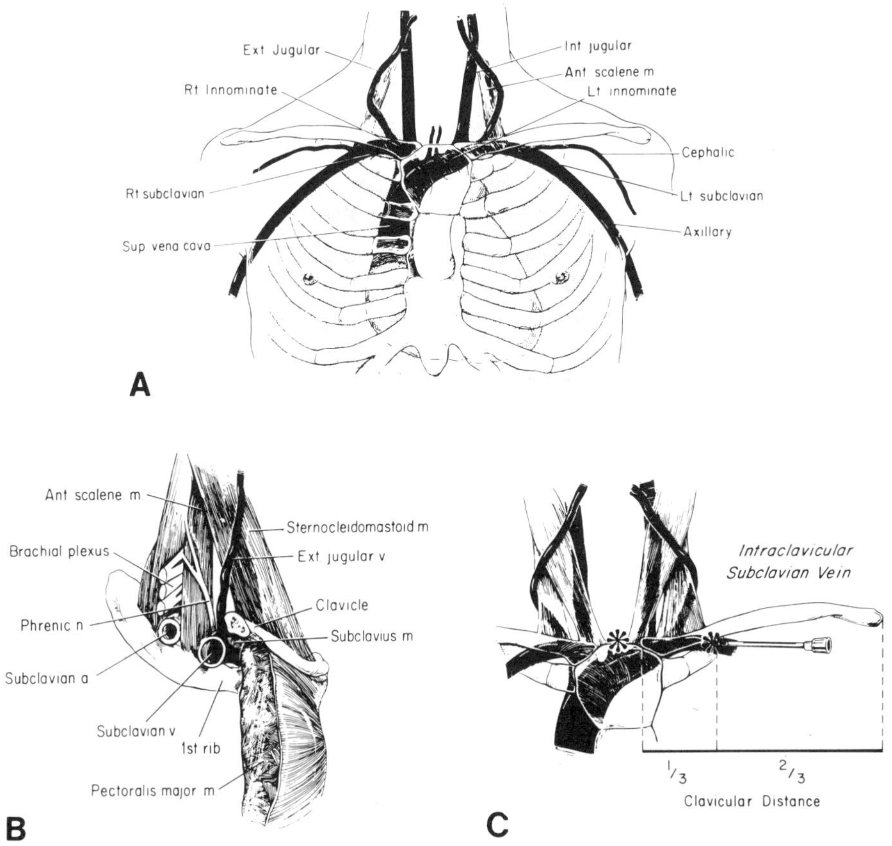

FIGURE 5. A, Normal venous anatomy of thoracic inlet and its relationship to bony cage. B, Relationship of subclavian vein to clavicle and first rib. C, The subclavian catheter is inserted one-third of the clavicular distance from the sternoclavicular joint. From Fischer, JE.[2]

washed with acetone to remove skin oil and debris and then scrubbed with a solution containing iodine. A double application of iodine paint is then applied and allowed to dry. The surgeon should then change his gloves. After selecting the site of insertion (which is medial to the midpoint of the clavicle), the skin and subcutaneous tissue is infiltrated with local anesthetic. The needle should be advanced toward a finger placed in the sternal notch, while the barrel of the syringe is kept in a plane almost parallel to the chest. To facilitate entry of blood into the syringe, negative pressure is applied to the barrel. Once the vein is entered, as evidenced by a "pop" and a rush of blood into the syringe, the needle should be advanced 3 to 4 ml. The needle is then held with a snap. The patient should then perform a Valsalva maneuver, about which he has been instructed prior to the actual insertion procedure. The syringe is then removed from the needle. The catheter is advanced using instruments to avoid bacterial contamination. The needle should be withdrawn from the subcutaneous tissue and a guard placed over the needle to avoid shearing and laceration of the catheter at this junction. The catheter is connected to a bottle of standard intravenous solution (5% dextrose in water) *which should not be the hyperalimentation solution.* To avoid two major complications during insertion, (1) shearing-off of the catheter and (2) pneumothorax, the needle and catheter should be withdrawn together if entry of the vein is unsuccessful, and a chest x-ray should be obtained before attempting cannulation of the contralateral, subclavian vein. With unsuccessful catheterization, the catheter should never be withdrawn through the needle or shearing-off of the catheter may occur. Verification of the intravascular location of the catheter is established by (1) lowering the intravenous fluid bottle below the level of the right atrium and observing retrograde flow of blood along the intravenous line and (2) plain chest x-ray, which should show the radiopaque catheter along the course of the superior vena cava. It should be realized that a false positive x-ray can result from inadvertent cannulation of the internal mammary vein. Misdirection of the catheter from the subclavian vein into the internal jugular vein is the most frequent placement error. The incidence of this problem can be reduced by having the patient look as far away from the surgeon during the placement of the catheter as possible. Once the catheter is verified to be in an appropriate position, the catheter is fixed in place by either a No. 2-0 or No. 0 monofilament suture or alternatively by steri-strips.

INITIATION OF TPN INFUSION AND METABOLIC MONITORING

Once the correct location of the central venous catheter has been verified by x-ray, infusion of TPN solution can be started. Two considerations are important in initiating infusion of this hypertonic solution: (1) glucose load and (2) water tolerance. Unfortunately, many patients receiving TPN may not have an appropriate increase in insulin release in response to the increased glucose load. Important studies relative to glucose metabolism during TPN administration by Sanderson and Deitel[157,158] demonstrated that the pancreatic islet cells appeared to adapt to the increased glucose load of TPN but still remained sensitive to changes in serum glucose levels. Patients on TPN had serum levels of insulin which were appropriate to the given glucose load, and they also responded appropriately to an intravenous glucose tolerance test with increased insulin release. Hypoglycemia occurred only if the patient received a glucose pulse, and then the TPN solution was rapidly decreased. *The abrupt cessation of TPN per se did not result in hypoglycemia.* While hypoglycemia occurred only if the TPN solution's rate of infusion was increased and decreased suddenly in Sanderson and Deitel's study, most protocols dictate a progressive decrease in the infusion rate prior to discontinuing TPN solution. Indeed, at least one episode of hypoglycemia occurred in nearly 10 percent of the patients receiving hyperalimentation solution in Ryan's study.[161] The majority of these instances of hypoglycemia occurred when the TPN solution had been stopped without tapering. If the TPN solution must be discontinued immediately, the patient is given 10 percent dextrose solution by a peripheral vein. If TPN is to be discontinued, the infusion rate is decreased over a three day period.

In a recent study,[159] we addressed two important questions: (1) What is the appropriate infusion rate for maximum utilization of glucose, the major caloric source in TPN? and (2) Does the patient adapt to a given infusion rate of glucose with increased glucose utilization? Five patients undergoing major abdominal surgery received ^{13}C-labelled glucose infusions as a method of determining glucose oxidation at three different infusion rates: (1) 4 mg/kg/minute on postoperative days three to five, (2) 7 mg/kg/minute on postoperative days five to seven, and (3) 9 mg/kg/minute on postoperative days seven to nine. Measurement of ^{13}C-CO_2 in the expired air and the plasma ^{13}C-glucose levels permitted calculation of the percentage of glucose oxidized. Figure 6 shows a typical response of patients to the three rates of glucose infusions. The 7 mg/kg/minute

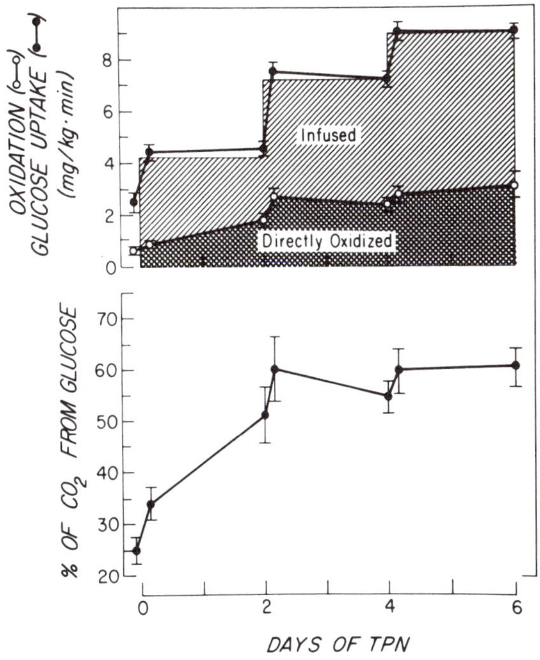

FIGURE 6. Top panel demonstrates a progressive increase in the amount of glucose directly oxidized at infusion rates of 4 mg/kg/minute to 7 mg/kg/minute. By contrast the 9 mg/kg/minute infusion is not accompanied by a significant increase in direct glucose oxidation. The excess glucose administered at the latter rate may be converted to hepatic fat. From Wolfe, RR, O'Donnell, TF, Jr., Stone, et al.[159]

infusion rate appeared to be the infusion rate associated with the maximal degree of glucose oxidation. A 9 mg/kg/minute infusion rate led to no increase in glucose oxidation, but a larger percentage of glucose was converted to fat. The 7 mg/kg/minute infusion rate is roughly comparable to 125 ml/hour or 3.0 L/24 hour which provides 35 kcal/kg/24 hour to a 70 kg individual. If the infusion rate were increased above this level, no greater percentage of glucose would be oxidized but more would be converted to hepatic lipid. Thus, an infusion rate of 3500 to 4000 kcal/24 hour would seem inappropriate in mildly stressed patients. One other finding of the study was that the plasma glucose level did not correlate with the percentage of glucose oxidized. Thus, it would appear that the main value of plasma glucose determinations is to avoid the hyperosmolar state.

The usual water requirement in the postsurgical 70 kg man is approximately 2500 ml/24 hour. Obviously, in an elderly 50 kg patient who may have underlying cardiac or renal disease, this water load may be sufficient to precipitate heart failure. Therefore, attention has to be paid to avoiding hypervolemic pulmonary edema. The occasional, judicious use of diuretics and a slow step by step increase in the TPN volume infused should be employed. For practical purposes, we generally initiate the infusion rate of TPN at 50 ml/hour during the first 12 hours. If the patient's plasma glucose levels remain less than 170 mg/dl, the rate of infusion is advanced to 75 ml/hour. As our studies have shown, the plasma glucose, as a guide to increases in the infusion rate, serves principally to avoid hyperosmolar states. The plasma glucose does not correlate with glucose-oxidation rates. The infusion rate should be progressively increased while maintaining a plasma glucose level of less than 200 mg/dl. The total caloric goal should be 1.76 to 2.5 times BEE and is dependent on the degree of stress (see Table 14).

COMPLICATIONS WITH TPN

The complications of TPN can be categorized into three general areas: (1) mechanical, (2) septic, and (3) metabolic (Table 21).

MECHANICAL COMPLICATIONS

The section on catheter placement addressed the important and compulsive steps which must be followed to minimize mechanical complications. Early studies on the complications of subclavian line insertions conducted at Bellevue Hospital[160] showed that the incidence of mechanical complications was directly related to the experience of the individual inserting the catheter. It should be noted that these insertions were not primarily for TPN administration. Pneumothorax is the most frequent acute mechanical complication associated with central-line insertion for TPN, and its incidence averaged 2 percent in Ryan and associates' series of 200 catheter insertions.[161] It is imperative that an upright chest x-ray be obtained if the initial cannulation of one subclavian vein is unsuccessful before attempting cannulation of the opposite side. The chest x-ray may prevent the catastrophic occurrence of bilateral pneumothoraces. If pneumothorax occurs, its management depends on the degree. Usually, a small-gauge French catheter, connected to an underwater seal, will allow resolution within 24 to 36 hours. The next

TABLE 21. Complications of Total Parenteral Nutrition

Complications	*Etiology*	*Diagnosis*	*Treatment*	*Prevention*
Mechanical Complications				
Hydrothorax	Incorrect needle trajectory	Dyspnea, chest pain, cyanosis, shock, chest x-ray	Aspiration	Careful catheter insertion technique; check placement with x-ray
Pneumothorax	Incorrect needle trajectory, air in syringe at puncture	Dyspnea, chest pain, cyanosis, shock, resonance to percussion, chest x-ray	Aspiration, tube thoracostomy	Careful catheter insertion technique; check placement with x-ray
Catheter embolism	Needle cuts off catheter tip	Cardiac arrhythmias, thrombosis, chest x-ray	Transvenous retrieval with guidewire snare	Withdraw needle simultaneously with catheter
Arterial puncture	Incorrect needle trajectory	Hematoma, bright red blood with high pressure in syringe	Pressure at site of puncture, observe for possible surgical intervention	Careful catheter insertion technique
Air embolism	Air leaks into catheter after removal of needle, at tubing changes, at detachment of IV lines	Dyspnea, chest pain, disorientation, tachypnea, tachycardia, cyanosis, elevated central venous pressure, cardiac arrest, coma, "mill-wheel churning" sound over anterior precordium	Cover catheter, raise right heart to force air out pulmonary artery (Durant maneuver)	Patient performs Valsalva maneuver in Trendelenburg position at insertion; occlude catheter site by air-tight dressing on removal of catheter
Myocardial perforation	Catheter tip in heart	Thrombosis, irritation of tricuspid valve, atrial or ventricular irritability, chest x-ray	Remove catheter	Careful catheter insertion technique; use Silastic catheter; check placement with chest x-ray
Metabolic Complications				
Hyperglycemia	High infusion rate of glucose in TPN fluid relative to renal clearance and pancreatic insulin response; stress, infections and medications	High blood and urine levels of glucose	Add insulin to infusate	Close monitoring of urine and blood glucose levels

TABLE 21 *Continued*

Complications	*Etiology*	*Diagnosis*	*Treatment*	*Prevention*
Hyperosmolar hyperglycemic nonketotic coma	Undetected maturity onset diabetes; excessive glucose load or large volume of TPN fluid delivered too rapidly	Confusion, disorientation, focal and grand mal seizures, lethargy, dehydration, glucosuria, coma, osmotic diuresis	Stop infusion; give hypo-osmolar glucose and saline; give insulin	Monitor blood and urine sugar levels; give insulin when necessary; increase glucose infusion rate by steps; do not exceed glucose tolerance
Hypomagnesemia	Often accompanies hypocalcemia; intracellular deposition during anabolic state induced by TPN	Tingling sensation around mouth, paresthesias in fingers, mental confusion, agitation, hyperreflexia	Increase magnesium sulfate in infusate	Monitor serum magnesium levels
Hypophosphatemia	Intracellular deposition during anabolic state induced by TPN; related to hypercalcemia or hyperthyroidism	Lethargy, altered speech, "thickened tongue," coma, anemia, peripheral paresthesias; depressed erythrocyte 2,3 DBG levels	Supplement diet with phosphate salts	Monitor serum phosphate levels
Hypocalcemia	Intracellular deposition during anabolic state induced by TPN; related to phosphate and albumin levels	Paresthesias, twitching; positive Chvostek's sign, convulsions	Supplement diet with calcium gluceptate, calcium gluconate	Regular monitoring of serum calcium; replace calcium when replacing phosphate
Hypokalemia	Related to nitrogen losses; intracellular deposition during anabolic state induced by TPN	Muscular weakness; paralysis and respiratory insufficiency; cardiac arrhythmias; ECG abnormalities	Supplement infusate with potassium salts	Monitor serum potassium levels
Hypovitaminosis		Various symptoms depending on which vitamin levels are deficient	Supplement diet with the deficient vitamins	Add a multiple vitamin injection to diet regularly

most common mechanical complication is puncture of the subclavian artery, which may or may not be accompanied by hemothorax. Direct compression over the supraclavicular area for 10 to 15 minutes usually permits sealing of the puncture site. If laceration of the artery has occurred, as evidenced by a pulsatile hematoma and hemothorax, surgical exploration may be required. It is important to obtain serial chest x-rays if this complication is suspected. Injuries to the brachial plexus, carotid artery, or thoracic duct, as well as air embolus, are less frequent mechanical complications of central-line insertion.[161,162] It should be remembered that any anatomic structure located within the proximity of the catheter insertion site may be damaged. Risk of air embolus, a potentially fatal mechanical complication, can be minimized by: (1) employing the Trendelenburg position and the Valsalva maneuver during catheter insertion and (2) providing adequate hydration prior to insertion to increase the central venous pressure. Finally, "shearing-off" the catheter by withdrawing it through the needle may require surgical exploration to remove the fragment. Fortunately, the catheter is radiopaque and x-ray localization in three planes is very useful. For the intravascular foreign body, extraction by an intravenous snare under fluoroscopy has been employed successfully as an alternative to open thoracotomy.[163]

Septic Complications

Infection of the central line generally occurs by migration of the bacteria from the skin insertion site along the catheter. The presence of sepsis distant from the site, such as an intra-abdominal abscess, does not appear to increase the incidence of catheter sepsis, even with known bacteremia.[164] Indeed, a septic complication rate of approximately 3 percent was achieved in one study in which greater than 75 percent of the patients had some form of infection at one time during the study. Therefore, stringent aseptic techniques must be followed during insertion of the catheter and in caring for the catheter. Alternate day cleansing of the catheter site with acetone and a compound containing iodine and redressing, all performed with sterile techniques, should minimize septic complications to approximately 3 percent,[165] although they may average up to 7 percent.[164] Skin organisms such as *Staphylococcus albus* or *aureus* are the most common. *Escherichia coli,* other enteric flora, and the various fungi follow in incidence as organisms frequently isolated from contaminated catheters. The increased relative incidence of fungi, principally *Candida,* may be related to the compromised state of the host (altered T cell function), concurrent antibiotics, and the nature of TPN solution, which is an ideal nutrient medium for fungi.[166]

One should adhere to an established protocol for deciding when to remove a TPN line in the case of suspected sepsis. Septic lines are life threatening complications, but inappropriate removal of the lines leads to relatively expensive reinsertion. The fever is generally not hectic but steady and low grade with only a rare spike. Usually, no specific source other than the line can be identified. If a patient on TPN develops a temperature, the following steps should be taken: (1) culture the solution and tubing and hang a new bottle or 20 percent dextrose solution, (2) draw blood cultures from the arm and line, (3) locate any obvious source of significant fever ($>$ 38°C) (e.g., abscess, urinary tract, infection). A central line for TPN *should be removed* from the septic patient and the tip cultured: (1) if no source of sepsis is defined in the face of 24 hours of fever, (2) if septic shock is present, (3) if positive cultures are returned from the central line, (4) if there is obvious local purulence and inflammation at the infraclavicular site, and (5) if there is evidence of supracardiac venous thrombosis. In general, antibiotics are not required for line sepsis and the temperature will usually disappear in 24 to 48 hours. A new line should be restarted *after* a 24 hour wait.

Metabolic Complications

Metabolic complications are usually related to a deficiency or an excess amount of the individual components of the TPN solution and thus can be grouped into carbohydrate, protein (amino acid), ionic, free-water, and vitamin related complications.

HYPERGLYCEMIA. Hyperglycemia is the most frequent and perhaps most dangerous metabolic complication of TPN. In the Tufts New England Medical Center series of 125 patients followed prospectively with sequential monitoring of blood sugar, mild hyperglycemia (defined as plasma glucose levels of 200 to 400 mg/dl on two successive blood glucose determinations) occurred in 9 percent of patients, while severe hyperglycemia (blood glucose greater than 400 mg/dl) was observed in 3 percent of patients.[167]

Mild hyperglycemia generally arises from too rapid an increase in the rate of glucose infusion and thus is more frequent during the initiation of TPN therapy. Alternatively, mild hyperglycemia may be related to glucose intolerance, usually induced by sepsis or unrecognized diabetes mellitus. Indeed, hyperglycemia following the initiation phase of TPN may be the first indication of occult sepsis. By contrast, severe hyperglycemia generally occurs with diseases which predispose to glucose intolerance. For example, of our 4 patients with severe hyperglycemia, 2 had sepsis, 1 had recently undergone a pancreatectomy, and 1 had diabetes mellitus. Thus, severe hyperglycemia should be a preventable complication if careful steps are taken to avoid too rapid a glucose infusion in disease states which predispose to hyperglycemia. As shown in Table 22, routine metabolic monitoring should be carried out more frequently at the onset of TPN therapy. Mild elevations in blood glucose are generally treated by decreasing the infusion rate. Persistent elevation of glucose to the mild range (200 to 400 mg/dl) or even severe hyperglycemia (>450 mg/dl) should be treated by the subcutaneous or intravenous administration of regular insulin. Once the daily insulin requirements are determined,

TABLE 22. Metabolic Monitoring

PRIOR TO INITIATING TPN AND DAILY FOR FIRST FIVE DAYS, THEREAFTER TWICE WEEKLY
Sodium, Potassium, Chloride, Carbon Dioxide, BUN, Creatinine, Glucose,* Urine Glucose and Specific Gravity
PRIOR TO INITIATING TPN THEN WEEKLY
Hemoglobin, White blood cell count Alkaline Phosphatase, Calcium, Bilirubin, Magnesium, Platelets, Phosphorus, Cholesterol, Albumin/Total Protein

*May be required more frequently.

regular insulin may be added to the TPN solution. The amount of insulin bound to the IV tubing and to the bottle wall is clinically inconsequential. It should be noted, however, that less than 10 percent of patients will require exogenous insulin administration during TPN. As discussed previously, Sanderson and Deitel[157,158] showed no real incidence of profound hypoglycemia upon cessation of TPN solution in these relatively healthy subjects, but most authorities recommend tapering of the TPN solution.[168] An infusion of 5 percent dextrose is started after cessation to avoid "rebound" hypoglycemia.

HYPOKALEMIA. The second most common metabolic abnormality in our series was ionic-hypokalemia. Increased protein synthesis and glucose uptake associated with anabolism lead to increased cellular uptake of potassium (3 mEq/gm nitrogen retained). Therefore, potassium administration should be adequate. In addition, potassium losses appear to be related to a fixed ratio of nitrogen loss.[169] Although each liter of TPN solution contains 40 mEq of potassium, additional potassium may be required for catabolic patients (sepsis, burns) or for those patients with abnormally high exogenous losses of protein such as intestinal fistulae. Daily or more frequent monitoring of the serum potassium with subsequent verification of the serum potassium by serial electrocardiograms is required. Hypokalemia and hyperkalemia occurred in only 4 percent of our patients.

HYPONATREMIA AND HYPERNATREMIA. The next two most frequent cation abnormalities are hyponatremia and hypernatremia. Hyponatremia may be related to the "sick-cell syndrome," excess free water administration, or external losses of sodium associated with hypotonic replacement. The "sick-cell syndrome" and associated hyponatremia is thought to be related to a defective sodium-potassium pump which permits an *intracellular* shift of sodium and water. By contrast, hypernatremia is associated with either hyperosmolar states in which osmotic diuresis has occurred or with external losses of hypotonic fluid, such as with intestinal fistulae. Inadequate free water replacement compounds this abnormality. Free water restriction is usually all that is required to correct hyponatremia. If the patient is dehydrated, isotonic saline administration may also be necessary. Hypertonic saline should be given only when severe hyponatremia is associated with disordered mental function (Chap. 15, Fluid, Electrolyte and Acid-Base Disorders). Free-water replacement (5% dextrose in water or hypotonic saline) should be administered when hypernatremia occurs (see Chap. 15). Physical examination, daily weighing, and careful recording of input and output will usually resolve issues regarding the causes of hypernatremia or hyponatremia and fluid balance.

HYPOPHOSPHATEMIA. Hypophosphatemia generally results from the entry of phosphate into cells associated with glucose and amino acid transport and utilization,[170] because phosphate is utilized intercellularly during protein, phospholipid, deoxyribonucleic acid (DNA), and adenosine triphosphate (ATP) synthesis. Symptoms of peroral or digital parethesias, neuromuscular weakness, respiratory failure, and obtundation may occur. Hypophosphatemia may be associated with decreased levels of 2,3-diphosphoroglycerate and red cell ATP, which shifts the oxyhemaglobin dissociation curve to the left.[171] Release of oxygen at the tissue level is inhibited by this phenomenon. Although up to 90 to 100 mEq of elemental phosphorus may be required per day, the routine addition of phosphate at 10 mEq KPO_4/L of TPN solution has prevented hypophosphatemia in our series. Similarly, abnormalities of magnesium and calcium have occurred less frequently with routine addition of these ions to TPN solutions (8 mEq Mg^{++} and 5 mEq Ca^{++}/L of TPN solution), as well as sequential monitoring for their deficiency.

TRACE METAL DEFICIENCIES. Although gross deficiencies of trace metal have been prevented in the past by administration of 1 U of fresh frozen plasma per week, the newer technique of adding trace metals to TPN solutions has obviated this routine[172] (Table 23). Zinc is an important trace metal in wound healing, and the proteolysis associated with trauma and sepsis encourages increased urinary zinc excretion. Chromium deficiency has been related to abnormal glucose tolerance and this metal appears essential for appropriate glucose utilization. Finally, copper deficiency may be characterized by a macrocytic anemia, but this is rare and occurs only after prolonged (>1 year) administration of TPN solution.

ESSENTIAL FATTY ACID DEFICIENCY. Essential fatty acid deficiency may be prevented by the administration of two 500 ml bottles of 10 percent intravenous fat per week. The data on essential fatty-acid deficiency developing as a complication of prolonged fat-free TPN administration is confusing. Due to preventitive measures, clinical evidence of essential fatty acid deficiency, characterized by eczematous, desquamative skin changes, thrombocytopenia, and anemia rarely develops,[173] but biochemical abnormalities have occurred as early as one month after initiation of TPN. The biochemical changes (abnormal serum ratios of fatty acids (C 20:3/20:4 >0.4) are related to the appearance of the abnormal fatty acid Δ5,8,11-eicosatrenoic acid (C 20:3) and the decrease in both linoleic (C 18:2) and arachidonic (C 20:4) acids and may develop by the third week of fat-free TPN therapy.[174] Although the daily application to the skin of safflower oil, a rich source of linoleic acid, may prevent fatty acid deficiency,[175] this is most effective in the pediatric patient. Alternatively, one or two 500 ml bottles of

TABLE 23. Trace Elements Included in TPN Solutions

	Adult Solution	*Pediatric Solution*	
	per 1000 ml	*per 1000 ml*	*per 125 ml*
Zinc	1 mg	800 μg	100 μg
Copper	400μg	160 μg	20 μg
Chromium	4 μg	1.4 μg	0.2 μg
Manganese	100 μg	50 μg	6.3 μg

*Trace elements are included in all total parenteral nutrition solutions except renal failure solution. They are added in quantities designed to prevent a deficiency. Unlike vitamins, exact prophylactic dosages of trace elements have not been determined.

intravenous fat may be infused weekly. Jeejeebhoy and his associates,[186] however, recommend a daily infusion of one 500 ml bottle of intravenous fat to prevent reversal of the normal ratio of linoleate, an essential fatty acid, to oleate, a nonessential fatty acid, in erythrocyte membrane phospholipids.

HYPERCHLOREMIC METABOLIC ACIDOSIS. The final, but infrequently encountered, metabolic complication, is related to the amino acid component of TPN. Hyperchloremic metabolic acidosis, which is secondary to the release of hydrochloric acid as amino acids are utilized, may be minimized by the addition of potassium acetate and sodium acetate to TPN solutions.[176] Newer amino acid formulations which contain greater amounts of acetate also have decreased the incidence of this complication. Elevated serum ammonia levels are more common in infants and patients with liver disease such as cirrhotics.[177] Sensitivity to amino acid compounds is quite rare in our experience although it is more common with protein hydrolysate solutions.

TPN SOLUTIONS FOR SPECIFIC APPLICATIONS (Table 24)

Solutions for Renal Failure

Renal failure is a stress state associated with proteolysis and subsequent mobilization of amino acids from muscle. The pioneering work of Giordano[178] and Giovannetti and Maggiore[179] showed that blood urea nitrogen (BUN) and creatinine levels rose to a lesser degree in patients who were fed an oral diet high in essential amino acids. In a randomized propective study of patients with acute renal failure, Abel and his associates[180] confirmed the initial favorable report of Dudrick and coworkers[181] who had found that an intravenous solution of hypertonic dextrose and essential amino acids was associated with a lowering of the BUN. In Abel's study, there was a slower rise in BUN and creatinine levels in the group treated with "renal failure solution" than in the control group. Even though the regimen may be at times hypocaloric, the provision of calories (1400 Kcal/L) and the essential amino acids decreases proteolysis and mobilization of amino acids from muscle. The essential amino acids promote "recycling of urea," so that BUN may be lowered by this second mechanism and mortality lowered.

Treatment differs for those patients who are on dialysis and those who are not. The solution for patients not on dialysis, where fluid restriction is imperative, is made by mixing 70 percent dextrose and water with an essential amino acid solution (Nephramine) to yield a final glucose concentration of approximately 47 percent. The total nitrogen load is 1.46 g/L or 13.1 gm total of essential amino acids/L. This highly osmolar (2100 mOsm/L) solution is administered through a central catheter. Strict attention should be paid to prevention of sepsis because of the predeliction for sepsis in the patient with renal failure. Infusion of the solution is initiated at a rate of 30ml/hour, which should permit administration of at least 1 L of solution per 24 hours initially. The infusion rate can almost be doubled over a couple of days and the rate of increase is dependent upon glucose and free-water tolerance. Serum glucose measurements should be performed during the initial phase of therapy every 6 to 8 hours, especially in the

TABLE 24. Amino Acid Profiles in Special Solutions

	Freamine II 4.25%	*FO-80* 4%	*Nephramine* 1.28%
Essential Amino Acids			
L-isoleucine	.295	.450	.140
L-leucine	.385	.550	.220
L-valine	.280	.420	.162
L-lysine	.435	.380	.160
L-methionine	.225	.050	.220
L-phenylalanine	.240	.050	.220
L-threomine	.170	.225	.100
L-tryptophan	.065	.038	.050
Total g/L	*2.095*	*2.163*	*1.272*
Nonessential Amino Acids			
L-histidine	.120	.120	
L-arginine	.155	.300	
glycine	.850	.450	
L-proline	.475	.400	
L-alanine	.300	.375	
L-serine	.250	.250	
L-cysteine g/L	.010	.020	
Total	*4.245*	*4.078*	
Branched Chain(%)	23	35	
Aromatic Acids(%)	7	2	
Ratio	3.29	17.5	

oliguric patient. Blood glucose concentration should be kept below 250 to 300 mg/dl by adjustment of the rate first and then by administration of insulin. If acceptable glucose levels cannot be maintained at low infusion rates (30 ml/hour), regular insulin should be added to the intravenous infusion at 15 U/L.

In the dialysis patient where total fluid volume is not as pressing a concern, both essential *and nonessential* amino acids may be administered along with hypertonic glucose. Therefore, in these patients, it is easier to provide an appropriate amount of calories. Indeed, in these patients, administration of adequate caloric requirements should be the overall goal rather than concerns for fluid limitations. Excess water may be removed at subsequent hemodialysis.

Solution for Liver Failure

Fischer and his associates[150] have shown that there is a beneficial effect of administering a solution of branched-chain amino acids in the treatment of encephalopathy associated with liver failure. Although the patient with liver failure requires exogenous protein to preserve lean body mass, his tolerance of a protein load is limited. Tailoring the type of amino acids administered to the patient with liver failure, as with the patient with renal failure, is important. Branched-chain amino acids decrease peripheral muscle proteolysis because they are incorporated into the labile amino acid pool and used subsequently in protein synthesis. Branched-chain amino acids also normalize the plasma aromatic amino acid/branched chain amino acid imbalance. Fischer and his associates have shown that in the untreated patient with hepatic encephalopathy, the plasma aromatic amino acids are elevated in relationship to the branched-chain amino acids. This results in a high concentration of aromatic amino acids in the brain and subsequent abnormalities in neurotransmitter function. When an intravenous solution high in branched-chain amino acids (FO-80) is supplied, the abnormal plasma ratio was corrected. More importantly, the patient's encephalopathy lightened. The solution presently employed by Fischer is investigational and not available for general use. While 50 percent of patients with mild hepatic encephalopathy may lighten with infusion of hypertonic glucose and low concentrations of amino acids, 50 percent would require the specialized branched-chain amino acid solution. Until FO-80 becomes commercially available, we have used a commercial amino acid mixture (Freamine II 4.25%) which is relatively high in branched-chain amino acids (23% total branched-chain amino acids vs. FO-80's 35%) and low in the aromatic (7% vs. FO-80's 2%) (see Table 23).

Pediatric Solutions

The pediatric patient requires more calories (60 to 90 Kcal/kg of body weight/24 hours) and more nitrogen (250/450 mg N/kg/24 hours) than the adult patient. Because of immature enzyme systems, amino acids may be more toxic to the infant. In these patients there is also an increased need for lipid, because of its vital role in the development of the brain and insufficient delivery of lipid may be associated with mental retardation. TPN administration in the infant requires special access via an operative procedure. A Silastic catheter is tunnelled subcutaneously in the scalp to an external jugular vein cutdown site, where it is threaded into the superior vena cava. The isolation of the administration site from the operative site minimizes infections. Because of the special volume problems encountered in the infant, TPN administration should be carried out with a pump which has pressure and volume control. The unique indications for TPN in a pediatric patient are generally those clinical situations which cannot be managed by tube feeding: pseudomembranous colitis, gastroschisis, omphalocele, reduplication of the gastrointestinal tract, and tracheal esophageal fistula. The reader is referred to more extensive discussions of this specialized need in pediatric surgical texts.

Intravenous Fat Regimen

Fat has long been recognized as an excellent caloric source. During the 1940s, a cottonseed oil emulsion for intravenous use was developed. The side effects from administration of this fat emulsion, however, were quite frequent, prompting its withdrawal from clinical use in the early 1960s.[182] Following extensive clinical testing in Scandinavia, a different fat emulsion for intravenous use, composed of soybean oil, was introduced in the United States. Intralipid uses 10 percent soybean oil emulsion as its caloric source and is usually infused with both dextrose solution (5 or 10%) and 3 percent amino acids

(Table 25). It must be kept refrigerated. By contrast, Liposyn uses safflower oil as its lipid source and does not require refrigeration.

COMPOSITION

Fat emulsions contain particulate matter which is less than 0.5 mm in diameter. This diameter is comparable to that of naturally occurring chylomicrons. Since the osmolarity of Intralipid is 280 mOsm/kg and is comparable to plasma osmolarity, peripheral administration is possible. The fatty acid content of Intralipid is 54 percent linoleic, 26 percent oleic, 9 percent palmitic, 8 percent linolenic, and 3 percent other fats (see Table 25). Other components besides soybean oil are 1.2 percent phosphatized egg yolk, which acts as an emulsifying agent, and glycerin, which is also added in pyrogen-free water.

METABOLISM

A greater number of calories per unit volume are derived from intravenous fat than from carbohydrate or protein, because fat provides 9 Kcal/g rather than 4 Kcal/g. In practical terms, fat emulsions provide 1.1 Kcal/ml, but admixing it with 5 or 10 percent dextrose and 3 percent isotonic amino acids at a 2:1 ratio as it enters the body via a "Y" shaped tubing lowers its caloric content to 0.6 Kcal/ml. This is certainly less than standard TPN (hypertonic glucose and amino acids), which is 0.9 to 1 Kcal/ml. In addition, the admixture increases the osmolarity of the solution to approximately 600 mOsm/kg. The fat particles break down in the plasma, releasing triglycerides. Lipoprotein lipase which is found in the liver, adipose tissue, red blood cells, and muscle hydrolyzes these triglyce-

TABLE 25. Fat Emulsions

	g/L	
Soybean Oil (Intralipid)		
or	100	
Safflower Oil (Liposyn)		
plus		
Glycerin	22.5	
Phospholipids	12	
Individual Fatty-Acid Composition		
	Intralipid (%)	*Liposyn (%)*
Linoleic acid	54	77
Oleic acid	26	13
Palmitic acid	9	7
Others	11	2.5

rides to glycerol and free fatty acids.[184] The free fatty acids are then used for resynthesis of triglycerides for storage or for oxidation as energy fuel.

Intralipid emulsion has a half-life of approximately 15 minutes, similar to that of chylomicrons. The maximum elimination rate of Intralipid depends on the concentration of lipoprotein lipase enzyme and therefore follows standard enzyme kinetics. Thus, elimination of fat is dependent upon the concentration of hepatic lipoprotein lipase at low plasma concentrations of Intralipid. At higher plasma concentrations, when the binding sites have been saturated, clearance is no longer dependent upon enzyme concentration. The maximum rate of clearance in adults is 3.8 g/kg/24 hours or 35 Kcal/kg/24 hours.[184] To date, there have been few controlled studies measuring the direct oxidation of intravenous fat in postoperative patients. Indirect studies comparing isocaloric, isonitrogenous administration of Intralipid to conventional TPN solutions have demonstrated no significant improvement in nitrogen balance.[185] Unfortunately, most of the studies have a variable population which prevents cross comparison. It is obvious that the degree of metabolism influences the degree of nitrogen balance.

INDICATIONS

There are two principal indications for the use of Intralipid: (1) as a source of fat to avoid free fatty acid deficiency during prolonged central nutrition (TPN) and (2) as a source of calories for patients on a peripheral vein regimen with glucose and amino acids (Fig. 7). The osmolarity of intravenous fat permits the infusion of a concentrated source of calories through a peripheral vein. The obvious advantages of this regimen would be avoidance of the mechanical and septic complications of a central line. The metabolic complications associated with intravenous fat are not as life-threatening but appear as frequently.[167] Ideally, the intravenous fat regimen is designed for patients with no pre-existing or only mild malnutrition, as well as those patients in whom oral or enteral feeding is contraindicated. We have avoided the use of intravenous fat regimen in patients with severe malnutrition because of the lower caloric density of intravenous fat regimen compared to standard TPN. Thus, the indications for TPN (see Table 17) would also apply to the fat regimen. Use of the intravenous fat regimen in the pediatric population appears quite advantageous because it avoids the operative procedure of a central line insertion. By employing a dosage rate of 4 g/kg/24 hours in infants and 3 g/kg/24 hours in children, a weight gain was observed in 29 of 31 patients who were maintained on this regimen from 5 to 25 days. The incidence of complications was extremely low.

ADMINISTRATION

In adults, 10 percent intravenous fat should be infused initially at a rate of 0.25–0.5 ml/minute for the first one-half hour (Table 26). Patients should be observed for adverse reactions described below. The infusion rate may be increased by steps so that a maximum of 500 ml in the initial 24-hour period may be given. The daily dose in adults should not exceed 25 ml/kg/24 hours or 2.5 g/kg/24 hours. By contrast, in the pediatric patient, the infusion rate should be initiated at 0.1 ml/minute for 15 minutes and may

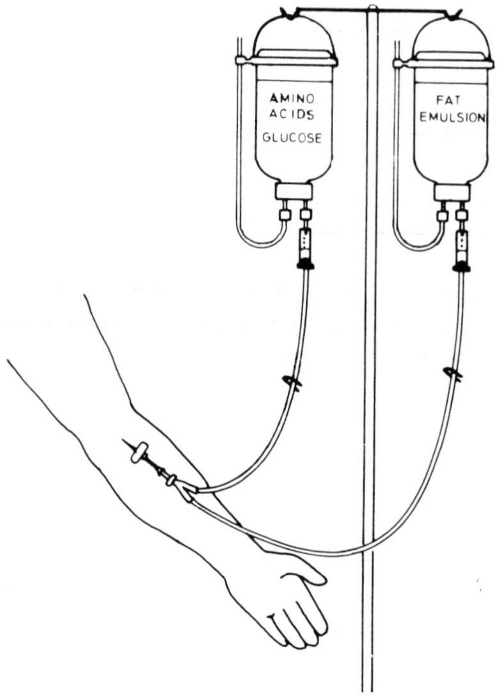

FIGURE 7. Y tubing for administration of intravenous fat emulsion. This allows simutaneous delivery of fat, amino acids, and glucose. From Fischer, JE.[2]

TABLE 26. Intravenous Fat Regimen

Infusion Rate	*Day 1*		*Day 3*	
Glucose/amino-acid solution	80 ml/hr	total: 2000 ml/24 hours	125 ml/hour max	total: 3000 ml/24 hours
10% lipid	0.25–0.5 ml/min × 30 minute then increase gradually	total: 500 ml/24 hour	125 ml/hour max 25 ml/kg/24 hours max	1500 ml/24 hours

Infuse lipid continuously over a 20 to 24 hour period simultaneously via Y tube with glucose/amino acid solution. *DO NOT USE FILTER.*

Lipid may comprise a maximum of 60% of the total daily calories.

Do not add antibiotics, electrolytes, or other infusates to the intravenous fat line. They may destroy emulsion and lead to fat emboli. Therefore, use separate line.

Change IV sites every 24 to 48 hours.

be increased to a maximum of 1 g/kg/24 hours on the first day. The maximum should not exceed 4 g/kg/24 hours.

CONTRAINDICATIONS (Table 27)

The following disorders are considered absolute contraindications to the use of intravenous fat: (1) pathologic hyperlipidemias, (2) lipoid nephroses, and (3) acute pancreatitis (if accompanied by hyperlipidemia). Hepatic disease, respiratory disease, anemia, and known coagulation disorders or fat emboli are *relative* contraindications to the use of intravenous fat. Thus, the selection of intravenous fat as a nutrition source must be individualized for each patient.

MONITORING (Table 28)

Liver function tests, including determination of SGOT, SGPT, LDH, and bilirubin, should be obtained on a three times a week. Coagulation screens should be obtained twice weekly. Arterial blood gases should be monitored frequently at the initiation of therapy, especially in patients with underlying respiratory disorders. The most important monitoring technique is that of determining plasma opacity. Following infusion of intravenous fat, 5 ml of blood is centrifuged and the opacity of the plasma checked. If a printed page cannot be read clearly through the plasma, the infusion rate should be decreased.

COMPLICATIONS

Use of intravenous fat has been associated with a very low incidence of acute toxicity. A curious syndrome, "the overloading syndrome," which is characterized by a viral-like complex of fever, chills, shivering, muscle pain, loss of appetite, and vomiting has been attributed to therapy with fat emulsions.[182] This syndrome was originally described with cottonseed oil emulsion, which has been withdrawn from the United States market, but has not been observed with the soybean oil emulsions. Intravenous fat interacts with a number of organs. Brown pigmentation has been described in the reticuloendothelial

TABLE 27. Contraindications to Use of Intravenous Fat Regimen

Absolute	*Relative*
Abnormal fat metabolism	Severe liver insufficiency
Pathologic hyperlipidemia	Pulmonary disease
Lipoid nephrosis	Anemia
Acute pancreatitis (if accompanied by hyperlipidemia)	Coagulation disorders
	Potential for fat embolism (e.g., fractures)
	Hemodialysis

TABLE 28. Monitoring Intravenous Fat Regimen

Special Tests	*Result*	*Action*
Plasma turbidity (daily)	Clear	Continue infusion
	Cloudy	Measure serum triglycerides
	Opaque	*Discontinue infusion* Measure triglycerides Reanalyze later for adequate clearing
Liver, function studies (3 × week)	Normal	Continue infusion
	Mildly elevated	? Causes sepsis, metastasis, excess calories
	Markedly elevated	Discontinue infusion
Coagulation studies (2 × week)	Normal	Continue infusion
	Abnormal	Discontinue infusion
Arterial blood gases (frequently initially and dependent upon respiratory condition)	Normal	Continue infusion
	Deterioration	Discontinue infusion

cells of the liver when liver function tests have remained normal. Initially, transient increases in values obtained from liver function studies may be observed, but they should subside by the third or fourth day of intravenous fat administration. Other causes of abnormal liver function may be related to excess caloric administration or to concomitant disease such as sepsis or liver metastases. Thus, abnormal liver function tests should prompt an evaluation for causes other than the intravenous fat. If no clear cause of the abnormal liver function tests is found, clinical judgment may dictate cessation of the intravenous fat administration. Changes in pulmonary function during the infusion of fat emulsion have also been documented. Pulmonary diffusion capacity may be decreased, but allegedly it is reversible by the use of heparin.[186] Elevated plasma triglyceride concentrations may aggravate an ischemic myocardium, so that the use of IV fat has been questioned in patients with recent myocardial infarction. Despite reports from animal experiments, no significant changes have been documented to occur in the coagulation system.[187] Clinical reports of hypercoaguability during the infusion of soybean oil emulsion have been poorly documented, and the data is conflicting. Recently, an association between intravenous fat and "sudden death" in patients on hemodialysis has been reported.[188] The cause and effect relationship, however, remains to be proven.

Protein-Sparing Intravenous Therapy

THEORY

In a series of provocative studies, Blackburn and his associates[189,190] challenged the benefits of the routine administration of hypocaloric 5 percent dextrose in water

(D5/W) to postoperative patients. These investigators showed that the infusion of 90 g of amino acids as a 3 percent isotonic solution was associated with less nitrogen imbalance than the conventional infusion of 5 percent dextrose in water. By measuring the levels of hormones and substrate-energy fuels, Blackburn and his colleagues demonstrated that D5/W administration was associated with higher insulin levels. Since insulin is a key antilipolytic hormone, endogenous fat release and subsequent ketone body formation by the liver were minimized on D5/W. Levels of free fatty acid and ketone bodies were low in patients receiving D5/W. By contrast, patients receiving dextrose-free, 3 percent isotonic amino acid solution had lower insulin levels, while levels of free fatty acid and ketone bodies were increased. The subsequent availability of fat, which could be oxidized as fuel, theoretically minimized protein oxidation and accounted for the more favorable nitrogen balance. Several subsequent studies[5,191] have verified the efficacy of peripheral protein-sparing solutions. A few investigators,[192,193] however, have stated that D5/W should be administered with 3 percent isotonic amino acids so that additional "caloric" benefits may be derived from the D5/W. Evidence against the combination of D5/W and 3 percent amino acid solutions has been developed by several investigators. Greenberg and his colleagues[196] have concluded that it was the amount of nitrogen infused, and not the nonprotein calories provided either as hypocaloric glucose or as lipid, which was associated with nitrogen sparing. Clinical experiments employing 3-methyl histidine as an index of peripheral protein catabolism showed that the combination of D5/W and isotonic amino acid mixture spared peripheral protein catabolism but at the expense of catabolism of the more valuable visceral protein.[195] Conversely, 3 percent isotonic amino acid solutions alone appeared to spare this visceral protein. This area remains controversial. We currently prefer 3 percent amino acids without glucose.

INDICATIONS

Peripheral protein-sparing solution should be used in patients who cannot use the enteral or oral routes for periods greater than 5 to 10 days (see Fig. 7). Protein-sparing solution may be used as a sole source of nutrition for up to two and a half weeks depending upon the patient's fat reserves. On nutritional evaluation, the patient should have evidence of adequate fat reserves without significant depletion of visceral protein stores to qualify for therapy with protein-sparing solution. Therefore, the patient with no or marginal depletion and who will be unable to take oral or enteral nutrition for at least five to seven days is the ideal candidate for protein-sparing therapy. Use of TPN or IV fat should be considered when parenteral nutrition is required for longer periods or the patient is significantly depleted. A simple rule of thumb for the use of protein-sparing regimen is that it should leave the patient at the same level of nutrition as was noted prior to the institution of therapy. Thus, the two major indications are: (1) patients who have the potential to become nutritionally depleted in association with the surgical procedure and the usual postoperative course and (2) patients on maintenance intravenous fluid therapy who are marginally depleted but do not fulfill the criteria for central total parenteral nutrition.[196]

CONTRAINDICATIONS

Patients without adequate fat stores or with severe visceral/peripheral protein depletion are not candidates for protein-sparing solutions (see Fig. 8). Use of protein-sparing solutions should be approached with caution in disease states where enhanced nitrogen breakdown occurs or where amino acid intolerance may develop. Thus, patients with kidney or liver failure and those in low-flow circulatory states are not optimal candidates for protein-sparing therapy.[197] Although sepsis and thermal injury are associated with mobilization of peripheral protein stores and subsequent ureagenesis, it has been our experience that this should not be an absolute contraindication but indeed may be an appropriate clinical role for protein-sparing solutions.

ADMINISTRATION (Table 29)

Postoperatively, administration of protein-sparing solution should be initiated in the adaptive phase following the acute phase.[196] During the acute phase, increased secretion of catecholamines, glucocorticoids, and glucagon are associated with the obligate protein catabolism and mobilization of all available fuel stores. Since fat mobilization is the

TABLE 29. Protein-Sparing Solution

ADMINISTRATION			
	3.5% Amino Acid (ml)	*Isotonic Saline ± Dextrose (ml)*	
Day 1	1000	1000–1500	
Day 2	1500–2000	500–1000	
Day 3	2500–300	500–1000	
MONITORING			
Test	*Frequency*	*Protein-Sparing Effect*	*Sepsis or Organ Failure*
BUN	Daily initially, then 2 × week	not >30–40 mg/dl* increase per 24 hr	>40 mg/dl increase per 24 hr
Blood glucose	Daily initially, then 2 × week	70–80 mg/dl	>100 mg/dl
Urine ketone	Daily	positive	negative
COMPLICATIONS			
Finding		*Possible Causes*	
↑BUN and confusion		Hepatic or renal insufficiency	
Hyperchloremic acidosis		Excess chloride as sodium or potassium salt	
Hyperammonemia		Excess amino acid administration or hepatic failure	

*Discontinue only if a 5 to 10 mg/dl rise/day × 3 consecutive days

predominant metabolic component during the adaptive phase, the use of protein-sparing solution should provide a favorable milieu for continued fat mobilization. The goal of intravenous therapy during the acute phase is to provide sufficient water and electrolytes to permit adaptation. Approximately 48 to 72 hours postoperatively, protein-sparing solution can be started.

The first step in any form of IV therapy is to estimate the water and electrolyte requirements (see also Chap 15, Fluid, Electrolyte and Acid-Base Disorders). Once the total amount of water and electrolytes are calculated for a 24 hour period, 3 or 3.5 percent isotonic amino acid solution can be initiated at a gradual rate. On the first day, 1 L of the solution should be infused in conjunction with the appropriate 1000 to 1500 ml of balanced electrolyte solution. On the second day, the patient may receive 1500 to 2000 ml of protein-sparing solution. Further water requirements may be met by the use of balanced electrolyte solution. Vitamins, minerals, and additional electrolytes may be added to the 3 or 3.5 percent amino acid solution. Three key signs guide an increase in the infusion rate of 3 percent amino acid to a total of 90 g maximum in a 24 hour period: (1) a BUN which is not elevated beyond 30 to 40 mg/dl, (2) a plasma glucose which falls below 100 mg/dl, and (3) a positive urine test for ketone bodies.[196] Because protein-sparing solution is isotonic, it can be infused safely and easily into peripheral veins without significant thrombophlebitis. The incidence of sepsis is low with a peripheral line; and additional IV fluids, blood products, and medication can be delivered through the same line if needed. This situation obviously contrasts with the centrally administered total parenteral nutrition solution. Table 18 shows the additives which should be included daily.

MONITORING (see Table 29)

BUN, blood sugar, and urinary ketones are obtained daily during the first four to five days of therapy. Ketone bodies should be observed in the urine within 48 to 72 hours after initiation of protein-sparing therapy. Since the renal threshold for ketone bodies is variable, use of protein-sparing solutions should be continued even if the urine is not positive for ketone bodies. The BUN should not rise to beyond 30 to 40 mg/dl nor should it increase precipitously. The blood sugar usually drops to the range of 70 to 80 mg/dl. The majority of patients will lose weight, which reflects principally the loss of body fat. Calculation of nitrogen balance by urinary urea measurements provides an adequate method for monitoring the "protein-sparing effect." Nitrogen intake can be calculated from the amount of 3 percent amino acid infused.

COMPLICATIONS (see Table 29)

An increased BUN and an increased blood glucose in the face of absent ketone bodies signifies stress associated with sepsis or organ failure. Such states prevent the favorable hormonal and substrate milieu associated with protein sparing. Patients with previously undetected liver disease may show amino acid intolerance characterized by a rising BUN and central nervous system signs. Hyperchloremic acidosis infrequently occurs and can be avoided by providing half the daily sodium and potassium as acetate or phosphate rather than chloride. Surprisingly enough, the fluid management of diabetes may be easier during the infusion of peripheral protein-sparing solution. Insulin requirements are lowered. Hyperammonemia may be encountered if large quantities of amino acids are infused. Since the effect of increased levels of free fatty acids on hypoxic myocardium is still controversial, protein-sparing solutions should not be selected for use in patients with a recent history of myocardial infarction.

REFERENCES

1. American College of Surgeons: Ballinger, W F (ed.): *Surgical Nutrition.* Philadelphia: W. B. Saunders Company, 1975.
2. Fischer, J E: *Total Parenteral Nutrition.* Boston: Little Brown and Company, 1976.
3. Schneider, H A, Anderson, C E, and Coursin, D B (eds.): *Nutritional Support of Medical Practice,* New York: Harper & Row, 1977.
4. Clowes, G H A, Jr., O'Donnell, T F, Ryan, N T, et al.: *Energy metabolism in sepsis: treatment based on different patterns in shock and high output state.* Ann Surg 175:584, 1974.
5. Blackburn, G L, Clowes, G H A, O'Donnell, T F, et al.: *Protein-sparing therapy during periods of starvation with sepsis or trauma.* Ann Surg 177:588, 1973.
6. O'Donnell, T F, Jr., Clowes, G H A, Jr., Blackburn, G L, et al.: *Proteolysis associated with a deficit of peripheral energy fuel states in septic man.* Surgery 80:192, 1976.
7. O'Donnell, T F, Jr., Clowes, G H A, Blackburn, G L, et al.: *Relationship of hind limb energy fuel metabolism to the circulatory responses in severe sepsis.* J Surg Res 16:112, 1974.
8. Butterworth, C E, and Blackburn, G L: *Hospital malnutrition.* Nutrition Today, 10:8, 1975.
9. Bistrian, B R, Blackburn, G L, Vitale, J, et al.: *Prevalence of protein-calorie malnutrition in general medical patients.* JAMA, 235:1567, 1976.
10. Dudrick, S J, and Duke, J H: *Nutritional complications in the surgical patient,* in Artz, C P, and Hardy, J D, (eds.): *Management of Surgical Complications,* ed. 3. Philadelphia: W. B. Saunders, 1975, p. 243.
11. Bollet, A J, and Owens, S O: *Evaluation of nutritional status of selected hospitalized patients.* Am J Clin Nutr, 26:931, 1973.
12. Bistrian, B R, Blackburn, G L, Hallowell, E, et al.: *Protein status of general surgical patients.* JAMA, 230:855, 1974.
13. Bistrian, B R, Blackburn, G L, Scrimshaw, N S, et al.: *Cellular immunity in semi-starved states in hospitalized adults.* Am J Clin Nutr 28:1148, 1975.
14. Bistrian, B R, Blackburn, G L, Sherman, M, et al.: *Therapeutic index of nutritional depletion in hospitalized adults.* Surg Gynecol Obstet, 141:512, 1975.
15. Blackburn, G L, Maini, B S, and Pierce, E C: *Nutrition in the critically ill patient.* Anesthesiology 47:181, 1977.
16. Blackburn, G L, and Bistrian, B R: *Nutritional care of the injured and/or septic patient.* Surg Clin North Am, 56:1195, 1976.
17. Blackburn, G L, and Flatt, J P: *Metabolic response to illness: role of protein sparing therapy.* Comp Ther 1:23, 1975.
18. Duke, J H, Jorgensen, S B, Broel, J R, et al.: *Contribution of protein to caloric expenditure following injury surgery.* Surgery, 68:168, 1970.
19. Elwyn, D H, Bryan-Brown, C W, and Shoemaker, W C: *Nutritional aspects of body water dislocations in postoperative and depleted patients.* Ann Surg 182:76, 1975.
20. Bergstrom, E V, and First, P., *Influence of the postoperative state on the intracellular free amino acids in human muscle tissue.* Ann Surg 182:665, 1975.
21. Moore, F D: *Metabolic Care of the Surgical Patient.* Philadelphia: W. B. Saunders, 1959, pp. 409–456.
22. Hill, G L, Blackett, R L, Pickford, I., et al.: *Malnutrition in surgical patients. An unrecognized problem.* Lancet 1:689, 1977.

23. HILL, G L, BLACKETT, R L, BURKENSHAW, L, ET AL.: *Proceedings: high incidence of malnutrition in hospitalized surgical patients.* Br J Surg 63:663, 1976.

24. MACFADYEN, B V, COPELAND, E M, AND DUDRICK, S J: *Surgery,* in SCHNEIDER, H A, ANDERSON, C E, AND COURSIN, D B (eds): *Nutritional Support of Medical Practice.* New York: Harper & Row, 1977, p. 485.

25. DOEKEL, R C, JR, ZWILLICH, C W, SCUGGIN, C H, ET AL.: *Clinical semistarvation: depression of hypoxic ventilatory response.* N Eng J Med 295:358, 1976.

26. KAMINSKI, M.: *Enteral hyperalimentation.* Surg Gynecol Obstet 143:12, 1976.

27. BISTRIAN, B R, AND BLACKBURN, G L: *Role of nutrition in the cellular immunity of hospitalized patients.* Fed Proc 33:691, 1974.

28. SOKOL, J: *Measurement of delayed skin test responses.* N Engl J Med 293:501, 1975.

29. LAW, D K, DUDRICK, S J, AND ABDOU, N I: *The effect of protein calorie malnutrition on immune competence.* Surg Gynecol Obstet 139:251, 1974.

30. MOSS, G, BIRENBAUM, A, BOVA, F, ET AL.: *Postoperative nutritional support: metabolic patterns following immediate total nutritional support: hormone levels, DNA synthesis, nitrogen balance, and accelerated wound healing.* J Surg Res, 21:383, 1970.

31. BYRD, H S, LAZARUS, H M, AND TORMA, M J: *Effects of parenteral alimentation in postoperative gastric function.* Am J Surg 130:688, 1975.

32. DINGMAN, R O: *Factors of clinical significance affecting wound healing.* Laryngyoscope, 83:1540, 1973.

33. MACLEAN, L D, MEAKINS, J L, TAGUCHI, K, ET AL.: *Host resistance in sepsis and trauma.* Ann Surg 182:207, 1975.

34. MACFADYEN, B V, DUDRICK, S J, RUBERG, R L: *Management of gastrointestinal fistulas with parenteral hyperalimentation.* Surgery 74:100, 1973.

35. COPELAND, E M, MACFAYDEN, B V, JR, AND DUDRICK, S J: *Effect of intravenous hyperalimentation on established delayed hypersensitivity in the cancer patient.* Ann Surg 184:60, 1976.

36. SCHWARTZ, G F, GREEN, H L, BENDON, M L, ET AL.: *Combined parenteral hyperalimentation and chemotherapy in the treatment of dissemenated solid tumors.* Am J Surg 121:169, 1971.

37. STRAUSS, R J, AND WISE, L: *Operative risks of obesity.* Surg Gynecol Obstet 146:286, 1978.

38. ANSELL, J E, KUMAR, R, AND DEYKIN, D: *The spectrum of vitamin K deficiency.* JAMA 238:40, 1977.

39. COSTA, G: *Cachexia and the systematic effects of tumors,* in HOLLAND, J F, AND FREI, E: *Cancer Medicine.* Philadelphia: Lea & Febiger, 1973.

40. THEOLOGIDES, A: *Pathogenesis of cachexia in cancer.* Cancer 29:484, 1972.

41. AXELROD, A E: *Nutrition in relation to acquired immunity,* in GOODHART, R S, AND SHILES, M E (eds.): *Modern Nutrition in Health and Disease,* ed. 5. Philadelphia: Lea & Febiger, 1973, p. 493.

42. TAYLOR, K B: *Gastroenterology,* in SCHNEIDER, H A, ANDERSON, C E, AND COURSIN, D B (eds.): *Nutritional Support of Medical Practice.* New York: Harper and Row. 1977, p. 332.

43. MOORE, F D, AND BRENNAN, M F: *Current concepts: intravenous feeding.* N Eng J Med, 287:862, 1972.

44. CUTHBERTSON, D P: *Postshock metabolic response.* Lancet 2:235, 1942.

45. KINNEY, J M: *Energy requirements of the surgical patient,* in BALLINGER, W F, COLLINS, J A, DRUEKER, W R, ET AL (eds.): *Manual of Surgical Nutrition.* Philadelphia: W. B. Saunders, 1975, p. 223.

46. WILMORE, D W, LONG, J M, MASON, A D, ET AL.: *Stress in surgical patients as a neurophysiologic reflex response.* Surg Gynecol Obstet 142:257, 1976.

47. GIDDINGS, A E: *The control of plasma glucose in the surgical patient.* Br J Surg 6:787, 1974.

48. GUMP, F E, LONG, C L, GEIGER, J W, ET AL.: *The significance of altered gluconeogenesis in surgical catabolism.* J Trauma, 15:704, 1975.

49. PAGE, G, BLACKBURN, G L, HEDDLE, R, ET AL.: *Crystalloid therapy in resuscitation during routine surgery and severe trauma.* Surg Forum 26:18, 1975.

50. RUTTEN, P, BLACKBURN, G L, FLATT, J P, ET AL.: *Determination of optional hyperalimentation infusion rate.* J Surg Res 18:477, 1975.

51. Wilmore, D W, Long, J M, Mason, A D, et al.: *Catecholamines, mediators of the hypometabolic response to thermal injury.* Ann Surg 180:653, 1974.

52. Calloway, D H, and Spector, H: *Nitrogen balance as related to caloric and protein intake in active young men.* Am J Clin Nutr 2:405, 1954.

53. Young, V R, Steffee, W, Pancherz, P, et al.: *Protein turnover in the whole body.* Nature (London) 253:157, 1975.

54. Harper, A E, Benevengen, N J, and Wohlnueter, R M: *Effects of ingestion of disproportionate amounts of amino acids.* Physiol Rev 50:428, 1970.

55. Blackburn, G L, and Bistrian, B R: *Curative nutrition: protein and calorie management,* in Schneider, H A, Anderson, C E, and Coursin, D B (eds.): *Nutritional Support in Medical Practice.* New York: Harper and Row, 1977, p. 80.

56. Blackburn, G L, Flatt, J P, and Hensle, T E: *Peripheral amino acid infusions* in Fischer, J (ed.): *Total Parenteral Nutrition.* Boston: Little Brown and Co., 1976, p. 363.

57. Hallowell, E, Sasvary, D, Bistrian, B R, et al.: *Factors determining optimal use of defined (elemental) formula diets.* Clin. Res. 24:500A, 1976.

58. Butterworth, C E: *Malnutrition in the hospital.* JAMA, 230:879, 1974.

59. Beisel, W R: *Nutrient wastage during infection,* in McKigney, J I, and Munro, H N (eds.): *Nutrient Requirements in Adolescence.* Cambridge: MIT Press, 1975, p. 257.

60. Beisel, W R: *Infectious diseases,* in Schneider, H A, Anderson, C E, and Coursin, D B (eds.): *Nutritional Support of Medical Practice,* New York: Harper and Row, 1977, p. 350

61. Long, C L: *Energy balance and carbohydrate metabolism in sepsis.* Am J Clin Nutr 30:1301, 1977.

62. Border, J R: *Metabolic response to short term starvation, sepsis and trauma.* Surg Ann 2:11, 1970.

63. Young, G A, Chem, C, and Hill, G L: *Assessment of protein calorie malnutrition in surgical patients from plasma proteins and anthropometric measurements.* Am J Clin Nutr 31:429, 1978.

64. Bistrian, B R: *Nutritional assessment and therapy of protein calorie malnutrition in the hospital.* J Am Diet Assoc, 71:393, 1977.

65. Waterlow, J C, Golden, J, and Picou, D: *The measurements of rates of protein turnover, synthesis and breakdown in man and the effects of nutritional status and surgical injury.* Am J Clin Nutr 30:1333, 1977.

66. Hoffenberg, R, Black, E, and Brock, J F: *Albumin and α globulin tracer studies in protein depletion states.* J Clin Invest 45:143, 1966.

67. MacKenzie, T, Blackburn, G L, and Flatt, J P: *Clinical assessment of nutritional status using nitrogen balance.* Fed Proc 33:683, 1974.

68. Munro, H N: *Basic concepts in the use of amino acids and protein hydrolysates for parenteral nutrition,* in *Symposium of Total Parenteral Nutrition.* American Medical Association Nashville, Tenn., 1972, p. 26.

69. Blackburn, G L, Bistrian, B R, Maini, B S, et al.: *Nutritional and metabolic assessment of the hospitalized patient.* J Parenteral Enteral Nutr 1:11, 1977.

70. Viteri, F E, and Alvarado, J: *The creatinine-height index: its use in the estimation of the degree of protein depletion and repletion in protein-calorie malnourished children.* Pediatrics 46:696, 1970.

71. Ryan, R J, Williams, J D, Ansell, B M, et al.: *The relationship of body composition or oxygen consumption and creatinine excretion in healthy and wasted man.* Metabolism 6:365, 1967.

72. Long, C L, Schiller, W R, Blakemore, W S, et al.: *Muscle protein catabolism in the septic patient as measured by 3-methylhistidine excretion.* Am J Clin Nutr 30:1349, 1977.

73. Frisancho, A R: *Triceps skinfold and upper arm size norms for the assessment of nutritional status.* Am J Clin Nutr 27:1052, 1974.

74. Bray, G A, Greenway, F L, Molitch, M E, et al.: *Use of anthropometric measures to assess weight loss.* Am J Clin Nutr 31:769, 1978.

75. Wilmore, D W: *The Metabolic Management of the Critically Ill.* New York: Plenum Medical Book Company, 1977, pp. 20–24.

76. Goldsmith, G A: *Curative nutrition: vitamins* in Schneider, H A, Anderson, C E, and Coursin, D B (eds.): *Nutritional Support of Medical Practice.* New York: Harper and Row, 1977, p. 101.

77. Theuer, R C, and Vitale, J J: *Drug and nutrient interactions,* in Schneider, H A, Anderson, C E, and Coursin, D B (eds.): *Nutritional Support of Medical Practice.* New York: Harper and Row, 1977, p. 257.

78. O'Neill, J A, Caldwell, M D, and Meng, H C: *Essential fatty acid deficiency in surgical patients.* Ann Surgery, 185:321, 1977.

79. Nichoalds, G E, Meng, H C, and Caldwell, M D: *Vitamin requirements in patients receiving total parenteral nutrition.* Arch Surg 112:361, 1977.

80. Law, D K, Dudrick, S J, and Abdou, N I: *Immunocompetence of patients with protein-calorie malnutrition.* Ann Intern Med 79:543, 1973.

81. Warren, J V, and Hill, G L: *T cells and protein nutrition in hospitalized surgical patients.* Br J Surg 12:897, 1977.

82. Lamberth, I E: *Obesity and anesthesia.* Clin Anesth 6(3):56, 1968.

83. Moore, F D, and Brennan, M F: *Surgical injury: body composition, protein metabolism and neuroendocrinology,* in Ballinger, W F, Collins, J A, Drucker, W R, et al. (eds.): *Manual of Surgical Nutrition.* Philadelphia: W. B. Saunders Co., 1975, p. 169.

84. Randall, H T: *Nutrition in surgical patients.* Amer J Surg 119:530, 1970.

85. Albanese, A, and Orto, L A: *The proteins and amino acids,* in Goodhart, R S, and Schills, M E (eds.): *Modern Nutrition in Health and Disease,* ed. 5. Philadelphia: Lea & Febiger, 1973, p. 28.

86. O'Keefe, S J D, and Sender, P M: *Catabolic loss of body nitrogen in response to surgery.* Lancet 2:1035, 1974.

87. Moore, F D: *Convalescence: the metabolic sequence after injury,* in *Manual of Preoperative and Postoperative Care.* Committee on Preoperative and Postoperative Care, American College of Surgery. Philadelphia: W. B. Saunders, 1971, p. 19.

88. Randall, H T: *Surgical Nutrition: parenteral and oral,* in *Manual of Preoperative and Postoperative Care.* Committee on Preoperative and Postoperative care, American College of Surgeons. Philadelphia: W. B. Saunders Company, 1971, p. 75.

89. Committee on Dietary Allowances and Committee on Interpretation of Recommended Dietary Allowances, Food and Nutrition Board, National Research Council: *Recommended Dietary Allowances.* Washington, D. C.: National Academy of Sciences, 1974, p. 37.

90. Close, J H: *The use of amino acid precursors in nitrogen accumulation diseases.* N Engl J Med 290:663, 1974.

91. Fischer, J E, Funovics, J M, Aguirre, A, et al.: *The role of plasma amino acids in hepatic encephalopathy.* Surgery 78:276, 1975.

92. Blackburn, G L, Maini, B S, and Pierce, E C: *Nutrition in the critically ill patient.* Anesthesiology 47:181, 1977.

93. Ghadimi, H (ed.): *Total Parenteral Nutrition: Premises and Promises.* New York: John Wiley and Sons, 1975.

94. Winters, R W, and Hasselmeyer, E G (eds.): *Intravenous Feeding in the High Risk Infant.* New York: John Wiley and Sons, 1975.

95. Wilmore, D W: *The Metabolic Management of the Critically Ill.* New York: Plenum Medical Books, 1977.

96. Clowes, G H A (ed.): *Response to infection and injury, I and II.* Surg Clin North Am, 56:802, 1976.

97. Hallowell, E, Sasvary, D, Bistrian, B R, et al.: *Factors determining optimal nutritional support in defined formula (elemental) diet therapy.* Clin Res 23:591A, 1976.

98. Ming, H C, and Wilmore, D W (eds.): *Proceedings of the American Medical Association Symposium on Fat Emulsions in Parenteral Nutrition.* Chicago: American Medical Association, 1975.

99. Zohrab, W J, McHattie, J D, and Jejeebhoy, K N: *Total parenteral alimentation with lipid.* Gastroenterology, 64:583, 1973.

100. Deitel, M, and Kaminsky, V: *Total nutrition by peripheral vein—the lipid system.* Can Med Assoc J 111:152, 1974.

101. Maini, B S, Smith, M F, Whittemore, S et al.: *Indications for the use of Intralipid.* J Parenteral Enteral Nutr, 1:5A, 1977.

102. Page, C P, Ryan, J A, and Haff, R C: *Continual catheter administration of an elemental diet.* Surg Gynecol Obstet 142:184, 1977.

103. Wade, J E: *Role of a clinical dietitian specialist on a nutrition support service.* J Am Diet Assoc 70:185, 1977.

104. Shils, M E, Block, A S, and Chernoff, R: *Liquid formulas for oral tube feeding.* Clinical Bulletin, 6:151, New York: Memorial Sloan Kettering Cancer Center, 1976.

105. Sandstead, H H, Carter, J P, and Darby, W J: *How to diagnose nutritional disorders in daily practice.* Nutrition Today 4:20, 1969.

106. Sandstead, H H, and Pearson, W N: *Clinical evaluation of nutrition status,* in Goodhart, R W, and Shils, M E (eds.): *Modern Nutrition in Health and Disease.* Philadelphia: Lea & Febiger, 1973, p. 572.

107. Kaminski, M.: *Parenteral hyperalimentation technique.* Am J IV Therapy December-January, 1975.

108. Sauberlich, H A: *Laboratory Tests for The Assessment of Nutritional Status.* Cleveland: CRC Press, 1974.

109. Hethcox, J M, and Stanazek, W F: *Interactions of drugs and diet.* Hosp Pharm 9:373, 1974.

110. Pierpaoli, P.: *Drug therapy and diet.* Drug Intill and Clin Pharm 6:89, 1972.

111. Hathcock, J: *Nutrition, toxicology and pharmacology.* Nutr Rev 34:65, 1976.

112. Masterton, J P, Dudley, H A F, and MacRae, S: *Design of tube feeds for surgical patients.* Br Med J 12:909. 1963.

113. White, P L, and Nagy, M E (eds.): *Total Parenteral Nutrition.* Acton, Maine: Publishing Sciences Group, 1974.

114. Abbott, W M: *Indications for parenteral nutrition,* in Fischer, J E (ed.): *Total Parenteral Nutrition.* Boston: Little Brown and Company, 1976, p. 3.

115. Johnson, E Q: *The therapeutic dietitian's role in the alimentation group.* J Am Dietet Assn 62:648, 1973.

116. Wade, J E: *Role of a clinical dietitian specialist on a nutrition support service.* J Am Dietet Assn 70:185, 1977.

117. Shils, M E: *Enternal nutrition by tube.* Cancer Research, 37:2432, 1977.

118. Randall, T H: *Enteric feeding,* in *Manual of Surgical Nutrition.* Bollinger, W F, Collins, J A, Drucker, W R, et al. (eds.): Philadelphia: W. B. Saunders, 1975, p. 267.

119. *Proceedings of the American Medical Association Conference on Defined Formula Diets.* Washington, D. C. Acton, Maine: Publishing Sciences Group, 1975.

120. Winitz, M, Adams, R F, Seedman, D A, et al.: *Studies of metabolic nutrition employing chemically defined diets, II. Effects of gut microflora populations.* Am J Clin Nutr 23:546, 1970.

121. Atteberry, H R, Sutter, V L, and Finegold, S M: *The effect of a partially chemically defined diet on normal human fecal flora.* Am J Clin Nutr 25:1391, 1972.

122. Bornside, G H, and Cohn, I: *Stability of normal fecal flora during a chemically defined, low residue liquid diet.* Ann Surg 181:58, 1975.

123. Cordaro, J T, Madson, R A, and Krieg, R E: *Effects of prototype space diet on bacterial fecal flora of humans.* Aerospace Med 41:734, 1970.

124. Crowther, J S, Draser, B S, Goddard, P, et al.: *The effect of a chemically defined diet on the fecal flora and fecal steroid concentration.* Gut 14:790, 1973.

125. Glatzer, D J, Boyle, P L, and Silen, W: *Preoperative preparation of the colon with an elemental diet.* Surgery 74:703, 1973.

126. Bradley, G P: *Oral antibiotic prophylaxis in protected environment units: effects of nonabsorbable and absorbable antibiotics on the fecal flora.* Antimicrob Agents Chemother 1:343, 1972.

127. Shils, M E: *Principles of nutritional therapy.* Cancer 43:2093, 1979.

128. Douglas, H O, Milliron, S, Nava, H, et al.: *Elemental diet as on adjunct for patients with locally advanced gastrointestinal cancer receiving radiation therapy: a prospectively randomised study.* J Parenteral Enteral Nutrition 2:676, 1978.

129. Dobbie, R P, and Butterick, O D: *Continuous pump/tube enteric hyperalimentation—use in esophageal disease.* J Parenteral Enteral Nutrition, 1:100, 1977.

130. Maini, B, Blackburn, G L, Bistrian, B R, et al.: *Cyclic hyperalimentation: an optimal technique for preservation of visceral protein.* J Surg Res 20:151, 1976.

131. Walker, W F: *Nutrition after injury.* World Rev Nutr Diet 19:173, 1974.

132. Clark, R B: *Caloric requirements after operation.* Proc Nutr Soc 30:158, 1971.

133. Organ, C H, and Finn, M P: *The importance of nutritional support for the geriatric surgical patient.* Geriatrics 32:77, 1977.

134. Neilen, T F, Grossi, C E, and Steier, M: *Use of elemental diets to correct catabolic states prior to surgery.* Ann Surg 180:9, 1974.

135. Bresner, M: *Nutrition for the surgical patient.* J Oral Surg 35:200, 1977.

136. Sorichon, E A, Englert, D, Duke, J H, et al.: *Intravenous hyperalimentation in 342 surgical patients.* Rev Surg 33:297, 1976.

137. Roe, C F: *Temperature regulation and energy metabolism in surgical patients.* Prog Surg 12:96, 1973.

138. Hartsuck, J W: *Fluid and electrolyte therapy.* Major Prob Clin Surg 17:39, 1975.

139. Heymsfield, S F, Bethel, R A, Ansley, J D, et al.: *Enteral hyperalimentation: an alternative to central venous hyperalimentation.* Ann Intern Med 90:63, 1979.

140. Shils, M E, Bloch, A S, and Chernoff, R: *Liquid formulas for oral and tube feeding.* J Parenteral Enteral Nutrition, 1:2, 1977.

141. Chawla, K K, and Wright, J: *A primer on liquid formula diets.* Practical Gastroenterology, 2:9, 1978.

142. Long, C L: *Energy and protein requirements in hospitalized patients.* J Parenteral Enteral Nutrition 3:69, 1979.

143. Kaminski, M V, Burke, W A, and Blackburn, G L: *Intravenous Hyperalimentation in Modern Hospital Practice.* Tuckahoe, N. Y.: USN Laboratories, 1977.

144. Rich, A J, and Wright, P O: *Ketosis and nitrogen excretion in undernourished surgical patients.* J Parenteral Enteral Nutrition 3:157, 1979.

145. Blackburn, G L, and Bothe, A: *Assessment of malnutrition.* Practical Gastroenterology 2:46, 1978.

146. Kinney, J N, Long, C L, and Duke, J H: *Carbohydrate and nitrogen metabolism after injury,* in Peters, R, and Knight, J (eds.): *Energy Metabolism and Trauma.* CIBA Foundation Symposium. London: J. and A. Churchill, 1970.

147. Law, D H: *Current concepts in nutrition: Total parenteral nutrition.* N Engl J Med 297:1104, 1977.

148. Sapir, D G, and Walser, M: *Nitrogen sparing induced early in starvation by infusion of branched-chain keto acids.* Metabolism 26:301, 1977.

149. Freund, H, Hoover, H C, Jr., Atamian, S, et al.: *Infusion of the branched-chain amino acids in postoperative patients: Anti-catabolic properties.* Ann Surg 190:18, 1979.

150. Fischer, J E, Funovics, J M, Agere, A, et al.: *The role of plasma amino acids in hepatic encephalopathy.* Surgery 78:276, 1975.

151. Peters, C, and Fischer, J E,: *Study on calorie:nitrogen ratio for total parenteral nutrition.* Surg Gynecol Obstet 151:1, 1980.

152. Studley, H O: *Percent weight loss: basic indicator of surgical risk.* JAMA 106:458, 1936.

153. Touloukian, R J, and Downing, S E: *Cholestasis associated with long-term parenteral hyperalimentation.* Arch Surg 106:58, 1973.

154. Stephens, R P, and Randall, H T: *Use of a concentrated, balanced, liquid elemental diet for nutritional management of catabolic states.* Ann Surg 170:642, 1969.

155. Dudrick, S J, and Ruberg, R L: *Principles in practice of parenteral nutrition.* Gastroenterology 61:901, 1971.

156. Abbott, W N: *Indications for parenteral nutrition in total parenteral nutrition,* in Fischer, J E (ed.): *Total Parenteral Nutrition.* Boston: Little, Brown and Company, 1977, p. 3.

157. Sanderson, I, and Deitel, M: *Insulin response in patients receiving concentrated infusions of glucose and caseine hydrolysate for complete parenteral nutrition.* Ann Surg 179:387, 1974.

158. Sanderson, I, and Deitel, M: *Insulin response in patients undergoing prolonged intravenous hyperalimentation.* Surg Forum 23:64, 1972.

159. Wolfe, R R, O'Donnell, T F, Jr., Stone, M D et al.: *Investigation of factors determining optimal glucose infusion rates in total parenteral nutrition.* Metabolism 29:892, 1980.

160. Bernard, R W, and Stahl, W N: *Subclavian vein catheterization. A prospective study: (1) Noninfectious complications.* Ann Surg 173:184, 1971.

161. Ryan, J A, Abel, R N, Abbott, W N, et al.: *Catheter complications in total parenteral nutrition. A prospective study of 200 consecutive patients.* N Engl J Med 290:757, 1974.

162. Flanagan, J P, Gradisar, I A, Gross, R J, et al.: *Air embolus—A lethal complication of subclavian venipuncture.* N Engl J Med 281:488, 1969.

163. Langston, C S: *The aberrant central venous catheter and its complications.* Radiology 100:55, 1974.

164. Goldmann, D A, and Maki, D G: *Infection control in total parenteral nutrition.* JAMA 223:1360, 1973.

165. Sanderson, I, and Deitel, N: *Intravenous hyperalimentation without sepsis.* Surg Gynecol Obstet 136:577, 1973.

166. Goldman, D A, Martin, W T, and Worthington, J W: *Growth of bacteria and fungi in total parenteral nutrition solutions.* Am J Surg 126:314, 1973.

167. Sceppa, L, and O'Donnell, T F: *Metabolic complications of total parenteral nutrition.* Presented at the American Society for Enternal and Parenteral Nutrition, Houston, Texas, Feb. 1978.

168. Ryan, J A: *Complications of total parenteral nutrition* in Fischer, J E (ed.): *Total Parenteral Nutrition.* Boston: Little, Brown and Company, 1976, p. 55.

169. Dudrick, S J, MacFayden, B V, Van Buren, C T, et al.: *Parenteral hyperalimentation, metabolic problems and solutions.* Ann Surg 176:259, 1972.

170. Ruberg, R L, Allen, T R, Goodman, M J, et al.: *Hypophosphatemia with hypophosphaturia in hyperalimentation.* Surg Forum 22:87, 1971.

171. Travis, S F, Sugerman, H J, and Ruberg, R L: *Alterations of red cell glycolytic intermediates and oxygen transport as a consequence of hypophosphatemia in patients receiving intravenous hyperalimentation.* N Engl J Med 285:763, 1971.

172. *The AMA Guidelines on Trace Elements.:* JAMA 241:2051, 1979.

173. Wilmore, D W, Moylan, J A, Helmkamp, G N, et al.: *Clinical evaluation of a 10 percent intravenous fat emulsion for total parenteral nutrition and thermally injured patients.* Ann Surg 178:503, 1973.

174. White, H B, Jr., Turner, M D, Turner, A C, et al.: *Blood lipid alterations in infants receiving intravenous fat-free alimentation.* J Pediat 83:305, 1973.

175. Press, M, Hartop, P J, and Protley, C: *Correction of essential fatty acid deficiency in man by the cutaneous application of sunflowerseed oil.* Lancet 1:597, 1974.

176. Heird, W C, Driscoll, J N, and Schullinger, J N: *Intravenous alimentation in pediatric patients.* J Pediat 80:351, 1972.

177. Heird, W C, Nicholson, J F, Driscoll, J N, et al.: *Hyperammonemia resulting from intravenous alimentation using a mixture of synthetic L-amino acids: A preliminary report.* J Pediat 81:162, 1972.

178. Giordano, C: *Use of exogenous and endogenous urea for protein synthesis in normal and uremic subjects.* J Lab Clin Med 62:231, 1963.

179. Giovannetti, S, and Maggiore, Q: *A low-nitrogen diet with protein of high biological value for severe chronic uremia.* Lancet 1:1000, 1964.

180. Abel, R M, Becks, C H, Jr., Abbott, W M, et al.: *Improved survival from acute renal failure following treatment with intravenous essential L-amino acids and glucose.* N Engl J Med 288:695, 1973.

181. Dudrick, S J, Steiger, E, and Long, J M: *Renal failure in surgical patients: treatment with intravenous essential amino acids in hypertonic dextrose.* Surgery 68:180, 1970.

182. Alexander, C S, and Zieve, L: *Fat infusions. Toxic effects and alterations in fasting serum lipids following prolonged use.* Arch Intern Med 107:514, 1961.

183. Clowes, G H A, Jr., O'Donnell, T F, Jr., Blackburn, G L, et al.: *Energy metabolism and proteolysis in traumatized and septic man.* Surg Clin North Am. 56:5, 1976.

184. Scow, R O, Hamosh, N, Blanchette-Mackie, J, et al.: *Uptake of blood triglycerides by various tissues.* Lipids 7:497, 1972.

185. Meng, H C: *Fat emulsions in parenteral nutrition,* in Fischer, J E (ed.): *Total Parenteral Nutrition.* Boston: Little, Brown and Co., 1975, p. 305.

186. Jeejeebhoy, K N, Anderson, G H, Nakhooda, A F, et al.: *Metabolic studies in parenteral nutrition with lipid in man. Comparison with glucose.* J Clin Invest 57:125, 1976.

187. Zohrab, W J, McHattie, J D, and Jeejeebhoy, K N: *Total parenteral alimentation with lipid.* Gastroenterology 64:583, 1973.

188. Greene, H L, Hazlett, D, Herman, R H, et al.: *Effect of Intralipid® on pulmonary membrane diffusing capacity (Dm) and pulmonary capillary blood volume (Vc).* Clin Res 19:677, 1971.

189. Duckert, F, and Hartmann, G: *Intravenose fettinfusion und blutgerinnung.* Schweiz Med Wochenschr 96:1205, 1966.

190. Blackburn, G L, and Flatt, J P: *Substrate profile in protein nutrition states,* in Brown, H (ed.): *Protein Nutrition.* Charles C Thomas, Springfield, Ill., 1974, p. 201.

191. Blackburn, G L, Flatt, J P, Clowes, G H A, et al.: *Peripheral intravenous feeding with isotonic amino acid solutions.* Am J Surg 125:447, 1973.

192. Hoover, H C, Grant, J P, Gorschboth, C, et al.: *Nitrogen sparing intravenous fluids in postoperative patients.* N Engl J Med 295:172, 1975.

193. Freeman, J B, Stegink, L D, Meyer, P D, et al.: *Metabolic effects of amino acids versus dextrose infusion in surgical patients.* Arch Surg 110:916, 1975.

194. Ching, N, Mills, C J, Gross, I C, et al.: *The absence of protein-sparing effects utilizing crystalline amino acids in stress patients.* Ann Surg 190:565, 1979.

195. Tweedle, D E, Fitzpatrick, G F, Brennan, N F, et al.: *Intravenous amino acids as a sole nutritional substrate.* Ann Surg 186:16, 1977.

196. Greenberg, G R, Marliss, E B, Anderson, G H, et al.: *Protein-sparing therapy in postoperative patients.* N Engl J Med 294:1411, 1976.

197. Kaminski, M V, Dunn, N P, Wannemacher, R W, et al.: *Specific muscle protein-sparing postoperative dextrose—free amino acid infusions.* J Parent Ent Nutr 1:147, 1977.

198. Blackburn, G L, and Bistrian, B R: *Nutritional care in the injured and/or septic patient.* Surg Clin North Am 56:1195, 1976.

199. Freeman, J B, Stegink, L D, Wittine, M F, et al.: *The current status of protein sparing.* Surg Gynecol Obstet 144:843, 1977.

ABBOTT, WM. NUTRITIONAL CARE OF THE TRAUMA PATIENT, S.G.&O, 157:585, DEC 1983.
DUDRICK, 100 PATIENT-YEARS OF AMBULATORY HOME TOTAL PARENTERAL NUTRITION, ANN. SURG, 199:770, 1984.

CHAPTER 17

ANESTHESIOLOGY

Paul R. Levesque, M.D.

To the countless considerations presented in the preceding sixteen chapters, we wish to add the anesthesiologist's logic, which on occasion will be found to depart from the internist's reasoning because of the very pragmatic aspect of anesthesia. Undoubtedly, more science is involved at present in managing a well conducted anesthetic than 10 or 20 years ago; nonetheless, the choice of anesthesia is still largely based on the skill and the practical experience of each anesthesiologist. For example, it might seem prudent for a patient with a history of asthma to have an inguinal herniorrhaphy done under spinal anesthesia, but experience has shown that these patients often develop severe bronchospasm due to sympathetic blockade or to the emotion of being awake during surgery. With the latest general anesthetics, some with bronchodilator properties, a well conducted general anesthetic is usually more satisfactory.

Preparing for the most remote possibility truly typifies the approach to a well administered anesthetic and will permit successful recovery of even the sickest patient. The preanesthetic visit is medically and legally essential. It includes a thorough scrutiny of the patient's chart, searching for instability of the patient's condition, current medication, history of adverse response to drugs, and past anesthetic experience. In seeing the patient, the anesthesiologist concentrates on items such as body build and malformations, anatomy of the upper airway, pattern of breathing, level of arousal, and degree of apprehension.

The American Society of Anesthesia (ASA) classification of physical status and risk should be familiar to all physicians involved in caring for the surgical patient. It is as follows:

Class 1. The patient has no organic, physiologic, biochemical, or psychiatric disturbance. The pathologic process requiring surgery does not entail a systemic disturbance. Example: a fit patient with inguinal hernia.

Class 2. The patient has mild to moderate systemic disturbance caused either by the condition requiring surgery or by other pathophysiologic processes such as slightly limiting organic heart disease, essential hypertension, or anemia. Some might include patients at the extremes of age here.

Class 3. Patients with a severe systemic disturbance from whatever cause, such as severe organic heart disease, severe diabetes with vascular complications, or healed myocardial infarction.

Class 4. The presence of life-threatening systemic disorders not always correctable by operation place patients in this class. Examples: marked decompensated cardiac disease, or persistent advanced degrees of pulmonary, hepatic, renal, or endocrine insufficiency.

Class 5. The moribund patient submitted to surgery in desperation. Example: the patient with burst abdominal aneurysm with profound shock.

Emergency Operation (E). Any patient in one of the classes above who is operated upon as an emergency. The letter E is placed beside the numerical classification. Thus, the patient with uncomplicated incarcerated hernia is classified 1E if operated upon on an emergency basis.

Although the above classification is widely used and is a good predictor of complications, the index proposed by Goldman is more accurate in predicting the outcome of anesthesia and surgery in patients with cardiac disease (Table 1).

On occasion the anesthesiologist is the first physician to see the patient preoperatively or the first physician to evaluate his or her general status. If the patient presents with an unstable medical condition, the anesthesiologist will seek consultation from the internist from whom he expects a clear diagnosis, an evaluation of the severity of the condition, and a regimen to establish preoperative stability of the patient's condition. More often than not, however, the internist will also express an opinion as to the choice of anesthesia and in so doing assumes a responsibility he does not have to shoulder. It is only with a solid understanding of the patient's preoperative medical condition coupled with the knowledge of pathophysiology of the contemplated surgical procedure that the decision can be made whether or not to proceed and what anesthesia should be chosen. The anesthesiologist is in an ideal position to make that decision.

UPTAKE, DISTRIBUTION, AND METABOLISM OF ANESTHETIC AGENTS

The precision and predictability of recovery from general anesthesia still amazes many. The ability to arouse a patient almost on command comes from an understanding of uptake and distribution of anesthetic agents, especially inhalational agents. The laws governing the precision of anesthetic induction also direct its reversibility. More accurate vaporizers and better choice of circuitry permit precise delivery of a known concentration of anesthetic.

Foster, Risk of Non Cardiac Operations in Patients with Defined Coronary Disease: Coronary Artery Surgery Study (CASS) Registry Experience, Ann. Thor. Surg. 41:42, Jan. 1986.

TABLE 1. Cardiac Risk Index Score*

Factors		*Points*
1 History:	Age > 70 years	5
	Myocardial Infarction < 6 months previously	10
2 Physical exam:	S_3 or jugular vein distention	11
3 ECG:	Any rhythm other than sinus	7
4 General information:	$Po_2 < 60$; $Pco_2 > 50$; $K^+ < 3$; BUN > 50; Creatinine > 3.0; Bedridden	3
5 Operation:	Emergency	4
	Intrathoracic or Intra-abdominal or Aortic surgery	3
	Total	50

Class: 1 = 0–5 points
2 = 6–12 points
3 = 13–25 points
4 = 26–50 points

*Goldman, L, Caldera, DL, Nussbaum, SB, et al.: *Multifactorial index of cardiac risk in non-cardiac surgical procedures.* N Engl J Med 297:845, 1977.

Consideration of the patient's size and body build plus understanding of the pathophysiology of diseases permit accurate predictability of outcome. For example, the functional residual capacity (FRC) serves to dilute the inspired concentration of inhalational anesthetic and to prevent sudden change in blood concentration. However, this effect will be enhanced with centrolobular emphysema due to an increased FRC. On the other hand, a patient with pulmonary fibrosis and decreased FRC will respond more rapidly to a change in anesthetic concentration. A variation in pulmonary or systemic blood volume will produce similar effects on the time constant of induction.

The anemic patient is known to respond more rapidly to induction. This is probably because most drugs including anesthetics are bound to red cells and plasma proteins.[1] It is conceivable that in a state of anemia and hypoproteinemia, less drug is bound and more is set free to enter the brain and produce its anesthetic effect. An increase in cardiac output due to anemia also contributes to hasten the time constant of induction. The scope of this book does not permit discussion of all factors affecting the action of anesthetics, but the above examples serve to illustrate the approach to the proper management of anesthesia.

CLINICAL SIGNIFICANCE OF BIOTRANSFORMATION OF INHALATIONAL ANESTHETICS

Although it was formerly thought that inhalational anesthetics were not metabolized in the body, it is now known that the liver plays an important role in the breakdown of anesthetic molecules producing secondary moieties which are potentially toxic to certain organs, particularly the kidney and the liver.[2] For example, as much as 70 percent of absorbed methoxyflurane and 20 percent of absorbed halothane and fluroxene is metabolized in man but only 2 to 3 percent of enflurane (Ethrane) is broken down. Reports of renal damage caused by prolonged administration of methoxyflurane have appeared in the literature.[3] We now know conclusively that this agent is converted to free fluoride in a dose-dependent manner. Furthermore, this effect can be induced by previous administration of drugs such as phenobarbital. Enflurane can also liberate free fluoride but does so to a much lesser extent and no well documented case of renal damage has been reported so far.[4] However, we avoid administering enflurane to patients with known renal dysfunction.

ANESTHESIA ON HEALTHY VOLUNTEERS

In this country, from 1955 to the late 1960s, numerous studies were conducted on healthy volunteers in which a single inhalational anesthetic was administered to evaluate its effect on respiratory or cardiac functions. Premedicants, surgery, or any adjuvant drugs were avoided. The paucity of side effects and the rapid recovery of these volunteers was astonishing. We personally conducted such studies to evaluate the circulatory effect of enflurane on 12 healthy volunteers. A constant concentration of 5 percent enflurane (i.e., more than three times the minimum alveolar anesthetic concentration) was administered for as long as four hours, and cardiac function, as measured by ventricular stroke work, cardiac output, and maximum velocity of contraction, was markedly lowered.[5] However, within 15 to 20 minutes following cessation of anesthetic administration, some of these volunteers would walk to their rooms unaided and would request their meal.

This anecdote is not cited to sell the innocuity of general anesthesia but to focus attention on all other factors that explain the postoperative status of some of our patients. No doubt surgery itself, blood loss, and the use of premedicants and muscle relaxants have a major effect on how well a patient will recover from a surgical procedure. Clearly the preoperative medical status has a strong influence on postanesthetic recovery. The nutritional status, the long immobility of the bedridden patient, and the wasting effect of chronic systemic diseases will affect the patient's sensitivity to anesthetic agents, the speed of recovery, and the severity of postoperative complications. Anesthesia cannot be routinely administered employing a basic recipe but has to be managed with a dose-response approach, as one cannot always predict the individual effect of a given drug at a given dose.

DRUG INTERACTIONS

During the preanesthetic visit, few items are of more concern to the anesthesiologist than the interaction between medications currently being administered and anesthetic agents or other adjuvant drugs. In spite of preanesthetic scrutiny, it is not always possible to identify the drugs involved in instances of illicit or over the counter drug use, especially when the patient comes through the emergency room in a comatose state and is rushed to surgery for massive bleeding or severe injury. Consequently, it is essential for both the internist and the anesthesiologist to be familiar with possible deleterious interactions between these drugs and anesthetic agents. The following discussion is not intended to be comprehensive but includes the most frequently encountered situations.

Tricyclic Antidepressants

Imipramine and amitriptyline are the most frequently used tricyclic antidepressants. These drugs often give rise to arterial pressure instability, tachycardia, and exquisite sensitivity to vasopressors.[6] If the patient is known to be taking these agents, the anesthesiologist will titrate the level of anesthesia using an inhalational anesthetic to provide better control of vital signs (see Chap. 11, Psychiatry).

Lithium Carbonate

Lithium carbonate is used to treat manic depressive states. It may cause prolongation of action of all muscle relaxants and may cause cardiac arrythmias. Use of succinylcholine should be avoided and competitive muscle relaxants should be titrated using nerve stimulator monitoring (see Chap. 11, Psychiatry).

Levodopa

Levodopa is frequently administered to parkinsonian patients. Levodopa has adrenergic activity and may interact with anesthetic agents like ether, cyclopropane, halothane, and ketamine to produce severe arrythmia and unpredictable episodes of hypotension and hypertension. Patients taking levodopa who receive narcotics may develop severe chest-wall rigidity which may cause marked hypoventilation and necessitate the use of muscle relaxants. Succinylcholine is best avoided because of its nicotinic properties, which when added to the adrenergic activity of levodopa may give rise to severe ventricular arrythmias (see Chap. 9, Neurology).

Monoamine Oxidase (MAO) Inhibitors

Phenelzine and nialamide used in certain types of depressions interact with meperidine to produce convulsions and coma by an unknown mechanism. Use of other opiates should be avoided. Vasopressors given to patients taking MAO inhibitors can cause severe hypertensive crisis. MAO inhibitors should be discontinued for at least two weeks before surgery (see Chap. 11, Psychiatry).

Phenothiazines

Because of their multiple sites of action and nonspecificity of effect, phenothiazines have been nearly abandoned by the anesthesiologist. Chlorpromazine has a potent antiadrenergic effect of long duration and is a strong central nervous system depressant that potentiates the action of premedicants and anesthetic agents such as opiate-anesthetics, barbiturates, and droperidol. Phenothiazines also inhibit central dopaminergic receptors and may cause muscle rigidity, parkinsonism, and other dystonic syndromes (see Chap. 11, Psychiatry).

Opiates

Patients receiving opiate medication chronically are resistant to most sedatives and anesthetic agents. However, the preanesthetic period is not the time for withdrawal of the opiate. Addicted patients should be given their usual daily requirements to prevent withdrawal syndrome and surgery should be managed under regional anesthesia or inhalational agents. Pentazocine (Talwin) is not a substitute for opiates as it may produce a full withdrawal syndrome and should be avoided (see Chap. 11, Psychiatry).

Anticonvulsants

Phenytoin, trimethadione, phenobarbital and other anticonvulsants are all central nervous system depressants and also will induce tolerance to sedatives and anesthetic agents by enzyme induction in the liver. This induced tolerance does not necessarily affect the cardiovascular system and the increased concentration of anesthetic needed to produce a surgical level of anesthesia may cause marked cardiovascular depression.

Beta-Adrenergic Blocking Agents

Propranolol may be useful in treating many acute situations including severe ventricular and supraventricular arrhythmias, hyperthyroid crisis, and acute myocardial ischemia. However, it may engender myocardial failure and bronchospasm. For the healthy patient taking propranolol for migraine, the tapering off before anesthesia is of no serious consequence. If propranolol is being administered to treat severe angina, it should not be discontinued. If hypotension from myocardial failure occurs during surgery in the patient receiving propranolol, it will often be refractory to most sympathomimetic amines. Recently we have observed two patients taking propranolol who displayed exquisite sensitivity to norepinephrine in whom large doses of dopamine had produced no effect. Recent data showing the inability of beta blockers to antagonize norepinephrine in rat postganglionic neurons would support this clinical finding.[7] The use of intravenous calcium or glucagon is an effective alternative in managing the above situation (see Chap. 3, Cardiology).

Quinidine

Quinidine directly depresses skeletal muscle tone and may potentiate the effect of muscle relaxants.

Digitalis

Although the positive inotropic effect of digitalis counteracts the negative inotropism of certain anesthetics like halothane and ether,[8] together they may have additive effects on cardiac conduction and rhythm. As does digitalis, halothane slows the heart rate and is arrhythmogenic at higher concentrations even in healthy young patients. Intravenous calcium, frequently used during anesthesia either as an inotropic agent or following multiple blood transfusions, might trigger ventricular arrhythmias in the digitalized patient, especially if hypokalemia coexists.

Nitroglycerin

Intravenous nitroglycerin is increasingly being used not only to treat coronary insufficiency but also to control ventricular preload and afterload in certain cardiovascular hyperkinetic states. Used in excess it produces methemoglobinemia which in turn will add to the methemoglobinemia due to other apparently benign maneuvers such as benzocaine spray used as a topical anesthetic before endoscopic procedures. The diagnosis is made by the typical brown color of the blood or by co-oxymetry. The treatment consists of intravenous methylene blue (1 to 2 mg/kg of body weight) which acts rapidly and efficiently.

Anticholinesterases

Pyridostigmine and neostigmine are widely used to treat myasthenia gravis. These agents are cholinergic and may promote vomiting and aspiration in patients in precarious respiratory status with weak or absent cough and gag reflexes. Administration of most anesthetics will accentuate muscle weakness permitting even extensive abdominal surgery without the use of muscle relaxants. Atropine will counteract the muscarinic effect of anticholinesterase drugs without affecting the nicotinic property for which they are used (see Chap. 9, Neurology).

Organophosphates

Echothiophate and isoflurophate are currently employed in the treatment of glaucoma. These drugs often prolong the effect of succinylcholine and procaine by inhibiting plasma pseudocholinesterase which hydrolyses acetylcholine as well as succinylcholine and procaine. Use of succinylcholine, procaine, and procainamide should be avoided in patients dependent on these organophosphates as their action might be markedly prolonged.

Antibiotics

Parenteral aminoglycoside antibiotics (e.g., neomycin, kanamycin, gentamicin, streptomycin, amikacin) have been shown to prolong the action of muscle relaxants and also to have a relaxant property of their own in normal and myasthenic patients. The action of these drugs can be antagonized by intravenous administration of neostigmine or calcium gluconate.

Because the tetracyclines have been shown to aggravate methoxyflurane nephrotoxicity, this agent should be avoided in patients taking any of the tetracyclines.

Many other esoteric drug interactions have been described, but those mentioned above are the most frequently encountered in surgical patients (Table 2).

PHYSIOLOGIC EFFECTS OF PATIENT'S POSITIONING DURING SURGERY

Awkward positioning during certain surgical procedures will sometimes produce physiologic changes that are poorly tolerated by patients having limited respiratory or cardiovascular reserve. During the preoperative visit, the anesthesiologist may test the effect of positioning on comfort as in the case of the arthritic patient or on the patient's ability to ventilate or maintain the level of blood pressure. An elderly patient suffering from right lower lobe pneumonia for instance might not tolerate lying on his right side as perfusion of the pneumonic lobe would be markedly increased and ventilation impaired, creating severe abnormality of the ventilation-perfusion ratio and hypoxia. In such cases, general anesthesia and respiratory assistance might be preferable to regional anesthesia.

ACID-BASE BALANCE

Preoperative conditions causing acid-base disturbances are discussed in Chapter 15, Fluid, Electrolyte, and Acid-Base Disorders. Observations frequently made during the perioperative period are discussed below.

Dilutional acidosis may be observed following overnight overhydration in preparation for major abdominal surgery. A large volume of fluid may be administered to compensate for possible dehydration due to bowel preparation but this may be overdone. Withholding fluids during the first hour of surgery will usually suffice to reestablish normal acid-base balance. The patient experiencing massive vomiting (acute intestinal obstruction) is frequently dehydrated and ketoacidotic with positive urine acetone measurements. Induction of anesthesia should be delayed until the acidosis is corrected. Indeed, true metabolic acidosis increases anesthetic requirements and diminishes the response to vasopressors and should be corrected preoperatively.

The patient with head trauma or acute cerebrovascular accident frequently presents a mixed acid-base imbalance composed of an acute or sometimes chronic hypocarbia from spontaneous hyperventilation with Pa_{CO_2} as low as 18 or 20 mm Hg added to a mild metabolic alkalosis from vomiting or from steroid therapy given prophylactically or therapeutically for intracranial hypertension. Hypocarbia is easily corrected with muscle relaxants and controlled respiration. The metabolic alkalosis is usually mild and rarely requires treatment.

Despite preoperative sedation, we have observed that about 40 percent of patients show acute respiratory alkalosis on induction, probably due to persistent anxiety and stimulation from insertion of invasive monitoring catheters. On the other hand, pro-

TABLE 2. Drug Interactions of Concern to the Anesthesiologist

Agents	*Known Drug Interaction*	*Specific Toxicity*	*Specific Disease Indication*	*Specific Disease Contraindication*
Inhalational Anesthetics				
Ether	Competitive muscle relaxants, L-dopa		Bronchospasm, asthma	Acidosis, dehydration, fever
Cyclopropane	Catecholamines, levodopa	Respiratory depression	Noncardiogenic hypotension	Thyrotoxicosis, pheochromocytoma, acidosis
Nitrous oxide		Pulmonary hypertension		Air emboli—bends, pneumothorax, abdominal distention
Halothane	Catecholamines, L-dopa	Liver?	Bronchospasm, asthma, hypertensive crisis	Drug-hepatitis, intracranial hypertension
Enflurane	Competitive muscle relaxants	Kidney?	Pheochromocytoma	Renal failure, seizures
Isoflurane	Competitive muscle relaxants		Pheochromocytoma	
Methoxyflurane	Competitive muscle relaxants	Kidney and liver		Renal failure, prolonged administration
Intravenous Anesthetics				
Thiopental, thiamylal methohexital	Anticonvulsants	Respiratory depressant	Intracranial hypertension, seizures	Bronchial asthma, acute intermittent porphyria
Neuroleptics	Monoamine oxidase inhibitors, pentazocine	Respiratory depressant		
Ketamine	Levodopa	Respiratory stimulant	Bronchospasm, asthma, full stomach hypovolemia	Intracranial hypertension, systemic hypertension, confusion states, coronary artery disease
Meperidine	Monoamine oxidase inhibitors, pentazocine	Potent respiratory depressant		
Morphine	Monoamine oxidase inhibitors, pentazocine	Potent respiratory depressant	Visceral pain, cardiac surgery	Asthma, histaminergic states hypovolemia

TABLE 2 *Continued*

Agents	*Known Drug Interaction*	*Specific Toxicity*	*Specific Disease Indication*	*Specific Disease Contraindication*
Muscle Relaxants				
Succinylcholine	Levodopa echothiopate, trimetaphan	Potassium release states	Sphincter spasms	Hypoxia (acute) hyperkalemia, liver disease myasthenic states
d-tubocurarine	Quinidine, lithium, propranolol, antibiotics	Histamine release	Tetanus, hypertonic states	Myasthenic states, hypotensive states
Pancuronium	Quinidine, lithium, propranolol, antibiotics		Tetanus, hypertonic states	Supraventricular tachycardia, myasthenic states
Medicants				
Atropine, scopolamine	Beta-agonist	Central nervous system	Vagotonic state, anxiety	Hyperthermia, myocardial irritability
Phenothiazines	Opiates, anesthetic agents, sedatives, gallamine	Cholangitis, Parkinsonism	Thyroid storm, hypertensive states	Parkinsonism, dystonic syndromes
Diazapam			Coronary insufficiency, muscle rigidity, tetanus	respiratory depression

longed intravenous induction with continuous intravenous drip of large doses of narcotics in well oxygenated patients usually produces marked bradypnea and acute respiratory acidosis ($Paco_2$ of 50 to 60 mm Hg). This technique is frequently used before cardiac surgery in adult patients, does not seem to be arrhythmogenic and does not seem to aggravate pre-existing arrhythmias. These observation are supported by similar findings by Rogers and coworkers in dogs.[9] Although the presence of coronary or pulmonary impairment might influence the findings of Rogers, we still view moderate respiratory acidosis as a benign if not beneficial occurrence in well oxygenated patients. There is good evidence to believe that acute respiratory acidosis producing a pH of 7.28 to 7.32 lowers myocardial and total body oxygen consumption and, conversely, respiratory alkalosis increases it.[10–12] Normal sleep is accompanied by respiratory acidosis ($Paco_2$ of 48 to 50 mm Hg) and decreases oxygen consumption in healthy individuals.[13,14]

ARTIFICIAL VENTILATION

Controlled, artificial ventilation and the use of muscle relaxants gives the anesthetist the ability to adjust arterial Pco_2 at will. Indeed, hyperventilation is often used to lower cerebral blood flow during brain surgery or to minimize the dose of intravenous or inhalational anesthetic. However, positive pressure breathing may cause changes in the distribution of pulmonary blood flow and the distribution of ventilation producing a disturbance in the ventilation-perfusion ratio in all regions of the lung and causing increased physiologic dead-space and shunting.[15] Positive pressure breathing may also produce a decreased urine output probably by increased renal vascular afterload.[16] It also has been shown that acute respiratory alkalosis increases myocardial and total body oxygen consumption, which might not be desirable, especially in a patient with coronary artery disease.[10–12]

MANAGEMENT OF PATIENTS WITH LUNG DISEASE

Pneumonia

In the case of an emergency procedure on a patient with pneumonia, a well conducted general anesthetic may have some benefits. Several pulmonary function tests can be performed during anesthesia including measurement of the alveolar-arterial oxygen pressure gradient ($P[A\text{-}a]O_2$), dead space to tidal volume ratio, and total pulmonary compliance, thereby augmenting the patient assessment. The act of intubating the trachea and producing hyperinflation of the lung can reopen atelectatic and pneumonitic areas. These maneuvers help evaluate the degree of pulmonary involvement and sometimes will improve oxygenation and other functions. A Swan-Ganz catheter inserted into such a patient permits the evaluation of right and left heart function and by measuring mixed venous and arterial PO_2 can give an estimate of cardiac output. However, these advantages have to be weighed against the possibility of bacterial dissemination and the lowering of pulmonary defense mechanisms caused by high oxygen inhalation, introduction of an endotracheal tube, and administration of an inhalational agent.[21] Thus, postponement of elective procedures until clinical and radiographic signs of pneumonia are eradicated is preferred.

Pneumoconiosis

The patient with severe pulmonary fibrosis secondary to pneumoconiosis usually tolerates general anesthesia well as long as the anesthesiologist understands the changes in pulmonary mechanics and right heart function. The low pulmonary compliance (stiff lung) often seen in these patients should be managed by low tidal volume and faster frequency of breathing. Also, central venous pressure and pulmonary wedge pressure monitoring are of great help in managing these patients.

Chronic Obstructive Pulmonary Disease (COPD)

To care for patients suffering from COPD with chronic hypercarbia is the ultimate challenge to anesthesiologists preoperatively, intraoperatively, and postoperatively. This condition increases respiratory complications by a factor of 4 to 20 during recovery.[22]

Preoperatively, the severe "blue bloater" is hypoxic, and the hypoxia is more severe than would be expected from hypoventilation alone. The patients ventilatory capacity is markedly reduced and his response to CO_2 challenge is diminished. The mechanics of breathing are impaired mainly because of hyperinflation from emphysema and increased small airway resistance (air trapping). He is often hypertensive with a variable degree of right ventricular failure and liver congestion. The patient may frequently be agitated which further increases an already elevated oxygen consumption caused by dyspnea. Preoperative preparation consists of the following: (1) smoking should be stopped for 10 to 15 days, (2) pulmonary function tests should be performed including response to bronchodilators, (3) antibiotic treatment should be instituted for several days before anesthesia if there are signs of bacterial infection, (4) physiotherapy of the chest with coughing exercises should be performed especially if large amounts of sputum are present, (5) cardiology and pulmonary consultations may be indicated to evaluate right and left heart and lung function, and (6) digitalis may be indicated in some patients. The patient should be informed of the nature of postoperative care including endotracheal intubation and respiratory assistance possibly for several days during recovery.

The type of anesthesia and the operative risk is very much dependent on the site of surgery. For surgery of the extremities, regional anesthesia is advisable, but for abdominal and thoracic procedures, general anesthesia by a skilled and informed anesthesiologist is essential.

Endotracheal intubation followed with artificial ventilation should be accompanied by the judicious use of proper settings allowing complete expiratory phase to occur and the use of positive end expiratory pressure (PEEP) to prevent air trapping. Long-acting muscle relaxants should be used sparingly if at all because these patients are often elderly with low muscle tone. Most abdominal procedures can be performed without using muscle relaxants if the level of anesthesia is adequate. This approach permits more rapid recovery of muscle strength and better pulmonary mechanics in the recovery room. Chronic hypercarbia is preserved, thus avoiding acute alkalemia and possibly further increase in oxygen consumption.[12] The heart should be monitored through a Swan-Ganz catheter and an EKG with chest lead, and urine output should be closely measured.

Postoperatively, the use of mechanical ventilation overnight is a wise approach, especially if the surgical procedure ends in late afternoon. The patient is then evaluated the next morning and the trachea extubated if at all possible. If the patient cannot be extubated, the prognosis for prolonged respiratory assistance is poor, because these patients will often have altered respiratory patterns with discoordination of respiratory muscles, abdominal distention, abundant bronchial secretions, and most of all, hypoxemia with $P(A\text{-}a)O_2$ exceeding 400 to 500 mm Hg for several days following surgery which most often reflects a reduced functional residual capacity (FRC) and an increased closing volume.[23,24] Incisional pain can be dealt with by using continuous epidural segmental block with diluted lidocaine or intrathecal narcotics. This approach permits good analgesia and preservation of muscle strength and avoids the systemic use of narcotic analgesics. The criteria utilized to determine whether a patient can be weaned from ventilatory assistance do not apply to patients with severe COPD. The postoperative value of respiratory rate, static pulmonary compliance, inspiratory force, dead-space to tidal-volume ratio (VD/VT), and $P(A\text{-}a)O_2$ should be compared to preoperative values and not to normal values.

Asthma

It is generally thought that surgery on asthmatic patients should be done under regional anesthesia. However, our experience in handling asthmatic patients under spinal anesthesia has not been happy. Unless asthma has been under good control for several weeks to several months preceding surgery, the asthmatic patient is better managed under general anesthesia where the use of muscle relaxants, a bronchodilator, and a judicious choice of anesthetic agents permits good control of respiratory function. Indeed, the emotion of having surgery is enough to trigger bronchospasm while a patient is under regional anesthesia. Such an episode is the more difficult to treat and one often ends up having to use general anesthesia anyway. The slightest effect of spinal anesthesia on the abdominal wall musculature will weaken the patient's ability to cough and will sometimes produce dyspnea which generates more anxiety followed by a full blown asthmatic attack. The use of agents like halothane, enflurane or isoflurane sometimes preceded by intravenous aminophylline will usually produce a quiet and uneventful anesthesia in these patients. Narcotics, especially morphine, are best avoided as these analgesics are known to trigger histamine release.

Oat Cell Carcinoma of the Lung (Eaton-Lambert Syndrome)

This specific pathology is mentioned here because a patient suffering from oat cell carcinoma of the lung can be very sensitive to muscle relaxants. Indeed, it seems that oat cell tumors produce a substance with myoneural junction blocking effect, and the use of usual competitive agents, like curare and pancuronium might cause prolonged apnea postoperatively.

Pneumothorax, Pleural Effusion, Hemomediastinum and Pneumomediastinum

A large pneumothorax and pleural effusions of cardiac, hepatic, or renal origin should be corrected preoperatively to improve pulmonary mechanics during and following surgery. The same can be said of pneumomediastinum or hemomediastinum and pneumopericardium or hemopericardium especially if there is evidence of cardiac tamponade. A further discussion of the management of patients with pulmonary disease may be found in Chapter 12, Pulmonary Diseases.

MANAGEMENT OF PATIENTS WITH CARDIOVASCULAR DISEASE

Effect of Controlled Ventilation on Cardiovascular System

Intermittent positive pressure ventilation (IPPV) lowers arterial blood pressure and cardiac output in healthy animal preparations and human volunteers.[16] The fall in arterial pressure is usually transient and is compensated for by an increase in systemic vascular resistance. The decrease in oxygen consumption during IPPV results from the decline in the work of breathing and compensates for the lower cardiac output.[17] For a given increase in airway pressure, there is a lesser increase in mean pleural pressure and consequently in pulmonary vascular pressure.

In myocardial or valvular diseases, the cardiovascular response to IPPV will be dependent on the type and degree of cardiac impairment. In the case of severe left ventricular failure and pulmonary vascular congestion, an increase in arterial pressure analogous to a square wave response to the Valsalva maneuver may be expected. In severe mitral stenosis accompanied by severe pulmonary hypertension, IPPV may produce minimal or no change. In a patient suffering from idiopathic hypertrophic subaortic stenosis (IHSS), pericarditis, or cardiac tamponade, IPPV may result in further decrease in ventricular compliance and alarming circulatory collapse.

Portal venous flow may be decreased by 27 to 62 percent during IPPV and splanchnic blood flow may also be seriously impaired.[18] Although renal blood flow seems unaffected, a redistribution causing a shift of blood flow from cortical to medullary tissue has been demonstrated, producing a fall in urine output, creatine clearance, and sodium excretion.[19] These changes could be explained by increase in renal vascular afterload as recently reported.[20]

Arrhythmias and Anesthesia

A stable treated ventricular dysrhythmia in older patients is not of great concern preoperatively as it usually vanishes following induction of anesthesia and reappears in the recovery room.

Although the interpretation of the preoperative abnormal EKG is within the realm of the cardiologist, the arrhythmias encountered during induction of anesthesia and during surgery would sometimes baffle him. Intraoperative arrhythmias are usually benign or readily preventable and reversible, including the multifocal premature ventricular contractions caused by cardiac manipulation; the sinus tachycardia seen with Enflurane, gallamine, droperidol, and succinylcholine (in atropinized patients); the marked bradycardia of hypothermia or of deep cyclopropane anesthesia; the frequent junctional tachycardia seen during halothane and Enflurane administration; the bouts of ventricular tachycardia sometimes seen during brain exploration; and the supraventricular arrhythmias seen during endotracheal intubation under light anesthesia. Anesthesiologists have learned to diagnose and treat these situations with confidence. Also, anesthesiologists have learned to diagnose artifactual changes such as an ST segment shift caused by certain oscilloscopes, the patient's position, or the mechanical faults of the pen on certain paper tracings. By experience, the anesthesiologist will make the differential diagnosis between these pseudoarrhythmias and the more serious changes seen during acute hypoxia or marked acid-base changes.

The situations described above are within the realm of the competent anesthesiologist. This statement is by no means meant to minimize the crucial role of the cardiologist in evaluating and preparing preoperative patients with heart disease or in assisting in the treatment of persistent arrhythmias or heart failure during the recovery period (see Chap. 3, Cardiology).

Management of Hypertensive Patients

In the 1920s, more than 30 percent of patients with hypertensive heart disease died during or shortly following surgery under general anesthesia, half of them from cardiac failure.[25]

A recent report by Goldman and Caldera[26] depicts a different picture. Multivariate analysis of data for patients with histories of hypertension shows that whether these patients are treated or not, neither the preoperative in-hospital diastolic nor systolic blood pressure measurements independently correlate with intraoperative blood pressure liability, incidence of arrhythmia, myocardial ischemia and failure, or postoperative renal failure. Their data demonstrates that effective intraoperative management may be more important than preoperative hypertensive control in terms of the incidence of cardiovascular complications in patients with moderate hypertension. However, these optimistic findings should not deter the screening and treatment of patients with a preoperative history of hypertension, since the postoperative incidence of hypertensive episodes is less in patients who were taking antihypertensive agents preoperatively. Prys-Roberts is of the opinion that the use of antihypertensive medication prior to anesthesia should be continued up to and including the day of surgery to minimize postoperative hypertension.[27]

The management of anesthesia in hypertensive patients at present seems to favor the use of a narcotic analgesic, muscle relaxants, nitrous oxide mixture with the judicious use of short-acting sympathomimetic amines and nitroprusside. If ST changes are noticed during a hypertensive episode, intravenous administration of nitroglycerin is indicated. Vascular surgery is frequently performed on these patients, and clamping of the aorta is often used, which will surely test the skill of the anesthetist in handling vasoactive substances. Intraoperative urine production may be severely impaired following clamping of the aorta, but urinary output usually recovers within 24 hours after surgery.[26] Detection of elevation in left ventricular filling pressure by means of pulmonary wedge pressure measurement through a Swan-Ganz catheter usually preceds ST segment changes as a sign of left ventricular strain.[26] The product of heart rate by systolic pressure (HR × SP) should be kept below 15,000 in these patients. The monitoring of the supply to demand ratio has been useful. It is determined by the diastolic pressure time index (DPTI) over the systolic pressure time index. It should be kept at 0.7 or above.

In summary, the patient with severe hypertension should be thoroughly evaluated for renal and cardiac function and controlled with appropriate antihypertensive and antianginal medications up to and including the day of surgery. (For further discussion of the management of the hypertensive patient see Chap. 13, Renal Disease and Hypertension.)

Management of Patients with Cardiac Disease

The diversity of cardiac dysfunctions seen preoperatively will usually respond to manipulation of preload, afterload, myocardial oxygen consumption, heart rate, and coronary perfusion by means of vasoactive drugs, modification of pulmonary mechanics, or fluid administration or restriction. For instance, nitrous oxide increases the mean pulmonary vascular pressure, whereas nitroprusside lowers preload and afterload and may cause coronary vasodilation.[28] Using the thermodilution Swan-Ganz catheter the anesthesiologist monitors cardiac output; estimates ventricular compliance, myocardial oxygen supply and demand, and valvular competence; and assisted by the rich pharmacopoeia available today, can modify these variables almost at will.

The anesthesiologist's handling of cardiac patients will frequently depart from the cardiologist's management. This is so because of the anesthesiologist's monitoring of the patient on a minute to minute basis; the use of potent, short-acting, immediately reversible cardiotonic and vasoactive drugs; the anesthesiologist's skill in manipulating pulmonary mechanics and the patient's position to produce the desired effects on the cardiovascular system on a moment to moment basis; and his knowledge of the cardiovascular effect of the surgical procedures. The anesthesiologist usually will shy away from using digitalis as it is too long acting, makes diagnosis of arrhythmias more difficult when so many other factors can be arrhythmogenic, and has been shown to cause coronary vasoconstriction[29] supposedly by stimulating alpha-adrenergic receptors. Furthermore, the combination of digitalis and furosemide has been shown to aggravate mesenteric insufficiency during abdominal surgery.[30]

The scope of this discussion does not permit a comprehensive review of the anesthetic management of all cardiac pathologic entities. However, to call the anesthetic approach to management of patients undergoing cardiac surgery "cardiac anesthesia," as is frequently done, is to employ a misnomer, because we believe that any patient with severe cardiac impairment who is scheduled for major surgery should be given at least similar treatment. "Cardiac anesthesia" includes more thorough preoperative preparedness and readiness to care rapidly for any sudden changes in the patient's cardiovascular status. It entails full monitoring of cardiovascular function with thermodilation Swan-Ganz catheters, arterial cannulae, two or three large intravenous catheters, multilead electrocardiogram including I, II, III, aVR, aVF, and V_5 leads, bipolar electroencephalogram and frequent measurements of blood gases. "Cardiac anesthesia" also demands immediate availability of a long list of vasoactive drugs already diluted and ready for prompt intravenous administration plus the immediate availability of apparatus such as a pacemaker, a defibrillator, and an intra-aortic balloon. The induction of anesthesia avoids the familiar thiopental-succinylcholine combination and usually consists of a balance technique using administration of large doses of morphine (1 to 3 mg/kg) given in a slow intravenous drip supplemented with diazepam, droperidol, or other sedatives or tranquilizers. Generous doses of pancuronium or *d*-tubocurarine are administered early to counteract the increased muscle tone frequently produced by morphine. This regimen is accompanied by early respiratory assistance before and following endotracheal intubation. The postoperative course is managed in a similar manner, and the patient is kept intubated and on the ventilator until the next morning when all variables are re-evaluated.

The patient with severe cardiac impairment who is scheduled for major noncardiac surgery is at a great disadvantage over the patient scheduled for cardiac surgery in that his cardiac anomaly will not be improved by the procedure often causing a more prolonged and difficult postoperative course. For additional discussion of the management of cardiac patients see Chapter 3, Cardiology.

MANAGEMENT OF PATIENTS IN LIVER FAILURE

The patient in hepatic coma or severe liver failure requiring emergency portocaval or splenorenal vascular bypass will often be in respiratory failure, and this association has a mortality of more than 95 percent.[31] The complex gastrointestinal and metabolic changes found in these patients will influence the absorption and therefore the dosage and duration of action of most anesthetic agents and adjuvant drugs. For instance, succinylcholine, whose duration of action is mainly influenced by hydrolytic breakdown in plasma by pseudocholinesterase produced by the liver, is either avoided or carefully titrated in order to prevent prolonged apnea.

Clinically these patients are metabolically hyperactive with hyperthermia, hyperventilation, increased cardiac output, and low peripheral resistance largely due to diffuse arteriovenous shunting. Some of the clinical changes, including the so-called hepatic encephalopathy, have been attributed to the accumulation of false neurotransmitters such as octopamine.[32] In spite of this metabolic hyperactivity, hypersensitivity to all drugs is usually expected. The hypoglycemia, hypokalemia, hypocalcemia, renal failure, bleeding, and disseminated intravascular coagulation that occur commonly in advanced liver failure will participate in creating a picture so complex that only symptomatic management can be expected.

If delirium tremens is present, the management should be aimed at lowering oxygen consumption by deep sedation, cooling blanket, cold intravenous fluids, muscle relaxants, and controlled ventilation as in any extreme hyperactive state. (For additional discussion of the management of patients with liver disease see Chap. 6, Gastroenterology.)

MANAGEMENT OF THE ALCOHOLIC PATIENT

Although ethanol causes hepatic enzyme induction producing tolerance to sedatives and anesthetics, this is usually not clinically important. The alcoholic patient is, in fact, likely to suffer from multiorgan failure of varied degree including alcoholic cardiomyopathy rendering the heart sensitive to anesthetic depressant effect. To dry out an alcoholic preoperatively is as risky as to withdraw the addictive drug from the narcotic addict. The use of intravenous alcohol should be considered in treating signs of delirium before anesthesia in patients needing emergency surgery.

Several drugs administered preoperatively to the alcoholic patient may produce unexpected effects. Chloral hydrate may cause marked vasodilation, tachycardia, palpitations, facial flushing, and dysphoria. Increased doses of phenytoin are needed to control seizures. Use of salicylates causes an increased incidence of gastrointestinal bleeding and enhances the inhibition of blood platelet aggregation. Alcohol potentiates the hypotensive effect of reserpine, methyldopa, hydralazine, guanethidine, and nitroglycerin, whereas propranolol may mask the symptoms of alcoholic hypoglycemia. Tricyclic antidepressants may render the alcoholic patient more prone to delirium tremens, whereas MAO inhibitors associated with Chianti wines (which contain tyramine) may produce serious hypertensive crisis. Antidiabetic oral medication may create fluctuating glucose blood levels and tolbutamide may produce a withdrawal syndrome[33] similar to that seen with disulfiram.

Chronic alcohol intake may produce a cross-tolerance to inhalational anesthetics in their effects on the central nervous system but may have a synergistic effect on the heart and circulation. Also the dose of barbiturates or narcotics necessary to produce apnea is 50 percent lower in the alcoholic patient. Finally, phenothiazine derivatives may cause signs of parkinsonism and respiratory depression more frequently in the alcoholic patient.[33]

If severe liver failure and malnutrition are present, the alcoholic patient may show sensitivity to succinylcholine, resulting in prolonged apnea which might necessitate respiratory assistance during the recovery period.

It is evident that the management of anesthesia for major surgery on the alcoholic patient should consist of full monitoring of all functions and should be conducted with meticulous attention to prevent respiratory and circulatory failure.

MANAGEMENT OF PATIENTS WITH ENDOCRINE DISEASES

Adrenal Cortical Disease

Acute adrenal insufficiency during anesthesia and surgery can cause rapid progression of symptoms leading to persistent hypotension, coma, and death. Fortunately, this is rarely seen at present.

The effect of anesthesia on adrenocortical function is minimal compared to that of surgery. Morphine, barbiturates, and Enflurane depress cortical secretion but not to a clinically significant extent.[34] Ether and cyclopropane, both rapidly vanishing from the anesthesia pharmacopoeia, increase cortisol as does halothane which has been reported to decrease the response to adrenocorticotropic hormone (ACTH) for as long as four hours postoperatively.[35,36]

Patients who have received glucocorticoid therapy within a year of surgery should receive increased doses of glucocorticoid during anesthesia because of potential adrenal suppression (see Chap. 5, Endocrinology).

Patients with adrenal insufficiency are exquisitely sensitive to narcotics, barbiturates, and general anesthetics and should never come to surgery untreated. If emergency surgery is unavoidable, such patients should be rapidly prepared with appropriate cortisol administration and the electrolytes and acid-base status evaluated and corrected if required (see Chap. 5). The anesthetic management should be based on a dose-response technique.

Cushing's syndrome is due to glucocorticoid excess. These patients often suffer from diabetes, hypertension, osteoporosis, weakness, central obesity, aberrant behavior, and hypokalemic alkalosis. They do not require preanesthetic administration of steroids, but following adrenalectomy, high doses of steroids are required as for patients with adrenal insufficiency. Care has to be used in mobilizing these patients under anesthesia because of bone fragility due to osteoporosis.

Patients with hyperaldosteronism (Conn's syndrome) often present a history of arrhythmias and are sensitive to nondepolarizing muscle relaxants due to hypokalemia and metabolic alkalosis. There has been report of tonic muscle contracture during induction of anesthesia attributed to the effect of potassium on muscle membrane potential.[34]

Pheochromocytoma

Increased understanding of the pathophysiology of pheochromocytomas and their operative management has led to a decline in the surgical mortality. About 25 to 45 percent of patients with these tumors died at surgery prior to 1950, this figure was reduced to 13 percent from 1950 to 1960, after which time the percentage has decreased to 1 to 5 percent.[37]

The preoperative preparation of patients with pheochromocytomas is fully discussed in Chapter 5, Endocrinology, and we will not add to this. However, as a general rule we prefer these patients to be weaned from long acting alpha- or beta- blocking agents preceding induction of anesthesia, since the anesthetist prefers to work with drugs that can be reversed within 1 to 2 minutes—controllability based on reversibility being a priority in anesthesia. This can be achieved either by rapid redistribution as with thiopental, rapid breakdown as with succinycholine, or by rapid action of antagonist drugs like curare-neostigmine or narcotic-naloxone combinations. Use of long acting phenoxybenzamine and chlorpromazine should be phased out in favor of shorter acting phentolamine or nitroprusside or even intravenous nitroglycerin in order to assure reversibility and controllability. The effect of these intravenous medications should be closely monitored, and at present a Swan-Ganz catheter is inserted the day preceding surgery before short acting agents are administered so that right and left ventricular filling pressures and performances can be assessed before, during, and following surgery. Moderate to heavy sedation is indicated in most patients preoperatively using short acting barbiturates or diazepam. We personally avoid the use of narcotics as, on occasion, they produce an elevation in blood pressure and, in excess, cause hypoventilation with secondary hypercarbia and hypoxia which per se are sympathetic stimulants. Atropine or scopolamine can be used if definite indication warrants it. Some of these patients come to surgery on full propranolol therapy given mainly to control arrhythmias or anginal pain. These patients may be completely refractory to vasopressors except for norepinephrine to which they may be exquisitely sensitive.[38] If administered, the usual concentrations of norepinephrine should be diluted by a factor of ten and administered slowly (0.4 mg/ml). Intravenous calcium or glucagon are effective alternatives.

Monitoring should consist of pulmonary arterial and wedge pressure and central venous pressure through a Swan-Ganz catheter inserted the preceding day and EKG with V_5 lead to detect any ST changes if hypertensive episodes occur, especially in older patients. A nerve stimulator to follow the need for muscle relaxants, central temperature probes, an arterial line for arterial pressure and blood gas monitoring, and three intravenous cannullae (one of which should be size #14 gauge to facilitate rapid infusion of fluid or blood) are normally employed.

Induction of anesthesia should be as gentle as possible to prevent any acute discomfort or changes in vital signs. Better control is achieved with slow inhalation induction assisted with minimal infusion of thiopental followed by intermittent infusion of *d*-tubocurarine up to a dose sufficient to intubate the trachea without the use of succinylcholine. Gallamine and pancuronium are parasympatholytic and may cause troublesome tachycardia. Use of succinylcholine is best avoided because of its muscarinic effect on the nonatropinized patient (i.e., bradycardia, hypotension) and its nicotinic effect on atropinized patients (i.e., hypertension, tachycardia, and arrhythmia). Topical anesthesia of the trachea using lidocaine 4 percent spray is essential. Indeed, the insertion of an endotracheal tube frequently produces severe hypertension and tachycardia in the healthiest patient and can be disastrous in the patient with pheochromocytoma. Once the proper level of enflurane anesthesia is established, surgery usually proceeds uneventfully until the tumor is exposed. Enflurane is preferable to halothane as it has a definite antiarrhythmic effect (cyclopropane and ether being contraindicated because of their stimulating effect on the sympathetic system).

During surgical manipulation of the tumor, hypertensive crisis and ventricular arrhythmias can occur. When halothane is the anesthetic, an arrhythmia can appear without a hypertensive response and this is where propranolol can be of great help. It is administered in small boluses of 0.25 mg until a sinus rhythm is re-established. When enflurane is the agent, a hypertensive response may occur without ventricular arrhythmia, and then phentolamine or nitroprusside are very effective. If the V_5 lead of the EKG shows signs of myocardial ischemia, intravenous nitroglycerin will serve to control the hypertension, myocardial ischemia, and arrhythmia as there is evidence that nitroglycerin has genuine antiarrhythmic properties.[39]

If a hypertensive crisis or arrhythmia occurs, we request that the surgeon quickly identify the venous drainage of the gland and ligate it, preventing further liberation of catecholamines into the circulation and eliminating any further crisis per se. Once this is done, marked vasodilation will often occur and rapid infusion of crystalloid and colloid will usually prevent severe hypotension. From this point, the management become symptomatic and most often uneventful. The postoperative course has been discussed in Chapter 5, Endocrinology.

Sipple's Syndrome

We have had the opportunity to administer anesthesia to twelve members of a kindred with Sipple's syndrome (phenochromocytoma, medullary carcinoma of the thyroid, and hyperparathyroidism). In these patients, symptoms were mild and the anesthetic and surgical management was uneventful. They were all managed as above with enflurane which might explain in part the absence of arrhythmias and severe hypertensive crises. The only arrhythmia seen in these patients was an occasional junctional tachycardia which responded rapidly to small doses of anticholinesterase agents like neostigmine or edrophonium.

Hyperthyroidism

In 1943, Astwood established a new era in medicine by using antithyroid drugs to treat hyperthyroidism. Since then, very few hyperthyroid patients reach the operating room without being well controlled. With present therapy, most patients are euthyroid before surgery.

Atropine is best avoided as a premedicant since it interferes with sweating and temperature control and may produce disturbing tachycardias. The preferred induction agent is thiopental because of its antithyroid activity.[40] The same care should be taken in using muscle relaxants and in intubating the trachea in patients with hyperthyroidism as in patients with pheochromocytoma. Cyclopropane and diethyl ether stimulate the sympathetic system and are contraindicated. Ketamine and halothane are arrhythmogenic and should be avoided. Enflurane, despite its tendency to increase heart rate,[5] is a suitable agent. Narcotic-curare, nitrous-oxide balance technique is satisfactory if light anesthesia is avoided as it might induce catecholamine release from surgical stimulation. Temperature monitoring and use of a cooling blanket are essential.

If emergency surgery is indicated on a thyrotoxic patient, heavy sedation and deep anesthesia must be achieved. Propranolol, steroids, injectable iodine, thionamide antithyroid drugs, and cold intravenous solutions must be available in case of "thyroid storm." If thyroid storm develops, the treatment is not unlike that of malignant hyperthermia, and although no report of cooling by extracorporeal circulatory bypass has appeared in the literature, it should be kept in mind if other means fail. (See Chap. 5, Endocrinology.)

Hypothyroidism

Mild hypothyroidism is an easier problem for the anesthesiologist to solve than is hyperthyroidism. The hypothyroid patient's central nervous system's reactivity is low, permitting low doses or concentration of anesthetic to achieve surgical anesthesia. Muscle tone is decreased allowing good surgical relaxation with administration of little or no muscle relaxants. The time constant of biotransformation is increased, permitting augmented duration of action of most agents. However, this last phenomenon impedes controllability of recovery, and narcotic and other sedatives should be used frugally if at all postoperatively.

The myxedematous patient may present with cardiac enlargement, myocardial depression, angina, and adrenal insufficiency. The indiscriminate use of vasoactive drugs in such patients can create confusing cardiovascular episodes including ventricular arrhythmia and fibrillation. These patients also develop hypothermia during surgery and a heating blanket is a must for prolonged procedures.

Patients who exhibit airway obstruction from a large goiter will require endotracheal intubation under topical anesthesia and the tube will be placed beyond the obstructed site as determined by preoperative x-rays of the neck and upper chest. Immediately following thyroid surgery and extubation, the anesthesiologist will do a direct laryngoscopy to verify normal mobility of the vocal cords and patency of the airway thereby ruling out damage to the recurrent laryngeal nerve which occasionally occurs during neck surgery. (For further discussion, see Chap. 5, Endocrinology.)

Diabetes

The patient with diabetes mellitus may present with an instability generated by variable stresses during anesthesia and surgery. The signs of hypoglycemia may be masked under general anesthesia, so it is preferable to withhold or reduce the dose of insulin, the morning of surgery. Frequent blood glucose determinations are taken during the procedure and 5 to 7 U of regular insulin are administered to keep serum glucose between 200 and 300 mg/dl.

In adult onset diabetes mellitus, ketoacidosis is rare, but hyperglycemia is common and should be treated as above. Hypoxia, burns, and surgical manipulations increase circulating catecholamines, glucagon, cortisol, and growth hormone and thus inhibit insulin secretion, increase glycogenolysis, and increase gluconeogenesis, elevating the blood glucose. If hyperglycemia is very marked (700 to 900 mg/dl), it should be treated slowly with 2 to 5 U of insulin per hour intravenously. During cardiopulmonary bypass, insulin release is decreased and hyperglycemia follows but insulin should not be administered unless blood glucose is increased to more than 300 mg/dl as the process rapidly reverses itself following weaning from cardiopulmonary perfusion. (See Chap. 5, Endocrinology for further details on the management of the diabetic patient.)

In managing the diabetic patient, the anesthesiologist is mainly concerned with the secondary effect of diabetes on the heart, the blood vessels, the kidney, and the peripheral nerves and will manage anesthesia accordingly.

MANAGEMENT OF PATIENTS WITH RENAL FAILURE AND RENAL TRANSPLANT DONORS

Until the mid-1960s, the anesthesiologist had little opportunity to care for patients with chronic, terminal renal failure. However, the recent improvement of the "artificial kidney" and government involvement in financing care of patients with renal failure has augmented enormously the number of such patients undergoing elective surgery of all kinds. Many of these patients have undergone several procedures such as the creation of an arteriovenous shunt, renal biopsy, nephrectomy, kidney transplant, transplant removal, and other surgical procedures unrelated to their renal impairment.

It is not unusual for these patients to have hemoglobin concentrations of 5 to 7 g/dl. In the face of normovolemia, this degree of anemia is well tolerated and does not necessitate preoperative transfusion.

The existence of an arteriovenous shunt might be assumed to increase the already elevated cardiac output of these anemic patients, but it seems that the lowering of arterial peripheral resistance overshadows the probable increase in preload and the shunt is usually well tolerated.[41] As reported by Lichtman,[42] in spite of the increase in 2, 3-diphosphoglycerate (2,3-DPG) in the anemic patient, the P_{50} value is unchanged adding to the confusion already existent in the attempt to attach clinical significance to these measurements.

In 1954, the first kidney transplantation between identical twins was performed at Peter Bent Brigham Hospital in Boston. Since then, this procedure has become routine in many teaching and private hospitals throughout the country. According to the Renal Transplant Registry of the National Institutes of Health, approximately 35,000 transplants have been registered and analyzed since 1963.

A nephrectomy is a major procedure that is not infrequently accompanied by major blood loss, pneumothorax, and postoperative infection and is of concern even in a healthy donor. The donor's history and physical examination should be conducted meticulously, and anesthesia should be planned according to any uncovered pathology in order to assure the most nearly perfect anesthetic. The left kidney is usually chosen as it is more accessible and contains a longer renal pedicle. As for any nephrectomy, blood should be readily available for transfusion because of possible slipping of the aortic side-clamp. Frequent monitoring of urine output is necessary to assure adequate perfusion to the kidney. Proper hydration is mandatory for continuous diuresis during mobilization of the kidney. Transdiaphragmatic pneumothorax is controlled with simple catheter drainage during closure.

The recipient is usually dialyzed the day preceding surgery. Arterial cannulation is avoided to preserve the arteries for future arteriovenous shunts. One venous catheter connected to 500 ml of 5 percent dextrose with one-half normal saline is sufficient. Even if the recipient is anemic, transfusion is avoided.

The left kidney of the donor is usually transplanted into either the left or right inguinal region. The transplant procedure usually requires general anesthesia with good muscle relaxation. Halothane or ether are the drugs of choice. Methoxyflurane and fluroxene have been shown to be nephrotoxic and should be avoided. Enflurane and isoflurane should also be avoided until better data is available. Intravenous anesthetic agents should be avoided as most of them are largely excreted by the kidney. If requested by the patient, a well managed spinal anesthesia will provide excellent working conditions for the surgeon. It is also the least toxic technique for the patient and the transplanted kidney.

Mannitol 12.5 gm and furosemide 40 mg are usually administered immediately preceding the opening of the arterial anastomosis. Hypotension should be treated with fluid infusion, but usually hypertension presents more of a problem and an alpha blocking agent or nitroprusside are sometimes necessary (for further discussion of renal transplantation see Chap. 13, Renal Disease and Hypertension).

PHYSIOLOGIC AND MEDICAL ASPECTS OF SPINAL AND EPIDURAL ANESTHESIA

The hypotensive effect of spinal anesthesia is often misunderstood. Other than the usual factors cited such as the state of the patient's hydration, the status of the cardiovascular system, or presence of full term pregnancy or large abdominal mass, one factor causing hypotension stands out in our experience and that is the speed of onset of anesthesia following injections of the drug into the subarachnoid space. This fact came to our attention during studies aimed at uncovering the effect of spinal anesthesia on the cardiovascular system in healthy volunteers.[43] We were using Nupercaine, an agent producing a slow onset of spinal block and the level was raised slowly up to the second thoracic dermatome. However, we were often unsuccessful in generating any lowering of the blood pressure or in altering cardiovascular parameters in spite of a high level of anesthesia. We substituted lidocaine, an agent producing rapid onset of spinal block, for Nupercaine and marked hypotension occurred even at a low level of anesthesia. Similarly, in clinical situations, severe hypotension can be prevented by using drugs and techniques that will produce a slow onset of anesthesia.

Morbidity secondary to a properly performed spinal block is low. Since the introduction of the small gauge spinal needles (25 gauge or smaller) the incidence of true spinal headache in our institution is less than 2 percent. The incidence of urinary retention is not any greater than following general anesthesia. As for permanent motor impairment, no case out of 10,098 studied by Dripps was identified.[44] However, minor neurologic sequelae are still reported. They are either transient, the symptoms disappearing within a few weeks or months or related to the uncovering of a previously unrecognized disease.

Epidural anesthesia has become more popular, especially in obstetrics for labor pain and delivery, because prolonged anesthesia can be achieved by inserting an indwelling catheter into the epidural space which permits the use of repeated injections. It also prevents the puncture of the dura and eliminates the occurrence of headache. The physiologic effect is similar to that of spinal anesthesia.

In certain situations, spinal or epidural anesthesia presents several advantages over general anesthesia. A case in point is the use of spinal block for transurethral resection of the prostate (TURP). TURP is often accompanied by water overload and intoxication toward the end of the resection, producing severe hyponatremia, left ventricular failure, and even cardiac standstill. The first sign of this eventuality is mental confusion and restlessness which could not be detected if surgery were performed under general anesthesia. Spinal anesthesia also prevents postoperative bladder spasm and pain for several hours during recovery.

SUMMARY

Interaction between surgeon, anesthesiologist, and internist has improved during the last decade. Not only has this resulted in better general patient care but it has also permitted patients to undergo surgery who would have been considered too poor a risk 10 years ago.

However, this improved relationship is not universal yet, and we believe it appropriate to recapitulate the objectives the anesthesiologist has in caring for his patients.

Overall, the anesthesiologist's intention is to see the patient safely through the operation and the perioperative period. To do this, he or she has to be fully aware of the patient's pathophysiologic derangements, understand their consequences for anesthesia as well as the effects, if any, that concurrent drug therapy will have on anesthesia management, and be satisfied that the patient's given circumstances cannot be otherwise improved. This last concern needs some clarification.

Should a patient with a severe derangement of his physiology, such as acute bronchitis, heart failure, pneumonia, or electrolyte imbalance, be scheduled for an elective operation, it is the anesthesiologist's duty to determine (in consultation with the surgeon and internist) if the patient's status can be improved before surgery. No rigid protocol in these matters can be established, since the overall condition of the patient as well as the urgency of surgery vary so much. Needless to say, the final decision in these matters is not an easy one, and frequently the situation is clouded by various pressures such as the schedules of the surgeons and the anesthesiologist or the internist's availability. In resolving such issues, the patient's welfare must be kept in everyone's mind at all times.

REFERENCES

1. ARONSON, HB, LEVESQUE, PR, CHARM, S, ET AL.: *Influence of anaesthetics on rheology of human blood.* Can Anaesth Soc J 15:244, 1968.
2. BROWN, BR, JR.: *Hepatic microsomal lipoperoxidation and inhalation anesthetics: a biochemical and morphologic study in the rat.* Anesthesiology 36:458, 1972.
3. MAZZE, RI, AND COUSINS, MJ: *Renal effects of anesthetics with special reference to the nephrotoxicity of methoxyflurane.* Can Anesth Soc J 20:64, 1973.
4. MAZZE, RI, COUSINS, MJ, AND BARR, GA: *Renal effects and metabolism of isoflurane in man.* Anesthesiology 40:536, 1974.
5. LEVESQUE, PR, NANAGAS, V, SHANKS, C, ET AL.: *Circulatory effects of enflurane in normocarbic human volunteers.* Can Anaesth Soc J 21:580, 1974.
6. CASCORBI, HF: *Peri-anesthetic problems with non-anesthetic drugs:* ASA Annual Refresher Course, Chicago, 1978, p. 212.
7. HORN, JP, AND MCAFEE, DA: *Nor-epinephrine inhibits calcium-dependent potentials in rat sympathetic neurons.* Science 204:1233, 1979.
8. SHIMOSATO, S, AND ETSTEN, BE: *The role of venous system in cardio-circulatory dynamics during spinal anesthesia in man.* Anesthesiology 30:619, 1979.
9. ROGERS, RM, SPEAR, JF, MOORE, EN, ET AL.: *Vulnerability of canine ventricle to fibrillation during hypoxia and respiratory acidosis.* Chest 63:986, 1973.
10. SPRINGER, RR, CLARK, DK, LEA, AS, ET AL: *Effects of changes in arterial carbon dioxide tension on oxygen consumption during cardiopulmonary bypass.* Chest 75:548, 1979.
11. THEYE, RA, AND MICHENFELDER, JD: *Whole-body and organ* V_{O2} *changes with enflurane, isoflurane, and halothane.* Br J Anaesth 47:813, 1975.
12. CAIN, SM: *Increased oxygen uptake with passive hyperventilation of dogs.* J Appl Physiol 28:4, 1970.
13. ROBIN, E, AND TRAVIS, K: *Alveolar gas tensions, pulmonary ventilation and blood pH during physiological sleep in normal subjects.* J Clin Invest 37:981, 1958.
14. INGVAR, DH, AND BULOW, KB: *Respiratory regulation in sleep.* Ann NY Acad Sci 109:870, 1963.
15. NUNN, JF, BERGMAN, NA, AND COLEMAN, AJ: *Factors influencing the arterial oxygen tension during anaesthesia with artificial ventilation.* Br J Anaesth 37:981, 1958.
16. COLGAN, FJ, BARROWN, RE, AND FAMMING, GL: *Constant positive pressure breathing and cardio-respiratory function.* Anesthesiology 34:145, 1971.
17. HEDLEY-WHYTE, J, BURGESS, GE, III, FEELEY, TW, ET AL.: *Applied Physiology of Respiratory Care.* Boston: Little, Brown and Co., 1976, p. 20.
18. COOPERMAN, LH, WARDEN, JC, AND PRICE, HL: *Splanchic circulation during nitrous-oxide anesthesia and hypocarbia in normal man.* Anesthesiology 29:254, 1978.
19. HALL, SV, JOHNSON, EE, AND HEDLEY-WHYTE, J: *Renal hemodynamics and function with continuous positive pressure ventilation in dogs.* Anesthesiology 41:452, 1974.
20. MARQUEZ, JM, DOUGLAS, ME, AND DOWNS, JB: *Renal function and cardiovascular responses during positive airway pressure.* Anesthesiology 50:393, 1979.
21. BRAIN, JD: *Anesthesia and respiratory defense mechanism.* Int Anesthesiol. Clin 15:169, 1977.
22. COLLINS, CD, DRAKE, CS, AND KNOWELDEN, J: *Chest complications after abdominal surgery: their anticipation and prevention.* Br J Anaesth 40:401, 1968.
23. KITAMURA, H. SAWA, T, AND IKEZONO, E: *Postoperative hypoxemia. The contribution of age to the maldistribution of ventilation.* Anesthesiology 36:244, 1972.
24. MILIC-EMILI, J, HENDERSON, JAM, DOLOVICH, MB, ET AL.: *Regional distribution of inspired gas in the lung.* J Appl Physiol 21:749, 1966.

25. Sprague, HB: *The heart in surgery. An analysis of the results of surgery on cardiac patients during the past ten years at Massachusetts General Hospital.* Surg Gynecol Obstet 49:54, 1929.
26. Goldman, L, and Caldera, DL: *Risks of general anesthesia and elective operation in the hypertensive patient.* Anesthesiology 50:285, 1979.
27. Prys-Roberts, C: *Hypertension and anesthesia fifty years on.* Anesthesiology 50:281, 1979.
28. Rowe, GG, and Henderson, RH: *Systemic and coronary hemodynamic effect of sodium nitroprusside.* Am Heart J 87:83, 1974.
29. Garan, H, Smith, TW, and Powell, WJ, Jr.: *The central nervous system as a site of action for the coronary vasoconstrictor effect of digoxin.* J Clin Invest 54:1365, 1974.
30. Adar, R, Franklin, A, and Salzman, EW: *Effect of furosemide on mesenteric blood flow in dogs.* Pharmacol Res Commun 6:485, 1974.
31. Hedley-Whyte, J, Burgess, GE, III, Feeley, TW, et al.: *Applied Physiology of Respiratory Care.* Boston: Little-Brown and Co., 1976, p. 225.
32. Molinoff, PB, Landsberg, L, and Axelrod, J: *An enzymatic assay for octopamine and other B-hydroxylated phenylethylamine.* J Pharmacol Exp Ther 170:253, 1969.
33. *Alcohol-drug interactions.* FDA Bulletin 9(2):39, 1979.
34. Ballinger, CM: *Endocrine and Enzymes in Anesthesiology.* Springfield, Illinois: Charles C Thomas, 1973.
35. Oyama, L: *Anesthesia Management of Endocrine Diseases.* New York: Springer-Verlag, 1973.
36. Plimpton, FG: *Corticosteroid treatment and surgery.* Anesthesia 24:3, 1969.
37. Engelman, K.: *Pheochromocytoma.* Clin Endocrinol Metab 6:769, 1977.
38. Braunwald, E: *Mechanisms of Contraction of the Normal and Failing Heart,* ed. 2. Boston: Little, Brown and Co., 1976, pp. 235, 339.
39. Stockman, MB, Verrier, RL, and Lown, B: *Effect of nitroglycerin on vulnerability to ventricular fibrillation during myocardial ischemia and reperfusion.* Am J Cardiol 43:233, 1979.
40. Stehling, LC: *Anesthetic management of the patient with hyperthyroidism.* Anesthesiology 41:585, 1974.
41. Zauder, HL: *Anesthesia for patients who have terminal renal disease.* Can Anaesth Soc J 14:255, 1967.
42. Lichtman, MA, Murphy, MS, Byer, BJ, et al.: *Hemoglobin affinity for oxygen in chronic renal disease: effect of hemodialysis.* Blood 43:417, 1974.
43. Li, TH, Shimosato, S, and Etsten, BE: *Methoxamine and cardiac output in non-anesthetized man and during spinal anesthesia.* Anesthesiology 26:21, 1965.
44. Vandam, LD, and Dripps, RD: *Long-term follow-up of patients who received 10098 spinal anesthetics.* JAMA 172:1483, 1960.

INDEX

A *t* following a page number indicates a table.